IRTEEN PAIRS OF DRUGS THAT CAN CAUSE LIFE-THREATENING REACTIONS IF USED TOGETHER:

Celecoxib (CELEBREX)—Warfarin (COUMADIN)

Citalop (CELEXA)—monoamine oxidase (MAO) inhibitor antidepressants

Garlic—Warfarin (COUMADIN)

Fenofibrate (TRICOR)—Atorvastatin (LIPITOR)

Gatifloxacin (TEQUIN)—Sotalol (BETAPACE)

Moxifloxacin (AVELOX)—Quinidine

Sildenafil (VIAGRA)—Nitroglycerin

Thidazine (MELLARIL)—Fluoxetine (PROZAC)

Lo statin (MEVACOR)—Gemfibrozil (LOPID)

Tramadol with cetaminophen (ULTRACET)—Paroxetine (PAXIL)

rapamil (CALAN SR)—Quinidine

Ziprasione (GEODON)—Sparfloxacin (ZAGAM)

Meperidi (DEMEROL)—Phenelzine (NARDIL)

St. Jon's Wort—Oral Contraceptives

. . . and hundreds of other pairs of dangerously interacting drugs listed inside

WORST PILLS, BEST PILLS

A Consumer's Guide to
Avoiding Drug-Induced Death or Illness

Sidney M. Wolfe, M.D.;

Larry D. Sasich, Pharm.D., M.P.H.; Peter Lurie, M.D., M.P.H.;

Rose-Ellen Hope, R.Ph.; Elizabeth Barbehenn, Ph.D.;

Deanne E. Knapp, Ph.D.; Amer Ardati, M.D.;

Sherri Shubin, M.D., M.P.H.; Diana B. Ku, Pharm.D.;

and Public Citizen's Health Research Group

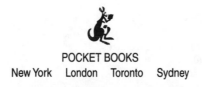

POCKET BOOKS
New York   London   Toronto   Sydney

Publisher's Note

The drug information contained in this book is based on product labeling published in current editions of *Physicians' Desk Reference*®, supplemented with facts from other sources the publisher believes reliable. While diligent efforts have been made to assure the accuracy of this information, the book does not list every possible adverse reaction, interaction, precaution, and effect of a drug; and all information is presented without guarantees by the authors, consultants, and publisher, who disclaim all liability in connection with its use.

This book is intended only as a reference for use in an ongoing partnership between doctor and patient in the vigilant management of the patient's health. It is not a substitute for a doctor's professional judgment, and serves only as a reminder of concerns that may need discussion. All readers are urged to consult with a physician before beginning or discontinuing use of any prescription drug or undertaking any form of self-treatment.

Brand names listed in this book are intended to represent only the more commonly used products. Inclusion of a brand name does not signify endorsement of the product; absence of a name does not imply a criticism or rejection of the product. The publisher is not advocating the use of any product described in this book, does not warrant or guarantee any of these products, and has not performed any independent analysis in connection with the product information contained herein.

 POCKET BOOKS, a division of Simon & Schuster, Inc.
1230 Avenue of the Americas, New York, NY 10020

ISBN: 0-7434-9256-0

This Pocket Books trade paperback edition January 2005

10   9   8   7   6   5   4

POCKET and colophon are registered trademarks
of Simon & Schuster, Inc.

Manufactured in the United States of America

For information regarding special discounts for bulk purchases,
please contact Simon & Schuster Special Sales at
1-800-456-6798 or business@simonandschuster.com

This book is dedicated to the memory of Phyllis McCarthy,
Office Manager and Managing Editor of Public Citizen's Health Research Group
publications for twenty-five years, who passed away in the planning stages of this book.
This edition could not exist without the previous editions, and none of those
could have been completed without her resourcefulness and dedication.

PREFACE

Worst Pills, Best Pills is an extraordinarily useful book. Starting with its first edition in 1988, it has consistently served as a reliable reference for people who wish to avoid drug-induced illnesses and injuries. The arrival of this new and up-to-date edition occurs at a critical time for all people who want to stay as healthy as possible.

Years of experience and, now, published research indicate that people who play an active, well-informed role in taking care of themselves are healthier. Recent studies prove what many experts have suspected all along: the so-called activated patient is better at preventing disease and getting over acute illnesses. For people of any age with a chronic illness, assuming the role of an involved, knowledgeable patient is critical to achieving the best outcomes.

When it comes to drugs, seeking out reliable information is more important now than ever. Patients have always asked for advice about their medications from doctors, pharmacists, nurses, friends, and family members. But today, pharmaceutical companies provide information directly to consumers through television, radio, print, and Web site advertising. While some consumers may welcome this direct influx of information from drug makers, it's important to remember that the primary purpose of these ads is to sell products rather than to inform. In fact, prescription drug ads have literally resuscitated the advertising industry after losses experienced when tobacco ads were outlawed. Even on the Internet—where drug information abounds—the vast majority of drug-related content is designed for commerce rather than education, making it extremely difficult for consumers to sort the best pills from the worst pills.

So, if your goal is to be an activated, well-informed consumer, you really do need to actively seek out information about the drugs you might use. Passively waiting to find out about your medications is not a good idea. Indeed, it is likely to be unsafe. As *Worst Pills, Best Pills* has taught for years, the drugs available to us can offer unparalleled health benefits, but they also have great potential to cause harm and even death.

Most physicians and nurses become aware of the dangers of improper drug use as soon as they enter the field of health care. As a physician/researcher, I became even more attuned to these hazards some 20 years ago when my colleagues and I discovered that adverse effects of prescribed drugs are the most common reversible cause of dementia and delirium in older people who were thought to have "irreversible" Alzheimer's disease. Since that discovery, health care providers have become increasingly aware of the potential ill effects of drugs. But there's more that the average patient can do to be alert as well. Using a reliable reference such as *Worst Pills, Best Pills*—along with common-sense advice from your health care providers—you can benefit from the best drug therapies modern medicine offers, while avoiding the hazards of improper or unsafe drug use.

As an experienced physician, I am always pleased when my patients ask questions about their medications. It shows they are actively seeking out information; they're not just passively accepting messages they hear in television ads or elsewhere about drugs that may or may not be right for them. This proactive, involved stance gives me confidence that they'll do well both in terms of preventing disease and managing any chronic conditions they may have.

So I encourage you to keep this book handy, using it as a reliable reference as you work with your doctor—ideally in an open, ongoing partnership that ultimately relies on shared knowledge and free flow of information.

Although its critiques of many drugs are often appropriately harsh, *Worst Pills, Best Pills* should not lead you to a hopeless or cynical attitude about all drugs. Today's patients have access to an array of effective medications that can be powerful and lifesaving. The opportunities for the effective cure of many acute illnesses and for reducing the effects of chronic disease have never been better—usually through a combination of medications, knowledge, and active self-care such as exercise, good nutrition, and nonmedication therapies.

The challenge is to distinguish useful and reasonably safe drugs from drugs best avoided, and to use effective and lifesaving drugs properly and safely. This remarkably useful book can help you to do just that.

Eric B. Larson, M.D., M.P.H., F.A.C.P.
Director, Group Health Cooperative's Center
for Health Studies
Clinical Professor, Medicine and Health
Services, University of Washington

ACKNOWLEDGMENTS

Worst Pills, Best Pills is the result of the talent, time, labor, and dedication of many people, including past and present members of the staff of Public Citizen's Health Research Group as well as many others outside the group.

While the health professionals and health scientists are the named authors of this book, many others made contributions of equal importance.

• Lynn Miller is the Health Research Group's office manager and designated copy editor. She labored mightily over the preparation of the manuscript, checking hundreds of references, proofreading attentively, communicating with the publishers, and shepherding the book through innumerable steps on the way to publication.

• Benita Marcus brought a new eye to the project, helping to reconceptualize it in an effort to make it more consumer-friendly. Her organizational skills and attention to detail are unmatched; she also offered extremely helpful proofreading and editorial suggestions.

• Meredith Larson only started working at Public Citizen late in the process of writing this book, but proved to be a quick study. Without her many trips to the library, quick mastery of the Reference Manager program, and unfailing sense of humor, this book could never have been completed as rapidly as it was.

We also wish to thank Paul Levy, an attorney with Public Citizen's Litigation Group, for a review of the manuscript.

Lisa Fugate, Elizabeth P. Hulstrand, and Laurie E. Kamimoto contributed to the original (1988) edition of this book. Several of their chapters remain in the present edition and were the foundation upon which the reviews of certain drugs were built.

We would also like to thank our editor, Kevin Smith, and his colleagues at Pocket Books and Simon & Schuster, who demonstrated patience with the complexity of the project while assuring that the process was moving forward. Special thanks to our copy editor, Jane Elias, whose attention to detail rivaled even Benita's but still allowed us the freedom to write the book we wanted. And thanks to Kelly Farley and Monica Hopkins at dix! for their helpfulness and patience in the final crunch. Finally, a heartfelt thanks to all our colleagues at Public Citizen, particularly Joe Zillo, who encouraged us from start to finish and ensured that we kept at least a tenuous grip on reality.

CONTENTS

INTRODUCTION

- A 40-year-old woman who dies from a heart arrhythmia (rhythm disturbance)
- A 58-year-old man who has just developed parkinsonism
- A 68-year-old woman with a hip fracture
- A 63-year-old woman whose memory and ability to think clearly are slipping, according to her daughter
- A 62-year-old man with recent onset of extreme dizziness and occasional fainting when he first gets up
- A 52-year-old woman who suddenly dies while having some dental work done

What Do These People Have in Common?

They are all tragic victims of serious but entirely preventable adverse reactions to prescription drugs. In each case, the drug was too dangerous to be used at all or was misprescribed. (See Chapter 3, "Drug-Induced Diseases," p. 17.) In fact, a study in the *Journal of the American Medical Association* found that adverse drug reactions are responsible for 100,000 fatalities a year and afflicting 2.2 million people with serious drug-induced diseases.[1] Drug-induced illness is one of the five leading causes of preventable disease and death in the United States. By reading and using *Worst Pills, Best Pills,* you can help protect yourself and your family from the preventable dangers of misprescribed drugs. But first, you may have some questions. Here are the answers to some frequently asked ones.

Question: **Sure, once in a while prescription drugs, whether prescribed properly or not, can cause adverse drug reactions. But the six cases above are unusual, aren't they?**

Answer: Unfortunately, they are all too common. In addition to the fact that there are 100,000 deaths a year from adverse drug reactions, each year approximately 1.5 million people in the United States are injured so seriously by adverse drug reactions that they require hospitalization. Seven hundred thousand people a year develop adverse drug reactions *after* they have been hospitalized for other reasons. Also, there are *61,000 people with drug-induced parkinsonism; 32,000 with hip fractures, including 1,500 deaths attributable to drug-induced falls; 16,000 with injuries from car crashes caused by adverse drug reactions; 163,000 with drug-induced or drug-worsened memory loss; 41,000 with hospitalizations—3,300 of whom died—from ulcers caused by non-steroidal anti-inflammatory drugs (NSAIDs), usually for arthritis; and hundreds of thousands of people with drug-induced dizziness or fainting.*

Other drug reactions can also lead to death. Older drugs such as digoxin (see p. 144), a heart medicine, cause 28,000 cases of life-threatening or fatal adverse reactions each year in hospitals alone, often because the prescribed dose is too high or the drug is given to people who do not need to be taking it in the first place. Newer drugs, such as the powerful sedative/tranquilizer Versed, can also be extremely dangerous if not used carefully. Used for so-called conscious sedation during oral surgery or during diagnostic procedures such as gastroscopy, this drug has caused dozens of preventable deaths when the dose was needlessly high.

Question: But why are so many people getting adverse drug reactions and how can they be prevented?

Answer: First: Often, the "disease" for which a drug is prescribed is actually an adverse reaction to another drug, masquerading as a disease. Second: Many times a drug is used to treat a problem that, although susceptible in some cases to a pharmaceutical solution, should first be treated with commonsense lifestyle changes. Third: The medical problem—as with viral infections such as colds and bronchitis in otherwise healthy children or adults—is both self-limited and completely unresponsive to treatments such as antibiotics or does not merit treatment with certain drugs. Fourth: A drug is the preferred treatment for the medical problem, but instead of using the safest, most effective—and often least expensive—treatment, one of the 181 **Do Not Use** drugs listed in this book—or another, much less preferable alternative—is prescribed. Fifth: Different prescription drugs, each of which on its own may be safe and effective, together can interact to cause serious injury or death (see examples in box on this page). Sixth: Adverse reactions can occur when two or more drugs in the same therapeutic category are used, even though the additional ones do not add to the effectiveness of the first but clearly increase the risk to the patient. Seventh: Many times the right drug is prescribed, but the dose is dangerously high.

Question: Why do older adults suffer more, and more serious, adverse drug reactions than younger people?

Answer: In Chapter 2 "Adverse Drug Reactions," p. 10, we discuss nine reasons, including

---

DRUGS THAT CAN CAUSE LIFE-THREATENING REACTIONS IF USED TOGETHER

TRICOR with LIPITOR	MEVACOR with LOPID
insulin with INDERAL	ULTRACET with PAXIL
COUMADIN with CELEBREX	TEGRETOL with FLAGYL
INSPRA with potassium	CALAN SR with quinidine
PROZAC with DESYREL	theophylline with TAGAMET
GEODON with ZAGAM	TEQUIN with BETAPACE
LANOXIN with CALAN SR	DEMEROL with NARDIL
TAGAMET with DILANTIN	COUMADIN with TAGAMET

---

both physical differences and differences and deficiencies in doctors' prescribing habits.

Studies have found that:

• Seventy percent of doctors treating Medicare patients flunked an exam concerning their knowledge of prescribing to older adults.

• Between 40 and 50% of drugs prescribed for older adults outside the hospital were overused.

• Among older patients being given three or more prescriptions upon leaving the hospital, 88% had prescriptions with one or more problems and 22% had prescription errors that were potentially serious or life-threatening. A closer look at these frequent, often serious prescribing mistakes showed that:

- Fifty-nine percent of patients were prescribed a less-than-optimal drug or one not effective for their disease.
- Twenty-eight percent of patients were given doses that were too high.
- Forty-eight percent of patients were given drugs with one or more potential harmful interactions with other drugs.

But, according to the World Health Organization, *"Quite often, the history and clinical examination of patients with side effects reveal that no valid indication [purpose] for the drug has been present."*[2]

Question: **Are you and the World Health Organization saying that if older people used fewer drugs, more selectively, most adverse reactions would be prevented?**
Answer: Yes, that is exactly what we are saying. Most older people and many younger people are using too many drugs, often for problems that are better treated with nondrug therapy. (See sections on sleeping pills and tranquilizers, p. 166, diabetes, p. 405, and hypertension, p. 60.)

Question: **Since more of these problems occur in older people, if I am not 60 or over, do I really need to worry about them?**
Answer: You certainly do, for two reasons. First, serious problems with prescription drugs do not suddenly start at age 60. Beginning in our thirties, the output of the heart and the ability of the liver to metabolize drugs, and even more important, the ability of the kidney to clear drugs out of the body, begin to decrease. Since most people in their thirties or forties are not given many prescription drugs, these changes alone do not usually lead to as large a number of drug-induced medical problems as they do in older adults. **But most of the adverse reactions discussed in this book can occur in anyone at any age. They just occur more often in older adults.** However, as people enter their fifties, the amount of prescription drug use starts increasing significantly, and the odds of getting an adverse drug reaction also increase.

For most of the categories of problems that can be caused by drugs, such as depression, sexual dysfunction, memory loss, hallucinations, insomnia, parkinsonism, constipation, and many others, we include lists of frequently prescribed drugs that can cause these problems in people of any age (see Chapter 3, p. 21). Only for the categories of hip fractures and of drug-induced automobile crashes resulting in injuries do the drug lists apply mainly to people 60 and older.

If you do not learn how to reduce (or keep low, if not at zero) the number of prescription drugs you are taking when you are in your thirties, forties, and fifties, you will be in great danger of becoming another overmedicated person at unnecessary risk of adverse drug reactions.

The second reason for concern, even though you may be less than 60 years old, is that all people under 60 have parents, grandparents, brothers, sisters, or friends who are over 60 and who could use some of your help in better coping with the onslaught of drugs and other treatments that most doctors are inclined to prescribe. (See Chapter 29, "Protecting Yourself and Your Family from Preventable Drug-Induced Injury," p. 862, for specific ways you can help yourself and others with the information in this book.)

Question: **How many of the drugs in this book should not be used?**
Answer: According to published studies and/or the Public Citizen's Health Research Group or its medical consultants, 181 of the 549 commonly prescribed drugs discussed in this book—approximately one-third—should not be used because safer alternative drugs are available. (See Chapters 4 through 28 for the 181 **Do Not Use** drugs and their safer alternatives.)

*The list of **Do Not Use** drugs includes widely used sleeping pills and tranquilizers such as Valium, Restoril, Ativan, and Tranxene; antidepressants such as Serzone and Elavil; painkillers or arthritis drugs such as Vioxx, Celebrex, Bextra, Darvocet-N and Darvon, and Ultram and Feldene; heart drugs such as Persantine, Lopid, Dyrenium, and Catapres; gastrointestinal drugs such as Bentyl, Donnatal, Librax, Lomotil, and Tigan; the widely used diabetes drugs Diabinese, Actos, Avandia, and Glucophage; birth control pills such as Yasmin, Desogen, and Ortho-Cept; and the toenail-fungus drug Lamisil. (The drugs are listed by their present or former brand name even if some are now big sellers as generic versions.)*

These 30 Do Not Use drugs alone account for more than 228 million prescriptions filled a year, at a cost of well in excess of $12 billion a year.

In several major categories of drugs, a large proportion are categorized as **Do Not Use** by our medical experts. They include:

- 22 of 51, or 43%, of the mind drugs (tranquilizers, sleeping pills, etc.)
- 22 of 109, or 20%, of the heart drugs
- 15 of 48, or 31%, of the gastrointestinal drugs
- 22 of 59, or 37%, of the pain/arthritis drugs

Overall, 53 of the 181 **Do Not Use** drugs, for which we list safer alternatives (29%), are among the 200 top-selling brand-name or generic drugs. These drugs had 370 million prescriptions filled in 2003 at a cost of $22.2 billion.[3]

Question: **What can be done about this serious epidemic of preventable drug-induced illness?**
Answer: The solution to this problem, a difficult one, will have to involve you, your doctor(s), and your pharmacist.

A good way to start is by being aware of the extraordinary variety of "illnesses" that are often written off to old age or to nervous problems but can be drug-induced. For example, all of the following medical problems have been found, in a significant number of instances, to occur as adverse drug reactions. The number of different drugs listed by name in the tables in Chapter 3 that can cause each type of adverse reaction is included:

- 166 drugs can cause depression
- 156 drugs can cause hallucinations or psychoses
- 129 drugs can cause sexual dysfunction
- 77 drugs can cause dementia
- 59 drugs can cause falls and hip fractures
- 28 drugs can cause auto accidents resulting in injuries

- 35 drugs can cause insomnia
- 107 drugs can cause constipation
- 40 drugs can cause parkinsonism

This list does not include those kinds of adverse reactions that are more difficult for patients or their friends to detect, such as early evidence of liver or lung damage, nor does it contain every drug, no matter how few prescriptions there are, which can cause the adverse effects listed here.

Further specific details of how to significantly reduce the risks of drug-induced death and injury are discussed in Chapter 29, including ten rules for safer drug use.

The first step is to take an inventory of all the drugs you, your parents, or other loved ones have used in the last month, including over-the-counter and prescription drugs. The most accurate way to do this is to **put all the drugs in a brown bag** and, the next time you or your parents go to the doctor, bring all of them along and **get the doctor to help you fill out the Drug Worksheet for Patients, Family, Doctor, and Pharmacist** (sample on p. 922). For each drug you or your parents are using, you will need to list the doses, how often the drug is taken and for how long, the medical conditions for which the doctor says each drug is being used, the adverse effects you or your parents are having from any of these drugs, and other information shown on the drug worksheet. Then you, your parents, and the doctor can begin the process of reducing the number of drugs being taken by eliminating the ones that are not absolutely necessary or are unnecessarily dangerous. At the same time, the dosage of drugs that are thought to be necessary can be reduced, if possible, to further decrease the risk of adverse drug reactions.

Question: **When I finally get down to the smallest number of drugs I really need to be taking and the lowest dose of each, is there any way that I can further cut down**

on the $1,200 a year I am now spending on prescription drugs?

Answer: As discussed in much more detail in Chapter 30, "Saving Money When Buying Prescription Drugs: Often Using Safer Alternatives as an Additional Benefit" (p. 874), each year a larger percentage of the most commonly used drugs are available in generic form—which is usually much less expensive—as the brand-name versions come off patent. In this chapter, we also discuss and rebut the myths that brand-name companies are using to frighten doctors and patients from using these much less expensive drugs.

In addition, many times you'll find that more expensive but not safer or more effective drugs are prescribed because they are heavily promoted to doctors.

In the drug profiles in Chapters 4 through 28, the availability of a generic version of each drug is listed at the top (except for those in the **Do Not Use** category).

One last thought: When we hear the phrase "drug abuse" these days, the first thing that comes to mind is heroin, cocaine, crack, or whatever drug is currently in the headlines. But what about drug abuse in older people? Well, older people do not use those kinds of drugs. That problem mainly has to do with younger people. But that is taking the narrow view that drug abuse means the drug-abusing person "chooses" to take drugs such as heroin and cocaine. If instead we broaden the definition of drug abuse to include older or younger victims of the drug choices of others—such as patients of doctors—then **the greatest epidemic of drug abuse in American society is among those patients who are the victims of misprescribing or overprescribing.** Like other epidemics, it is preventable. This book will help you start that process.

REFERENCES

1. Lazarou J, Pomeranz BH, Corey PN. Incidence of adverse drug reactions in hospitalized patients: A meta-analysis of prospective studies. *Journal of the American Medical Association* 1998; 279:1200–5.

2. *Drugs for the Elderly.* 2nd ed. Copenhagen, Denmark: World Health Organization, 1997.

3. Information compiled from http://www.drugtopics.com.

4. Lasser KE, Allen PD, Woolhandler SJ, et al. Timing of new black-box warnings and withdrawals for prescription medications. *Journal of the American Medical Association* 2002; 287:2215–20.

HOW THIS BOOK WAS COMPILED

Which Drugs Are Included in the Book?

The decision as to which drugs were to be included in the book was based in part on data from the *Drug Topics* list of the 200 most commonly prescribed drugs in the United States in 2003, all of which are included in the book. We also added a number of drugs that have only recently come on the market but that are likely soon to become among the most often prescribed drugs. In addition, we included many drugs that, although not in the top 200, are often used by older adults and were in earlier editions of *Worst Pills, Best Pills*. We did not include in the book any drug if more than 50% of its use was in the hospital, such as a number of antibiotics, drugs for general anesthesia, and other drugs. Nor did we include most drugs used primarily for the treatment of cancer.

The total number of drugs listed in the book is 549 and the names appear in the Index. The generic names are in lowercase letters, and the brand names are in capital letters.

What Information Goes into the Discussions of Specific Drugs?

In addition to information that is referenced in the listed medical journal articles and books, much of the other information comes from the current *Physicians' Desk Reference (PDR)* and the *United States Pharmacopeia Drug Information (USP DI)*, 2003 edition.

On What Basis Is a Drug Listed as "Do Not Use?"

All drugs were initially reviewed by Public Citizen's Health Research Group staff to decide which ones should be listed as **Do Not Use.** Subsequently, most drugs were also reviewed, depending on their therapeutic category, by at least one specialist in areas including cardiology, diabetology, gastroenterology, infectious diseases, neurology, and psychiatry. Each drug met at least one of the criteria listed above for **Do Not Use** and/or was thought by Public Citizen's Health Research Group staff and at least one of the above consultants to merit a **Do Not Use** designation. (The names and affiliations of these consultants are listed on p. xxxiii.)

For each of the 181 drugs listed as **Do Not Use,** at least one or more of the following reasons was used as the basis for the decision:

1. Published references explicitly stating not to use the drug in older adults and other information advising against use in younger people.

2. Single-ingredient drugs that, in the opinion of Public Citizen's Health Research Group and its consultants, are not as safe as the alternative drug or other treatment that is always listed on the page to the right of the **Do Not Use.**

3. Lack of evidence of effectiveness of the drug in the opinion of Public Citizen's Health Research Group and its consultants. This was most commonly seen in combination drugs in which at least one ingredient has not been proven to be effective or the second ingredient has not been proven significantly to add to the effectiveness of the first. Therefore the combination drug is more dangerous than an alternative without the unproven ingredient because it has increased risks posed by the extra ingredient without any increased benefit.

4. Fixed-combination drugs that do not, in the opinion of Public Citizen's Health Research Group and its consultants, meet the criteria for justifying their use. Use fixed combinations of drugs only when they are logical and well studied and they either aid compliance or improve tolerance or efficacy obtained with a single ingredient. **Few fixed combinations meet this standard.**

5. Smoke and Mirrors Drugs. These drugs, such as Lexapro, Nexium, and Clarinex, are the desperate ways drug companies try to cope with the expiration of a patent on one of their big-selling drugs. Instead of just throwing in the towel to lower-priced generic equivalents, they patent an optical isomer or metabolite that is certain to function in an identical fashion as the original drug. These few drugs are **Do Not Use** for economic reasons.

On What Basis Is a Drug Listed as "Limited Use"?

Drugs were designated for "Limited Use" on the basis of one or more of the following criteria:

1. Published studies stating that the drug should only be used as a second-line drug if another drug does not work.

2. Published studies showing that the drug is more dangerous than another, preferable drug but not so much so that it merits being listed as **Do Not Use.**

3. Published evidence that the drug, although effective and safe enough for the treatment of certain conditions, is widely used for inappropriate and therefore unnecessarily unsafe purposes. The widespread use of antipsy-

chotic drugs for treating older adults who are not psychotic (see p. 183) is an example of this serious problem.

4. Combination drugs that should be reserved for second-choice use. (Most are **Do Not Use.**) Examples are many combination high blood pressure drugs that are required to carry a warning label. The label states that because it is a fixed-combination drug, the drug is not indicated for initial treatment of high blood pressure.

On What Basis Is a Drug Listed as "Do Not Use Until Seven Years After Release"?

Safety dictates the designation of a new drug as "Do Not Use Until Seven Years After Release." The exception to this rule is a rare "breakthrough" drug that offers a documented therapeutic benefit over older proven drugs. The "Do Not Use Until Seven Years After Release" designation is made for the following reasons:

1. New drugs are the most dangerous because we know the least about their safety.

2. New drugs are tested in a relatively small number of people before they are approved, and much more is known about their effectiveness than their safety.

3. Though more is known about the effectiveness of new drugs, it is rarely known if they are more or less effective than older drugs.

4. Serious adverse effects or life-threatening drug interactions may not be detected until a new drug has been taken by hundreds of thousands of people.

5. A number of new drugs have been withdrawn from the market, or serious new adverse reaction warnings have been added to their labeling, usually within seven years after they have been released.

In a recent study, the estimated probability of acquiring a new black-box warn-

ing or being withdrawn from the market over a period of 25 years was 20%. Half of these black-box warning changes occurred within seven years of drug introduction; half of the withdrawals occurred within two years. The safety of new agents cannot be known with certainty until a drug has been on the market for many years.[4]

The problem has become more serious in recent years because of the record numbers of new drugs that have been approved in the United States due to intense political pressure exerted by the pharmaceutical industry through Congress on a weakened Food and Drug Administration (FDA). In a period of only nine months, between September 1997 and June 1998, three new drugs with known safety problems were withdrawn, all on the market for less than five years. They should not have been approved but were approved by the FDA. Tragically, in each of these cases, there were multiple other older proven drugs available for treating the same conditions that these drugs were approved for, and hundreds of people were needlessly killed or injured.

What Is the Basis for the Warnings About Pregnancy and Breast-feeding?

We derived the information for the pregnancy and breast-feeding warnings primarily from the most recent drug labels, available from the 2004 *PDR* or the manufacturer. For a few older drugs that had been dropped from the most recent *PDR,* we used the 2000 *PDR* as our source.

HOW TO USE THIS BOOK

This book gives a profile of 538 drugs commonly used by consumers. The profiles are divided into 25 chapters based on the type of problem treated: Drugs for Heart Conditions, Mind Drugs, Drugs for Pain and Arthritis, etc.

These chapters have (1) discussions of the most important medical problems (for example, high blood pressure) and the types of treatment available, and (2) the drug profiles.

Before looking up any of the drugs in this book, please read the following guide to the format of the drug and supplement profiles.

GUIDE TO THE DRUG AND SUPPLEMENT PROFILES

This page, showing the format of our drug profiles, will help you understand the information provided about each of the 549 drugs in this book. If a drug profile lacks any of the sections described below, it means there is no relevant information.

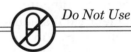 *Do Not Use*

We recommend that these drugs not be used and we suggest an alternative treatment. Listings for these drugs do not include information on whether or not a generic version is available, or the sections titled Before You Use This Drug, When You Use This Drug, How to Use This Drug, Interactions with Other Drugs, Adverse Effects, and Periodic Tests.

Do Not Use Until Seven Years After Release

We recommend that these drugs not be used for at least seven years from date of release unless it is one of those rare "breakthrough" drugs that offer you a documented therapeutic advantage over older, proven drugs. (The year in which the drug will have been on the market for seven years is given in the profile of each drug with this designation.)

Last Choice

We believe that these drugs should be used only if other drugs are ineffective or cannot be used to treat your medical condition.

Limited Use

We believe that these drugs offer limited benefit or benefit only certain people or conditions.

Generic Name

This is the chemical name of the active ingredient(s).

BRAND NAME (Manufacturer)

These are the brand names used by the manufacturers. The names are those of the most frequently prescribed drugs. In most cases, no more than five brand names appear because of space limitations. You always should learn both the brand and the generic names of your drug.

GENERIC: Tells if a generic product is available that is sold under the chemical name of the drug.

FAMILY: This is the class of similar drugs.

PREGNANCY AND BREAST FEEDING WARNINGS
Describes human and animal evidence of potential harm with such uses.

The text section describes the drug's actions and effects, in older adults in particular, and the conditions for which the drug is prescribed. It explains how and why the drug should or should not be used.

Before You Use This Drug

• Presents information that your doctor should know before you start to use the drug, such as your past and present health conditions and prescription and nonprescription drugs that you use.

When You Use This Drug

• Presents information that will ensure your safety and maximum benefit while using the drug.

How to Use This Drug

• Tells you what to do about a missed dose and how to take the drug.

Interactions with Other Drugs

Alphabetically lists the names of the drugs that may interact most harmfully with the drug profiled if they are used at the same time. The generic drugs are in lowercase letters and the brand names are in CAPITAL LETTERS. Make sure you know the generic name of your drugs, since only one or two brand names are listed for each generic drug.

Adverse Effects

• Presents the unwanted adverse effects that may occur while you use the drug (and sometimes after you stop). There are two categories of adverse effects: (1) those that require immediate medical attention, including signs of overdose for many drugs, and (2) signs that do not require immediate attention but should be brought to your doctor's attention if they persist.

Periodic Tests

• Names the medical tests that should or might need to be done during the time that you use this drug, such as complete blood count, complete urine test, electrocardiogram (ECG, EKG), or eye pressure exam. You should ask your doctor which of these tests you need.

Boxed Warnings

The drug profiles contain various kinds of warnings, including FDA-mandated black boxes, usually warning about the dangers of the drug; warnings about drugs that should not be used if you are pregnant or breast-feeding; warnings about drugs that can pose a risk if it is hot outside, because they may decrease your ability to sweat; drugs that are addicting; and drugs that pose special mental and physical adverse effects, specifically drugs having an anticholinergic effect.

Talk to your doctor before deciding to make any changes in your prescription drugs based on the information in this book.

MEDICAL CONSULTANTS

The following physicians, with expertise in various medical subspecialties, gave generously of their time to read and make helpful suggestions about the parts of the book that fell into their area of expertise.

Frank Calia, M.D., Professor Emeritus of Medicine, Microbiology, and Immunology, University of Maryland School of Medicine, Baltimore, Maryland (Drugs for Infections for all four editions)

Charles Gerson, M.D., physician in private practice of gastroenterology, New York City, and attending physician, Mount Sinai School of Medicine, New York (Drugs for Gastrointestinal Disorders for all four editions)

Louis Rakita, M.D., Department of Cardiology, Cleveland Metropolitan General Hospital and Professor of Medicine, Case Western Reserve University School of Medicine, Cleveland, Ohio (Drugs for Heart Conditions for all four editions)

Fredric Solomon, M.D., Clinical Professor of Psychiatry and Behavioral Sciences, George Washington University School of Medicine (Sleeping Pills, Minor Tranquilizers, Antidepressants, and Antipsychotic Drugs for all four editions; Drugs for Attention Deficit Hyperactivity Disorder, this edition)

E. Fuller Torrey, M.D., author of *Surviving Schizophrenia,* former director of chronic psychiatric disease wards, St. Elizabeth's Hospital, Washington, D.C., staff member, Public Citizen's Health Research Group, and Deputy Director for Laboratory Research, Stanley Medical Research Institute (Antipsychotic Drugs and Antidepressants for first, third, and fourth editions)

Jonathan Trobe, M.D., Professor of Ophthalmology and Neurology, University of Michigan School of Medicine, Ann Arbor, Michigan (Eye Drugs, this edition)

Patrick Walsh, M.D., Professor of Surgery and Director, Brady Urological Institute, Johns Hopkins University School of Medicine, Baltimore, Maryland (Drugs for Enlarged Prostate, this edition)

1

MISPRESCRIBING AND OVERPRESCRIBING OF DRUGS

The numbers are staggering: in 2003, an estimated 3.4 billion prescriptions were filled in retail drugstores and by mail order in the United States. That averages out to 11.7 prescriptions filled for each of the 290 million people in this country.[1] But many people do not get any prescriptions filled in a given year, so it is also important to find out how many prescriptions are filled by those who fill one or more prescriptions. In a study based on data from 2000, more than twice as many prescriptions were filled for those 65 and older (23.5 prescriptions per year) than for those younger than 65 (10.1 prescriptions per year).[2] Another way of looking at the high rate of prescriptions among older people is the government finding that although Medicare beneficiaries comprise only 14% of the community population, they account for more than 41% of prescription medicine expenses.[3]

There is no dispute that for many people, prescriptions are beneficial, even lifesaving in many instances. But hundreds of millions of these prescriptions are wrong, either entirely unnecessary or unnecessarily dangerous. Inappropriate prescribing is an academically gentle euphemism for prescriptions for which the risks outweigh the benefits, thus conferring a negative health impact on the patient. A recent comprehensive review of studies of such inappropriate prescribing in older patients found that 21.3% of community-dwelling patients 65 years or older were using at least one drug inappropriately prescribed. Much more so than age, per se, the total number of drugs being pre-

scribed was an important predictor of inappropriate prescribing, as was female gender.[4] Another study found that, conservatively—using very narrow criteria for inappropriate prescribing—elderly United States patients were prescribed at least one inappropriate drug at an estimated 16.7 million visits to physician offices or hospital outpatient departments in the year 2000.[5] Examples of specific drugs that have been inappropriately prescribed, including studies involving younger adults and children, are given later in this chapter.

At the very least, misprescribing wastes tens of billions of dollars, barely affordable by many people who pay for their own prescriptions. But there are much more serious consequences. As discussed in Chapter 2, p. 10, more than 1.5 million people are hospitalized and more than 100,000 die each year from largely preventable adverse reactions to drugs that should not have been prescribed as they were in the first place.[6] What follows is a summary of the **seven all-too-often-deadly sins of prescribing.**

First: The "disease" for which a drug is prescribed is actually an adverse reaction to another drug, masquerading as a disease but unfortunately not recognized by doctor and patient as such. Instead of lowering the dose of the offending drug or replacing it with a safer alternative, the physician adds a second drug to the regimen to "treat" the adverse drug reaction caused by the first drug. Examples discussed in this book (see later in this chapter and in Chapter 3) include drug-induced parkinsonism, depression, sexual dysfunction, insomnia, psychoses, constipation, and many other problems.

Second: A drug is used to treat a problem that, although in some cases susceptible to a pharmaceutical solution, should first be treated with commonsense lifestyle changes. Problems such as insomnia and abdominal pain often have causes that respond very well to nondrug treatment, and often the physician can uncover these causes by taking a careful history. Other examples include medical problems such as high blood pressure, mild adult-onset diabetes, obesity, anxiety, and situational depression. Doctors should recommend lifestyle changes as the first approach for these conditions, rather than automatically reach for the prescription pad.

Third: The medical problem is both self-limited and completely unresponsive to treatments such as antibiotics or does not merit treatment with certain drugs. This is seen most clearly with viral infections such as colds and bronchitis in otherwise healthy children or adults.

Fourth: A drug *is* the preferred treatment for the medical problem, but instead of the safest, most effective—and often least expensive—treatment, the physician prescribes one of the 181 Do Not Use drugs listed in this book or another, much less preferable alternative. An example of a less preferable alternative would be a drug to which the patient has a known allergy that the physician did not ask about.

Fifth: Two drugs interact. Each on its own may be safe and effective, but together they can cause serious injury or death.

Sixth: Two or more drugs in the same therapeutic category are used, the additional one(s) not adding to the effectiveness of the first but clearly increasing the risk to the patient. Sometimes the drugs come in a fixed combination pill, sometimes

as two different pills. Often heart drugs or mind-affecting drugs are prescribed in this manner.

Seventh: The right drug is prescribed, but the dose is dangerously high. This problem is seen most often in older adults, who cannot metabolize or excrete drugs as rapidly as younger people. This problem is also seen in small people who are usually prescribed the same dose as that prescribed to people weighing two to three times as much as they do. Thus, per pound, they are getting two to three times as much medicine as the larger person.

Evidence of Misprescribing and Overprescribing

Here are some examples from recent studies by a growing number of medical researchers documenting misprescribing and overprescribing of specific types of drugs:

Treating Adverse Drug Reactions with More Drugs

Researchers at the University of Toronto and at Harvard have clearly documented and articulated what they call the *prescribing cascade*. It begins when an adverse drug reaction is misinterpreted as a new medical condition. Another drug is then prescribed, and the patient is placed at risk of developing additional adverse effects relating to this potentially unnecessary treatment.[7] To prevent this prescribing cascade, doctors—and patients—should follow what we call Rule 7 of the Ten Rules for Safer Drug Use (see p. 864): Assume that any new symptom you develop after starting a new drug might be caused by the drug. If you have a new symptom, report it to your doctor.

Some of the instances of the prescribing cascade that these and other researchers have documented include:

• The increased use of anti-Parkinson's drugs to treat drug-induced parkinsonism caused by the heartburn drug metoclopramide[7] (REGLAN) or by some of the older antipsychotic drugs.

• A sharply increased use of laxatives in people with decreased bowel activity that has been caused by antihistamines such as diphenhydramine (BENADRYL), antidepressants such as amitriptyline (ELAVIL)—a **Do Not Use** drug—or some antipsychotic drugs such as thioridazine (MELLARIL).[8]

• An increased use of antihypertensive drugs in people with high blood pressure that was caused or increased by very high doses of nonsteroidal anti-inflammatory drugs (NSAIDs), used as painkillers or for arthritis.[9]

Failing to Treat Certain Problems with Nondrug Treatments

Research has shown that many doctors are too quick to pull the prescription trigger. In one study, in which doctors and nurse practitioners were presented with part of a clinical scenario—as would occur when first seeing a patient with a medical problem—and then encouraged to ask to find out more about the source of the problem, 65% of doctors recommended that a patient complaining of insomnia be treated with sleeping pills even though, had they asked more questions about the patient, they would have found that the patient was not exercising, was drinking coffee in the evening, and, although awakening at 4 A.M., was actually getting seven hours of sleep by then.[10]

In a similar study, doctors were presented with a patient who complained of abdominal pain and whose endoscopy showed diffuse irritation in the stomach. Sixty-five percent of the doctors recommended treating the problem with a drug—a histamine antagonist (such as Zantac, Pepcid, or Tagamet). Had they asked more questions they would have discovered that the patient was using aspirin, drinking a lot of coffee, smoking cigarettes, and was under considerable emotional stress—all potential contributing factors to abdominal pain and stomach irritation.

In summarizing the origin of this overprescribing problem, the authors stated: "Apparently quite early in the formulation of the problem, the conceptual focus [of the doctor] appears to shift from broader questions like 'What is wrong with this patient?' or 'What can I do to help?' to the much narrower concern, 'Which prescription shall I write?' " They argued that this approach was supported by the "barrage" of promotional materials that only address drug treatment, not the more sensible lifestyle changes to prevent the problem.[11]

In both of the above scenarios, nurse practitioners were much more likely than doctors to take an adequate history that elicited the causes of the problems and, not surprisingly, were only one-third as likely as the doctors to decide on a prescription as the remedy instead of suggesting changes in the patient's habits.

Throughout the book, in the discussions about insomnia, high blood pressure, situational depression, mild adult-onset diabetes, and other problems, you will find out about the proven-effective nondrug remedies that should first be pursued before yielding to the riskier pharmaceutical solutions.

Treating Viral Infections with Antibiotics or Treating Other Diseases with Drugs That Are Not Effective for Those Problems

Two recently published studies, based on nationwide data from office visits for children and adults, have decisively documented the expensive and dangerous massive overprescribing of antibiotics for conditions that, because of their viral origin, do not respond to these drugs. Forty-four percent of children under 18 years old were given antibiotics for treatment of a cold and 75% for treatment of bronchitis. Similarly, 51% of people 18 or older were treated with antibiotics for colds and 66% for bronchitis. Despite the lack of evidence of any benefit for most people from these treatments, more than 23 million prescriptions a year were written for colds, bronchitis, and upper respiratory infections. This accounted for approximately one-fifth of all prescriptions for antibiotics written for children or adults.[12,13] An accompanying editorial warned of "increased costs from unnecessary prescriptions, adverse drug reactions, and [subsequent] treatment failures in patients with antibiotic-resistant infections" as the reasons to try to reduce this epidemic of unnecessary antibiotic prescribing.[14]

Similar misprescribing of a drug useful and important for certain problems, but not necessary or effective, and often dangerous, for other problems can be seen in another recent study. In this case, 47% of the people admitted to a nursing home who were taking digoxin, an important drug for treating an abnormal heart rhythm called atrial fibrillation or for treating severe congestive heart failure, did not have either of these medical problems and were thereby being put at risk for life-threatening digitalis toxicity without the possibility of any benefit.[15]

A final example in this category involves the overuse of a certain class of drugs, in this case calcium channel blockers, which have not been established as effective for treating people who have had a recent heart attack. The study shows that this prescribing pattern actually did indirect damage to patients because their use was replacing the use of beta-blockers, drugs shown to be very effective for reducing the subsequent risk of death or hospitalization following a heart attack. Use of a calcium channel blocker instead of a beta-blocker was associated with a doubled risk of death, and beta-blocker recipients were hospitalized 22% less often than nonrecipients.[16]

The Prescribing of More Dangerous and/or Less Effective Do Not Use Drugs Instead of Safer Alternatives

There are 181 **Do Not Use** drugs listed in this book for which we recommend safer alternatives. Twenty-two of these **Do Not Use** drugs are for heart disease or high blood pressure and make up 20% of all the drugs in the book for these problems. Twenty-two of the **Do Not Use** drugs are for treating insomnia, anxiety, depression, or other mental problems, and make up 43% of the drugs in the book for these problems. Another 22 of the **Do Not Use** drugs are for treating pain, and make up 37% of the drugs in the book for these problems. Fifteen of the **Do Not Use** drugs are for treating gastrointestinal problems and make up 31% of the drugs in the book for these problems. Twenty-two of the **Do Not Use** drugs are for treating coughs, colds, allergies, or asthma, and make up 47% of the drugs in the book for these problems. Twenty of the **Do Not Use** drugs are for treating infections and make up 31% of the drugs in the book for these problems. Although the original determinations for these **Do Not Use** drugs were based on their use by older adults, we have concluded that the same warnings apply to use by anyone.

Included in this book are 19 drugs we label **Do Not Use Until Seven Years After Release.** We have applied this warning to drugs that have only recently appeared on the market, for which there is no evidence of their superiority over older drugs about which we have much more information as to long-term safety and effectiveness. Because of incomplete and worrisome safety information, there is a risk that some of these newer drugs will have to be banned. But by the time they have been on the market for seven years, it is much less likely that they will be banned, and it is much more likely that, if they are still being used, there will be much better information about their safety and effectiveness, such as a new black-box warning not present when the drugs were first marketed.

Another category of drugs that is misprescribed even though there are safer alternatives are drugs to which patients are known to be allergic, but about which their physicians have not taken a careful medical history.

The Causes of Misprescribing and Overprescribing

The Drug Industry

The primary culprit in promoting the misprescribing and overprescribing of drugs is the pharmaceutical industry, which now sells about $216 billion worth of drugs in the United States alone.[1] The industry uses loopholes in the law not requiring proof of superiority over existing drugs for approval, and otherwise intimidates the Food and Drug Administration (FDA) into approving record numbers of me-too drugs (drugs that offer no significant benefit over drugs already on the market) that often have dangerous adverse effects. In addition, the industry spends well in excess of $21 billion a year to promote drugs[17] using advertising and promotional tricks that push at or through the envelope of being false and misleading. This industry has been extremely successful in distorting, in a profitable but dangerous way, the rational processes for approving and prescribing drugs. Two studies of the accuracy of ads for prescription drugs widely circulated to doctors both concluded that a substantial proportion of these ads contained information that was false or misleading and violated FDA laws and regulations concerning advertising.[18,19]

The fastest-growing segment of drug advertising is directed not at doctors but at patients. It has been estimated that from 1991 to 2002 DTC (direct-to-consumer) advertising expenditures in the United States grew from about $60 million a year to $3 billion a year,[17] an increase of 50-fold in just eleven years, employing mis-

leading advertising campaigns similar to those used for doctors. A study by *Consumer Reports* of 28 such ads found that "only half were judged to convey important information on side effects in the main promotional text," only 40% were "honest about efficacy and fairly described the benefits and risks in the main text," and 39% of the ads were considered "more harmful than helpful" by at least one reviewer.[20] This campaign has been extremely successful. According to a drug industry spokesman, "There's a strong correlation between the amount of money pharmaceutical companies spend on DTC advertising and what drugs patients are most often requesting from physicians." The advertising "is definitely driving patients to the doctor's office, and in many cases, leading patients to request the drugs by name."[21] The problems with DTC advertising are best summed up in an article written by a physician more than 15 years ago in the *New England Journal of Medicine*, before the current binge had really begun: "If direct [to consumer] advertising should prevail, the use of prescription medication would be warped by misleading commercials and hucksterism. The choice of a patient's medication, even of his or her physician, could then come to depend more on the attractiveness of a full-page spread or prime-time commercial than on medical merit . . . such advertising would serve only the ad-makers and the media, and might well harm our patients."[22]

The Food and Drug Administration (FDA)

Attempting to fend off FDA-weakening legislation even worse than that which was signed into law in 1997, the FDA has bent over backwards to approve more drugs, culminating in 1996 and 1997 when the agency approved a larger number than had ever been approved in any two-year period. Thousands of people were injured or killed after taking one of three such recently approved drugs (which have subsequently been recalled from the market). These drugs were the weight-loss drug dexfenflu-ramine (REDUX), the heart drug mibefradil (POSICOR), and the painkiller bromfenac (DURACT). Other drugs that would not have gotten approved in a more cautious era at the FDA have also been approved, but are likely either to be banned or to be forced to carry severe warnings that will substantially reduce their use. Many of these are included in this book and listed as **Do Not Use** drugs.

In the 33 years since the Public Citizen's Health Research Group started monitoring the FDA and the drug industry, the current pro-industry attitude at the FDA is as bad and dangerous as it has ever been. In addition to record numbers of approvals of questionable drugs, FDA enforcement over advertising has all but disappeared. From a peak number of 157 enforcement actions to stop illegal prescription drug ads that understate risks and/or overstate benefits in 1998, the number has decreased to only 24—an 85% decrease—in 2003.[23] There is no evidence that the accuracy or legality of these ads has increased during this interval, and the amount of such advertising has clearly increased. The division at FDA responsible for policing prescription drug advertising has never been given adequate resources to keep up with the torrent of newly approved drugs. More recently, however, it has also been thwarted by marching orders from higher up in the agency to, effectively, go easy on prescription drug advertising. As a result, the drug industry correctly believes it can get away with more violative advertising than in the past. The role of the United States Congress in pushing the FDA into approving more drugs, and passing, with the FDA's reluctant approval, legislation to further weaken the FDA's ability to protect the public, cannot be overlooked.

Physicians

The well-financed promotional campaigns by drug companies would not have as much of an impact as they do were there not such an educational vacuum about proper prescribing of drugs, a serious problem that must be laid at the feet of medical school and residency training. The varieties of overprescribing and misprescribing of drugs by doctors—**the seven all-too-often-deadly sins of prescribing** referred to on pp. 1–2—are all strongly enhanced by the mind-altering properties of drug promotion. The best doctors, of whom there are many, do not waste their time talking to drug sales people, toss promotional materials away, and ignore drug ads in medical journals. Too many other doctors, however, are heavily influenced by drug companies, accepting free meals, free drinks, and free medical books in exchange for letting the drug companies "educate" them at symposia in which the virtues of certain drugs are extolled. Unfortunately, many of these doctors are too arrogant to realize that there is no such thing as a free lunch. The majority of doctors attending such functions have been found to increase their prescriptions for the targeted drugs following attendance at the "teach-in."[24]

Beyond traditional advertising and promotion and their influence, bias of drug-company-sponsored research, as published in medical journals, also can sway doctors toward more favorable impressions about drugs. An analysis was done of 56 trials that were paid for by drug companies and reported in 52 medical journals about drugs for arthritis and pain—NSAIDs. (These drug-company-sponsored studies represented 85% of those that the researchers originally looked at.) In studies identifying the company's drug as less toxic than another drug, in barely one-half of the studies was there justification for the finding of less toxicity. This certainly explains why, contrary to fact, newer arthritis drugs almost always "seem" safer than older, usually much less expensive ones.[25]

A final example demonstrates the ignorance of many physicians, especially in dealing with prescribing drugs to older adults. A study of physicians who treat Medicare patients found that 70% of the doctors who took an examination concerning their knowledge of prescribing for older adults failed to pass the test. The majority of physicians who were contacted for participation in the study refused to take the test, often giving as their reason that they had a "lack of interest in the subject." The authors concluded "many of these physicians [who failed the exam] had . . . not made good use of the best information on prescribing for the elderly."[26]

Pharmacists

A small fraction of pharmacists have, in our view, betrayed their professional ethics and are working for drug companies, engaging in such activities as calling doctors to get them to switch patients from drugs made by a company other than the one the pharmacist works for to the pharmacist's employer's drugs. In addition, pharmacy organizations such as the American Pharmaceutical Association and others have fought hard to prevent the FDA from requiring accurate patient package information to be dispensed with each prescription filled.

Too many pharmacists, despite having computers to aid them, have been willing to fill prescriptions for pairs of drugs that, because of life-threatening adverse drug interactions if used at the same time, should never be dispensed to the same person.

• Sixteen (32%) of 50 pharmacies in Washington, D.C., filled prescriptions for erythromycin and the now-banned terfenadine (SELDANE) without comment.[27] These two drugs, if used in combination, can cause fatal heart arrhythmias.

• In another study, of 245 pharmacists in seven cities, about one-third of pharmacists did not alert consumers to the potentially fatal and widely publicized interaction between Hismanal, a commonly used but now banned antihistamine, and Nizoral, an often-prescribed antifungal drug. Only 4 out of 17 pharmacists warned of the interaction between oral contraceptives and Rimactane, an antibiotic that could decrease the effectiveness of the oral contraceptive. Only 3 out of 61 pharmacists issued any verbal warnings about the interaction between Vasotec and Dyazide—two drugs for treating hypertension—which may lead to dangerously high levels of potassium in the blood.[28]

• In yet another study, concurrent use of terfenadine (SELDANE) and contraindicated drugs declined over time. The rate of same-day dispensing declined by 84%, from an average of 2.5 per 100 persons receiving terfenadine in 1990 to 0.4 per 100 persons during the first six months of 1994, while the rate of overlapping use declined by 57% (from 5.4 to 2.3 per 100 persons). Most cases involved erythromycin. Despite substantial declines following reports of serious drug-drug interactions and changes in product labeling, concurrent use of terfenadine and contraindicated antibiotics such as erythromycin and clarithromycin (BIAXIN) and antifungals such as ketoconazole (NIZORAL) continued to occur.[29]

Patients

For too many patients, the system is stacked against you—drug companies, doctors, and pharmacists are too often making decisions that ultimately derive from what is best for the drug companies, doctors, and pharmacists, and not necessarily from what is best for you. This book has been researched and written to help you come out ahead in the struggle with our health care industry.

In Chapter 3, concerning adverse drug reactions, you can learn which common medical problems—depression, insomnia, sexual disorders, parkinsonism, falls and hip fractures, constipation, and many others—can actually be caused by drugs. Once you recognize these problems, you will be enabled to better take care of yourself and your family, and bring such problems to an end by discussing safer alternatives with your physician.

Chapters 4 through 28, the largest section of the book, discuss 538 drugs, including 181 that we and our consultants think you should not use. For each of these, we recommend safer alternatives. In addition, Chapters 4 through 28 list hundreds of drug combinations that should not be used because of serious interactions.

Chapter 29 presents a detailed strategy, beyond information on specific adverse effects and drugs, to help you to use drugs more safely, including Ten Rules for Safer Drug Use and how to use and maintain your own Drug Worksheet for Patient, Family, Doctor, and Pharmacist. This is your personalized plan for avoiding becoming a victim of overprescribing or misprescribing.

Chapter 30 discusses the latest information about generic drugs and shows you how and why you can and should save hundreds of dollars a year or more. In short, this book is intended to help you and your family to improve your health by using drugs, if necessary, more carefully and recognizing those you should avoid.

REFERENCES

1. Ukens C. How mail order pharmacy gained in market share in 2003. *Drug Topics* 2004:148.

2. Stagnitti MN. Trends in outpatient prescription drug utilization and expenditures: 1997–2000: AHRQ Statistical Brief #21. Available at: http://www.meps.ahrq.gov/papers/st21/stat21.htm 2004.

3. Stagnitti MN, Miller GE, and Moeller JF. Outpatient prescription drug expenses, 1999: MEPS Chartbook No. 12, ARHQ Pub. No. 04-0001. Rockville, Md.: Agency for Healthcare Research and Quality; 2003.

4. Liu GG, Christensen DB. The continuing challenge of inappropriate prescribing in the elderly: An update of the evidence. *Journal of the American Pharmaceutical Association* 2002; 42:847–57.

5. Goulding MR. Inappropriate medication prescribing for elderly ambulatory care patients. *Archives of Internal Medicine* 2004; 164:305–12.

6. Lazarou J, Pomeranz BH, Corey PN. Incidence of adverse drug reactions in hospitalized patients: A meta-analysis of prospective studies. *Journal of the American Medical Association* 1998; 279:1200–5.

7. Rochon PA, Gurwitz JH. Optimising drug treatment for elderly people: The prescribing cascade. *British Medical Journal* 1997; 315:1096–9.

8. Monane M, Avorn J, Beers MH, et al. Anticholinergic drug use and bowel function in nursing home patients. *Archives of Internal Medicine* 1993; 153:633–8.

9. Rochon PA, Gurwitz JH. Drug therapy. *The Lancet* 1995; 346:32–6.

10. Everitt DE, Avorn J, Baker MW. Clinical decision-making in the evaluation and treatment of insomnia. *American Journal of Medicine* 1990; 89:357–62.

11. Avorn J, Everitt DE, Baker MW. The neglected medical history and therapeutic choices for abdominal pain: A nationwide study of 799 physicians and nurses. *Archives of Internal Medicine* 1991; 151:694–8.

12. Nyquist AC, Gonzales R, Steiner JF, et al. Antibiotic prescribing for children with colds, upper respiratory tract infections, and bronchitis. *Journal of the American Medical Association* 1998; 279:875–7.

13. Gonzales R, Steiner JF, Sande MA. Antibiotic prescribing for adults with colds, upper respiratory tract infections, and bronchitis by ambulatory care physicians. *Journal of the American Medical Association* 1997; 278:901–4.

14. Schwartz B, Mainous AG III, Marcy SM. Why do physicians prescribe antibiotics for children with upper respiratory tract infections? *Journal of the American Medical Association* 1998; 279:881–2.

15. Aronow WS. Prevalence of appropriate and inappropriate indications for use of digoxin in older patients at the time of admission to a nursing home. *Journal of the American Geriatric Society* 1996; 44:588–90.

16. Soumerai SB, McLaughlin TJ, Spiegelman D, et al. Adverse outcomes of underuse of beta-blockers in elderly survivors of acute myocardial infarction. *Journal of the American Medical Association* 1997; 277:115–21.

17. This data is from PhRMA, the prescription drug industry's U.S. trade association, and is based on data from 2002. Available at: http://www.phrma.org/publications/2003-10-07.892.pdf.

18. Wilkes MS, Doblin BH, Shapiro MF. Pharmaceutical advertisements in leading medical journals: experts' assessments. *Annals of Internal Medicine* 1992; 116:912–9.

19. Stryer D, Bero LA. Characteristics of materials distributed by drug companies: An evaluation of appropriateness. *Journal of General Internal Medicine* 1996; 11:575–83.

20. Drug advertising: Is this good medicine? *Consumer Reports* 1996; 61:62–3.

21. The top 200 drugs. *American Druggist* 1998; 46–53.

22. Cohen EP. Direct-to-the-public advertisement of prescription drugs. *New England Journal of Medicine* 1988; 318:373–6.

23. The data on FDA enforcement actions are derived from the FDA Web site at http://www.fda.gov/cder/warn/index.htm.

24. *Medical Marketing and Media* 1990.

25. Rochon PA, Gurwitz JH, Simms RW, et al. A study of manufacturer-supported trials of nonsteroidal anti-inflammatory drugs in the treatment of arthritis. *Archives of Internal Medicine* 1994; 154:157–63.

26. Ferry ME, Lamy PP, Becker LA. Physicians' knowledge of prescribing for the elderly: A study of primary care physicians in Pennsylvania. *Journal of the American Geriatric Society* 1985; 33:616–25.

27. Cavuto NJ, Woosley RL, Sale M. Pharmacies and prevention of potentially fatal drug interactions. *Journal of the American Medical Association* 1996; 275:1086–7.

28. Headden S. Danger at the Drugstore. *U.S. News and World Report* 1996; 46–53.

29. Thompson D, Oster G. Use of terfenadine and contraindicated drugs. *Journal of the American Medical Association* 1996; 275:1339–41.

2

ADVERSE DRUG REACTIONS

How Serious Is the Problem and How Often and Why Does It Occur?

Although some adverse drug reactions (ADR) are not very serious, others cause the death, hospitalization, or serious injury of more than 2 million people in the United States each year, including more than 100,000 fatalities. In fact, adverse drug reactions are one of the leading causes of death in the United States.[1] Most of the time, these dangerous events could and should have been avoided. Even the less drastic reactions, such as change in mood, loss of appetite, and nausea, may seriously diminish the quality of life.

Despite the fact that more adverse reactions occur in patients 60 or older, the odds of suffering an adverse drug reaction really begin to increase even before age 50. Almost half (49.5%) of Food and Drug Administration (FDA) reports of deaths from adverse drug reactions and 61% of hospitalizations from adverse drug reactions were in people younger than 60.[2] Many physical changes that affect the way the body can handle drugs actually begin in people in their thirties, but the increased prescribing of drugs does not begin for most people until they enter their fifties. By then, the amount of prescription drug use starts increasing significantly, and therefore the odds of having an adverse drug reaction also increase. **The risk of an adverse drug reaction is about 33% higher in people aged 50 to 59 than it is in people aged 40 to 49.**[3, 4]

Adverse Reactions to Drugs Cause Hospitalization of 1.5 Million Americans Each Year

An analysis of numerous studies in which the cause of hospitalization was determined found that approximately 1.5 million hospitalizations a year were caused by adverse drug reactions.[1] This means that every day more than 4,000 patients have adverse drug reactions so serious that they need to be admitted to American hospitals.

A review of patients admitted to medical wards of a hospital found that although for 3.8% of hospital admissions, adverse drug reactions led directly to hospitalization, 57% of these adverse drug reactions were not recognized by the attending physician at the time of admission. As in numerous other studies, many of these admissions should have been prevented. In fact, 18.6% of all drugs prescribed prior to admission were contraindicated.[5]

Another review of studies of the percentage of hospital admissions related to adverse drug reactions found that up to 88% of ADR-related hospitalizations in the elderly are preventable. In addition, elderly people were four times more likely to be hospitalized by ADR-related problems than nonelderly.[6]

Although the rate of drug-induced hospitalization is higher in older adults (an average of about 10% of all hospitalizations for older adults are caused by adverse drug reactions) because they use more drugs, a significant proportion of hospitalizations for children are also caused by adverse drug reactions.

A recent review of all studies concerning the reasons for pediatric hospitalization (children under the age of 19) found that 2.09% of all pediatric hospitalizations were caused by adverse drug reactions and that 39% of these were life-threatening.[7] Using the most recent published data on pediatric hospitalizations,[8] there were 3.8 million children under the age of 19 hospitalized in the United States in 1997. This means that in one year, there are 79,000 children (2.09% × 3.8 million children) admitted to the hospital because of adverse drug reactions, 31,000 of these children having life-threatening adverse reactions.

Adverse Reactions as a Major Cause of Emergency Room Visits

A recent review of studies concerning the causes of people going to hospital emergency rooms found that as many as 28% of all emergency department visits were drug-related, including a large proportion due to adverse drug reactions and inappropriate prescriptions. Of all of the drug-related visits, the authors found that 70% were preventable.[9]

Adverse Reactions Occur During Hospitalization to 770,000 People a Year

In addition to the 1.5 million people a year who are admitted to the hospital because of adverse drug reactions, an additional three-quarters of a million people a year develop an adverse reaction after they are hospitalized. According to national projections based on a study involving adverse drug reactions developing in patients in the hospital, 770,000 additional patients a year—more than 2,000 patients a day—suffer an adverse event caused by drugs once they are admitted. Many of the reactions in the patients studied were serious, even life-threatening, and included cardiac arrhythmias, kidney failure, bleeding, and dangerously low blood pressure. People with these adverse reactions had an almost twofold higher risk of death compared to other otherwise comparable hospitalized patients who did not have a drug reaction. Most important, according to the researchers, almost 50% of these adverse reactions were preventable. Among the kinds of preventable problems were adverse interactions between drugs that should not have been prescribed together (hundreds of these are listed in Chapter 3 of this book), known allergies to drugs that had not been asked about before the patients got a prescription, and excessively high doses of drugs prescribed without considering the patient's weight and kidney function.[10]

Thus, adding the number of people with adverse drug reactions so serious that they require hospitalization to those in which the adverse reaction was "caused" by the hospitalization, more than 2.2 million people a year, or 6,000 patients a day, suffer these adverse reactions. In both situations, many of these drug-induced problems should have been prevented.

Dangerous Prescribing Outside the Hospital for 6.6 Million Older Adults a Year

Based on the **Do Not Use** principle we have advocated concerning certain drugs for more than 16 years in our *Worst Pills, Best Pills* books and monthly newsletter, several published studies have examined the extent to which people are prescribed drugs that are contraindicated because there are safer alternatives. One study, whose authors stated that *"Worst Pills, Best Pills* stimulated this research," found that almost one out of four older adults living at home— 6.6 million people a year—were prescribed a "potentially inappropriate" drug or drugs, placing them at risk of such adverse drug effects as mental impairment and sedation, even though the study only examined the use of a relatively short list of needlessly dangerous drugs (fewer than the number listed as **Do Not Use** drugs in this book).[11]

Other researchers looked not only at people for whom a contraindicated drug was prescribed, but also at prescriptions for older people involving two other categories: questionable combinations of drugs and excessive treatment duration. The authors categorized all of this as "high-risk prescribing" and limited their analysis to just the three classes of drugs most commonly causing drug-related illness: cardiovascular drugs, psychotropic drugs (ones that act on the mind) such as tranquilizers and antidepressants, and anti-inflammatory drugs. They found that 52.6% of all people 65 or older were given one or more prescriptions for a high-risk drug.[12] Thus, more than twice as many older adults were the victims of high-risk prescribing when these two additional categories were added.

Nine Reasons Why Older Adults Are More Likely Than Younger Adults to Have Adverse Drug Reactions

Many of the studies and much of the information concerning the epidemic of drug-induced disease focuses on people 60 and over. As we have mentioned previously, some of the changes that eventually lead to great numbers of adverse reactions in older adults (in combination with increased drug use) really begin to occur in the mid-thirties. In connection with the idea that drug-induced disease begins to get more common before age 60, it is interesting to note that in a number of studies comparing the way "older" people clear drugs out of the body with the way younger people do, the definition of older is above 50, and younger is below 50.[3]

1. Smaller Bodies and Different Body Composition: Older adults generally weigh less and have a smaller amount of water and a larger proportion of fat than younger adults. Body weight increases from age 40 to 60, mainly due to increased fat, then decreases from age 60 to 70,

with even sharper declines from 70 on. Therefore, the amount of a drug per pound of body weight or per pound of body water will often be much higher in an older adult than it would be if the same amount of the drug were given to a younger person. In addition, drugs that concentrate in fat tissue may stay in the body longer because there is more fat for them to accumulate in.

2. Decreased Ability of the Liver to Process Drugs: Because the liver does not work as well in older adults, they are less able than younger people to process certain drugs so that they can be excreted from the body. This has important consequences for a large proportion of the drugs used to treat heart conditions and high blood pressure, as well as many other drugs processed by the liver. The ability of the body to rid itself of drugs such as Valium, Librium, and many others is affected by this decrease in liver function.

3. Decreased Ability of the Kidneys to Clear Drugs Out of the Body: The ability of the kidneys to clear many drugs out of the body decreases steadily from age 35 to 40 on. By age 65, the filtering ability of the kidneys has already decreased by 30%. Other aspects of kidney function also decline progressively as people age. This has an effect on the safety of a large number of drugs.

4. Increased Sensitivity to Many Drugs: The problems of decreased body size, altered body composition (more fat, less water), and decreased liver and kidney function cause many drugs to accumulate in older people's bodies at dangerously higher levels and for longer times than in younger people. These age-related problems are further worsened by the fact that even at "normal" blood levels of many drugs, older adults have an increased sensitivity to their effects, often resulting in harm. This is seen most clearly with drugs that act on the central nervous system, such as many **sleeping pills, alcohol, tranquilizers, strong painkillers such as morphine or pentazocine (TALWIN), and most drugs that have anti-**

cholinergic effects (see *Anticholinergic* in the Glossary, p. 889). This latter group includes antidepressants, antipsychotic drugs, antihistamines, drugs used to calm the intestinal tract (for treating ulcers or some kinds of colitis) such as Donnatal, atropine, and Librax, antiparkinsonian drugs, and other drugs such as Norpace.

For all of the drugs in the above-mentioned groups that are listed in this book, we include an "anticholinergic" warning as follows:

WARNING

[Name of drug] can cause or worsen high blood pressure. It is especially dangerous for people who have high blood pressure, heart disease, diabetes, or thyroid disease. People over 60 are more likely than younger people to experience effects on the heart and blood pressure, restlessness, nervousness, and confusion.

ANTICHOLINERGIC EFFECTS

WARNING: SPECIAL MENTAL AND PHYSICAL ADVERSE EFFECTS

Older adults are especially sensitive to the harmful anticholinergic (see Glossary, p. 889) effects of [name of drug class]. These drugs should not be used unless absolutely necessary.

Mental effects: confusion, delirium, short-term memory problems, disorientation, and impaired attention.

Physical effects: dry mouth, constipation, difficulty urinating (especially for a man with an enlarged prostate), blurred vision, decreased sweating with increased body temperature, sexual dysfunction, and worsening of glaucoma.

Yet another example of the marked increase in the sensitivity of older adults to drugs has to do with stimulant drugs that are in the same family as amphetamines, or "speed." Despite the dangers of these drugs for anyone, especially older adults, they are widely promoted and prescribed, including Ornade, Tavist-D, Entex LA, and Actifed. All of these contain amphetamine-like drugs such as pseudoephedrine. For any of these drugs discussed in this book, most of which are listed as **Do Not Use** drugs, the following warning is given:

5. Decreased Blood-Pressure-Maintaining Ability: Because older adults are less able to compensate for some of the effects of drugs, there is yet another reason why they are more vulnerable to adverse effects of drugs and more sensitive to the intended effects. The most widespread example of older adults' decreased ability to compensate is seen when they get out of bed and/or suddenly rise from a seated position. As you rise, your blood pressure normally falls, decreasing the blood flow to your head and resulting in less blood flow to the brain. Younger people's bodies can compensate for this: receptors in the neck, sensing that the blood pressure is falling as the person rises, tighten up the blood vessels in other parts of the body, thus keeping the overall blood pressure high enough. In older adults, these receptors do not work as well. Often, upon standing, older adults feel giddy, lightheaded, and dizzy. They may even faint because the blood pressure in the head falls too rapidly.

The ability to maintain a proper blood pressure is further weakened when you use any of a very long list of drugs, **the most common examples being high blood pressure drugs. Other categories of drugs that cause an exaggerated blood pressure drop include sleeping pills, tranquilizers, antidepressants, antipsychotic drugs, antihistamines, drugs for heart pain (angina), and**

antiarrhythmics. (See p. 31 for a full list of drugs that can cause this difficulty.)

This problem of so-called postural hypotension—the sudden fall in blood pressure on standing, brought about by a combination of aging and drugs—can be catastrophic. The falls that often result can end in hip fractures, a leading cause of death in older adults, or other serious injuries.

6. Decreased Temperature Compensation: Younger adults are more easily able than older people to withstand very high or very low temperatures. They sweat and dilate (widen) blood vessels to get rid of excess heat when it is hot, and constrict (narrow) blood vessels to conserve heat when it is cold. Older adults' bodies are less able to do this. As in the case of blood pressure compensation, this "normal" temperature-regulating problem of older adults can be significantly worsened by any of a large number of prescription and over-the-counter drugs, resulting in fatal or life-threatening changes in body temperature. **Many older adults' deaths during heat waves or prolonged cold spells can be attributed to drugs that interfere with temperature regulation. Most of these people did not know they were at increased risk.** All drugs in this book that contain a warning about anticholinergic effects can have this harmful effect on withstanding heat waves.

7. More Diseases That Affect the Response to Drugs: Older adults are much more likely than younger adults to have at least one disease—such as liver or kidney damage (not just the decreased function of older age), poor circulation, and other chronic conditions—that alters their response to drugs. Little is known about the influence of multiple diseases on drug effects in the elderly.

One well-understood example, however, is the effect of heart failure on the way people can handle drugs. When the heart is not able to pump as much blood as it used to, the change that occurs in heart failure, there is also a decrease in the flow of blood to the kidneys. For the same reasons discussed in reason number 3, the reduced flow of blood to the kidneys decreases the kidneys' ability to rid drugs from the blood and excrete them in the urine.

8. More Drugs and, Therefore, More Adverse Drug Reactions and Interactions: Since older adults use significantly more prescription drugs than younger people, they have greatly increased odds of having a drug reaction caused by the dangerous interaction between two drugs. Often, older adults take one or more over-the-counter drugs in addition to their prescription drugs. This further increases the likelihood of adverse drug interactions. One of the more common kinds of adverse drug interactions is the ability of some drug to cause a second drug to accumulate to dangerous levels in the body. At the end of the discussion of each drug in Chapters 4 through 28, except for the 181 **Do Not Use** drugs, there is a list of other drugs that can cause serious adverse interactions.

PARTIAL LIST OF DRUG INTERACTIONS

Some of these interactions are life-threatening or of great potential harm to patients. (See individual drug profiles for complete lists of interactions.)

TRICOR	with	LIPITOR
INSPRA	with	potassium
CELEBREX	with	warfarin (COUMADIN)
MEVACOR	with	LOPID
TEQUIN	with	BETAPACE
ALDACTONE	with	potassium
PROZAC	with	DESYREL
ULTRACET	with	PAXIL
insulin	with	INDERAL
TEGRETOL	with	erythromycin
TAGAMET	with	DILANTIN
GEODON	with	ZAGAM
INDERAL	with	TAGAMET
DEMEROL	with	NARDIL
CALAN SR	with	quinidine
theophylline	with	TAGAMET
warfarin (COUMADIN)	with	TAGAMET
LANOXIN	with	CALAN SR

9. Inadequate Testing of Drugs in Older Adults Before Approval: Although older adults use a disproportionate share of prescription drugs, few of these drugs are adequately tested in older adults before being approved by the FDA.

Dr. Peter Lamy of the University of Maryland School of Pharmacy has stated, "We test drugs in young people for three months; we give them to old people for 15 years." The FDA is slowly remedying this serious problem by requiring that the people on whom a drug is tested be representative of those who will use the drug if it is approved. Nonetheless, most drugs on the market today, which are heavily used by older adults, were not adequately tested in this age group.

In summary, there are significant differences between younger and older patients, often not realized by doctors or patients. Increasing awareness of these differences will result in the prescription of far fewer drugs to older adults, and those that are prescribed will be given at lower doses in most instances.

REFERENCES

1. Lazarou J, Pomeranz BH, Corey PN. Incidence of adverse drug reactions in hospitalized patients: A meta-analysis of prospective studies. *Journal of the American Medical Association* 1998; 279:1200–5.

2. Food and Drug Administration. Second Annual Adverse Drug/Biologic Reaction Report: 1986, 1987.

3. Vestal RE, ed. *Drug Treatment in the Elderly.* Sydney, Australia: ADIS Health Service Press, 1984.

4. Calculation of 33% increase in risk of adverse reaction (age 50–59 vs. 40–49) is based on an average of all three studies listed on page 32 of the Vestal reference.

5. Dormann H, Criegee-Rieck M, Neubert A, et al. Lack of awareness of community-acquired adverse drug reactions upon hospital admission: Dimensions and consequences of a dilemma. *Drug Safety* 2003; 26:353–62.

6. Beijer HJ, de Blaey CJ. Hospitalisations caused by adverse drug reactions (ADR): A meta-analysis of observational studies. *Pharmacy World and Science* 2002; 24:46–54.

7. Impicciatore P, Choonara I, Clarkson A, et al. Incidence of adverse drug reactions in paediatric in/out-patients: A systematic review and meta-analysis of prospective studies. *British Journal of Clinical Pharmacology* 2001; 52:77–83.

8. Miller MR, Elixhauser A, Zhan C. Patient safety events during pediatric hospitalizations. *Pediatrics* 2003; 111:1358–66.

9. Patel P, Zed PJ. Drug-related visits to the emergency department: How big is the problem? *Pharmacotherapy* 2002; 22:915–23.

10. Classen DC, Pestotnik SL, Evans RS, et al. Adverse drug events in hospitalized patients: Excess length of stay, extra costs, and attributable mortality. *Journal of the American Medical Association* 1997; 277:301–6.

11. Willcox SM, Himmelstein DU, Woolhandler S. Inappropriate drug prescribing for the community-dwelling elderly. *Journal of the American Medical Association* 1994; 272:292–6.

12. Tamblyn RM, McLeod PJ, Abrahamowicz M, et al. Questionable prescribing for elderly patients in Quebec. *Canadian Medical Association Journal* 1994; 150:1801–9.

3

DRUG-INDUCED DISEASES

How Extensive Is the Problem of Specific Adverse Drug Reactions?

Each year, more than 9.6 million adverse drug reactions occur in older Americans. The referenced study found that 37% of these adverse reactions were not reported to the doctor, presumably because patients did not realize the reactions were due to the drug. This is not too surprising considering that most doctors admitted they did not explain possible adverse effects to their patients.[1]

The following national estimates are based on well-conducted studies, mainly in the United States:

• *Each year, in hospitals alone, there are 28,000 cases of life-threatening heart toxicity from adverse reactions to digoxin,* the most commonly used form of digitalis in older adults.[2] Since as many as 40% or more of these people are using this drug unnecessarily (see discussion on p. 144), many of these injuries are preventable.

• *Each year 41,000 older adults are hospitalized—and 3,300 of these die from ulcers caused by NSAIDs* (nonsteroidal anti-inflammatory drugs, usually for treatment of arthritis).[3] Thousands of younger adults are hospitalized. (For a list of drugs that can cause gastrointestinal bleeding, see p. 37.)

• *At least 16,000 injuries from auto crashes each year involving older drivers are attributable to the use of psychoactive drugs,* specifically benzodiazepines and tricyclic antidepressants.[4] Psychoactive drugs are those that affect the mind or behavior. (For a list of drugs that can cause auto crashes, see p. 34.)

• *Each year 32,000 older adults suffer from hip fractures—contributing to more than 1,500 deaths—attributable to drug-induced falls.*[5,6] In one study, the main categories of drugs responsible for the falls leading to hip fractures were sleeping pills and minor tranquilizers (30%), antipsychotic drugs (52%), and antidepressants (17%). All of these categories of drugs are often prescribed unnecessarily, especially in older adults. (See section on minor tranquilizers and sleeping pills, antipsychotic drugs, and antidepressants, p. 166.) The in-hospital death rate for hip fractures in older adults is 4.9%.[7] Multiplying this times the 32,000 hip fractures a year in older adults attributable to drug-induced falls, 1,568 older adults die each year from adverse drug reactions that cause hip fractures. (For a list of drugs that can cause hip fractures because of drug-induced falls, see p. 33.)

• *Approximately 163,000 older Americans suffer from serious mental impairment (memory loss, dementia) either caused or worsened by drugs.*[8,9] In a study in the state of Washington, in 46% of the patients with drug-induced mental impairment, the problem was caused by minor tranquilizers or sleeping pills; in 14%, by high blood pressure drugs; and in 11%, by antipsychotic drugs. (For a list of drugs that can cause or worsen dementia, see p. 28.)

• *Two million older Americans are addicted or at risk of addiction to minor tran-*

17

quilizers or sleeping pills because they have used them daily for at least one year, even though there is no acceptable evidence that the tranquilizers are effective for more than four months, and the sleeping pills for more than 30 days.[10]

• *Drug-induced tardive dyskinesia has developed in 73,000 older adults; this condition is the most serious and common adverse reaction to antipsychotic drugs, and it is often irreversible.* Tardive dyskinesia is characterized by involuntary movements of the lips, tongue, and sometimes the fingers, toes, and trunk. Since most of the older people taking these drugs were not actually psychotic, they have a serious side effect from antipsychotic drugs prescribed without justification.[11] (For a list of drugs that can cause tardive dyskinesia or other movement disorders, see p. 31.)

• *Drug-induced parkinsonism has developed in 61,000 older adults due to the use of antipsychotic drugs such as Haldol, Thorazine, Mellaril, Stelazine, and Prolixin.* There are also other parkinsonism-inducing drugs, such as Reglan, Compazine, and Phenergan, prescribed for gastrointestinal problems.[12] As mentioned above, most (about 80%) older adults receiving antipsychotic drugs do not have schizophrenia or other conditions that justify the use of such powerful drugs. (For a list of drugs that can cause parkinsonism, see p. 30.)

A serious problem exists because both doctors and patients do not realize that practically any symptom in older adults and in many younger adults can be caused or worsened by drugs.[13] Some doctors and patients assume that what are actually adverse drug reactions are simply signs of aging. As a result, many serious adverse reactions are entirely overlooked or not recognized until they have caused significant harm.

The drugs responsible for the most serious adverse reactions in older adults are tranquilizers, sleeping pills, and other mind-affecting

Mental Adverse Drug Reactions: depression, hallucinations, confusion, delirium, memory loss, impaired thinking

Nervous System Adverse Drug Reactions: parkinsonism, involuntary movements of the face, arms, legs (tardive dyskinesia), sexual dysfunction

Dizziness on Standing, Falls Sometimes Resulting in Hip Fractures, Automobile Accidents Resulting in Injury

Gastrointestinal Adverse Drug Reactions: loss of appetite, constipation

Urinary Problems: difficulty urinating, leaking of urine

drugs; cardiovascular drugs such as high blood pressure drugs, digoxin, and drugs for abnormal heart rhythms;[14] and drugs for treating intestinal problems.

Specific Patient Examples of Drug-Induced Diseases

Fifty-four-Year-Old Woman Homebound from Lung Toxicity due to a Heart Drug Never Approved to Treat Her Condition

Liz was prescribed the drug Cordarone to treat a common heart condition. She was not told that the drug was not approved by the FDA for her condition. The pharmacy leaflet mentioned nausea and dizziness with the drug, but not death from lung toxicity. She is now dependent on an oxygen tank to breathe and does not have the strength to clean her house. It is estimated that as many as 17% of patients experience lung toxicity from amiodarone, and about 10% of them die.

Fifty-eight-Year-Old Man Develops Parkinsonism from Antipsychotic Drug Being Used to Treat His "Irritable Bowel" Problem

Larry, an otherwise healthy 58-year-old man with diarrhea believed to be due to "irritable bowel syndrome," was given Stelazine, a powerful antipsychotic tranquilizer to "calm down" his intestinal tract. Stelazine is not even approved for treating such medical problems. Six months after starting Stelazine, Larry developed severe parkinsonism and was started on L-dopa, a drug for treating Parkinson's disease. Presumably, the doctor did not realize the parkinsonism was drug-induced, and the Stelazine was continued. For seven years, Larry took both drugs. Then a neurologist specializing in Parkinson's disease saw Larry, recognized the real cause of his problem, stopped the Stelazine, and slowly withdrew the L-dopa over a six-month period. Larry's severe, disabling parkinsonism cleared completely.

As mentioned above, 61,000 older adults develop drug-induced parkinsonism each year. At least 80% of them, like Larry, should never have been put on the drugs causing the parkinsonism in the first place. Also, as in Larry's situation, a large proportion of these people have doctors who think that their parkinsonism developed spontaneously.

The doctors not only fail to suspect that it is caused by a drug such as Stelazine, or other antipsychotic drugs (Reglan, Compazine, or Phenergan), but they add a second drug to treat the disease that has been caused by the first drug.

The same neurologist who "cured" Larry of his drug-induced parkinsonism saw, in just three years, 38 other patients with drug-induced parkinsonism and 28 with drug-induced tardive dyskinesia.

None of these people were psychotic, the one justification for antipsychotic medications. Rather, the most common reasons for using the parkinsonism-inducing drugs were chronic anxiety and gastrointestinal complaints. The most frequent culprit (in 19 of these 39 patients) was metoclopramide (REGLAN), usually prescribed for heartburn, or for nausea and vomiting. Doctors often prescribe Reglan before trying other more conservative and safer methods. (See alternative treatment of nausea and

vomiting, p. 560.) Other drugs that brought on parkinsonism included Compazine, Haldol, and Thorazine.[15]

Sarah's 80-Year-Old Father's Confusion and Hallucinations Were Induced by His Ulcer Drugs

Sarah wrote us about her father, saying that she had to repeatedly nag his doctor about the possible role of her dad's ulcer drugs in causing confusion and hallucinations before the doctor listened. Three different drugs—Tagamet, Zantac, and Pepcid—had been tried for her father's ulcers, and each had caused these adverse reactions. When the doctor finally switched Sarah's father to an antacid, Maalox, his mind completely cleared and he was his old self, no longer confused or hallucinating.

Seventy-nine-Year-Old Woman Has Reversible Mental Impairment

Sally, the mother-in-law of a physician, was noted by her son-in-law, who had not seen her for several months, to have suffered severe impairment of her otherwise sharp mind. She was acting confused and, for the first time in her life, was unable to balance her checkbook. When questioned by her son-in-law, she was able to remember that her problem had started around the time she was put on a tranquilizer, Ativan. After this link was discovered, the drug was slowly discontinued and all of the mental impairment that had begun when the drug was started disappeared.

Sixty-four-Year-Old Man Has Auto Accident After One Dose of Tranquilizer

Ben, the 64-year-old uncle of a physician, was scheduled to have a biopsy done at a local hospital at eight in the morning. So that he would be relaxed for the biopsy, four days before it was to be done the doctor gave him a free sample of a tranquilizer, Xanax, to take an hour or so before the procedure. Ben was not told that he should not use drugs like this if he was going to drive and, while driving to the hospital for the biopsy, he blacked out. The car went over a fence and sustained $6,000 worth of damage, but fortunately Ben was unhurt. (See Drugs That Can Cause Automobile Accidents, p. 34.)

Sixty-three-Year-Old Gets into "Drug-Illness" Cycle

Nancy, a healthy 63-year-old woman, complained about difficulty going to sleep. Instead of taking a careful history and finding out that she had recently started drinking several cups of coffee at dinner, her doctor prescribed a sleeping pill. A subsequent referral was also made to a psychiatrist because of depression (possibly partly induced by the sleeping pill), and an antidepressant drug was also prescribed. If this patient also took an antihistamine-containing drug for a cold (not an effective treatment), she would be using three drugs, all of which have powerful sedative effects, which could make her so groggy that standing would be difficult, and falling would be easy.

Sixty-Year-Old Woman Given "Overdose" of Propranolol

Elsie, a 60-year-old woman who worked as an assistant at a senior citizens' center, was started on propranolol to treat her high blood pressure. Unfortunately, her doctor did not realize that the dose of this sometimes useful drug (see p. 87) must be reduced in older adults, and she was prescribed 80 milligrams twice a day. Two days after she started taking the drug, she began feeling very weak—so much so that by the third day, she went to a hospital emergency room, where her pulse rate was found to be 36 beats per minute. This dangerously low rate fully explained her weakness. The drug was stopped and Elsie's heart rate re-turned to normal. Later a low dose of a different drug was prescribed and had no adverse effects.

Seven-Year-Old Boy Dies from Drug Prescribed for Attention Deficit Hyperactivity Disorder

Bernie, a bright 7-year-old, was prescribed an antidepressant, imipramine (TOFRANIL), to treat attention deficit hyperactivity disorder. Because his parents were not provided with accurate, complete information about the drug, they were unaware that the drug could cause life-threatening heart arrhythmias, that the dose prescribed was too high, and that the tremor and convulsions that Bernie began to have were actually adverse drug reactions to imipramine. Treatment with the drug was continued, and one day, while at school, he collapsed and died of a heart arrhythmia. If his parents had been adequately warned about this drug, Bernie would be alive today.

In discussing the problem of adverse drug reactions in the elderly, the World Health Organization has stated some principles applicable to people of all ages: *"Quite often, the history and clinical examination of patients with side effects reveal that no valid indication [purpose] for the offending drug has been present . . . Adverse reactions can to a large extent be avoided in the elderly by choosing safe and effective drugs and applying sound therapeutic principles in prescribing, such as starting with a small dose, observing the patient frequently, and avoiding excessive polypharmacy [the use of multiple drugs at the same time]."* [16]

In other words, according to the World Health Organization, patients who suffer adverse drug reactions are very often victims of drugs that there is no valid reason for them to take.

A carefully controlled study examined the details of prescriptions of people being discharged from a community hospital with three or more prescriptions to treat chronic illnesses.[17] The results of this study are quite disturbing, both in what they say about the doctors' prescribing practices and in the evidence as to the potential damage that could be done to older adults as a result of these practices. Of the 236 people intensively studied:

• Eighty-eight percent of the people had one or more prescribing problems with the prescriptions they were given. At least one potentially serious, life-threatening problem occurred, which could have been as a result of the prescriptions written for 22% of these patients.

When the specific problems with the prescriptions were examined, the results were as follows:

• Fifty-nine percent of the patients had been given one or more prescriptions for a drug that was an inappropriate choice of therapy because it was either "less than optimal medication given the patient's diagnosis" or there was no established indication for it;
• Twenty-eight percent of the patients were given too high a dose of the drug, an "overdose";
• Forty-eight percent of the patients were given a combination of drugs that can result in one or more harmful drug interactions;
• Twenty percent of the patients were given drugs that unnecessarily duplicated the therapeutic effect of another drug they were taking.

The good news from this study, however, was that a consultant pharmacist, involved in the care of more than 50% of these patients, was able to reduce the risks by making recommendations to the prescribing physicians.

In the remaining part of this chapter, we will provide lists of the most common drug-induced adverse effects along with the drugs that can cause them. In the box below are some of the symptoms that, although they are frequently caused by drugs, are the kinds of problems that you or many doctors might first attribute simply to "growing old" or "getting nervous" instead of to a drug.

Which Adverse Effects Can Be Caused by Which Drugs?

The following charts are to be used by patients who have any of a variety of medical problems (or by doctors) to find out which drugs, especially ones they are using or are considering using, can cause specific adverse reactions. The lists are compiled from a variety of sources.[16,18–23]

Although some of these adverse effects occur most commonly in older adults, all of them have also been documented in younger people, although not as often in some instances.

SUMMARY OF ADVERSE REACTIONS AND THE DRUGS THAT CAUSE THEM

Only the most easily detectable problems are considered, and only the most common drugs causing each problem are listed.

Adverse Drug Reaction	(Number of Drugs)	Examples of Brand Names
Depression	166	Accutane, Advil, Catapres, Cipro, Dalmane, Factive, Inderal, Naprosyn, Norpace, Pepcid, Reglan, Tagamet, Talwin, Ultracet, Valium, Xanax, Zantac
Psychoses/ hallucinations	156	Aldomet, Benadryl, Catapres, Celebrex, Cipro, Dexatrim, Elavil, Halcion, Inderal, Lanoxin, Procanbid, Sonata, Tagamet, Ultracet, Valium, Vioxx
Confusion/ delirium	147	Amaryl, Ambien, Benadryl, Catapres, Cipro, Compazine, Diabeta, Diabinese, Dymelor, Elavil, Mellaril, Sinemet, Tagamet, Valium, Xanax, Zantac
Dementia	76	Aldomet, Inderal, Maxzide, Mellaril, Regroton, Restoril, Ser-Ap-Es, Tagamet, Valium, Xanax, Zantac
Insomnia	35	Avelox, Floxin, Inderal, Lasix, Mevacor, Nicorette, Sudafed, Synthroid, Theo-24

Adverse Drug Reaction	(Number of Drugs)	Examples of Brand Names
Parkinsonism	40	Abilify, Aldomet, Asendin, Cardizem, Compazine, Elavil, Geodon, Haldol, Mellaril, Prozac, Reglan, Regroton, Risperdal, Thorazine
Tardive dyskinesia	19	Abilify, Asendin, Buspar, Compazine, Geodon, Haldol, Mellaril, Risperdal, Thorazine, Wellbutrin, Zyban, Zyprexa
Dizziness on standing	154	Abilify, Calan SR, Cardizem CD, Cardura, Catapres, Compazine, Elavil, Geodon, Haldol, Hytrin, Inderal, Isordil, Lasix, Minipress, Nitro-Bid, Prinivil, Procardia, Sonata, Tenormin, Valium, Xanax
Falls/hip fracture	59	Ambien, Celexa, Compazine, Dalmane, Elavil, Haldol, Isordil, Lexapro, Navane, Nembutal, Prozac, Restoril, Sinequan, Valium, Xanax
Automobile accidents	28	Ambien, Asendin, Ativan, Celexa, Elavil, Lexapro, Norpramin, Pamelor, Paxil, Prozac, Sinequan, Tofranil, Valium, Xanax, Zoloft
Sexual dysfunction	127	Abilify, Calan SR, Geodon, Lopid, Lopressor, Norpace, Pepcid, Proscar, Prozac, Sarafem, Tagamet, Tegretol, Transderm-Scop, Zantac

Adverse Drug Reaction	(Number of Drugs)	Examples of Brand Names
Loss of appetite, nausea, vomiting	63	Advil, Avelox, Daypro, Demerol, EES, Feldene, Feosol, K-Lor, Lanoxin, Levaquin, Relafen, Sumycin, Theo-24, Ultracet, Ultram
Abdominal pain, ulcers, GI bleeding	48	Advil, Anaprox, Celebrex, Cortone, Daypro, Decadron, Feldene, Indocin, Motrin, Relafen, Somophyllin, Theo-24, Ultracet, Vioxx, Zithromax
Constipation	107	Amphojel, Benadryl, Caltrate, Cogentin, Inderal, Lotronex, Maalox, Talwin, Tylenol No. 3, Tylox, Ultram, Urised
Diarrhea	56	Aciphex, Aldomet, Avelox, Cipro, Dulcolax, Maalox, Phillips' Milk of Magnesia, Nexium, Peri-Colace, Precose, Prilosec, Sporanox, Sumycin, Zelnorm
Lung toxicity	59	Cordarone, Feldene, Inderal, Prinivil, Tegretol, Vasotec, Visken
Blocked urination	56	Antivert, Artane, Benadryl, Bentyl, Compazine, Duragesic, Elavil, Felbatol, Haldol, Sinequan, Tavist, Ultram, Zyban
Urine leakage	84	Aricept, Celexa, Esidrix, Hytrin, Inderal, Lasix, Lexapro, Lithobid, Minipress, Neurontin, Paxil, Restoril, Tenormin, Valium, Xanax, Zaroxolyn, Ziac, Zoloft

Drugs That Can Affect the Mind

Drugs That Can Cause Depression

BRAND NAME	GENERIC NAME

Acne/Psoriasis Drugs

ACCUTANE	isotretinoin
SORIATANE	acitretin

Antibiotics and other anti-infective agents

	dapsone
	sulfonamides
AVELOX	moxifloxacin
BACTRIM	trimethoprim/ sulfamethoxazole
CHIBROXIN, NOROXIN	norfloxacin
CILOXAN, CIPRO	ciprofloxacin
FACTIVE	gemifloxacin
FLAGYL	metronidazole
FLOXIN, OCUFLOX	ofloxacin
INH	isoniazid
LARIAM	mefloquine
LEVAQUIN	levofloxacin
MAXAQUIN	lomefloxacin
PENETREX	enoxacin
SEROMYCIN	cycloserine
SYMMETREL	amantadine
TEQUIN	gatifloxacin
TROVAN	trovafloxacin
TRECATOR-SC	ethionamide
ZAGAM	sparfloxacin
ZOVIRAX	acyclovir

Corticosteroids, systemic

ACTHAR	corticotropin (ACTH)
AZMACORT	triamcinolone
CORTEF	hydrocortisone
Cortone	cortisone
DECADRON, HEXADROL	dexamethasone
DELTASONE, METICORTEN	prednisone
DIPROLENE, VALISONE	betamethasone
MEDROL	methylprednisolone
METRETON, PRED FORTE	prednisolone

Eye drugs

BETAGAN	levobunolol
CARTROL	carteolol
DIAMOX	acetazolamide
OPTIPRANOLOL	metipranolol
TIMOPTIC	timolol

Gastrointestinal drugs

AXID	nizatidine
PEPCID	famotidine
REGLAN	metoclopramide
TAGAMET	cimetidine
ZANTAC	ranitidine

BRAND NAME	GENERIC NAME

Heart and blood vessel drugs
Antiarrhythmics

LANOXIN	digoxin
NORPACE	disopyramide
PROCANBID	procainamide

Cholesterol-lowering drugs

LESCOL	fluvastatin
LIPITOR	atorvastatin
MEVACOR	lovastatin
PRAVACHOL	pravastatin
ZOCOR	simvastatin

High blood pressure drugs (beta-blockers)

BLOCADREN	timolol
CARTROL	carteolol
COREG	carvedilol
CORGARD	nadolol
INDERAL, INDERAL LA	propranolol
KERLONE	betaxolol
LEVATOL	penbutolol
LOPRESSOR, TOPROL XL	metoprolol
NORMODYNE, TRANDATE	labetalol
SECTRAL	acebutolol
TENORMIN	atenolol
VISKEN	pindolol
ZEBETA	bisoprolol

High blood pressure drugs (beta-blockers with diuretics)

CORZIDE	nadolol/ bendroflumethiazide
INDERIDE LA	propranolol/ hydrochlorothiazide
LOPRESSOR HCT	metoprolol/ hydrochlorothiazide
TENORETIC	atenolol/chlorthalidone
TIMOLIDE	timolol/ hydrochlorothiazide
ZIAC	bisoprolol/ hydrochlorothiazide

High blood pressure drugs (calcium channel blockers)

ADALAT, PROCARDIA, ADALAT CC, PROCARDIA XL	nifedipine
CALAN SR, COVERA-HS, ISOPTIN SR, VERELAN	verapamil
CARDENE, CARDENE SR	nicardipine
CARDIZEM CD, DILACOR XR, TIAZAC	diltiazem
DYNACIRC, DYNACIRC CR	isradipine
NORVASC	amlodipine
PLENDIL	felodipine
SULAR	nisoldipine

Drugs That Can Cause Depression (continued)

BRAND NAME	GENERIC NAME

High blood pressure drugs (calcium channel blockers with ACE inhibitors)

LEXXEL	felodipine/enalapril
LOTREL	amlodipine/benazepril
TARKA	verapamil/trandolapril
TECZEM	diltiazem/enalapril

High blood pressure drugs (thiazide diuretics)

DIURIL	chlorothiazide
HYDRODIURIL, MICROZIDE	hydrochlorothiazide
HYGROTON	chlorthalidone
RENESE	polythiazide

High blood pressure drugs (thiazide diuretic combinations)

DIUPRES	reserpine/chlorothiazide
ENDURONYL	deserpidine/ methyclothiazide
HYDROPRES	reserpine/ hydrochlorothiazide
REGROTON, DEMI-REGROTON	reserpine/chlorthalidone
SALUTENSIN	reserpine/ hydroflumethiazide
SER-AP-ES	reserpine/hydralazine/ hydrochlorothiazide

High blood pressure drugs (other)

	reserpine
ALDOMET	methyldopa
CATAPRES	clonidine
HYTRIN	terazosin
MINIPRESS	prazosin
TENEX	guanfacine

Mind-Affecting Drugs
Antidepressants

WELLBUTRIN	bupropion

Barbiturates

BUTISOL	butabarbital
LUMINAL, SOLFOTON	phenobarbital
NEMBUTAL	pentobarbital
SECONAL	secobarbital

Tranquilizers or sleeping pills

ATIVAN	lorazepam
BUSPAR	buspirone
CENTRAX	prazepam
DALMANE	flurazepam
HALCION	triazolam
LIBRIUM	chlordiazepoxide
LIMBITROL	amitriptyline/ chlordiazepoxide
NOLUDAR	methyprylon
RESTORIL	temazepam
SERAX	oxazepam
TRANXENE	clorazepate

BRAND NAME	GENERIC NAME
VALIUM	diazepam
XANAX	alprazolam

Neurological drugs
Anticonvulsants

DEPAKENE/DEPAKOTE	divalproex, valproate, valproic acid
DILANTIN	phenytoin
KEPPRA	levetiracetam
KLONOPIN	clonazepam
LUMINAL, SOLFOTON	phenobarbital
MYSOLINE	primidone
TEGRETOL	carbamazepine
TOPAMAX	topiramate
ZARONTIN	ethosuximide

Antiparkinsonians

ELDEPRYL	selegiline, deprenyl
LARODOPA	levodopa
PARLODEL	bromocriptine
PERMAX	pergolide
SINEMET	levodopa/carbidopa

Painkillers/narcotics

ADVIL, MOTRIN	ibuprofen
ALEVE, ANAPROX, NAPROSYN	naproxen
ANSAID, OCUFEN	flurbiprofen
CLINORIL	sulindac
DAYPRO	oxaprozin
DEMEROL	meperidine
DOLOBID	diflunisal
FELDENE	piroxicam
INDOCIN	indomethacin
LODINE	etodolac
MECLOMEN	meclofenamate
MS CONTIN, ROXANOL	morphine
NALFON	fenoprofen
ORUDIS	ketoprofen
RELAFEN	nabumetone
TALWIN	pentazocine
TALWIN-NX	pentazocine/naloxone
TOLECTIN	tolmetin
ULTRACET	tramadol/acetominophen
ULTRAM	tramadol
VOLTAREN	diclofenac

Dietary supplements

	ephedra

Other drugs

	amphetamines (during withdrawal)
	progestins
AMIPAQUE	metrizamide
ANTABUSE	disulfiram
ELSPAR	asparaginase
ERGAMISOL	levamisole
LIORESAL	baclofen

Drugs That Can Cause Depression (continued)

BRAND NAME	GENERIC NAME
NORPLANT	levonorgestrel implant
ONCOVIN	vincristine
ROFERON-A, INTRON A	interferon alfa
SANSERT	methysergide
SEROMYCIN	cycloserine
SUSTIVA	efavirenz
VELBAN	vinblastine
ZYBAN	bupropion

Drugs That Can Cause Psychoses, Such as Hallucinations

BRAND NAME	GENERIC NAME
Antibiotics and other anti-infective agents	
	dapsone
	sulfonamides
ARALEN	chloroquine
ATABRINE	quinacrine
AVELOX	moxifloxacin
BACTRIM	trimethoprim/ sulfamethoxazole
CHIBROXIN, NOROXIN	norfloxacin
CILOXAN, CIPRO	ciprofloxacin
FACTIVE	gemifloxacin
FLAGYL	metronidazole
FLOXIN, OCUFLOX	ofloxacin
FUNGIZONE	amphotericin B
INH	isoniazid
LARIAM	mefloquine
LEVAQUIN	levofloxacin
MAXAQUIN	lomefloxacin
MINTEZOL	thiabendazole
NEGGRAM	nalidixic acid
OFF	deet
PENETREX	enoxacin
PODOFIN	podophyllum
SEROMYCIN	cycloserine
SUSTIVA	efavirenz
SYMMETREL	amantadine
TEQUIN	gatifloxacin
TRECATOR-SC	ethionamide
TROVAN	trovafloxacin
VALTREX	valacyclovir
VIRAMUNE	nevirapine
WYCILLIN	penicillin G procaine
ZAGAM	sparfloxacin
ZOVIRAX	acyclovir
Cold, cough, allergy, and asthma drugs	
Antihistamines	
ALERMINE, CHLOR-TRIMETON	chlorpheniramine

BRAND NAME	GENERIC NAME
ATARAX, VISTARIL	hydroxyzine
BENADRYL, SOMINEX	diphenhydramine
DIMETANE	brompheniramine
MYIDIL	tripolidine
OPTIMINE	azatadine
PERIACTIN	cyproheptadine
TAVIST, TAVIST-1	clemastine
Asthma drugs	
MAXAIR	pirbuterol
PROVENTIL, VENTOLIN	albuterol
Nasal decongestants	
	ephedrine
AFRIN	oxymetazoline
NALDECON	phenylephrine
SUDAFED	pseudoephedrine
Corticosteroids, systemic	
ACTHAR	corticotropin (ACTH)
AZMACORT	triamcinolone
CORTEF	hydrocortisone
CORTONE	cortisone
DECADRON, HEXADROL	dexamethasone
DELTASONE, METICORTEN	prednisone
DIPROLENE, VALISONE	betamethasone
MEDROL	methylprednisolone
METRETON, PRED FORTE	prednisolone
Eye drugs	
BETAGAN	levobunolol
TIMOPTIC	timolol
Gastrointestinal drugs	
TAGAMET	cimetidine
Heart and blood vessel drugs	
LANOXICAPS, LANOXIN	digoxin
Antiarrhythmics	
MEXITIL	mexiletine
PROCANBID	procainamide
NORPACE	disopyramide
TONOCARD	tocainide
XYLOCAINE	lidocaine
High blood pressure drugs	
ALDOMET	methyldopa
CAPOTEN	captopril
CARTROL	carteolol
CATAPRES	clonidine
COREG	carvedilol
CORGARD	nadolol
HYTRIN	terazosin
INDERAL, INDERAL LA	propranolol
KERLONE	betaxolol
LEVATOL	penbutolol
LOPRESSOR, TOPROL XL	metoprolol
MINIPRESS	prazosin
NORMODYNE, TRANDATE	labetalol
SECTRAL	acebutolol
TENEX	guanfacine

Drugs That Can Cause Psychoses, Such as Hallucinations (continued)

BRAND NAME	GENERIC NAME
TENORMIN	atenolol
VISKEN	pindolol
ZEBETA	bisoprolol

Mind-affecting drugs
Antidepressants

BRAND NAME	GENERIC NAME
ASENDIN	amoxapine
AVENTYL, PAMELOR	nortriptyline
DESYREL	trazodone
ELAVIL	amitriptyline
LIMBITROL	amitriptyline/ chlordiazepoxide
LUDIOMIL	maprotiline
NORPRAMIN	desipramine
SINEQUAN	doxepin
TOFRANIL	imipramine
TRIAVIL	amitriptyline/ perphenazine
WELLBUTRIN	bupropion

Tranquilizers or sleeping pills

BRAND NAME	GENERIC NAME
AMBIEN	zolpidem
DESYREL	trazodone
BUSPAR	buspirone
EFFEXOR	venlafaxine
HALCION	triazolam
NOLUDAR	methyprylon
PLACIDYL	ethchlorvynol
SONATA	zaleplon
VALIUM	diazepam

Neurological drugs
Anticonvulsants

BRAND NAME	GENERIC NAME
DILANTIN	phenytoin
KEPPRA	levetiracetam
KLONOPIN	clonazepam
MYSOLINE	primidone
TEGRETOL	carbamazepine
ZARONTIN	ethosuximide

Antiparkinsonians

BRAND NAME	GENERIC NAME
COMTAN	entacapone
ELDEPRYL	selegiline, deprenyl
LARODOPA	levodopa
PARLODEL	bromocriptine
PERMAX	pergolide
SINEMET	levodopa/carbidopa

Painkillers/narcotics

BRAND NAME	GENERIC NAME
ACTIQ, DURAGESIC	fentanyl
ARTHROPAN*	choline salicylate*
ASCRIPTIN*, BUFFERIN*	buffered aspirin*
ECOTRIN*, GENUINE BAYER ASPIRIN*	aspirin*
CELEBREX	celecoxib
DARVON, DARVON-N	propoxyphene
DISALCID*	salsalate*
DOAN'S PILLS*	magnesium salicylate*
INDOCIN	indomethacin
KETALAR	ketamine
MS CONTIN, ROXANOL	morphine
ORUDIS	ketoprofen
TALWIN	pentazocine
TALWIN-NX	pentazocine/naloxone
TRILISATE*	choline and magnesium salicylates
ULTRACET	tramadol/acetaminophen
ULTRAM	tramadol
VIOXX	rofecoxib

Other drugs

BRAND NAME	GENERIC NAME
	amphetamines
	atropine
	barbiturates
	cocaine
AMICAR	aminocaproic acid
AMIPAQUE	metrizamide
ANTABUSE	disulfiram
ARALEN	chloroquin
EPOGEN	erythropoietin
FLEXERIL	cyclobenzaprine
IFEX	ifosfamide
KETALAR	ketamine
LEUKERAN	chlorambucil
LEVOTHROID, SYNTHROID	levothyroxine
LIORESAL	baclofen
NARDIL	phenelzine
ONCOVIN	vincristine
PROLEUKIN	interleukin-2
RITALIN	methylphenidate
SANSERT	methysergide
SYMMETREL	amantadine
VIAGRA	sildenafil
XYLOCAINE	lidocaine
ZANAFLEX	tizanidine
ZYBAN	bupropion

*Salicylates can cause psychoses when they are used in high doses.

*Salicylates can cause psychoses when they are used in high doses.

Drugs That Can Cause Sudden Onset of Confusion or Delirium

BRAND NAME	GENERIC NAME
Antibiotics and other anti-infective agents	
AVELOX	moxifloxacin
BACTRIM	trimethoprim/ sulfamethoxazole
CHIBROXIN, NOROXIN	norfloxacin
CILOXAN, CIPRO	ciprofloxacin
CYTOVENE	ganciclovir
FACTIVE	gemifloxacin
FLOXIN, OCUFLOX	ofloxacin
LEVAQUIN	levofloxacin
MAXAQUIN	lomefloxacin
PENETREX	enoxacin
SYMMETREL	amantadine
TEQUIN	gatifloxacin
TROVAN	trovafloxacin
URISED	atropine/hyoscyamine/ methenamine/methylene blue/phenylsalicylate/ benzoic acid
VIRAMUNE	nevirapine
ZAGAM	sparfloxacin
ZOVIRAX	acyclovir
Cold, cough, allergy, and asthma drugs	
ALERMINE, CHLOR-TRIMETON	chlorpheniramine
ATARAX, VISTARIL	hydroxyzine
BENADRYL, SOMINEX FORMULA	diphenhydramine
DIMETANE	brompheniramine
MYIDIL	triprolidine
OPTIMINE	azatadine
PERIACTIN	cyproheptadine
TAVIST, TAVIST-1	clemastine
Corticosteroids, systemic	
ACTHAR	corticotropin (ACTH)
AZMACORT	triamcinolone
CORTEF	hydrocortisone
CORTONE	cortisone
DECADRON, HEXADROL	dexamethasone
DELTASONE, METICORTEN	prednisone
DIPROLENE, VALISONE	betamethasone
MEDROL	methylprednisolone
METRETON, PRED FORTE	prednisolone
Diabetes drugs	
AMARYL	glimepiride
DIABETA, MICRONASE	glyburide
DIABINESE	chlorpropamide
DYMELOR	acetohexamide
GLUCOTROL	glipizide

BRAND NAME	GENERIC NAME
HUMALOG, HUMULIN	insulin
ORINASE	tolbutamide
TOLINASE	tolazamide
Gastrointestinal drugs	
	atropine
ANTIVERT	meclizine
AXID	nizatidine
BENTYL	dicyclomine
COMPAZINE	prochlorperazine
DITROPAN	oxybutynin
DONNATAL	atropine/hyoscyamine/ scopolamine/ phenobarbital
LIBRAX	chlordiazepoxide/clidinium
LOMOTIL	diphenoxylate/atropine
PEPCID	famotidine
PHENERGAN	promethazine
TAGAMET	cimetidine
TIGAN	trimethobenzamide
ZANTAC	ranitidine
Heart and blood vessel drugs	
CATAPRES	clonidine
DURAQUIN, QUINAGLUTE DURA-TABS, QUINIDEX	quinidine
LANOXICAPS, LANOXIN	digoxin
NORPACE	disopyramide
TENEX	guanfacine
Mind-affecting drugs	
Antidepressants	
ASENDIN	amoxapine
AVENTYL, PAMELOR	nortriptyline
DESYREL	trazodone
ELAVIL	amitriptyline
Lithobid, Lithonate	lithium
LIMBITROL	amitriptyline/ chlordiazepoxide
LUDIOMIL	maprotiline
NORPRAMIN	desipramine
PROZAC	fluoxetine
SINEQUAN	doxepin
TOFRANIL	imipramine
TRIAVIL	amitriptyline/perphenazine
WELLBUTRIN	bupropion
Antipsychotics	
CLOZARIL	clozapine
COMPAZINE	prochlorperazine
HALDOL	haloperidol
MELLARIL	thioridazine
NAVANE	thiothixene
PROLIXIN	fluphenazine
REGLAN	metoclopramide
STELAZINE	trifluoperazine
THORAZINE	chlorpromazine
TRIAVIL	amitriptyline/perphenazine

Drugs That Can Cause Sudden Onset of Confusion or Delirium (continued)

BRAND NAME	GENERIC NAME
Barbiturates	
BUTISOL	butabarbital
LUMINAL, SOLFOTON	phenobarbital
NEMBUTAL	pentobarbital
Tranquilizers or sleeping pills	
AMBIEN	zolpidem
ATARAX, VISTARIL	hydroxyzine
ATIVAN	lorazepam
BUSPAR	buspirone
CENTRAX	prazepam
DALMANE	flurazepam
DORIDEN	glutethimide
HALCION	triazolam
LIBRIUM	chlordiazepoxide
MILTOWN, EQUANIL	meprobamate
NOCTEC	chloral hydrate
NOLUDAR	methyprylon
RESTORIL	temazepam
SERAX	oxazepam
TRANXENE	clorazepate
VALIUM	diazepam
XANAX	alprazolam
Neurological drugs	
Anticonvulsants	
DILANTIN	phenytoin
KLONOPIN	clonazepam
Antiparkinsonians	
ARTANE	trihexyphenidyl
COGENTIN	benztropine
LARODOPA	levodopa
PARLODEL	bromocriptine
PERMAX	pergolide
SINEMET	levodopa/carbidopa
Painkillers/narcotics	
ADVIL, MOTRIN	ibuprofen
ALEVE, ANAPROX, NAPROSYN	naproxen
ANSAID, OCUFEN	flurbiprofen
ARTHROPAN*	choline salicylate*
ASCRIPTIN*, BUFFERIN*	buffered aspirin*
ECOTRIN*, GENUINE BAYER ASPIRIN*	aspirin*
CLINORIL	sulindac
DAYPRO	oxaprozin
DISALCID*	salsalate*
DOAN'S PILLS*	magnesium salicylate*
DOLOBID	diflunisal

BRAND NAME	GENERIC NAME
FELDENE	piroxicam
INDOCIN	indomethacin
LODINE	etodolac
MECLOMEN	meclofenamate
NALFON	fenoprofen
ORUDIS	ketoprofen
RELAFEN	nabumetone
TALWIN	pentazocine
TALWIN-NX	pentazocine/naloxone
TOLECTIN	tolmetin
TORADOL	ketorolac
TRILISATE*	choline and magnesium salicylates*
VOLTAREN	diclofenac
Dietary supplements	
	St. John's wort
Other drugs	
ADSORBOCARPINE, ISOPTO CARPINE	pilocarpine
AMIPAQUE	metrizamide
ANTABUSE	disulfiram
CATAPRES	clonidine
CYTOSAR-U	cytarabine
DIAMOX	acetazolamide
ELSPAR	asparaginase
KETALAR	ketamine
LIORESAL	baclofen
ZYBAN	bupropion

Drugs That Can Cause or Worsen Dementia (Mental Impairment—Forgetfulness, Slow Thinking, Inability to Care for Oneself, Confusion)

Unlike the drugs listed on p. 27, which cause sudden confusion and/or delirium, these drugs cause mental impairment that is much slower and more subtle in onset.[24] **The categories of drugs with the biggest risk for mental impairment are the sleeping pills and so-called minor tranquilizers.**

BRAND NAME	GENERIC NAME
Gastrointestinal drugs	
AXID	nizatidine
PEPCID	famotidine
TAGAMET	cimetidine
ZANTAC	ranitidine

---

*Salicylates can cause psychoses when they are used in high doses.

---

*Salicylates can cause psychoses when they are used in high doses.

Drugs That Can Cause or Worsen Dementia (continued)

BRAND NAME	GENERIC NAME

Heart and blood vessel drugs
High blood pressure drugs (beta-blockers)

BRAND NAME	GENERIC NAME
BLOCADREN	timolol
CARTROL	carteolol
COREG	carvedilol
CORGARD	nadolol
CORZIDE	nadolol/ bendroflumethiazide
INDERAL, INDERAL LA	propranolol
INDERIDE LA	propranolol/ hydrochlorothiazide
KERLONE	betaxolol
LEVATOL	penbutolol
LOPRESSOR, TOPROL XL	metoprolol
LOPRESSOR HCT	metoprolol/ hydrochlorothiazide
NORMODYNE, TRANDATE	labetalol
SECTRAL	acebutolol
TENORETIC	atenolol/chlorthalidone
TENORMIN	atenolol
VISKEN	pindolol
ZEBETA	bisoprolol
ZIAC	bisoprolol/ hydrochlorothiazide

High blood pressure drugs (diuretics)

BRAND NAME	GENERIC NAME
ALDACTAZIDE	spironolactone/ hydrochlorothiazide
ALDORIL	methyldopa/ hydrochlorothiazide
APRESAZIDE	hydralazine/ hydrochlorothiazide
BUMEX	bumetanide
COMBIPRES	clonidine/chlorthalidone
DEMADEX	torsemide
DIUPRES	reserpine/chlorothiazide
DIURIL	chlorothiazide
DYAZIDE, MAXZIDE	triamterene/ hydrochlorothiazide
ENDURON	methyclothiazide
ENDURONYL	deserpidine/ methyclothiazide
ESIDRIX, HYDRODIURIL	hydrochlorothiazide
HYDROPRES	reserpine/ hydrochlorothiazide
HYGROTON	chlorthalidone
INDERIDE LA	propranolol/ hydrochlorothiazide
LOZOL	indapamide
METAHYDRIN, NAQUA	trichlormethiazide
MODURETIC	amiloride/ hydrochlorothiazide

BRAND NAME	GENERIC NAME
REGROTON	reserpine/chlorthalidone
SALUTENSIN	reserpine/ hydroflumethiazide
SER-AP-ES	reserpine/hydralazine/ hydrochlorothiazide
TENORETIC	atenolol/chlorthalidone
ZAROXOLYN, DIULO	metolazone

High blood pressure drugs (other)

	reserpine
ALDOMET	methyldopa

Mind-affecting drugs
Antidepressants

Prozac	fluoxetine

Antipsychotics

COMPAZINE	prochlorperazine
HALDOL	haloperidol
MELLARIL	thioridazine
NAVANE	thiothixene
PROLIXIN	fluphenazine
STELAZINE	trifluoperazine
THORAZINE	chlorpromazine
TRIAVIL	amitriptyline/perphenazine

Barbiturates

BUTISOL	butabarbital
LUMINAL, SOLFOTON	phenobarbital
NEMBUTAL	pentobarbital

Tranquilizers or sleeping pills

ATARAX, VISTARIL	hydroxyzine
ATIVAN	lorazepam
BUSPAR	buspirone
CENTRAX	prazepam
DALMANE	flurazepam
DORIDEN	glutethimide
HALCION	triazolam
LIBRIUM	chlordiazepoxide
MILTOWN, EQUANIL	meprobamate
NOCTEC	chloral hydrate
NOLUDAR	methyprylon
RESTORIL	temazepam
SERAX	oxazepam
TRANXENE	clorazepate
VALIUM	diazepam
XANAX	alprazolam

Neurological drugs

KLONOPIN	clonazepam

Drugs That Can Cause Insomnia

BRAND NAME	GENERIC NAME

Antibiotics and other anti-infective agents

	dapsone
AVELOX	moxifloxacin
FLOXIN, OCUFLOX	ofloxacin

Drugs That Can Cause Insomnia (continued)

BRAND NAME	GENERIC NAME
FLUMADINE	rimantadine
LEVAQUIN	levofloxacin
SYMMETREL	amantadine
ZOVIRAX	acyclovir
ZYVOX	linezolid

Cold, cough, allergy, and asthma drugs
ELIXOPHYLLIN, SLO-BID, THEO-24	theophylline
SUDAFED	pseudoephedrine

Gastrointestinal drugs
TAGAMET	cimetidine

Heart and blood vessel drugs
ALDOMET	methyldopa
DURAQUIN, QUINAGLUTE DURA-TABS, QUINIDEX	quinidine
ESIDRIX, HYDRODIURIL	hydrochlorothiazide
INDERAL, INDERAL LA	propranolol
LASIX	furosemide
MEVACOR	lovastatin

Mind-affecting drugs
**Tranquilizers or sleeping pills
(Note: These drugs may cause rebound insomnia.)**
DALMANE	flurazepam
HALCION	triazolam

Antidepressants
BUSPAR	buspirone
EFFEXOR	venlafaxine

Antipsychotics
RISPERDAL	risperidone

Neurological drugs
DILANTIN	phenytoin
LARODOPA	levodopa
FELBATOL	felbamate
NEURONTIN	gabapentin
TOPAMAX	topiramate

Other drugs
	alcohol
	caffeine
	interferons
DELTASONE	prednisone
LEVOTHROID, SYNTHROID	levothyroxine
METRETON	prednisolone
NICORETTE, NICODERM	nicotine
RITALIN	methylphenidate

Drugs That Can Cause Abnormal, Involuntary Movements

Drugs That Can Induce Parkinsonism

The following drugs can cause a tremor often indistinguishable from Parkinson's disease. If signs of the disease develop after one begins to use one of these drugs, discontinuing the drug will often result in the disappearance of the parkinsonism. Unfortunately, doctors often do not recognize the drug-induced nature of this problem, and instead of discontinuing the drug that caused the problem, they add another drug to treat the parkinsonism.

BRAND NAME	GENERIC NAME

Heart and blood vessel drugs
High blood pressure drugs (diuretics)
DIUPRES	reserpine/chlorothiazide
ENDURONYL	deserpidine/methyclothiazide
HYDROPRES	reserpine/hydrochlorothiazide
REGROTON, DEMI-REGROTON	reserpine/chlorthalidone
SALUTENSIN	reserpine/hydroflumethiazide
SER-AP-ES	reserpine/hydralazine/hydrochlorothiazide

High blood pressure drugs (other)
	reserpine
ALDOMET	methyldopa
CARDIZEM CD, DILACOR XR, TIAZAC	diltiazem

Mind-affecting drugs
Antidepressants
ASENDIN	amoxapine
AVENTYL, PAMELOR	nortriptyline
DESYREL	trazodone
ELAVIL	amitriptyline
LIMBITROL	amitriptyline/chlordiazepoxide
LUDIOMIL	maprotiline
LUVOX	fluvoxamine
NORPRAMIN	desipramine
PAXIL	paroxetine
PROZAC	fluoxetine
SINEQUAN	doxepin
TOFRANIL	imipramine
TRIAVIL	amitriptyline/perphenazine

Drugs That Can Induce Parkinsonism (continued)

BRAND NAME	GENERIC NAME
WELLBUTRIN	bupropion
ZOLOFT	sertraline
Antipsychotics	
ABILIFY	aripiprazole
COMPAZINE	prochlorperazine
GEODON	ziprasidone
HALDOL	haloperidol
MELLARIL	thioridazine
NAVANE	thiothixene
PROLIXIN	fluphenazine
RISPERDAL	risperidone
STELAZINE	trifluoperazine
THORAZINE	chlorpromazine
TRIAVIL	amitriptyline/perphenazine
ZYPREXA	olanzapine
Tranquilizers	
BUSPAR	buspirone
Dietary supplements	
	kava-kava
Other drugs	
REGLAN	metoclopramide
ZYBAN	bupropion

Drugs That Can Induce Tardive Dyskinesia

Tardive dyskinesia is the most common and serious adverse effect of antipsychotic drugs and is often irreversible. It is characterized by involuntary movements of the lips, tongue, and sometimes the fingers, toes, and trunk. It may occur in as many as 40% of people over the age of 60 taking antipsychotic drugs. **Tardive dyskinesia is more common and more severe in older adults, and antipsychotic drugs are quite often prescribed unnecessarily in this age group. (See discussion of this in *Antipsychotic Drugs*, p. 176.)**

BRAND NAME	GENERIC NAME
Mind-affecting drugs	
Antidepressants	
ASENDIN	amoxapine
PROZAC	fluoxetine
WELLBUTRIN	bupropion
Antipsychotics	
ABILIFY	aripiprazole
COMPAZINE	prochlorperazine
GEODON	ziprasidone
HALDOL	haloperidol

BRAND NAME	GENERIC NAME
MELLARIL	thioridazine
NAVANE	thiothixene
PHENERGAN	promethazine
PROLIXIN	fluphenazine
RISPERDAL	risperidone
STELAZINE	trifluoperazine
THORAZINE	chlorpromazine
TRIAVIL	amitriptyline/perphenazine
ZYPREXA	olanzapine
Tranquilizers	
BUSPAR	buspirone
Neurological drugs	
ELDEPRYL	selegiline, deprenyl
Other drugs	
ZYBAN	bupropion

Drugs That Can Disturb Balance

Drugs That Can Cause Dizziness on Standing (Postural Hypotension)

BRAND NAME	GENERIC NAME
Antibiotics and other anti-infective agents	
AVELOX	moxifloxacin
CHIBROXIN, NOROXIN	norfloxacin
CILOXAN, CIPRO	ciprofloxacin
FACTIVE	gemifloxacin
FLOXIN, OCUFLOX	ofloxacin
LEVAQUIN	levofloxacin
MAXAQUIN	lomefloxacin
PENETREX	enoxacin
VERMOX	mebendazole
ZAGAM	sparfloxacin
Cold, cough, allergy, and asthma drugs	
ALERMINE, CHLOR-TRIMETON	chlorpheniramine
ATARAX, VISTARIL	hydroxyzine
BENADRYL, SOMINEX FORMULA	diphenhydramine
DELSYM	dextromethorphan
DIMETANE	brompheniramine
MYIDIL	triprolidine
OPTIMINE	azatadine
PERIACTIN	cyproheptadine
TAVIST, TAVIST-1	clemastine
Eye drugs	
BETAGAN	levobunolol
CARTROL	carteolol
NEPTAZANE	methazolamide
OPTIPRANOLOL	metipranolol
TIMOPTIC	timolol

Drugs That Can Cause Dizziness on Standing (continued)

BRAND NAME	GENERIC NAME

Heart and blood vessel drugs
Antianginal drugs

BRAND NAME	GENERIC NAME
ISMO, IMDUR	isosorbide-5-mononitrate
ISORDIL, SORBITRATE	isosorbide dinitrate
NITRO-BID, NITROSTAT, TRANSDERM-NITRO	nitroglycerin

High blood pressure drugs (beta-blockers)

BRAND NAME	GENERIC NAME
BLOCADREN	timolol
CARTROL	carteolol
COREG	carvedilol
CORGARD	nadolol
CORZIDE	nadolol/ bendroflumethiazide
INDERAL, INDERAL LA	propranolol
INDERIDE LA	propranolol/ hydrochlorothiazide
KERLONE	betaxolol
LEVATOL	penbutolol
LOPRESSOR, TOPROL XL	metoprolol
LOPRESSOR HCT	metoprolol/ hydrochlorothiazide
NORMODYNE, TRANDATE	labetalol
SECTRAL	acebutolol
TENORETIC	atenolol/chlorthalidone
TENORMIN	atenolol
VISKEN	pindolol
ZEBETA	bisoprolol
ZIAC	bisoprolol/ hydrochlorothiazide

High blood pressure drugs (diuretics)

BRAND NAME	GENERIC NAME
ALDACTAZIDE	spironolactone/ hydrochlorothiazide
ALDORIL	methyldopa/ hydrochlorothiazide
APRESAZIDE	hydralazine/ hydrochlorothiazide
BUMEX	bumetanide
COMBIPRES	clonidine/chlorthalidone
DEMADEX	torsemide
DIUPRES	reserpine/chlorothiazide
DIURIL	chlorothiazide
DYAZIDE, MAXZIDE	triamterene/ hydrochlorothiazide
ENDURON	methyclothiazide
ENDURONYL	deserpidine/ methyclothiazide
ESIDRIX, HYDRODIURIL	hydrochlorothiazide
HYDROPRES	reserpine/ hydrochlorothiazide
HYGROTON	chlorthalidone

BRAND NAME	GENERIC NAME
INDERIDE LA	propranolol/ hydrochlorothiazide
LASIX	furosemide
LOZOL	indapamide
METAHYDRIN, NAQUA	trichlormethiazide
MODURETIC	amiloride/ hydrochlorothiazide
REGROTON, DEMI- REGROTON	reserpine/chlorthalidone
SALUTENSIN	reserpine/ hydroflumethiazide
SER-AP-ES	reserpine/hydralazine/ hydrochlorothiazide
TENORETIC	atenolol/chlorthalidone
ZAROXOLYN, DIULO	metolazone

High blood pressure drugs (other)

BRAND NAME	GENERIC NAME
	reserpine
ACCUPRIL	quinapril
ADALAT, ADALAT CC, PROCARDIA, PROCARDIA XL	nifedipine
ALDACTONE	spironolactone
ALDOMET	methyldopa
ALTACE	ramipril
APRESOLINE	hydralazine
CALAN SR, COVERA-HS, ISOPTIN SR, VERELAN	verapamil
CAPOTEN	captopril
CARDENE, CARDENE SR	nicardipine
CARDIZEM CD, DILACOR XR, TIAZAC	diltiazem
CARDURA	doxazosin
CATAPRES	clonidine
DYNACIRC, DYNACIRC CR	isradipine
HYTRIN	terazosin
ISMELIN	guanethidine
LEXXEL	felodipine/enalapril
LOTENSIN	benazepril
LOTREL	amlodipine/benazepril
MAVIK	trandolapril
MINIPRESS	prazosin
MONOPRIL	fosinopril
NORVASC	amlodipine
PLENDIL	felodipine
PRINIVIL, ZESTRIL	lisinopril
SULAR	nisoldipine
TARKA	verapamil/trandolapril
TENEX	guanfacine
UNIVASC	moexipril
VASOTEC	enalapril
WYTENSIN	guanabenz

Drugs That Can Cause Dizziness on Standing (continued)

BRAND NAME	GENERIC NAME
Mind-affecting drugs	
Antidepressants	
ASENDIN	amoxapine
AVENTYL, PAMELOR	nortriptyline
DESYREL	trazodone
EFFEXOR	venlafaxine
ELAVIL	amitriptyline
LIMBITROL	amitriptyline/ chlordiazepoxide
LUDIOMIL	maprotiline
LUVOX	fluvoxamine
NORPRAMIN	desipramine
PAXIL	paroxetine
PROZAC	fluoxetine
SERZONE	nefazodone
SINEQUAN	doxepin
TOFRANIL	imipramine
TRIAVIL	amitriptyline/perphenazine
ZOLOFT	sertraline
Antipsychotics	
ABILIFY	aripiprazole
CLOZARIL	clozapine
COMPAZINE	prochlorperazine
GEODON	ziprasidone
HALDOL	haloperidol
MELLARIL	thioridazine
NAVANE	thiothixene
PROLIXIN	fluphenazine
RISPERDAL	risperidone
STELAZINE	trifluoperazine
THORAZINE	chlorpromazine
TRIAVIL	amitriptyline/perphenazine
ZYPREXA	olanzapine
Tranquilizers or sleeping pills	
AMBIEN	zolpidem
ATARAX, VISTARIL	hydroxyzine
ATIVAN	lorazepam
CENTRAX	prazepam
DALMANE	flurazepam
DORIDEN	glutethimide
HALCION	triazolam
LIBRIUM	chlordiazepoxide
MILTOWN, EQUANIL	meprobamate
NOCTEC	chloral hydrate
NOLUDAR	methyprylon
PLACIDYL	ethchlorvynol
RESTORIL	temazepam
SERAX	oxazepam
SONATA	zaleplon
TRANXENE	clorazepate
VALIUM	diazepam

BRAND NAME	GENERIC NAME
VERSED	midazolam
XANAX	alprazolam
Neurological drugs	
Anticonvulsants	
KLONOPIN	clonazepam
Antiparkinsonians	
ELDEPRYL	selegiline, deprenyl
LARODOPA	levodopa
PARLODEL	bromocriptine
SINEMET	levodopa/carbidopa

Drugs That Can Cause Falls/Hip Fractures

A study found that a significant proportion of hip fractures in older adults could be attributed to the use of four classes of drugs: sleeping pills, tranquilizers, antipsychotics, and antidepressant drugs. The following are examples of such drugs as well as others that have been associated with falls, which could also increase the risk of hip fractures. In addition to these drugs, all of the drugs listed above as causing dizziness on standing can also cause falls.

BRAND NAME	GENERIC NAME
Heart and blood vessel drugs	
ISMO, IMDUR	isosorbide-5-mononitrate
ISORDIL, SORBITRATE	isosorbide dinitrate
NITRO-BID, NITROSTAT, TRANSDERM-NITRO	nitroglycerin
Mind-affecting drugs	
Antidepressants	
ASENDIN	amoxapine
AVENTYL, PAMELOR	nortriptyline
CELEXA	citalopram
DESYREL	trazodone
ELAVIL	amitriptyline
LEXAPRO	escitalopram
LIMBITROL	amitriptyline/ chlordiazepoxide
LUDIOMIL	maprotiline
LUVOX	fluvoxamine
NORPRAMIN	desipramine
PAXIL	paroxetine
PROZAC, SARAFEM	fluoxetine
SINEQUAN	doxepin
TOFRANIL	imipramine
TRIAVIL	amitriptyline/perphenazine
WELLBUTRIN	bupropion
ZOLOFT	sertraline

Drugs That Can Cause Falls/Hip Fractures (continued)

BRAND NAME	GENERIC NAME
Antipsychotics	
ABILIFY	aripiprazole
GEODON	ziprasidone
COMPAZINE	prochlorperazine
HALDOL	haloperidol
MELLARIL	thioridazine
NAVANE	thiothixene
PROLIXIN	fluphenazine
RISPERDAL	risperidone
STELAZINE	trifluoperazine
THORAZINE	chlorpromazine
TRIAVIL	amitriptyline/perphenazine
ZYPREXA	olanzapine
Barbiturates	
BUTISOL	butabarbital
LUMINAL, SOLFOTON	phenobarbital
NEMBUTAL	pentobarbital
Tranquilizers or sleeping pills	
AMBIEN	zolpidem
ATARAX, VISTARIL	hydroxyzine
ATIVAN	lorazepam
BUSPAR	buspirone
CENTRAX	prazepam
DALMANE	flurazepam
DORIDEN	glutethimide
HALCION	triazolam
LIBRIUM	chlordiazepoxide
MILTOWN, EQUANIL	meprobamate
NOCTEC	chloral hydrate
NOLUDAR	methyprylon
PLACIDYL	ethchlorvynol
RESTORIL	temazepam
SERAX	oxazepam
SONATA	zaleplon
TRANXENE	clorazepate
VALIUM	diazepam
XANAX	alprazolam
Neurological drugs	
DILANTIN	phenytoin
KLONOPIN	clonazepam
LUMINAL, SOLFOTON	phenobarbital
TEGRETOL	carbamazepine
Other drugs	
ZYBAN	bupropion

Drugs That Can Cause Automobile Accidents

BRAND NAME	GENERIC NAME
Mind-affecting drugs	
Antidepressants	
ANAFRANIL	clomipramine
ASENDIN	amoxapine
AVENTYL, PAMELOR	nortriptyline
CELEXA	citalopram
ELAVIL	amitriptyline
LEXAPRO	escitalopram
LIMBITROL	amitriptyline/ chlordiazepoxide
LUDIOMIL	maprotiline
LUVOX	fluvoxamine
NORPRAMIN	desipramine
PAXIL	paroxetine
PROZAC, SARAFEM	fluoxetine
SINEQUAN	doxepin
SURMONTIL	trimipramine
TOFRANIL	imipramine
TRIAVIL	amitriptyline/ perphenazine
VIVACTIL	protriptyline
ZOLOFT	sertraline
Tranquilizers and sleeping pills	
AMBIEN	zolpidem
ATIVAN	lorazepam
CENTRAX	prazepam
LIBRIUM	chlordiazepoxide
PAXIPAM	halazepam
SERAX	oxazepam
TRANXENE	clorazepate
VALIUM	diazepam
XANAX	alprazolam
SONATA	zaleplon

Drugs That Can Cause Sexual Dysfunction

BRAND NAME	GENERIC NAME
Antibiotics and other anti-infective agents	
NIZORAL	ketoconazole
TEGISON	etretinate
Anticholinergics	
BANTHINE	methantheline
BENTYL	dicyclomine
CANTIL	mepenzolate
DARBID	isopropamide
DITROPAN	oxybutynin
HOMAPIN	homatropine
PAMINE	methscopolamine
PATHILON	tridihexethyl
PRO-BANTHINE	propantheline

Drugs That Can Cause Sexual Dysfunction (continued)

BRAND NAME	GENERIC NAME
QUARZAN	clidinium
ROBINUL	glycopyrrolate
TRAL	hexocyclium
TRANSDERM-SCOP	scopolamine
VALPIN	anisotropine

Cancer drugs

INTRON A, ROFERON-A	interferon alfa
LUPRON	leuprolide
NOLVADEX	tamoxifen
RHEUMATREX DOSE PACK	methotrexate

Eye drugs

DARANIDE	dichlorphenamide
DIAMOX	acetazolamide
NEPTAZANE	methazolamide

Gastrointestinal drugs

AXID	nizatidine
AZULFIDINE	sulfasalazine
PEPCID	famotidine
PRILOSEC	omeprazole
REGLAN	metoclopramide
TAGAMET	cimetidine
ZANTAC	ranitidine

Heart and blood vessel drugs
Antianginal drugs

ADALAT, ADALAT CC, PROCARDIA, PROCARDIA XL	nifedipine
CALAN SR, COVERA-HS, ISOPTIN SR, VERELAN	verapamil
LANOXICAPS, LANOXIN	digoxin

Antiarrhythmics

CORDARONE	amiodarone
MEXITIL	mexiletine
NORPACE	disopyramide

Blood vessel dilators

CERESPAN, PAVABID	papaverine

Cholesterol-lowering drugs

ATROMID-S	clofibrate
LOPID	gemfibrozil

High blood pressure drugs (beta-blockers)

BLOCADREN	timolol
CARTROL	carteolol
COREG	carvedilol
INDERAL, INDERAL LA	propranolol
KERLONE	betaxolol
LEVATOL	penbutolol
LOPRESSOR, TOPROL XL	metoprolol
NORMODYNE, TRANDATE	labetalol
TENORMIN	atenolol
ZEBETA	bisoprolol

BRAND NAME	GENERIC NAME

High blood pressure drugs (diuretics)

ESIDRIX, HYDRODIURIL	hydrochlorothiazide
HYGROTON	chlorthalidone
LOZOL	indapamide
MIDAMOR	amiloride

High blood pressure drugs (other)

	reserpine
ALDACTONE	spironolactone
ALDOMET	methyldopa
APRESOLINE	hydralazine
CATAPRES	clonidine
DEMSER	metyrosine
HYLOREL	guanadrel
INVERSINE	mecamylamine
ISMELIN	guanethidine
MINIPRESS	prazosin
TENEX	guanfacine
WYTENSIN	guanabenz

Mind-affecting drugs
Antidepressants

ASENDIN	amoxapine
AVENTYL, PAMELOR	nortriptyline
DESYREL	trazodone
EFFEXOR	venlafaxine
ELAVIL	amitriptyline
LEXAPRO	escitalopram
LITHOBID, LITHONATE	lithium
LUDIOMIL	maprotiline
LUVOX	fluvoxamine
MARPLAN	isocarboxazid
NARDIL	phenelzine
NORPRAMIN	desipramine
PARNATE	tranylcypromine
PAXIL	paroxetine
PROZAC, SARAFEM	fluoxetine
SERZONE	nefazodone
SINEQUAN	doxepin
TOFRANIL	imipramine
VIVACTIL	protriptyline
ZOLOFT	sertraline

Antipsychotics

ABILIFY	aripiprazole
GEODON	ziprasidone
CLOZARIL	clozapine
HALDOL	haloperidol
MELLARIL	thioridazine
MOBAN	molindone
NAVANE	thiothixene
ORAP	pimozide
PROLIXIN	fluphenazine
RISPERDAL	risperidone
SERENTIL	mesoridazine
STELAZINE	trifluoperazine
TARACTAN	chlorprothixene

Drugs That Can Cause Sexual Dysfunction (continued)

BRAND NAME	GENERIC NAME
THORAZINE	chlorpromazine
TRILAFON	perphenazine
ZYPREXA	olanzapine

Barbiturates

NEMBUTAL	pentobarbital

Tranquilizers

BUSPAR	buspirone
VALIUM	diazepam
XANAX	alprazolam

Neurological drugs
Anticonvulsants

DILANTIN	phenytoin
TEGRETOL	carbamazepine
ZARONTIN	ethosuximide

Antiparkinsonians

LARODOPA	levodopa
PARLODEL	bromocriptine
PERMAX	pergolide

Painkillers/narcotics

ALEVE, ANAPROX, NAPROSYN	naproxen
DOLOPHINE, METHADOSE	methadone
INDOCIN	indomethacin
REVIA, TREXAN	naltrexone

Other drugs

	alcohol
	amphetamines
	cocaine
ANTABUSE	disulfiram
DANOCRINE	danazol
DEPO-TESTOSTERONE	testosterone
DIPRIVAN	propofol
FASTIN	phentermine
INTRALIPID	fat emulsion
LIORESAL	baclofen
MAZANOR, SANOREX	mazindol
PLEGINE	phendimetrazine
PROSCAR	finasteride
SYNAREL	nafarelin
TENUATE, TEPANIL	diethylpropion

Drugs That Can Affect the Gastrointestinal (GI) Tract

Drugs That Can Cause Loss of Appetite, Nausea, or Vomiting

BRAND NAME	GENERIC NAME

Antibiotics and other anti-infective agents

AVELOX	moxifloxacin
ACHROMYCIN, PANMYCIN, SUMYCIN	tetracycline
BIAXIN	clarithromycin
CHIBROXIN, NOROXIN	norfloxacin
DIFLUCAN	fluconazole
ERYTHROCIN, EES	erythromycin
FLAGYL	metronidazole
FLOXIN, OCUFLOX	ofloxacin
LEVAQUIN	levofloxacin
SPORANOX	itraconazole
TAMIFLU	oseltamivir
ZITHROMAX	azithromycin
ZYVOX	linezolid

Cancer drugs

Many anticancer drugs affect the gastrointestinal tract. They are not listed in this book.

Cold, cough, allergy, and asthma drugs

CHOLEDYL	oxtriphylline
ELIXOPHYLLIN, SLO-BID, THEO-24	theophylline
SOMOPHYLLIN, SOMOPHYLLIN-DF	aminophylline

Heart and blood vessel drugs

KATO, K-LOR, SLOW-K	potassium supplements
LANOXICAPS, LANOXIN	digoxin
LOCHOLEST, QUESTRAN	cholestyramine
MEVACOR	lovastatin

Mind-affecting drugs

BUSPAR	buspirone
EFFEXOR	venlafaxine
LUVOX	fluvoxamine
PAXIL	paroxetine
PROZAC	fluoxetine
RISPERDAL	risperidone
SERZONE	nefazodone
WELLBUTRIN	bupropion
ZOLOFT	sertraline

Neurological drugs

ELDEPRYL	selegiline, deprenyl
LARODOPA	levodopa
SINEMET	levodopa/carbidopa

Drugs That Can Cause Loss of Appetite, Nausea, or Vomiting (continued)

BRAND NAME	GENERIC NAME

Painkillers/narcotics

BRAND NAME	GENERIC NAME
	codeine
ADVIL, MOTRIN	ibuprofen
ALEVE, ANAPROX, NAPROSYN	naproxen
ANSAID, OCUFEN	flurbiprofen
CLINORIL	sulindac
DAYPRO	oxaprozin
DEMEROL	meperidine
DOLOBID	diflunisal
DURAGESIC	fentanyl
FELDENE	piroxicam
IMURAN	azathioprine
INDOCIN	indomethacin
LODINE	etodolac
MECLOMEN	meclofenamate
NALFON	fenoprofen
ORUDIS	ketoprofen
RELAFEN	nabumetone
ROXANOL, MS CONTIN	morphine
STADOL, STADOL NS	butorphanol
TALWIN	pentazocine
TALWIN-NX	pentazocine/naloxone
TOLECTIN	tolmetin
ULTRACET	tramadol/acetaminophen
ULTRAM	tramadol
VOLTAREN	diclofenac

Other drugs

BRAND NAME	GENERIC NAME
	estrogens
ESTRADERM, ESTRACE	estradiol
FEOSOL, SLOW FE	ferrous sulfate
FEOSTAT	ferrous fumarate
FERGON	ferrous gluconate
ZYBAN	bupropion

Drugs That Can Cause Abdominal Pain, Ulcers, or Gastrointestinal Bleeding

Although all of these drugs can cause abdominal pain, bleeding, and ulcers, **piroxicam (FELDENE) and indomethacin (INDOCIN) are more dangerous than the others and should not be used by older adults.**

BRAND NAME	GENERIC NAME

Antibiotics and other anti-infective agents

BRAND NAME	GENERIC NAME
DIFLUCAN	fluconazole
TAMIFLU	oseltamivir
ZITHROMAX	azithromycin

BRAND NAME	GENERIC NAME

Cold, cough, allergy, and asthma drugs

BRAND NAME	GENERIC NAME
CHOLEDYL	oxtriphylline
ELIXOPHYLLIN, SLO-BID, THEO-24	theophylline
SOMOPHYLLIN, SOMOPHYLLIN-DF	aminophylline

Corticosteroids, systemic

ACTHAR	corticotropin (ACTH)
AZMACORT	triamcinolone
CORTEF	hydrocortisone
CORTONE	cortisone
DECADRON, HEXADROL	dexamethasone
DELTASONE, METICORTEN	prednisone
DIPROLENE, VALISONE	betamethasone
MEDROL	methylprednisolone
METRETON, PRED FORTE	prednisolone

Mind-affecting drugs

BUSPAR	buspirone
WELLBUTRIN	bupropion

Neurological drugs

ELDEPRYL	selegiline, deprenyl

Painkillers/narcotics

ACTIQ, DURAGESIC	fentanyl
ADVIL, MOTRIN	ibuprofen
ALEVE, ANAPROX, NAPROSYN	naproxen
ANSAID, OCUFEN	flurbiprofen
ARTHROPAN	choline salicylate
ASCRIPTIN, BUFFERIN	buffered aspirin
BEXTRA	valdecoxib
CELEBREX	celecoxib
GENUINE BAYER ASPIRIN, ECOTRIN	aspirin
CLINORIL	sulindac
DAYPRO	oxaprozin
DISALCID	salsalate
DOAN'S PILLS	magnesium salicylate
DOLOBID	diflunisal
FELDENE	piroxicam
INDOCIN	indomethacin
LODINE	etodolac
MECLOMEN	meclofenamate
NALFON	fenoprofen
ORUDIS	ketoprofen
RELAFEN	nabumetone
TOLECTIN	tolmetin
TORADOL	ketorolac
TRILISATE	choline and magnesium salicylates
ULTRACET	tramadol/acetaminophen
ULTRAM	tramadol
VIOXX	rofecoxib
VOLTAREN	diclofenac

Drugs That Can Cause Abdominal Pain, Ulcers, or Gastrointestinal Bleeding (continued)

BRAND NAME	GENERIC NAME

Other drugs

REMICADE	infliximab
ZYBAN	bupropion

Drugs That Can Cause Constipation

BRAND NAME	GENERIC NAME

Antibiotics and anti-infective agents

URISED	atropine/hyoscyamine/ methenamine/methylene blue/phenyl salicylate/ benzoic acid
ZYVOX	linezolid

Cold, cough, allergy, and asthma drugs

ALERMINE, CHLOR-TRIMETON	chlorpheniramine
ATARAX, VISTARIL	hydroxyzine
BENADRYL, SOMINEX FORMULA	diphenhydramine
DIMETANE	brompheniramine
MYIDIL	triprolidine
OPTIMINE	azatadine
PERIACTIN	cyproheptadine
TAVIST, TAVIST-1	clemastine

Eye drugs

BETAGAN	levobunolol

Gastrointestinal drugs

	atropine
AMPHOJEL	aluminum hydroxide
ANTIVERT	meclizine
BENTYL	dicyclomine
CALTRATE, OS-CAL 500	calcium carbonate
COMPAZINE	prochlorperazine
DONNATAL	atropine/hyoscyamine/ scopolamine/ phenobarbital
DULCOLAX*	bisacodyl*
GAVISCON, GAVISCON-2	aluminum hydroxide and magnesium carbonate
LIBRAX	chlordiazepoxide/clidinium
LOMOTIL	diphenoxylate/atropine
LOTRONEX	alosetron
MAALOX, MAALOX TC	aluminum and magnesium hydroxide
MYLANTA, MYLANTA II	magnesium hydroxide/ aluminum hydroxide/ simethicone

*Constipation can occur with prolonged use.

BRAND NAME	GENERIC NAME
PHENERGAN	promethazine
REGLAN	metoclopramide
TIGAN	trimethobenzamide

Heart and blood vessel drugs
Antiarrhythmics

MEXITIL	mexiletine
NORPACE	disopyramide

Cholesterol-lowering drugs

LOCHOLEST, QUESTRAN	cholestyramine
MEVACOR	lovastatin

High blood pressure drugs (beta-blockers)

BLOCADREN	timolol
CARTROL	carteolol
COREG	carvedilol
CORGARD	nadolol
CORZIDE	nadolol/ bendroflumethiazide
INDERAL, INDERAL LA	propranolol
INDERIDE LA	propranolol/ hydrochlorothiazide
KERLONE	betaxolol
LEVATOL	penbutolol
LOPRESSOR, TOPROL XL	metoprolol
LOPRESSOR HCT	metoprolol/ hydrochlorothiazide
NORMODYNE, TRANDATE	labetalol
SECTRAL	acebutolol
TENORETIC	atenolol/chlorthalidone
TENORMIN	atenolol
VISKEN	pindolol
ZEBETA	bisoprolol
ZIAC	bisoprolol/ hydrochlorothiazide

High blood pressure drugs (other)

ADALAT, ADALAT CC, PROCARDIA, PROCARDIA XL	nifedipine
CALAN SR, COVERA-HS, ISOPTIN SR, VERELAN	verapamil
CARDENE, CARDENE SR	nicardipine
DYNACIRC, DYNACIRC CR	isradipine
LEXXEL	felodipine/enalapril
LOTREL	amlodipine/benazepril
NORVASC	amlodipine
PLENDIL	felodipine
SULAR	nisoldipine
TARKA	verapamil/trandolapril
TECZEM	diltiazem/enalapril

Mind-affecting drugs
Antidepressants

ASENDIN	amoxapine
AVENTYL, PAMELOR	nortriptyline
DESYREL	trazodone
ELAVIL	amitriptyline

Drugs That Can Cause Constipation (continued)

BRAND NAME	GENERIC NAME
LIMBITROL	amitriptyline/ chlordiazepoxide
LUDIOMIL	maprotiline
NORPRAMIN	desipramine
SINEQUAN	doxepin
TOFRANIL	imipramine
TRIAVIL	perphenazine/ amitriptyline
WELLBUTRIN	bupropion

Antipsychotics

CLOZARIL	clozapine
COMPAZINE	prochlorperazine
HALDOL	haloperidol
MELLARIL	thioridazine
NAVANE	thiothixene
PROLIXIN	fluphenazine
RISPERDAL	risperidone
STELAZINE	trifluoperazine
THORAZINE	chlorpromazine
TRIAVIL	amitriptyline/ perphenazine
ZYPREXA	olanzapine

Tranquilizers and sleeping pills

BUSPAR	buspirone
DORIDEN	glutethimide

Neurological drugs

Anticonvulsants

KLONOPIN	clonazepam

Antiparkinsonians

ARTANE	trihexyphenidyl
COGENTIN	benztropine

Painkillers/narcotics

ACTIQ, DURAGESIC	fentanyl
DARVOCET-N, WYGESIC	propoxyphene/ acetaminophen
DARVON, DARVON-N	propoxyphene
DARVON COMPOUND, DARVON COMPOUND-65	propoxyphene/ aspirin/caffeine
DEMEROL	meperidine
DILAUDID	hydromorphone
EMPIRIN WITH CODEINE	aspirin/codeine
PERCODAN, PERCODAN-DEMI	aspirin/oxycodone
ROXANOL, MS CONTIN	morphine
SYNALGOS-DC	dihydrocodeine/ aspirin/caffeine
TALWIN	pentazocine
TALWIN-NX	pentazocine/naloxone
TYLENOL NO. 3	acetaminophen/codeine
TYLOX, PERCOCET	acetaminophen/ oxycodone

BRAND NAME	GENERIC NAME
ULTRACET	tramadol/acetaminophen
ULTRAM	tramadol
VICODIN	acetaminophen/ hydrocodone

Other drugs

DITROPAN	oxybutynin
REGLAN	metoclopramide

Drugs That Can Cause Diarrhea

BRAND NAME	GENERIC NAME

Antibiotics and other anti-infective agents

AVELOX	moxifloxacin
ACHROMYCIN, PANMYCIN, SUMYCIN	tetracycline
BIAXIN	clarithromycin
CEFTIN	cefuroxime axetil
CEFZIL	cefprozil
CHIBROXIN, NOROXIN	norfloxacin
CILOXAN, CIPRO	ciprofloxacin
CLEOCIN	clindamycin
FLOXIN, OCUFLOX	ofloxacin
ILOSONE	erythromycin estolate
LEVAQUIN	levofloxacin
LINCOCIN	lincomycin
LORABID	loracarbef
MAXAQUIN	lomefloxacin
OMNIPEN	ampicillin
PENETREX	enoxacin
SUPRAX	cefixime
SPORANOX	itraconazole
VERMOX	mebendazole
ZAGAM	sparfloxacin
ZITHROMAX	azithromycin
ZYVOX	linezolid

Diabetes drugs

GLUCOPHAGE	metformin

Gastrointestinal drugs

ACIPHEX	rabeprazole
CYTOTEC	misoprostol
DIALOSE PLUS, PERI-COLACE	docusate/casanthranol
DULCOLAX	bisacodyl
MAALOX, MAALOX TC	aluminum hydroxide and magnesium hydroxide
MYLANTA, MYLANTA-II	magnesium hydroxide/ aluminum hydroxide/ simethicone
NEXIUM	esomeprazole
PHILLIPS' MILK OF MAGNESIA	magnesium hydroxide
PRILOSEC	omeprazole

Drugs That Can Cause Diarrhea (continued)

BRAND NAME	GENERIC NAME

Heart and blood vessel drugs

LANOXICAPS, LANOXIN	digoxin
PERSANTINE	dipyridamole
PLETAL	cilostazol

Antiarrhythmics

DURAQUIN, QUINAGLUTE DURA-TABS, QUINIDEX	quinidine
MEXITIL	mexiletine

High blood pressure drugs (diuretics)

DIUPRES	reserpine/chlorothiazide
ENDURONYL	deserpidine/methyclothiazide
HYDROPRES	reserpine/hydrochlorothiazide
REGROTON, DEMI-REGROTON	reserpine/chlorthalidone
SALUTENSIN	reserpine/hydroflumethiazide
SER-AP-ES	reserpine/hydralazine/hydrochlorothiazide

High blood pressure drugs (other)

	reserpine
ALDOMET	methyldopa
ISMELIN	guanethidine

Mind-affecting drugs

BUSPAR	buspirone
LUVOX	fluvoxamine
PAXIL	paroxetine
PROZAC	fluoxetine
WELLBUTRIN	bupropion
ZOLOFT	sertraline

Other drugs

IMURAN	azathioprine
NICORETTE, NICODERM	nicotine
PRECOSE	acarbose
ZYBAN	bupropion

Drugs That Can Cause Lung Toxicity

BRAND NAME	GENERIC NAME

Antibiotics and other anti-infective agents

FANSIDAR	pyrimethamine-sulfadoxine
FURADANTIN, MACROBID, MACRODANTIN	nitrofurantoin

Cancer drugs

ALKERAN	melphalan
BICNU	carmustine
BLENOXANE	bleomycin
CEENU	lomustine
CYTOSAR-U	cytarabine

BRAND NAME	GENERIC NAME
CYTOXAN	cyclophosphamide
ELDISINE	vindesine
LEUKERAN	chlorambucil
MATULANE	procarbazine
MUTAMYCIN	mitomycin
MYLERAN	busulfan
PROLEUKIN	aldesleukin/interleukin-2
RHEUMATREX DOSE PACK	methotrexate
VELBAN	vinblastine

Cold, cough, allergy, and asthma drugs

BRETHAIRE, BRETHINE, BRICANYL	terbutaline

Eye drugs

ADSORBOCARPINE, ISOPTO CARPINE	pilocarpine

Gastrointestinal drugs

AZULFIDINE	sulfasalazine

Heart and blood vessel drugs
Antiarrhythmics

CORDARONE	amiodarone
RYTHMOL	propafenone
TONOCARD	tocainide
XYLOCAINE	lidocaine

High blood pressure drugs (beta-blockers)

BLOCADREN	timolol
INDERAL, INDERAL LA	propranolol
VISKEN	pindolol

High blood pressure drugs (diuretics)

ESIDRIX, HYDRODIURIL	hydrochlorothiazide

High blood pressure drugs (other)

CAPOTEN	captopril
PRINIVIL, ZESTRIL	lisinopril
VASOTEC	enalapril

Mind-affecting drugs

PLACIDYL	ethchlorvynol

Neurological drugs
Anticonvulsants

DILANTIN	phenytoin

Antiparkinsonians

PARLODEL	bromocriptine

Painkillers/narcotics

ADVIL, MOTRIN	ibuprofen
ALEVE, ANAPROX, NAPROSYN	naproxen
GENUINE BAYER ASPIRIN, ECOTRIN	aspirin
CLINORIL	sulindac
CUPRIMINE, DEPEN	penicillamine
DARVON, DARVON-N	propoxyphene
DOLOPHINE, METHADOSE	methadone
FELDENE	piroxicam

Drugs That Can Cause Lung Toxicity (continued)

BRAND NAME	GENERIC NAME
IMURAN	azathioprine
INDOCIN	indomethacin
MYOCHRYSINE	gold sodium thiomalate
NARCAN	naloxone
SANSERT	methysergide
SOLGANAL	aurothioglucose
VOLTAREN	diclofenac

Other drugs

BRAND NAME	GENERIC NAME
	cocaine
	protamine
	tryptophan
ANECTINE	succinylcholine
DANTRIUM	dantrolene
NORCURON	vercuronium
PAVULON	pancuronium
TEGRETOL	carbamazepine
TRACRIUM	atracurium
TUBARINE	tubocurarine
YUTOPAR	ritodrine

Drugs That Can Affect the Urinary Tract

Drugs That Can Block Urination

All of the following drugs can cause urinary retention, the inability to urinate or difficulty in urinating, particularly in men with enlarged prostate glands.

BRAND NAME	GENERIC NAME
Antibiotics and other anti-infective agents	
URISED	atropine/hyoscyamine/ methenamine/methylene blue/phenyl salicylate/ benzoic acid
Cold, cough, allergy, and asthma drugs	
ALERMINE, CHLORTRIMETON	chlorpheniramine
ATARAX, VISTARIL	hydroxyzine
ATROVENT	ipratropium
BENADRYL, SOMINEX FORMULA	diphenhydramine
DIMETANE	brompheniramine
MYIDIL	triprolidine
OPTIMINE	azatadine
PERIACTIN	cyproheptadine
TAVIST, TAVIST-1	clemastine
Eye drugs	
NEPTAZANE	methazolamide

BRAND NAME	GENERIC NAME
Gastrointestinal drugs	
	atropine
ANTIVERT	meclizine
BENTYL	dicyclomine
COMPAZINE	prochlorperazine
DONNATAL	atropine/hyoscyamine/ scopolamine/ phenobarbital
LIBRAX	chlordiazepoxide/clidinium
LOMOTIL	diphenoxylate/atropine
PHENERGAN	promethazine
REGLAN	metoclopramide
TIGAN	trimethobenzamide
Heart and blood vessel drugs	
Antiarrhythmics	
NORPACE	disopyramide
High blood pressure drugs	
ADALAT, ADALAT CC, PROCARDIA, PROCARDIA XL	nifedipine
CARDENE, CARDENE SR	nicardipine
DYNACIRC, DYNACIRC CR	isradipine
Mind-affecting drugs	
Antidepressants	
ASENDIN	amoxapine
AVENTYL, PAMELOR	nortriptyline
DESYREL	trazodone
ELAVIL	amitriptyline
LIMBITROL	amitriptyline/ chlordiazepoxide
LUDIOMIL	maprotiline
NORPRAMIN	desipramine
PROZAC	fluoxetine
SINEQUAN	doxepin
TOFRANIL	imipramine
TRIAVIL	amitriptyline/perphenazine
WELLBUTRIN	bupropion
Antipsychotics	
COMPAZINE	prochlorperazine
HALDOL	haloperidol
MELLARIL	thioridazine
NAVANE	thiothixene
PROLIXIN	fluphenazine
REGLAN	metoclopramide
STELAZINE	trifluoperazine
THORAZINE	chlorpromazine
TRIAVIL	amitriptyline/perphenazine
Tranquilizers	
BUSPAR	buspirone
Neurological drugs	
ARTANE	trihexyphenidyl
COGENTIN	benztropine
ELDEPRYL	selegiline, deprenyl
FELBATOL	felbamate

Drugs That Can Block Urination (continued)

BRAND NAME	GENERIC NAME
Other drugs	
ACTIQ, DURAGESIC	fentanyl
DITROPAN	oxybutynin
PROAMATINE	midodrine
ULTRAM	tramadol
ZYBAN	bupropion

Drugs That Can Cause Loss of Bladder Control (Incontinence)

All of the drugs listed above that may block urination can, when the bladder gets too full, cause "overflow" leakage. In addition, the following drugs can also cause urine to leak:

BRAND NAME	GENERIC NAME
Antibiotics and other anti-infective agents	
URISED	atropine/hyoscyamine/ methenamine/methylene blue/phenyl salicylate/ benzoic acid
Eye drugs	
BETAGAN	levobunolol
Gastrointestinal drugs	
CYTOTEC	misoprostol
Heart and blood vessel drugs	
High blood pressure drugs (beta-blockers)	
BLOCADREN	timolol
CARTROL	carteolol
COREG	carvedilol
CORGARD	nadolol
CORZIDE	nadolol/ bendroflumethiazide
INDERAL, INDERAL LA	propranolol
INDERIDE LA	propranolol/ hydrochlorothiazide
KERLONE	betaxolol
LEVATOL	penbutolol
LOPRESSOR, TOPROL XL	metoprolol
LOPRESSOR HCT	metoprolol/ hydrochlorothiazide
NORMODYNE, TRANDATE	labetalol
SECTRAL	acebutolol
TENORETIC	atenolol/chlorthalidone
TENORMIN	atenolol
VISKEN	pindolol
ZEBETA	bisoprolol
ZIAC	bisoprolol/ hydrochlorothiazide

BRAND NAME	GENERIC NAME
High blood pressure drugs (diuretics)	
ALDACTAZIDE	spironolactone/ hydrochlorothiazide
ALDORIL	methyldopa/ hydrochlorothiazide
APRESAZIDE	hydralazine/ hydrochlorothiazide
BUMEX	bumetanide
COMBIPRES	clonidine/chlorthalidone
DEMADEX	torsemide
DIUPRES	reserpine/chlorthalidone
DIURIL	chlorothiazide
DYAZIDE, MAXZIDE	triamterene/ hydrochlorothiazide
ENDURON	methyclothiazide
ENDURONYL	deserpidine/ methyclothiazide
ESIDRIX, HYDRODIURIL	hydrochlorothiazide
HYDROPRES	reserpine/ hydrochlorothiazide
HYGROTON	chlorthalidone
INDERIDE LA	propranolol/ hydrochlorothiazide
LASIX	furosemide
LOZOL	indapamide
METAHYDRIN, NAQUA	trichlormethiazide
MODURETIC	amiloride/ hydrochlorothiazide
REGROTON, DEMI- REGROTON	reserpine/chlorthalidone
SALUTENSIN	reserpine/ hydroflumethiazide
SER-AP-ES	reserpine/hydralazine/ hydrochlorothiazide
TENORETIC	atenolol/chlorthalidone
ZAROXOLYN, DIULO	metolazone
High blood pressure drugs (other)	
ADALAT, ADALAT CC, PROCARDIA, PROCARDIA XL	nifedipine
ALDACTONE	spironolactone
CARDENE, CARDENE SR	nicardipine
CARDURA	doxazosin
DYNACIRC, DYNACIRC CR	isradipine
HYTRIN	terazosin
MINIPRESS	prazosin
Mind-affecting drugs	
Antidepressants	
CELEXA	citalopram
LEXAPRO	escitalopram
LITHOBID, LITHONATE	lithium
LUVOX	fluvoxamine
PAXIL	paroxetine
PROZAC	fluoxetine

Drugs That Can Cause Loss of Bladder Control (continued)

BRAND NAME	GENERIC NAME
WELLBUTRIN	bupropion
ZOLOFT	sertraline

Antipsychotics

CLOZARIL	clozapine
RISPERDAL	risperidone
ZYPREXA	olanzapine

Tranquilizers or sleeping pills

ATARAX, VISTARIL	hydroxyzine
ATIVAN	lorazepam
BUSPAR	buspirone
CENTRAX	prazepam
DALMANE	flurazepam
DORIDEN	glutethimide
HALCION	triazolam

BRAND NAME	GENERIC NAME
LIBRIUM	chlordiazepoxide
MILTOWN, EQUANIL	meprobamate
NOCTEC	chloral hydrate
NOLUDAR	methyprylon
PLACIDYL	ethchlorvynol
RESTORIL	temazepam
SERAX	oxazepam
TRANXENE	clorazepate
VALIUM	diazepam
XANAX	alprazolam

Neurological drugs

ARICEPT	donepezil
KLONOPIN	clonazepam
NEURONTIN	gabapentin

Other drugs

ZYBAN	bupropion

REFERENCES

1. Of the 42.34 million Americans 60 and older (*Statistical Abstracts of the United States* 1992, 1991 population data), approximately 90% are taking one or more medications for a total of 37.83 million older people. According to a study of verified adverse drug reactions (German PS, Klein LE. Adverse drug experience among the elderly. *Pharmaceuticals for the Elderly*. Pharmaceutical Manufacturers Association, November 1986), 25.4% of the elderly patients 60 and older had at least one adverse drug reaction during the six-month interval that the study encompassed. Twenty-five and four-tenths percent of 37.83 million people is 9.61 million adverse reactions for the six-month period. The number of adverse reactions in a year would certainly be higher. The actual number of adverse reactions is also much higher, since this calculation assumes all patients were being seen outside of the hospital or nursing home. Because the use of drugs in nursing homes and hospitals is much higher than in clinics, the number of adverse reactions is also higher.

2. Using the basis for estimating the number of admissions to medical wards of hospitals of 6.05 million in 1990 (see reference 1 in the previous chapter for the basis of this estimate), and the estimate that in 22.4% of medical admissions the patients are using digoxin and that 2.06% of these suffer life-threatening heart toxicity from digoxin (both are from Miller RR, Greenblatt DJ. *Drug Effects in Hospitalized Patients*. New York: John Wiley and Sons, 1976), this amounts to 6.05 million times 22.4% times 2.06%, or 27,917 older adults in hospitals who suffer from life-threatening heart toxicity from digoxin. This estimate understates the magnitude of the problem because the proportion of patients in the Miller/Greenblatt book using digoxin and experiencing life-threatening heart toxicity is based on all patients of all ages, whereas the rate of digoxin use and therefore the rate of life-threatening reactions is higher in older adults. The estimate is also lower because it does not include cases of digoxin toxicity that occur in surgical patients.

3. Ray WA, Griffin MR, Shorr RI. Adverse drug reactions and the elderly. *Health Affairs* 1990; 9:114–22.

4. Ray WA, Fought RL, Decker MD. Psychoactive drugs and the risk of injurious motor vehicle crashes in elderly drivers. *American Journal of Epidemiology* 1992; 136:873–83.

5. Ray WA, Griffin MR, Schaffner W, et al. Psychotropic drug use and the risk of hip fracture. *New England Journal of Medicine* 1987; 316:363–9.

6. The estimate of 32,000 hip fractures in older adults is based on projecting the findings of this study of drug-induced hip fractures in older Michigan Medicaid patients to the entire country.

7. Myers AH, Robinson EG, Van Natta MI, et al. Hip fractures among the elderly: Factors associated with in-hospital mortality. *American Journal of Epidemiology* 1991; 134:1128–37.

8. Larson EB, Kukull WA, Buchner D, et al. Adverse drug reactions associated with global cognitive impairment in elderly persons. *Annals of Internal Medicine* 1987; 107:169–73.

9. This estimate is based on projecting the findings of the Larson study on the 1.43 million Americans 65 and older who have dementia. See discussion on sleeping pills and tranquilizers (p. 166) for more details about this serious problem.

10. See discussion on sleeping pills and tranquilizers (p. 166) for more details on this estimate.

11. See discussion on antipsychotic drugs (p. 268) for more details about drug-induced tardive dyskinesia and misprescribing of antipsychotic drugs.

12. The estimate of 61,000 older adults suffering from drug-induced parkinsonism is derived as follows: As described in detail in the chapter on antipsychotic drugs (see p. 268), there are an estimated 750,000 people 65 and older in nursing homes or living in the community who are regularly (for three or four months or longer) being prescribed antipsychotic drugs. According to a survey in 1981 of 5,000 patients being treated with antipsychotic drugs, 13.2% had parkinsonism [see reference 15 below and p. 179 in chapter 5, Mind Drugs, for further discussion of this problem]. Another study by the same researchers found that 62% became better (no longer had parkinsonism) within 30 days of discontinuing the drug. Thus, at least 62% of the 13.2% of patients getting antipsychotic drugs or 7.92% of all patients getting these drugs suffer from drug-induced parkinsonism. Calculating 7.92% of 750,000 patients getting these drugs for at least several months yields 61,380 patients with drug-induced parkinsonism. This is a very conservative estimate because it does not include either those patients using antipsychotic drugs for less than three to four months (an additional 1.16 million people) who are also at risk for drug-induced parkinsonism (because 90% of the cases occur within 72 days after beginning the drug) or those who get drug-induced parkinsonism from the related drugs metoclopramide (REGLAN), prochlorperazine (COMPAZINE), promethazine (PHENERGAN), usually prescribed for nausea.

13. Vestal RE, ed. *Drug Treatment in the Elderly*. Sydney, Australia: ADIS Health Service Press, 1984.

14. Ouslander JG. Drug therapy in the elderly. *Annals of Internal Medicine* 1981; 95:711–22.

15. Grimes JD. Drug-induced parkinsonism and tardive dyskinesia in nonpsychiatric patients. *Canadian Medical Association Journal* 1982; 126:468.

16. *Drugs for the Elderly*. 2nd edition. Copenhagen, Denmark: World Health Organization, 1997:28.

17. Lipton HL, Bero LA, Bird JA, et al. The impact of clinical pharmacists' consultations on physicians' geriatric drug prescribing: A randomized controlled trial. *Medical Care* 1992; 30:646–58.

18. Drugs that may cause psychiatric symptoms. *Medical Letter on Drugs and Therapeutics* 2002; 44:59–62.

19. Davies DM, ed. *Textbook of Adverse Drug Reactions*. New York: Oxford University Press, 1977.

20. Aronson JK, VanBoxtel CJ, eds. *Side Effects of Drugs Annual* 18. Amsterdam: Elsevier, 1995.

21. Aronson JK, ed. *Side Effects of Drugs Annual* 24. Amsterdam: Elsevier, 2001.

22. Aronson JK, ed. *Side Effects of Drugs Annual* 25. Amsterdam: Elsevier, 2002.

23. Other sources included the *Physicians' Desk Reference* and outside consultants.

24. See reference 8 above. Although this study found specific drugs in certain therapeutic classes to cause an increased risk of mental impairment, we list all of the drugs in that class here, since for benzodiazepines, beta-blockers, and major tranquilizers (antipsychotic drugs), for example, there is no reason to believe that the whole class would not have this adverse effect.

4

DRUGS FOR HEART CONDITIONS

HIGH BLOOD PRESSURE

High blood pressure, or hypertension, is a major contributing factor to the development of strokes, heart attacks, kidney disease, and circulation disorders. Elevated cholesterol levels can also result in an increase in heart attacks and strokes. Heart disease and stroke remain the first and third leading causes of death in the

United States. More than 33 million Americans are estimated to have high blood pressure; this includes more than 14 million persons between the ages of 45 and 64.[1] Many people with increased blood pressure also have other risk factors such as elevated cholesterol, diabetes, and smoking. But many do not. Conversely, many people with higher cholesterol levels also have high blood pressure, smoke, or are diabetic, but many have only elevated cholesterol levels. In addition, the risk of cardiovascular disease—such as heart attacks and strokes—increases with age. Thus, it is extremely important to look at the global risk of cardiovascular disease rather than focusing on just the blood pressure or just the cholesterol level.[155]

High Blood Pressure in Pregnancy

Antihypertensive drugs may directly or indirectly harm the fetus. If the maternal placental circulation is reduced by lowering the mother's blood pressure too much, there is the danger of immediate harm to the fetus by depriving it of an adequate supply of blood and thus of essential nourishment.

The Merck Manual[156,157] recommends that women with preexisting mild hypertension (140/90 to 150/100 millimeters of mercury) discontinue antihypertensive drugs as soon as pregnancy is confirmed and monitor their blood pressure regularly. For patients with preexisting moderate hypertension (150/100 to 180/110 millimeters of mercury), methyldopa (ALDOMET) is the drug of choice. Women with severe hypertension (greater than or equal to 180/110 millimeters of mercury) represent a much more complicated medical condition in which less desirable drugs may be appropriate.

Leg Swelling (Edema) in Pregnancy

The routine use of diuretics (see p. 60) in pregnancy is inappropriate and exposes the mother and fetus to unnecessary hazards. Edema occurs in a majority of pregnant women and is not harmful to either the mother or fetus. It can often be relieved by lying down or elevating the legs.

Diuretics, a group of drugs used to treat hypertension and edema, can cause harm by reducing the mother's circulating blood volume. This reduces the amount of oxygen and nutrition available to the fetus. Diuretics can also cause low levels of sodium and potassium as well as yellow skin (jaundice) and bleeding in the newborn and have, in addition, the potential for some of the adverse effects seen in the adult (see p. 60). Diuretics do not prevent the development of nor are they useful in the treatment of preeclampsia (toxemia of pregnancy). Thiazide diuretics can also cross the placenta and thus have the added potential for direct adverse effects.

Regardless of your age, reducing your blood pressure using diet and exercise, or diuretics or beta-blockers if drug treatment is necessary, reduces your risk of heart attack and stroke.

When your blood pressure is taken, you are given two numbers, which represent the systolic pressure and the diastolic pressure—140/90 (mm Hg—millimeters of mercury, under pressure), for example. Systolic pressure, the upper number (140), reflects the pressure in the arteries as the heart contracts, pumps blood, and the blood vessels fill with blood. As the arteries harden with age (arteriosclerosis), the systolic pressure increases. Diastolic pressure, the lower number (90), reflects the pressure in the arteries as the heart relaxes and fills with blood. This is associated with a run-off of blood from the blood vessels.

A person's blood pressure can be higher when measured at the doctor's office than when measured at home; feeling nervous probably contributes to the higher reading. Ask your doctor about the various methods available for home monitoring of blood pressure, so you can see if yours is lower at home. If so, it is possible that you actually do not have high blood pressure and do not have to be treated.

Either your systolic or your diastolic pressure can be elevated. Elevations of either one or both of these pressures may significantly increase your chance of having a stroke or heart attack, much more so in the presence of other risk factors as discussed above.

Nondrug Treatment of High Blood Pressure

A healthy lifestyle is critical for the prevention of high blood pressure and is an essential part of the management of those with hypertension. Major lifestyle modifications shown to lower high blood pressure include weight reduction in those who are overweight or obese.[23] In addition, sodium reduction and a diet rich in vegetables, fruits, and low-fat dairy products lowers blood pressure in both those with and without hypertension.[45] For example, a 1,600 milligram sodium restriction has effects similar to treatment with a single blood-pressure-lowering drug.[4] Exercise[67] and moderate alcohol intake are also beneficial in maintaining a healthy blood pressure.[8]

A study of nutritional therapy showed that over one-third of people who previously needed drug treatment for high blood pressure were able to adequately control their blood pressure with nutritional therapy alone.[9] In addition, these methods are safer than using medication, since they have no adverse effects. Trying them will often make other beneficial contributions to your health.

1. **Lose weight:** Nearly two-thirds of adults in the United States are overweight, and 30.5 percent are obese, according to data from a 1999–2000 National Institutes of Health survey. Many people in this category who lose weight can reduce their blood pressure by 15%.

2. **Reduce your salt intake:** Changing your diet by not using your salt shaker and reducing your in-take of processed and salty foods is a good first step.

3. **Restrict alcohol:** Cutting alcohol intake to, at most, one drink a day also can reduce blood pressure.

4. **Exercise:** Mild aerobic exercise such as walking 15 or 20 minutes a day at a comfortable pace will have a beneficial effect on heart and blood pressure.

5. **Decrease your fat intake:** Decreasing the amount of animal fat in your diet has a beneficial effect on blood pressure. Furthermore, a high-fat diet is a risk factor for heart disease independent of high blood pressure. Decreasing the amount of fat in your diet will therefore help reduce your overall risk of developing heart disease.

6. **Increase the fiber in your diet:** Diets with a high fiber content can lower blood pressure.[10] One study showed a drop of 10 mm Hg in systolic pressure and 5 mm Hg of diastolic pressure in people who took fiber supplements for two months, without any other dietary changes.[11] Fiber can be increased by eating more fruits, vegetables, and whole grains.

In a clinical trial performed on people 60 to 80 years old with well-controlled blood pressures, who had been taking a high-blood-pressure-lowering drug for years, found that keeping salt intake to 1,800 milligrams per day or less and losing a moderate amount of weight (on the order of 10 pounds) were responsible for further significant decreases in blood pressure while continuing drug treatment. At the end of the study more than 30% of the patients had lowered their blood pressure enough through salt reduction and weight loss to no longer require blood-pressure-lowering drugs. Salt reduction was equally effective in overweight and non-overweight participants and was as effective as weight reduction in preventing recurrence of high blood pressure, need for a blood-pressure-lowering drug, or a cardiovascular event such as a stroke, heart attack, or chest pain (angina).

Salt reduction combined with weight loss was more effective than either alone for control of high blood pressure, with or without the use of a blood-pressure-lowering drug.[12]

Decades of extensive research now make it possible to speak in terms of preventing high blood pressure rather than treating it with drugs, which is defensive, mainly reactive, time-consuming, associated with adverse drug effects, costly, only partially successful, endless, and is not a cure. In the editorial that accompanied the study the author said: *"Hence, there is now evidence for a 'fare for all seasons,' to be consumed from post weaning through older age, to prevent adverse BP [blood pressure] levels, other major risk factors, and cardiovascular and other chronic diseases. This fare is delectably high in fruits and vegetables; high in legumes and whole grains; high in fat-free and low-fat dairy products, poultry, fish, shellfish, and meats; high in all essential nutrients; reduced in salt; reduced in total fat, saturated fat, and cholesterol; with no more than 2 drinks per day for those who choose to ingest alcohol; and controlled in calories to prevent or correct obesity."*[13]

When Is Drug Treatment Necessary?

Several factors should be taken into account when considering whether your high blood pressure should be treated. One is the benefits of the treatment for your blood pressure, which vary significantly depending on how high it is, your age, and whether you have other risk factors such as high cholesterol or are a smoker or a diabetic, and whether you have had a heart attack, heart failure, a stroke, or have kidney damage. The other consideration is the risks or the adverse effects of the treatment, which will vary depending on what is being considered.

Several studies have shown that the treatment of an elevated diastolic pressure does decrease your chance of having a stroke or heart attack. However, if only your systolic pressure is elevated, which often occurs in older adults, it is controversial as to what benefits are gained by treatment. Doctors generally agree that systolic blood pressure readings above a certain level—such as 160—are dangerous enough so that they require treatment. Treatment of systolic blood pressure below these levels is more controversial.

The following examples are applicable to people who do not have cardiovascular diseases such as a heart attack, angina, heart failure, or a stroke and who are between the ages of 30 and 74. The results are from an online cardiovascular risk calculator that can be found at www.widebay dgp.org.au/Resources/5yrRiskCalc.xls.[158]

Example A: John is a 50-year-old man with a blood pressure of 160/90. With the upper limit of normal being 140/90, he has what is referred to as **isolated systolic hypertension** because of his systolic pressure of 160. However, John has a normal total cholesterol of 193 and a normal HDL (the "good" cholesterol) of 50. HDL is referred to as "good" cholesterol because it protects against coronary artery disease. He does not have diabetes, is not a smoker, has never had angina, a heart attack or heart failure, and does not have kidney damage. John turns out to have a 5-year risk of having a cardiovascular event (heart attack, stroke, etc.) of 6.2%, well under the 5-year risk of over 10% that might merit drug treatment.[155] It would be a good idea for John—or most people, for that matter—to adopt the nondrug approaches to lowering his blood pressure discussed above, but since his **global risk** is as low as it is, drug treatment is not indicated even if his blood pressure stays the same.

Example B: Mary is a 60-year-old woman, also with a blood pressure of 160/90. Like John, Mary has a normal total cholesterol of 193 and a normal HDL (the "good" cholesterol) of 50. She also does not have diabetes, is not a smoker, and has never had angina, a heart attack, heart failure, or kidney damage. Using the same risk calculator, Mary's 5-year risk of having a cardiovascular event is 6.8%, about the same as John's even though she is 10 years older. Again, there is no reason for her to have drug treatment for her isolated systolic hypertension because her global risk is low.

There is little doubt that many Marys and Johns are being treated with drugs for high blood pressure even though their risk of strokes and heart attacks is as low as it is. This is because most doctors focus on just one risk factor—in this case blood pressure—instead of examining the total picture.

Example C: Larry is a 50-year-old man who also has a blood pressure of 160/90, but he is a diabetic and although his total cholesterol is also 193, his HDL is only 40 (less of the "good cholesterol"). Though his blood pressure is the same as that of John and Mary, his 5-year cardiovascular risk is 17.6%, more than twice as high as theirs. He should start a program of exercise and diet to see if his blood pressure can be lowered that way, and then, if it still remains elevated, a drug to treat the hypertension such as a thiazide diuretic should be tried. (See p. 60.)

Are many people being given antihypertensive drugs unnecessarily? One study found that 41% of patients 50 and older who were carefully taken off their high blood pressure medications did not need them, having normal blood pressure 11 months after the drug was stopped.[14]

Which Drug to Use?

Regardless of your age, much of the time high blood pressure can be controlled with just one drug. The National Institutes of Health's National Heart, Lung and Blood Institute recommends beginning treatment with a mild water pill (diuretic) at a low dose. The safest and best

studied of the diuretics is hydrochlorothiazide (see p. 60). The starting dose should be low: 12.5 to 25 milligrams per day or even every other day. Confirming the advice we have been giving to readers of this book since 1988 is a large definitive study (named ALLHAT) involving more than 33,000 patients aged 55 or older that found "compelling evidence that thiazide diuretics (such as hydrochlorothiazide or chlorthalidone) should be the initial drug of choice for patients with hypertension." Thus, the widespread prescribing practice—spurred on by massive advertising—of starting people with newly diagnosed hypertension with calcium channel blockers (such as Norvasc, Cardizem, or Procardia), ACE inhibitors (such as Zestril, Accupril, or Vasotec), or other drugs that are not thiazides lacks any scientific rationale.

For older adults, in general, the rule for treating high blood pressure, as with so many other drug treatments, is "start low and go slow." According to experts in prescribing for older adults, for mild hypertension (or heart failure) start with half the standard starting dose and increase gradually.

If a second drug is needed the National Heart, Lung, and Blood Institute recommends beta-blockers (see p. 87), although they are not as effective in older adults as they are in younger adults. Because of this, beta-blockers should never be used as the first drug in treating high blood pressure in older adults. **ACE inhibitors are also effective drugs to use as a second agent.** It is rarely necessary to take more than two drugs to treat high blood pressure. If you are taking more than two, a reassessment is indicated.

Common Adverse Effects of High Blood Pressure Drugs

The decision to use drugs to treat high blood pressure should be based on a consideration of both the benefits and the risks of the treatment.

Therefore it is very important that you report any adverse effects of the drugs to your doctor, so that your situation can be reassessed. These are some of the possible adverse effects of the various antihypertensive drugs.[15]

• Depression—especially with beta-blockers, reserpine, methyldopa, and clonidine (see *Drugs That Can Cause Depression, in Chapter 3,* p. 23).
• Sedation and fatigue—especially with beta-blockers, reserpine, methyldopa, and clonidine.
• Impotence and sexual dysfunction—especially with beta-blockers, methyldopa, and many other heart drugs (see *Drugs That Can Cause Sexual Dysfunction, in Chapter 3,* p. 34).
• Dizziness (from a drop in blood pressure after standing up, which can result in accidental falls and broken bones)—seen with all high blood pressure drugs to some degree, and especially with guanethidine, prazosin, and methyldopa. Older adults are more prone to this adverse effect because the internal blood pressure regulation system works more slowly as we age (see *Drugs That Can Cause Dizziness on Standing, in Chapter 3,* p. 31).
• Loss of appetite and nausea—especially with hydrochlorothiazide, digoxin, and potassium supplements (see *Drugs That Can Cause Loss of Appetite, Nausea, or Vomiting, in Chapter 3,* p. 36).

These and other adverse effects can occur with any medication for high blood pressure. Those listed occur most often. If you experience any effects, or just feel worse in general, tell your doctor. It is often better to tolerate a slightly higher blood pressure with no adverse effects from medication than to have a lower blood pressure along with serious effects from medication that will adversely affect your life.

For example, let's consider the steps in devising a treatment for a 75-year-old woman whose baseline blood pressure is 200/90 mm Hg:

1. She is first treated with 12.5 milligrams of hydrochlorothiazide. This results in a blood pressure of 170/90, and she feels quite well.
2. Her doctor attempts to lower her blood pressure further by adding another drug, propranolol, to her treatment. This results in a blood pressure of 160/90, but she "feels awful" and complains of fatigue and confusion.
3. Her doctor might consider discontinuing the propranolol and using another drug. A better idea might be to accept a blood pressure of 170/90 using hydrochlorothiazide alone or to lower it further with nondrug therapy.

Stopping Drug Treatment

Historically, patients have been taught that hypertension means treatment for life, although countless thousands of patients have abandoned their treatment without their doctors' knowledge or consent. For some patients, this may be a dangerous idea, but for many others the treatment may no longer be needed. Two large studies in Australia and Britain have shown that one-third to one-half of patients with mild hypertension for whom treatment was stopped had normal blood pressures a year or more later.[16]

An editorial in the *British Medical Journal* stated, *"Treatment of hypertension is part of preventive medicine and like all preventive strategies, its progress should be regularly reviewed by whoever initiates it. Many problems could be avoided by not starting antihypertensive treatment until after prolonged observation. . . . Patients should no longer be told that treatment is necessarily for life: the possibility of reducing or stopping treatment should be mentioned at the outset."*[16]

This view is shared by American experts in hypertension who have stated that "once blood pressure has been normal for a year or more, a cautious decrease in antihypertensive dosage and renewed attention to nonpharmacologic treatment may be worth trying."[17]

Drugs Used to Treat High Blood Pressure

Diuretics

Eighteen different diuretics are available in the U.S., falling into three general categories: (1) the thiazide type, the best-known member of which is hydrochlorothiazide (ESIDREX, HYDRODIURIL); (2) loop diuretics, which include furosemide (LASIX) (the "loop" pertains to the part of the kidney in which the drug works) and are more potent than the thiazide type for removing sodium and fluid, but are not first-choice drugs for the treatment of high blood pressure; and (3) potassium-sparing diuretics, which, as the name implies, cut down on the loss of potassium in the minority of patients whose blood levels of potassium decrease when taking thiazides or loop diuretics.

The latest revision of the National Institutes of Health's guidelines on high blood pressure, the Seventh Report of the Joint National Committee, or JNC VII, again recommends that thiazide diuretics should be used in the drug treatment for most patients with uncomplicated high blood pressure, either alone or in combination with other drugs.[18]

The thiazide-type diuretics improve survival in patients with high blood pressure. They also have been shown to reduce incidence of stroke and cardiovascular events in elderly people with a type of high blood pressure known as isolated systolic hypertension. The most widely used thiazide diuretics are hydrochlorothiazide and chlorthalidone (HYGROTON).

We have long recommended, as does JNC VII, that the starting dose of hydrochlorothiazide should be 12.5 milligrams per day. For years the lowest strength available was a 25 milligram tablet that had to be broken in half to achieve the 12.5 milligram dose. There is now a 12.5 milligram capsule of hydrochlorothiazide available with the brand name Microzide.

There is growing evidence that thiazide diuretics, such as hydrochlorothiazide, significantly decrease the rate of bone mineral loss in both men and women because they reduce the amount of calcium lost in the urine. Research now suggests that thiazide diuretics may protect against hip fracture.

The loop diuretics can be used to treat high blood pressure in patients with kidney insufficiency. In those without kidney insufficiency, they may be less effective than the thiazides for the treatment of high blood pressure.

DIURETICS

Generic Drug Name (Brand Name)

Thiazide Type
bendroflumethiazide (NATURETIN)
chlorothiazide (DIURIL)
hydrochlorothiazide (ESIDREX, MICROZIDE)
hydroflumethiazide (SALURON, DIUCARDIN)
chlorthalidone (HYGROTON)
indapamide (LOZOL)
methyclothiazide (ENDURON)
metolazone (ZAROXOLYN, MYKROX)
polythiazide (RENESE)
trichlormethiazide (NAQUA)

Loop Type
bumetanide (BUMEX)
ethacrynic acid (EDECRIN)
furosemide (LASIX)
torsemide (DEMADEX)

Potassium-Sparing
amiloride (MIDAMOR)
eplerenone (INSPIRA)
spironolactone (ALDACTONE)
triamterene (DYRENIUM)

The potassium-sparing diuretics can cause dangerously elevated blood levels of potassium, particularly in patients with kidney impairment and in those taking ACE inhibitors, angiotensin receptor blockers (ARBs), or using potassium supplements.

Beta-blockers

Currently, there are 13 beta-blockers on the U.S. market. In addition to high blood pressure, some of the beta-blockers are also used to treat chest pain (angina), heart attacks, irregular heart rhythms, glaucoma, and migraine headaches.

Beta-blockers should not be taken if you have asthma, emphysema, chronic bronchitis, bronchospasm, allergies, or heart block. If you have heart failure, beta-blockers can cause dramatic improvement but must be taken under careful supervision. A baseline electrocardiogram (ECG, EKG) should be taken before a beta-blocker is first prescribed to be sure that you do not have heart block. Do not smoke while taking a beta-blocker (you shouldn't be smoking anyway). If you smoke, you might as well stop taking the beta-blocker. Not only will smoking aggravate some of the respiratory adverse effects, but it greatly reduces the level of drug in your body.

Beta-blockers can cause a spasm in the air passages of the lungs (bronchospasm) and bring on asthmatic wheezing even when beta-blocker eye drops are used to treat glaucoma. Therefore, beta-blockers should not be used if you have asthma, bronchospasm, chronic bronchitis, or emphysema. If you are experiencing breathing difficulty while taking a beta-blocker, call your doctor immediately.

The following table lists the beta-blockers currently available on the U.S. market.

BETA-BLOCKERS

Generic Drug Name (Brand Name)

acebutolol (SECTRAL)
atenolol (TENORMIN)
betaxolol (KERLONE)
bisoprolol (ZEBETA)
carteolol (CARTROL)
carvedilol (COREG)
labetalol (NORMODYNE, TRANDATE)
metoprolol (LOPRESSOR, TOPROL XL)
nadolol (CORGARD)
penbutolol (LEVATOL)
pindolol (VISKEN)
propranolol (INDERAL)
timolol (BLOCADREN)

Alpha-blockers

This family of drugs includes doxazosin (CARDURA; see p. 102), prazosin (MINIPRESS; see p. 102), and terazosin (HYTRIN; see p. 102). The alpha-blockers are also used to treat benign prostatic hyperplasia, or an enlarged prostate gland.

The National Institutes of Health (NIH) no longer recommends the routine use of alpha-blockers for the treatment of high blood pressure.[18]

In March 2000, the NIH announced that it had stopped one part of a large high blood pressure study because the alpha-blocker doxazosin proved to be less effective than the old thiazide diuretic chlorthalidone (HYGROTON; see p. 60) in reducing some forms of cardiovascular disease. The study, called the Antihypertensive and Lipid Lowering Treatment to Prevent Heart Attack Trial (ALLHAT), found users of doxazosin had 25% more cardiovascular events and were twice as likely to be hospitalized for congestive heart failure as users of chlorthalidone.[19]

Angiotensin Converting Enzyme (ACE) Inhibitors

There are now 10 angiotensin converting enzyme (ACE) inhibitors on the U.S. market. The ACE inhibitors work to lower blood pressure by preventing the production of angiotensin II, a potent, naturally occurring hormone that raises blood pressure.

The two most-studied ACE inhibitors, captopril (CAPOTEN) and enalapril (VASOTEC), are available at lower cost as generics.

All ACE inhibitors reduce blood pressure and various ACE inhibitors reduce mortality in patients with coronary artery disease. They prolong the survival of patients with heart failure after a heart attack, and preserve kidney function in those with diabetes. The ACE inhibitors may also preserve kidney function in nondiabetic patients with a kidney disorder.[20] The table below lists the available ACE inhibitors and their FDA-approved uses.

When used in pregnancy during the second and third trimesters, ACE inhibitors can cause injury and even death to the developing fetus. You should always tell your doctor if you are pregnant or thinking of becoming pregnant before you use an ACE inhibitor.

A common adverse effect, after taking ACE inhibitors for a few weeks, is a dry, hacking cough, especially in women. Check with your doctor about a four-day withdrawal from your ACE inhibitor to determine if this is the cause of your cough. This trial withdrawal can prevent unnecessary and sometimes costly tests and treatments to determine other causes of cough.

Angiotensin Receptor Blockers (ARBs)

Seven ARBs are now on the market in the United States. These drugs work by blocking the effect of angiotensin II, a potent, naturally occurring hormone that raises blood pressure. In contrast, the previously mentioned ACE inhibitors prevent the production of angiotensin II in the body.

The best therapeutic role for the ARBs appears to be in patients in whom ACE inhibitors are indicated but who are unable to tolerate them.

The development of the dry, hacking cough often seen with the use of ACE inhibitors does not appear to be as frequent with the angiotensin receptor antagonists. This family of drugs carries the same warning as ACE inhibitors about use in pregnancy.

FDA-APPROVED USES FOR ACE INHIBITORS

Generic Drug Name (Brand Name)	High Blood Pressure	Heart Failure	Left Ventrical Dysfunction after Heart Attack	Asymptomatic Left Ventricular Dysfunction	Acute Heart Attack	Risk Reduction of Heart Attack, Stroke, Cardiovascular Death
benazepril (LOTENSIN)	yes					
captopril (CAPOTEN)	yes	yes	yes			
enalapril (VASOTEC)	yes	yes		yes		
fosinopril (MONOPRIL)	yes	yes				
lisinopril (PRINIVIL, ZESTRIL)	yes	yes			yes	
moexipril (UNIVASC)	yes					
perindopril (ACEON)	yes					
quinapril (ACCUPRIL)	yes	yes				
ramipril (ALTACE)	yes	yes				yes
trandolapril (MAVIK)	yes	yes	yes			

FDA-APPROVED USES FOR ANGIOTENSIN RECEPTOR BLOCKERS

Generic Drug Name (Brand)	High Blood Pressure	Reduce the Risk of Stroke	Prevent Kidney Damage in Diabetics with High Blood Pressure	Heart Failure in Those That Can't Take ACE Inhibitors
candesartan (ATACAND)	yes			
eprosartan (TEVETEN)	yes			
irbesartan (AVAPRO)	yes			
losartan (COZAAR)	yes	yes	yes	
olmesartan (BENICAR)	yes			
telmisartan (MICARDIS)	yes			
valsartan (DIOVAN)	yes			yes

The table above lists the available ARBs and their FDA-approved uses.

Calcium Channel Blockers

There are currently eight calcium channel blockers on the market in the United States. Despite recommendations of the National Institutes of Health's National Heart, Lung and Blood Institute dating back to 1993 that diuretics and beta-blockers should be used first in the treatment of mild to moderate high blood pressure, the calcium channel blockers remained the largest-selling family of high-blood-pressure-lowering drugs in the United States during the 1990s.[21] In 2002, the calcium channel blocker amlodipine (NORVASC) was the fourth most frequently dispensed drug in the United States, with over 30 million prescriptions being dispensed.

The calcium channel blocker mibefradil (POSICOR) was withdrawn from the market because of harmful drug interactions.

In 1995, Public Citizen's Health Research Group filed a petition with the Food and Drug Administration to add warnings to the labeling of all calcium channel blockers about the increased risk of heart attack and death. Our petition was based on three well-conducted observational research studies.[22–24]

Observational studies are frequently criticized by doctors who do not understand this type of research. Most of what we know about adverse drug reactions and what we are likely to learn in the future about them comes from observational research. This type of research was used to show the link between cigarette smoking and lung cancer.

Our petition helped to bring about important labeling changes in February 1996 on one of the calcium channel blockers, the short-acting form of nifedipine. The labeling for this form of nifedipine now warns doctors that this product should not be used for the treatment of high blood pressure because of sudden, life-threatening decreases in blood pressure that can occur.

The calcium channel blockers currently marketed in the United States are listed in the following table.

CALCIUM CHANNEL BLOCKERS

amlodipine (NORVASC)
diltiazem (CARDIZEM, CARDIZEM CD)
felodipine (PLENDIL)
isradipine (DYNACIRC)
nicardipine (CARDENE)
nifedipine (PROCARDIA XL)
nisoldipine (SULAR)
verapamil (COVERA HS)

ELEVATED CHOLESTEROL LEVELS

Nondrug Lowering of Cholesterol

In addition to exercise to lower cholesterol, another safe and less costly measure is to eat a low-fat diet, using mostly polyunsaturated fats (such as canola, corn, safflower, and sunflower oils) or monounsaturated fats (such as olive oil). A change from animal to vegetable proteins often corrects high cholesterol. However, it is inadvisable to go on a very low-fat diet. The main focus on cholesterol-lowering diets has been on saturated fat and cholesterol content, not soluble fiber. (When added to the diet, psyllium or oat bran is a safe, effective way of lowering cholesterol.) Exercise and weight reduction are also recommended. Conditions that aggravate high cholesterol, such as dependence on alcohol or tobacco, diabetes, high blood pressure, low magnesium or potassium, and thyroid disease, should be corrected before adding a cholesterol-reducing drug. If cholesterol remains high despite diet, add 10 grams of psyllium a day (see p. 566). Numerous studies have shown that psyllium, for example five grams twice a day, can significantly lower total cholesterol and LDL cholesterol.[25] Psyllium, a naturally occurring vegetable fiber, is clearly safer than any of the cholesterol-lowering drugs.

Cholesterol-Lowering[26] Drugs for People 70 and Older

It is clear that the relationship between moderately elevated cholesterol levels and increased risk of heart disease is not as clear as people get older.[26] As geriatricians Fran Kaiser and John Morely have written: *"Given the uncertainty of the effects of cholesterol manipulation in older individuals, what should be the approach of the prudent geriatrician to hypercholesterolemia [elevated blood cholesterol levels]? In persons over 70 years of age, life-long dietary habits are often difficult to change and overzealous dietary manipulation may lead to failure to eat and subsequent malnutrition. Thus in this group minor dietary manipulations such as the addition of some oatmeal [or other sources of oat bran or soluble fiber] and beans and modest increases in the amount of fish eaten, may represent a rational approach. Recommending a modest increase in exercise would also seem appropriate. Beyond this, it would seem best to remember that the geriatrician's dictum is to use no drug for which there is not a clear indication."*[27]

The use of cholesterol-lowering drugs in people 70 or older should be limited to patients with very high cholesterol levels (greater than 300 milligrams) and those who manifest cardiovascular disease (previous history of heart attack or angina).[28]

The only large clinical trial looking exclusively at the effect of statins on people over the age of 70 provides clear evidence for avoiding these drugs for use in primary prevention of cardiovascular disease in older people who have not had a previous heart attack, stroke, angina, or other cardiovascular diseases or family history. Five thousand eight hundred and four people aged 70 through 82 were randomized to get a statin or a placebo and were followed for an average of 3.2 years. For the more than 3,200 people in this study without prior cardiovascular disease, the statin had no beneficial effect in preventing subsequent cardiovascular disease. There was, however, a significant 25% increased amount of cancer in those getting the statin, particularly gastrointestinal cancers, the cancer predicted in the animal studies of these drugs (see below). The increase was larger the greater the number of years the drug was being used. No other study analyzing cancer exclusively in large numbers of older patients getting statins has refuted this finding of increased gastrointestinal cancer.[29]

In summary, people over 70 using statins for

primary prevention of cardiovascular disease have no benefit, compared to a placebo, but an increased risk of muscle damage (rhabdomyolysis), liver damage, and, as found in the study described above, an increased risk of cancer. It needs to be emphasized, however, that for those over 70 who have had previous cardiovascular disease, the use of statins may be beneficial.

There are even questions as to whether elderly people who are hypertensive should have their cholesterol lowered by drugs. One review concluded, *"Further trials are required before routinely suggesting that it is advantageous to lower cholesterol in an elderly hypertensive who does not have pre-existing evidence of coronary heart disease."* [30]

Cholesterol-Lowering Drugs and Cancer

Researchers from the University of California [31] have raised questions about the correlation between an increased risk of cancer and lifelong use of cholesterol-lowering drugs by millions of people who have no signs of illness other than an elevated blood cholesterol level. This research is based on animal studies and is sure to be controversial.

Animal studies consistently show a cancer-causing effect for the two most popular classes of cholesterol-lowering drugs, the fibrates or fibric acid derivatives, which include clofibrate (ATROMID-S) and gemfibrozil (LOPID), and the widely used statin drugs, fluvastatin (LESCOL), lovastatin (MEVACOR), pravastatin (PRAVACHOL), and simvastatin (ZOCOR). Evidence of a cancer-causing effect from these drugs based on clinical trials in humans is inconclusive because of inconsistent results and a follow-up period that, to date, is too short to detect some cancers that can take years to develop. The ultimate effect of cholesterol-lowering drugs in humans may not be known for decades.

As part of the Food and Drug Administration's requirements for getting a new drug approved, companies are required to report the result of cancer experiments on rodents (rats and mice). The most common technique is to give three groups of rodents different doses of a new drug for two years and then compare the incidence of cancer among these groups as well as with a fourth group that received a dummy drug called a placebo. Rats and mice are used because almost all known agents that cause cancer in humans have been found to cause it in these animals. The results of rodent studies are generally published in scientific journals, but are summarized in a product information sheet, or "package insert," distributed to the pharmacist with each prescription drug. You can get a package insert for any drug you are taking by asking your pharmacist for one.

Researchers have taken the rodent cancer data from the 1992 and 1994 editions of the *Physicians' Desk Reference (PDR,* a compilation of package inserts available in many public libraries). The package inserts for cholesterol-lowering drugs show that all the fibrates and statins cause cancer in rats and mice. In most instances, cancer-causing dose levels corresponded to maximums recommended for humans.

How should consumers weigh the worrisome but uncertain risk of cancer based on animal studies against the demonstrated benefits of lowering cholesterol? With some caution.

On the one hand, the study's authors clearly state that they do not know whether treatment with these cholesterol-lowering drugs will lead to an increased rate of cancer in coming decades. They believe that, for patients with known heart disease, the recent studies suggest that benefits of cholesterol-lowering drugs exceed their risks, at least in men and in the short term (five years). Given the strength of this evidence, it is reasonable to treat high blood cholesterol with drugs in patients with heart or other atherosclerotic disease. On the other hand, for patients not at high short-term risk of heart disease (especially patients with life expectancies of more than 10 to 20 years), drug treatment should probably be avoided. For this group, the benefits of treatment are smaller and the potential risk of increased cancer in the decades after treatment is of greater concern. The authors suggest that cholesterol-lowering drug treatment should be avoided except in patients at high short-term risk of coronary heart disease.

This question of whether the risks of cancer may outweigh the benefits has been answered, at least for older people, in a study published six years after the above-mentioned review of animal evidence of carcinogenicity was published. For those over 70 without previous cardiovascular disease, there was no benefit but there was an increased risk of cancer, especially gastrointestinal cancer as discussed in the section on cholesterol-lowering drugs for people 70 or older (p. 55).

When Is Drug Treatment Necessary?

Several factors should be taken into account when considering whether people with elevated cholesterol levels should be treated. One is the benefits of the treatment, which vary significantly depending on how abnormal the levels are. Other factors include your age and whether you have other risk factors such as high blood pressure, smoking, or diabetes, and whether you have had a heart attack, heart failure, a stroke, or have kidney damage. The other consideration is the risks or the adverse effects of the treatment, which will vary depending on what is being considered.

Although there is clear evidence that certain of the statin drugs (see p. 109) not only lower total cholesterol and LDL cholesterol (the "bad" cholesterol) but also decrease the risk of heart attacks and strokes, this evidence is strongest for people who are at much higher risk of these diseases because they have already had a heart attack, angina, bypass surgery or angioplasty,

or a stroke. The treatment of such people to reduce the chance of further cardiovascular disease is known as **secondary prevention.**

The evidence for treatment, especially with cholesterol-lowering drugs, is much weaker for people who have not yet had the cardiovascular disease described above, known as **primary prevention.** This is especially so for those people who do not have more than one of the following risk factors: hypertension, diabetes, smoking, obesity, or a close family history of premature heart attacks or strokes. Other predisposing risk factors include a sedentary lifestyle and a high-fat diet. It is likely that millions of people being given cholesterol-lowering drugs such as statins for **primary prevention** do not have more than one of these risk factors and are only being treated because of their total cholesterol or LDH cholesterol levels.

The following examples are applicable to people who do not have cardiovascular diseases such as heart attack, angina, heart failure, or stroke and who are between the ages of 30 and 74. The results are from an on-line cardiovascular risk calculator that can be found at www.widebay dgp.org.au/Resources/5yrRiskCalc.xls.[158]

Example A: Ben is a 55-year-old man with a total cholesterol of 240 and an HDL of 50. However, his blood pressure is a normal 120/90 and he is neither a diabetic nor does he smoke. Ben turns out to have a 5-year risk of having a cardiovascular event (heart attack, stroke, etc.) of only 5.1%, about one-half of the 5-year risk of over 10% that might merit drug treatment.[155] It would be a good idea for Ben—or most people, for that matter—to adopt the nondrug approaches to lowering his cholesterol discussed above, but since his **global risk** is as low as it is, drug treatment is not indicated even if his total cholesterol and HDL cholesterol stay the same.

Example B: Sally is a 65-year-old woman who, like Ben above, has a total cholesterol of 240, an

HDL of 50, a normal blood pressure of 120/90 and is neither a diabetic nor smokes. She turns out to have a 5-year risk of having a cardiovascular event (heart attack, stroke, etc.) of only 5.0%, similar to Ben's even though she is 10 years older, and she also has one-half of the 5-year risk of over 10% that might merit drug treatment.[155]

There is little doubt that many Sallys and Bens are being treated with drugs to lower their cholesterol even though their global risk of having a heart attack or stroke over the next five years is as low as it is. This is because most doctors focus on just one risk factor—in this case cholesterol—instead of examining the total picture including blood pressure and other factors.

Example C: David is a 55-year-old man who, like Ben above, has a total cholesterol of 240, but a lower HDL of 30, a slightly higher blood pressure of 130/90, and does not smoke but is a diabetic. David turns out to have a 5-year risk of having a cardiovascular event (heart attack, stroke, etc.) of 16.1%, more than three times higher than that of either Ben or Sally and well above the 5-year risk of over 10% that might merit drug treatment.[155] If this has not already been done in the context of treating his diabetes, David should start a program of exercise and diet to see if his total cholesterol can be lowered (and HDL—the "good cholesterol"—increased), and then, if total cholesterol still remains elevated, a drug to lower cholesterol, such as niacin-containing drugs or statins (see p. 109) should be tried. It is likely that an exercise and diet program would also lower his mildly elevated blood pressure.

POTASSIUM SUPPLEMENTATION

Who Needs Nondietary Potassium Supplementation?

Very few people actually need to take a potassium supplement or a potassium-sparing diuretic (amiloride, spironolactone, triamterene). If, however, you take digoxin, have severe liver disease, or take large doses of diuretics (water pills) for heart disease, eating a potassium-rich diet may not be sufficient to replace the potassium that you are losing. If you fall into one of these categories, it is very important for your doctor to precisely monitor and regulate the amount of potassium in your bloodstream. A potassium supplement or a potassium-sparing diuretic may be necessary. Read about the methods of increasing the potassium in your body discussed below and consult with your doctor about which will be best for you.

Who Does Not Need It?

Most people taking a thiazide diuretic (hydrochlorothiazide or metolazone, for example) for high blood pressure (hypertension) do not need potassium-sparing diuretics[32] or potassium supplements. This is especially true if treatment is started at a low dose (12.5 milligrams of hydrochlorothiazide for treatment of mild hypertension). Supplementing the diet with potassium-rich foods or beverages (see tables below) is sufficient to prevent low levels of potassium.[33]

Mild potassium deficiency (between 3.0 and 3.5 millimoles of potassium per liter of blood) can occur during diuretic therapy, but it usually has no symptoms and requires no treatment other than eating foods that are rich in potassium. Most people do not get severe potassium deficiency (less than 3.0 millimoles per liter) from treatment with diuretics. Comparisons of

POTASSIUM LEVELS IN MILLIEQUIVALENTS (MEQ) OF SELECTED FOODS AND POTASSIUM SUPPLEMENTS

Potassium Source	Amount	(mEq)
Peaches, dried, uncooked	1 cup	39
Raisins, dried, uncooked	1 cup	31
Dates, dried, cut	1 cup, pitted	29
Apricots, dried, uncooked	17 large halves	25
Figs, dried	7 medium	23
Prune juice, canned	1 cup	15
Watermelon	1 slice (1½ inches)	15
Banana	1 medium	14
Beef round	4 ounces	14
Cantaloupe	½ (5 inches in diameter)	13
Orange juice, fresh	1 cup	13
Turkey, roasted	3½ ounces	13
Klotrix Tabs	1 tablet	10
Kaon Cl-10	1 tablet	10
Milk, whole, 3.5% fat	1 cup	9
Slow-K	1 tablet	8
Kaon-Cl	1 tablet	6.7

FOODS HIGH IN POTASSIUM

All-bran cereals	Lentils
Almonds	Liver, beef
Apricots (dried)	Milk
Avocado	Molasses
Bananas	Peaches
Beans	Peanut butter
Beef	Peas
Broccoli	Pork
Brussels sprouts	Potatoes
Cantaloupe	Prunes (dried)
Carrots (raw)	Raisins
Chicken	Shellfish
Citrus fruits	Spinach
Coconut	Tomato juice
Crackers (rye)	Turkey
Dates and figs (dried)	Veal
Fish, fresh	Watermelon
Ham	Yams

people eating a potassium-rich diet, people taking potassium supplements, and people taking potassium-sparing drugs have shown that (1) diet is the safest method of replacing potassium and (2) potassium supplements and potassium-sparing drugs return potassium levels to normal in only 50% of the users. Therefore, if you have mild potassium deficiency, eat a few bananas before risking the adverse effects of potassium supplements or potassium-sparing drugs. Ask your doctor what your potassium levels were before and after you started diuretic treatment. You probably do not need a non-dietary potassium supplement or potassium-sparing drug.

Three Ways to Increase Your Potassium Levels

The safest and least expensive way is to increase the amount of potassium-rich food in your daily diet. This will provide sufficient potassium replacement for the overwhelming majority of people taking diuretics (people who also take digoxin or who have liver disease may be exceptions).

Restricting sodium (salt) intake also helps to maintain potassium levels while lowering sodium levels. In fact, salt substitutes containing potassium chloride may be an additional source of potassium intake.[33] If you are already taking potassium supplements or potassium-sparing diuretics, consult your doctor before using salt substitutes. A dosage adjustment may be necessary to prevent too much potassium in the body, a potentially fatal condition.

Potassium supplements are a second method for replacing potassium, but these can cause serious adverse reactions. Potassium is an irritant to the mucous membranes that line the mouth, throat, stomach, and intestines. If not properly dissolved and dispersed in the digestive tract, potassium can come in contact with these membranes and cause bleeding, ulcers, and perforations. Use of potassium supplements, because of serious potential adverse effects, should be restricted to people who are eating plenty of potassium-rich foods, yet still have a low level of potassium in their blood (less than 3.0 millimoles per liter).[34]

There are several kinds of potassium supplements:

- **Liquids:** Liquid supplements are safer than tablets[32] because, when taken in a diluted form over a five- to ten-minute period, potassium is effectively dispersed in the digestive tract, and thus causes less stomach and intestinal irritation and ulceration. Packaged as a liquid, powder, or dissolvable tablet, all forms must be completely dissolved in at least one-half cup of cold water or juice before drinking, and then sipped slowly over five to ten minutes.

- **Extended-release tablets or capsules:** Although liquid supplements are safest, tablets and capsules are widely used to avoid the unpleasant taste of the liquids.[32] Rarely, but often unpredictably, these tablets and capsules can cause stomach and intestinal ulcers, bleeding, blockage, and perforation when the potassium in the tablets and capsules does not dissolve and comes in contact with the lining of the digestive tract. Abdominal pain, diarrhea, nausea, vomiting, and heartburn have also been reported. Because the amount of time required for food to be digested and travel through the digestive tract increases with age, older people are more likely to experience adverse effects with these tablets or capsules.[32] Increased transit time leaves more opportunity for an undissolved or partially dissolved tablet or capsule to damage mucous lining.

- **Enteric-coated tablets:** Avoid these. "Enteric-coated" potassium tablets are not reliably absorbed and have frequently been blamed for intestinal ulceration.[35]

The last method for increasing potassium levels is with a class of drugs called potassium-sparing diuretics. Examples of these drugs are spironolactone (ALDACTONE), triamterene (DYRENIUM), and amiloride (MIDAMOR). Potassium-sparing diuretics are also found in combination products such as Moduretic and Aldactazide. These should not be used for older adults. These drugs can cause potentially fatal adverse effects such as kidney failure and the retention of too much potassium, which causes irregular heartbeats and heart rhythm. Studies have shown that the potassium supplements discussed above are equally effective and less dangerous than potassium-sparing diuretics, if nondietary potassium replacement is required.

If you are taking a potassium-sparing diuretic, you should never also use a potassium supplement or salt substitute containing potassium.[32] You also should not use an ACE inhibitor such as captopril (see p. 91) with potassium supplements because of the risk of high levels of potassium. Too-high levels of potassium, a potentially fatal condition that may not produce warning symptoms, may develop rapidly.

DRUG PROFILES

High Blood Pressure

Thiazide Diuretics

Chlorthalidone (klor *thal* i done)
HYGROTON (Aventis)

Hydrochlorothiazide
(hye dro klor oh *thye* a zide)
ESIDRIX (Novartis)
HYDRODIURIL (Merck)
MICROZIDE (Watson)

Limited Use

Chlorothiazide (klor oh *thye* a zide)
DIURIL (Merck)

Methyclothiazide (meth ee kloe *thye* a zide)
ENDURON (Abbott)

Metolazone (me *tole* a zone)
DIULO (Searle)
ZAROXOLYN (CellTech)

Polythiazide (pol e *thye* a zide)
RENESE (Pfizer)

GENERIC: available
FAMILY: Thiazide Diuretics (see p. 51)

PREGNANCY WARNING

Thiazides cross the placenta and expose the fetus to the drug. Hazards include fetal or newborn liver damage and bleeding as well as other adverse reactions that have occurred in adults. Because of the potential for serious adverse effects to the fetus, these drugs should not be used by pregnant women for hypertension or the normal edema of pregnancy.

BREAST-FEEDING WARNING

Thiazides are excreted in human milk. Because of the potential for serious adverse effects in nursing infants, you should not take these drugs while nursing.

Diuretics, commonly called "water pills," are used to treat high blood pressure (hypertension), congestive heart failure, and other conditions in which the body holds too much fluid. The routine use of diuretics in otherwise healthy pregnant women is inappropriate and exposes the mother and fetus to unnecessary hazard.[36]

All diuretics have potential adverse effects, commonly including loss of potassium and sodium from the body, harmful interactions with other drugs, and allergic reactions. Diuretics in this family (thiazide diuretics) are mild, which reduces the risk of dizziness, falling, and other adverse effects that you may suffer if your

---

HEAT STRESS ALERT

These drugs can affect your body's ability to adjust to heat, putting you at risk of "heat stress." If you live alone, ask a friend to check on you several times during the day. Early signs of heat stress are dizziness, lightheadedness, faintness, and slightly high temperature. Call your doctor if you have any of these signs. Drink more fluids (water, fruit and vegetable juices) than usual—even if you're not thirsty—unless your doctor has told you otherwise. Do not drink alcohol.

---

body loses too much fluid. It has recently been stated by an expert on hypertension in older adults that "thiazide diuretics [as the ones discussed on this page] are almost certainly safer than any of the other drugs available to treat hypertension."[37]

If you have high blood pressure, the best way to reduce or eliminate your need for medication is by improving your diet, losing weight, exercising, and decreasing your salt and alcohol intake. Mild hypertension can be controlled by proper nutrition and exercise. If these measures do not lower your blood pressure enough and you need medication, **hydrochlorothiazide, a water pill (see thiazide diuretics, p. 60), is the drug of choice, starting with a low dose of 12.5 milligrams daily.** It also costs less than other blood pressure drugs.

There is growing evidence that thiazide diuretics, such as hydrochlorothiazide, significantly decrease the rate of bone mineral loss in both men and women because they reduce the amount of calcium lost in the urine.[38] Research now suggests that thiazide diuretics may protect against hip fracture.[39]

Hydrochlorothiazide has been studied more than the other diuretics in this family, is available in a generic form, usually costs less, and is just as effective as the other thiazide diuretics. If you are taking a thiazide diuretic other than hydrochlorothiazide, compare cost and then ask your doctor about switching.

If you are taking hydrochlorothiazide, you should not—in most cases—be taking more than 50 milligrams per day. Daily doses higher than 50 milligrams do not significantly improve blood pressure control and can make adverse effects worse.[40]

If your hypertension is severe, rather than mild, and has not responded to a drug in this family, you may need a stronger drug. See p. 49 for a discussion of the alternatives.

Whatever drugs you take for high blood pressure, once your blood pressure has been normal for a year or more, a cautious decrease in dose and renewed attention to nondrug treatment may be worth trying, according to *The Medical Letter.*[17]

And an editorial in the *British Medical Journal* stated: *"Treatment of hypertension is part of preventive medicine and like all preventive strategies, its progress should be regularly reviewed by whoever initiates it. Many problems could be avoided by not starting antihypertensive treatment until after prolonged observation. . . . Patients should no longer be told that treatment is necessarily for life: the possibility of reducing or stopping treatment should be mentioned at the outset."*[16]

Before You Use This Drug

Do not use if you have or have had:

- a sensitivity to sulfa drugs (sulfonamides) or thiazide drugs

Tell your doctor if you have or have had:

- allergies to drugs
- diabetes
- gout
- kidney, liver, or pancreas problems
- lupus erythematosus
- a salt- or sugar-restricted diet
- pregnancy or are breast-feeding

- high calcium in your blood
- high cholesterol or triglycerides

Tell your doctor about any other drugs you take, including aspirin, herbs, vitamins, and other nonprescription products.

When You Use This Drug

- **Because these drugs help you lose water, you may become dehydrated. Check with your doctor to make certain your fluid intake is adequate and appropriate especially if you have vomiting or diarrhea.**
- Stay out of the sun as much as possible, and call your doctor if you get a rash, hives, or skin reaction. These drugs can make you more sensitive to the sun.
- **These drugs may cause your body to lose potassium, an important mineral.** Potassium loss is worse when there is too much salt in your diet. See p. 58 for information on how to make sure you get enough potassium.
- You may feel dizzy when rising from a lying or sitting position. When getting out of bed, hang your legs over the side of the bed for a few minutes, then get up slowly. When getting up from a chair, stay beside the chair until you are sure that you are not dizzy. (See p. 13.)
- If you plan to have any surgery, including dental, tell your doctor that you take a thiazide diuretic.
- **Do not take any other drugs without first talking to your doctor—especially nonprescription drugs for appetite control, asthma, colds, coughs, hay fever, or sinus problems.**

How to Use This Drug

- If you miss a dose, take it as soon as you remember, but skip it if it is almost time for the next dose. **Do not take double doses.**
- Do not share your medicine with others.

- Take the drug(s) at the same time each day.
- Take with food or milk to avoid stomach irritation. Tablet may be crushed and mixed with food or drink.
- If you are taking a thiazide diuretic more than once a day, try to take the last dose before 6 P.M. This will help you avoid interrupting your sleep to go to the bathroom.
- Store at room temperature with lid on tightly. Do not store in the bathroom. Do not expose to heat, moisture, or strong light. Keep out of reach of children.

Interactions with Other Drugs

The following drugs, biologics (e.g., vaccines, therapeutic antibodies), or foods are listed in *Evaluations of Drug Interactions* 2003 as causing "highly clinically significant" or "clinically significant" interactions when used together with any of the drugs in this section. In some sections with multiple drugs, the interaction may have been reported for one but not all drugs in this section, but we include the interaction because the drugs in this section are similar to one another. We have also included potentially serious interactions listed in the drug's FDA-approved professional package insert or in published medical journal articles. There may be other drugs, especially those in the families of drugs listed below, that also will react with this drug to cause severe adverse effects. Make sure to tell your doctor and pharmacist the drugs you are taking and tell them if you are taking any of these interacting drugs:

Other blood pressure lowering drugs.

Nonsteroidal anti-inflammatory drugs such as celecoxib (CELEBREX) and ibuprofen (MOTRIN) (see p. 288).

ACTH, acarbose, ACTOS, ALFENTA, alfentanil, anisindione, ANSAID, aprobarbital, aspirin, AVANDAMET, AVANDIA, betamethasone, BEXTRA, bumetanide,

BUMEX, BUPRENEX, buprenorphine, butabarbital, butalbital, BUTISOL SODIUM, CARDIOQUIN, CELESTONE, chlorpropamide, cholestyramine, choline magnesium trisalicylate, CLINORIL, codeine, COUMADIN, DARVON, DAYPRO, DEMADEX, DEMEROL, deslanoside, dezocine, DIABETA, DIABINESE, diclofenac, dicumarol, diflunisal, digoxin, DILAUDID, dofetilide, DOLOBID, DOLOPHINE HCL, DURAGESIC, ESKALITH, etodolac, FELDENE, fenoprofen, fentanyl, FIORICET, flurbiprofen, furosemide, glimepiride, glipizide, GLUCOPHAGE, GLUCOTROL XL, glyburide, GLYSET, guanethidine, HYDRO-CET, hydrocodone, hydromorphone, IN-DOCIN, indomethacin, insulin, ISMELIN, ketoprofen, ketorolac, LANOXICAPS, LANOXIN, LASIX, LEVO-DROMORAN, levorphanol, lithium, LODINE, magnesium salicylate, meclofenamate, mefenamic acid, meloxicam, mephobarbital, mepiridine, METAGLIP, metformin, methadone, methenamine, miglitol, MIRADON, MOBIC, morphine, nabumetone, NAPROSYN, naproxen, NEMBUTAL SODIUM, NITRO-DUR, nitroglycerin, norepinephrine, ORU-VAIL, oxaprozin, oxycodone, OXYCONTIN, pentobarbital, phenobarbital, pioglitazone, piroxicam, PONSTEL, PRANDIN, PRE-COSE, propoxyphene, QUESTRAN, QUINIDEX, quinidine, QUINAGLUTE, RELAFEN, remifentanil, repaglinide, rofecoxib, rosiglitazone, salsalate, secobarbital, SECONAL SODIUM, sufentanil, sulindac, TIKOSYN, tolazamide, tobutamide,

> The drugs listed above have reported interactions with hydrochlorothiazide. Not all of these interactions may have been reported for the other thiazide diuretics listed in this section. Always ask your doctor and pharmacist about specific interactions for the thiazide diuretic you are taking.

TOLECTIN, TOLINASE, tolmetin, TORADOL, torsemide, ULTIVA, UREX, valdecoxib, VIOXX, warfarin.

Adverse Effects

Call your doctor immediately if you experience:

- coughing, wheezing, or hoarseness
- difficulty breathing
- dry mouth or increased thirst that does not go away quickly after you take a drink
- fever, chills
- irregular heartbeat, chest pain
- mood or mental changes
- confusion, convulsions, or irritability
- muscle cramps, pain
- nausea, vomiting
- unusual tiredness or weakness
- weak pulse
- black, tarry stools
- blood in urine or stools
- joint, lower back, or side pain
- painful or difficult urination
- skin rash or hives
- yellow eyes or skin
- unusual bleeding or bruising

Call your doctor if these symptoms continue:

- dizziness, lightheadedness
- diarrhea
- loss of appetite, upset stomach
- headache
- blurred vision or "halo" effect
- premature ejaculation or difficulty with erection
- increased sensitivity of skin to sunlight

Periodic Tests

Ask your doctor which of these tests should be done periodically while you are taking this drug:

- blood pressure
- complete blood count
- blood levels of sodium, potassium, chloride, calcium, sugar, and uric acid
- liver function tests
- kidney function tests
- cholesterol or triglyceride tests

Thiazide-Like Diuretics

 Do Not Use

ALTERNATIVE TREATMENT:
See Hydrochlorothiazide, p. 60.

Indapamide (in *dap* a mide)
LOZOL (Aventis)

FAMILY: Thiazide-Like Diuretics (see p. 51)

Indapamide was approved in the United States in July 1983 for the treatment of high blood pressure alone or in combination with other blood-pressure-lowering drugs. The drug was listed as a limited use drug in the 1999 edition of *Worst Pills, Best Pills*. We changed this classification as a result of adverse drug reaction reports from Australia.

The August 2002 issue of the *Australian Adverse Drug Reactions Bulletin* reviewed reports of low blood levels of sodium (hyponatremia) induced by indapamide.

Indapamide was first marketed in Australia in the mid-1980s and is the drug most commonly implicated in causing hyponatremia, with 164 cases being reported to the Australian authorities. Of these 164 reports, 68 also described low blood levels of potassium (hypokalemia). Over half (92) of the reports described symptoms including confusion, nausea, vomiting, dizziness, loss of appetite, malaise, fatigue, fainting, somnolence, and convulsions. Most patients, 88%, were 65 years or over and 82% were female.

The main symptoms of hyponatremia involve the central nervous system and include lethargy, confusion, stupor, or coma.

Our search of the FDA adverse drug reaction database through the first quarter of 2002 found 222 reports of hyponatremia associated with the use of indapamide. The FDA conservatively estimates that for each adverse reaction reported, 10 go unreported.

The Australian authorities recommend that indapamide should be used cautiously and changes in conscious or mental state should prompt measurement of the blood sodium concentration. Our advice is that indapamide should not be used.

We can think of no reason why a patient should be placed at risk of developing hyponatremia when more effective, safer water pills that are less likely to cause hyponatremia are available to treat high blood pressure such as hydrochlorothiazide (HYDRODIURIL).

If you have high blood pressure, the best way to reduce or eliminate your need for medication is by improving your diet, losing weight, exercising, and decreasing your salt and alcohol intake (see p. 47). If these measures do not lower your blood pressure enough and you need medication, **hydrochlorothiazide, a water pill (see thiazide diuretics, p. 60), is the drug of choice, starting with a low dose of 12.5 milligrams daily.** It also costs less than other blood pressure drugs.

There is growing evidence that thiazide diuretics, such as hydrochlorothiazide, significantly decrease the rate of bone mineral loss in both men and women because they reduce the amount of calcium lost in the urine.[38] Research now suggests that thiazide diuretics may protect against hip fracture.[39]

If your high blood pressure is more severe, and hydrochlorothiazide alone does not control it, the best treatment is a combination of hydrochlorothiazide and a second type of drug called a beta-blocker, such as propranolol (see p. 87). If you can't take a drug in the beta-blocker family,

another family of high-blood-pressure-lowering drugs may be added to your treatment. In either case, your doctor would prescribe the hydrochlorothiazide and the second drug separately, with the dose of each drug adjusted to meet your needs, rather than using a product that combines the drug in a fixed combination.

Whatever drugs you take for high blood pressure, once your blood pressure has been normal for a year or more, a cautious decrease in dose and renewed attention to nondrug treatment may be worth trying, according to *The Medical Letter.*[17]

And an editorial in the *British Medical Journal* stated: *"Treatment of hypertension is part of preventive medicine and like all preventive strategies, its progress should be regularly reviewed by whoever initiates it. Many problems could be avoided by not starting antihypertensive treatment until after prolonged observation. . . . Patients should no longer be told that treatment is necessarily for life: the possibility of reducing or stopping treatment should be mentioned at the outset."*[16]

Loop Diuretics

Limited Use

Bumetanide (byoo *met* a nide)
BUMEX (Roche)

Furosemide (fur *oh* se mide)
LASIX (Aventis)

GENERIC: not available
FAMILY: Loop Diuretics (see p. 51)

PREGNANCY WARNING

These drugs caused fetal harm in animal studies, including growth retardation, delayed development of the bones in the spine, problems with kidney function, and death. Because of the potential for serious adverse effects to the fetus, these drugs should not be used by pregnant women.

These drugs are known to be excreted either in animal or human milk. Because of the potential for serious adverse effects in nursing infants, you should not take these drugs while nursing.

HEAT STRESS ALERT

These drugs can affect your body's ability to adjust to heat, putting you at risk of "heat stress." If you live alone, ask a friend to check on you several times during the day. Early signs of heat stress are dizziness, lightheadedness, faintness, and slightly high temperature. Call your doctor if you have any of these signs. Drink more fluids (water, fruit and vegetable juices) than usual—even if you're not thirsty—unless your doctor has told you otherwise. Do not drink alcohol.

WARNING: THIAMINE DEFICIENCY WITH FUROSEMIDE

Studies have shown that significant amounts of thiamine (vitamin B₁) are lost in the urine of people using furosemide (LASIX) and that patients therefore become thiamine deficient. The researchers found that replenishing thiamine, by taking one 100 milligram pill of thiamine hydrochloride daily for seven weeks, significantly improved heart function in patients who were using furosemide.[42, 43]

It is likely that after replacing the significant thiamine losses with these larger doses, the daily maintenence dose will be less. For now, however, we recommend the use of 100 milligrams of thiamine hydrochloride a day for at least seven weeks in people who have used furosemide chronically. If there seems to be an improvement in your heart status, and your physician agrees, you should continue with a daily dose of about 50 milligrams of thiamine as long as you are taking furosemide.

Bumetanide and furosemide are very strong "water pills" (diuretics) with many adverse effects. They are used to treat fluid retention and high blood pressure. If you are over 60, you should use bumetanide only for reducing fluid retention, and then only if you have decreased kidney function[44] and have already tried a milder drug such as hydrochlorothiazide (see p. 60) or the more proven and less expensive furosemide without success.[45] People over 60 years old who have normal kidney function should rarely, if ever, use bumetanide or furosemide.[15]

The World Health Organization recommends that furosemide should not be used for the treatment of high blood pressure in older adults because it has been associated with the occurrence of stroke.[46] Older adults are more likely than others to develop blood clots, shock, dizziness, confusion, and insomnia, and to have an increased risk of falling while taking bumetanide or furosemide.[47]

If you have high blood pressure, the best way to reduce or eliminate your need for medication is by improving your diet, losing weight, exercising, and decreasing your salt and alcohol intake. Mild hypertension can be controlled by proper nutrition and exercise. If these measures do not lower your blood pressure enough and you need medication, **hydrochlorothiazide, a water pill (see thiazide diuretics, p. 60), is the drug of choice, starting with a low dose of 12.5 milligrams daily.** It also costs less than other blood pressure drugs.

There is growing evidence that thiazide diuretics, such as hydrochlorothiazide, significantly decrease the rate of bone mineral loss in both men and women because they reduce the amount of calcium lost in the urine.[38] Research now suggests that thiazide diuretics may protect against hip fracture.[39]

If your high blood pressure is more severe, and hydrochlorothiazide alone does not control it, the best treatment is a combination of hydrochlorothiazide and a second type of drug called a beta-blocker, such as propranolol (see p. 87). If you can't take a drug in the beta-blocker family, another family of high-blood-pressure-lowering drugs may be added to your treatment. In either case, your doctor would prescribe the hydrochlorothiazide and the second drug separately, with the dose of each drug adjusted to meet your needs, rather than using a product that combines the drug in a fixed combination.

Whatever drugs you take for high blood pressure, once your blood pressure has been normal for a year or more, a cautious decrease in dose and renewed attention to nondrug treatment may be worth trying, according to *The Medical Letter.*[17]

And an editorial in the *British Medical Journal* stated: *"Treatment of hypertension is part of preventive medicine and like all preventive strategies, its progress should be regularly reviewed by whoever initiates it. Many problems could be avoided by not starting antihypertensive treatment until after prolonged observation. . . . Patients should no longer be told that treatment is necessarily for life: the possibility of reducing or stopping treatment should be mentioned at the outset."*[16]

Before You Use This Drug

Do not use if you have or have had:

- a sensitivity to sulfa drugs (sulfonamides) or yellow dye #5

Tell your doctor if you have or have had:

- allergies to drugs
- diabetes
- kidney, liver, or pancreas problems
- gout
- hearing loss
- recent heart attack
- history of irregular heartbeats
- lupus erythematosus
- salt- or sugar-restricted diet
- pregnancy or are breast-feeding

- have diarrhea
- low urine output

Tell your doctor about any other drugs you take, including aspirin, herbs, vitamins, and other nonprescription products.

When You Use This Drug

- **Check with your doctor to make certain your fluid intake is adequate and appropriate. Because bumetanide is a very strong water pill, you are in danger of becoming dehydrated.**
- You may feel dizzy when rising from a lying or sitting position. When getting up from bed, hang your legs over the side of the bed for a few minutes, then get up slowly. When getting up from a chair, stay beside the chair until you are sure that you are not dizzy. (See p. 13.)
- **Bumetanide and furosemide will cause your body to lose potassium, an important mineral.** See p. 58 for information on how to make sure you get enough potassium.
- Bumetanide can cause a loss of hearing, which is usually temporary but may be permanent. The risk of hearing loss is greater if you are also using amphotericin B or an antibiotic from the aminoglycoside family (see p. 617 for two examples).
- If you plan to have any surgery, including dental, tell your doctor that you take this drug.
- **Do not take other drugs without first talking to your doctor—especially nonprescription drugs for appetite control, asthma, colds, coughs, hay fever, or sinus problems.**

How to Use This Drug

- If you miss a dose, take it as soon as you remember, but skip it if it is almost time for the next dose. **Do not take double doses.**

- Do not share your medication with others.
- Take the drug at the same time(s) each day.
- Take with food or milk to avoid stomach irritation.
- Tablet may be crushed and mixed with food or drink.
- If you are taking bumetanide more than once a day, try to take the last dose before 6 P.M. This will help you avoid interrupting your sleep to go to the bathroom.
- Store at room temperature with lid on tightly. Do not store in the bathroom. Do not expose to heat, moisture, or strong light. Keep out of reach of children.

Interactions with Other Drugs

The following drugs, biologics (e.g., vaccines, therapeutic antibodies), or foods are listed in *Evaluations of Drug Interactions* 2003 as causing "highly clinically significant" or "clinically significant" interactions when used together with any of the drugs in this section. In some sections with multiple drugs, the interaction may have been reported for one but not all drugs in this section, but we include the interaction because the drugs in this section are similar to one another. We have also included potentially serious interactions listed in the drug's FDA-approved professional package insert or in published medical journal articles. There may be other drugs, especially those in the families of drugs listed below, that also will react with this drug to cause severe adverse effects. Make sure to tell your doctor and pharmacist the drugs you are taking and tell them if you are taking any of these interacting drugs:

ACTH, acebutolol, ALFENTA, alfentanil, amlodipine, CAPOTEN, captopril, cephalexin, charcoal, chlorpropamide, cholestyramine, cisplatin, DIABINESE, digoxin, ELIXOPHYLLIN, ESKALITH, INDERAL, INDERAL LA, KEFLEX, LANOXICAPS, LANOXIN, lithium, LITHOBID, LITHONATE, LOCHOLEST, NEBCIN, NORVASC, PLATINOL, propranolol, QUESTRAN, SECTRAL, SLO-BID, THEO-24, theophylline.

Adverse Effects

Call your doctor immediately if you experience:

- signs of potassium loss: dry mouth, increased thirst, irregular heartbeat, mood or mental changes, muscle cramps or pain, nausea, vomiting, unusual tiredness or weakness, weak pulse
- skin rash or hives
- chest pain
- nipple tenderness
- black, tarry stools
- blood in urine or stools
- cough or hoarseness
- fever
- chills
- joint, lower back, or side pain
- painful or difficult urination
- pinpoint red spots on skin
- ringing or buzzing in ears or hearing loss
- dizziness or lightheadedness
- severe stomach pain with nausea or vomiting
- unusual bleeding or bruising
- yellow eyes or skin
- yellow vision

Call your doctor if these symptoms continue:

- dizziness, lightheadedness
- diarrhea
- loss of appetite
- upset stomach
- headache
- blurred vision

- premature ejaculation or difficulty with erection
- chest pain

Periodic Tests

Ask your doctor which of these tests should be done periodically while you are taking this drug:

- blood pressure
- complete blood count
- blood levels of sodium, potassium, chloride, calcium, sugar, and uric acid
- liver function tests
- kidney function tests
- weight measurement
- carbon dioxide measurement

Potassium-Sparing Diuretics

 Do Not Use

ALTERNATIVE TREATMENT:
See Hydrochlorothiazide, p. 60

Amiloride and Hydrochlorothiazide
(a *mill* oh ride and hye dro klor o *thye* azide)
MODURETIC (Merck)

FAMILY: Potassium-Sparing Diuretics
Thiazide Diuretics (see p. 51)

PREGNANCY WARNING

Amiloride crossed the placenta in animal studies. These studies were not done at high enough doses to know what the potential adverse effects on the fetus might be.

BREAST-FEEDING WARNING

Amiloride is excreted in the breast milk of animals. There were adverse effects in animal studies on growth and survival. No studies were done on humans but many drugs are excreted in human milk. Because of the potential for serious adverse effects in nursing infants, you should not take amiloride while nursing.

FDA BLACK BOX WARNING

Like other potassium-conserving diuretic combinations, MODURETIC may cause hyperkalemia (serum potassium levels greater than 5.5 mEq per liter). In patients without renal impairment or diabetes mellitus, the risk of hyperkalemia with MODURETIC is about 1–2 percent. This risk is higher in patients with renal [kidney] impairment or diabetes mellitus (even without recognized diabetic nephropathy). Since hyperkalemia, if uncorrected, is potentially fatal, it is essential to monitor serum potassium levels carefully in any patient receiving MODURETIC, particularly when it is first introduced, at the time of dosage adjustment, and during any illness that could affect renal function.[48]

This product, a combination of amiloride and hydrochlorothiazide (see p. 60), is used to treat high blood pressure (hypertension). Older adults should not use drugs that contain a fixed combination of amiloride and hydrochlorothiazide. Thiazides with amiloride may produce high potassium in the blood and substantial sodium depletion.[46]

There are good reasons not to use any fixed-combination drug for high blood pressure. A single drug is often enough to control high blood pressure. If a combination drug like this one is controlling your high blood pressure, it is quite possible that one drug alone would do the same job. There is no reason to put yourself at extra risk by taking drugs you do not need.

The FDA-approved professional product labeling for this drug carries the following warning in bold type:

This fixed combination drug is not indicated for the initial therapy of edema or hypertension except in individuals in

whom the development of hypokalemia cannot be risked.[48]

If you have high blood pressure, the best way to reduce or eliminate your need for medication is by improving your diet, losing weight, exercising, and decreasing your salt and alcohol intake. Mild hypertension can be controlled by proper nutrition and exercise. If these measures do not lower your blood pressure enough and you need medication, **hydrochlorothiazide, a water pill (see thiazide diuretics, p. 60), is the drug of choice, starting with a low dose of 12.5 milligrams daily.** It also costs less than other blood pressure drugs.

There is growing evidence that thiazide diuretics, such as hydrochlorothiazide, significantly decrease the rate of bone mineral loss in both men and women because they reduce the amount of calcium lost in the urine.[38] Research now suggests that thiazide diuretics may protect against hip fracture.[39]

If your high blood pressure is more severe, and hydrochlorothiazide alone does not control it, the best treatment is a combination of hydrochlorothiazide and a second type of drug called a beta-blocker, such as propranolol (see p. 87). If you can't take a drug in the beta-blocker family, another family of high-blood-pressure-lowering drugs may be added to your treatment. In either case, your doctor would prescribe the hydrochlorothiazide and the second drug separately, with the dose of each drug adjusted to meet your needs, rather than using a product that combines the drug in a fixed combination.

Whatever drugs you take for high blood pressure, once your blood pressure has been normal for a year or more, a cautious decrease in dose and renewed attention to nondrug treatment may be worth trying, according to *The Medical Letter.*[17]

And an editorial in the *British Medical Journal* stated: *"Treatment of hypertension is part of preventive medicine and like all preventive strategies, its progress should be regularly reviewed by whoever initiates it. Many problems could be avoided by not starting antihypertensive treatment until after prolonged observation. . . . Patients should no longer be told that treatment is necessarily for life: the possibility of reducing or stopping treatment should be mentioned at the outset."*[16]

Do Not Use Until Seven Years After Release

Eplerenone (e *plare* e none)
(Do Not Use Until 2011)
INSPRA (Searle)

GENERIC: not available

FAMILY: Potassium-Sparing Diuretics (see p. 51)

PREGNANCY WARNING

Eplerenone increased fetal resorptions in animal studies. Tell your doctor if you are pregnant or thinking of becoming pregnant before you use this drug.

BREAST-FEEDING WARNING

Eplerenone was excreted in animal milk. It is likely that this drug is also excreted in human milk. Because of the potential for serious adverse effects in nursing infants, you should not take this drug while nursing.

Eplerenone was initially approved by the FDA in September 2002 to treat high blood pressure, but the drug's manufacturer chose not to put the product on the market at that time. Rather, the company opted to wait to market eplerenone until it had also gained approval for improving the survival of stable patients with a damaged left ventricle (large chamber of the heart) and evidence of congestive heart failure after a heart attack. This approval was granted in October 2003.

This additional approved use for the drug allows it to be legally advertised as more than just another high-blood-pressure-lowering drug. This is important because the marketplace for

THE HEALTH RESEARCH GROUP'S SEVEN-YEAR RULE

You should wait at least seven years from the date of release to take any new drug unless it is one of those rare "breakthrough" drugs that offers you a documented therapeutic advantage over older proven drugs. New drugs are tested in a relatively small number of people before being released, and serious adverse effects or life-threatening drug interactions may not be detected until the new drug has been taken by hundreds of thousands of people. A number of new drugs have been withdrawn within their first seven years after release. Also, warnings about serious new adverse reactions have been added to the labeling of a number of drugs, or new drug interactions have been detected, usually within the first seven years after a drug's release.

high-blood-pressure-lowering drugs is crowded, with dozens of competing agents, and eplerenone is not very distinguished as a high-blood-pressure-lowering drug.

Eplerenone belongs to the family of water pills, or diuretics, known as potassium-sparing diuretics and is most similar to the older drug spironolactone (ALDACTONE, see p. 74). One of the major concerns of potassium-sparing diuretics such as spironolactone and eplerenone is that they can lead to dangerously high levels of potassium (hyperkalemia) that can potentially cause death in the elderly and in persons with poor kidney function.

This statement appears in the professional product labeling, or package insert, for eplerenone: "The principal risk of INSPRA is hyperkalemia. Hyperkalemia can cause serious, sometimes fatal, arrhythmias (heart rhythm disturbances)."[49]

As mentioned above, eplerenone is not much of a high-blood-pressure-lowering drug. A senior FDA scientist wrote in a September 27, 2002, memo, about the drug's effectiveness and the risk of increasing potassium blood levels: *"We have no reason to think eplerenone is anything but a garden-variety antihypertensive [blood-pressure-lowering drug] of ordinary effectiveness; i.e., there is no reason to accept increased risk [elevated potassium levels] compared to alternative agents."*[50]

The FDA reviewed a number of clinical trials in which eplerenone was compared directly to other high-blood-pressure-lowering drugs. Eplerenone was found comparable to spironolactone, the thiazide diuretic hydrochlorothiazide (HYDRODIURIL) (see p. 60), and the angiotensin converting enzyme (ACE) inhibitor enalapril (VASOTEC) (see p. 91). Nothing special was found with eplerenone.

The Medical Letter on Drugs and Therapeutics, a publication we frequently cite because of its reputation as an independent source of drug information, concluded its review of eplerenone by saying the drug is "modestly effective for treatment of hypertension."[51]

A large clinical trial found the addition of the drug to the best standard therapy improved the survival of patients who had a heart attack complicated by a damaged left ventricle and heart failure.[52]

This study found that death from all causes was lower in those taking eplerenone compared to patients receiving a placebo. In the placebo group, 16.7% of patients died. This was decreased to 14.4% in the eplerenone group. The absolute difference in risk of dying between the two groups was 2.3%. Knowing the absolute risk allows calculation of the number of patients that need to be treated with eplerenone to prevent one death. This number is 44 patients for a period of 16 months.

The downside of eplerenone, as alluded to above, is the risk of developing a serious elevation in blood potassium level, or hyperkalemia. In those taking eplerenone, 5.5% of the patients experienced a serious elevation in their potassium blood level. Whereas in those given the placebo, only 3.9% had a serious episode of hyperkalemia. This is an absolute difference of 1.6% in risk of developing hyperkalemia with eplerenone. With this percentage, the number of patients taking eplerenone that must be treated before there is one case of hyperkalemia that develops can be calculated. This is referred to as the number needed to harm and is 63 patients on eplerenone treated for over 16 months.

On its face it appears that the benefits of eplerenone outweigh the risk of hyperkalemia and not all cases of hyperkalemia result in death. Although the patients in this study were carefully watched by the researchers, this is not always the case in the everyday practice of medicine. In addition, patients were excluded from entering the study if they were taking a potassium-sparing diuretic or had decreased kidney function, both of which increase the risk of hyperkalemia. If, for example, once eplerenone is widely prescribed and the percentage of patients who develop hyperkalemia increases by a modest 1.0%, from 5.5% to 6.5%, the number needed to harm drops to 38 patients on eplerenone for 16 months.

Before You Use This Drug

Do not use if you have or have had:

- allergies
- diabetes
- kidney problems
- microalbuminuria (albumin protein in the urine)
- potassium that is high (hyperkalemia)
- pregnancy or are breast-feeding

Tell your doctor if you have or have had:

- liver disease
- allergy to eplerenone

Tell your doctor about any other drugs you take, including antifungals, diuretics, potassium, herbs, over-the-counter medications, and vitamins.

When You Use This Drug

- Do not take any potassium supplements or use salt substitutes containing potassium.
- Limit intake of sodium salts.
- Be aware that eplerenone may cause dizziness.
- Tell any doctor, dentist, emergency help, or pharmacist you see that you take this drug.

How to Use This Drug

- If you miss a dose, take it as soon as possible, unless it is almost time for the next dose. **Do not take double doses.**
- Do not share your medication with others.
- Take the drug at the same time(s) each day.
- Swallow tablet(s) with or without food.
- Do not break, chew, or crush this drug.
- Avoid taking with grapefruit juice.
- Store tablets at room temperature with lid on tightly. Do not store in the bathroom. Do not expose to heat, moisture, or strong light. Keep out of reach of children.

Interactions with Other Drugs

The following drugs, biologics (e.g., vaccines, therapeutic antibodies), or foods are listed in *Evaluations of Drug Interactions* 2003 as causing "highly clinically significant" or "clinically significant" interactions when used together with any of the drugs in this section. In some sections with multiple drugs, the interaction may have been reported for one but not all drugs in this section, but we include the interaction because the drugs in this section are similar to one another. We have also included potentially serious interactions listed in the drug's FDA-approved professional package insert or in published medical journal articles. There may be other drugs, especially those in the families of drugs listed below, that also will react with this drug to cause severe adverse effects. Make sure to tell your doctor and pharmacist the drugs you are taking and tell them if you are taking any of these interacting drugs:

ACCUPRIL, ACCURETIC, ACEON, ADVIL, ALDACTONE, ALEVE, ALTACE, amiloride, ANSAID, benazepril, BIAXIN, CALAN, CAPOTEN, CAPOZIDE, captopril, cilazapril, clarithromycin, CLINORIL, COZAAR, DAYPRO, diclofenac, DIFLUCAN, diflunisal, DIOVAN, DIOVAN HCT, DOLOBID, DYAZIDE, DYRENIUM, EES, EFFER-K, E-MYCIN, enalapril, ERYBID, ERYC, ERYPED, ERY-TAB, ERYTHROCIN, ERYTHROCOT, erythromycin, ESKALITH, etodolac, fenoprofen, floctafenine, fluconazole, flurbiprofen, fosinopril, GLU-K, grapefruit juice, hypercium, HYZAAR, ibuprofen, ILOSONE, ILOTYCIN, INDOCIN, indomethacin, INHIBASE, INVIRASE, ISOPTIN, itraconazole, K+CARE, KALETRA, KAON-CL, KAYLIXIR, K-DUR, K-ELECTROLYTE, ketoconazole, ketoprofen, KLEASE, KLOR-CON, KLORVESS, K-LYTE, K-NORM, KOLYUM, K-TABS, lisinopril, lithium, LITHOBID, LODINE, losartan, LOTENSIN, LOTENSIN HCT, MAVIK, MAXZIDE, meclofenamate, MECLOMEN, mefanamicacid, meloxicam, MICRO-K, MIDAMOR, MOBIC, MODURETIC, moexipril, MONOPRIL, MOTRIN, MY-E, nambutenone, NAPROSYN, naproxen, nefazodone, nelfinavir, NIZORAL, NORVIR, ORUDIS, oxaprozin, PCE, perindopril, piroxicam, PONSTEL, potassium salt substitutes that contain potassium, PRINIVIL, PRINZIDE, quinapril, ramipril, RELAFEN, ritonavir, saquinavir, SERZONE, spironolactone, SPORANOX, SPRIOZIDE, St. John's wort, sulindac, TAO, TEN-K, tenoxicam, tiaprofenic acid, TOLECTIN, tolmetin, trandolapril, triamterene, TRI-K, troleandomycin, TWIN-K, UNIRETIC, UNIVASC, valsartan, VASERETIC, VASOTEC, verapamil, VIRACEPT, VOLTAREN, WINTROCIN, ZESTORETIC, ZESTRIL.

Adverse Effects

Call your doctor immediately if you experience:

- cloudy urine
- high cholesterol or triglyceride levels in the blood
- chest pain or discomfort
- dizziness
- confusion
- nervousness
- weakness or heaviness of legs
- arm, back, or jaw pain
- chest tightness
- fast or irregular heartbeat
- shortness of breath
- sweating
- nausea or vomiting
- headache
- abdominal pain

Call your doctor if these symptoms continue:

- stomach pain
- breast enlargement in men
- breast swelling or pain in men or women
- cough
- chills
- diarrhea
- fever
- fatigue
- flulike symptoms
- headache
- menstrual changes or abnormal vaginal bleeding
- joint pain
- loss of appetite
- muscle aches and pains

Periodic Tests

Ask your doctor which of these tests should be done periodically while you are taking this drug:

- blood pressure
- blood test for potassium
- kidney function tests such as creatinine clearance

———

Limited Use

Spironolactone (speer on oh *lak* tone)
ALDACTONE (Searle)

GENERIC: available

FAMILY: Potassium-Sparing Diuretics (see p. 51)

PREGNANCY WARNING

Spironolactone caused fetal harm in animal studies. Because of the potential for serious adverse effects to the fetus, this drug should not be used by pregnant women.

BREAST-FEEDING WARNING

Spironolactone is excreted in human milk. Because of the potential for serious adverse effects in nursing infants including spironolactone's ability to produce tumors, you should not take this drug while nursing.

FDA BLACK BOX WARNING

Spironolactone has been shown to be a tumorigen in chronic toxicity studies in rats. Aldactone should be used only in those conditions described under Indications and Usage. Unnecessary use of this drug should be avoided.

Spironolactone is a water pill (diuretic) that removes less of the mineral potassium from your body than other types of diuretics do. Doctors sometimes prescribe it for high blood pressure,

HEAT STRESS ALERT

This drug can affect your body's ability to adjust to heat, putting you at risk of "heat stress." If you live alone, ask a friend to check on you several times during the day. Early signs of heat stress are dizziness, lightheadedness, faintness, and slightly high temperature. Call your doctor if you have any of these signs. Drink more fluids (water, fruit and vegetable juices) than usual—even if you're not thirsty—unless your doctor has told you otherwise. Do not drink alcohol.

instead of another diuretic, in the hope that it will prevent a potassium imbalance, but there is no guarantee that this will work.

Spironolactone can cause severe adverse effects. It is especially dangerous for people with kidney disease.[53,54] **It can cause kidney failure, retention of too much potassium,[53,55–57] muscle paralysis,[58] and mental confusion[53] in older adults.** These effects may be fatal.

Because of its dangers, spironolactone is not the best drug for treating high blood pressure or water retention. Older adults should not use spironolactone just for its ability to keep potassium in the body. If you need extra potassium, you can adjust your diet or take potassium supplements. Both methods are equally effective[59] (see p. 58) and are safer than using spironolactone. The only reason for an older adult to use this drug is to control a rare condition in which the body releases too much aldosterone (a hormone that regulates potassium and sodium levels).

If you have high blood pressure, the best way to reduce or eliminate your need for medication is by improving your diet, losing weight, exercising, and decreasing your salt and alcohol intake. Mild hypertension can be controlled by proper nutrition and exercise. If these measures do not lower your blood pressure enough and you need medication, **hydrochlorothiazide, a water pill (see thiazide diuretics, p. 60), is the drug of choice, starting with a low dose of 12.5 milligrams daily.** It also costs less than other blood pressure drugs.

There is growing evidence that thiazide diuretics, such as hydrochlorothiazide, significantly decrease the rate of bone mineral loss in both men and women because they reduce the amount of calcium lost in the urine.[38] Research now suggests that thiazide diuretics may protect against hip fracture.[39]

If your high blood pressure is more severe, and hydrochlorothiazide alone does not control it, the best treatment is a combination of hydrochlorothiazide and a second type of drug called a beta-blocker, such as propranolol (see p. 87). If you can't take a drug in the beta-blocker family, another family of high-blood-pressure-lowering drugs may be added to your treatment. In either case, your doctor would prescribe the hydrochlorothiazide and the second drug separately, with the dose of each drug adjusted to meet your needs, rather than using a product that combines the drug in a fixed combination.

Whatever drugs you take for high blood pressure, once your blood pressure has been normal for a year or more, a cautious decrease in dose and renewed attention to nondrug treatment may be worth trying, according to *The Medical Letter.*[17]

And an editorial in the *British Medical Journal* stated: *"Treatment of hypertension is part of preventive medicine and like all preventive strategies, its progress should be regularly reviewed by whoever initiates it. Many problems could be avoided by not starting antihypertensive treatment until after prolonged observation. . . . Patients should no longer be told that treatment is necessarily for life: the possibility of reducing or stopping treatment should be mentioned at the outset."*[16]

Before You Use This Drug

Tell your doctor if you have or have had:

- allergies to drugs
- diabetes
- heart, kidney, or liver problems
- menstrual problems
- breast enlargement
- pregnancy or are breast-feeding
- high potassium levels
- gout
- kidney stones

Tell your doctor about any other drugs you take, including aspirin, herbs, vitamins, and other nonprescription products.

When You Use This Drug

- Do not use potassium supplements, salt substitutes (potassium chloride), or potassium-rich foods.
- If you plan to have any surgery, including dental, tell your doctor that you take this drug.
- **Do not take any other drugs without first talking to your doctor—especially nonprescription drugs for appetite control, asthma, colds, coughs, hay fever, or sinus problems.**

How to Use This Drug

- If you miss a dose, take it as soon as you remember, but skip it if it is almost time for the next dose. **Do not take double doses.**
- Do not share your medication with others.
- Take it at the same time each day. If a single dose, take it in the morning after breakfast; if more than one dose, take the last no later than 6 P.M. unless your doctor states otherwise.
- Take with food or milk to avoid stomach irritation.
- Store at room temperature with lid on tightly. Do not store in the bathroom. Do not ex-

pose to heat, moisture, or strong light. Keep out of reach of children.

Interactions with Other Drugs

The following drugs, biologics (e.g., vaccines, therapeutic antibodies), or foods are listed in *Evaluations of Drug Interactions* 2003 as causing "highly clinically significant" or "clinically significant" interactions when used together with any of the drugs in this section. In some sections with multiple drugs, the interaction may have been reported for one but not all drugs in this section, but we include the interaction because the drugs in this section are similar to one another. We have also included potentially serious interactions listed in the drug's FDA-approved professional package insert or in published medical journal articles. There may be other drugs, especially those in the families of drugs listed below, that also will react with this drug to cause severe adverse effects. Make sure to tell your doctor and pharmacist the drugs you are taking and tell them if you are taking any of these interacting drugs:

ATACAND, AVAPRO, benazepril, BENICAR, candesartan, CAPOTEN, captopril, cholestyramine, COZAAR, cyclosporine, digoxin, DIOVAN, enalapril, eprosartan, ESKALITH, fosinopril, irbesartan, IS-MELIN, KATO, K-LOR, KLOTRIX, LANOXICAPS, LANOXIN, lisinopril, LITHANE, lithium, LOCHOLEST, losartan, LOTENSIN, MAVIK, MICARDIS, moexipril, MONOPRIL, olmesartan, potassium chloride, PRINIVIL, QUESTRAN, SANDIMMUNE, SLOW-K, telmisartan, TEVETEN, trandolapril, UNIVASC, valsartan, VASOTEC, ZESTRIL

Adverse Effects

Call your doctor immediately if you experience:

- signs of potassium imbalance: confusion; anxiety; irregular heartbeat; numbness or tingling in hands, feet, lips; difficulty breathing; unusual tiredness or weakness; heavy legs
- sore throat and fever
- skin rash or itching
- cough or hoarseness
- fever
- chills
- lower back or side pain
- painful or difficult urination
- severe or continuing nausea or vomiting
- diarrhea
- postmenopausal bleeding
- breast enlargement or tenderness

Call your doctor if these symptoms continue:

- drowsiness
- stomach cramps
- diarrhea
- inability to get or keep an erection
- unusual sweating
- voice deepening and breast tenderness
- increased hair growth in women
- enlarged breasts in men
- irregular menstrual periods
- dry mouth, increased thirst
- nausea, vomiting
- mental confusion
- stumbling, clumsiness
- dizziness
- headache
- decreased sexual ability

Periodic Tests

Ask your doctor which of these tests should be done periodically while you are taking this drug:

- blood pressure
- complete blood count
- kidney function tests

- blood levels of potassium and sodium (weekly when first starting to use the drug)
- electrocardiograms

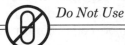 *Do Not Use*

ALTERNATIVE TREATMENT:
See Hydrochlorothiazide, p. 60.

Spironolactone and Hydrochlorothiazide
(speer on oh *lak* tone and hye dro klor oh *thye* a zide)
ALDACTAZIDE (Searle)

FAMILY: Potassium-Sparing Diuretics
Thiazide Diuretics (see p. 51)

FDA BLACK BOX WARNING

Spironolactone, an ingredient of Aldactazide, has been shown to be a tumorigen in chronic toxicity studies in rats. Aldactazide should be used only in those conditions described under Indications and Usage. Unnecessary use of this drug should be avoided.

Fixed-dose combination drugs are not indicated for initial therapy of edema or hypertension. Edema or hypertension requires therapy titrated to the individual patient. If the fixed combination represents the dosage so determined, its use may be more convenient in patient management. The treatment of hypertension and edema is not static but must be reevaluated as conditions in each patient warrant.

This product, a combination of spironolactone (see p. 74) and hydrochlorothiazide (see p. 60), is used to treat high blood pressure (hypertension). **Older adults should not use drugs that contain a fixed combination of spironolactone and hydrochlorothiazide.**

Spironolactone can cause severe adverse effects. It is especially dangerous for people with kidney disease.[53, 54] **It can cause kidney failure, retention of too much potassium,**[53, 55–57] **muscle paralysis,**[58] **and mental confusion in older adults.** These effects may be fatal.

In addition to spironolactone's dangers, there are good reasons not to use any fixed-combination drug for high blood pressure. A single drug is often enough to control high blood pressure. If a combination drug like this one is controlling your high blood pressure, it is quite possible that one drug alone would do the same job. There is no reason to put yourself at extra risk by taking drugs you do not need.

If you have high blood pressure, the best way to reduce or eliminate your need for medication is by improving your diet, losing weight, exercising, and decreasing your salt and alcohol intake. Mild hypertension can be controlled by proper nutrition and exercise. If these measures do not lower your blood pressure enough and you need medication, **hydrochlorothiazide, a water pill (see thiazide diuretics, p. 60), is the drug of choice, starting with a low dose of 12.5 milligrams daily.** It also costs less than other blood pressure drugs.

There is growing evidence that thiazide diuretics, such as hydrochlorothiazide, significantly decrease the rate of bone mineral loss in both men and women because they reduce the amount of calcium lost in the urine.[38] Research now suggests that thiazide diuretics may protect against hip fracture.[39]

If your high blood pressure is more severe, and hydrochlorothiazide alone does not control it, the best treatment is a combination of hydrochlorothiazide and a second type of drug called a beta-blocker, such as propranolol (see p. 87). If you can't take a drug in the beta-blocker family, another family of high-blood-pressure-lowering drugs may be added to your treatment. In either case, your doctor would prescribe the hydrochlorothiazide and the second drug separately, with the dose of each drug adjusted to meet your needs, rather than using a product that combines the drug in a fixed combination.

Whatever drugs you take for high blood pressure, once your blood pressure has been normal for a year or more, a cautious decrease in dose and renewed attention to nondrug treatment may be worth trying, according to *The Medical Letter.*[17]

And an editorial in the *British Medical Journal* stated: *"Treatment of hypertension is part of preventive medicine and like all preventive strategies, its progress should be regularly reviewed by whoever initiates it. Many problems could be avoided by not starting antihypertensive treatment until after prolonged observation. . . . Patients should no longer be told that treatment is necessarily for life: the possibility of reducing or stopping treatment should be mentioned at the outset."*[16]

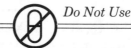

Do Not Use

ALTERNATIVE TREATMENT:
See Hydrochlorothiazide, p. 60.

Triamterene (trye *am* ter een)
DYRENIUM (Wellspring Pharm)

FAMILY: Potassium-Sparing Diuretics (see p. 51)

PREGNANCY WARNING

Triamterene crosses the placenta and exposes the fetus to the drug. Because of the potential for serious adverse effects to the fetus, this drug should not be used by pregnant women.

BREAST-FEEDING WARNING

Triamterene is excreted in animal milk and this may occur in humans. Because of the potential for serious adverse effects in nursing infants, you should not take triamterene while nursing.

Triamterene is a water pill (diuretic) that removes less potassium from your body than other types of diuretics do. Doctors sometimes prescribe it for high blood pressure, instead of another diuretic, in the hope that it will prevent a potassium imbalance. **It should not be used by older adults.** It can cause serious and sometimes fatal adverse effects such as kidney stones, kidney failure, retention of too much potassium in your body, and a drop in your body's production of blood cells (bone marrow depression).[44,35]

If you have high blood pressure, the best way to reduce or eliminate your need for medication is by improving your diet, losing weight, exercising, and decreasing your salt and alcohol intake. If these measures do not lower your blood pressure enough and you need medication, **hydrochlorothiazide, a water pill (see thiazide diuretics, p. 60), is the drug of choice, starting, with a low dose of 12.5 milligrams daily.** It also costs less than other blood pressure drugs.

There is growing evidence that thiazide diuretics, such as hydrochlorothiazide, significantly decrease the rate of bone mineral loss in both men and women because they reduce the amount of calcium lost in the urine.[38] Research now suggests that thiazide diuretics may protect against hip fracture.[39]

If your high blood pressure is more severe, and hydrochlorothiazide alone does not control it, the best treatment is a combination of hydrochlorothiazide and a second type of drug called a beta-blocker, such as propranolol (see p. 87). If you can't take a drug in the beta-blocker family, another family of high-blood-pressure-lowering drugs may be added to your treatment. In either case, your doctor would prescribe the hydrochlorothiazide and the second drug separately, with the dose of each drug adjusted to meet your needs, rather than using a product that combines the drug in a fixed combination.

If you are taking triamterene, ask your doctor about switching to hydrochlorothiazide (see p. 60). If you need to replace potassium in your body because of potassium losses from other drugs, certain potassium supplements are less dangerous than a drug such as triamterene and are equally effective[59] (see p. 58).

Whatever drugs you take for high blood pressure, once your blood pressure has been normal for a year or more, a cautious decrease in dose and renewed attention to nondrug treatment may be worth trying, according to *The Medical Letter*.[17]

And an editorial in the *British Medical Journal* stated: *"Treatment of hypertension is part of preventive medicine and like all preventive strategies, its progress should be regularly reviewed by whoever initiates it. Many problems could be avoided by not starting antihypertensive treatment until after prolonged observation. . . . Patients should no longer be told that treatment is necessarily for life: the possibility of reducing or stopping treatment should be mentioned at the outset."*[16]

───────

Limited Use

Triamterene and Hydrochlorothiazide
(trye *am* ter een and hye dro klor oh *thye* a zide)
DYAZIDE (GlaxoSmithKline)
MAXZIDE (Mylan)

GENERIC: available

FAMILY: Potassium-Sparing Diuretics
Thiazide Diuretics (see p. 51)

PREGNANCY WARNING
Triamterene crosses the placenta and exposes the fetus to the drug. Because of the potential for serious adverse effects to the fetus, this drug should not be used by pregnant women.

BREAST-FEEDING WARNING
Triamterene is excreted in animal milk and this may occur in humans. Because of the potential for serious adverse effects in nursing infants, you should not take triamterene while nursing.

FDA BLACK BOX WARNING

Abnormal elevation of serum potassium levels (greater than or equal to 5.5 mEq/liter) can occur with all potassium-sparing diuretic combinations, including these drugs. Hyperkalemia [elevated serum potassium levels] is more likely to occur in patients with renal [kidney] impairment and diabetes (even without evidence of renal impairment), and in the elderly or severely ill. Since uncorrected hyperkalemia may be fatal, serum potassium levels must be monitored at frequent intervals, especially in patients first receiving these drugs, when dosages are changed, or with any illness that may influence renal function.

HEAT STRESS ALERT

This drug can affect your body's ability to adjust to heat, putting you at risk of "heat stress." If you live alone, ask a friend to check on you several times during the day. Early signs of heat stress are dizziness, lightheadedness, faintness, and slightly high temperature. Call your doctor if you have any of these signs. Drink more fluids (water, fruit and vegetable juices) than usual—even if you're not thirsty—unless your doctor has told you otherwise. Do not drink alcohol.

These products are a combination of triamterene (see p. 78) and hydrochlorothiazide (see p. 60) and are used to treat high blood pressure (hypertension). **Older adults should never use drugs that contain a fixed combination of triamterene and hydrochlorothiazide as a first-choice drug.** Triamterene can cause kidney stones, kidney failure, and retention of too much potassium (especially if potassium supplements are also given), adverse effects that may be fatal.[44, 55] Because of these

---

WARNING

A fixed-combination drug should not be the first drug used to treat your high blood pressure. You may not need more than one drug. If you do need two drugs, the fixed-combination product may not contain the dose of each drug that is right for you. Your doctor has to regularly check your condition and reevaluate the effect of the drug(s) you take. This may mean adjusting doses, and even changing drugs, to ensure proper treatment. This fixed-combination drug may be the best drug for you, but it should be used only after you have tried each of its ingredients separately, in varying doses. If the doses that you need to control your high blood pressure match those in this fixed-combination product, use it if the combination drug is more convenient.

---

effects, we do not recommend that any older adult use triamterene alone.

In addition to triamterene's dangers, there are good reasons not to use any fixed-combination drug for high blood pressure. A single drug is often enough to control high blood pressure. If a combination drug like this one is controlling your high blood pressure, it is quite possible that one drug alone would do the same job. There is no reason to put yourself at extra risk by taking drugs you do not need.

If you have high blood pressure, the best way to reduce or eliminate your need for medication is by improving your diet, losing weight, exercising, and decreasing your salt and alcohol intake. Mild hypertension can be controlled by proper nutrition and exercise. If these measures do not lower your blood pressure enough and you need medication, **hydrochlorothiazide, a water pill (see thiazide diuretics, p. 60), is the drug of choice, starting with a low dose of 12.5 milligrams daily.** It also costs less than other blood pressure drugs.

There is growing evidence that thiazide diuretics, such as hydrochlorothiazide, significantly decrease the rate of bone mineral loss in both men and women because they reduce the amount of calcium lost in the urine.[38] Research now suggests that thiazide diuretics may protect against hip fracture.[39]

Since Dyazide and Maxzide contain 25 milligrams and 50 milligrams of hydrochlorothiazide respectively, it is not possible for older adults to start with a lower starting dose of 12.5 milligrams if either of these products is used. People responding to 12.5 milligrams of hydrochlorothiazide alone will have a lower risk of adverse effects and less need to use potassium supplements or a potassium-saving drug such as triamterene.

If hydrochlorothiazide alone would control your high blood pressure, there is no reason to take the extra risk of using triamterene as well.

If your high blood pressure is more severe, and hydrochlorothiazide alone does not control it, there are still better drug treatments than this combination product. The best treatment in this case is a combination of hydrochlorothiazide and a second type of drug called a beta-blocker, such as propranolol (see p. 87). If you can't take a drug in the beta-blocker family, another may be used instead. In either case, your doctor would prescribe the hydrochlorothiazide and the second drug separately, with the dose of each drug adjusted to meet your needs, rather than using a product that combines the drugs in advance in a fixed combination.

If you are taking this fixed-combination drug, ask your doctor about changing your prescription.

Whatever drugs you take for high blood pressure, once your blood pressure has been normal for a year or more, a cautious decrease in dose and renewed attention to nondrug treatment may be worth trying, according to *The Medical Letter.*[17]

And an editorial in the *British Medical Journal* stated: "*Treatment of hypertension is part of preventive medicine and like all preventive strategies, its progress should be regularly reviewed by whoever initiates it. Many problems could be avoided by not starting antihypertensive treatment until after prolonged observation. . . . Patients should no longer be told that treatment is necessarily for life: the possibility of reducing or stopping treatment should be mentioned at the outset."*[16]

Before You Use This Drug

Do not use if you have or have had:

- high potassium levels
- pregnancy or are breast-feeding

Tell your doctor if you have or have had:

- kidney or liver problems
- diabetes
- small urine volume

Tell your doctor about any other drugs you take, including aspirin, herbs, vitamins, and other nonprescription products.

When You Use This Drug

- Do not use potassium supplements, salt substitutes (potassium chloride), or potassium-rich foods.
- If you plan to have any surgery, including dental, tell your doctor that you take this drug.
- Do not take any other drugs without first talking to your doctor—especially nonprescription drugs for appetite control, asthma, colds, coughs, hay fever, or sinus problems.
- Because these drugs help you lose water, you may become dehydrated. Check with your doctor to make certain your fluid intake is adequate and appropriate, especially if you have vomiting or diarrhea.
- Stay out of the sun as much as possible, and call your doctor if you get a rash, hives, or skin reaction. These drugs can make you more sensitive to the sun.
- You may feel dizzy when rising from a lying or sitting position. When getting out of bed, hang your legs over the side of the bed for a few minutes, then get up slowly. When getting up from a chair, stay beside the chair until you are sure that you are not dizzy. (See p. 13.)
- If you plan to have any surgery, including dental, tell your doctor that you take this drug.
- **Do not take any other drugs without first talking to your doctor—especially nonprescription drugs for appetite control, asthma, colds, coughs, hay fever, or sinus problems.**

How to Use This Drug

- If you miss a dose, take it as soon as you remember, but skip it if it is almost time for your next scheduled dose. **Do not take double doses.**
- Do not share your medication with others.
- Take the drug at the same time(s) each day.
- Take the drug with food or drink.
- Swallow extended-release tablets whole. Do not crush or break them. Take with a full glass (eight ounces) of water. Take your last dose of the day with a full glass of water at least an hour before bedtime.
- Store at room temperature with lid on tightly. Do not store in the bathroom. Do not expose to heat, moisture, or strong light. Keep out of reach of children.

Interactions with Other Drugs

The following drugs, biologics (e.g., vaccines, therapeutic antibodies), or foods are listed in *Evaluations of Drug Interactions* 2003 as causing "highly clinically significant" or "clinically significant" interactions when used together with any of the drugs in this section. In some sections with multiple drugs, the interaction may have been reported for one but not all drugs in this section, but we include the interaction because the drugs in this section are similar to one another. We have also included potentially serious interactions listed in the drug's FDA-approved professional package insert or in published medical journal articles. There may be other drugs, especially those in the families of drugs listed below, that also will react with this drug to cause severe adverse effects. Make sure to tell your doctor and pharmacist the drugs you are taking and tell them if you are taking any of these interacting drugs:

> alcohol, barbiturates, cholestyramine, COLESTID, colestipol, corticosteroids, dofetilide, lithium, narcotics, norepineph-rine, NSAIDs, other drugs for lowering blood pressure, QUESTRAN, skeletal muscle relaxants (these are for both triamterene and hydrochlorothiazide), TIKOSYN.

Adverse Effects

Call your doctor immediately if you experience:

- difficulty breathing
- coughing or hoarseness
- dry mouth or increased thirst that does not go away quickly after you take a drink
- fever
- chills
- irregular heartbeat, chest pain
- weak pulse
- mood or mental changes
- confusion, convulsions, or irritability
- muscle cramps, pain
- unusual tiredness or weakness
- black, tarry stools
- blood in urine or stools
- severe stomach pain with nausea and vomiting
- joint, lower back, or side pain
- painful or difficult urination
- skin rash or hives
- yellow eyes or skin
- unusual bleeding or bruising

Call your doctor if these symptoms continue:

- headache
- dizziness
- nausea or vomiting
- stomach cramps and diarrhea
- drowsiness
- dry mouth
- increased thirst
- lack of energy
- increased sensitivity to sunlight

Periodic Tests

Ask your doctor which of these tests should be done periodically while you are taking this drug:

- blood pressure
- blood counts
- blood potassium concentration
- ECG

Angiotensin Receptor Blockers

Limited Use

Irbesartan (ir be *sar* tan)
AVAPRO (Sanofi)

Losartan (loe *sar* tan)
COZAAR (Merck)

Telmisartan (tel mi *sar* tan)
MICARDIS (Boehringer Ingelheim)

Valsartan (val *sar* tan)
DIOVAN (Novartis)

Do Not Use Until Seven Years After Release

Candesartan (kan de *sar*tan)
(Do Not Use Until 2007)
ATACAND (AstraZeneca)

Eprosartan (ep roe *sar*tan)
(Do Not Use Until 2006)
TEVETEN (Unimed)

Olmesartan (ol me *sar*tan)
(Do Not Use Until 2009)
BENICAR (Forest)

Combination Drugs Containing Angiotensin Receptor Blockers

If you are taking any of the angiotensin receptor blockers–hydrochlorothiazide combination products listed below, also read the additional information pertaining to hydrochlorothiazide on p. 60.

Limited Use

Irbesartan and Hydrochlorothiazide
(ir be *sar*tan and hye dro klor o *thye* a zide)
AVALIDE (Sanofi)

Losartan and Hydrochlorothiazide
(loe *sar*tan and hye dro klor o *thye* a zide)
HYZAAR (Merck)

Telmisartan and Hydrochlorothiazide
(tel mi *sar*tan and hye dro klor o *thye* a zide)
MICARDIS HCT (Boehringer Ingelheim)

Valsartan and Hydrochlorothiazide
(val *sar*tan and hye dro klor o *thye* a zide)
DIOVAN HCT (Novartis)

Do Not Use Until Seven Years After Release

Candesartan and Hydrochlorothiazide
(kan de *sar*tan and hye dro klor o *thye* a zide)
(Do Not Use Until 2007)
ATACAND HCT (AstraZeneca)

Olmesartan and Hydrochlorothiazide
(ol me *sar*tan and hye dro klor o *thye* a zide)
(Do Not Use Until 2009)
BENICAR-HCT (Forest)

GENERIC: not available

FAMILY: Angiotensin Receptor Blockers (see p. 53)
Thiazide Diuretics (see p. 51)

PREGNANCY WARNING

When used in pregnancy during the second and third trimesters, drugs that act directly on the renin-angiotensin system can cause injury and even death to the developing fetus. When pregnancy is detected, angiotensin receptor blockers should be discontinued as soon as possible.

BREAST-FEEDING WARNING

These drugs are excreted in animal milk and this may occur in humans. Because of the potential for serious adverse effects in nursing infants, you should not take these drugs while nursing.

THE HEALTH RESEARCH GROUP'S SEVEN-YEAR RULE

You should wait at least seven years from the date of release to take any new drug unless it is one of those rare "breakthrough" drugs that offers you a documented therapeutic advantage over older proven drugs. New drugs are tested in a relatively small number of people before being approved, and serious adverse effects or life-threatening drug interactions may not be detected until the new drug has been taken by hundreds of thousands of people. A number of new drugs have been withdrawn in their first seven years after release. Also, serious new adverse reaction warnings have been added to the labeling of a number of drugs, or new drug interactions have been detected, often within the first seven years after a drug's release.

WARNING

A fixed-combination drug should not be the first drug used to treat your high blood pressure. You may not need more than one drug. If you do need two drugs, the fixed-combination product may not contain the dose of each drug that is right for you. Your doctor has to regularly check your condition and reevaluate the effect of the drug(s) you take. This may mean adjusting doses, and even changing drugs, to ensure proper treatment. This fixed-combination drug may be the best drug for you, but it should be used only after you have tried each of its ingredients separately, in varying doses. If the doses that you need to control your high blood pressure match those in this fixed-combination product, use it if the combination drug is more convenient.

There are now eight angiotensin receptor blockers (see p. 53) on the market in the U.S. The primary use of this family of drugs is to lower high blood pressure.

Angiotensin receptor blockers as well as angiotensin converting enzyme (ACE) inhibitors (see p. 91) have an effect on a natural substance called angiotensin that can raise blood pressure. Like ACE inhibitors, angiotensin receptor blockers appear to be less effective in lowering blood pressure in most African-Americans than other blood-pressure-lowering drugs.[20]

Like the ACE inhibitors, these drugs also have the adverse effect of causing too high a potassium level in the blood. The angiotensin receptor blockers do not cause a dry, hacking cough as often as the ACE inhibitors.

The ACE inhibitors have a long-term protective benefit on the heart and kidneys, and information is now becoming available on the effect of the angiotensin receptor blockers in these conditions. A study comparing the addition of the older angiotensin receptor blocker valsartan (DIOVAN) or a placebo to standard treatment in patients with heart failure found that more people died taking valsartan than taking the placebo, though the difference was not statistically significant. A disturbing finding of this study is that in patients taking an ACE inhibitor plus a beta-blocker such as atenolol (TENORMIN; see p. 87) who were given valsartan were significantly more likely to do worse or die than those taking the placebo.[60]

The angiotensin receptor blocker losartan (COZAAR) was compared to the ACE inhibitor captopril (CAPOTEN) to assess their effect on survival in patients with heart failure. Captopril was found superior to losartan in improving survival in these elderly heart failure patients.[61]

The FDA's Cardiovascular and Renal Drugs Advisory Committee voted not to recommend the approval of the angiotensin receptor blocker irbesartan (AVAPRO) to curb kidney damage in patients with type-2 diabetes.[62]

If you have high blood pressure, the best way to reduce or eliminate your need for medication is by improving your diet, losing weight, exercising, and decreasing your salt and alcohol intake. Mild hypertension can be controlled by proper nutrition and exercise. If these measures do not lower your blood pressure enough and you need medication, **hydrochlorothiazide or chlorthalidone, water pills (see thiazide diuretics, p. 60), should be used first, starting with a low dose.** These drugs also cost much less than other blood pressure drugs.

There is growing evidence that thiazide diuretics, such as hydrochlorothiazide, significantly decrease the rate of bone mineral loss in both men and women because they reduce the amount of calcium lost in the urine.[38] Research now suggests that thiazide diuretics may protect against hip fracture.[39]

If your high blood pressure is more severe, and hydrochlorothiazide alone does not control it, the best treatment is a combination of hydrochlorothiazide and a second type of drug called a beta-blocker, such as propranolol (see p. 87). If you can't take a drug in the beta-blocker family, another family of high-blood-pressure-lowering drugs may be added to your treatment. In either case, your doctor would prescribe the hydrochlorothiazide and the second drug separately, with the dose of each drug adjusted to meet your needs, rather than using a product that combines the drug in a fixed combination.

Whatever drugs you take for high blood pressure, once your blood pressure has been normal for a year or more, a cautious decrease in dose and renewed attention to nondrug treatment may be worth trying, according to *The Medical Letter.*[17]

And an editorial in the *British Medical Journal* stated: *"Treatment of hypertension is part of preventive medicine and like all preventive strategies, its progress should be regularly reviewed by whoever initiates it. Many problems could be avoided by not starting antihypertensive treatment until after prolonged observation. . . . Patients should no longer be told that treatment is necessarily for life: the possibility of reducing or stopping treatment should be mentioned at the outset."*[16]

Before You Use This Drug

Tell your doctor if you have or have had:

- allergy to these drugs
- diabetes
- heart, kidney, or liver problems
- sodium deficiency
- dehydration due to excessive perspiration, vomiting, diarrhea, dialysis, dietary salt restriction
- pregnancy or are breast-feeding

Tell your doctor about any other drugs you take, including aspirin, herbs, vitamins, and other nonprescription products.

When You Use This Drug

- Continue to follow your diet, exercise regularly, and avoid undue stress. Do not use salt substitutes or salt-free milk.

- Use caution when exercising or in hot weather due to risk of dehydration.
- Drink fluids to prevent dehydration, especially when exercising during hot weather, or if you develop nausea, vomiting, or diarrhea.
- Do not drink alcohol, which can cause dehydration.
- The first time you take this drug, have a friend stay with you until you know how you react.
- You may feel dizzy when rising from a lying or sitting position. When getting out of bed, hang your legs over the side of the bed for a few minutes, then get up slowly. When getting up from a chair, stay beside the chair until you are sure that you are not dizzy (see p. 13).
- Until you know how you react to this drug, do not drive or perform other activities that require alertness.
- Monitor your blood pressure periodically.
- **Do not take any other drugs without first talking to your doctor especially nonprescription drugs for appetite control, asthma, colds, coughs, hay fever, or sinus problems.**
- Notify your doctor immediately if pregnancy is suspected.
- Check with your doctor if severe nausea, vomiting, or diarrhea continues.

How to Use This Drug

- If you miss a dose, take it as soon as you remember, but skip it if it is almost time for the next dose. **Do not take double doses.**
- Do not share your medication with others.
- Take the drug at the same time(s) each day.
- Take with or without food. Do not break, chew, or crush this drug.
- Do not suddenly stop taking without checking with your doctor to find out if you need to taper off these drugs.
- Store at room temperature with lid on tightly. Do not store in the bathroom. Do not ex-

pose to heat, moisture, or strong light. Keep out of reach of children.

Interactions with Other Drugs

The following drugs, biologics (e.g., vaccines, therapeutic antibodies), or foods are listed in *Evaluations of Drug Interactions* 2003 as causing "highly clinically significant" or "clinically significant" interactions when used together with any of the drugs in this section. In some sections with multiple drugs, the interaction may have been reported for one but not all drugs in this section, but we include the interaction because the drugs in this section are similar to one another. We have also included potentially serious interactions listed in the drug's FDA-approved professional package insert or in published medical journal articles. There may be other drugs, especially those in the families of drugs listed below, that also will react with this drug to cause severe adverse effects. Make sure to tell your doctor and pharmacist the drugs you are taking and tell them if you are taking any of these interacting drugs:

ALDACTONE, amiloride, DYRENIUM, ESKALITH, INDOCIN, indomethacin, KLOTRIX, lithium, MIDAMOR, NORVIR, potassium supplements, RIFADIN, rifampin, ritonavir, spironolactone, triamterene.

Adverse Effects

Call your doctor immediately if you experience:

- cough
- bronchitis
- dizziness, lightheadedness, or fainting
- fever
- chills
- confusion
- headache

- hoarseness
- cold
- joint, lower back, or side pain
- sore throat
- nosebleeds
- bleeding gums
- skin rash
- swelling of lips, eyes, face, tongue, hands, or feet
- sudden trouble swallowing or breathing
- painful, burning, or bloody urination or changes in frequency
- unusual tiredness or weakness
- changes in vision
- fast or irregular heartbeat
- large hives
- numbness or tingling in hands, feet, or lips
- itching
- loss of appetite
- heartburn
- pain in legs (rhabdomyolysis as class action in olmesartan label)
- stomach pain or bloating
- loss of voice
- yellow eyes or skin

Call your doctor if these symptoms continue:

- back pain
- cold symptoms
- abdominal pain or heartburn (telmisartan)
- flatulence, bloating, or gas (telmisartan)
- coughing
- ear congestion or pain
- diarrhea
- nausea (telmisartan)
- fatigue, weakness
- headache
- indigestion
- leg pain
- muscle cramps or pain
- nasal or sinus congestion
- sleep disturbance
- anxiety or nervousness

Periodic Testing

Ask your doctor which of these tests should be done periodically while you are taking this drug:

- blood pressure
- digoxin levels (with telmisartan)
- renal function determinations
- liver function tests
- potassium levels
- blood counts

Beta-blockers

Acebutolol (ace ah *butte* o lole)
SECTRAL (ESP Pharma)

Atenolol (a *ten* ah lole)
TENORMIN (AstraZeneca)

Betaxolol (bait *ax* o lole)
KERLONE (Lorex)

Bisoprolol (bis *oh* proe lole)
ZEBETA (Duramed)

Carvedilol (car *veh* di lole)
COREG (GlaxoSmithKline)

Metoprolol (me toe *proe* lole)
LOPRESSOR (Novartis)
TOPROL XL (Astra)

Nadolol (nay *doe* lole)
CORGARD (Apothecon)

Penbutolol (pen *hyoo* toe lole)
LEVATOL (Schwarz)

Pindolol (pin *doe* lole)
VISKEN (Novartis)

Propranolol (proe *pran* oh lole)
INDERAL, INDERAL LA (Wyeth-Ayerst)

Timolol (*tye* mo lole)
BLOCADREN (Merck)

Limited Use

Labetalol (la *bet* a lole)
NORMODYNE (Schering)
TRANDATE (Glaxo Wellcome)

Combination Drugs Containing Beta-blockers

If you are taking any of the beta blocker–hydrochlorothiazide combination products listed below, also read the additional information pertaining to hydrochlorothiazide on p. 60.

Bisoprolol and Hydrochlorothiazide
(bis *oh* proe lole and hye dro klor o *thye* a zide)
ZIAC (Duramed)

Metoprolol and Hydrochlorothiazide
(me toe *proe* lole and hye dro klor o *thye* a zide)
LOPRESSOR HCT (Novartis)

Propranolol (extended release) and Hydrochlorothiazide
(proe *pran* oh lole and hye dro klor o *thye* a zide)
INDERIDE LA (Wyeth-Ayerst)

Timolol and Hydrochlorothiazide
(*tye* mo lole and hye dro klor o *thye* a zide)
TIMOLIDE (Merck)

If you are taking the beta-blocker–chlorthalidone combination products listed below, also read the additional information pertaining to chlorthalidone on p. 60.

Atenolol and Chlorthalidone
(a *ten* oh lole and klor *thal* i done)
TENORETIC (AstraZeneca)

GENERIC: available

FAMILY: Beta-blockers (see p. 52)
              Thiazide Diuretics (see p. 51)

PREGNANCY WARNING

These drugs cross the placenta and expose the fetus to the drug. Because of the potential for serious adverse effects to the fetus, these drugs should not be used by pregnant women.

BREAST-FEEDING WARNING

These drugs are known to be excreted either in animal or human milk. Because of the potential for serious adverse effects in nursing infants, you should not take these drugs while nursing.

HEAT STRESS ALERT

This drug can affect your body's ability to adjust to heat, putting you at risk of "heat stress." If you live alone, ask a friend to check on you several times during the day. Early signs of heat stress are dizziness, lightheadedness, faintness, and slightly high temperature. Call your doctor if you have any of these signs. Drink more fluids (water, fruit and vegetable juices) than usual—even if you're not thirsty—unless your doctor has told you otherwise. Do not drink alcohol.

The drugs listed above have reported interactions with propranolol. Always ask your doctor and pharmacist about specific interactions for the beta-blocker you are taking.

WARNING

A fixed-combination drug should not be the first drug used to treat your high blood pressure. You may not need more than one drug. If you do need two drugs, the fixed-combination product may not contain the dose of each drug that is right for you. Your doctor has to regularly check your condition and reevaluate the effect of the drug(s) you take. This may mean adjusting doses, and even changing drugs, to ensure proper treatment. This fixed-combination drug may be the best drug for you, but it should be used only after you have tried each of its ingredients separately, in varying doses. If the doses that you need to control your high blood pressure match those in this fixed-combination product, use it if the combination drug is more convenient.

Beta-blocking drugs are used to treat high blood pressure (hypertension), chest pain (angina), heart attacks, irregular heartbeats (arrhythmias), to decrease the frequency of migraine headaches, and for tremor of unknown origin. If you are over 60, you will generally need to take less than the usual adult dose, especially if your kidney function is impaired.

For young adults with high blood pressure, doctors usually prescribe a drug in this family before any other drug. But for African-Americans and older adults, these drugs are less effective as the sole treatment. For these groups of people, doctors usually prescribe another type of drug called a diuretic (water pill) to lower blood pressure, and add a beta-blocker as a second drug if the diuretic alone is not enough.

If you have high blood pressure, the best way to reduce or eliminate your need for medication is by improving your diet, losing weight, exercising, and decreasing your salt and alcohol intake. Mild hypertension can be controlled by proper nutrition and exercise. If these measures do not lower your blood pressure enough and you need medication, **hydrochlorothiazide, a water pill (see thiazide diuretics, p. 60), is the drug of choice, starting with a low dose of 12.5 milligrams daily.** It also costs less than other blood pressure drugs.

There is growing evidence that thiazide diuretics, such as hydrochlorothiazide, significantly decrease the rate of bone mineral loss in both men and women because they reduce the amount of calcium lost in the urine.[38] Research now suggests that thiazide diuretics may protect against hip fracture.[39]

If your high blood pressure is more severe, and hydrochlorothiazide alone does not control it, the best treatment is a combination of hydrochlorothiazide and a second type of drug called a beta-blocker, such as propranolol (see p. 87). If you can't take a drug in the beta-blocker family, another family of high-blood-pressure-lowering drugs may be added to your treatment. In either case, your doctor would prescribe the hydrochlorothiazide and the second drug separately, with the dose of each drug adjusted to meet your needs, rather than using a product that combines the drug in a fixed combination.

Whatever drugs you take for high blood pressure, once your blood pressure has been normal for a year or more, a cautious decrease in dose and renewed attention to nondrug treatment may be worth trying, according to *The Medical Letter.*[17]

And an editorial in the *British Medical Journal* stated: *"Treatment of hypertension is part of preventive medicine and like all preventive strategies, its progress should be regularly reviewed by whoever initiates it. Many problems could be avoided by not starting antihypertensive treatment until after prolonged observation. . . . Patients should no longer be told that treatment is necessarily for life: the possibility of reducing or stopping treatment should be mentioned at the outset."*[16]

Before You Use This Drug

Do not use if you have or have had:

- heart failure
- low blood pressure
- heart block
- slow heart rate
- asthma
- emphysema or chronic bronchitis

Tell your doctor if you have or have had:

- allergies to drugs, foods, or insects
- pregnancy or are breast-feeding
- angina
- gout
- alcohol dependence
- mental depression
- kidney, liver, lung, or pancreas disease
- diabetes
- lupus erythematosus
- difficulty breathing
- poor blood circulation
- Raynaud's syndrome
- thyroid problems
- myasthenia gravis
- psoriasis

Tell your doctor about any other drugs you take, including aspirin, herbs, vitamins, and other nonprescription products.

When You Use This Drug

- **Learn to take your pulse, and get immediate medical help if your pulse slows to 50 beats per minute or slower, even if you are feeling well. Some people have suffered from slowed heart rate and heart failure while taking these drugs.**
- Until you know how you react to this drug, do not drive or perform other activities requiring alertness.
- Be careful not to overexert yourself, even though your chest pain may feel better.
- **Do not stop taking this drug suddenly.** Your doctor must give you a schedule to decrease your dose gradually, to prevent chest pain and possible heart attack. Have enough medication on hand to get through weekends, holidays, and vacations.
- You may feel dizzy when rising from a lying or sitting position. When getting out of bed, hang your legs over the side of the bed for a few minutes, then get up slowly. When getting up from a chair, get up slowly and stay beside the

chair until you are sure that you are not dizzy. (See p. 13.)

- Caution diabetics (see p. 405).
- If you plan to have any surgery, including dental, tell your doctor that you take this drug.
- **Do not take other drugs without talking to your doctor first—especially nonprescription drugs for appetite control, asthma, colds, coughs, hay fever, sinus problems, or alcohol.**

How to Use This Drug

- If you miss a dose, take it as soon as you remember, but skip it if it is less than eight hours until your next scheduled dose or if it is less than four hours for acebutolol, bisoprolol, metoprolol, pindolol, or timolol. **Do not take double doses.**
- Do not share your medication with others.
- Take the drug at the same time(s) each day.
- Ask your doctor whether to take your drug with food or on an empty stomach.
- Extended-release dosage forms must not be crushed; others can be crushed and mixed with water, or swallowed whole with water.
- Store at room temperature with lid on tightly. Do not store in the bathroom. Do not expose to heat, moisture, or strong light. Keep out of reach of children.
- Ask your doctor if you should check your pulse.

Interactions with Other Drugs

The following drugs, biologics (e.g., vaccines, therapeutic antibodies), or foods are listed in *Evaluations of Drug Interactions* 2003 as causing "highly clinically significant" or "clinically significant" interactions when used together with any of the drugs in this section. In some sections with multiple drugs, the interaction may have been reported for one but not all drugs in this section, but we include the inter-action because the drugs in this section are similar to one another. We have also included potentially serious interactions listed in the drug's FDA-approved professional package insert or in published medical journal articles. There may be other drugs, especially those in the families of drugs listed below, that also will react with this drug to cause severe adverse effects. Make sure to tell your doctor and pharmacist the drugs you are taking and tell them if you are taking any of these interacting drugs:

ALDOMET, AMARYL, amiodarone, ANZEMET, arbutamine, CALAN SR, CATAPRES, chlorpromazine, cimetidine, clonidine, cocaine, CORDARONE, COUMADIN, COVERA-HS, dolasetron, ELIXOPHYLLIN, ephedrine, FLUOTHANE, fluoxetine, furosemide, glimepiride, GLYSET, halothane, HUMALOG, HUMULIN, INDOCIN, indomethacin, insulin, ISOPTIN SR, LASIX, lidocaine, LITHOBID, LITHONATE, MAXALT, methyldopa, miglitol, MINIPRESS, moxisylyte, NORVIR, prazosin, PROZAC, RIFADIN, rifampin, ritonavir, rizatriptan, SLO-BID, TAGAMET, theophylline, THEO-24, THORAZINE, thioridazine, THYROID STRONG, tobacco, TUBARINE, tubocurarine, verapamil, VERELAN, warfarin, XYLOCAINE, zileuton, zolmitriptan, ZOMIG, ZYFLO.

Adverse Effects

Call your doctor immediately if you experience:

- difficulty breathing and/or wheezing
- dizziness
- weight increase
- cold hands or feet
- depression
- skin rash
- swelling of ankles, feet, or legs
- slow pulse

- back or joint pain
- chest pain
- confusion
- dark urine
- fever and sore throat
- hallucinations
- irregular heartbeat
- red, scaling, or crusted skin
- unusual bleeding and bruising
- yellow eyes or skin
- convulsions
- bluish-colored fingernails or palms

Call your doctor if these symptoms continue:

- headache
- dizziness, lightheadedness
- nausea, vomiting, stomachache
- diarrhea
- unusual tiredness or weakness
- disturbed sleep, nightmares
- decreased sexual ability
- anxiety or nervousness
- constipation
- stuffy nose
- dry, sore eyes, changes in taste, frequent urination (acebutolol and carteolol)
- itching skin; numbness; tingling fingers, toes, skin; nightmares (labetolol)

Call your doctor if these symptoms continue after you stop using the medication:

- fast or irregular heartbeat
- chest pain
- headache
- shortness of breath
- sweating
- trembling
- feelings of discomfort, weakness, or illness

Periodic Tests

Ask your doctor which of these tests should be done periodically while you are taking this drug:

- complete blood count
- blood pressure and pulse rate
- heart function tests, such as electrocardiogram (ECG, EKG)
- kidney function tests
- liver function tests
- blood glucose levels

ACE Inhibitors

Limited Use

Benazepril (ben *ay* ze pril)
LOTENSIN (Novartis)

Captopril (*kap* toe pril)
CAPOTEN (Bristol-Myers Squibb)

Enalapril (n *al* ap ril)
VASOTEC (Merck)

Fosinopril (foe *sin* oh pril)
MONOPRIL (Bristol-Myers Squibb)

Lisinopril (liss *sin* o pril)
PRINIVIL (Merck)
ZESTRIL (AstraZeneca)

Moexipril (moe *ex* i pril)
UNIVASC (Schwarz)

Perindopril (per *in* doe pril)
ACEON (Solvay)

Quinapril (*kwin* a pril)
ACCUPRIL (Pfizer)

Ramipril (*ra* mi pril)
ALTACE (King)

Trandolapril (tran *dol* ap ril)
MAVIK (Abbott)

Combination Drugs Containing ACE inhibitors

If you are taking any of the ACE inhibitor–hydrochlorothiazide combination products listed below, also read the additional information pertaining to hydrochlorothiazide on p. 60.

Limited Use

Benazepril and Hydrochlorothiazide
(ben *ay* ze pril and hy dro klor o *thye* a zide)
LOTENSIN HCT (Novartis)

Captopril and Hydrochlorothiazide
(*kap* toe pril and hy dro klor o *thye* a zide)
CAPOZIDE (Bristol-Myers Squibb)

Enalapril and Hydrochlorothiazide
(n *al* ap ril and hy dro klor o *thye* a zide)
VASERETIC (Merck)

Lisinopril and Hydrochlorothiazide
(liss *sin* oh pril and hy dro klor o *thye* a zide)
PRINZIDE (Merck)
ZESTORETIC (AstraZeneca)

GENERIC: not available
FAMILY: Angiotensin Converting Enzyme (ACE) Inhibitors
(see p. 53)
Thiazide Diuretics (see p. 51)

PREGNANCY WARNING
When used in pregnancy during the second and third trimesters, ACE inhibitors can cause injury and even death to the developing fetus. When pregnancy is detected, ACE inhibitors should be discontinued as soon as possible.

BREAST-FEEDING WARNING
These drugs are known to be excreted either in animal or human milk. Because of the potential for serious adverse effects in nursing infants, you should not take these drugs while nursing.

These drugs belong to a group of drugs for high blood pressure called angiotensin converting enzyme (ACE) inhibitors. Captopril, lisinopril, and enalapril are the preferred ACE inhibitors

---

HEAT STRESS ALERT

This drug can affect your body's ability to adjust to heat, putting you at risk of "heat stress." If you live alone, ask a friend to check on you several times during the day. Early signs of heat stress are dizziness, lightheadedness, faintness, and slightly high temperature. Call your doctor if you have any of these signs. Drink more fluids (water, fruit and vegetable juices) than usual—even if you're not thirsty—unless your doctor has told you otherwise. Do not drink alcohol.

COUGH ALERT

A common adverse effect, after taking ACE inhibitors for a few weeks, is a dry, hacking cough, especially in women. Check with your doctor about a four-day withdrawal from your ACE inhibitor to determine if this is the cause of your cough. This trial withdrawal can prevent unnecessary and sometimes costly tests and treatments.

---

because they have been on the market the longest.

ACE inhibitors are effective drugs for the treatment of high blood pressure (hypertension) and congestive heart failure in older adults. After a heart attack, treatment with some ACE inhibitors prevents subsequent heart failure and reduces morbidity and mortality.[63] In people with high blood pressure and kidney disease, ACE inhibitors, along with water pills, slow progressive kidney failure.[64–66]

ACE inhibitors may also be the preferred class of drugs to control blood pressure in those people with kidney damage from diabetes.[64,67,68] They can cause dangerous adverse effects such as bone marrow depression and kidney disease, and therefore should be taken in lower doses by

---

WARNING

A fixed-combination drug should not be the first drug used to treat your high blood pressure. You may not need more than one drug. If you do need two drugs, the fixed-combination product may not contain the dose of each drug that is right for you. Your doctor has to regularly check your condition and reevaluate the effect of the drug(s) you take. This may mean adjusting doses, and even changing drugs, to ensure proper treatment. This fixed-combination drug may be the best drug for you, but it should be used only after you have tried each of its ingredients separately, in varying doses. If the doses that you need to control your high blood pressure match those in this fixed-combination product, use it if the combination drug is more convenient.

---

older adults. This may amount to less than one-third the doses used in the past.

You are more likely to suffer harmful effects from ACE inhibitors if you have decreased kidney function, especially if you are dehydrated. Since older adults generally have some decrease in kidney function, these drugs may be especially dangerous for them. For this reason, they should not be the first choice for patients with kidney disease. In addition, patients taking a diuretic (water pill) should be watched carefully or, at their physician's discretion, be taken off that medication when an ACE inhibitor is started. Patients using potassium-sparing drugs (see below) should not use ACE inhibitors.

At times when using ACE inhibitors, the blood pressure goes too low, especially with the first dose. Older people are more likely to be sensitive to low blood pressure. A rare but potentially life-threatening reaction is angioedema, a sudden swelling of the face, lips, and particularly the tongue, which may last three days.[69, 70] While this reaction usually occurs with the first dose, it can occur years later. Once angioedema occurs, all ACE inhibitors should be stopped.[70] In general, if you are over 60, you should be taking less than the usual adult dose. Since enalapril stays in the body longer than captopril, its adverse effects may last longer.

If you have high blood pressure, the best way to reduce or eliminate your need for medication is by improving your diet, losing weight, exercising, and decreasing your salt and alcohol intake. Mild hypertension can be controlled by proper nutrition and exercise. If these measures do not lower your blood pressure enough and you need medication, **hydrochlorothiazide, a water pill (see thiazide diuretics, p. 60), is the drug of choice, starting with a low dose of 12.5 milligrams daily.** It also costs less than other blood pressure drugs.

If your high blood pressure is more severe, and hydrochlorothiazide alone does not control it, the best treatment is a combination of hydrochlorothiazide and a second type of drug called a beta-blocker, such as propranolol (see p. 87). If you can't take a drug in the beta-blocker family, another family of high-blood-pressure-lowering drugs may be added to your treatment. In either case, your doctor would prescribe the hydrochlorothiazide and the second drug separately, with the dose of each drug adjusted to meet your needs, rather than using a product that combines the drug in a fixed combination.

Whatever drugs you take for high blood pressure, once your blood pressure has been normal for a year or more, a cautious decrease in dose and renewed attention to nondrug treatment may be worth trying, according to *The Medical Letter.*[17]

And an editorial in the *British Medical Journal* stated: *"Treatment of hypertension is part of preventive medicine and like all preventive strategies, its progress should be regularly re-*

viewed by whoever initiates it. Many problems could be avoided by not starting antihypertensive treatment until after prolonged observation. . . . Patients should no longer be told that treatment is necessarily for life: the possibility of reducing or stopping treatment should be mentioned at the outset." [16]

Before You Use This Drug

Do not use if you have or have had:

- angioedema [70]
- severe kidney disease
- high blood potassium levels
- liver disease
- a potassium-sparing drug such as spironolactone (ALDACTONE), triamterene (DYRENIUM—a **Do Not Use** drug) or triamterene and hydrochlorothiazide (DYAZIDE/MAXZIDE)
- pregnancy or are breast-feeding

Tell your doctor if you have or have had:

- allergies to drugs
- an autoimmune disease such as lupus or scleroderma
- renal artery stenosis or generalized arteriosclerosis [71]
- asthma or other lung problems
- bone marrow depression
- cerebrovascular accident
- diabetes
- salt-restricted diet
- heart, kidney, or liver problems

Tell your doctor about any other drugs you take, including aspirin, herbs, vitamins, alcohol, and other nonprescription products.

When You Use This Drug

- If you take a diuretic, your doctor may taper you off of it, or lower your dose, a few days prior to starting one of these drugs. Take the first dose of any of these drugs under medical supervision. For hypertension, treatment supervision should last at least two hours and then an additional hour after your blood pressure has stabilized. Usually, this will be at a doctor's office. Have a companion stay with you until at least six hours has elapsed from your first dose.
- When taken for congestive heart failure, supervision should continue at least six hours. Many doctors prefer to start these drugs in a hospital. You should be watched closely for two weeks.
- You should also be closely supervised whenever your dose of any of these drugs or diuretics is changed.
- You may feel dizzy when rising from a lying or sitting position. If you are lying down, hang your legs over the side of the bed for a few minutes, then get up slowly. When getting up from a chair, stay by the chair until you are sure that you are not dizzy. (See p. 13).
- Drink plenty of fluids to avoid dehydration, especially when exercising, during spells of hot weather, or if you have nausea, vomiting, or diarrhea. Call your doctor if any of these conditions continue or become severe.
- **Do not take other drugs without talking to your doctor first—especially nonprescription drugs for appetite control, asthma, colds, coughs, hay fever, or sinus problems.**
- Be careful not to overexert yourself, even though your chest pain may feel better. Talk to your doctor about a safe exercise program.
- Until you know how you react to these drugs, do not drive or perform other activities requiring alertness. Do not drive after taking the first dose, or any time your dose changes.
- Maintain some sodium (salt) in your diet, but avoid excess salt. Do not use low-salt milk, or salt substitutes containing potassium. Check with your doctor before going on any kind of diet. [72] Do not drink alcohol.
- Take your blood pressure periodically. Having your blood pressure checked away from the

doctor's office is good practice. If possible, have your own automatic blood pressure measuring device, but be sure to have both your blood pressure and the device checked by your doctor.

• If you plan to have any surgery, including dental, tell your doctor that you take one of these drugs.

• **Do not stop taking this drug suddenly.** Your doctor must give you a schedule to lower your dose gradually.

• Tell your doctor immediately if you suspect you are pregnant.

• Tell your doctor if you have chills, fever, or sore throat.

How to Use This Drug

• If you miss a dose, take it as soon as you remember but skip it if it is almost time for the next dose. **Do not take double doses.**

• Do not share your medication with others.

• Take at the same time(s) each day, with the last dose at bedtime to control blood pressure overnight and decrease daytime drowsiness.

• Take with or without food except for captopril and moexipril, which are to be taken on an empty stomach at least one hour before meals.

• Swallow tablets whole or break in half as prescribed.

• Continue to take, even if you feel well.

• Store at room temperature with lid on tightly. Do not store in the bathroom. Do not expose to heat, moisture, or strong light. Keep out of reach of children.

Interactions with Other Drugs

The following drugs, biologics (e.g., vaccines, therapeutic antibodies), or foods are listed in *Evaluations of Drug Interactions* 2003 as causing "highly clinically significant" or "clinically significant" interactions when used together with any of the drugs in this section. In some sections with multiple drugs, the interaction may have been reported for one but not all drugs in this section, but we include the interaction because the drugs in this section are similar to one another. We have also included potentially serious interactions listed in the drug's FDA-approved professional package insert or in published medical journal articles. There may be other drugs, especially those in the families of drugs listed below, that also will react with this drug to cause severe adverse effects. Make sure to tell your doctor and pharmacist the drugs you are taking and tell them if you are taking any of these interacting drugs:

The blood-pressure-lowering effects of the ACE inhibitors are enhanced when used with other blood-pressure-lowering drugs such as the thiazide diuretics (see p. 60).

Fosinopril may interact with antacids such as Maalox.

Quinapril may interact with tetracycline (ACHROMYCIN, SUMYCIN).

Ramipril may interact with the oral drugs used for type-2 diabetes (see p. 406) or insulin.

ACE inhibitors may interact with nonsteroidal anti-inflammatory drugs (NSAIDs), such as ibuprofen (MOTRIN). See page 488 for a list of NSAIDs.

Other interacting drugs are:

ADVIL, alcohol, ALDACTONE, amiloride, aspirin, chlorpromazine, digoxin, DYRENIUM, ECOTRIN, furosemide, GENUINE BAYER ASPIRIN, ibuprofen, INDOCIN, indomethacin, KATO, K-LOR, LANOXICAPS, LANOXIN, LASIX, lithium, LITHOBID, LITHONATE, MIDAMOR, MOTRIN, potassium chloride, salt substitutes, rofecoxib, SLOW-K, spironolactone, triamterene, THORAZINE, VIOXX.

Adverse Effects

Seek emergency help if you experience:

- difficulty breathing
- sudden swelling of eyes, face, lips, throat, tongue

Call your doctor immediately if you experience:

- chest pain or angina
- confusion
- dizziness, lightheadedness
- fainting
- fever or chills
- irregular heartbeat
- hoarseness
- joint pain
- a feeling of heaviness or weakness in your legs, awkwardness when walking
- nervousness
- numbness or tingling in hands, feet, lips
- skin rash with or without itching
- difficulty swallowing
- swelling of hands, face, mouth, ankles, feet
- stomach pain, nausea, vomiting
- itchiness
- yellow eyes or skin

Call your doctor if these symptoms continue:

- diarrhea
- cough or dry, tickling sensation in throat
- fatigue, unusual tiredness
- headache
- nausea, vomiting
- altered or lost sense of taste, loss of appetite
- urinary pain, or change in frequency or quantity of urine

Periodic Tests

Ask your doctor which of these tests should be done periodically while you are taking this drug:

- blood pressure
- kidney function tests
- liver function tests
- urinary protein
- white blood cell count
- potassium levels

Calcium Channel Blockers, Short-Acting

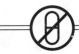 *Do Not Use*

ALTERNATIVE TREATMENT:
See Hydrochlorothiazade, p. 60.

Nifedipine, Short-Acting Forms
(nye *feh* di peen)
ADALAT (Bayer)
PROCARDIA (Pfizer)

FAMILY: Calcium Channel Blockers (see p. 54)
               Drugs for Angina

PREGNANCY WARNING

Nifedipine causes severe adverse effects including fetal death in animal studies. This drug should not be used by pregnant women.

BREAST-FEEDING WARNING

There is no information in the drug label about excretion in milk. However, because many drugs are excreted in milk and because of the potential for serious adverse effects in nursing infants, you should not take nifedipine while nursing.

The short-acting form of nifedipine is approved by the FDA only for the treatment of chest pain (angina). It has never been approved to treat any type of high blood pressure, including high blood pressure emergencies. In fact, in 1985 an FDA advisory committee voted unanimously not to recommend that short-acting nifedipine be approved to treat high blood pressure emergencies.[73]

The National Heart, Lung and Blood Institute, part of the National Institutes of Health, declared in August 1995 that "short-acting nifedipine should be used with great caution (if at all), especially at higher doses, in the treatment of hypertension, angina, and MI (heart attack)."[74]

An article appearing in the *Journal of the American Medical Association* in 1996 called for a moratorium on the use of short-acting nifedipine to treat high blood pressure emergencies due to its cardiovascular adverse effects.[75]

The countless injuries and deaths that occurred when short-acting nifedipine was used to treat chronic high blood pressure or high blood pressure emergencies were preventable tragedies.

If you have high blood pressure, the best way to reduce or eliminate your need for medication is by improving your diet, losing weight, exercising, and decreasing your salt and alcohol intake. Mild hypertension can be controlled by proper nutrition and exercise. If these measures do not lower your blood pressure enough and you need medication, **hydrochlorothiazide, a water pill (see thiazide diuretics, p. 60), is the drug of choice, starting with a low dose of 12.5 milligrams daily.** It also costs less than other blood pressure drugs.

There is growing evidence that thiazide diuretics, such as hydrochlorothiazide, significantly decrease the rate of bone mineral loss in both men and women because they reduce the amount of calcium lost in the urine.[38] Research now suggests that thiazide diuretics may protect against hip fracture.[39]

If your high blood pressure is more severe, and hydrochlorothiazide alone does not control it, the best treatment is a combination of hydrochlorothiazide and a second type of drug called a beta-blocker, such as propranolol (see p. 87). If you can't take a drug in the beta-blocker family, another family of high-blood-pressure-lowering drug may be added to your treatment. In either case, your doctor would prescribe the hydrochlorothiazide and the second drug separately, with the dose of each drug

adjusted to meet your needs, rather than using a product that combines the drug in a fixed combination.

Whatever drugs you take for high blood pressure, once your blood pressure has been normal for a year or more, a cautious decrease in dose and renewed attention to nondrug treatment may be worth trying, according to *The Medical Letter.*[17]

And an editorial in the *British Medical Journal* stated: *"Treatment of hypertension is part of preventive medicine and like all preventive strategies, its progress should be regularly reviewed by whoever initiates it. Many problems could be avoided by not starting antihypertensive treatment until after prolonged observation. . . . Patients should no longer be told that treatment is necessarily for life: the possibility of reducing or stopping treatment should be mentioned at the outset."*[16]

Calcium Channel Blockers, Long-Acting

Limited Use

Amlodipine (am *loe* di peen)
NORVASC (Pfizer)

Diltiazem (dil *tee* a zem)
CARDIZEM (Aventis)
CARDIZEM CD (Biovail)
DILACOR XR (Watson)
TIAZAC (Biovail)

Felodipine (fe *loe* di peen)
PLENDIL (AstraZeneca)

Isradipine (is *rad* ip ene)
DYNACIRC, DYNACIRC CR (Reliant)

Nicardipine (nick *card* ip ene)
CARDENE, CARDENE SR (Roche)

Nifedipine (nye *fed* i peen)
ADALAT CC (Bayer)
PROCARDIA XL (Pfizer)

Nisoldipine (nis *old* i peen)
SULAR (First Horizon)

Verapamil (ver *ap* a mil)
CALAN, CALAN SR, COVERA-HS (Searle)
ISOPTIN, ISOPTIN SR (Abbott)
VERELAN (Elan)

GENERIC: In some strengths of nifedipine only
FAMILY: Calcium Channel Blockers (see p. 54)

PREGNANCY WARNING

These drugs caused fetal harm in animal studies, including delays in growth and development and death. Because of the potential for serious adverse effects to the fetus, these drugs should not be used by pregnant women.

BREAST-FEEDING WARNING

These drugs are excreted in human milk. Because of the potential for serious adverse effects in nursing infants, you should not take these drugs while nursing.

These drugs belong to a family of antihypertensive drugs called calcium channel blockers. They are used primarily to treat chest pain (angina) and also to lower blood pressure (hypertension). Calcium channel blockers control, but do not cure, high blood pressure.

In 1995, Public Citizen's Health Research Group filed a petition with the FDA to add warnings to the labeling of all calcium channel blockers about the increased risk of heart attack and death. Our petition was based on three well-conducted observational research studies.[22–24, 72] Observational studies are frequently criticized by doctors who do not understand this type of research. Most of what we know about adverse drug reactions and what we are likely to learn in the future comes from observational research. This type of research was used to show the link between cigarette smoking and lung cancer.

Our petition helped to bring about important labeling changes in February 1996 on one of the calcium channel blockers, the short-acting form of nifedipine (see p. 96). The labeling for this form of nifedipine now warns doctors that this product should not be used for the treatment of high blood pressure.

Despite the recommendations of the National Institutes of Health's National Heart, Lung and Blood Institute that diuretics and beta-blockers should be used first in the treatment of mild to moderate high blood pressure, the calcium channel blockers have been the largest-selling family of high-blood-pressure-lowering drugs in the U.S.[21] Over 30 million prescriptions were dispensed in 2002 for the calcium channel blocker amlodipine.

A major study published in 2002 known as the Antihypertensive and Lipid-Lowering Treatment to Prevent Heart Attack Trial (ALLHAT for short) found that the older thiazide diuretic chlorthalidone (HYGROTON) (see p. 60) was found to be the superior drug compared to the calcium channel blocker amlodipine in the treatment of high blood pressure. This was the largest and longest trial of its kind, with patients being followed for four to eight years.[76]

Each calcium channel blocker differs in the likelihood of harmful adverse effects. Although this group of calcium channel blockers is less likely than verapamil to cause constipation, it is more apt to cause dizziness, flushing, headaches, rapid heartbeat, and swelling of legs and feet compared to other calcium channel blockers.[77] These adverse effects can seriously limit use.

If you have high blood pressure, the best way to reduce or eliminate your need for medication is by improving your diet, losing weight, exercising, and decreasing your salt and alcohol intake. Mild hypertension can be controlled by proper nutrition and exercise. If these measures do not lower your blood pressure enough and you need medication, **hydrochlorothiazide, a water pill (see thiazide diuretics, p. 60), is the drug of choice, starting with**

a low dose of 12.5 milligrams daily. It also costs less than other blood pressure drugs.

There is growing evidence that thiazide diuretics, such as hydrochlorothiazide, significantly decrease the rate of bone mineral loss in both men and women because they reduce the amount of calcium lost in the urine.[38] Research now suggests that thiazide diuretics may protect against hip fracture.[39]

If your high blood pressure is more severe, and hydrochlorothiazide alone does not control it, the best treatment is a combination of hydrochlorothiazide and a second type of drug called a beta-blocker, such as propranolol (see p. 87). If you can't take a drug in the beta-blocker family, another family of high-blood-pressure-lowering drugs may be added to your treatment. In either case, your doctor would prescribe the hydrochlorothiazide and the second drug separately, with the dose of each drug adjusted to meet your needs, rather than using a product that combines the drug in a fixed combination.

Whatever drugs you take for high blood pressure, once your blood pressure has been normal for a year or more, a cautious decrease in dose and renewed attention to nondrug treatment may be worth trying, according to *The Medical Letter.*[17]

And an editorial in the *British Medical Journal* stated: *"Treatment of hypertension is part of preventive medicine and like all preventive strategies, its progress should be regularly reviewed by whoever initiates it. Many problems could be avoided by not starting antihypertensive treatment until after prolonged observation. . . . Patients should no longer be told that treatment is necessarily for life: the possibility of reducing or stopping treatment should be mentioned at the outset."*[16]

Before You Use This Drug

Do not use if you have or have had:

- severe hypotension

Tell your doctor if you have or have had:

- allergies to drugs
- aortic stenosis
- diabetes
- heart, kidney, or liver problems
- low potassium levels in your blood
- mental depression
- narrowing of GI tract (with nifedipine only)
- low blood pressure
- pregnancy or are breast-feeding

Tell your doctor about any other drugs you take, including aspirin, herbs, vitamins, and other nonprescription products. Be sure to include the name of any eye drops that you use.

If you are taking a beta-blocker, your doctor may gradually take you off of it before starting a calcium channel blocker.

When You Use This Drug

- **Learn to take your pulse, and get immediate help if your pulse slows to 50 beats per minute or slower, even if you are feeling well.**
- Periodically check your blood pressure one or two hours after you take a dose, and again eight hours after your last dose.
- Follow a diet recommended by your doctor.
- Have your doctor suggest exercises that avoid overexertion.
- **Do not stop taking calcium channel blockers suddenly. Contact your doctor for a schedule to decrease your drug gradually.**
- You may feel dizzy when rising from a lying or sitting position. If you are lying down, hang your legs over the side of the bed for a few minutes, then get up slowly. When getting up from a chair, stay by the chair until you are sure that you are not dizzy. (See p. 13.)
- If you plan to have any surgery, including dental, tell your doctor that you take this drug.

- See your dentist frequently for teeth cleaning to prevent gum problems.
- **Do not take other drugs without talking to your doctor first—especially drugs for asthma, colds, cough, diet, hay fever, or sinus problems.**

How to Use This Drug

- If you miss a dose, take it as soon as you remember, but skip it if it is almost time for the next dose. **Do not take double doses.**
- Do not share your medication with others.
- Take the drug at the same time(s) each day.
- Swallow capsule or tablet whole. Do not break, chew, or crush long-acting forms of this drug.
- Be aware that the shell, empty of the drug, of some forms will pass in your stool.
- Store at room temperature with lid on tightly. Do not store in the bathroom. Do not expose to heat, moisture, or strong light. Keep out of reach of children.

Interactions with Other Drugs

The following drugs, biologics (e.g., vaccines, therapeutic antibodies), or foods are listed in *Evaluations of Drug Interactions* 2003 as causing "highly clinically significant" or "clinically significant" interactions when used together with any of the drugs in this section. In some sections with multiple drugs, the interaction may have been reported for one but not all drugs in this section, but we include the interaction because the drugs in this section are similar to one another. We have also included potentially serious interactions listed in the drug's FDA-approved professional package insert or in published medical journal articles. There may be other drugs, especially those in the families of drugs listed below, that also will react with this drug to cause severe adverse effects. Make sure to tell your doctor and pharmacist the drugs you are taking and tell them if you are taking any of these interacting drugs:

The use of beta-blockers (see p. 52) may increase the likelihood of congestive heart failure, severe low blood pressure, or worsening of chest pain (angina).

AGENERASE, alfuzosin, amprenavir, cimetidine, delavirdine, DILANTIN, LANOXICAPS, LANOXIN, mizolastine, phenytoin, RESCRIPTOR, UROXATRAL.

The drugs listed above have reported interactions with nifedipine. Not all of these interactions may have been reported for the other, newer calcium channel blockers listed in this section. Always ask your doctor and pharmacist about specific interactions for the calcium channel blocker you are taking.

Adverse Effects

Call your doctor immediately if you experience:

- chest pain
- dizziness
- irregular heartbeat
- pounding headache [78]
- fiery-red discoloration of knees or ankles [78]
- swelling of legs, ankles, or feet
- yellowing of skin or eyes
- problems urinating [79]
- breathing difficulty
- coughing or wheezing
- skin rash
- bleeding, tender, or swollen gums
- fainting
- painful swollen joints (with nifedipine only; unknown for others)
- trouble seeing (with nifedipine only; unknown for others)

Call your doctor if these symptoms continue:

- drowsiness
- dry mouth
- flushing and feeling of warmth

- headache
- indigestion
- muscle cramps
- nausea
- numbness
- redness, heat, or pain in the fingers (This is more apt to happen during warm weather or while in bed at night.[80] If this occurs, dip your hands in cold water.)
- skin rash
- feeling of weakness
- constipation
- diarrhea
- dizziness, lightheadedness
- increased appetite and/or weight gain

Periodic Tests

Ask your doctor which of these tests should be done periodically while you are taking this drug:

- blood pressure
- heart function tests, such as electrocardiogram (ECG, EKG)
- heart rate
- kidney function tests
- liver function tests
- potassium blood levels
- neurological tests

 Do Not Use

ALTERNATIVE TREATMENT:
See Hydrochlorothiazide, p. 60.

Amlodipine and Benazepril
(am *loh* di peen and ben *ay* ze pril)
LOTREL (Novartis)

Diltiazem and Enalapril
(dil *tye* a zem and e *nal* a pril)
TECZEM (Biovail)

Felodipine and Enalapril
(fe *loe* di peen and e *nal* a pril)
LEXXEL (AstraZeneca)

Verapamil and Trandolapril
(ver *ap* a mil and tran *doe* la pril)
TARKA (Abbott)

FAMILY: Calcium Channel Blockers (see p. 54)
Angiotensin Converting Enzyme (ACE) Inhibitors (see p. 53)

See Pregnancy and Breast-Feeding Warnings for Calcium Channel Blockers (p. 96) and Angiotensin Converting Enzyme (ACE) Inhibitors (p. 91)

These products are fixed combinations of a calcium channel blocker and an angiotensin converting enzyme (ACE) inhibitor drug. We have listed these drugs as **Do Not Use** because they are combinations that do not contain a first-choice drug for the treatment of high blood pressure such as a diuretic or beta-blocker.

There are good reasons not to use any fixed-combination drug for high blood pressure. A single drug is often enough to control high blood pressure. If a combination drug like this one is controlling your high blood pressure, it is quite possible that one drug alone would do the same job. There is no reason to put yourself at extra risk by taking drugs you do not need.

If you have high blood pressure, the best way to reduce or eliminate your need for medication is by improving your diet, losing weight, exercising, and decreasing your salt and alcohol intake. Mild hypertension can be controlled by proper nutrition and exercise. If these measures do not lower your blood pressure enough and you need medication, **hydrochlorothiazide, a water pill (see thiazide diuretics, p. 60), is the drug of choice, starting with a low dose of 12.5 milligrams daily.** It also costs less than other blood pressure drugs.

There is growing evidence that thiazide diuretics, such as hydrochlorothiazide, significantly decrease the rate of bone mineral loss in both men and women because they reduce the amount of calcium lost in the urine.[38] Research now suggests that thiazide diuretics may protect against hip fracture.[39]

If your high blood pressure is more severe, and hydrochlorothiazide alone does not control it, the best treatment is a combination of hydrochlorothiazide and a second type of drug called a beta-blocker, such as propranolol (see p. 87). If you can't take a drug in the beta-blocker family, another family of high-blood-pressure-lowering drugs may be added to your treatment. In either case, your doctor would prescribe the hydrochlorothiazide and the second drug separately, with the dose of each drug adjusted to meet your needs, rather than using a product that combines the drug in a fixed combination.

Whatever drugs you take for high blood pressure, once your blood pressure has been normal for a year or more, a cautious decrease in dose and renewed attention to nondrug treatment may be worth trying, according to *The Medical Letter.*[17]

And an editorial in the *British Medical Journal* stated: *"Treatment of hypertension is part of preventive medicine and like all preventive strategies, its progress should be regularly reviewed by whoever initiates it. Many problems could be avoided by not starting antihypertensive treatment until after prolonged observation. ... Patients should no longer be told that treatment is necessarily for life: the possibility of reducing or stopping treatment should be mentioned at the outset."*[16]

Alpha-blockers

Do Not Use (for high blood pressure)

ALTERNATIVE TREATMENT:
See Hydrochlorothiazide, p. 60.

Doxazosin (dox *ay* zo sin)
CARDURA (Pfizer)

Prazosin (*prae* zo sin)
MINIPRESS (Pfizer)

Terazosin (ter *ay* zo sin)
HYTRIN (Abbott)

FAMILY: Alpha-blockers (see p. 102)

PREGNANCY WARNING

These drugs caused fetal harm in animal studies, including stillbirths and prolonged gestation. Because of the potential for serious adverse effects to the fetus, these drugs should not be used by pregnant women.

BREAST-FEEDING WARNING

These drugs are known to be excreted either in animal or human milk. Because of the potential for serious adverse effects in nursing infants, you should not take these drugs while nursing.

The alpha-blocker family includes five drugs, alfuzosin (UROXATRAL), doxazosin (CARDURA), prazosin (MINIPRESS), tamsulosin (FLOMAX), and terazosin (HYTRIN). Three of these drugs, doxazosin, prazosin, and terazosin, are approved by the FDA to treat high blood

The **Do Not Use** classification for these three drugs only applies to their use in the treatment of high blood pressure, not when they are used to manage the symptoms of an enlarged prostate gland.

Information on the use of the alpha-blockers in the treatment of an enlarged prostate gland can be found in the chapter on prostate drugs (see p. 489).

pressure. Alfuzosin and tamsulosin are FDA-approved to treat benign prostatic hyperplasia (BPH), or an enlarged prostate gland. Terazosin and doxazosin are approved for both high blood pressure and enlarged prostate.

The National Heart, Lung, and Blood Institute, a part of the National Institutes of Health, announced in early March 2000 that it had stopped one part of a large high blood pressure study because one of the drugs being tested, the alpha-blocker doxazosin, was found less effective than the old water pill (diuretic) chlorthalidone (see p. 60) in reducing some forms of cardiovascular disease.[19]

The study, called the Antihypertensive and Lipid Lowering Treatment to Prevent Heart Attack Trial (or ALLHAT for short), found that users of doxazosin had 25 percent more cardiovascular events and were twice as likely to be hospitalized for congestive heart failure as users of the thiazide diuretic chlorthalidone. The drugs were similarly effective in preventing heart attacks and in reducing the risk of death from all causes. The doxazosin group also had poorer compliance with treatment—only 75 percent were still on the drug or another alpha-blocker after four years, compared with 86 percent still taking chlorthalidone or another diuretic.

Overall, chlorthalidone was found to be superior to doxazosin for blood pressure control, drug compliance, and in reducing cardiovascular complications. In addition, chlorthalidone is much less expensive than doxazosin.

In light of the ALLHAT results, the American College of Cardiology recommended on March 15, 2000, that physicians reassess the use of alpha-blockers for the treatment of high blood pressure.

If you have high blood pressure, the best way to reduce or eliminate your need for medication is by improving your diet, losing weight, exercising, and decreasing your salt and alcohol intake. Mild hypertension can be controlled by proper nutrition and exercise. If these measures do not lower your blood pressure enough and you need medication, **hydrochlorothiazide or chlorthalidone, water pills (see thiazide diuretics, p. 60), should be used first, starting with a low dose.** These drugs also cost much less than other blood pressure drugs.

There is growing evidence that thiazide diuretics, such as hydrochlorothiazide, significantly decrease the rate of bone mineral loss in both men and women because they reduce the amount of calcium lost in the urine.[38] Research now suggests that thiazide diuretics may protect against hip fracture.[39]

If your high blood pressure is more severe, and hydrochlorothiazide alone does not control it, the best treatment is a combination of hydrochlorothiazide and a second type of drug called a beta-blocker, such as propranolol (see p. 87). If you can't take a drug in the beta-blocker family, another family of high-blood-pressure-lowering drugs may be added to your treatment. In either case, your doctor would prescribe the hydrochlorothiazide and the second drug separately, with the dose of each drug adjusted to meet your needs, rather than using a product that combines the drug in a fixed combination.

Whatever drugs you take for high blood pressure, once your blood pressure has been normal for a year or more, a cautious decrease in dose and renewed attention to nondrug treatment may be worth trying, according to *The Medical Letter.*[17]

And an editorial in the *British Medical Journal* stated: *"Treatment of hypertension is part of preventive medicine and like all preventive strategies, its progress should be regularly reviewed by whoever initiates it. Many problems could be avoided by not starting antihypertensive treatment until after prolonged observation. . . . Patients should no longer be told that treatment is necessarily for life: the possibility of reducing or stopping treatment should be mentioned at the outset."*[16]

Other Drugs for High Blood Pressure

Limited Use

Hydralazine (hy *dral* a zeen)
APRESOLINE (Novartis)

GENERIC: available

If you are taking the combination product listed below, also read the information pertaining to hydrochlorothiazide on p. 60.

Hydralazine and Hydrochlorothiazide
(hy *dral* a zeen and hye dro klor o *thye* a zide)
APRESOLINE ESIDREX (Novartis)

GENERIC: available

FAMILY: Other Drugs for High Blood Pressure

PREGNANCY WARNING

Hydralazine caused fetal harm in animal studies, including malformation of the bones of the face and head as well as cleft palate. Because of the potential for serious adverse effects to the fetus, this drug should not be used by pregnant women.

BREAST-FEEDING WARNING

No information is available from either human or animal studies. However, it is likely that this drug, like many others, is excreted in human milk, and because of the potential for serious adverse effects in nursing infants, you should not take this drug while nursing.

Hydralazine was first approved for marketing in the U.S. in 1953. It is used to treat high blood pressure (hypertension), but it is not the first-choice drug for this purpose. People with coronary artery disease should not use hydralazine at all.[20]

Frequent severe adverse effects seen with hydralazine include rapid heart rate, worsening of chest pain, headache, dizziness, fluid retention, nasal congestion, lupuslike syndrome, and inflammation of the liver (hepatitis).[20]

WARNING

A fixed-combination drug should not be the first drug used to treat your high blood pressure. You may not need more than one drug. If you do need two drugs, the fixed-combination product may not contain the dose of each drug that is right for you. Your doctor has to regularly check your condition and reevaluate the effect of the drug(s) you take. This may mean adjusting doses, and even changing drugs, to ensure proper treatment. This fixed-combination drug may be the best drug for you, but it should be used only after you have tried each of its ingredients separately, in varying doses. If the doses that you need to control your high blood pressure match those in this fixed-combination product, use it if the combination drug is more convenient.

The starting dose of hydralazine should be between 10 and 12.5 milligrams, four times a day. The total daily dose should not go over 150 to 200 milligrams.[15] If you have impaired kidney function, you should be taking a smaller dose.

If you have high blood pressure, the best way to reduce or eliminate your need for medication is by improving your diet, losing weight, exercising, and decreasing your salt and alcohol intake. Mild hypertension can be controlled by proper nutrition and exercise. If these measures do not lower your blood pressure enough and you need medication, **hydrochlorothiazide or chlorthalidone, water pills (see thiazide diuretics, p. 60), should be used first, starting with a low dose.** These drugs also cost much less than other blood pressure drugs.

There is growing evidence that thiazide diuretics, such as hydrochlorothiazide, significantly decrease the rate of bone mineral loss in both men and women because they reduce the amount of calcium lost in the urine.[38] Research now suggests that thiazide diuretics may protect against hip fracture.[39]

If your high blood pressure is more severe, and hydrochlorothiazide alone does not control it, the best treatment is a combination of hydrochlorothiazide and a second type of drug called a beta-blocker, such as propranolol (see p. 87). If you can't take a drug in the beta-blocker family, another family of high-blood-pressure-lowering drugs may be added to your treatment. In either case, your doctor would prescribe the hydrochlorothiazide and the second drug separately, with the dose of each drug adjusted to meet your needs, rather than using a product that combines the drug in a fixed combination.

Whatever drugs you take for high blood pressure, once your blood pressure has been normal for a year or more, a cautious decrease in dose and renewed attention to nondrug treatment may be worth trying, according to *The Medical Letter.*[17]

And an editorial in the *British Medical Journal* stated: *"Treatment of hypertension is part of preventive medicine and like all preventive strategies, its progress should be regularly reviewed by whoever initiates it. Many problems could be avoided by not starting antihypertensive treatment until after prolonged observation. . . . Patients should no longer be told that treatment is necessarily for life: the possibility of reducing or stopping treatment should be mentioned at the outset."*[16]

Before You Use This Drug

Do not use if you have or have had:

- aortic aneurysm
- disease of the arteries that nourish the heart
- disease of the blood vessels that nourish the brain
- rheumatic heart disease
- severe heart disease

- severe kidney disease
- pregnancy or are breast-feeding
- phenylketonuria (if you take the solution)

Tell your doctor if you have or have had:

- allergies to drugs
- heart or blood vessel disease
- kidney disease
- stroke

Tell your doctor about any other drugs you take, including aspirin, herbs, vitamins, and other nonprescription products.

When You Use This Drug

- Until you know how you react to this drug, do not drive or perform other activities requiring alertness.
- **Do not stop taking this drug suddenly. Your doctor must give you a schedule to decrease your dose gradually.**
- You may feel dizzy when rising from a lying or sitting position. When getting out of bed, hang your legs over the side of the bed for a few minutes, then get up slowly. When getting up from a chair, get up slowly and stay beside the chair until you are sure that you are not dizzy. (See p. 13.)
- If you plan to have any surgery, including dental, tell your doctor that you take this drug.
- **Do not take other drugs without talking to your doctor first—especially nonprescription drugs for appetite control, asthma, colds, coughs, hay fever, or sinus problems.**
- You may need more vitamin B_6 (pyridoxine) than usual. Ask your doctor about getting more vitamin B_6 in your diet or about taking a supplement.
- Do not drink alcohol.

How to Use This Drug

• If you miss a dose, take it as soon as you remember, but skip it if it is almost time for the next dose. **Do not take double doses.**
• Do not share your medication with others.
• Take the drug at the same time(s) each day.
• Take with food.
• This medication can be taken whole or broken, chewed or crushed.
• Crush tablet and mix with food or drink, or swallow whole with water. The liquid form of the drug may be mixed with fruit juice or applesauce just prior to use.
• Keep the liquid form in the refrigerator. Do not use it after 14 days or if its color changes; replace it.
• Do not store tablets in the bathroom. Do not expose to heat, moisture, or strong light.
• Call your doctor if you miss two doses in a row.

Interactions with Other Drugs

The following drugs, biologics (e.g., vaccines, therapeutic antibodies), or foods are listed in *Evaluations of Drug Interactions* 2003 as causing "highly clinically significant" or "clinically significant" interactions when used together with any of the drugs in this section. In some sections with multiple drugs, the interaction may have been reported for one but not all drugs in this section, but we include the interaction because the drugs in this section are similar to one another. We have also included potentially serious interactions listed in the drug's FDA-approved professional package insert or in published medical journal articles. There may be other drugs, especially those in the families of drugs listed below, that also will react with this drug to cause severe adverse effects. Make sure to tell your doctor and pharmacist the drugs you are taking and tell them if you are taking any of these interacting drugs:

Promethazine.

Adverse Effects

Call your doctor immediately if you experience:

• blisters on skin
• chest pain
• general discomfort or weakness
• muscle or joint pain
• numbness, tingling, pain, or weakness in hands and feet
• skin rash or itching
• sore throat and fever
• swelling of feet or lower legs
• swelling of lymph glands
• fever

Call your doctor if these symptoms continue:

• diarrhea
• constipation
• loss of appetite
• nausea, vomiting
• rapid or irregular heartbeat
• redness or flushing of face
• shortness of breath on exertion
• dizziness, lightheadedness
• watering or irritated eyes
• headache
• stuffy nose (do not take any medication for this)

Periodic Tests

Ask your doctor which of these tests should be done periodically while you are taking this drug:

• blood pressure
• antinuclear antibody titer
• complete blood count
• direct Coombs' test
• lupus erythematosus (LE) cell preparation

Do Not Use

ALTERNATIVE TREATMENT:
See Hydrochlorothiazide, p. 60.

Clonidine (*kloe* ni deen)
CATAPRES (Boehringer Ingelheim)

Clonidine and Chlorthalidone
(*kloe* ni deen and klor *thal* i done)
COMBIPRES (Boehringer Ingelheim)

Clonidine Transdermal Therapeutic System
CATAPRES-TTS (Boehringer Ingelheim)

FAMILY: Other Drugs for High Blood Pressure

PREGNANCY WARNING

Clonidine caused fetal harm in animal studies, including increased resorptions. Because of the potential for serious adverse effects to the fetus, these drugs should not be used by pregnant women.

BREAST-FEEDING WARNING

Clonidine is excreted in human milk. Because of the potential for serious adverse effects in nursing infants, you should not take this drug while nursing.

Do not suddenly stop using these drugs. Sudden withdrawal from clonidine can cause sweating, tremors, flushing, and even severe high blood pressure. This dangerous reaction may occur after missing only one or two doses. Ask your doctor for a schedule that reduces your dose of clonidine gradually over at least 10 days, and even more slowly if symptoms occur. At the same time as you are reducing your dose of clonidine, your doctor should start you on another drug for high blood pressure.

Clonidine, a so-called alpha agonist, and the combination of clonidine and chlorthalidone (see p. 60) are used to treat high blood pressure (hypertension). Clonidine has severe adverse effects and should not be used.

The main problem with clonidine is that missing only one or two doses of the drug can have serious effects, including sweating, tremors, flushing, and severe high blood pressure. Clonidine can also cause severe depression and is particularly dangerous for anyone with a history of depression. Nearly one-fourth of the people who use the patch form have a skin reaction.

If you have high blood pressure, the best way to reduce or eliminate your need for medication is by improving your diet, losing weight, exercising, and decreasing your salt and alcohol intake. If these measures do not lower your blood pressure enough and you need medication, **hydrochlorothiazide, a water pill (see thiazide diuretics, p. 60), is the drug of choice, starting with a low dose of 12.5 milligrams daily.** It also costs less than other blood pressure drugs.

There is growing evidence that thiazide diuretics, such as hydrochlorothiazide, significantly decrease the rate of bone mineral loss in both men and women because they reduce the amount of calcium lost in the urine.[38] Research now suggests that thiazide diuretics may protect against hip fracture.[39]

If your high blood pressure is more severe, and hydrochlorothiazide alone does not control it, the best treatment is a combination of hydrochlorothiazide and a second type of drug called a beta-blocker, such as propranolol (see p. 87). If you can't take a drug in the beta-blocker family, another family of high-blood-pressure-lowering drugs may be added to your treatment. In either case, your doctor would prescribe the hydrochlorothiazide and the second drug separately, with the dose of each drug adjusted to meet your needs, rather than using a product that combines the drug in a fixed combination.

Whatever drugs you take for high blood pressure, once your blood pressure has been normal for a year or more, a cautious decrease in dose and renewed attention to nondrug treatment may be worth trying, according to *The Medical Letter.*[17]

And an editorial in the *British Medical Journal* stated: *"Treatment of hypertension is part of preventive medicine and like all preventive strategies, its progress should be regularly reviewed by whoever initiates it. Many problems could be avoided by not starting antihypertensive treatment until after prolonged observation. . . . Patients should no longer be told that treatment is necessarily for life: the possibility of reducing or stopping treatment should be mentioned at the outset."*[16]

High Cholesterol

Fibrates

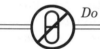 *Do Not Use*

ALTERNATIVE TREATMENT:
See Cholesterol-Lowering Drugs, p. 55.

Gemfibrozil (gem *fi* broe zil)
LOPID (Pfizer)

FAMILY: Fibrates

PREGNANCY WARNING

Gemfibrozil caused fetal harm in animal studies, including increased incidence of stillbirths and abnormal bone and eye formation. Because of the potential for serious adverse effects to the fetus, gemfibrozil should not be used by pregnant women.

BREAST-FEEDING WARNING

Gemfibrozil caused decreases in pup growth during nursing, suggesting its transfer to milk. Gemfibrozil is likely excreted in human milk. Because of the potential for serious adverse effects in nursing infants, you should not take this drug while nursing.

Gemfibrozil is given to people who have high levels of cholesterol or fats in their blood, to lower those levels in the hope of preventing heart disease. Although gemfibrozil does lower the level of fats in your blood, it has little effect on cholesterol levels. More importantly, there is no evidence that it decreases your risk of sickness or death from heart disease. In fact, there is no proof that gemfibrozil has any health benefit, such as lowering the chance of having a heart attack, for most people with high blood cholesterol or fat levels.

Referring to a study in which some patients who had had a previous heart attack were given gemfibrozil, and some were given a placebo, an FDA physician summarized the results: *"showed adverse trends with higher total mortality, higher coronary deaths and higher coronary heart disease events in the gemfibrozil (LOPID) group compared to the placebo group. . . . Studies have repeatedly shown increased gallbladder toxicity and statistically increased appendectomies with gemfibrozil. . . . We are concerned about the potential for human carcinogenesis induced by long-term treatment with fibrates [such as gemfibrozil] based on animal findings at doses equal to those used with humans."*[81]

Other serious problems with this drug are seen if it is used in combination with the statin drugs, such as lovastatin (MEVACOR), pravastatin (PRAVACHOL), or simvastatin (ZOCOR) (see p. 113). There are numerous reports of severe muscle damage, sometimes accompanied by life-threatening destruction of muscle and subsequent kidney damage.[82] Therefore, gemfibrozil and the "statin" drugs should not be used together.

The use of cholesterol-lowering drugs in people 70 or older should be limited to patients with very high cholesterol levels (greater than 300 milligrams) and those who manifest cardiovascular disease (previous history of heart attack or angina).[28] (See p. 55.)

The first, safer, and less costly measure to lower cholesterol for people under 70 is to eat a low-fat diet, using mostly polyunsaturated fats (such as canola, corn, safflower, and sunflower oils) or monounsaturated fats (such as olive oil). A change from animal to vegetable proteins often corrects high cholesterol. However, it is inadvisable to go on a very low-fat diet. The main focus on cholesterol-lowering diets has been on saturated fat and cholesterol content, not soluble fiber. (When added to the diet, psyllium or oat bran is a safe, effective way of lowering cholesterol.) Exercise and weight reduction are also recommended. Conditions that aggravate high cholesterol, such as dependence on alcohol or tobacco, diabetes, high blood pressure, low magnesium or potassium, and thyroid disease, should be corrected before adding a cholesterol-reducing drug. If cholesterol remains high despite diet, add 10 grams of psyllium a day (see p. 566).

Do Not Use

ALTERNATIVE TREATMENT:
See Niaspan, p. 120.

Fenofibrate (fen o *fi* brate)
TRICOR (Abbott)

FAMILY: Fibrates

PREGNANCY WARNING

Fenofibrate caused fetal harm in animal studies, including death and malformations. Because of the potential for serious adverse effects to the fetus, fenofibrate should not be used by pregnant women.

BREAST-FEEDING WARNING

Fenofibrate caused harm in nursing animals. Because of the potential for serious adverse effects in nursing infants, including the potential for producing tumors, you should not take fenofibrate while nursing.

Fenofibrate was first marketed in France in 1975.[83] The drug was approved in the U.S. in 1993 but the manufacturer chose not to market it until clearance was granted by the FDA in February 1998 for a micronized (the drug ground into a smaller particle size) version of fenofibrate. There is no known therapeutic advantage of the micronized product over the older nonmicronized one, but the new patent on this new dosage form has allowed Abbott to extend its period of patent exclusivity.

Fenofibrate is approved by the FDA for treatment of people with specific types of high cholesterol and triglycerides, another type of blood fat. Studies in people using two drugs in the same family as fenofibrate (clofibrate and gemfibrozil) showed that drugs in this class increase the risk of cancer, pancreatitis (inflammation of the pancreas), gallstones, and problems from gallstone surgery; most importantly, they caused an overall increase in mortality. Long-term human studies have not been done with fenofibrate, but studies in rats found an increased risk of liver, pancreatic, and testicular tumors. Niaspan, an intermediate-release dosage form of the vitamin niacin, is effective for treating elevated triglycerides but is not as dangerous as fenofibrate.

Statins

Limited Use

Atorvastatin (a *tore* va stat in)
LIPITOR (Pfizer)

GENERIC: not available

Fluvastatin (*flu* va stat in)
LESCOL (Novartis)
LESCOL XL (Novartis)

GENERIC: not available
FAMILY: Statins

Atorvastatin and fluvastatin are members of the statin family of cholesterol-lowering drugs.

BREAST-FEEDING WARNING

Some drugs in this class have been shown to be excreted in breast milk in animal studies. Because of the potential for serious adverse effects in nursing infants, you should not take these drugs while nursing.

PREGNANCY WARNING

These drugs should not be used if you are pregnant or are thinking of becoming pregnant. The risk of use of these drugs in pregnant women clearly outweighs any possible benefit.

Any person with elevated LDL cholesterol or other form of elevated blood fats (hyperlipidemia) should undergo medical evaluation to rule out other causes before drug treatment is begun.

Secondary causes include:
- diabetes
- hypothyroidism (low thyroid activity)
- chronic kidney failure
- drugs that increase LDL cholesterol and decrease HDL cholesterol: progestins, anabolic steroids, and corticosteroids[84]

The statin drugs work by inhibiting an enzyme that is responsible for the production of cholesterol in the body. Like all cholesterol-lowering drugs, atorvastatin and fluvastatin should be used in addition to a diet restricted in saturated fat and cholesterol only when the response to diet and other nondrug treatment measures, including exercise, have been inadequate.

The manufacturer of atorvastatin has not presented scientific evidence acceptable to the FDA so that the drug can be advertised as reducing the risk of a serious cardiovascular event such as a heart attack or stroke. Before any claim of such a health benefit for a drug can be advertised it must be included in the drug's FDA-approved professional product labeling, or package insert. Thus, no claim is made for the health benefit of reducing strokes or heart attacks in the professional product labeling for atorvastatin.[85]

In early 2003, a highly publicized study comparing a high dose of atorvastatin to a standard dose of pravastatin (PRAVACHOL) found that atorvastatin was better in reducing a combination of adverse cardiovascular events in people who had recently been hospitalized with a heart attack or angina. Although a combination of subsequent events was reduced by atorvastatin (compared with pravastatin), there was no significant reduction in the incidence of heart attacks alone or strokes alone.[86] As of the time this book went to press, the FDA had not yet approved atorvastatin for reducing the risk of heart attacks.

The FDA cited atorvastatin's manufacturer in 1998 for violating the advertising provisions of the Food, Drug, and Cosmetic Act because of a misleading TV ad implying that "Lipitor as a treatment option . . . is likely to have long-term benefits on disease and survival." The citation was issued despite the fact the ad header had to read "The effect of Lipitor on cardiovascular morbidity and mortality has not been determined."[87]

Fluvastatin has FDA-approved uses similar to atorvastatin, namely to lower cholesterol, except this statin can also be promoted in patients with coronary heart disease to reduce the chance of undergoing coronary revascularization procedures such as balloon or bypass surgery.[88] Reducing the chance of undergoing a coronary revascularization procedure is not the same as reducing the risk of a heart attack or stroke.

In contrast, the manufacturers of pravastatin (PRAVACHOL), simvastatin (ZOCOR), and lovastatin (MEVACOR) can make health claims of reducing the risk of heart attack and stroke because they have conducted studies demonstrating these benefits (see p. 113).

Drug-induced muscle injury, or rhabdomyolysis, is a known adverse effect of all statin cholesterol-lowering drugs. Rhabdomyolysis is usually accompanied by pain, tenderness, and weakness in the affected muscles. The most important consequences of rhabdomyolysis, however, are not those on the muscles themselves. As muscle cells break down, they release substances that can cause injury to the kidneys, sometimes permanent but even when reversible, sometimes requiring temporary hemodialysis (mechanical filtering of the blood). If muscle cells break down rapidly enough, released potassium can cause lethal heart rhythm disturbances. A number of drugs can interact with the statin drugs that can increase the likelihood of drug-induced muscle injury. See the section on interactions with other drugs (p. 112).

Cases of fatal rhabdomyolysis led to the withdrawal of the statin drug cerivastatin (BAYCOL) in August 2001.[89] The newest statin, rosuvastatin (CRESTOR), is listed as a **Do Not Use** drug because of cases of rhabdomyolysis and kidney toxicity seen in clinical trials before the drug was approved (see p. 117).

Liver toxicity is another potential problem with the statin drugs. The current labeling for these drugs states that elevations in liver function tests, an early indication of possible liver toxicity, have been seen with the use of statins. The labeling also warns, "It is recommended that liver function tests be performed prior to and at 12 weeks following initiation of therapy or the elevation of dose." No mention is made of possible liver failure.

The FDA undertook an evaluation of reports of potential liver failure associated with the use of the statin drugs in May 2000. A total of 90 cases of liver failure had been reported to the FDA for the six statin drugs on the market at the time. Of the 90 cases, 62 were consistent with the FDA's definition of liver failure and more than half of these 62 patients died.[90]

Before You Use This Drug

Do not use if you have or have had:

- allergy to atorvastatin or fluvastatin
- alcoholism or alcohol abuse
- active liver problems
- pregnancy or are breast-feeding

Tell your doctor if you have or have had:

- low blood pressure
- electrolyte imbalance, such as low magnesium, potassium
- endocrine disorder
- infection (severe)
- organ transplant
- seizures
- surgery (major)
- trauma
- history of liver disease

Tell your doctor about any other drugs you take, including antibiotics, anticoagulants, antifungals, heart drugs, herbs, over-the-counter medicines, and vitamins.

When You Use This Drug

- Have regular visits with your doctor to check your progress.
- Limit alcohol.
- Eat a diet low in saturated fats. Restrict carbohydrates to lower triglycerides. Lose weight if necessary.
- Avoid dehydration. Drink adequate water.
- Exercise regularly, as aerobic exercise, walking, or running.
- Tell any doctor, dentist, emergency help, pharmacist, or surgeon you see that you use a statin drug.
- Notify your doctor immediately if you have muscle pain, tenderness, or weakness.

• Don't take over-the-counter niacin without checking with your doctor.

• Tell your doctor immediately if you suspect that you are pregnant.

How to Use This Drug

• If you miss a dose, take it as soon as possible, unless it is almost time for the next dose. **Do not take double doses.**

• Do not share your medication with others.

• Take the drug at the same time(s) each day.

• Do not take atorvastatin with large amounts of grapefruit juice.

• Take atorvastatin of fluvastatin with or without food, but it is best to be consistent.

• Wait at least one hour before taking cholestyramine or colestipol.

• Store at room temperature with lid on tightly. Do not expose to heat, moisture, or strong light. Do not store in the bathroom. Keep out of the reach of children.

Interactions With Other Drugs

The following drugs, biologics (e.g., vaccines, therapeutic antibodies), or foods are listed in *Evaluations of Drug Interactions* 2003 as causing "highly clinically significant" or "clinically significant" interactions when used together with any of the drugs in this section. In some sections with multiple drugs, the interaction may have been reported for one but not all drugs in this section, but we include the interaction because the drugs in this section are similar to one another. We have also included potentially serious interactions listed in the drug's FDA-approved professional package insert or in published medical journal articles. There may be other drugs, especially those in the families of drugs listed below, that also will react with this drug to cause severe adverse effects. Make sure to tell your doctor and pharmacist the drugs you are taking and tell them if you are taking any of these interacting drugs:

Statins can increase risk of muscle toxicity when used with certain drugs. This occurs with all doses of atorvastatin, and with fluvastatin over 40 milligrams: cyclosporine, SANDIMMUNE.

Risk of muscle toxicity may also be increased by taking statins with certain other drugs. Your doctor should monitor you closely when taking: fibrates, gemfibrozil, LOPID, niacin (in high doses), NIASPAN, nicotinic acid.

Statins can increase risk of muscle toxicity when used with certain antibiotics. This does not occur with fluvastatin, but atorvastatin doses should be reduced 50% when taken with: EES, E-MYCIN, ERYTHROCIN, erythromycin, ERYZOLE, ILOSONE, ILOTYCIN, PCE, PEDIAZOLE.

Fluvastatin is not affected by antifungals. However, atorvastatin should be temporarily stopped or dose reduced by 50% when used with certain antifungals: itraconazole, SPORANOX.

Atorvastatin may increase the blood levels of oral contraceptives that contain ethinyl estradiol and norethindrone.

Do not take atorvastatin or fluvastatin within one hour of: cholestyramine, COLESTID, colestipol, QUESTRAN.

Both atrovastatin and fluvastatin may require extra monitoring and dose adjustment if used with anticoagulants and digitalis: fluvastatin may require adjustment with certain anticonvulsants: COUMADIN, digoxin, DILANTIN, LANOXIN, phenytoin, warfarin.

The dose of fluvastatin may need to be reduced when taken with: RIFADIN, RIFAMATE, rifampin, RIFATER, RIMACTANE.

Adverse Effects

Call your doctor immediately if you experience:

- fever
- muscle aches, pain, stiffness, cramps, tenderness, or weakness
- pain in abdomen
- tiredness or weakness that is unusual
- urine that appears dark

Call your doctor if these symptoms continue:

- constipation
- diarrhea
- dizziness
- gas
- belching
- heartburn
- indigestion
- impotence
- pain in stomach
- skin rash

Periodic Tests

Ask your doctor which of these tests should be done periodically while you are taking this drug:

- cholesterol
- creatinine phosphokinase (CPK)
- kidney function
- lipid profile
- liver function

Lovastatin (*low* vah stat in)
MEVACOR (Merck)

Lovastatin Extended-Release
ALTOCOR (Andrix)

Pravastatin (*prav* ah stat in)
PRAVACHOL (Bristol-Myers Squibb)

Simvastatin (sim va stat in)
ZOCOR (Merck)

GENERIC: not available except for lovastatin
FAMILY: Statins

Lovastatin, pravastatin, and simvastatin are members of the statin family of cholesterol-lowering drugs. The statin drugs work by inhibiting an enzyme that is responsible for the production of cholesterol in the body. Like all cholesterol-lowering drugs, these drugs should

---

PREGNANCY WARNING

These drugs should not be used if you are pregnant or are thinking of becoming pregnant. The risk of use of these drugs in pregnant women clearly outweighs any possible benefit.

BREAST-FEEDING WARNING

Some drugs in this class have been shown to be excreted in breast milk in animal studies. Because of the potential for serious adverse effects in nursing infants, you should not take these drugs while nursing.

Any person with elevated LDL cholesterol or other form of elevated blood fats (hyperlipidemia) should undergo medical evaluation to rule out other causes before drug treatment is begun.

Secondary causes are:
- diabetes
- hypothyroidism (low thyroid activity)
- chronic kidney failure
- drugs that increase LDL cholesterol and decrease HDL cholesterol: progestins, anabolic steroids, and corticosteroids [84]

be used in addition to a diet restricted in saturated fat and cholesterol only when the response to diet and other nondrug-treatment measures, including exercise, have been inadequate.

Lovastatin, pravastatin, and simvastatin are sometimes referred to as "natural statins" because they are similar to chemicals produced naturally by fungi.[91]

The manufacturers of these three drugs have presented sufficient scientific evidence to the FDA so that these drugs can legally be advertised as reducing the risk of serious cardiovascular events such as a heart attack or stroke. Before any claim of a health benefit for a drug can be advertised, it must be included in the drug's FDA-approved professional product labeling, or package insert.

The major FDA-approved uses for lovastatin are to reduce the risk in individuals without symptomatic cardiovascular disease, and with moderately elevated cholesterol levels, of heart attack, unstable angina (chest pain), and the need for coronary revascularization procedures such as angioplasty or heart bypass surgery.[92]

Pravastatin was approved by the FDA as the primary drug for individuals without clinically evident coronary heart disease to reduce the risks of heart attack, revascularization procedures such as angioplasty and heart bypass surgery, and cardiovascular mortality, without increasing the risk of death from noncardiovascular causes.[93]

Pravastatin is also approved for the secondary prevention of cardiovascular events. Secondary prevention refers to reducing the risk of a serious outcome in individuals who already have clinically evident coronary heart disease. Pravastatin is approved to reduce the risk of coronary death, heart attack, coronary revascularization procedures, stroke and stroke/transient ischemic attack (TIA), and to slow the progression of coronary atherosclerosis.[93]

The FDA has approved simvastatin for use in individuals at high risk of coronary events because of existing coronary heart disease, diabetes, peripheral vessel disease, history of stroke, or other cerebrovascular disease. In this group of patients this statin is approved to reduce the risk of coronary heart disease death, nonfatal heart attack and stroke, coronary and noncoronary revascularization procedures.[94]

The consumer's "gold standard" for knowing the health benefits, if any, of a prescription drug is the FDA-approved professional product labeling for that drug. It is clear from the FDA-approved labeling for the statins that lovastatin, pravastatin, and simvastatin should be used before either atorvastatin (LIPITOR) or fluvastatin (LESCOL) because of acceptable scientific evidence of a health benefit, rather than just the ability to lower cholesterol (atorvastatin and fluvastatin).

The question of whether, in general, the statin drugs have a role in the primary prevention of cardiovascular disease remains controversial, even though pravastatin has been approved for this purpose. Primary prevention is the use of the statin drugs to prevent a serious cardiovascular event in otherwise healthy individuals with mildly elevated cholesterol levels. We tend to agree with the experts that given the present evidence, the statins have not been shown to provide an overall health benefit in primary prevention studies.[95] The health benefit of using lovastatin, pravastatin, or simvastatin in secondary prevention, or in those that have had heart attacks or strokes, is much clearer.

Drug-induced muscle injury, or rhabdomyolysis, is a known adverse effect of all statin cholesterol-lowering drugs. Rhabdomyolysis is usually accompanied by pain, tenderness, and weakness in the affected muscles. The most important consequences of rhabdomyolysis, however, are not those on the muscles themselves. As muscle cells break down, they release substances that can cause injury to the kidneys, sometimes permanent but even when reversible, sometimes requiring temporary kidney dialysis (mechanical filtering of the blood).

If muscle cells break down rapidly enough, released potassium can cause lethal heart rhythm disturbances. A number of drugs can interact with the statin drugs that can increase the likelihood of drug-induced muscle injury. See the section on interactions with other drugs, p. 116.

A large number of cases of fatal rhabdomyolysis led to the withdrawal of the statin drug cerivastatin (BAYCOL) in August 2001.[89] The newest statin, rosuvastatin (CRESTOR), is listed as a **Do Not Use** drug because of cases of rhabdomyolysis and direct kidney toxicity (not just from rhabdomyolysis) seen in clinical trials before the drug was approved (see p. 117).

Liver toxicity is another potential problem with the statin drugs. The current labeling for these drugs states that elevations in liver function tests, an early indication of possible liver toxicity, have been seen with the use of statins. The labeling also warns, "It is recommended that liver function tests be performed prior to and at 12 weeks following initiation of therapy or the elevation of dose." No mention is made of possible liver failure.

The FDA undertook an evaluation of reports of potential liver failure associated with the use of the statin drugs in May 2000. A total of 90 cases of liver failure had been reported to the FDA for the six statin drugs on the market at the time. Of the 90 cases, 62 were consistent with the FDA's definition of liver failure and more than half of these 62 patients died.[90]

If you take statins with other drugs, the warnings, contraindications, adverse effects, and drug interactions of those drugs must be added to those for statins.

Before You Use This Drug

Do not use if you have or have had:

- liver disease

Tell your doctor if you have or have had:

- allergies
- alcoholism or alcohol abuse
- low blood pressure
- endocrine disorder
- electrolyte imbalance such as low magnesium, potassium
- infection (severe)
- liver problems
- organ transplant with immunosuppressant therapy
- pregnancy or are breast-feeding
- seizures
- surgery (major)
- trauma

Tell your doctor about any other drugs you take, including immunosuppressants, herbs, over-the-counter medications, or vitamins.

When You Use This Drug

- Limit alcohol.
- Eat a diet low in saturated fats. Restrict sugar and carbohydrates to lower triglycerides.
- Lose weight if necessary.
- Avoid dehydration. Drink adequate water.
- Exercise regularly, such as aerobic exercise, walking, or running.
- Protect yourself from sunburn with sunscreen or protective clothing.
- Tell any doctor, dentist, dental surgeon, emergency help, pharmacist, or surgeon you see that you take a natural statin drug.

How to Use This Drug

- If you miss a dose, take it as soon as possible, unless it is almost time for the next dose. **Do not take double doses.**
- Do not share your medication with others.
- Take the drug at the same time(s) each day.
- Take lovastatin with meals. Pravastatin and simvastatin may be taken with or without food, but be consistent. It is best to take simvastatin at night.[96] It is advisable to be consistent about the time you take it. Take Altocor at bedtime with a low-fat snack.

• If your dosage requires you to split tablets, and your eyesight is poor or you have limited physical ability, ask your pharmacy if they provide a service to split the tablets.

• If you take extended-release tablets, swallow these whole. Do not break, chew, or crush the tablet.

• If you take aspirin with a statin, check that the aspirin does not have an odor of vinegar or that the tablet is disintegrating.

• Take grapefruit, pomelos, or Seville oranges at a different time of the day from lovastatin or simvastatin. Even then, limit grapefruit juice to one eight-ounce glass or one-half fresh grapefruit.[97]

• Do not take cholestyramine or colestipol within one hour of taking pravastatin.

• Store tablets in a container at room temperature with the lid on tightly. Do not store in the bathroom. Do not expose to heat, moisture, or strong light. Keep out of reach of children.

Interactions with Other Drugs

The following drugs, biologics (e.g., vaccines, therapeutic antibodies), or foods are listed in *Evaluations of Drug Interactions* 2003 as causing "highly clinically significant" or "clinically significant" interactions when used together with any of the drugs in this section. In some sections with multiple drugs, the interaction may have been reported for one but not all drugs in this section, but we include the interaction because the drugs in this section are similar to one another. We have also included potentially serious interactions listed in the drug's FDA-approved professional package insert or in published medical journal articles. There may be other drugs, especially those in the families of drugs listed below, that also will react with this drug to cause severe adverse effects. Make sure to tell your doctor and pharmacist the drugs you are taking and tell them if you are taking any of these interacting drugs:

With lovastatin, pravastatin, and simvastatin, risk of muscle toxicity increases when taken with certain drugs. Avoid taking with gemfibrozil, LOPID.

With simvastatin and lovastatin, risk of muscle toxicity increases when taken with other drugs, especially ones also broken down by enzymes CYP34A: BIAXIN, clarithromycin, cyclosporine, EES, E-MYCIN, ERYTHROCIN, erythromycin, fibrates, ILOSONE, ILOTYCIN, itraconazole, ketoconazole, niacin over 1 gram per day, NIASPAN, NIZORAL, NORVIR, PCE, PEDIAZOLE, protease inhibitors, ritonavir, SANDIMMUNE, SERZONE, SPORANOX.

Avoid doses of lovastatin higher than 40 milligrams per day or simvastatin higher than 20 milligrams per day when also using: amiodarone, CALAN, CORDARONE, ISOPTIN, verapamil, VERELAN.

Pravastatin effectiveness can be reduced by these drugs. Do not take within one hour of pravastatin: cholestyramine, COLESTID, colestipol, QUESTRAN.

Taking simvastatin may cause toxicity of some drugs. Your doctor may do extra tests and adjust doses when you are also using: digoxin, LANOXIN.

Simvastatin effectiveness may be reduced by certain anticonvulsants. Your doctor may do more tests and adjust doses if you also use: DILANTIN, phenytoin.

If you use a natural statin, especially lovastatin, your doctor may do more tests and adjust doses of: COUMADIN, warfarin.

Adverse Effects

Call your doctor immediately if you experience:

- fever
- muscle aches, cramps, pain, tenderness, or weakness
- tiredness or weakness that is unusual

Call your doctor if these symptoms continue:

- constipation
- diarrhea
- dizziness
- gas
- headache
- heartburn
- problems with sexual function
- insomnia
- nausea
- pain in stomach
- skin rash

Periodic Testing

Ask your doctor which of these tests should be done periodically while you are taking this drug:

- cholesterol levels
- creatinine kinase (CK)
- eye tests
- kidney function tests
- liver function tests
- prothrombin (blood-clotting) times

 Do Not Use

ALTERNATIVE TREATMENT:
See Cholesterol-Lowering Drugs, p. 55.

Rosuvastatin (rahs *yew* va statin)
CRESTOR (AstraZeneca)

FAMILY: Statins

PREGNANCY WARNING

The statins should not be used if you are pregnant or are thinking of becoming pregnant. The risk of use of the statins in pregnant women clearly outweighs any possible benefit.

BREAST-FEEDING WARNING

Some drugs in this class have been shown to be excreted in breast milk in animal studies. Because of the potential for serious adverse effects in nursing infants, you should not take this drug while nursing.

Rosuvastatin became the sixth cholesterol-lowering statin drug on the U.S. market when it was approved by the FDA on August 13, 2003. The other members of the statin family are atorvastatin (LIPITOR), fluvastatin (LESCOL), lovastatin (MEVACOR), pravastatin (PRAVACHOL), and simvastatin (ZOCOR). These drugs are only approved to be used along with a low-cholesterol diet and an exercise program to lower cholesterol.

One of the statins, cerivastatin (BAYCOL), was removed from the market because of at least 31 reports of fatal rhabdomyolysis, an adverse reaction involving the destruction of muscle tissue that can lead to kidney failure. We had warned patients not to use this drug more than three years before it was removed from the market.

AstraZeneca originally filed its application with the FDA to market rosuvastatin in June 2001. The application was delayed when the company halted clinical trials worldwide after reports of kidney damage and muscle weakness (an early signal for rhabdomyolysis) in clinical trials in patients taking 80 milligrams of the drug per day. The FDA asked AstraZeneca for more data and the company stopped development of the 80 milligram dose because of the safety problems. Rosuvastatin will only be sold in 5, 10, 20, and 40 milligram strengths. Because of safety concerns there will be special restrictions on the distribution of the 40 milligram strength that will be discussed further below.

The Health Research Group made a formal presentation before the FDA's Endocrinologic and Metabolic Drugs Advisory Committee on July 19, 2003, strongly opposing the approval of rosuvastatin because of its unique kidney toxicity. We were also seriously concerned because of seven cases of rhabdomyolysis that were common enough to have shown up in the preapproval clinical trials of rosuvastatin in which the 80 milligram dose was used. Not one case of rhabdomyolysis appeared in any of the preapproval studies of the previously approved statins, including cerivastatin, which was removed from the market because of rhabdomyolysis.

We testified before the advisory committee that a major factor that distinguishes rosuvastatin from the other five statins remaining on the market is the drug's potential to cause kidney toxicity. In the FDA review documents posted on the agency's Web site before the Endocrinologic and Metabolic Drugs Advisory Committee, it was noted, "In contrast to currently approved statins, rosuvastatin was also associated with renal [kidney] findings not previously reported with other statins."[98]

A number of patients taking primarily the 80 and 40 milligram doses of rosuvastatin had an increased frequency of persistent protein in the urine (proteinuria) and blood in the urine (hematuria), which in some subjects was also associated with another abnormal test result, the serum creatinine level, that is an early signal for kidney toxicity. The FDA documents pointed out that there were two cases of kidney failure and one case of kidney insufficiency with

80 milligrams of rosuvastatin, in which these patients also had experienced both protein and blood in the urine.

An FDA medical officer reviewing rosuvastatin had sobering comments on the cases of kidney problems with the drug: *"These three cases of renal insufficiency of unknown etiology are of concern because they present with a clinical pattern, which is similar to the renal disease seen with rosuvastatin in these clinical trials. There is mild proteinuria associated with hematuria and the suggestion of tubular inflammation or necrosis [death of cells]. All cases occurred at the 80 mg dose which was also associated with the greatest number of patients with abnormal renal findings in these clinical trials. Proteinuria and hematuria could be potentially managed with regular urinalysis screening. However, if they are the signals for the potential progression to renal failure in a small number of patients, this may represent an unacceptable risk since currently approved statins do not have similar renal effects."*[98]

PUBLIC CITIZEN PETITION TO BAN ROSUVASTATIN (CRESTOR)

Our concerns prior to approval about rhabdomyolysis and kidney toxicity have been confirmed in the results of the first year of marketing in the UK and Canada and in the first six months of marketing in the U.S. Data obtained from the U.S., the UK and Canada show that seven cases of rhabdomyolysis and nine cases of kidney damage or failure occurred after FDA approval. On the basis of this information, confirming the fact that the drug has the unique risks we were concerned with prior to its approval, we filed a petition in March 2004 asking the FDA to take the drug off the market. Major U.S. insurers, including WellPoint/Blue Cross, with 16 million beneficiaries, have refused to reimburse for the drug because of safety concerns.

AstraZeneca attempted to "spin" the drug's potential for causing elevated protein levels in the urine by claiming that it was due to a previously unobserved effect of the statin family of drugs. However, the research submitted by Astra-Zeneca to the FDA did not show a similar degree of urine protein elevation with any of the other statins.

A popular buzzword frequently used by the FDA these days is "risk management"—assessing public health risks, analyzing methods for reducing them, and taking appropriate action. The FDA's risk-management strategy for the safety problems associated with rosuvastatin can hardly be called appropriate. The 40 milligram tablet will not be stocked in retail pharmacies and the pharmacy would need to go through a wholesaler to obtain the 40 milligram tablets. This would take an extra day before the tablets arrived at the pharmacy. Somehow the FDA believes that "these steps will help to ensure that the 40-mg dose is available only to patients who truly need this dose." To easily beat this restriction, there is nothing to prevent a physician from writing a prescription for 20 milligram tablets and instructing the patient to take two tablets of rosuvastatin daily.

Clearly, the only "appropriate" and safe risk-management strategy for rosuvastatin would have been not to have approved the drug in the first place.

Rosuvastatin's professional labeling also carries warnings about elevated liver enzymes, an early signal for possible liver toxicity, and muscle pain and weakness that may be precursors to rhabdomyolysis. These warnings appear in the labeling for all statin drugs:

It is recommended that liver function tests be performed before and at 12 weeks following both the initiation of therapy and any elevation of dose, and periodically (e.g., semiannually) thereafter.

Rare cases of rhabdomyolysis with acute renal failure secondary to myoglobinuria [a protein from muscle] have been reported with rosuvastatin and with other drugs in this class.

The professional product labeling goes on to instruct physicians to tell patients "to promptly report unexplained muscle pain, tenderness, or weakness, particularly if accompanied by malaise or fever."

The risk of muscle damage leading to rhabdomyolysis during treatment with rosuvastatin may be increased when it is used together with other cholesterol-lowering drugs and cyclosporine (NEORAL, SANDIMMUNE), a drug used after transplantation to prevent organ rejection.

A single rosuvastatin dose given to healthy volunteers on the cholesterol-lowering drug gemfibrozil (LOPID) resulted in a significant increase in the amount of rosuvastatin in the body. There is a bold statement in the Warnings section of rosuvastatin's labeling that states: **"Combination therapy with rosuvastatin and gemfibrozil should generally be avoided."** The risk of muscle problems possibly leading to rhabdomyolysis is also increased when niacin is used to lower cholesterol in combination with rosuvastatin.

When rosuvastatin was given together with cyclosporine in heart transplant patients, the amount of rosuvastatin increased significantly in the blood compared with healthy volunteers. This increase is considered to be clinically significant.

When rosuvastatin was given to patients on stable warfarin (COUMADIN) treatment to prevent blood clots, there was a clinically significant rise in the International Normalized Ratio (INR), the laboratory test used to monitor warfarin therapy that can increase the risk of bleeding.

A number of factors went into our decision to list rosuvastatin as a **Do Not Use** drug:

1. Rosuvastatin joins atorvastatin and fluvastatin (see p. 109) as the statins that have not

been approved by the FDA to confer a health benefit to the patients who use them, in terms of reducing the serious cardiovascular consequences of high cholesterol such as a first or second heart attack or stroke. Lovastatin, pravastatin, and simvastatin have shown such benefits to patients in addition to their cholesterol-lowering properties, and this is reflected in the professional product labels and advertising for these drugs.

The only reliable, valid indicator that consumers can use that a drug has a demonstrated health benefit is if that information is contained in the drug's FDA-approved product labeling. Advertising claims for drugs cannot be made unless research showing that the drug will actually do what a manufacturer claims it will do has been submitted to and approved by the FDA.

2. Rosuvastatin causes abnormal elevations in urine protein and blood that are signals for serious kidney toxicity, and several cases of renal failure have now been reported after its approval; other statins are not associated with this risk of kidney toxicity.

3. Rosuvastatin is the only statin that has shown life-threatening rhabdomyolysis in pre-approval clinical trials, and seven additional cases have occurred after its approval.

Rosuvastatin was approved for use in both the UK and Canada in February 2003, six months before the drug's approval in this country. Through the end of October 2003, cases of kidney failure and rhabdomyolysis have been reported in the UK. In Canada, through September 2003 there had been reports of kidney toxicity in five patients taking rosuvastatin.

In summary, rosuvastatin has no proven health benefit. As discussed above, it has caused potentially serious kidney toxicity that is not seen with the other statins, it is the only statin that caused rhabdomyolysis, a life-threatening adverse drug reaction, in preapproval clinical trials, and there are already three statins on the market that are safer than

rosuvastatin and have demonstrated a health benefit to patients.

Other Drugs for High Cholesterol

Niacin Extended [intermediate] Release
NIASPAN (KOS)

GENERIC: not available

FAMILY: Other Drugs for High Cholesterol

PREGNANCY WARNING

Animal studies have not been done. However, because of the potential for serious adverse effects to the fetus, Niaspan should not be used by pregnant women.

BREAST-FEEDING WARNING

Niacin is excreted in human milk. Because of the potential for serious adverse effects in nursing infants, you should not take Niaspan while nursing.

Niacin intermediate-release tablets contain niacin, one of the B-complex family of vitamins. Niacin is also known as nicotinic acid or vitamin B_3. Niacin in proper doses reduces total cholesterol (TC), low-density lipoprotein cholesterol (LDL-C), and triglycerides (TG), and increases high-density lipoprotein cholesterol (HDL-C).[99]

Niacin intermediate-release tablets are approved by the FDA to reduce cholesterol and to reduce the risk of recurrent nonfatal heart attack in patients with a history of a previous heart attack and elevated cholesterol levels. Niacin and other cholesterol-lowering drugs are approved as an adjunct to diet when the response to a diet restricted in saturated fat and cholesterol and other nondrug measures alone have been inadequate.[99]

Niacin's ability to reduce mortality and the risk of nonfatal heart attack was shown in the Coronary Drug Project,[100] completed in 1975. This study was designed to assess the safety and efficacy of niacin and other lipid-altering

WARNING

NIASPAN preparations should not simply be substituted for equivalent doses of immediate-release (crystalline) niacin. For patients switching from immediate-release niacin to NIASPAN, therapy with NIASPAN should be initiated with low doses (i.e., 500 milligrams at bedtime), and the NIASPAN dose should then be titrated to the desired therapeutic response.

LIVER DYSFUNCTION

Cases of severe hepatic (liver) toxicity, including widespread destruction of liver cells, have occurred in patients who have substituted sustained-release (modified-release, timed-release, extended-release) niacin products for immediate-release (crystalline) niacin at equivalent doses.

NIASPAN should be used with caution in patients who consume substantial quantities of alcohol and/or have a past history of liver disease. Active liver diseases or unexplained transaminase elevations are contraindications to the use of NIASPAN.

Any person with elevated LDL cholesterol or other form of elevated blood fats (hyperlipidemia) should undergo medical evaluation to rule out other causes before drug treatment is begun.

Secondary causes include:
• diabetes
• hypothyroidism (low thyroid activity)
• chronic kidney failure
• drugs that increase LDL cholesterol and decrease HDL cholesterol: progestins, anabolic steroids, and corticosteroids[84]

---

drugs in men 30 to 64 years old with a history of a previous heart attack. Over an observation period of 5 years, niacin treatment was associated with a statistically significant reduction in nonfatal, recurrent heart attacks. The incidence of nonfatal heart attack was 8.9% for the 1,119 patients randomized to niacin versus 12.2% for the 2,789 patients who received a placebo. This is an absolute risk difference of 3.3%, which means that 30 patients would need to be treated with niacin for 5 years to prevent one nonfatal heart attack. Total mortality was similar in the two groups at 5 years (24.4% with niacin versus 25.4% in those taking the placebo).[99]

Sustained-release forms of niacin (lasting longer in the body than intermediate-release Niaspan) are available as unregulated dietary supplements, have not been approved for lowering cholesterol, and should not be used. Also called extended-release, modified-release, or time-released, these forms of niacin can have occurrences of severe liver toxicity that can lead to liver failure. This is much less of a problem with Niaspan, available only on prescription, which is released into the blood at a rate between the immediate- and extended-release forms.

Liver function tests should be performed on all patients during therapy with Niaspan. These tests should be conducted before treatment begins, every 6 to 12 weeks for the first year of treatment, and periodically thereafter, for example at approximately 6-month intervals. If the liver function tests show evidence of progression, particularly if they rise to three times the upper limit of normal or are associated with the symptoms of liver toxicity—nausea, fever, and/or malaise—Niaspan should be stopped.

Flushing is a common adverse effect of niacin treatment that usually subsides after several weeks of consistent niacin use. Flushing may vary in severity, may last for several hours after dosing, and will, if Niaspan is taken at bedtime, most likely occur during sleep. If you are awakened by flushing at night, get up slowly, especially if you feel dizzy, feel faint, or are

taking blood-pressure-lowering medications. Taking aspirin approximately 30 minutes before taking Niaspan or a nonsteroidal anti-inflammatory drug (NSAID) such as ibuprofen (MOTRIN) may minimize the flushing.[99]

Before You Take This Drug

Do not use if you have or have had:

- allergies to niacin or niacinamide
- bleeding
- liver problems
- pregnancy or are breast-feeding
- peptic ulcer

Tell your doctor if you have or have had:

- low blood pressure
- diabetes
- glaucoma
- gout
- history of liver problems
- kidney disease

Tell your doctor about any other drugs you take, including herbs, over-the-counter medications, and other vitamins.

When You Use This Drug

- Avoid alcohol and hot liquids around the time of taking niacin to reduce flushing.
- Consider additional soluble fiber to lower cholesterol, such as hydroxypropylmethylcellulose, oats, or psyllium, as well as spreads with plant sterols.
- Lose weight if indicated.
- Stop smoking.
- Exercise regularly, such as aerobic exercise, running, or walking.
- Reduce stress.
- Check with your doctor before you stop taking the drug.
- If you develop dizziness, feel faint, also take medications to lower blood pressure, or

awaken due to flushing, then change positions gradually from lying down to sitting, and sitting to standing.
- If you are diabetic and your blood glucose increases while taking niacin, notify your doctor.
- Tell any doctor, dentist, emergency help, or pharmacist you see that you use extended-release niacin.

How to Use This Drug

- If you miss a dose, take it as soon as possible, unless it is almost time for the next dose. **Do not take double doses.**
- Do not share your drug with others.
- Take the drug at the same time(s) each day.
- Swallow tablets whole with milk, in the middle of a meal, or after a low-fat snack to prevent upset stomach. Do not take on an empty stomach.
- Extended-release capsules may be opened and the contents mixed with applesauce, jelly, or ketchup, then swallowed without chewing.
- Do not drink alcohol or hot liquids (such as coffee) with or immediately following taking niacin to reduce possibility of flushing.
- To minimize flushing, take aspirin or a nonsteroidal anti-inflammatory drug (NSAID) about 30 minutes before extended-release niacin.
- Store tablets at room temperature with the lid on tightly. Do not expose to heat, moisture, or strong light. Keep out of reach of children.
- Take exactly as ordered by your doctor.

Interactions with Other Drugs

The following drugs, biologics (e.g., vaccines, therapeutic antibodies), or foods are listed in *Evaluations of Drug Interactions* 2003 as causing "highly clinically significant" or "clinically significant" interactions when used together with any of the drugs in this section. In some sections with multiple drugs, the interaction may have been reported for one but not all drugs in this section, but we include the interaction because the drugs in this section are similar to one another. We have also included potentially serious interactions listed in the drug's FDA-approved professional package insert or in published medical journal articles. There may be other drugs, especially those in the families of drugs listed below, that also will react with this drug to cause severe adverse effects. Make sure to tell your doctor and pharmacist the drugs you are taking and tell them if you are taking any of these interacting drugs:

Niacin used with statins has been reported to increase risk of rhabdomyolysis, a condition of destruction of skeletal muscle that can be fatal, and acute kidney failure. If used together, careful monitoring should be done for muscle pain, tenderness, or weakness: ALTOCOR, atorvastatin, CRESTOR, fluvastatin, LIPITOR, lovastatin, MEVACOR, PRAVACHOL, pravastatin, rosuvastatin, simvastatin, ZOCOR.

The effect of niacin may be reduced by: ACTIGALL, chenodiol, ursodiol.

Niacin may add to the effects of vasoactive drugs: adrenergic blocking agents, calcium channel blockers, nitrates, nitroglycerin.

Niacin increase of HDL may be blocked by antioxidants:[101] Avoid especially combinations and high doses of: betacarotene, probucol, selenium, vitamin C, vitamin E.

Niacin interactions can be beneficially used to reduce the severity of flushing: aspirin 325 milligrams before each niacin dose, or one aspirin before breakfast for 14 days.

Adverse Effects

Call your doctor immediately if you experience:

- appetite decrease
- severe stomach pain
- yellow eyes
- itchy, rashy, or yellowish skin
- light gray stools
- dark urine
- wheezing (occurs more with injection)

Call your doctor if these symptoms continue:

- feeling of warmth
- flushing or red skin
- headache
- stomachache
- rash
- stuffy nose, runny nose, sneezing
- irregular heartbeat
- diarrhea
- dizziness or faintness
- dry skin or eyes
- frequent urination or unusual thirst
- joint, side, or lower back pain
- swelling of feet or lower legs
- muscle ache
- unusual tiredness
- nausea or vomiting

Periodic Testing

Ask your doctor which of these tests should be done periodically while you are taking this drug:

- cholesterol
- blood glucose, phosphorus, or potassium
- kidney function
- liver function
- prothrombin time (blood clotting)
- uric acid

Do Not Use Until Seven Years After Release

Ezetimibe (eh *zet* i meeb)
(Do Not Use Until 2009)
ZETIA (Merck/Schering Plough)

GENERIC: not available

FAMILY: Other Drugs for High Cholesterol

PREGNANCY WARNING

Ezetimibe crossed the placenta and caused an increase in misshapen skeletons in animal studies. Because of the potential for serious adverse effects to the fetus, ezetimibe should not be used by pregnant women.

BREAST-FEEDING WARNING

Ezetimibe is excreted in animal milk. It is likely that this drug, like many others, is also excreted in human milk and, because of the potential for serious adverse effects in nursing infants, you should not take ezetimibe while nursing.

Ezetimibe is a drug that lowers cholesterol. It is approved to treat high cholesterol due to high low-density lipoprotein cholesterol (LDL-C), due to heredity, or due to high blood levels of sitosterol and campesterol.[102] Ezetimibe belongs to a new class of drugs called azetidinones.

All cholesterol-lowering drugs are intended to be part of a therapy that also includes a diet low in saturated fat and cholesterol, and exercise. Drugs should be prescribed only after diet alone proves inadequate.

Ezetimibe works by partially blocking the absorption of cholesterol in the small intestine.[94] If you have moderate to severe liver disease you should not use ezetimibe.[103] Unlike the statin drugs (see p. 109), ezetimibe does not lower production of cholesterol by your liver. In fact, your liver may compensate by increasing cholesterol production, yet overall LDL declines. Although ezetimibe lowers cholesterol levels, there is no evidence that it reduces the risk of heart attacks or strokes.

Ezetimibe also enhances lowering of cholesterol when used with some other cholesterol-lowering drugs, such as statins.[104–107] However, adding ezetimibe to statins increases the risk of serious liver adverse events compared with either drug used alone.[159] Ezetimibe should not be used with fibric acid drugs such as gemfibrozil (LOPID) and fenofibrate (TRICOR).

If you take ezetimibe with other cholesterol-lowering drugs, these drugs have contraindications, warnings, and adverse effects that must be considered in addition to ones for ezetimibe (see Cholesterol-Lowering Drugs, p. 55).

Before You Take This Drug

Tell your doctor if you have or have had:

- allergies
- heart problems
- liver problems
- muscle pain, tenderness, or weakness
- pregnancy or are breast-feeding

Tell your doctor about any other drugs you take, including herbs, over-the-counter drugs, progestins, steroids, and vitamins.

While You Take This Drug

- Eat a diet low in saturated fats and cholesterol, such as the Step 1 diet of the National Cholesterol Education Program. Eat whole grains, legumes, fruits, vegetables, nuts, and fish. Limit cholesterol to 100 milligrams per day, fat to 20% of calories, and saturated fats to 6% of diet. Limit soluble fibers.
- Exercise regularly.
- Tell your doctor if you plan to become pregnant.
- Tell any doctor, dentist, or pharmacist you see that you take this drug.

How to Use This Drug

- If you miss a dose of ezetimibe, take it as soon as possible, but do not take two doses during the same day. **Do not take double doses.**
- Do not share your medication with others.

- Take the drug at the same time(s) each day.
- Swallow tablets with or without food.
- Take ezetimibe at least two hours before or four hours after any bile acid sequestrant.
- Store tablets at room temperature with lid on tightly. Do not store in the bathroom. Do not expose to heat, moisture, or strong light. Keep out of reach of children.

Interactions with Other Drugs

The following drugs, biologics (e.g., vaccines, therapeutic antibodies), or foods are listed in *Evaluations of Drug Interactions* 2003 as causing "highly clinically significant" or "clinically significant" interactions when used together with any of the drugs in this section. In some sections with multiple drugs, the interaction may have been reported for one but not all drugs in this section, but we include the interaction because the drugs in this section are similar to one another. We have also included potentially serious interactions listed in the drug's FDA-approved professional package insert or in published medical journal articles. There may be other drugs, especially those in the families of drugs listed below, that also will react with this drug to cause severe adverse effects. Make sure to tell your doctor and pharmacist the drugs you are taking and tell them if you are taking any of these interacting drugs:

Risk of gall bladder disease could increase if ezetimibe is taken with: fenofibrate, fibric acid, gemfibrozil, LOFIBRA, LOPID, TRICOR.

Bile acid sequestrants interfere with absorption of ezetimibe. Take ezetimibe at least two hours before or four hours after: cholestyramine, COLESTID, colestipol, PREVALITE, QUESTRAN, WELCHOL.

If you use ezetimibe with this drug, your doctor should monitor you closely: cyclosporine, SANDIMMUNE.

Adverse Effects

Call your doctor immediately if you experience:

- large, hive-like swelling on face, lips, eyelids, tongue, throat, hands, legs, feet, sex organs
- Skin rash

Call your doctor if these symptoms continue:

- dizziness
- pain in abdomen, back, chest, joints, or stomach
- muscle pain
- chest pain
- trouble breathing
- trouble swallowing
- hoarseness
- dry or sore throat
- chills or fever
- cold symptoms, such as congested sinus or runny nose
- coughing
- diarrhea
- fatigue
- headache

Other adverse effects are possible, especially if you take additional drugs. Check any concerns with your doctor.

Periodic Testing

Ask your doctor which of these tests should be done periodically while you are taking this drug:

- cholesterol levels (especially LDL and total cholesterol)
- liver function tests (ALT or AST)

Limited Use

Cholestyramine (coal es *tire* am ene)
LOCHOLEST (Eon)
QUESTRAN, QUESTRAN LIGHT
(Bristol-Myers Squibb)

GENERIC: not available

FAMILY: Other Drugs for High Cholesterol

PREGNANCY WARNING

Cholestyramine is known to interfere with the absorption of fat-soluble vitamins, and even vitamin supplementation may not be adequate. Because of the potential for serious adverse effects to the fetus, this drug should not be used by pregnant women.

BREAST-FEEDING WARNING

Because the lack of proper vitamin absorption by the mother could have a harmful effect on a nursing infant, you should not take cholestyramine while nursing.

Cholestyramine was first marketed in the U.S. in 1973. It is used primarily to lower cholesterol, specifically low-density lipoprotein (LDL). It works by binding bile acid in the intestines and therefore increasing the breakdown of cholesterol in the body. In middle-aged people it is clear that lowering cholesterol lessens the risk of coronary artery disease, but no cholesterol-lowering drug has been shown to lower overall death rates in this age group. In older adults the extent to which higher cholesterol levels contribute to heart disease and should be treated with drugs is much less clear. Cholestyramine helps control high cholesterol, but does not cure the condition. Besides removing cholesterol, cholestyramine may remove needed nutrients and medicines from your body, and actually increase triglycerides.[108] People over age 60 and those who take high doses are more likely to experience harmful effects from cholestyramine.

The first, safer, and less costly measure to lower cholesterol for people under 70 is to eat a low-fat diet, using mostly polyunsaturated fats (such as canola, corn, safflower, and sunflower oils) or monounsaturated fats (such as olive oil). A change from animal to vegetable proteins often corrects high cholesterol. However, it is inadvisable to go on a very low-fat diet. The main focus on cholesterol-lowering diets has been on saturated fat and cholesterol content, not soluble fiber. (When added to the diet, psyllium or oat bran is a safe, effective way of lowering cholesterol.) Exercise and weight reduction are also recommended. Conditions that aggravate high cholesterol, such as dependence on alcohol or tobacco, diabetes, high blood pressure, low magnesium or potassium, and thyroid disease should be corrected before adding a cholesterol-reducing drug. If cholesterol remains high despite diet, add 10 grams of psyllium a day (see p. 566).

Before You Use This Drug

Do not use if you have or have had:

- complete biliary obstruction
- constipation

Tell your doctor if you have or have had:

- allergies to drugs
- bleeding disorders
- chronic constipation or other gastrointestinal problems
- diabetes
- gallbladder problems
- heart, kidney, or liver problems
- hemorrhoids
- osteoporosis
- phenylketonuria (PKU)
- thyroid disorder
- gastrointestinal ulcers
- pregnancy or are breast-feeding (impaired absorption of vitamins and nutrients)

Tell your doctor about any other drugs you take, including aspirin, herbs, vitamins, and other nonprescription products. When taking cholestyramine it is important that your doctor knows all the drugs you take.

When You Use This Drug

• Tell any other doctor, dentist, nurse practitioner, or surgeon you see that you take cholestyramine.

• Tell your doctor whenever you start any new medication.

• If you take other medications, check with your doctor.

• Continue to follow a low-fat diet.

• Avoid constipation. Increase your fiber with more bran, fluids, fruits, or psyllium. If constipation persists, try a stool softener.

How to Use This Drug

• If you miss a dose, take it as soon as you remember but skip it if it is almost time for the next dose. **Do not take double doses.**

• Do not share your medication with others.

• Take the drug at the same time(s) each day.

• Take cholestyramine within half an hour of meals,[109] preferably before meals.[110]

• If you take the bar form of cholestyramine, chew thoroughly before swallowing. Drink plenty of fluids.

• If you take the powder form of cholestyramine, measure the dose, unless you use premeasured packets. The color of the powder varies from batch to batch. Never swallow the dry form, but mix the powder in two or more ounces of water, milk, or apple or orange juice. Stir vigorously, then shake. However, the mixture will not dissolve. To further improve flavor, try stirring in a heavy fruit juice or pulpy fruits (applesauce, fruit cocktail, crushed pineapple), thin soups, or mix it with milk in cold or hot cereal. Chilling the mixture may aid the flavor. If you use a carbonated beverage, stir slowly to reduce foaming. Avoid taking with highly acidic drinks, such as Kool-Aid.[111] Swallow immediately. Do not hold or swish the mixture in your mouth.[111] To be sure all the medication is taken, rinse the container thoroughly and drink the remaining contents.

• If you take any other medications, separate the times as far apart from cholestyramine as possible, but at least one hour before you take the cholestyramine, or four to eight hours after you take the cholestyramine.

• Store at room temperature with the lid of bulk powder closed tightly.

• Do not store in the bathroom. Do not expose to heat, moisture, or strong light. Keep out of reach of children.

Interactions with Other Drugs

The following drugs, biologics (e.g., vaccines, therapeutic antibodies), or foods are listed in *Evaluations of Drug Interactions* 2003 as causing "highly clinically significant" or "clinically significant" interactions when used together with any of the drugs in this section. In some sections with multiple drugs, the interaction may have been reported for one but not all drugs in this section, but we include the interaction because the drugs in this section are similar to one another. We have also included potentially serious interactions listed in the drug's FDA-approved professional package insert or in published medical journal articles. There may be other drugs, especially those in the families of drugs listed below, that also will react with this drug to cause severe adverse effects. Make sure to tell your doctor and pharmacist the drugs you are taking and tell them if you are taking any of these interacting drugs:

ARAVA, CELLCEPT, COUMADIN, CRYSTODIGIN, digitoxin, EVISTA, furosemide, glipizide, GLUCOTROL, LASIX, leflunomide, mycophenolate, raloxifene, THYROID STRONG, warfarin.

If you stop taking cholestyramine, your doctor will again review doses of your other drugs. Serious harm may occur if you stop taking cholestyramine while taking other medicines.

Adverse Effects

Call your doctor immediately if you experience:

- unusual bleeding or bruising
- black, tarry stools
- constipation
- severe stomach pain with nausea and vomiting
- sudden weight loss

Call your doctor if these symptoms continue:

- belching or hiccups
- bloating
- diarrhea
- dizziness
- headache
- heartburn, indigestion, stomach pain
- irritation of skin, tongue, or anal area
- nausea or vomiting

Periodic Testing

Ask your doctor which of these tests should be done periodically while you are taking this drug:

- blood calcium, cholesterol, and triglyceride levels
- prothrombin time
- blood pressure

Abnormal Heart Rhythm

Limited Use

Disopyramide (dye soe *peer* a mide)
NORPACE (Searle)

GENERIC: available

FAMILY: Drugs for Abnormal Heart Rhythm

PREGNANCY WARNING

This drug caused harm to developing fetuses in animal studies, including decreased implantation, growth, and survival. Use during pregnancy only for clear medical reasons. Tell your doctor if you are pregnant or thinking of becoming pregnant before you take this drug.

BREAST-FEEDING WARNING

Disopyramide is excreted in human milk. Because of the potential for serious adverse effects in nursing infants, you should not take this drug while nursing.

FDA BLACK BOX WARNING

When this drug was used to treat rhythm disturbances of the small chambers of the heart (atria), it provided no survival advantage and a higher risk of serious adverse effects than older drugs such as digoxin (see p. 144), the beta-blockers (see p. 87), and the calcium channel blockers diltiazem and verapamil (see p. 97).[112, 113]

This drug is not approved by the FDA to treat rhythm disturbances of the atria.

ANTICHOLINERGIC EFFECTS

WARNING: SPECIAL MENTAL AND PHYSICAL ADVERSE EFFECTS

Older adults are especially sensitive to the harmful anticholinergic (see Glossary, p. 889), effects of disopyramide. Drugs in this family should not be used unless absolutely necessary.

Mental Effects: confusion, delirium, short-term memory problems, disorientation, and impaired attention

Physical Effects: dry mouth, constipation, difficulty urinating (especially for a man with an enlarged prostate), blurred vision, decreased sweating with increased body temperature, sexual dysfunction, and worsening of glaucoma

---

WARNING! INCREASED RISK OF DEATH

In the National Heart, Lung, and Blood Institute's Cardiac Arrhythmia Suppression Trial (CAST) (a long-term, multicentered, randomized, double-blind study), in patients with asymptomatic non-life-threatening ventricular (the large chambers of the heart) arrhythmias (rhythm disturbances) who had a heart attack more than six days but less than two years previous, deaths or nonfatal cardiac arrest were seen in 7.7% of those patients treated with encainide or flecainide, members of the Class 1 group of antiarrhythmic drugs, compared to 3.0% in patients receiving an inactive sugar pill or placebo.

Because of the known ability of the Class 1 drugs, such as quinidine, to cause rhythm disturbances, and the lack of evidence of improved survival for any antiarrhythmic drug in patients without life-threatening heart rhythm disturbances, the use of the Class 1 drugs should be reserved for patients with life-threatening rhythm disturbances of the ventricles. These warnings now appear in the FDA-approved product labeling, or package insert, for all Class 1 drugs, including: disopyramide (NORPACE and generics), flecainide (TAMBOCOR), mexiletine (MEXITIL and generics), moricizine (ETHMOZINE), procainamide (PROCANBID and generics), propafenone (RYTHMOL), quinidine (DURAQUIN, QUINAGLUTE DURA-TABS, QUINIDEX, and generics), and tocainide (TONOCARD).

Disopyramide slows the heart rate and stabilizes irregular heartbeats (arrhythmias).

Disopyramide is linked to a high incidence of congestive heart failure and problems with urination, so people with these medical problems should not use the drug. [15] Since there is a narrow range between a helpful and a harmful amount of this drug in your body, call your doctor immediately if you experience these adverse effects or any of those listed under Adverse Effects. **If you have decreased kidney function, you should be taking less than the usual dose of disopyramide.**[15]

Many people who are taking disopyramide or another drug in its family have relatively mild disturbances in their heart rhythm and no symptoms of underlying heart disease. The vast majority of these people do not need these drugs, and there is no evidence that using them improves health. In fact, most of the drugs in this family have severe adverse effects that are sometimes worse and even more life-threatening than the irregular heartbeats they treat. All of these drugs can also cause new irregularities in your heartbeat.

If you have an irregular heartbeat without any symptoms of underlying heart disease, you should not be exposed to the dangers of a drug that has no health benefit for your condition.[114] If you are taking disopyramide or another drug in its family for an irregular heartbeat (arrhythmia), talk to your doctor and find out whether you also have symptoms of underlying heart disease. If not, discuss the possibility of stopping the drug.

Disopyramide remains on a well-recognized list of drugs that are inappropriate for use in older adults because it may induce heart failure in older adults and is strongly anticholinergic.[115]

Before You Use This Drug

Do not use if you have or have had:

- complete heart block
- shock due to heart failure
- QT interval prolongation (congenital)

Tell your doctor if you have or have had:

- allergies to drugs
- diabetes
- any heart problems

- enlarged prostate gland
- glaucoma
- kidney function impairment
- liver function impairment
- too much or too little blood potassium or magnesium
- myasthenia gravis
- urinary obstruction
- pregnancy or are breast-feeding
- low blood pressure

Tell your doctor about any other drugs you take, including aspirin, herbs, vitamins, and other nonprescription products.

When You Use This Drug

- Until you know how you react to this drug, do not drive or perform other activities requiring alertness. Disopyramide may cause dizziness.
- You may feel dizzy when rising from a lying or sitting position. When getting out of bed, hang your legs over the side of the bed for a few minutes, then get up slowly. When getting up from a chair, get up slowly and stay beside the chair until you are sure that you are not dizzy. (See p. 13.)
- Notify your physician and take sugar if symptoms of low blood sugar appear.
- Take precautions during exercise or hot weather because of possible reduced sweating.
- **Do not stop taking this drug suddenly. Your doctor must give you a schedule to lower your dose gradually, to prevent serious changes in heart function.**
- Wear a medical identification bracelet or carry a card stating that you take this drug.
- If you plan to have any surgery, including dental, tell your doctor that you take this drug.

How to Use This Drug

- If you miss a dose, take it as soon as you remember, but skip it if it is less than four hours (eight hours if you are taking extended-release capsules) until your next scheduled dose. **Do not take double doses.**
- Do not share your medication with others.
- Take the drug at the same time(s) each day.
- Take with food or milk.
- Swallow extended-release tablets whole. Do not crush or break.
- Store at room temperature with lid on tightly. Do not store in the bathroom. Do not expose to heat, moisture, or strong light. Keep out of reach of children.

Interactions with Other Drugs

The following drugs, biologics (e.g., vaccines, therapeutic antibodies), or foods are listed in *Evaluations of Drug Interactions* 2003 as causing "highly clinically significant" or "clinically significant" interactions when used together with any of the drugs in this section. In some sections with multiple drugs, the interaction may have been reported for one but not all drugs in this section, but we include the interaction because the drugs in this section are similar to one another. We have also included potentially serious interactions listed in the drug's FDA-approved professional package insert or in published medical journal articles. There may be other drugs, especially those in the families of drugs listed below, that also will react with this drug to cause severe adverse effects. Make sure to tell your doctor and pharmacist the drugs you are taking and tell them if you are taking any of these interacting drugs:

AVELOX, BETAPACE, charcoal, DILANTIN, EES, ERYTHROCIN, erythromycin, halofantrine, ISORDIL, isosorbide dinitrate, mizolastine, moxifloxacin, NORVIR, ORAP, phenytoin, pimozide, PRIFTIN, rifapentine, ritonavir, SORBITRATE, sotalol, sparfloxacin, ZAGAM, zotepine.

Adverse Effects

Call your doctor immediately if you experience:

- difficulty urinating
- chest pains
- confusion
- dizziness, lightheadedness, or fainting
- unusual tiredness
- muscle weakness
- shortness of breath
- swelling of feet or lower legs
- unusually fast or slow heartbeat
- rapid weight gain
- rash and/or itching
- enlargement of breasts in men
- nosebleeds or bleeding gums
- depression
- sore throat and fever
- yellow eyes and skin
- signs of low blood sugar: anxious feeling, chills, cold sweats, confusion, cool pale skin, drowsiness, headache, excessive hunger, nausea, nervousness, rapid heartbeat, shakiness, unsteady walk, unusual tiredness or weakness

Call your doctor if these symptoms continue:

- dry mouth, throat, eyes, or nose (relieve by sucking ice or chewing sugarless gum)
- bloating or stomach pain
- blurred vision
- decreased sexual ability
- loss of appetite
- nausea
- nervousness
- frequent urge to urinate
- constipation
- diarrhea
- headache
- trouble sleeping

Periodic Tests

Ask your doctor which of these tests should be done periodically while you are taking this drug:

- blood pressure
- heart function tests, such as electrocardiogram (ECG, EKG)
- kidney function tests
- liver function tests
- blood levels of glucose and potassium
- eye pressure exams

Limited Use

Procainamide (proe *kane* a mide)
PROCANBID (King)

GENERIC: available

FAMILY: Drugs for Abnormal Heart Rhythm

PREGNANCY WARNING

Animal studies were not done. However, because of the potential for serious adverse effects to the fetus (see boxes below), procainamide should not be used by pregnant women.

BREAST-FEEDING WARNING

Procainamide is excreted in human milk and absorbed by the nursing infant. Because of the potential for serious adverse effects in nursing infants, you should not take this drug while nursing.

FDA BLACK BOX WARNING

Positive ANA Titer: The prolonged administration of procainamide often leads to the development of a positive antinuclear antibody (ANA) test, with or without symptoms of lupus erythematosus-like syndrome. If a positive ANA titer develops, the benefits versus risks of continued procainamide therapy should be assessed.

FDA BLACK BOX WARNING
BLOOD DYSCRASIAS
(DISORDERS)

Agranulocytosis, bone marrow depression, neutropenia, hypoplastic anemia, and thrombocytopenia have been reported in patients receiving procainamide hydrochloride at a rate of approximately 0.5%. Most patients received procainamide hydrochloride within the recommended dosage range. Fatalities have occurred (with approximately 20–25% mortality in reported cases of agranulocytosis). Since most of these events have been noted during the first 12 weeks of therapy, it is recommended that complete blood counts, including white cell, differential, and platelet counts, be performed at weekly intervals for the first 3 months of therapy, and periodically thereafter. Complete blood counts should be performed promptly if the patient develops any signs of infection (such as fever, chills, sore throat, or stomatitis), bruising, or bleeding. If any of these hematologic disorders are identified, procainamide hydrochloride should be discontinued. Blood counts usually return to normal within 1 month of discontinuation. Caution should be used in patients with preexisting marrow failure or cytopenia of any type.

WARNING

When this drug was used to treat rhythm disturbances of the small chambers of the heart (atria), it provided no survival advantage and a higher risk of serious adverse effects than older drugs such as digoxin (see p. 144), the beta-blockers (see p. 87), and the calcium channel blockers diltiazem and verapamil (see p. 97).[112, 113]

This drug is not approved by the FDA to treat rhythm disturbances of the atria.

Procainamide slows the heart rate and stabilizes irregular heartbeats (arrhythmias) of the large chambers of the heart (ventricles). Since this drug frequently causes a disease called lupus erythematosus, as well as other adverse effects, it is not the best choice for long-term treatment of irregular heartbeats. **If your kidney or liver function is impaired, you should be taking less than the usual dose.**[116]

Many people who are taking procainamide or another drug in its family have relatively mild disturbances in their heart rhythm and no symptoms of underlying heart disease. The vast majority of these people do not need these drugs, and there is no evidence that using them improves health. In fact, most of the drugs in this family have severe adverse effects that are sometimes worse and even more life-threatening than the irregular heartbeats they treat. All of these drugs can also cause new irregularities in your heartbeat.

If you have an irregular heartbeat without any symptoms of underlying heart disease, you should not be exposed to the dangers of a drug that has no health benefit for your condition.[114] If you are taking procainamide or another drug in its family for an irregular heartbeat (arrhythmia), talk to your doctor and find out whether you also have symptoms of underlying heart disease. If not, discuss the possibility of stopping the drug.

Since there is a narrow range between a helpful and a harmful amount of this drug in your body, call your doctor immediately if you experience adverse effects (see Adverse Effects).

Before You Use This Drug

Do not use if you have or have had:

- complete heart block
- digitalis toxicity with heart block
- a particular heart arrhythmia called Torsades de pointes

Tell your doctor if you have or have had:

- allergies to drugs
- asthma or emphysema

WARNING! INCREASED RISK OF DEATH

In the National Heart, Lung, and Blood Institute's Cardiac Arrhythmia Suppression Trial (CAST) (a long-term, multicentered, randomized, double-blind study), in patients with asymptomatic non-life-threatening ventricular (the large chambers of the heart) arrhythmias (rhythm disturbances) who had a heart attack more than six days but less than two years previous, deaths or nonfatal cardiac arrest were seen in 7.7% of those patients treated with encainide or flecainide, members of the Class 1 group of antiarrhythmic drugs, compared to 3.0% in patients receiving an inactive sugar pill or placebo.

Because of the known ability of the Class 1 drugs, such as quinidine, to cause rhythm disturbances, and the lack of evidence of improved survival for any antiarrhythmic drug in patients without life-threatening heart rhythm disturbances, the use of the Class 1 drugs should be reserved for patients with life-threatening rhythm disturbances of the ventricles. These warnings now appear in the FDA-approved product labeling, or package insert, for all Class 1 drugs, including: disopyramide (NORPACE and generics), flecainide (TAMBOCOR), mexiletine (MEXITIL and generics), moricizine (ETHMOZINE), procainamide (PROCANBID and generics), propafenone (RYTHMOL), quinidine (DURAQUIN, QUINAGLUTE DURA-TABS, QUINIDEX, and generics), and tocainide (TONOCARD).

- digitalis toxicity
- incomplete heart block or other heart problems
- kidney or liver problems
- lupus erythematosus
- myasthenia gravis
- pregnancy or are breast feeding

Tell your doctor about any other drugs you take, including aspirin, herbs, vitamins, and other nonprescription products.

When You Use This Drug

- Until you know how you react to this drug, do not drive or perform other activities requiring alertness. Procainamide may cause dizziness.
- **Do not stop taking this drug suddenly. Your doctor must give you a schedule to lower your dose gradually, to prevent serious changes in heart function.**
- Wear a medical identification bracelet or carry a card stating that you take procainamide.
- If you plan to have any surgery, including dental, tell your doctor that you take this drug.

How to Use This Drug

- If you miss a dose, take it as soon as you remember, but skip it if it is less than two hours until your next scheduled dose. **Do not take double doses.**
- Do not share your medication with others.
- Take the drug at the same time(s) each day.
- Take with food or milk.
- Swallow extended-release tablets whole. Do not crush or break them.
- Store at room temperature with the lid on tightly. Do not store in the bathroom. Do not expose to heat, moisture, or strong light. Keep out of reach of children.

Interactions with Other Drugs

The following drugs, biologics (e.g., vaccines, therapeutic antibodies), or foods are listed in *Evaluations of Drug Interactions* 2003 as causing "highly clinically significant" or "clinically significant" interactions when used together with any of the drugs in this section. In some sections with multiple drugs, the interaction may have been reported for one but not all drugs in this section, but we include the interaction because the drugs in this section are similar to one another. We have also included potentially serious interactions listed in the drug's FDA-approved professional package insert or in published medical journal articles. There may be other drugs, especially those in the families of drugs listed below, that also will react with this drug to cause severe adverse effects. Make sure to tell your doctor and pharmacist the drugs you are taking and tell them if you are taking any of these interacting drugs:

amiodarone, AVELOX, BETAPACE, cimetidine, CORDARONE, cyclosporine, GLUCOVANCE, halofantrine, metformin, mizolastine, moxifloxacin, NEORAL, ORAP, pimozide, sotalol, SANDIMMUNE, sparfloxacin, TAGAMET, ZAGAM, zotepine.

Adverse Effects

Call your doctor immediately if you experience:

- **signs of lupuslike syndrome:** fever, chills, joint pain or swelling, pain with breathing, skin rash or itching
- hallucinations
- depression
- sore mouth, gums, or throat
- unusual bleeding or bruising
- unusual tiredness or weakness

Call your doctor if these symptoms continue:

- diarrhea
- loss of appetite
- dizziness or lightheadedness

Signs of overdose:

- confusion, dizziness, fainting
- drowsiness
- nausea and vomiting
- unusual decrease in urination
- unusually fast or irregular heartbeat

If you suspect an overdose, call this number to contact your poison control center: (800) 222-1222.

Periodic Tests

Ask your doctor which of these tests should be done periodically while you are taking this drug:

- complete blood count
- heart function tests, such as electrocardiogram (ECG, EKG)
- blood pressure
- liver function tests
- blood levels of procainamide and NAPA (a metabolite of procainamide)
- antinuclear antibody test (if this is positive, ask your doctor about changing your drug, since a positive value is often linked with a lupuslike syndrome)

Limited Use

Mexiletine (mex *ill* et een)
MEXITIL (Boehringer Ingelheim)

GENERIC: not available
FAMILY: Drugs for Abnormal Heart Rhythm

PREGNANCY WARNING

No data is available for mexiletine, as it was not tested properly in animal studies. Use during pregnancy only for clear medical reasons. Tell your doctor if you are pregnant or thinking of becoming pregnant before you take this drug.

BREAST-FEEDING WARNING

Mexiletine is excreted in human milk. Because of the potential for serious adverse effects in nursing infants, you should not take this drug while nursing.

Mexiletine slows rapid heartbeat and stabilizes irregular heartbeats (arrhythmias). Mexiletine prevents recurrence of ventricular arrhythmias, such as premature heartbeats.

WARNING! INCREASED RISK OF DEATH

In the National Heart, Lung, and Blood Institute's Cardiac Arrhythmia Suppression Trial (CAST) (a long-term, multicentered, randomized, double-blind study), in patients with asymptomatic non-life-threatening ventricular (the large chambers of the heart) arrhythmias (rhythm disturbances) who had a heart attack more than six days but less than two years previous, deaths or nonfatal cardiac arrest were seen in 7.7% of those patients treated with encainide or flecainide, members of the Class 1 group of antiarrhythmic drugs, compared to 3.0% in patients receiving an inactive sugar pill or placebo.

Because of the known ability of the Class 1 drugs, such as quinidine, to cause rhythm disturbances, and the lack of evidence of improved survival for any antiarrhythmic drug in patients without life-threatening heart rhythm disturbances, the use of the Class 1 drugs should be reserved for patients with life-threatening rhythm disturbances of the ventricles. These warnings now appear in the FDA-approved product labeling, or package insert, for all Class 1 drugs, including: disopyramide (NORPACE and generics), flecainide (TAMBOCOR), mexiletine (MEXITIL and generics), moricizine (ETHMOZINE), procainamide (PROCANBID and generics), propafenone (RYTHMOL), quinidine (DURAQUIN, QUINAGLUTE DURA-TABS, QUINIDEX, and generics), and tocainide (TONOCARD).

It is as effective as quinidine for some, but not all, arrhythmias[111] and sometimes is used with quinidine.[118] Mexiletine has little risk of organ toxicity but has a high risk of noncardiac adverse effects.[119] However, these adverse effects often cause people to stop taking mexiletine.[117, 118] Lower doses can reduce unwanted effects. People with decreased liver function should take a lower dose. At times mexiletine actually worsens some types of arrhythmias. It is not for use in minor arrhythmias. Use of mexiletine with procainamide (PROCANBID) is of little or no value.[120]

Before You Use This Drug

Do not use if you have or have had:

- cardiogenic shock
- heart block of second or third degree without a pacemaker

Tell your doctor if you have or have had:

- allergies to drugs
- angina
- congestive heart failure[121]
- heart block or other heart problems
- kidney[118] or liver problems

- low blood pressure
- myocardial infarction
- pacemaker
- seizures
- pregnancy or are breast-feeding

Tell your doctor about any other drugs you take, including aspirin, herbs, vitamins, and other nonprescription products.

When You Use This Drug

- Until you know how you react to this drug, do not drive or perform other activities requiring alertness. This drug may cause blurred vision and drowsiness.
- You may feel dizzy when rising from a lying or sitting position. If you are lying down, hang your legs over the side of the bed for a few minutes, then get up slowly. When getting up from a chair, stay by the chair until you are sure that you are not dizzy. (See p. 13.)
- Ask your doctor to recommend exercises suitable to your condition.
- Quit smoking, or at least try to cut down on smoking.
- Carry identification stating that you take mexiletine.

• If you plan to have any surgery, including dental, tell your doctor that you take this drug.

How to Use This Drug

• If you miss a dose, take it as soon as you remember but skip it if it is less than four hours until your next scheduled dose. **Do not take double doses.**
• Do not share your medication with others.
• Take the drug at the same time(s) each day.
• Take with food, milk, or antacids to lessen stomach upset. Space doses evenly apart. Antacids with calcium or magnesium may slow absorption of mexiletine. If you use these antacids, be consistent in usage, and avoid large doses.
• Swallow capsule whole.
• Store at room temperature with lid on firmly. Do not store in the bathroom. Do not expose to heat, moisture, or strong light. Keep out of reach of children.

Interactions with Other Drugs

The following drugs, biologics (e.g., vaccines, therapeutic antibodies), or foods are listed in *Evaluations of Drug Interactions* 2003 as causing "highly clinically significant" or "clinically significant" interactions when used together with any of the drugs in this section. In some sections with multiple drugs, the interaction may have been reported for one but not all drugs in this section, but we include the interaction because the drugs in this section are similar to one another. We have also included potentially serious interactions listed in the drug's FDA-approved professional package insert or in published medical journal articles. There may be other drugs, especially those in the families of drugs listed below, that also will react with this drug to cause severe adverse effects. Make sure to tell your doctor and pharmacist the drugs you are taking and tell them if you are taking any of these interacting drugs:

cimetidine, NORVIR, PRIFTIN, rifapentine, ritonavir, SLO-BID, SLO-PHYLLIN, TAGA-MET, THEO-DUR, theophylline.

Mexiletine intensifies the effect of caffeine. Eliminate or reduce your intake of beverages containing caffeine.

Adverse Effects

Call your doctor immediately if you experience:

• unusual bleeding or bruising
• difficulty breathing
• chest pain
• fainting
• fever, chills
• unusually fast or slow heartbeat
• seizures

Call your doctor if these symptoms continue:

• abdominal pain
• confusion
• constipation
• diarrhea
• depression
• dizziness, lightheadedness
• dry mouth
• headache
• heartburn
• impotence
• nausea, vomiting, loss of appetite
• nervousness
• numbness or tingling of fingers, toes
• pain in joints
• ringing in ears
• skin rash, yellowing of skin
• problems sleeping
• slurred speech
• swelling of hands or feet
• trembling or shaking of hands

- unsteadiness, trouble walking
- unusual tiredness or weakness
- decrease in urination
- blurred vision

Periodic Tests

Ask your doctor which of these tests should be done periodically while you are taking this drug:

- blood pressure
- blood mexiletine levels
- electrocardiogram (ECG, EKG)
- liver function tests

Last Choice

Amiodarone (am ee *oh* da rone)
CORDARONE (Wyeth)
PACERONE (Upsher-Smith)

GENERIC: available
FAMILY: Drugs for Abnormal Heart Rhythm

PREGNANCY WARNING
Amiodarone caused malfunctioning thyroids in human infants. Amiodarone also caused malformations in animal studies. This drug should not be used by pregnant women.

BREAST-FEEDING WARNING
Amiodarone is excreted in human milk. Because of the potential for serious adverse effects in nursing infants, you should not take this drug while nursing.

Amiodarone is used to treat and prevent life-threatening irregular heartbeats, especially ventricular arrhythmias. It should be used only when other drugs or devices are ineffective or cannot be tolerated. It is best to start amiodarone in a hospital.

Amiodarone accumulates in the body, leading to a substantial number of potential adverse effects. More than 80% of people who take amiodarone experience adverse, sometimes fatal, effects. Amiodarone can cause toxic reactions in the liver, lung, thyroid, and, ironically, the heart. People with advanced heart failure who take amiodarone are at extremely high risk for early sudden death.[122] Changes in vision are common.[123] Women are more prone to adverse effects. So are those who develop low potassium. Injectable amiodarone can lower the blood pressure too much. Older people may be more sensitive to adverse effects on the thyroid,[124] while people under age 60 are more apt to develop skin reactions, including sunburn.[125] Fair-skinned individuals' skin may turn blue-gray in color.[124] Adverse effects are not dose related and most are not predictable. Many studies of amiodarone are small. One study shows a trend toward a lower mortality with amiodarone.[126]

Amiodarone remains on a well-recognized list of drugs that are inappropriate for use in older adults because of causing heart rhythm disturbances and lack of effectiveness in this age group.[115]

Before You Use This Drug

Tell your doctor if you have or have had:

- allergies including iodine and lactose
- asthma
- high or low blood pressure
- other heart problems, such as bradycardia, congestive heart failure, heart block, or sinus node impairment
- liver problems
- thyroid problems
- pregnancy or are breast-feeding

Tell your doctor about any other drugs you take, including aspirin, herbs, vitamins, and other nonprescription products. Before you start this drug, request a thyroid test.

When You Use This Drug

- Wear identification that you take amiodarone.

FDA BLACK BOX WARNING

Cordarone (AMIODARONE) is intended for use only in patients with the indicated life-threatening arrhythmias because its use is accompanied by substantial toxicity.

Cordarone has several potentially fatal toxicities, the most important of which is pulmonary toxicity (hypersensitivity pneumonitis or interstitial/alveolar pneumonitis) that has resulted in clinically manifest disease at rates as high as 10% to 17% in some series of patients with ventricular arrhythmias given doses around 400 mg/day, and as abnormal diffusion capacity without symptoms in a much higher percentage of patients. Pulmonary toxicity has been fatal about 10% of the time. Liver injury is common with Cordarone, but is usually mild and evidenced only by abnormal liver enzymes. Overt liver disease can occur, however, and has been fatal in a few cases. Like other antiarrhythmics, Cordarone can exacerbate the arrhythmia, e.g., by making the arrhythmia less well tolerated or more difficult to reverse. This has occurred in 2 to 5% of patients in various series, and significant heart block or sinus bradycardia has been seen in 2 to 5%. All of these events should be manageable in the proper clinical setting in most cases. Although the frequency of such proarrhythmic events does not appear greater with Cordarone than with many other agents used in this population, the effects are prolonged when they occur.

Even in patients at high risk of arrhythmic death, in whom the toxicity of Cordarone is an acceptable risk, Cordarone poses major management problems that could be life-threatening in a population at risk of sudden death, so that every effort should be made to utilize alternative agents first. The difficulty of using Cordarone effectively and safely itself poses a significant risk to patients. Patients with the indicated arrhythmias must be hospitalized while the loading dose of Cordarone is given, and a response generally requires at least one week, usually two or more. Because absorption and elimination are variable, maintenance-dose selection is difficult, and it is not unusual to require dosage decrease or discontinuation of treatment. In a retrospective survey of 192 patients with ventricular tachyarrhythmias, 84 required dose reduction and 18 required at least temporary discontinuation because of adverse effects, and several series have reported 15 to 20% overall frequencies of discontinuation due to adverse reactions. The time at which a previously controlled life-threatening arrhythmia will recur after discontinuation or dose adjustment is unpredictable, ranging from weeks to months.

The patient is obviously at great risk during this time and may need prolonged hospitalization. Attempts to substitute other antiarrhythmic agents when Cordarone must be stopped will be made difficult by the gradually, but unpredictably, changing amiodarone body burden. A similar problem exists when Cordarone is not effective; it still poses the risk of an interaction with whatever subsequent treatment is tried.

• Protect yourself from sunburn during and for several months following stopping treatment, using a sunblock. Wear protective brimmed hats, long sleeves, and pants.

• If you plan to have any surgery, including dental, tell your doctor that you take this drug.

How to Use This Drug

• If you miss a dose, take it as soon as you remember, but skip it if it is almost time for your next scheduled dose. Notify your doctor if you miss two or more doses in a row. **Do not take double doses.**

• Do not share your medication with others.

• Take the drug at the same time(s) each day.

• Tablet must always be taken the same way, either with or without food.

• Do not break, chew, or crush this drug.

• Injection should be given by a health professional.

• If you stop taking this medication, remember that adverse effects can still last for several weeks or months.

WARNING

When this drug was used to treat rhythm disturbances of the small chambers of the heart (atria), it provided no survival advantage and a higher risk of serious adverse effects than older drugs such as digoxin (see p. 144), the beta-blockers (see p. 87), and the calcium channel blockers diltiazem and verapamil (see p. 97).[112,113]

This drug is not approved by the FDA to treat rhythm disturbances of the atria.

---

sections with multiple drugs, the interaction may have been reported for one but not all drugs in this section, but we include the interaction because the drugs in this section are similar to one another. We have also included potentially serious interactions listed in the drug's FDA-approved professional package insert or in published medical journal articles. There may be other drugs, especially those in the families of drugs listed below, that also will react with this drug to cause severe adverse effects. Make sure to tell your doctor and pharmacist the drugs you are taking and tell them if you are taking any of these interacting drugs:

• Store tablets at room temperature with lid on tightly. Do not store in the bathroom. Do not expose to heat, moisture, or strong light. Keep out of reach of children.

Interactions with Other Drugs

The following drugs, biologics (e.g., vaccines, therapeutic antibodies), or foods are listed in *Evaluations of Drug Interactions* 2003 as causing "highly clinically significant" or "clinically significant" interactions when used together with any of the drugs in this section. In some

antihistamines, antipsychotics, AVELOX, beta-blockers, BETAPACE, calcium channel blockers, COUMADIN, CRIXIVAN, cyclosporine, digoxin, DILANTIN, diuretics, DURAQUIN, flecainide, grapefruit juice, halofantrine, indinavir, LANOXICAPS, LANOXIN, lidocaine, LOPRESSOR, metoprolol, mexiletine, MEXITIL, mizolastine, moxifloxacin, NORVIR, ORAP, phenytoin, pimozide, procainamide, PROCANBID, propafenone, QUINAGLUTE DURA-TABS, QUINIDEX, quinidine, RIFADIN, rifampin,

---

WARNING! INCREASED RISK OF DEATH

In the National Heart, Lung, and Blood Institute's Cardiac Arrhythmia Suppression Trial (CAST) (a long-term, multicentered, randomized, double-blind study), in patients with asymptomatic non-life-threatening ventricular (the large chambers of the heart) arrhythmias (rhythm disturbances) who had a heart attack more than six days but less than two years previous, deaths or nonfatal cardiac arrest were seen in 7.7% of those patients treated with encainide or flecainide, members of the Class 1 group of antiarrhythmic drugs, compared to 3.0% in patients receiving an inactive sugar pill or placebo.

Because of the known ability of the Class 1 drugs, such as quinidine, to cause rhythm disturbances, and the lack of evidence of improved survival for any antiarrhythmic drug in patients without life-threatening heart rhythm disturbances, the use of the Class 1 drugs should be reserved for patients with life-threatening rhythm disturbances of the ventricles. These warnings now appear in the FDA-approved product labeling, or package insert, for all Class 1 drugs, including: disopyramide (NORPACE and generics), flecainide (TAMBOCOR), mexiletine (MEXITIL and generics), moricizine (ETHMOZINE), procainamide (PROCANBID and generics), propafenone (RYTHMOL), quinidine (DURAQUIN, QUINAGLUTE DURA-TABS, QUINIDEX, and generics), and tocainide (TONOCARD).

---

ritonavir, RYTHMOL, SANDIMMUNE, sotalol, sparfloxacin, TAMBOCOR, warfarin,
ZAGAM, zotepine.

*Interactions with amiodarone can occur months
after you stop taking amiodarone because it
stays in the body for months after stopping treatment.*

Adverse Effects

Call your doctor immediately if you experi-ence:

- difficulty breathing
- dizziness, lightheadedness, or fainting
- fever
- cough
- unusual and uncontrolled movements of the body
- coldness
- dry eyes, sensitivity of eyes to light
- heartbeat becoming faster, slower, or irreg-ular
- nervousness
- numbness or tingling in fingers or toes
- trembling or shaking of hands
- weakness of arms or legs
- swelling or painful scrotum
- sensitivity to heat or sunlight
- skin rash, blue-gray color, coldness, puffi-ness, or irritation at site of injection
- difficulty sleeping
- sweating
- swelling of legs or feet
- tiredness
- vision changes, blurred or blue-green halos around objects
- difficulty walking (weak arms and legs)
- undesired weight loss or gain
- yellowing of skin or eyes

Call your doctor if these symptoms con-tinue:

- appetite loss
- constipation
- dizziness
- flushing of face
- hair loss
- headache
- nausea or vomiting
- decreased sexual ability and interest
- sunburn
- bitter or metallic taste

Call your doctor if these symptoms occur after you stop treatment:

- cough
- slight fever
- painful breathing
- shortness of breath

Periodic Testing

Ask your doctor which of these tests should be done periodically while you are taking this drug:

- liver function tests
- chest examination
- broncoscopy
- chest X-ray
- heart function tests, such as electrocardio-gram (ECG, EKG)
- gallium radionuclide scan
- eye examination
- plasma amiodarone determinations
- lung function determinations
- thyroid function determinations

Limited Use

Quinidine (*kwin* i deen)
DURAQUIN (Parke-Davis)
QUINAGLUTE DURA-TABS (Berlex)
QUINIDEX (Wyeth)

GENERIC: available
FAMILY: Drugs for Abnormal Heart Rhythm

PREGNANCY WARNING

No data are available for quinidine. Use during pregnancy only for clear medical reasons. Tell your doctor if you are pregnant or thinking of becoming pregnant before you take this drug.

BREAST-FEEDING WARNING

Quinidine is excreted in human milk. Because of the potential for serious adverse effects in nursing infants, you should not take this drug while nursing.

FDA BLACK BOX WARNING

In many trials of antiarrhythmic therapy for non-life-threatening arrhythmias, active antiarrhythmic therapy has resulted in increased mortality; the risk of active therapy is probably greatest in patients with structural heart disease.

In the case of quinidine used to prevent or defer recurrence of atrial [small chambers of the heart] flutter/fibrillation, the best available data come from a meta-analysis [statistical summary] described under CLINICAL PHARMACOLOGY—Clinical Effects [a section of the drug's professional product labeling]. In the patients studied, the mortality associated with the use of quinidine was more than three times as great as the mortality associated with the use of placebo.

Another meta-analysis, also described under CLINICAL PHARMACOLOGY—Clinical Effects, showed that in patients with various non-life-threatening ventricular arrhythmias, the mortality associated with the use of quinidine was consistently greater than that associated with the use of any of a variety of alternative antiarrhythmics.

WARNING

When this drug was used to treat rhythm disturbances of the small chambers of the heart (atria), it provided no survival advantage and a higher risk of serious adverse effects than older drugs such as digoxin (see p. 144), the beta-blockers (see p. 87), and the calcium channel blockers diltiazem and verapamil (see p. 97).[112, 113]

Quinidine slows the heart rate and decreases irregular heartbeats (arrhythmias). **If your kidney function is impaired, you will need to take less than the usual dose.**

Many people who are taking quinidine or another drug in its family have relatively mild disturbances in their heart rhythm and no symptoms of underlying heart disease. The vast majority of these people do not need these drugs, and there is no evidence that using them improves health. In fact, most of the drugs in this family have severe adverse effects that are sometimes worse, and even more life-threatening, than the irregular heartbeats they treat. All of these drugs can also cause new irregularities in your heartbeat.

If you have an irregular heartbeat, without any symptoms of underlying heart disease, you should not be exposed to the dangers of a drug that has no health benefit for your condition.[114] If you are taking quinidine or another drug in its family for an irregular heartbeat (arrhythmia), talk to your doctor and find out whether you also have symptoms of underlying heart disease. If not, discuss the possibility of stopping the drug.

Some people are very sensitive to quinidine and may have difficulty breathing, changes in vision, dizziness, fever, headache, ringing in ears, or skin rash when taking this drug. Since there is a narrow range between a helpful and a harmful amount of this drug, call your doctor immediately if you experience these adverse effects (as well as any of those listed under Adverse Effects).

Before You Use This Drug

Do not use if you have or have had:

- complete heart block
- digitalis toxicity with heart block

WARNING! INCREASED RISK OF DEATH

In the National Heart, Lung, and Blood Institute's Cardiac Arrhythmia Suppression Trial (CAST) (a long-term, multicentered, randomized, double-blind study), in patients with asymptomatic non-life-threatening ventricular (the large chambers of the heart) arrhythmias (rhythm disturbances) who had a heart attack more than six days but less than two years previous, deaths or nonfatal cardiac arrest were seen in 7.7% of those patients treated with encainide or flecainide, members of the Class 1 group of antiarrhythmic drugs, compared to 3.0% in patients receiving an inactive sugar pill or placebo.

Because of the known ability of the Class 1 drugs, such as quinidine, to cause rhythm disturbances, and the lack of evidence of improved survival for any antiarrhythmic drug in patients without life-threatening heart rhythm disturbances, the use of the Class 1 drugs should be reserved for patients with life-threatening rhythm disturbances of the ventricles. These warnings now appear in the FDA-approved product labeling, or package insert, for all Class 1 drugs, including: disopyramide (NORPACE and generics), flecainide (TAMBOCOR), mexiletine (MEXITIL and generics), moricizine (ETHMOZINE), procainamide (PROCANBID and generics), propafenone (RYTHMOL), quinidine (DURAQUIN, QUINAGLUTE DURA-TABS, QUINIDEX, and generics), and tocainide (TONOCARD).

- pregnancy or are planning to become pregnant, or are breast-feeding

Tell your doctor if you have or have had:

- allergies to drugs
- asthma or emphysema
- incomplete heart block or other heart problems
- digitalis toxicity
- kidney or liver problems
- increased secretion of thyroid hormones
- low blood potassium or other electrolyte disorders that can result from severe diarrhea or vomiting, or dialysis
- myasthenia gravis
- psoriasis
- difficulty stopping bleeding

Tell your doctor about any other drugs you take, including aspirin, herbs, vitamins, and other nonprescription products.

When You Use This Drug

- **Do not stop taking this drug suddenly. Your doctor must give you a schedule to lower your dose gradually, to prevent serious changes in heart function.**

- Wear a medical identification bracelet or carry a card stating that you take quinidine.
- If you plan to have any surgery, including dental, tell your doctor that you take this drug.

How to Use This Drug

- If you miss a dose, take it as soon as you remember, but skip it if it is almost time for your next scheduled dose. **Do not take double doses.**
- Do not share your medication with others.
- Take the drug at the same time(s) each day.
- Take with food or milk.
- Do not break, chew, or crush this drug. Take your last dose of the day at least an hour before bedtime.
- Store at room temperature with lid on tightly. Do not store in the bathroom. Do not expose to heat, moisture, or strong light. Keep out of reach of children.

Interactions with Other Drugs

The following drugs, biologics (e.g., vaccines, therapeutic antibodies), or foods are listed in

Evaluations of Drug Interactions 2003 as causing "highly clinically significant" or "clinically significant" interactions when used together with any of the drugs in this section. In some sections with multiple drugs, the interaction may have been reported for one but not all drugs in this section, but we include the interaction because the drugs in this section are similar to one another. We have also included potentially serious interactions listed in the drug's FDA-approved professional package insert or in published medical journal articles. There may be other drugs, especially those in the families of drugs listed below, that also will react with this drug to cause severe adverse effects. Make sure to tell your doctor and pharmacist the drugs you are taking and tell them if you are taking any of these interacting drugs:

acetazolamide, amiodarone, arbutamine, AVELOX, AZOPT, bendroflumethiazide, benzthiazide, brinzolamide, CALAN SR, chlorothiazide, cimetidine, codeine, CORDARONE, COUMADIN, COVERA-HS, cyclopenthiazide, cyclosporine, cyclothiazide, delavirdine, DIAMOX, dichlorphenamide, digoxin, DILANTIN, DIURIL, dorzolamide, ENDURON, flumethazide, fluvoxamine, FORTOVASE, GLUCOVANCE, halofantrine, hydrochlorothiazide, hydroflumethiazide, ISOPTIN SR, itraconazole, ketoconazole, LANOXICAPS, LANOXIN, LUMINAL, metformin, methazolamide, methyclothiazide, mizolastine, moxifloxacin, NAQUA, NATURETIN-5, NEORAL, NIZORAL, NORVIR, phenobarbital, phenytoin, polythiazide, potassium citrate, PRIFTIN, propafenone, RENESE, RESCRIPTOR, RIFADIN, rifampin, rifapentine, RIMACTANE, ritonavir, RYTHMOL, SANDIMMUNE, saquinavir, SERLECT, sertindole, sodium acetate, sodium bicarbonate, SOLFOTON, sparfloxacin, SPORANOX, TAGAMET, THAM, trichlormethiazide, tromethamine, TRUSOPT, TUBARINE, tubocurarine, verapamil, VERELAN, warfarin, xipamide, zotepine, ZAGAM.

Adverse Effects

Call your doctor immediately if you experience:

- blurred—or any change in—vision
- abdominal pain and/or yellow eyes or skin
- confusion or delirium
- disturbed color perception
- intolerance of light
- dizziness or fainting
- fever
- severe headache
- ringing in ears or loss of hearing
- skin rash, hives, or itching
- painful joints
- wheezing, shortness of breath
- unusual bleeding or bruising
- unusually fast heartbeat
- unusual tiredness or weakness

Call your doctor if these symptoms continue:

- bitter taste in mouth
- confusion
- diarrhea
- flushing or itching skin
- loss of appetite
- muscle weakness
- nausea, vomiting, stomach pain

Periodic Tests

Ask your doctor which of these tests should be done periodically while you are taking this drug:

- blood pressure
- complete blood count
- heart function tests, such as electrocardiogram (ECG, EKG)
- kidney function tests
- liver function tests
- blood levels of potassium and quinidine

Heart Failure and Angina

Do Not Use
(Except After Valve Replacement)

ALTERNATIVE TREATMENT:
ALTERNATIVE TREATMENT FOR ANGINA:
See Propranolol, p. 87.

Dipyridamole (dye peer *id* a mole)
PERSANTINE (Boehringer Ingelheim)

FAMILY: Blood-Clotting Inhibitor

PREGNANCY WARNING

No valid data are available for dipyridamole, as it was not tested properly in animal studies. Because of the lack of health benefit to the mother, there is no reason to use dipyridamole during pregnancy.

BREAST-FEEDING WARNING

Dipyridamole is excreted in human milk. Because of the potential for serious adverse effects in nursing infants, you should not take this drug while nursing.

Dipyridamole is approved by the FDA for use in combination with warfarin (see p. 152) after heart valve replacement to prevent blood clots.[127]

This drug has not been proven to have any health benefit except in one study involving a certain type of heart surgery—heart valve replacement. It is also sometimes given in combination with aspirin to prevent a stroke, but there is no proof that this combination works any better than aspirin alone. There is no convincing evidence that dipyridamole will prevent or relieve any disease of the blood vessels supplying the brain, decrease the severity or frequency of chest pain (angina), or improve the mental or physical state of older or senile people.

Dipyridamole remains on a well-recognized list of drugs that are inappropriate for use in

older adults because it may cause a rapid lowering of blood pressure when a patient stands up (orthostatic hypotension) that could lead to fainting and falling.[115]

Digoxin (di *jox* in)
LANOXIN, LANOXICAPS (GlaxoSmithKline)

GENERIC: available

FAMILY: Drugs for Abnormal Heart Rhythm
Drugs for Heart Failure

PREGNANCY WARNING

No data are available for digoxin as it was not tested in animal studies. Use during pregnancy only for clear medical reasons. Tell your doctor if you are pregnant or thinking of becoming pregnant before you take this drug.

BREAST-FEEDING WARNING

Digoxin is excreted in human milk with the concentration in the milk about the same as in the mother's blood. Because of the potential for serious adverse effects in nursing infants, you should not take this drug while nursing.

Digoxin is approved by the FDA for the treatment of mild to moderate heart failure. It is often used in combination with a thiazide diuretic, or water pill (see p. 60), and an angiotensin converting enzyme (ACE) inhibitor (see p. 91). Digoxin is also approved to control the rate of beating of the large chambers of the heart (ventricles) in people with a chronic rapid beating of the small chambers of the heart (atria).[128]

The symptoms of heart failure are fatigue, difficulty breathing, swelling (especially in the legs and ankles), and rapid or "galloping" heartbeats.

Before prescribing digoxin for heart failure, your doctor should first try giving you another type of drug called a thiazide diuretic (water pill) (see p. 60). You should only switch to digoxin if the diuretic does not control your symptoms well enough. **In general, if you are over 60, you should be taking a smaller daily**

dose than the usual 0.25 milligrams,[116] **especially if you have impaired kidney function.**

Anyone taking digoxin is at risk of toxic effects (digitalis toxicity). While you are taking digoxin, your doctor should regularly check the levels of the drug in your blood. You and your doctor should also watch for the subtle symptoms of toxicity: fatigue, loss of appetite, nausea and vomiting, problems with vision, bad dreams, nervousness, drowsiness, and hallucinations.[129] Other signs of toxicity are changes in heart rhythm, slow pulse, and lethargy. Since there is a narrow range between a helpful and a harmful amount of digoxin in your body, you should take the drug daily in the exact amount prescribed. If you get too much digoxin in your body, you may develop the effects listed above; if you get too little, you may develop symptoms of heart failure or a rapid heart rate.

Digoxin is often overprescribed for older adults.[130] One study of people using digoxin outside the hospital found that four out of ten were getting no benefit from the drug.[131] Because of digoxin's toxic effects, taking the drug when it has no benefit is not only wasteful but also dangerous. As many as one in five digoxin users develop signs of toxic effects,[35] and much of this could be prevented if the people who did not need digoxin were taken off the drug. Evidence shows that **up to eight out of ten long-term digoxin users can stop using the drug successfully, under close supervision by a doctor, with no harmful results.**[132] This is partly due to digoxin being wrongly prescribed in the first place.

If you have used digoxin regularly for some time, ask your doctor if you might be able to try withdrawing from the drug. You are more likely to be able to stop taking digoxin if you meet the following conditions:

1. You have used digoxin for a long time without your initial symptoms of heart failure coming back.

2. You have a normal heart rhythm.

3. You are not using digoxin to control an irregular heart rhythm.

There is no good way of knowing in advance who can stop taking digoxin. People taking digoxin to correct an irregular heart rhythm should not attempt to stop taking the drug, but most other people will benefit from a trial of withdrawal under close supervision by a doctor.

Before You Use This Drug

Do not use if you have or have had:

- toxic effects from other digitalis preparations
- ventricular fibrillation
- pregnancy or are breast-feeding

Tell your doctor if you have or have had:

- allergies to drugs
- decreased thyroid hormones
- rheumatic fever
- heart block
- carotid sinus hypersensitivity
- high or low blood potassium, magnesium, or calcium levels
- insufficient oxygen supply to the heart
- irregular or rapid heartbeat
- kidney or liver problems
- heart attack
- severe lung disease
- heart disease in which enlargement of the heart muscle decreases the heart's ability to pump blood (IHSS)

Tell your doctor about any other drugs you take including aspirin, herbs, vitamins, and other nonprescription products.

When You Use This Drug

- **Learn to take your pulse, and get immediate medical help if your pulse slows to 60 beats per minute or less. Some people**

have suffered a slow heart rate and heart failure while using digoxin.

• **Do not stop taking this drug suddenly.** Your doctor must give you a schedule to lower your dose gradually, to prevent serious changes in your heart function.

• Wear a medical identification bracelet or carry a card saying that you take digoxin.

• Eat a diet that is rich in potassium, adequate in magnesium, and low in salt and dietary fiber (see p. 58).

• **Do not take other drugs without talking to your doctor first—especially nonprescription drugs for appetite control, asthma, colds, coughs, hay fever, or sinus problems.**

• If you plan to have any surgery, including dental, tell your doctor that you take this drug.

How to Use This Drug

• If you miss a dose, either take within 12 hours or wait until your next scheduled dose. **Do not take double doses.** If you miss two or more doses in a row, call your doctor.

• Do not share your medication with others.

• Take the drug at the same time(s) each day.

• Crush tablets and mix with water, or swallow whole with water.

• Measure the liquid form only with the specially marked dropper.

• Store at room temperature with lid on tightly. Do not store in the bathroom. Do not expose to heat, moisture, or strong light. Keep out of reach of children.

Interactions with Other Drugs

The following drugs, biologics (e.g., vaccines, therapeutic antibodies), or foods are listed in *Evaluations of Drug Interactions* 2003 as causing "highly clinically significant" or "clinically significant" interactions when used together with any of the drugs in this section. In some sections with multiple drugs, the interaction may have been reported for one but not all drugs in this section, but we include the interaction because the drugs in this section are similar to one another. We have also included potentially serious interactions listed in the drug's FDA-approved professional package insert or in published medical journal articles. There may be other drugs, especially those in the families of drugs listed below, that also will react with this drug to cause severe adverse effects. Make sure to tell your doctor and pharmacist the drugs you are taking and tell them if you are taking any of these interacting drugs:

ACHROMYCIN, ADVIL, ALDACTONE, alprazolam, aluminum hydroxide, amiodarone, AMPHOJEL, ANECTINE, antacids, arbutamine hydrochloride, atorvastatin, AZULFIDINE, BIAXIN, CALAN SR, CALCIJECT, calcium chloride injection, CAPOTEN, captopril, cholestyramine, clarithromycin, CORDARONE, COVERA HS, CUPRIMINE, cyclophosphamide, cyclosporine, CYTOXAN, DELTASONE, DEPEN, diazepam, DILANTIN, diphenoxylate, DURAQUIN, EES, ERYTHROCIN, erythromycin, furosemide, GAVISCON, GLUCOVANCE, hydroxychloroquine, ibuprofen, INDOCIN, indomethacin, ISOPTIN SR, itraconazole, kaolin and pectin, KAO-SPEN, KAPECTOLIN, LASIX, LIPITOR, LOCHOLEST, LOMOTIL, magnesium hydroxide, magnesium trisilicate, MATULANE, metformin, METICORTEN, metoclopramide, MICARDIS, MINIPRESS, MOTRIN, neomycin, NEORAL, NEO-RX, ONCOVIN, PANMYCIN, paricalcitol, penicillamine, phenytoin, PHILLIPS' MILK OF MAGNESIA, PLAQUENIL, potassium-depleting diuretics, prazosin, prednisone, PRO-BANTHINE, procarbazine, propafenone, propantheline, QUESTRAN, QUINAGLUTE DURA-TABS, QUINIDEX, quinidine, REGLAN, RYTHMOL, SANDIM-MUNE, spironolactone, SPORANOX, succinylcholine, sulfasalazine, telmisartan, tetracycline, THYROID STRONG, tramadol, ULTRAM, VALIUM, VERELAN, verapamil, vincristine, XANAX, ZEMPLAR.

Adverse Effects

Call your doctor immediately if you experience:

- loss of appetite
- nausea or vomiting
- lower stomach pain
- diarrhea
- slow and/or irregular heartbeats
- slow pulse
- unusual tiredness or weakness
- blurred vision or colored "halos"
- depression or confusion
- anxiety
- drowsiness
- headache
- bad dreams, hallucinations, nervousness
- skin rash or hives
- fainting
- dizziness

Periodic Tests

Ask your doctor which of these tests should be done periodically while you are taking this drug:

- blood pressure and pulse rate
- heart function tests, such as electrocardiogram (ECG, EKG)
- kidney function tests
- liver function tests
- blood levels of potassium, magnesium, and calcium
- blood levels of digoxin

Isosorbide Dinitrate
(eye soe *sor* bide dye nye trate)
ISORDIL (Wyeth-Ayerst)
SORBITRATE (AstraZeneca)

Isosorbide-5-mononitrate
(eye soe *sor* byde five mon oh *ni* trate)
ISMO (Wyeth-Ayerst)
IMDUR (Schering-Plough)

Nitroglycerin (nye troe *gli* ser in)
MINITRAN (3M)
NITRO-BID (Aventis)
NITRO-DUR (Key)
NITROSTAT (Parke-Davis)
TRANSDERM-NITRO (Novartis)

GENERIC: available
FAMILY: Drugs for Angina
Nitrates

PREGNANCY WARNING

Nitroglycerin caused liver tumors in an animal carcinogenicity study and was positive in the Ames test (a test for DNA damage). It also caused death in rabbit pups whose mothers were treated with the drug. Use during pregnancy only for clear medical reasons. Tell your doctor if you are pregnant or thinking of becoming pregnant before you take this drug.

BREAST-FEEDING WARNING

There are no data from either human or animal studies. It is likely that this drug, like many others, is excreted in human milk. Because of the potential for serious adverse effects in nursing infants, it is advisable not to take this drug while nursing.

WARNING

If you are taking any member of the nitrate family of drugs, you should not take sildenafil (VIAGRA), vardenafil (LEVITRA), or tadalafil (CIALIS), which are drugs used for sexual dysfunction. The use of these erectile dysfunction drugs in men who were treated with a nitrate has resulted in deaths.

```
┌─────────────────────────────────────────────┐
│               HEAT STRESS ALERT               │
│  ───────────────────────────────────────────  │
│                                               │
│    These drugs can affect your body's abil-  │
│  ity to adjust to heat, putting you at risk  │
│  of "heat stress." If you live alone, ask a  │
│  friend to check on you several times dur-   │
│  ing the day. Early signs of heat stress are │
│  dizziness, lightheadedness, faintness, and  │
│  slightly high temperature. Call your doctor │
│  if you have any of these signs. Drink more  │
│  fluids (water, fruit and vegetable juices)  │
│  than usual—even if you're not thirsty—      │
│  unless your doctor has told you otherwise.  │
│  Do not drink alcohol.                        │
└─────────────────────────────────────────────┘
```

Isosorbide dinitrate, isosorbide-5-mononitrate—the major breakdown product of isosorbide dinitrate—and nitroglycerin are used to treat sudden severe attacks of chest pain (acute angina). They come in several different forms: tablets that dissolve under the tongue (sublingual), chewable tablets, tablets and capsules to be swallowed, ointments and patches to be applied to the skin, and oral spray. For treating sudden attacks of chest pain, only the sublingual tablets and certain chewable tablets are effective. The other dosage forms are used on a regular basis to prevent angina attacks from occurring, although the high doses of oral tablets and capsules needed to be effective make them less useful.

Wearing nitroglycerin patches continuously can lead to tolerance to nitroglycerin, which can be prevented or slowed by wearing patches for only 10 to 12 hours, instead of continuously. However, the nitrate-free interval may be associated with decreased tolerance to exercise, and the possibility of increased angina.[133]

Before You Use This Drug

Tell your doctor if you have or have had:

- allergies to any adhesives, drugs, or other materials
- glaucoma

- hemorrhage of a blood vessel supplying the head
- food absorption problem
- recent heart attack or stroke or enlarged heart
- severe anemia
- trauma to the head
- kidney or liver problems
- overactive thyroid
- pregnancy or are breast-feeding

Tell your doctor about any other drugs you take, including aspirin, herbs, vitamins, and other nonprescription products.

When You Use This Drug

- You may feel dizzy for a time, or faint, after taking these drugs, especially if you are upright and standing still. If you feel dizzy, put your head between your knees, breathe deeply, and move your arms and legs.
- You may develop a headache from the drug, but it can usually be relieved with aspirin.
- Be careful not to overexert yourself, even though your chest pain may feel better.
- Do not drink alcohol.
- **If you are taking this drug regularly, do not stop taking it suddenly.** Your doctor must give you a schedule to lower your dose gradually, to prevent chest pain and possible heart attack.
- Until you know how you react to this drug, do not drive or perform other activities requiring alertness.
- If applicable carry identification that you use nitroglycerin patches.
- If you seek emergency care, or have surgery, including dental, tell your doctor that you take nitroglycerin and the form you use.

How to Use This Drug

For sublingual form:

- Place tablet under tongue and allow it to dissolve. Do not chew, crush, or swallow.

While tablet is dissolving, do not eat, drink, or smoke.

• Store tablets only in the original container with the lid on tightly. Nitroglycerin is very sensitive and can lose strength rapidly if not stored properly. Do not add any other drug, material, or object to the container that was not there originally. Protect from air, heat, moisture, and sunlight. This includes times you carry nitroglycerin with you or store it away from home. Special stainless-steel containers are available to wear for emergency supplies of nitroglycerin. Once any container of nitroglycerin is opened, the supply should be replaced within six months.

• For isosorbide dinitrate and mononitrate: You should feel the drug's effect in five minutes. If the pain does not go away in 5 to 10 minutes, take a second tablet. If you still have chest pain after three tablets in 15 minutes, call your doctor or go to an emergency room immediately.

• For nitroglycerin: You should feel the drug's effect in 5 minutes. If the pain does not go away in 5 minutes, take a second tablet. If you still have chest pain after three tablets in 10 to 15 minutes, call your doctor or go to an emergency room immediately.

• **Do not take other drugs without talking to your doctor first—especially nonprescription drugs for appetite control, asthma, colds, coughs, hay fever, or sinus problems. Alcohol use may cause low blood pressure.**

For patch form:

• Open and prepare patch according to package instructions. Do not cut or trim the patch to adjust the dose.

• Select a site that is dry, on the chest, upper arm, or shoulders. Avoid areas that are broken, calloused, hairy, irritated, or shaved. Do not use sites below the knee or elbow, or areas where movement or clothing is apt to dislodge the patch. The need to rotate sites has recently been questioned.

• Press adhesive side of patch to skin firmly.

• Replace patch if it loosens or falls off.

• Leave on the amount of time specified by your doctor, then remove.

• Apply new patch at the same time each day.

• Discard used patch.

• Store unopened patches at room temperature. Do not expose to high temperatures or moisture. Do not store in a bathroom or refrigerator.

Interactions with Other Drugs

The following drugs, biologics (e.g., vaccines, therapeutic antibodies), or foods are listed in *Evaluations of Drug Interactions* 2003 as causing "highly clinically significant" or "clinically significant" interactions when used together with any of the drugs in this section. In some sections with multiple drugs, the interaction may have been reported for one but not all drugs in this section, but we include the interaction because the drugs in this section are similar to one another. We have also included potentially serious interactions listed in the drug's FDA-approved professional package insert or in published medical journal articles. There may be other drugs, especially those in the families of drugs listed below, that also will react with this drug to cause severe adverse effects. Make sure to tell your doctor and pharmacist the drugs you are taking and tell them if you are taking any of these interacting drugs:

alteplase, CIALIS, D.H.E.-45, dihydroergotamine, ERGOMAR, ergotamine, heparin, imipramine, LEVITRA, sildenafil, tadalafil, TOFRANIL, vardenafil, VIAGRA.

The blood-pressure-lowering effects of drugs such as beta-blockers (see p. 87), calcium channel blockers (see p. 97), and phenothiazines (see p. 268) are enhanced when taken with nitrates.

Adverse Effects

Call your doctor immediately if you experience:

- blurred vision
- dry mouth
- severe or prolonged headache
- skin rash

Call your doctor if these symptoms continue:

- dizziness, lightheadedness
- restlessness
- nausea or vomiting
- flushed face and neck
- rapid pulse or heartbeat
- burning, itching, or reddened skin

Signs of overdose:

- bluish lips, fingernails, or palms
- dizziness or fainting
- feeling of pressure in head
- shortness of breath
- unusual tiredness or weakness
- weak and unusually fast heartbeat
- fever
- seizures

If you suspect an overdose, call this number to contact your poison control center: (800) 222-1222.

Periodic Tests

Ask your doctor which of these tests should be done periodically while you are taking this drug:

- blood pressure and pulse
- heart function tests, such as electrocardiogram (ECG, EKG)

Other Heart Drugs

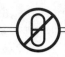 *Do Not Use*

ALTERNATIVE TREATMENT:
Mild exercise and no smoking.

Cilostazol (sil-*oh*-sta-zol)
PLETAL (Otsuka American Pharmaceutical)

FAMILY:　Blood Flow Improvers

PREGNANCY WARNING

Cilostazol caused fetal harm in animal studies, including damage to the heart, kidney, and skeleton. Because of the potential for serious adverse effects to the fetus, this drug should not be used by pregnant women.

BREAST-FEEDING WARNING

Cilostazol is excreted in animal milk. Because of the potential for serious adverse effects in nursing infants, you should not take this drug while nursing.

FDA BLACK BOX WARNING

Cilostazol and several of its metabolites [breakdown products] are inhibitors of phosphodiesterase III. Several drugs with this pharmacologic effect have caused decreased survival compared to placebo in patients with class III–IV congestive heart failure. PLETAL is contraindicated in patients with congestive heart failure of any severity.[134]

Cilostazol carries the above boxed warning at the beginning of its FDA-approved professional product labeling about the drug's use in patients with congestive heart failure.

Cilostazol was approved by the FDA in January 1999 for the reduction of the symptoms of intermittent claudication, a chronic debilitating, non-life-threatening disorder that causes pain, ache, cramping, numbness, or sense of fatigue in the leg muscles during exercise but is relieved with rest. The drug was approved despite the fact that it adds very little to the benefits of exercise alone and is associated with decreased survival in certain patients with heart failure.

Cilostazol is not a new drug. It has been sold in Japan since 1988 and is also available in Korea, Thailand, the Philippines, the People's Republic of China, Argentina, and Indonesia.

Prior to cilostazol's approval, Public Citizen's Health Research Group wrote the FDA on two occasions, to urge strongly that it not be approved.[135, 136] Cilostazol works by inhibiting an enzyme known as phosphodiesterase III. Other drugs that affect this enzyme and are used to treat conditions such as congestive heart failure have been associated with increased risk of death. In fact, one of these, flosequinan (MANOPLAX), was withdrawn from the market in 1993 for just this reason.[137] Also, a pooled safety analysis of clinical trials submitted to the FDA by Otsuka found a higher mortality rate at 30 days after treatment in patients taking cilostazol than in those taking an inactive dummy drug (placebo). This difference was not statistically significant.[138]

Cilostazol works by inhibiting the clumping of elements in the blood known as platelets. Because clumping of platelets is one of the body's first defenses against bleeding, cilostazol's effect on platelets has raised concerns about its use together with clopidogrel (PLAVIX, see p. 155), a drug that also affects platelets and is used to reduce the risk of heart attack and stroke in patients with atherosclerosis (documented by a recent stroke or heart attack) or peripheral arterial disease. Studies of the use of cilostazol together with clopidogrel are planned.

Interactions with Other Drugs

The following drugs, biologics (e.g., vaccines, therapeutic antibodies), or foods are listed in *Evaluations of Drug Interactions* 2003 as causing "highly clinically significant" or "clinically significant" interactions when used together with any of the drugs in this section. In some sections with multiple drugs, the interaction may have been reported for one but not all drugs in this section, but we include the interaction because the drugs in this section are similar to one another. We have also included potentially serious interactions listed in the drug's FDA-approved professional package insert or in published medical journal articles. There may be other drugs, especially those in the families of drugs listed below, that also will react with this drug to cause severe adverse effects. Make sure to tell your doctor and pharmacist the drugs you are taking and tell them if you are taking any of these interacting drugs:

BIAXIN, CARDIZEM, clarithromycin, COUMADIN, DIFLUCAN, DILACOR, diltiazem, EES, erythromycin, fluconazole, fluoxetine, fluvoxamine, itraconazole, ketoconazole, LUVOX, miconazole, MONISTAT IV, nefazodone, NIZORAL, omeprazole, PRILOSEC, PROZAC, sertraline, SERZONE, SPORANOX, warfarin, ZOLOFT.

A study published in the August 18, 1998, issue of the journal *Circulation* compared cilostazol to a placebo in patients with intermittent claudication.[139] At the beginning of this 12-week study, the patients in the placebo group could walk, on average, 184 yards and those in the cilostazol group could walk 155 yards before having to stop because of their symptoms. At the end of the 12 weeks, the distance that could be walked by placebo patients had dropped to an average of 166 yards, while cilostazol patients increased their maximum walking distance to 253 yards. The placebo group could walk an average of 18 yards less and the cilostazol patients could walk 98 yards farther. Overall, there was no statistically significant difference between cilostazol and placebo at the end of the study.

Otsuka submitted to the FDA eight large clinical trials comparing cilostazol to placebo to support its petition for the drug's approval. On average, cilostazol patients could walk only 65 yards farther than those patients taking a placebo after 12 to 24 weeks of treatment.[140]

Two studies were also provided to the FDA comparing cilostazol to pentoxifylline (TRENTAL), the only other drug approved for the treatment of intermittent claudication in the U.S. In the first of these studies the patients taking cilostazol were able to walk about 108 yards farther than those receiving pentoxifylline. In the second, walking distance was improved by only 41 yards in those taking cilostazol compared to the pentoxifylline group. Because of these conflicting results the FDA denied Otsuka America's request to allow them to claim that cilostazol is superior to pentoxifylline in the treatment of intermittent claudication.[138]

We have listed pentoxifylline as a **Do Not Use** drug since the first edition of *Worst Pills, Best Pills* (1988) because of its lack of significant effectiveness (see p. 152). Swedish drug regulatory authorities had refused to approve pentoxifylline in 1995.

Cilostazol has shown only a small effect in increasing walking distance in patients with intermittent claudication. There are unanswered and very worrisome questions about its safety, and combined with the increased risk of death that has been seen with other phosphodiesterase III–inhibiting drugs, cilostazol should be avoided.

Pentoxifylline was approved by the FDA in 1984 to reduce the symptoms of intermittent claudication, a chronic debilitating, non-life-threatening disorder that causes pain, ache, cramping, numbness, or sense of fatigue in the leg muscles during exercise but is relieved with rest. The manufacturer claims that the drug improves the flow of blood through the blood vessels by making red blood cells more flexible.

The editors of the highly respected *Medical Letter on Drugs and Therapeutics,* an independent source of drug information for pharmacists and physicians, concluded their 1984 review of the drug by saying:

"Pentoxifylline may increase walking distance in some patients with symptoms of intermittent claudication, but it appears to be less effective than physical training. The drug might be worth trying in patients who cannot follow an exercise program and are not good candidates for surgery."[141]

A recent review of the effects of exercise for leg pain due to intermittent claudication found that exercise is of significant benefit to patients with leg pain due to this disorder.[142]

Pentoxifylline may also have serious dangers. There is a report of two cases in which pentoxifylline caused fatal damage to patients' bone marrow.[143]

Swedish drug regulatory authorities refused to approve pentoxifylline in 1995.

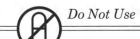 *Do Not Use*

ALTERNATIVE TREATMENT:
Mild exercise and no smoking.

Pentoxifylline (pen tox *if* i lin)
TRENTAL (Aventis)

FAMILY: Blood Flow Improvers

Warfarin (*war* far in)
COUMADIN (Bristol-Myers Squibb)

GENERIC: available
FAMILY: Blood-Clotting Inhibitors

Warfarin reduces the blood's ability to clot (coagulate) and prevents blood clots from forming in the arteries and veins. It is prescribed for

PREGNANCY WARNING

Warfarin should not be used if you are pregnant or are thinking of becoming pregnant. Severe malformations have occurred in infants of mothers taking this drug. The risk of use of warfarin in pregnant women clearly outweighs any possible benefit.

BREAST-FEEDING WARNING

There is no information from either human or animal studies. However, because of the potential for serious adverse effects in nursing infants, you should not take warfarin while nursing.

DRUG INTERACTION WARNING: INCREASED RISK OF BLEEDING WHEN ACETAMINOPHEN AND WARFARIN (COUMADIN) ARE TAKEN TOGETHER

Acetaminophen may interact with warfarin to increase the risk of bleeding. This risk increases with increasing doses of acetaminophen. The risk of bleeding has been found to increase tenfold in people who were taking 28 or more regular-strength acetaminophen tablets per week, or the equivalent of 18 or more extra-strength tablets per week, compared to those taking warfarin and no acetaminophen.[144] A regular-strength tablet contains 325 milligrams of acetaminophen and extra-strength tablets contain 500 milligrams each of the drug.

Warfarin is a drug of considerable benefit after heart valve replacement and in preventing blood clots from a type of heart rhythm disturbance known as atrial fibrillation. It also reduces the risk of death, recurrent heart attacks, and stroke after a heart attack.

Based on this new evidence, if you are taking warfarin you should notify your doctor before taking any product containing acetaminophen.

people with a history of abnormal blood clots or who are at high risk of having abnormal clots. **If you are over 60, you should generally be taking less than the usual adult dose,** to lower the risk of heavy bleeding (hemorrhage). Once you have taken warfarin for three months, your doctor should reevaluate your need to continue taking it.

If you do not take this drug properly, it can cause severe adverse effects (see Adverse Effects). **You must take warfarin exactly on schedule.** While taking warfarin, **your doctor should monitor your progress with regular blood tests to ensure that you are taking the most effective dose of the drug.**

Warfarin can interact with nearly all drugs. Its anticlotting action is very difficult to control when other drugs are added or subtracted, or when another drug's dose is changed. Another medication may either increase or decrease warfarin's action. **While taking warfarin, do not take any other drugs, including non-prescription drugs (such as aspirin, cold remedies, antacids, laxatives), or change** **the dose of any drug that you currently take, without consulting your doctor first.**

Before You Use This Drug

Do not use if you have or have had:

- recent surgery
- aneurysm or dissecting aorta
- threatened or incomplete abortion
- eclampsia or preeclampsia
- cerebrovascular hemorrhage, confirmed or suspected
- blood disorders
- active bleeding

- severe, uncontrolled high blood pressure
- pregnancy or are breast-feeding

Tell your doctor if you have or have had:

- allergies to drugs
- heart problems, including atrial fibrillation, myocardial infarction, or stroke
- thromboembolism
- severe allergies
- ulcers or other lesions of the gastrointestinal tract, respiratory tract, or urinary tract
- kidney or liver problems
- diverticulitis
- vasculitis
- infectious disease
- vitamin K deficiency
- alcohol dependence
- severe inflammation of blood vessels
- subacute bacterial endocarditis (infection of the heart)
- diabetes
- recent injury
- childbirth
- spinal puncture
- a fall or blow to the body or head
- wounds from trauma, ulcers, or surgery
- fever lasting more than a couple of days
- an intrauterine device (IUD)
- heavy or unusual menstrual bleeding
- medical or dental surgery
- severe or continuing diarrhea

Tell your doctor about any other drugs you take, including aspirin, herbs, vitamins, and other nonprescription products.

When You Use This Drug

- Wear a medical identification bracelet or carry a card stating that you take warfarin.
- Be very careful doing activities that may cause cuts or bleeding, such as shaving or cooking.
- Consult with your doctor immediately if any signs of bleeding occur.
- Do not drink alcohol.
- Eat a normal, balanced diet. **Do not change your diet or take nutritional supplements or vitamins without first checking with your doctor.**
- If you plan to have any surgery, including dental, tell your doctor that you take this drug.
- **Do not take any other drugs, including nonprescription products (aspirin, cold remedies, antacids, laxatives), or change the dose of drugs you are taking, without consulting your doctor.**
- **Be sure to schedule regular doctor visits for blood tests.**

How to Use This Drug

- If you miss a dose, take it as soon as you remember, but skip it if you don't remember until the next day. **Do not take double doses.** Keep a record of missed doses and give the list to your doctor at each visit.
- Do not share your medication with others.
- Take the drug at the same time(s) each day.
- Store at room temperature with lid on tightly. Do not store in the bathroom. Do not expose to heat, moisture, or strong light. Keep out of reach of children.

Interactions with Other Drugs

Warfarin can interact with nearly all drugs. Its anticlotting action is very difficult to control when other drugs are added or subtracted, or when another drug's dose is changed. Another medication may either increase or decrease warfarin's action. While taking warfarin, do not take any other drugs, including nonprescription drugs (such as aspirin, cold remedies, antacids, laxatives), or change the dose of any drug that you currently take, without consulting your doctor first.

Adverse Effects

Call your doctor immediately if you experience:

- abnormal bleeding
- bloody, cloudy, or dark urine
- difficult or painful urination or sudden decrease in amount of urine
- dizziness or fainting
- swelling of ankles, feet, or legs
- unusual weight gain
- blue or purple toes
- chills, fever, sore throat, or unusual tiredness
- yellow eyes or skin
- nausea or vomiting
- diarrhea
- skin rash, hives, or itching
- sores or white spots in mouth or throat
- sores on skin
- stomach cramps or pain
- loss of appetite
- nervousness
- confusion
- blurred vision
- chest pain
- difficulty breathing

Call your doctor if these symptoms continue:

- bloated stomach or gas
- cold intolerance
- diarrhea
- loss of appetite
- nausea or vomiting
- stomach cramps or pain

Not needing medical attention:

- loss of hair on scalp
- orange-red urine with anisindione

Signs of overdose:

- bleeding gums when brushing teeth
- nosebleeds
- unexplained bruising
- unusually heavy bleeding from cuts or wounds
- unusually heavy or unexpected menstrual bleeding

- abdominal pain or swelling
- sudden lightheadedness
- weakness
- loss of consciousness
- backaches
- blood in urine
- bloody or tarry stools
- constipation
- headache
- joint pain
- stiffness or swelling
- coughing up blood, vomiting blood or material that looks like coffee grounds
- pinpoint red spots on skin

If you suspect an overdose, call this number to contact your poison control center: (800) 222-1222.

Periodic Tests

Ask your doctor which of these tests should be done periodically while you are taking this drug:

- prothrombin time, now measured by the INR (measure of how long it takes your blood to clot): INR should be checked daily for the first week, weekly until a therapeutic level is achieved, and then monthly.
- complete blood count
- stool tests for possible blood loss
- urine tests for possible blood loss

Limited Use

Clopidogrel (kloh *pid* oh grel)
PLAVIX (Bristol-Myers Squibb)

GENERIC: not available

FAMILY: Blood-Clotting Inhibitors
Adenosine Diphosphate Blockers

PREGNANCY WARNING

There was no evidence of toxicity in animal studies. Use during pregnancy only for clear medical reasons. Tell your doctor if you are pregnant or thinking of becoming pregnant before you take this drug.

BREAST-FEEDING WARNING

Clopidogrel is excreted in animal milk. It is likely that this drug, like many others, is also excreted in human milk. Because of the potential for serious adverse effects in nursing infants, you should not take this drug while nursing.

Because the retail cost of clopidogrel is at least 100 times greater than the cost of aspirin and is no better than aspirin in preventing a second heart attack or stroke, its use should be limited to those who cannot take aspirin. The long-term use of clopidogrel in the management of patients with acute coronary syndromes is unclear. Long-term clopidogrel may be no better than aspirin.

CLOPIDOGREL AND THROMBOTIC THROMBOCYTOPENIC PURPURA (TTP)

TTP is a life-threatening adverse effect that is characterized by a breakdown of red blood cells, low levels of cells that help stop bleeding (platelets), fever, mental changes, and kidney problems.

Clopidogrel is approved by the FDA to reduce the risk of a new heart attack or stroke in patients with a history of a recent heart attack or stroke. The drug has also been approved by the FDA for a condition known as acute coronary syndrome in patients who may be treated medically or with a stent (a metal device placed in a coronary vessel to keep it open) or bypass surgery to reduce the rate of heart attack, stroke, and cardiovascular death. Acute coronary syndrome consists of unstable chest pain (angina) and changes in the electrocardiogram (EKG or ECG) that suggest a heart attack.

A single clinical trial was the basis for the FDA approving clopidogrel for preventing a second heart attack or stroke. In this trial, clopidogrel was directly compared to aspirin.[145] The difference between clopidogrel and aspirin was very small but statistically significant, favoring clopidogrel. A critique of the trial concluded by saying that the result "leaves open questions about whether such a difference is clinically meaningful, or in fact, reproducible."[146]

The trial mentioned above failed to show that clopidogrel was superior to aspirin in preventing a second heart attack or stroke. The fact that clopidogrel is no better than aspirin has not stopped its manufacturer from advertising it as a better drug. This resulted in the FDA warning Bristol-Myers Squibb/Sanofi in April 2001 about its false and misleading promotion of clopidogrel as being superior to aspirin.[147]

In a study examining the management of acute coronary syndromes, clopidogrel was found to be marginally better than aspirin by only 2.1 percent. However, there were statistically significantly more patients with major bleeding episodes (defined as needing a transfusion of at least two units of blood) in those taking clopidogrel. In this study, 1% more patients taking clopidogrel had a major bleeding episode compared to the aspirin-treated patients, but there was no statistical difference between those taking clopidogrel or aspirin in regard to episodes of life-threatening bleeding.[148]

A further analysis of the trial mentioned above found that in patients with acute coronary syndrome taking aspirin, adding clopidogrel was beneficial, compared to placebo, in reducing major cardiovascular events.[149] However, it has been noted that beyond 30 days there was no significant advantage to treatment with clopidogrel over placebo in regard to cardiovascular death or nonfatal heart attack. The long-term role of clopidogrel remains unclear.[150]

Ticlopidine (TICLID; see p. 158), a close chemical relative of clopidogrel, has been linked to a life-threatening blood disorder called thrombotic thrombocytopenic purpura (TTP).[151] Clopidogrel has also been linked to TTP. TTP was identified in 11 patients in a two-year period between March 1998 and March 2000 from an active surveillance program that involved blood banks around the U.S.[152] Between the end of 1997 and the fourth quarter of 2001 the FDA received 16 reports of TTP. It is not known if these 16 reports included the 11 mentioned above.

Before You Use This Drug

Do not use if you have or have had:

- intracranial hemorrhage
- peptic ulcer

Tell your doctor if you have or have had:

- allergy to this drug
- bleeding problems
- liver disease
- stomach ulcers
- pregnancy or are breast-feeding
- recent surgery or trauma

Tell your doctor about any other drugs you take, including aspirin, herbs, vitamins, and other nonprescription products.

When You Use This Drug

- Do not exceed the prescribed dose.
- Tell any doctor, dentist, emergency medical technician, pharmacist, or surgeon you see that you take clopidogrel. This is especially important for any surgery, including dental.

How to Use This Drug

- If you miss a dose, take it as soon as you remember, but skip it if it is almost time for the next dose. **Do not take double doses.**
- Do not share your medication with others.
- Take the drug at the same time(s) each day.
- Store at room temperature with the lid on tightly. Do not store in the bathroom. Do not ex-

pose to heat, moisture, or strong light. Keep out of reach of children.

Interactions with Other Drugs

The following drugs, biologics (e.g., vaccines, therapeutic antibodies), or foods are listed in *Evaluations of Drug Interactions* 2003 as causing "highly clinically significant" or "clinically significant" interactions when used together with any of the drugs in this section. In some sections with multiple drugs, the interaction may have been reported for one but not all drugs in this section, but we include the interaction because the drugs in this section are similar to one another. We have also included potentially serious interactions listed in the drug's FDA-approved professional package insert or in published medical journal articles. There may be other drugs, especially those in the families of drugs listed below, that also will react with this drug to cause severe adverse effects. Make sure to tell your doctor and pharmacist the drugs you are taking and tell them if you are taking any of these interacting drugs:

acemetacin, ANSAID, atorvastatin, CLINORIL, COUMADIN, DAYPRO, DEMADEX, diclofenac, DILANTIN, enoxaparin, eptifibatide, etodolac, fenbufen, fenoprofen, FELDENE, flurbiprofen, fluvastatin, ibuprofen, indomethacin, INTEGRILIN, ketoprofen, ketorolac, LESCOL, LIPITOR, LODINE, LOVENOX, meclofenamate, mefenamic acid, meloxicam, MOBIC, nadroparin, NALFON, naproxen, NOLVADEX, ORINASE, ORUVAIL, oxaprozin, phenytoin, piroxicam, PONSTEL, sulindac, tamoxifen, tiaprofenic acid, tolbutamide, TOLECTIN, tolfenamic acid, tolmetin, TORADOL, torsemide, VOLTAREN.

Adverse Effects

Call your doctor immediately if you experience:

- black, tarry stools
- blood in urine or stools
- chest pain
- cough
- fainting
- fever, chills, sneezing, or sore throat
- frequent, painful, or difficult urination
- generalized pain
- sudden or severe headache
- irregular heartbeat
- joint pain
- nosebleed
- red or purple spots on the skin
- runny nose
- shortness of breath
- skin blistering, flaking, or peeling
- sneezing
- severe stomach pain
- swelling of feet or lower legs
- ulcers, sores, or white spots in the mouth
- unusual bleeding or bruising
- vomiting of blood or material that looks like coffee grounds
- sudden weakness

Call your doctor if these symptoms continue:

- abdominal or stomach pain
- anxiety
- back pain
- constipation
- diarrhea
- depression
- dizziness
- fever
- chills
- headache
- heartburn
- insomnia
- itching
- joint pain
- leg cramps
- muscle aches
- nausea or vomiting
- numbness or tingling
- skin rash

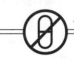 Do Not Use

ALTERNATIVE TREATMENT:
See clopidogrel, p. 155.

Ticlopidine (tye *kloe* pi deen)
TICLID (ROCHE)

FAMILY: Blood-Clotting Inhibitors
Adenosine Diphosphate Blockers

PREGNANCY WARNING

Ticlopidine caused fetal harm in animal studies. Because of the potential for serious adverse effects to the fetus, this drug should not be used by pregnant women.

BREAST-FEEDING WARMING

Ticlopidine is excreted in animal milk. It is likely that this drug, like many others, is also excreted in human milk. Because of the potential for serious adverse effects in nursing infants, you should not take this drug while nursing.

Ticlopidine is approved by the FDA to prevent stroke in people who already had strokes or have signs of developing a stroke. It should not be used by people who can take aspirin. It is also frequently used for prevention of stroke and clot formation after a procedure in which a thin tube called a stent is implanted to keep narrowed heart vessels open. However, this is not an FDA-approved use for this drug.

Ticlopidine prolongs bleeding time so blood clots are less apt to form. The dose of ticlopidine is adjusted according to bleeding time. Although somewhat more effective than aspirin in preventing strokes, ticlopidine causes significantly more adverse effects than aspirin, including life-threatening blood disorders. It lowers the white blood cell count, increasing

---

FDA BLACK BOX WARNING

TICLID can cause life-threatening hematological (blood) adverse reactions, including neutropenia/agranulocytosis, thrombotic throbocytopenia purpura (TTP) and aplastic anemia.

Neutropenia/Agranlocytosis: Among 2048 patients in clinical trials in stroke patients, there were 50 cases (2.4%) of neutropenia (less than 1200 neutrophils/mm^3), and the neutrophil count was below 450/mm^3 in 17 of these patients (0.8% of the total population).

TTP: One case of thrombotic thrombocytopenic purpura was reported during clinical trials in some patients. Based on postmarketing data, US physicians reported about 100 cases between 1992 and 1997. Based on an estimated patient exposure of 2 million to 4 million, and assuming an event reporting rate of 10% (the true rate is not known), the incidence of ticlopidine associated TTP may be as high as one case in 2000 to 4000 patients exposed.

Aplastic Anemia: Aplastic anemia was not seen during clinical trials in stroke patients, but US physicians reported about 50 cases between 1992 and 1998. Based on an estimated patient exposure of 2 million to 4 million, and assuming an event reporting rate of 10% (the true rate is not known), the incidence of ticlopidine associated aplastic anemia may be as high as one case in every 4000 to 8000 patients exposed.

Monitoring of Clinical Hematologic Status: Severe hematological adverse reactions may occur within a few days of the start of therapy. The incidence of TTP peaks after about 3 to 4 weeks of therapy and neutropenia peaks at approximately 4 to 6 weeks. The incidence of aplastic anemia peaks after about 4 to 8 weeks of therapy. The incidence of the hematologic adverse reactions declines thereafter. Only a few cases of neutropenia, TTP, or aplastic anemia have arisen after more than three months of therapy.

Hematological adverse reactions cannot be reliably predicted by any identified demographic or clinical characteristics. During the first 3 months of treatment, patients receiving TICLID must, therefore, be hematologically and clinically monitored for evidence of neutropenia or TTP. If any such evidence is seen, TICLID should be immediately discontinued.

---

risk of infections, and can injure the ability of bone marrow to make red blood cells. Ticlopidine also increases cholesterol about 10%. It should only be used by people who are allergic to aspirin. Ticlopidine should not be used by people who have had bleeding ulcers or liver disease. Anyone with kidney problems may need lower doses of ticlopidine.

Over half the individuals who take ticlopidine have had gastrointestinal adverse effects.[153] Older people are even more likely to experience adverse effects, especially gastrointestinal effects, such as nausea and diarrhea. Severe blood disorders have been reported, most frequently in women over 75 years of age.[154]

Worldwide, through 1994, a total of 645 cases of serious blood disorders had been associated with the use of ticlopidine. Of these 645 cases, 102 (16%) resulted in death. Since ticlopidine was first marketed in late 1991 through March 1995, the FDA had received 209 reports associating various types of blood disorders with this drug. Of 188 people for whom complete information was available, 36 (19%) had died. In reports to the FDA, onset of the blood disorder occurred about 30 to 45 days after starting ticlopidine. In some of the reports, people had been taking other drugs that can cause blood disorders, but most had no known causes other than ticlopidine. The bone marrow's ability to make blood cells returned to normal in most people after they stopped the drug.[154]

Potassium (poe *tass* ee um)
Supplements (Nondietary)

Packets for Suspension
MICRO-K LS (KV PHARM)

Limited Use

Extended-Release Potassium Supplements
K-DUR (Key)
K-TABS (Abbott)
KAON-CL (Savage)

GENERIC: available

FAMILY: Potassium Supplements (see p. 58)

PREGNANCY WARNING

No data is available on the use of potassium supplements during pregnancy. Use during pregnancy only for clear medical reasons. Tell your doctor if you are pregnant or thinking of becoming pregnant before you take this drug.

BREAST-FEEDING WARNING

There is no information on the use of potassium supplements during nursing. There should be no problem as long as the mother's potassium levels do not get too high.

If you need to get more of the mineral potassium, the safest and least expensive way is to eat more potassium-rich foods daily (see p. 58) for a discussion of dietary potassium). When researchers compared people eating a potassium-rich diet, people taking potassium supplements, and people taking drugs designed to keep potassium in the body, they found the following: (1) diet is the safest way to replace potassium and (2) potassium supplements and potassium-sparing drugs return potassium levels to normal in only half the people who use them.

Potassium supplements can cause stomach and intestinal ulcers, bleeding, blockage, and perforation. Because of these serious potential adverse effects, you should only take supplements if you have been eating plenty of potassium-rich foods yet still have a low level of potassium in your blood (less than 3 millimoles per liter of blood).[34] Also, you should only take potassium supplements if you have adequate kidney function. The safest form of potassium supplement is an oral solution (liquid) of potassium chloride, and you should only use other forms if you cannot tolerate the liquid. However, enteric-coated potassium products should never be taken.

Before You Use This Drug

Do not use if you have or have had:

- Addison's disease
- prolonged and severe diarrhea
- heart disease
- intestinal blockage
- kidney disease or decreased urine production
- stomach ulcer
- high blood potassium levels

Tell your doctor about any other drugs you take, including aspirin, herbs, vitamins, and other nonprescription products.

When You Use This Drug

- If you have black, tarry stools or bloody vomit, call your doctor immediately. These are signs of stomach or intestinal bleeding.
- Schedule regular appointments with your doctor to check your progress.
- Check with your doctor before using salt substitutes, low-salt milk, or other low-salt foods. Because these foods often contain potassium, your potassium supplement dose may have to be adjusted to avoid getting dangerously high levels of potassium in your blood.
- Ask your doctor whether you should supplement your diet with vitamin B_{12}. Your body may not be able to absorb this vitamin as well while you are taking potassium supplements.

How to Use This Drug

• If you miss a dose, take it within two hours of the time you were supposed to take it. **Do not take double doses.**

• Do not share your medication with others.

• Take the drug at the same time(s) each day.

• Take with, or immediately after, meals. If you are taking extended-release tablets or capsules, swallow them whole, without chewing or crushing them. Take tablets with a full glass (eight ounces) of water. Take your last dose of the day with a full glass of water at least an hour before bedtime. Taking this drug with food may help prevent stomach irritation. If you are taking a solution, dissolvable tablet, or powder, dissolve it completely in at least half a glass (four ounces) of juice or cold water, then sip slowly over a five- to ten-minute period. Do not use tomato juice, which has a high salt content.

• Store at room temperature with lid on tightly. Do not store in the bathroom. Do not expose to heat, moisture, or strong light. Do not allow the liquid form to freeze. Keep out of reach of children.

Interactions with Other Drugs

The following drugs, biologics (e.g., vaccines, therapeutic antibodies), or foods are listed in *Evaluations of Drug Interactions* 2003 as causing "highly clinically significant" or "clinically significant" interactions when used together with any of the drugs in this section. In some sections with multiple drugs, the interaction may have been reported for one but not all drugs in this section, but we include the interaction because the drugs in this section are similar to one another. We have also included potentially serious interactions listed in the drug's FDA-approved professional package insert or in published medical journal articles. There may be other drugs, especially those in the families of drugs listed below, that also will react with this drug to cause severe adverse effects. Make sure to tell your doctor and pharmacist the drugs you are taking and tell them if you are taking any of these interacting drugs:

angiotensin converting enzyme (ACE) inhibitors (see p. 91), angiotensin receptor blockers (see p. 82), potassium-sparing diuretics (see p. 69), salt substitutes.

Adverse Effects

Call your doctor immediately if you experience:

• confusion
• irregular heartbeat
• numbness or tingling in hands, feet, or lips
• unusual tiredness or weakness
• weakness or heaviness of legs
• difficulty breathing
• unexplained anxiety
• abdominal or stomach pain, cramping, or soreness
• chest or throat pain
• bloody or black tarry stools

Call your doctor if these symptoms continue:

• diarrhea
• nausea or vomiting
• stomach pain, discomfort, or gas

These adverse effects can be reduced by taking potassium with food or by using more liquid (water or juice) to dilute it.

Periodic Tests

Ask your doctor which of these tests should be done periodically while you are taking this drug:

• heart function tests, such as electrocardiogram (ECG, EKG)
• kidney function tests
• blood potassium or magnesium levels
• blood pH and bicarbonate levels

REFERENCES

1. U.S. Bureau of the Census. *Statistical Abstract of the United States: 2001.* 121st ed. Washington, D.C.: U.S. Bureau of the Census; 2001:109.

2. The Trials of Hypertension Prevention Collaborative Research Group. Effects of weight loss and sodium reduction intervention on blood pressure and hypertension incidence in overweight people with high-normal blood pressure. *Archives of Internal Medicine* 1997; 157:657–67.

3. He J, Whelton PK, Appel LJ, et al. Long-term effects of weight loss and dietary sodium reduction on incidence of hypertension. *Hypertension* 2000; 35:544–49.

4. Sacks FM, Svetkey LP, Vollmer WM, et al. Effects on blood pressure of reduced dietary sodium and the Dietary Approaches to Stop Hypertension (DASH) diet. DASH-Sodium Collaborative Research Group. *New England Journal of Medicine* 2001; 344:3–10.

5. Vollmer WM, Sacks FM, Ard J, et al. Effects of diet and sodium intake on blood pressure: subgroup analysis of the DASH-sodium trial. *Annals of Internal Medicine* 2001; 135:1019–28.

6. Kelley GA, Kelley KS. Progressive resistance exercise and resting blood pressure: A meta-analysis of randomized controlled trials. *Hypertension* 2000; 35:838–43.

7. Whelton SP, Chin A, Xin X, et al. Effect of aerobic exercise on blood pressure: A meta-analysis of randomized, controlled trials. *Annals of Internal Medicine* 2002; 136:493–503.

8. Xin X, He J, Frontini MG, et al. Effects of alcohol reduction on blood pressure: A meta-analysis of randomized controlled trials. *Hypertension* 2001; 38:1112–7.

9. Stamler R, Stamler J, Grimm R, et al. Nutritional therapy for high blood pressure. Final report of a four-year randomized controlled trial—the Hypertension Control Program. *Journal of the American Medical Association* 1987; 257:1484–91.

10. Nonpharmacological approaches to the control of high blood pressure. Final report of the Subcommittee on Nonpharmacological Therapy of the 1984 Joint National Committee on Detection, Evaluation, and Treatment of High Blood Pressure. *Hypertension* 1986; 8:444–67.

11. Schlamowitz P, Halberg T, Warnoe O, et al. Treatment of mild to moderate hypertension with dietary fibre. *The Lancet* 1987; 2:622–3.

12. Whelton PK, Appel LJ, Espeland MA, et al. Sodium reduction and weight loss in the treatment of hypertension in older persons: A randomized controlled trial of nonpharmacologic interventions in the elderly (TONE). TONE Collaborative Research Group. *Journal of the American Medical Association* 1998; 279:839–46.

13. Stamler J. Setting the TONE for ending the hypertension epidemic. *Journal of the American Medical Association* 1998; 279:878–9.

14. Hansen AG, Jensen H, Langesen LP, et al. Withdrawal of antihypertensive drugs in the elderly. *Acta Medica Scandivica* 1982; 676:178–85.

15. Vestal RE, ed. *Drug Treatment in the Elderly.* Sydney, Australia: ADIS Health Science Press, 1984:77–88.

16. Burton R. Withdrawing antihypertensive treatment. *British Medical Journal* 1991; 303:324–5.

17. Drugs for hypertension. *Medical Letter on Drugs and Therapeutics* 1991; 33:33–8.

18. National Institutes of Health. The Seventh Report of the Joint National Committee on Prevention, Detection, Evaluation, and Treatment of High Blood Pressure, 2003.

19. ALLHAT Collaborative Research Group. Major cardiovascular events in hypertensive patients randomized to doxazosin vs chlorthalidone: The antihypertensive and lipid-lowering treatment to prevent heart attack trial (ALLHAT). *Journal of the American Medical Association* 2000; 283:1967–75.

20. Drugs for hypertension. *Medical Letter on Drugs and Therapeutics* 2001; 43:17–22.

21. Siegel D, Lopez J. Trends in antihypertensive drug use in the United States: Do the JNC V recommendations affect prescribing? Fifth Joint National Commission on the Detection, Evaluation, and Treatment of High Blood Pressure. *Journal of the American Medical Association* 1997; 278:1745–8.

22. Psaty BM, Heckbert SR, Koepsell TD, et al. The risk of myocardial infarction associated with antihypertensive drug therapies. *Journal of the American Medical Association* 1995; 274:620–5.

23. Pahor M, Guralnik JM, Corti MC, et al. Long-term survival and use of antihypertensive medications in older persons. *Journal of the American Geriatrics Society* 1995; 43:1191–7.

24. Furberg CD, Psaty BM, Meyer JV. Nifedipine. Dose-related increase in mortality in patients with coronary heart disease. *Circulation* 1995; 92:1326–31.

25. Levin EG, Miller VT, Muesing RA, et al. Comparison of psyllium hydrophilic mucilloid and cellulose as adjuncts to a prudent diet in the treatment of mild to moderate hypercholesterolemia. *Archives of Internal Medicine* 1990; 150:1822–7.

26. Hall KM, Luepker RV. Is hypercholesterolemia a risk factor and should it be treated in the elderly? *American Journal of Health Promotion* 2000; 14:347–56.

27. Kaiser FE, Morley JE. Cholesterol can be lowered in older persons: Should we care? *Journal of the American Geriatrics Society* 1990; 38:84–5.

28. American College of Physicians. Geriatrics: Nutritional issues. Medical Knowledge Self-Assessment Program IX, 1991.

29. Shepherd J, Blauw GJ, Murphy MB, et al. Pravastatin in elderly individuals at risk of vascular disease (PROSPER): A randomised controlled trial. *The Lancet* 2002; 360:1623–30.

30. Beckett N, Nunes M, Bulpitt C. Is it advantageous to lower cholesterol in the elderly hypertensive? *Cardiovascular Drugs and Therapy* 2000; 14:397–405.

31. Newman TB, Hulley SB. Carcinogenicity of lipid-lowering drugs. *Journal of the American Medical Association* 1996; 275:55–60.

32. Klotrix and other slow-release potassium tablets. *Medical Letter on Drugs and Therapeutics* 1981; 23:3–4.

33. Slow-K—follow-up. *Medical Letter on Drugs and Therapeutics* 1978; 20:30–31.

34. Harrington JT, Isner JM, Kassirer JP. Our national obsession with potassium. *American Journal of Medicine* 1982; 73:155–9.

35. AMA Department of Drugs. *AMA Drug Evaluations.* 5th ed. Chicago: American Medical Association, 1983:66.

36. *Physicians' Desk Reference.* 58th ed. Montvale, N.J.: Thomson PDR, 2004:3348–9.

37. Morgan T, Adam W, Hodgson M. Adverse reactions to long-term diuretic therapy for hypertension. *Journal of Cardiovascular Pharmacology* 1984; 6(suppl 1):S269–73.

38. Wasnich R, Davis J, Ross P, et al. Effect of thiazide on rates of bone mineral loss: A longitudinal study. *British Medical Journal* 1990; 301:1303–5.

39. Schoofs MW, van der KM, Hofman A, et al. Thiazide diuretics and the risk for hip fracture. *Annals of Internal Medicine* 2003; 139:476–82.

40. Drugs for hypertension. *Medical Letter on Drugs and Therapeutics* 1984; 26:107–12.

41. Indapamide and hyponatremia. *Australian Adverse Drug Reactions Bulletin* 2002; 21:xx.

42. Seligmann H, Halkin H, Rauchfleisch S, et al. Thiamine deficiency in patients with congestive heart failure receiving long-term furosemide therapy: A pilot study. *American Journal of Medicine* 1991; 91:151–5.

43. Shimon I, Almog S, Vered Z, et al. Improved left ventricular function after thiamine supplementation in patients with congestive heart failure receiving long-term furosemide therapy. *American Journal of Medicine* 1995; 98:485–90.

44. Lynn KL, Bailey RR, Swainson CP, et al. Renal failure with potassium-sparing diuretics. *New Zealand Medical Journal* 1985; 98:629–33.

45. Bumetanide (Bumex)—a new "loop" diuretic. *Medical Letter on Drugs and Therapeutics* 1983; 25:61–3.

46. *Drugs for the Elderly.* Copenhagen, Denmark: World Health Organization, 1985.

47. Sobel KG, McCart GM. Drug use and accidental falls in an intermediate care facility. *Drug Intelligence and Clinical Pharmacy* 1983; 17:539–42.

48. *Physicians' Desk Reference.* 58th ed. Montvale, N.J.: Thomson PDR, 2004:2032–5.

49. Pfizer. Inspra (eplerenone) Professional Product Labeling, October 1, 2003. Available at: http://www.inspra.com/inspra.pdf. Accessed January 21, 2004.

50. Temple, R. Memo From: Director, Office of Drug Evaluation I, Food and Drug Administration—Eplerenone, September 27, 2002.

51. Eplerenone (Inspra). *Medical Letter on Drugs and Therapeutics* 2003; 45:39–40.

52. Pitt B, Remme W, Zannad F, et al. Eplerenone, a selective aldosterone blocker, in patients with left ventricular dysfunction after myocardial infarction. *New England Journal of Medicine* 2003; 348:1309–21.

53. Greenblatt DJ, Koch-Weser J. Adverse reactions to spironolactone: A report from the Boston Collaborative Drug Surveillance Program. *Journal of the American Medical Association* 1973; 225:40–43.

54. Neale TJ, Lynn KL, Bailey RR. Spironolactone-associated aggravation of renal functional impairment. *New Zealand Medical Journal* 1976; 83:147–9.

55. Davies DM, ed. *Textbook of Adverse Drug Reactions.* Oxford: Oxford University Press, 1977:237.

56. Yap V, Patel A, Thomsen J. Hyperkalemia with cardiac arrhythmia: Induction by salt substitutes, spironolactone, and azotemia. *Journal of the American Medical Association* 1976; 236:2775–6.

57. Pongpaew C, Songkhla RN, Kozam RL. Hyperkalemic cardiac arrhythmia secondary to spironolactone. *Chest* 1973; 63:1023–5.

58. Udezue EO, Harrold BP. Hyperkalaemic paralysis due to spironolactone. *Postgraduate Medical Journal* 1980; 56:254–5.

59. Papademetriou V, Burris J, Kukich S, et al. Effectiveness of potassium chloride or triamterene in thiazide hypokalemia. *Archives of Internal Medicine* 1985; 145:1986–90.

60. Cohn JN, Tognoni G. A randomized trial of the angiotensin-receptor blocker valsartan in chronic heart failure. *New England Journal of Medicine* 2001; 345:1667–75.

61. Pitt B, Poole-Wilson PA, Segal R, et al. Effect of losartan compared with captopril on mortality in patients with symptomatic heart failure: Randomised trial—the Losartan Heart Failure Survival Study ELITE II. *The Lancet* 2000; 355:1582–7.

62. Dickinson J. Cardiovascular Panel Votes Down Avapro sNDA (Supplemental New Drug Application). January 18, 2002. Available at: *Dickinson's FDA Webview,* http://www.fdaweb.com.

63. Pfeffer MA, Braunwald E, Moye LA, et al. Effect of captopril on mortality and morbidity in patients with left ventricular dysfunction after myocardial infarction: Results of the survival and ventricular enlargement trial. The SAVE Investigators. *New England Journal of Medicine* 1992; 327:669–77.

64. Lewis EJ, Hunsicker LG, Bain RP, et al. The effect of angiotensin-converting-enzyme inhibition on diabetic nephropathy. The Collaborative Study Group. *New England Journal of Medicine* 1993; 329:1456–62.

65. Maschio G, Alberti D, Janin G, et al. Effect of the angiotensin-converting-enzyme inhibitor benazepril on the progression of chronic renal insufficiency. The Angiotensin-Converting-Enzyme Inhibition in Progressive Renal Insufficiency Study Group. *New England Journal of Medicine* 1996; 334:939–45.

66. Giatras I, Lau J, Levey AS. Effect of angiotensin-converting enzyme inhibitors on the progression of nondiabetic renal disease: A meta-analysis of randomized trials. Angiotensin-Converting-Enzyme Inhibition and Progressive Renal Disease Study Group. *Annals of Internal Medicine* 1997; 127:337–45.

67. Ravid M, Lang R, Rachmani R, et al. Long-term renoprotective effect of angiotensin-converting enzyme inhibition in non-insulin-dependent diabetes mellitus: A 7-year follow-up study. *Archives of Internal Medicine* 1996; 156:286–9.

68. Kasiske BL, Kalil RS, Ma JZ, et al. Effect of antihypertensive therapy on the kidney in patients with diabetes: A meta-regression analysis. *Annals of Internal Medicine* 1993; 118:129–138.

69. Gannon TH, Eby TL. Angioedema from angiotensin converting enzyme inhibitors: A cause of upper airway obstruction. *Laryngoscope* 1990; 100:1156–60.

70. Roberts JR, Wuerz RC. Clinical characteristics of angiotensin-converting enzyme inhibitor-induced angioedema. *Annals of Emergency Medicine* 1991; 20:555–8.

71. Sterner G. Renal artery stenosis and ACE inhibitor. *Journal of Internal Medicine* 1990; 228:541.

72. Stoltz ML, Andrews CE Jr. Severe hyperkalemia during very-low-calorie diets and angiotensin converting enzyme use. *Journal of the American Medical Association* 1990; 264:2737–8.

73. Messerli FH, Kowey P, Grodzicki T. Sublingual nifedipine for hypertensive emergencies. *The Lancet* 1991; 338:881.

74. National Heart, Lung, and Blood Institute. New analyses regarding the safety of calcium channel blockers: A statement for health professionals, August 31, 1995.

75. Grossman E, Messerli FH, Grodzicki T, et al. Should a moratorium be placed on sublingual nifedipine capsules given for hypertensive emergencies and pseudoemergencies? *Journal of the American Medical Association* 1996; 276:1328–31.

76. Major outcomes in high-risk hypertensive patients randomized to angiotensin-converting enzyme inhibitor or calcium channel blocker vs diuretic: The Antihypertensive and Lipid-Lowering Treatment to Prevent Heart Attack Trial (ALLHAT). *Journal of the American Medical Association* 2002; 288:2981–97.

77. Lavarenne J. Side-effects of calcium inhibitors. *Therapie* 1989; 44:197–200.

78. Webster J, Petrie JC, Jeffers TA, et al. Nicardipine sustained release in hypertension. *British Journal of Clinical Pharmacology* 1991; 32:433–9.

79. Dukes MNG, Beeley L, eds. *Side Effects of Drugs Annual* 13. Amsterdam: Elsevier, 1989:158.

80. Dukes MNG, Beeley L, eds. *Side Effects of Drugs Annual* 14. Amsterdam: Elsevier, 1990:165.

81. Pierce R. Statement by Food and Drug Administration Supervisory Medical Officer to National Institutes of Health Consensus Development Conference Panel on Triglycerides, High Density Lipoprotein and Coronary Heart Disease, February 25, 1992.

82. Pierce LR, Wysowski DK, Gross TP. Myopathy and rhabdomyolysis associated with lovastatin-gemfibrozil combination therapy. *Journal of the American Medical Association* 1990; 264:71–5.

83. Fenofibrate. *Prescrire International* 1994; 3:140.

84. Executive Summary of the Third Report of The National Cholesterol Education Program (NCEP) Expert Panel on Detection, Evaluation, and Treatment of High Blood Cholesterol in Adults (Adult Treatment Panel III). *Journal of the American Medical Association* 2001; 285:2486–97.

85. *Physicians' Desk Reference.* 58th ed. Montvale, N.J.: Thomson PDR, 2004:2606–10.

86. Cannon CP, Braunwald E, McCabe CH, et al. Comparison of intensive and moderate lipid lowering with statins after acute coronary syndromes. *New England Journal of Medicine* 2004; 350:1495–1504.

87. Food and Drug Administration. Notice of Violation—Lipitor (atorvastatin calcium), December 23, 1998. Available at: http://www.fda.gov/cder/warn/nov98/7301.pdf. Accessed January 21, 2004.

88. *Physicians' Desk Reference.* 58th ed. Montvale, N.J.: Thomson PDR, 2004:2274–8.

89. Food and Drug Administration. FDA Talk Paper: Bayer Voluntarily Withdraws Baycol, August 8, 2001.

90. Ahmad SR. OPDRA [FDA] Safety Review: Statins and Hepatotoxicity, May 1, 2000.

91. Wierzbicki AS. Synthetic statins: More data on newer lipid-lowering agents. *Current Medical Research and Opinion* 2001; 17:74–7.

92. *Physicians' Desk Reference.* 58th ed. Montvale, N.J.: Thomson PDR, 2004:2025–30.

93. *Physicians' Desk Reference.* 58th ed. Montvale, N.J.: Thomson PDR, 2004:1069–74.

94. *Physicians' Desk Reference.* 58th ed. Montvale, N.J.: Thomson PDR, 2004:2113–8.

95. The University of British Columbia Department of Pharmacology & Therapeutics. Do Statins have a Role in Primary Prevention? June 1, 2003. Available at: http://www.ti.ubc.ca. Accessed January 26, 2004.

96. Wallace A, Chinn D, Rubin G. Taking simvastatin in the morning compared with in the evening: Randomised controlled trial. *British Medical Journal* 2003; 327:788.

97. Drug interactions with grapefruit juice. *Medical Letter on Drugs and Therapeutics* 2004; 46:2–4.

98. Food and Drug Administration. FDA Advisory Committee Meeting Briefing Document NDA 21–366 for the use of Crestor, June 11, 2003.

99. *Physicians' Desk Reference.* 58th ed. Montvale, N.J.: Thomson PDR, 2004:1797–1801.

100. Clofibrate and niacin in coronary heart disease. *Journal of the American Medical Association* 1975; 231:360–81.

101. Cheung MC, Zhao XQ, Chait A, et al. Antioxidant supplements block the response of HDL to simvastatin-niacin therapy in patients with coronary artery disease and low HDL. *Arteriosclerotic Thrombic and Vascular Biology* 2001; 21:1320–6.

102. *Physicians' Desk Reference.* 58th ed. Montvale, N.J.: Thomson PDR, 2004: 3085–9.

103. Three new drugs for hyperlipidemia. *Medical Letter on Drugs and Therapeutics* 2003; 45:17–9.

104. Ballantyne CM, Houri J, Notarbartolo A, et al. Effect of ezetimibe coadministered with atorvastatin in 628 patients with primary hypercholesterolemia: A prospective, randomized, double-blind trial. *Circulation* 2003; 107:2409–15.

105. Davidson MH, McGarry T, Bettis R, et al. Ezetimibe coadministered with simvastatin in patients with primary hypercholesterolemia. *Journal of the American College of Cardiology* 2002; 40:2125–34.

106. Gagne C, Bays HE, Weiss SR, et al. Efficacy and safety of ezetimibe added to ongoing statin therapy for treatment of patients with primary hypercholesterolemia. *American Journal of Cardiology* 2002; 90:1084–91.

107. Gagne C, Gaudet D, Bruckert E. Efficacy and safety of ezetimibe coadministered with atorvastatin or simvastatin in patients with homozygous familial hypercholesterolemia. *Circulation* 2002; 105:2469–75.

108. Jay RH, Rampling MW, Betteridge DJ. Abnormalities of blood rheology in familial hypercholesterolaemia: Effects of treatment. *Atherosclerosis* 1990; 85:249–56.

109. Dunagan, WC, Ridner, ML, eds. *Manual of Medical Therapeutics.* 26th ed. St. Louis: Washington University, 1989:421.

110. Choice of cholesterol-lowering drugs. *Medical Letter on Drugs and Therapeutics* 1991; 33:1–4.

111. Curtis DM, Driscoll DJ, Goldman DH, et al. Loss of dental enamel in a patient taking cholestyramine. *Mayo Clinic Proceedings* 1991; 66:1131.

112. Van Gelder IC, Hagens VE, Bosker HA, et al. A comparison of rate control and rhythm control in patients with recurrent persistent atrial fibrillation. *New England Journal of Medicine* 2002; 347:1834–40.

113. Wyse DG, Waldo AL, DiMarco JP, et al. A comparison of rate control and rhythm control in patients with atrial fibrillation. *New England Journal of Medicine* 2002; 347:1825–33.

114. Nygaard TW, Sellers TD, Cook TS, et al. Adverse reactions to antiarrhythmic drugs during therapy for ventricular arrhythmias. *Journal of the American Medical Association* 1986; 256:55–7.

115. Fick DM, Cooper JW, Wade WE, et al. Updating the Beers criteria for potentially inappropriate medication use in older adults: Results of a US consensus panel of experts. *Archives of Internal Medicine* 2003; 163:2716–24.

116. Vestal RE, ed. *Drug Treatment in the Elderly.* Sydney, Australia: ADIS Health Science Press, 1984:66.

117. Frank MJ, Watkins LO, Prisant LM, et al. Mexiletine versus quinidine as first-line antiarrhythmia therapy: Results from consecutive trials. *Journal of Clinical Pharmacology* 1991; 31:222–8.

118. Dukes MNG, Beeley L, eds. *Side Effects of Drugs Annual* 15. Amsterdam: Elsevier, 1991:178–80.

119. Podrid PJ, Kowey PR, Frishman WH, et al. Comparative cost-effectiveness analysis of quinidine, procainamide and mexiletine. *American Journal of Cardiology* 1991; 68:1662–7.

120. Widerhorn J, Sager PT, Rahimtoola SH, et al. The role of combination therapy with mexiletine and procainamide in patients with inducible sustained ventricular tachycardia refractory to intravenous procainamide. *Pacing Clinical Electrophysiology* 1991; 14:420–6.

121. Gottlieb SS, Weinberg M. Comparative hemodynamic effects of mexiletine and quinidine in patients with severe left ventricular dysfunction. *American Heart Journal* 1991; 122:1368–74.

122. Middlekauff HR, Stevenson WG, Saxon LA, et al. Amiodarone

and torsades de pointes in patients with advanced heart failure. *American Journal of Cardiology* 1995; 76:499–502.

123. Shukla R, Jowett NI, Thompson DR, et al. Side effects with amiodarone therapy. *Postgraduate Medical Journal* 1994; 70:492–8.

124. *USP DI, Drug Information for the Health Care Professional.* 16th ed. Rockville, Md.: The United States Pharmacopeial Convention, 1996:83–7.

125. Tisdale JE, Follin SL, Ordelova A, et al. Risk factors for the development of specific noncardiovascular adverse effects associated with amiodarone. *Journal of Clinical Pharmacology* 1995; 35:351–6.

126. Singh SN, Fletcher RD, Fisher SG, et al. Amiodarone in patients with congestive heart failure and asymptomatic ventricular arrhythmia: Survival Trial of Antiarrhythmic Therapy in Congestive Heart Failure. *New England Journal of Medicine* 1995; 333:77–82.

127. *Physicians' Desk Reference.* 58th ed. Montvale, N.J.: Thomson PDR, 2004:1019–20.

128. *Physicians' Desk Reference.* Montvale, N.J.: Thomson PDR, 2004:1558–62.

129. Drugs in the elderly. *Medical Letter on Drugs and Therapeutics* 1979; 21:43–4.

130. Carlson KJ, Lee DC, Goroll AH, et al. An analysis of physicians' reasons for prescribing long-term digitalis therapy in outpatients. *Journal of Chronic Diseases* 1985; 38:733–9.

131. Lee DC, Johnson RA, Bingham JB, et al. Heart failure in outpatients: A randomized trial of digoxin versus placebo. *New England Journal of Medicine* 1982; 306:699–705.

132. Fleg JL, Lakatta EG. How useful is digitalis in patients with congestive heart failure and sinus rhythm? *International Journal of Cardiology* 1984; 6:295–305.

133. Drugs for stable angina pectoris. *Medical Letter on Drugs and Therapeutics* 1994; 36:111–4.

134. *Physicians' Desk Reference.* 58th ed. Montvale, N.J.: Thomson PDR, 2004:2500–3.

135. Wolfe SM, Sasich LD, Barbehenn E. Letter to the Food and Drug Administration Concerning Cilostazol (Pletal), December 30, 1998. Available at: http://www.citizen.org/publications/release.cfm?ID=6666. Accessed January 8, 2004.

136. Barbehenn E, Wolfe SM. Letter to the Food and Drug Administration Concerning Cilostazol (Pletal), September 18, 1998. Available at: http://www.citizen.org/publications/release.cfm?ID=6656. Accessed January 8, 2004.

137. Mayor GH. Dear Health Professional Letter, Re: Withdrawal of Manoplax (flosequinan), July 20, 1993.

138. Rodin SM. Food and Drug Administration Medical Officer Review of Cilostazol, July 27, 1998:136–46.

139. Dawson DL, Cutler BS, Meissner MH, et al. Cilostazol has beneficial effects in treatment of intermittent claudication: Results from a multicenter, randomized, prospective, double-blind trial. *Circulation* 1998; 98:678–86.

140. Borer JS. Otsuka America's Presentation Before the Food and Drug Administration's Cardiovascular and Renal Drugs Advisory Committee, July 9, 1998.

141. Pentoxifylline for intermittent claudication. *Medical Letter on Drugs and Therapeutics* 1984; 26:103–4.

142. Leng GC, Fowler B, Ernst E. Exercise for intermittent claudication. *Cochrane Database of Systematic Reviews* 2000; CD000990.

143. Mass RD, Venook AP, Linker CA, et al. Pentoxifylline and aplastic anemia. *Annals of Internal Medicine* 1987; 107:427–8.

144. Hylek EM, Heiman H, Skates SJ, et al. Acetaminophen and other risk factors for excessive warfarin anticoagulation. *Journal of the American Medical Association* 1998; 279:657–62.

145. CAPRIE Steering Committee. A randomised, blinded, trial of clopidogrel versus aspirin in patients at risk of ischaemic events (CAPRIE). *The Lancet* 1996; 348:1329–39.

146. Gorelick PB, Born GV, D'Agostino RB, et al. Therapeutic benefit: Aspirin revisited in light of the introduction of clopidogrel. *Stroke* 1999; 30:1716–21.

147. Haffer AST. Food and Drug Administration Warning—Plavix (clopidogrel) Advertising, May 9, 2001.

148. Yusuf S, Zhao F, Mehta SR, et al. Effects of clopidogrel in addition to aspirin in patients with acute coronary syndromes without ST-segment elevation. *New England Journal of Medicine* 2001; 345:494–502.

149. Mehta SR, Yusuf S, Peters RJ, et al. Effects of pretreatment with clopidogrel and aspirin followed by long-term therapy in patients undergoing percutaneous coronary intervention: The PCI-CURE study. *The Lancet* 2001; 358:527–33.

150. Stables RH. Clopidogrel in invasive management of non-ST-elevation ACS. *The Lancet* 2001; 358:520–1.

151. Bennett CL, Davidson CJ, Raisch DW, et al. Thrombotic thrombocytopenic purpura associated with ticlopidine in the setting of coronary artery stents and stroke prevention. *Archives of Internal Medicine* 1999; 159:2524–8.

152. Bennett CL, Connors JM, Carwile JM, et al. Thrombotic thrombocytopenic purpura associated with clopidogrel. *New England Journal of Medicine* 2000; 342:1773–7.

153. Desager JP. Clinical pharmacokinetics of ticlopidine. *Clinical Pharmacokinetics* 1994; 26:347–55.

154. Wysowski DK, Bacsanyi J. Blood dycrasias and hematologic reactions in ticlopidine users. *Journal of the American Medical Association* 1996; 276:952.

155. Volpe M, Alderman MH, Furberg CD, et al. Beyond hypertension: Towards guidelines for cardiovascular risk reduction. *American Journal of Hypertension.* In Press.

156. Pregnancy Complicated by Disease. In *The Merck Manual of Medical Diagnosis and Therapy.* 17th ed. Beers MH, Berkow R, eds. 2004. Available at: http://www.merck.com/mrkshared/mmanual/section18/chapter251/2 51d.jsp.

157. Abnormalities of Pregnancy. In *The Merck Manual of Medical Diagnosis and Therapy.* 17th ed. Beers MH, Berkow R, eds. 2004. Available at http://www.merck.com/mrkshared/mmanual/section18/chapter252/2 52d.jsp.

158. Five-year cardiovascular risk calculator adapted by Rodney Jackson, MBChB, PhD, FRACP, Professor of Epidemiology, Department of Community Health, School of Medicine, University of Auckland, New Zealand, from the results of the Framingham Heart Study to evaluate cardiovascular risk. See Web site for reference: http://www.widebay-dgp.org.au/resources/5yrRiskCalc.xls.

159. Stadel B. FDA Medical Safety Review, 2002:43.

5

MIND DRUGS

SLEEPING PILLS AND TRANQUILIZERS

Tranquilizers (minor tranquilizers or antianxiety pills) and sleeping pills are discussed together because the most commonly used drugs in both classes belong to the same family of chemicals, called benzodiazepines. *Many of the benzodiazepines, along with another sleeping pill, zolpidem (AMBIEN), were among the 200 most dispensed drugs in community pharmacies in 2002. Although Zolpidem is not a benzodiazepine, it has many of the same effects, including the potential to cause drug-induced dependence and addiction.*

Older adults have a much more difficult time eliminating benzodiazepines and similar drugs from their bloodstreams and these drugs can thus accumulate in their bodies. Also, older adults are more sensitive to the effects of many of these drugs than are younger adults. For older adults the risk of serious adverse drug effects is significantly increased. Serious adverse effects may include: unsteady gait, dizziness, falling (causing an increased risk of hip fractures), increased risk of an auto accident, drug-induced or drug-worsened impairment of thinking, memory loss, and addiction.

Despite these significantly increased risks, sleeping pills and minor tranquilizers are prescribed much more often for older adults than they are for younger adults, for much longer periods of time, and usually not at the reduced dose that could decrease the risks. Commonly used sleeping pills or tranquilizers, in addition to the benzodiazepines, include the following:

Non-Benzodiazepine Sleeping Pills and Tranquilizers
- Buspirone (BUSPAR)
- Barbiturates: According to the World Health Organization, these drugs should not be used by older adults for anxiety or sleep disorders.[1] (Phenobarbital can be used for the treatment of convulsions or seizures.)
- Meprobamate (MILTOWN, EQUANIL)
- Hydroxyzine (ATARAX, VISTARIL) as a sleeping pill or tranquilizer
- Glutethimide (DORIDEN)
- Chloral hydrate (NOCTEC)
- Methyprylon (NOLUDAR)
- Diphenhydramine (BENADRYL, SOMINEX FORMULA)

How Often Are These Drugs Prescribed?

One study found that older adults, 65 or older, in good health were prescribed tranquilizers such as diazepam (VALIUM), sleeping pills, and sedatives 7.5 times more often than healthy people aged 18 to 64.[2]

In the United States, there was a large shift, between 1985 and 1997, in the use of psychotherapy to treat office visits in which patients had an anxiety disorder. In 1985, psychotherapy was offered, alone or in combination with prescription drugs, in 23% of office visits for anxiety disorders, but the use of psychotherapy dropped precipitously to only 5% of visits in 1997. This shift from psychotherapy to drug therapy was also accompanied by an extraordinary increase in the use of antidepressants in such visits. In 1985, in only 15.5% of visits by patients with anxiety disorders was an antidepressant prescribed, but by 1997, in 40.4% of such visits an antidepressant was prescribed, the increase mainly accounted for by the increased use of selective serotonin reuptake inhibitor (SSRI) antidepressants such as fluoxetine (PROZAC) and paroxetine (PAXIL).[3]

A survey in the United States of almost 6,000 people between the ages of 15 and 54 found that primary care physicians were much more likely than psychiatrists to prescribe antidepressants, tranquilizers, or sleeping pills for patients who did not have mood or anxiety disorders. Primary care doctors prescribed antidepressants to 22% of people, tranquilizers to 17% of people, and sleeping pills to 13% of people without mood or anxiety disorders. The author concluded that "primary care physicians are less selective in their use of psychoactive medicines, perhaps because of lower sensitivity and specificity of diagnoses in primary care settings."[4]

How Much Use Is Justified in View of the Significant Risks?

Minor Tranquilizers

Although minor tranquilizers are prescribed more often and for longer periods of time for older adults than for younger adults, studies have shown that, if anything, older adults have lower levels of "psychic distress" or serious "life crisis" than younger adults. Worse yet, since older adults usually take more prescription drugs for the direct treatment of physical diseases, the prescribing of tranquilizers is all the more dangerous because of possibly dangerous interactions.

In 1979, Roche, then the maker of Valium, Librium, and Dalmane, sent doctors brochures encouraging the use of Valium for older adults as "an important component of treatment programs for the relief of excessive geriatric anxiety and psychic tension."[5]

Faced with falling sales of Valium, the early 1980s saw Roche (and other drug makers) aggressively pursue the older adult market share. A series of handsomely illustrated brochures entitled *Roche Seminars on Aging* were mailed to doctors in 1982. Roche recommended Valium as appropriate for the elderly with "limited" coping skills, facing "not only the constraints brought about by their own reduced capabilities, but also those imposed by the social structure and environment."

In a discussion about the use of tranquilizers and sleeping pills by older adults, World Health Organization (WHO) experts said the following: *"Anxiety is a normal response to stress and only when it is severe and disabling should it lead to drug treatment. Long-term treatment . . . is rarely effective and should be avoided. . . . Short-term use (less than two weeks) will minimize the risk of dependence."*

They concluded by saying that *"discussion of the problems of sleeplessness and anxiety and the drawbacks of drug therapy will often help the patient to come to terms with his or her problem without the need to resort to drugs."*[1]

Two studies on alternatives to the use of minor tranquilizers further highlight how much of the present use is unnecessary. Ninety patients, suffering mainly from anxiety, were randomly divided into two groups when they went to see their family doctors. The first group was given the usual dose of one of the benzodiazepine tranquilizers. The other group was given a small dose of a much safer treatment consisting solely of "listening, explanation, advice, and reassurance." The two treatments were equally effective in relieving the anxiety, but those receiving the informal counseling were more satisfied with their treatment than those given minor tranquilizers.[6]

In a second study, patients with anxiety were given either one of three different tranquilizers or a placebo (sugar pill). At the end of a month, with weekly evaluations of their anxiety levels being made by the patients themselves and by professional evaluators, the results showed "all four treatments to be efficacious in their therapeutic effects on relieving anxiety."[7] That is, placebos worked as well as tranquilizers.

Sleeping Pills

The increases in the use of these drugs by older adults, noted above, flies strongly in the face of the conclusions and recommendations of an exhaustive study by the National Academy of Sciences' Institute of Medicine in 1979.[8,9]

Speaking generally about the use of sleeping pills, the study concluded that: *"hypnotics (sleeping medications) should have only a limited place in contemporary medical practice: it is difficult to justify much of the current prescribing of sleeping medication. As a standard of prudent ambulatory medical care, the committee favors the prescription of only very limited numbers of sleeping pills for use for a few nights at a time. . . . Hypnotic drugs should be selected carefully and prescribed cautiously, if at all, for patients . . . who are old."*

Commenting specifically on sleeping pill use

by older adults, the authors said: *"Of particular concern is the regular and prolonged use by this group of sleep-inducing medications that are of dubious value, and that add new hazards to their already complicated drug intake regimens."*

Although older people tend to complain more than younger people about sleeping problems, the study found that the time it takes to fall asleep does not increase with age, and that the total sleep time decreases very little, if at all. Older people who go to bed early and take catnaps during the daytime often do have sleeping problems. But, the study concluded, "it is this pattern of daytime sleep that must be changed instead of treating the night time insomnia that results from it."

According to Dr. Marshall Folstein, a Johns Hopkins psychiatrist and expert in Alzheimer's disease, *"it is extraordinarily rare to find an older person who actually requires them [sleeping pills]."* [10]

What Are the Main Risks of Sleeping Pills and Tranquilizers?

Drug-induced dependence, daytime sedation, confusion, memory loss, increased risk of an auto accident, poor coordination resulting in falls and hip fractures, impaired learning ability, slurred speech, and even death are adverse effects of these drugs. They are more likely to occur when these drugs are taken in combination with alcohol or other depressant drugs. They can happen to anyone at any age.

Older adults, however, cannot clear many of these drugs from their systems as rapidly as younger people can. They are also more sensitive to the drugs' adverse effects. Despite this evidence, older adults (1) are more likely to be given a prescription for tranquilizers or sleeping pills, (2) are not usually given the reduced dose that would at least diminish the odds of serious adverse effects, and (3) are prescribed these drugs for longer periods of time than are

younger people. Therefore, it is not surprising that older adults are at much greater risk of suffering from adverse effects, and, when they occur, they are much more serious.

One of the biggest impediments to discovering and eliminating these drug-induced problems is their frequent attribution to the aging process instead of to the drugs. The onset of impaired intelligence with memory loss, confusion, or impaired learning, or the onset of loss of coordination in a younger person will more likely prompt an inquiry leading to the drug as culprit. But the same symptoms in an older person, especially if they develop more slowly, are often dismissed with a familiar remark, "Well, he (or she) is just growing old, what do you expect?" This lack of suspicion allows the drug to keep doing damage because the doctor keeps up the prescription.

Hip Fractures

A study of 1,021 older adults with hip fractures found that 14% of these life-threatening injuries are attributable to the use of mind-affecting drugs, including sleeping pills and minor tranquilizers, antipsychotics, and antidepressants. [11]

There are approximately 227,000 hip fractures each year in the United States, virtually all in older adults. [12] Since the above study found that 14% of hip fractures are drug-induced, this means that if the results of the study are projected nationally, approximately 32,000 hip fractures a year in older adults are caused by the use of mind-affecting drugs. Of these, about 30%, or almost 10,000 hip fractures a year, are caused by sleeping pills and minor tranquilizers, particularly the long-acting drugs such as Valium, Librium, and Dalmane.

In a random sample of more than 4,000 people aged 20–89 followed for 12 years, 8.2% had suffered falls sufficiently serious as to cause hospitalization or death. People who had had one such injurious fall were 3.4 times more likely to have been daily users of sleeping pills and were 2.2 times more likely to have sometimes used these medicines. Even more striking, those people who had suffered two or more injurious falls were 8.2 times more likely to be daily users of sleeping pills and 3.9 times more likely to be occasional users of sleeping pills. This confirms and better quantifies earlier studies clearly linking the use of sleeping pills with falls and serious injuries.[13]

Especially in older people, injurious falls cause hip fractures that frequently lead to an increased risk of death.

Automobile Crashes That Caused Injuries

A study involving 495 automobile crashes by older drivers in which an injury occurred found that a significant number of such crashes by older adults aged 65–84 were attributable to the use of benzodiazepine tranquilizers and cyclic antidepressants. The study was particularly impressive because its findings were strengthened by observing that the rate of crashes that caused injuries increased in the same group of people when they were using these drugs as opposed to when they were not using the drugs. The majority of the excess number of auto crashes were attributable to the benzodiazepines. The authors, stating that the study findings may be generalizable to the population at large, found that if the association is causal, out of the 217,000 crashes that cause injuries that occur each year among elderly drivers, at least 16,000 are attributable to psychoactive drug use (specifically benzodiazepines and tricyclic antidepressants).[14]

Drug-Induced or Drug-Worsened Senility (Decreased Mental Functioning)

Drug-induced impairment of thinking is one of the most reversible, or treatable, forms of dementia. It is a by-product of the increased use of drugs during the past few decades. Among the 33 million people 65 and over in the United States, approximately 5 out of every 100 have dementia, with an estimated 1 of these 5 due to "reversible" conditions such as treatable diseases (thyroid disease, for example) or adverse effects of drugs.[15]

A study of 308 older adults with significant intellectual impairment found that in 11.4% of these people the problem was caused or worsened by a drug.[16] This study, the first ever to systematically analyze this problem, revealed that after stopping the use of the dementia-causing drugs, all persons had long-term improvement of their mental function. The most common class of drugs to cause the impairment of mental function was the sleeping pill/tranquilizer group. It accounted for 46% of the drug-induced or drug-worsened dementia.

The University of Washington researchers who did the study had two further observations:

1. "Most patients had used these drugs for years, and the side effect of cognitive (mental) impairment developed insidiously as a 'late' complication of a drug begun at an earlier age."
2. "The improvement experienced by patients in this study was usually surprising to family and caregivers. The patients noted an improved sense of well-being and were better able to care for themselves."

If these important findings are applied to all of the estimated 1.43 million Americans 65 and over who have dementia, there are 163,000 people whose mental impairment has either been entirely caused by or worsened by drugs. For approximately 75,000 older adults, their impaired mental functioning is caused by sleeping pills or minor tranquilizers.

Drug-Induced Dependence

Drug-induced dependence is often called addiction by drug companies and doctors who seek to shift blame to the patients who were prescribed a drug but were not told that the drug could cause physical dependence. The withdrawal from drug-induced dependence includes symptoms of sweating, nervousness, or when more severe, hallucinations or seizures that are often accompanied by psychological dependence.

The myth used to be that only people who were prone to addiction, as judged by a prior history of alcoholism or other drug problems, would possibly become addicted to benzodiazepine tranquilizers or sleeping pills. Even then they would have to use very large doses of these drugs for a long period of time before addiction could occur.

This attitude, intended to cover up a major national problem, was "pushed" by the president of Hoffman-la Roche, the world's biggest benzodiazepine maker (Valium, Librium, and Dalmane). Testifying in 1979 before U.S. Senate hearings on the abuse of these drugs, Robert Clark said that "true addiction is probably exceedingly unusual and, when it occurs, is probably confined to those individuals with abuse-prone personalities who ingest very large amounts."[17]

It was clear then and is now even clearer that a large fraction, probably the overwhelming majority, of people who use any of the benzodiazepines at the recommended dose for more than one or two months will become dependent.

Another study showed that a large proportion of people became *dependent* on these drugs and experienced an unpleasant withdrawal syndrome when they suddenly stopped taking the drug (as opposed to gradually tapering the dose to reduce, if not eliminate, the withdrawal symptoms). The only difference between addiction to the longer-acting drugs such as Valium and Dalmane, and the shorter-acting drugs such as Ativan and Serax, was the time, after the drug was suddenly stopped, that it took before withdrawal symptoms occurred. With the longer-acting drugs the day of worst symptoms was the tenth; for the shorter-acting drugs it was the first. Withdrawal symptoms included anxiety, headache, insomnia, tension, sweating, difficulty concentrating, tremor, fear, and fatigue.

The authors of the study concluded that *"when withdrawal was abrupt, symptoms were more frequent and more severe than when a gradual tapering technique was used. . . . there is little justification for abrupt withdrawal."*[18]

Serious Breathing Problems

Another serious adverse effect of the benzodiazepines is their effect on respiration. One effect of these drugs has to do with sleep apnea, a common condition in older adults in which, for varying periods of time while asleep, breathing stops. Dr. William Dement, an expert in sleep research, has found that older people with sleep apnea who use sleeping medications can stop breathing for much longer—dangerously longer—periods of time as a result of the respiration-suppressing effects of the drugs. He told a government task force on sleeping problems that people over 65 should not use Dalmane because of the risk of worsening sleep apnea.[19]

A second problem in this category affects people with severe lung disease. Anyone with severe lung disease should not use benzodiazepines because they decrease the urge to breathe, which can be life-threatening.[20] Asthmatics should also avoid benzodiazepine sleeping pills and tranquilizers.

Other Adverse Effects[21]

• **Frequent:** drowsiness and lack of coordination that can affect walking or driving a car.

• **Occasional:** confusion, forgetfulness, rebound insomnia (more difficulty sleeping when the drug wears off), or, especially with triazolam (HALCION), excitement instead of sedation.

• **Rare:** low blood pressure, bone marrow toxicity, liver disease, allergies, and rage reactions.

Reducing the Risks from Sleeping Pills and Tranquilizers

The best way to reduce the risks of these powerful drugs is to avoid using them for most of the conditions for which they are now prescribed, especially in older adults.

Alternatives for Anxiety

According to noted British psychiatrist Dr. Malcolm Lader: *"Until recently most anxious patients in the United Kingdom were treated with tranquilizers, usually a benzodiazepine. However, recognition that these drugs can cause dependence even at normal therapeutic dosages has led to a re-evaluation of drug therapy, and the value of non-pharmacologic treatments is increasingly being recognized."* [22]

Two British doctors use a nondrug alternative for the treatment of mild to moderate anxiety (and similar problems). They say that "the best treatment is likely to be brief counseling provided by the general practitioner or by another professional working in the practice. Such counseling need not be intensive or specially skilled. It should always include careful assessment of the causes of the patient's distress. Once these have been identified, anxiety may often be reduced to tolerable levels by means of explanation, exploration of feelings, reassurance, and encouragement." [6]

What else can be done? Talking to nonmedical people—a friend, a spouse, a relative, a member of the clergy, may help to identify causes of anxiety and potential solutions. Gathering the courage to talk about difficult concerns will generally be a better solution than taking pills. For some people, a specialized form of psychotherapy can treat anxiety. If indeed medication is needed, it is best to see a psychiatrist. Getting regular exercise can also help relieve anxiety.

In addition, the use of foods, beverages, and over-the-counter (nonprescription) or pre-scription drugs that have significant stimulant effects can also cause a chemically induced anxiety that can be remedied. (See the list of such substances below, under alternatives for sleeping problems.)

Alternatives for Sleeping Problems

Experts in sleep and aging have recently stated that:

• Many old people have exaggerated expectations of what sleep should be like and they "spend too much time in bed chasing sleep."
• Many older people use sleep as an escape from boredom.
• "It's extraordinarily rare to find an old person who actually requires [sleeping pills]." [10]

If the cause of the sleeping problem is depression (see p. 184 for other problems that go along with depression), the depression should be addressed rather than simply treating the symptom by prescribing sleeping medication. If the cause is a medical condition, with pain as one of the components, the pain has to be treated rather than using a sleeping pill to induce sleep despite the pain. In the case of senile brain disease, such as Alzheimer's, the sleep disturbance will probably not respond to sleeping medications. [8]

Drugs can produce stimulating effects and a chemically induced anxiety, making sleep more difficult:

• *Over-the-counter (nonprescription) drugs:* Sleeplessness can be caused by caffeine, found in Anacin and other drugs, the stimulants found in Actifed, Contac, Sudafed, and other decongestant products, and the ingredients in many asthma drugs.
• *Prescription drugs:* Sleeping problems may be caused by asthma drugs containing theophylline or aminophylline such as Slo-bid and Somophyllin, amphetamines such as Dexedrine and diet pills, steroids such as cortisone and

prednisone, thyroid drugs, and the withdrawal from the use of sleeping pills, tranquilizers, and antidepressants. (See p. 29 in Chapter 3 for a list of drugs that can cause insomnia.)

If you have a sleeping problem and use one of these drugs, or if the problem began when you started using another drug, talk to your doctor. Tell him or her all the drugs (over-the-counter and prescription) you are taking. It might be possible to change the drug or lower the dosage to help you sleep. Returning to sleeping pills to get past withdrawal effects will only place you in a vicious cycle.

An excellent review of nonpharmacologic approaches to managing insomnia offers suggestions far more sensible, less dangerous, and less expensive than reliance on prescription drugs. As the authors of this review stated, "Nonpharmacological treatments not only cause fewer side effects, but they can sustain long-term improvements more successfully than pharmacological treatments."[23]

We review some of the suggestions from this review below:

Stimulus Control

Instructions given to patients for this "treatment" include the following:

1. Go to bed only when you feel tired.

2. Use the bed and bedroom for sleep and sex. For example, do not read books or magazines, watch TV, eat, or worry while in bed.

3. Leave the room if you do not fall asleep within 15–20 minutes. Remain in the other room for as long as you wish or need. Return to bed only when you feel sleepy again.

4. If you still cannot sleep, repeat step 3. Do this as often as necessary throughout the night.

5. Get up at the same time every morning regardless of how much sleep you obtained the night before (use an alarm clock if necessary).

6. Avoid napping.

Sleep Hygiene Education

1. Avoid the use of caffeine-containing products (including tea, coffee, and chocolate), nicotine, and alcohol, especially later in the day.

2. Avoid heavy meals within two hours of bedtime.

3. Avoid drinking fluids after supper to prevent frequent nighttime urination.

4. Avoid environments that will make you really active after 5:00 P.M. (i.e., avoid noisy environments).

5. Only use your bed for sleep. Sit in your chair when you just want to relax.

6. Avoid watching television in bed (i.e., watch it in your chair).

7. Establish a routine for getting ready to go to bed.

8. Set time aside to relax before bed, and utilize relaxation techniques.

9. Create an atmosphere conducive to sleep: Keep yourself at a comfortable temperature by modifying the number of blankets you use. Use earplugs if it is too noisy. Make the room darker if there is too much light (e.g., close the door). Put an extra mattress on your bed if it is uncomfortable.

10. When in bed, relax and think pleasant thoughts to help you fall asleep.

11. Get up at the same time every day, including weekends. Use an alarm clock if it will help.

12. Avoid taking daytime naps. If you have to take them, make sure you do so before 3.00 P.M. and that the total time napping does not exceed one hour.

13. Pursue regular physical activity, such as walking or gardening, but avoid vigorous exercise too close to bedtime.

Which Tranquilizers or Sleeping Pills Should You Use, If Any?

Although we strongly discourage the use of these drugs in most situations, especially for older adults, there are some perfectly competent physicians who, in very well defined circumstances and for very short periods of time, will prescribe them. But even the labeling approved by the Food and Drug Administration for all of the tranquilizers has to state, "Anxiety or tension associated with the stress of everyday life usually does not require treatment with an anxiolytic [tranquilizer]."[125],[126] (See the six rules for safer use on p. 175.)

As mentioned at the beginning of this chapter, older adults should never use barbiturates as sleeping pills or tranquilizers. Other drugs such as meprobamate (MILTOWN, EQUANIL), hydroxyzine (VISTARIL, ATARAX) for sleep, glutethimide (DORIDEN), chloral hydrate (NOCTEC), and methyprylon (NOLUDAR) should also not be used.[24]

This leaves buspirone (BUSPAR, see p. 232) and the benzodiazepines, with the eight benzodiazepine drugs marketed primarily as tranquilizers and five as sleeping pills. All of these drugs are equally effective in tranquilizing or promoting sleep. "Calling some anti-anxiety drugs and others hypnotics (sleeping pills) has more to do with marketing than with pharmacology."[25]

These 13 benzodiazepine drugs are different from each other, and the difference has to do with the different ways in which they are dangerous for older adults. The World Health Organization specifically recommends that older adults should not use the sleeping pill DALMANE (flurazepam), "owing to a high incidence of adverse effects."[26]

Seven other benzodiazepines are also more slowly cleared out of the body, especially in older adults, and can therefore accumulate, leading to higher blood levels and increased risks. These drugs, which also should be avoided by older adults, are diazepam (VALIUM), chlordiazepoxide (LIBRIUM), clorazepate (TRANXENE), prazepam (CENTRAX), halazepam (PAXIPAM), quazepam (DORAL), and estazolam (PROSOM).

Another widely used sleeping pill, triazolam (HALCION), should also be avoided by older adults because it is so short-acting that it can cause rebound insomnia (increased sleeping problems when the drug effect has worn off), anxiety, serious amnesia (forgetfulness or memory loss in which long periods of time can completely disappear from memory), and violent, aggressive behavior. In 1992, Public Citizen's Health Research Group petitioned the Food and Drug Administration to ban Halcion. The sleeping pill estazolam (PROSOM) is in the same class as Halcion and, according to *The Medical Letter,* there is no reason to use it.[26] It also has the disadvantage of slow clearance from the body.

In a discussion of which of these drugs are best for older adults, it was stated that oxazepam (SERAX) and temazepam (RESTORIL) were the drugs of choice.[27] It has also been stated that "oxazepam (SERAX) may be the safest benzodiazepine for the older patient" because "oxazepam may offer the advantages of a short half-life and the absence of active metabolites" (that is, chemicals the body converts the drug into that can also have adverse effects).[24] In addition, studies have shown that oxazepam has much less of a "street" drug abuse potential than, for example, diazepam (VALIUM).[28],[29]

We do not recommend the use of any benzodiazepines other than oxazepam. Here is how the large proportion of older adults who are using these drugs to their physical and mental detriment can stop using them, more safely.

If you have been taking any of these drugs for longer than several weeks continuously, there is a good chance that you have become addicted. Stopping the drugs suddenly (going "cold turkey") is a bad idea. With the help of your doctor, work out a schedule for slowly tapering down the amount of tranquilizer or sleeping pill by an average of 5 to 10% each day. Keep a written record of the dosage reduction schedule with you. This will greatly reduce the difficulty of stopping the use of these drugs.

In an article on how 11 of these benzodiazepines compare with one another as far as memory loss (a serious problem especially in older adults), geriatric drug expert Dr. Peter Lamy stated that oxazepam had less memory impairment than all other benzodiazepines except clorazepate,[30] a long-acting tranquilizer that should not be used by older adults for the reasons mentioned above.

For other patients—not older adults—temazepam and clorazepate can also be used. In addition, the sleeping pill zolpidem (AMBIEN), discussed on p. 230, can also be used for those under 60. However, as mentioned in the profile on this drug, although it is technically not a benzodiazepine—the family containing Librium and Valium—it may still cause addiction and it should not be used for more than one to three weeks.

In summary, the only prescription tranquilizers or sleeping pills that we advise for limited use in the older adult are buspirone (BUSPAR) and oxazepam, available generically, and under the brand name of Serax.

RULES FOR SAFER USE OF OXAZEPAM

(This is the only benzodiazepine we believe should be prescribed for older adults.)

1. The dose should be one-third to one-half the dose for younger people. This means that the highest starting dose for older adults should be 7.5 milligrams, one to three times a day, if used as a tranquilizer, or 7.5 milligrams at bedtime, if used as a sleeping pill. (This is half of a 15 milligram tablet, generically available.)

2. Ask your doctor to limit the size of the prescription to seven days' worth of pills.

3. Ask your doctor to write NO REFILL on the prescription so that you will not be inclined (because of the "good chemical feelings" these pills may provide) to refill the prescription five times without seeing the doctor again. This dangerously lax refill policy is perfectly legal because oxazepam and other similar drugs are not very carefully controlled by the government. By urging your doctor to write NO REFILL, you are making sure that he or she will reevaluate your condition after you use oxazepam for a short time. You want to discuss how you are doing with your anxiety or sleeping problem, rather than continuing to take the drug without a reevaluation. Continuing to take oxazepam without talking to your doctor could be the first step to addiction or other drug-induced problems.

4. At the end of the first day, and every day you use oxazepam, evaluate what you have done, on your own or by talking to others, to find out what is making you anxious. This includes evaluation of what you have done to alter the internal or external circumstances causing your anxiety. Keep a record of these evaluations. As soon as possible, try reducing the dose, in consultation with your doctor. Since you only have enough medication for one week, it is unlikely you will have become addicted this quickly.

5. Do not drive a car or operate dangerous machinery while using oxazepam.

6. Do not drink alcohol. The combination of this drug with alcohol dangerously increases the effects of both. An overdose of oxazepam in combination with alcohol can be fatal.

Before using oxazepam, make sure that your doctor knows if you are taking other drugs with a sedative or "downer" effect, such as antidepressants, antipsychotics, antihistamines, narcotic painkillers, epilepsy medications, barbiturates, or other sleeping medications. Oxazepam taken with other drugs with sedative effects dangerously increases the risks of both.

ANTIPSYCHOTIC DRUGS: ANOTHER GROUP OF DANGEROUSLY OVERUSED DRUGS

Antipsychotic drugs, also called neuroleptic drugs or major tranquilizers, are properly and successfully used to treat serious psychotic mental disorders, the most common of which is schizophrenia. Schizophrenia is a disease in which people have lost touch with reality, often see or hear things that are not there (hallucinations), believe things that are not true (delusions), often have severe mood problems such as depression, lose their expressiveness of feeling ("flat affect"), and in general have disorders of thinking. Psychoses include other mental disorders which involve abnormal perceptions of reality such as hallucinations and delusions. Schizophrenia and the other psychoses are much less common in older adults than in younger adults, according to studies done by the National Institute of Mental Health.

Whereas about 1.12% of people aged 18 to 44 have been found to have active schizophrenia (symptoms in last six months) and 0.6% of 45- to 64-year-olds have this diagnosis, only 0.1% of people 65 and older are diagnosed as having active schizophrenia.[31] In other words, active schizophrenia is only one-tenth to one-fifth as common in older adults as in younger adults.

In younger adults, an alarming number of those with schizophrenia who could and often have previously benefited from antipsychotic drugs are not receiving them. They are seen, among other places, on the streets and in homeless shelters. In older adults, the problem is not underuse but, rather, gross overuse by people who are not psychotic.

Drugs That Can Cause Psychoses (Hallucinations) or Delirium

For anyone of any age who has recently become psychotic (has hallucinations, for example) or developed delirium, there should be careful questioning to see if this serious mental problem might have been drug-induced before the person is started on antipsychotic drugs. Drugs that may cause hallucinations or other symptoms of psychosis include many street drugs (e.g., PCP, LSD) as well as many prescribed drugs listed below. In someone who is 60 years old or older, there is a strong likelihood that the recent onset of hallucinations, delirium, or other behavior that is like schizophrenia is due either to the effects of the drugs listed below or withdrawal from addiction to alcohol, barbiturates, or other sleeping pills or tranquilizers. Commonly used drugs that may cause psychotic symptoms such as hallucinations or delirium include the following:[21]

- analgesics/narcotics such as indomethacin (INDOCIN), ketamine (KETALAR), morphine (ROXANOL), pentazocine (TALWIN), propoxyphene (DARVON), and salicylates (aspirin)
- antibiotics and other anti-infective agents such as acyclovir (ZOVIRAX), amantadine (SYMMETREL), amphotericin B (FUNGIZONE), chloroquine (ARALEN), cycloserine (SEROMYCIN), dapsone, ethionamide (TRECATOR-SC), isoniazid (INH), nalidixic acid (NEGGRAM), penicillin G, podophyllum (PODOFIN), quinacrine (ATABRINE), and thiabendazole (MINTEZOL)
- anticonvulsants such as ethosuximide (ZARONTIN), phenytoin (DILANTIN), and primidone (MYSOLINE)
- allergy drugs such as antihistamines (CHLOR-TRIMETON, DIMETANE, etc.)
- antiparkinsonians such as levodopa and carbidopa (SINEMET), bromocriptine (PARLODEL), and levodopa (LARODOPA)
- asthma drugs such as albuterol (PROVENTIL, VENTOLIN)

• drugs for depression such as trazodone (DESYREL) and tricyclic antidepressants such as amitriptyline (ELAVIL) and doxepin (SINEQUAN)

• heart drugs such as digitalis preparations (LANOXIN, etc.), lidocaine (XYLOCAINE), procainamide (PROCANBID), and tocainide (TONOCARD)

• high blood pressure drugs such as clonidine (CATAPRES), methyldopa (ALDOMET), prazosin (MINIPRESS), and propranolol (INDERAL)

• nasal decongestants such as ephedrine, oxymetazoline (AFRIN), phenylephrine (NALDECON), and pseudoephedrine (SUDAFED)

• drugs such as amphetamines, PCP, barbiturates, and powder and crack cocaine

• sedatives/tranquilizers such as alprazolam (XANAX), diazepam (VALIUM), ethchlorvynol (PLACIDYL), and triazolam (HALCION)

• steroids such as dexamethasone (DECADRON) and prednisone (DELTASONE)

• other drugs such as atropine, aminocaproic acid (AMICAR), baclofen (LIORESAL), cimetidine (TAGAMET), ranitidine (ZANTAC), disulfiram (ANTABUSE), methylphenidate (RITALIN), methysergide (SANSERT), metrizamide (AMIPAQUE), phenelzine (NARDIL), thyroid hormones, and vincristine (ONCOVIN)

How Often Are Antipsychotic Drugs Used in Older Adults?

There was more than a doubling of the number of prescriptions for antipsychotic drugs in U.S. doctors' offices between 1989 and 1997. In 1989, such prescriptions were written during 3.2 million office visits, but were written during 6.9 million office visits in 1997. Most of the increase was in the prescribing of the newer, so-called atypical antipsychotic drugs such as risperidone (RISPERDOL) and olanzapine (ZYPREXA). Although the proportions of the various diseases being treated with these drugs remained constant, with 78% of patients being treated for schizophrenia, affective disorders such as depression, or other psychiatric disorders, 22% of patients in 1997 were being prescribed these powerful drugs for a "nonpsychiatric disorder." The number of office visits in 1997 during which such a prescription was written was 1.5 million.[32]

In nursing homes in the United States, where misuse of antipsychotic drugs has been notorious, antipsychotic drugs were found to be the leading cause of adverse drug reactions, comprising 23% of all adverse drug reactions, and also were found to be the leading cause of preventable adverse drug reactions. Collectively, antipsychotic drugs, sleeping pills, and antidepressants accounted for 48% of all adverse drug reactions in nursing homes and 62% of the preventable adverse reactions.[33]

A recent study in the UK, with findings similar to those in the United States, found that only 17.8% of nursing home residents receiving antipsychotic drugs were getting them for appropriate reasons. The wise advice given by these authors needs to be taken seriously by those in charge of nursing homes worldwide and, moreover, by all who take care of elderly patients. "Before pharmacotherapy is considered for elderly patients with problem behaviour, physical causes, behavioural modification and environmental changes should be explored. [Antipsychotics] can be withdrawn in up to half of recipients with no deterioration or an improvement in resident cognition, memory, or behaviour."[34]

What Are These Antipsychotic Drugs Being Prescribed For, If Not for Schizophrenia and Other Psychoses?

A group of physicians and other health professionals who specialize in geriatric pharmacology have stated: *"The usefulness of antipsychotic medications in nonpsychotic, elderly patients has been questioned.... The high fre-*

quency of toxic reactions to these drugs is well documented, with many older patients who take them experiencing orthostatic hypotension [low blood pressure on sitting or standing], Parkinson's syndrome, tardive dyskinesia [see p. 897], akathisia [see p. 889], worsened confusion, dry mouth, constipation, oversedation, and urinary incontinence." [35]

One of the more common purposes for which antipsychotic drugs are blatantly misused is as a sedative in nursing home patients. [36] Other unjustifiable uses include controlling the overall level of disturbance in older demented (nonpsychotic) patients, [37] and for treating chronic anxiety. [38] Two different studies concluded that often the most mentally alert and least physically disabled people are given these drugs. [39,40] This is consistent with the charge that these drugs are being used more for the convenience of the nursing home staff or other caretakers than for the needs of the patients.

Another study found that "80% of elderly demented persons are receiving tranquilizers (antipsychotic drugs) unnecessarily." [41] Other researchers concluded that antipsychotics are "frequently prescribed inappropriately as sedatives to elderly patients" and that "using these drugs incorrectly or for unnecessarily prolonged periods enhances the probability of developing this virtually untreatable, disfiguring syndrome" (referring to tardive dyskinesia). [42]

In other words, medical professionals should attempt to find out what it is in the environment that may be causing or contributing to the problems older people are having and, if possible, change it, rather than endanger their health with these powerful drugs. A perfect example is the use of antipsychotic drugs at the end of the day to treat the so-called sundowner syndrome. As the end of the day approaches, some nursing home or hospital patients become agitated, restless, or confused and may wander about. A careful study of the characteristics of people with this problem found that they were much more likely to have been in their present room for less than one month, to have come to the nursing home or hospital recently, and to be awakened on the evening shift. The implication was that changes in the management of these patients by nurses and other staff could reduce the problem without resorting to the use of antipsychotic drugs. [43]

Has Federal Regulation Improved the Use of Antipsychotic Drugs in Nursing Homes?

The Omnibus Budget Reconciliation Act of 1987 (OBRA-87) included provisions for regulating the use of psychotropic medications, particularly antipsychotics, in long-term care facilities. Several surveys conducted since the enactment of OBRA-87 suggest that the use of these powerful drugs in elderly nursing home residents is being curtailed.

A review of prescription and medical records in eight nursing homes conducted between August 1994 and March 1996 found that of a total of 1,573 residents, 279 were taking antipsychotic drugs (17.7%). Of these 279, 70.9% were receiving the drug for an appropriate reason, 90.1% were prescribed the drug within the recommended dosage limits, and appropriate target symptoms were documented in 90.4% of these residents. [44]

Benefits and Risks of Antipsychotic Drugs

For the small fraction of older adults taking antipsychotic drugs appropriately, that is for the treatment of psychotic illnesses such as schizophrenia, the significant risks are more than balanced out by the proven benefits for those people who respond. But at least 80% of the use of these drugs in older adults is inappropriate. Either the drugs are ineffective, as in the treatment of senile dementia, or unnecessary, as in their frequent uses to sedate or control nonpsychotic behavior that is often responsive to nondrug approaches.

What Are the Main Adverse Effects of Antipsychotic Drugs?

Falls and hip fractures

Approximately 16,000 older adults a year suffer from drug-induced hip fractures, attributable to the use of antipsychotic drugs. In one study, the main category of drugs responsible for falls leading to hip fractures was antipsychotic drugs.[11] Fifty-two percent of those hip fractures attributable to the use of mind-affecting drugs were due to antipsychotic drug use. (Also, see section on minor tranquilizers and sleeping pills, p. 168.)

Nerve problems

Tardive dyskinesia: This is the most common, serious, and sometimes irreversible adverse effect of antipsychotic drugs. It is characterized by involuntary movements of the lips, tongue, and sometimes the fingers, toes, and trunk.[21] Older adults are at increased risk for this adverse effect, and it may occur in as many as 40% of people over the age of 60 taking antipsychotic drugs.[45]

Tardive dyskinesia is more common and more severe in older adults. The majority of cases are irreversible and often result in immobility, difficulty chewing and swallowing, and eventually weight loss and dehydration. None of the antipsychotic drugs has a lower chance of causing this problem than others.[41]

In most studies of elderly patients, the incidence of tardive dyskinesia in people taking antipsychotic medications is between 30 and 35%. However, a recent study found that in those elderly patients who had never before been given an antipsychotic drug, the incidence of tardive dyskinesia was 60% in those patients given the drugs for depression, significantly higher than in older adults getting these drugs for other purposes.[46] Most studies find that increased age and long duration of therapy are important predictors for increased rates of tardive dyskinesia. Another variable between studies is the differing definitions of tardive dyskinesia. The risk of tardive dyskinesia is somewhat less for the newer, atypical antipsychotic drugs.

Another study estimated that there were 192,718 people in the United States who had developed tardive dyskinesia attributable to antipsychotic drugs.[46] Of these, 54,284 cases occurred in nursing homes. If 80% of these exposures to antipsychotic drugs were unnecessary, more than 43,000 people in nursing homes developed tardive dyskinesia unnecessarily because they should not have been given these drugs. An additional 112,854 people not in an institution also suffered from tardive dyskinesia induced by antipsychotic drugs. According to national drug prescribing data, approximately 33% of the prescriptions for the drugs were in people over the age of 60.[36] Thus, an additional 37,000 noninstitutionalized older adults appear to have developed tardive dyskinesia from these drugs. If the prescriptions for 80% of these people are unnecessary, another 30,000 cases of tardive dyskinesia that should have been avoided have occurred. Thus, there are approximately 73,000 cases of tardive dyskinesia in older adults that are the result of poor prescribing practices by physicians.

To date, no drug has been found to be effective in treating tardive dyskinesia, thus making its prevention extremely important.

Drug-induced parkinsonism: Drug-induced parkinsonism involves the following symptoms: difficulty speaking or swallowing; loss of balance; masklike face; muscle spasms; stiffness of arms or legs; trembling and shaking; unusual twisting movements of body.

Although many people believe that parkinsonism is one of the inevitable consequences of growing old, a large proportion of the cases seen in older adults are caused by drugs. A study found that 51% of 93 patients referred for evaluation of newly developed parkinsonism had drug-induced diseases.[47] One-fourth of patients with drug-induced parkinsonism could not walk when first seen by their doctors, and 45% required hospital admission. The parkinsonism cleared in 66% of the patients, but 11% continued to have the disease a year after the drug was stopped. An additional 25% who had cleared initially went on to develop classic Parkinson's disease, leading the authors to speculate that, for this latter 25%, these drugs were "unmasking" a disease that might have showed up later.

Even more disturbing is the finding in another study in which 36% of patients with drug-induced parkinsonism had been started on antiparkinson drugs to treat the disease! Because the doctors had not considered the possibility that a drug was responsible for the disease, they assumed that the patients had classic Parkinson's disease and treated the parkinsonism with another drug instead of stopping the one responsible for the disease in the first place.[38]

Another way of looking at this serious problem is to ask what proportion of patients who take antipsychotic drugs or other drugs that can also cause these problems (Phenergan, Compazine, and Reglan) get drug-induced parkinsonism. In various groups of patients in whom this has been studied, the range is from 15 to 52%.[38] In one study, 26% of older adults (60 and over) taking haloperidol (HALDOL) developed drug-induced parkinsonism.[48] Other studies have shown an overall incidence of 15.4%, but among patients over 60, the incidence was approximately 40%.[49] In the same study, 90% of the cases of drug-induced parkinsonism began within 72 days after starting the drug.

In older persons the symptoms of an adverse drug reaction may be mistaken for a new disease or attributed to the normal process of aging. The chance of such misinterpretation is more likely when symptoms of an adverse reaction are indistinguishable from an illness common in the elderly, such as Parkinson's disease.

A study published in the *Journal of the American Medical Association* reported that the likelihood of being treated for Parkinson's disease increases threefold in elderly patients taking the antinausea drug metoclopramide. The most troubling finding of this study, according to the authors, was the extent to which adverse metoclopramide reactions were treated with levodopa-containing drugs, carrying increased risk of toxicity at greater cost, but offering little likelihood of benefit.[50]

Restless leg (akathisia): Another very common adverse effect of these drugs is the restless leg syndrome, in which the person restlessly paces around and describes having the "jitters." When seated, the patient often taps his or her feet. Not infrequently, this might be interpreted as needing more antipsychotic medicine. Instead of reducing the dose of the drug or stopping it entirely, more of the drug causing the problem may be used.

Weakness and muscle fatigue (akinesia): The most common of this group of drug-induced nerve problems (extrapyramidal reactions) is when the patient appears listless, disinterested, and depressed. This drug-induced problem is often misdiagnosed as primary depression, and the patient is put on antidepressant drugs. Giving these drugs along with the antipsychotic drugs even further increases the risk of serious adverse effects. Once again, instead of recognizing a drug-induced problem and either stopping or lowering the dose of the drug, another drug is added, making things even worse.

Although seen as a component of parkinsonism, akinesia can also occur on its own. Additional problems can include infrequent blinking, slower swallowing of saliva with subsequent drooling, and a lack of facial expression.

As a general rule, if any elderly person on psychoactive medication—sleeping pills, antianxiety tranquilizers, antidepressants, or antipsychotic drugs—appears to be doing poorly, first think about reducing the dose or stopping the drug rather than adding another drug.

Anticholinergic adverse effects

The two types of anticholinergic effects (see Glossary, p. 889) are those affecting the brain, such as confusion, delirium, short-term memory problems, disorientation, and impaired attention, and those affecting the rest of the body. The latter type includes dry mouth, constipation, retention of urine (especially in men with an enlarged prostate), blurred vision, decreased sweating with increased body temperature, sexual dysfunction, and worsening of glaucoma. These adverse effects are much more common in the so-called high-dose antipsychotic drugs (see chart below).

Sedation

Sedation is one of the most common adverse effects of the antipsychotic drugs, especially with the high-dose drugs. Since these drugs are often improperly prescribed as sleeping pills, older adults will often have a decreased level of functioning during the day. In nonpsychotic older adults, the largest group being given these drugs, the quality of sleep is extremely unpleasant. The frightening aspects of this drug-induced disturbed sleep can last up to 24 hours after a single dose.

Hypotensive effects: lowering of blood pressure to levels that are too low

Orthostatic (postural) hypotension, or the fall in blood pressure that occurs when someone stands up suddenly, is a common adverse effect of antipsychotic drugs, especially in older adults. It can be even more troublesome if the person is already at increased risk for this problem because he or she is taking other drugs to treat high blood pressure. As a result of such a drug-induced drop in blood pressure, falls that result in injury, heart attacks, and strokes can occur. For this reason, before starting one of these drugs, the person's blood pressure should be taken both in the lying position and after standing for two minutes. This should be repeated after the person has used the drug for several weeks. People taking these drugs should rise slowly from a lying position and wear supportive stockings to help prevent hy-

---

ADVERSE EFFECTS OF ANTIPSYCHOTIC DRUGS

Generic/Brand Name	Sedative	Anticholinergic (dry mouth, urine retention, confusion)	Extrapyramidal (parkinsonism, tardive dyskinesia)	Hypotensive
chlorpromazine/THORAZINE	strong	strong	moderate	strong
thioridazine/MELLARIL	strong	strong	mild	moderate
trifluoperazine/STELAZINE	mild	mild	strong	moderate
fluphenazine/PROLIXIN	mild	mild	strong	mild
haloperidol/HALDOL	mild	mild	strong	mild
loxapine/LOXITANE	mild	mild	strong	mild
thiothixene/NAVANE	mild	mild	strong	moderate
clozapine/CLOZARIL	strong	strong	mild	strong
olanzapine/ZYPREXA	mild	moderate	mild	strong
risperidone/RISPERDAL	strong	mild	strong	moderate

mild = mild adverse effects
moderate = moderate adverse effects
strong = strong adverse effects [24,51–55]

potension. This adverse effect is also seen more often with the use of the higher-dose drugs, such as chlorpromazine (THORAZINE), but occurs with all of the antipsychotic drugs.

Blood sugar elevation and diabetes mellitus

Elevations in blood sugar (glucose),[56–58] in some cases extreme and associated with ketoacidosis or hyperosmolar coma or death, has been reported in patients treated with atypical antipsychotics that include aripiprazole (ABILIFY), clozapine (CLOZARIL), olanzapine (ZYPREXA), quetiapine (SEROQUEL), risperidone (RISPERDAL), and ziprasidone (GEODON).

The relationship between atypical antipsychotic use and glucose abnormalities is complicated by the possibility of an increased background risk of diabetes mellitus in patients with schizophrenia and the increasing incidence of diabetes mellitus in the general population. Given these confounders, the relationship between atypical antipsychotic use and hyperglycemia-related adverse events is not completely understood. Precise risk estimates for hyperglycemia-related adverse events in patients treated with atypical antipsychotics are not available.

Patients with an established diagnosis of diabetes mellitus who are started on atypical antipsychotics should be monitored regularly for worsening of glucose control. Patients with risk factors for diabetes mellitus (e.g., obesity, family history of diabetes) who are starting treatment with atypical antipsychotics should undergo fasting blood glucose testing at the beginning of treatment and periodically during treatment. Any patient treated with atypical antipsychotics should be monitored for symptoms of hyperglycemia, including polydipsia (excessive thirst/drinking of liquids), polyuria (excessive urination), polyphagia (excessive eating), and weakness. Patients who develop symptoms of hyperglycemia during treatment with atypical antipsychotics should undergo fasting blood glucose testing. In some cases, hyperglycemia has resolved when the atypical antipsychotic was discontinued; however, some patients required continuation of antidiabetic treatment despite discontinuation of the suspect drug.

For a variety of reasons, including increased appetite, the newer, so-called atypical antipsychotic drugs commonly cause a significant increase in weight that can be troublesome to and dangerous for patients using these drugs. For various drugs in this group, the usual range of weight gain is from 5 to 20 pounds, but there are a large number of reports of people gaining much more than 20 pounds, especially with longer-term use of the drugs. In addition to and related to weight gain are metabolic disorders including elevated blood sugar, the onset of diabetes, and abnormalities of fat metabolism such as elevated triglyceride levels. Patients should be informed of these effects to help prevent excessive body weight gain.[110]

Cerebrovascular adverse events, including stroke, in elderly patients with dementia

Cerebrovascular adverse events (e.g., stroke, transient ischemic attack), including fatalities, were reported in patients in clinical trials of the atypical antipsychotics in elderly patients with dementia-related psychosis.[59] In placebo-controlled trials, there was a significantly higher incidence of cerebrovascular adverse events in patients treated with these drugs compared to patients treated with placebo. The atypical antipsychotics are not approved for the treatment of patients with dementia-related psychosis.

Other adverse effects

Other adverse effects include weight gain, poor ability to withstand high or low temperatures (because these drugs affect the body's temperature regulation center), increased sensitivity to sunlight and other skin problems, bone marrow toxicity, and abnormal heart rhythms.

How to Reduce the Risks of These Antipsychotic Drugs

• *Give antipsychotic drugs only to people who need them.* The majority, at least 80%, of older adults being prescribed these drugs should not be getting them, and the serious adverse effects are just as harmful in them as in the small fraction of people for whom the drugs are appropriate (people with schizophrenia). Thus, the most effective way of reducing the risk of these drugs for most older adults is to stop using them. Unless the patient has schizophrenia or another psychotic condition, beginning to use them or continuing to use them provides significant risks without compensating benefits. These drugs are also not effective for psychoses seen with senile dementia.[40] As discussed on p. 178, the use of these powerful drugs for older people who have depression is fraught with a high incidence—60%—of tardive dyskinesia.

Antipsychotic drugs should never be used as sleeping pills or to treat anxiety.

• *Start with the lowest possible dose.* For older adults this is usually one-tenth to two-fifths the dose for younger adults. Use the drug for as short a period of time as possible.[24] If, however, the use of antipsychotic drugs is indicated, the first thing to realize is that as is the case for many drugs for older adults, the starting dose and, very likely, the eventually used dose should be lower than the dose for younger adults. There are three reasons why this is so for the antipsychotic drugs:

First, kidney function in older adults decreases, which means that the drugs last longer in the body. They get more "mileage" out of a given dose. Second, because of a decrease in an important brain chemical—dopamine—as people age, there is an increased risk in older adults of the adverse effects, such as drug-induced parkinsonism or akinesia. Third, because of another change in brain metabolism with aging, there is an increased sensitivity to the anticholinergic (see Glossary, p. 889) effects of these drugs, such as confusion, delirium, dry mouth, difficulty urinating, constipation, and worsening of glaucoma.[60]

• *Pay attention to the adverse effect profile of the drugs* (see comparison chart on p. 181). As mentioned previously, the antipsychotic drugs are all quite similar in their effectiveness for treating psychoses, but differ mainly in the spectrum of their adverse effects. The chart shows a great difference in the severity of the adverse reactions, depending on whether the drug is a less potent or more potent one.

At the top of the list is the less potent, higher-dose chlorpromazine (THORAZINE). It causes more sedative, anticholinergic, and hypotensive effects but has a relatively lower risk of the extrapyramidal effects, such as restless leg and drug-induced parkinsonism. In the middle of the list are more potent, lower-dose drugs, such as haloperidol (HALDOL) and thiothixene (NAVANE). They cause fewer sedative, anticholinergic, and hypotensive adverse effects but have a higher risk of the extrapyramidal adverse effects, such as drug-induced parkinsonism. At the bottom of the list are drugs that have more recently come on the market.

Since all of these drugs are equally effective, the choice depends on which adverse effects would likely be or are most intolerable. For a person with a tendency to become faint or dizzy upon standing (orthostatic, postural hypotension), the addition of Thorazine, with its high risk of lowering blood pressure, would not be a good idea. Instead, if drug treatment is really necessary, one of the more potent drugs with fewer hypotensive and sedative effects might be a better choice. Similarly, people who already have trouble walking or who have trouble with their posture would be at much greater risk if they developed one of the extrapyramidal adverse effects of Haldol, Navane, or the other more potent antipsychotic drugs. Therefore, these people would probably do better on one of the less potent drugs with fewer extrapyramidal adverse effects, such as clozapine or olanza-pine. The most important consideration is to adjust the dose, or change or discontinue drugs when and if adverse effects occur. This is especially true when the adverse effects are as bad as or worse than the original reason for starting the drug.

DEPRESSION: WHEN ARE DRUGS CALLED FOR AND WHICH ONES SHOULD YOU USE?

Should Everyone Who Is Sad or Depressed Take Antidepressants?

Although depression is the most common mental illness in older adults, not everyone who is sad or depressed is a candidate for these powerful drugs.

Kinds of Depression

Drug-induced depression

Ironically, one of the kinds of depression that should not be treated with drugs is depression caused by other kinds of drugs. If someone is depressed and the depression started after beginning a new drug, it may well be drug-caused. Commonly used drugs known to cause depression include the following:

- barbiturates such as phenobarbital
- tranquilizers such as diazepam (VALIUM) and triazolam (HALCION)
- heart drugs containing reserpine (SER-AP-ES and others)
- beta-blockers such as propranolol (INDERAL)
- high blood pressure drugs such as clonidine (CATAPRES), methyldopa (ALDOMET), and prazosin (MINIPRESS)
- drugs for treating abnormal heart rhythms such as disopyramide (NORPACE)

- ulcer drugs such as cimetidine (TAGAMET) and ranitidine (ZANTAC)
- antiparkinsonians such as levodopa (LARODOPA) and bromocriptine (PARLODEL)
- corticosteroids such as cortisone (CORTONE) and prednisone (DELTASONE)
- anticonvulsants such as phenytoin (DILANTIN), ethosuximide (ZARONTIN), and primidone (MYSOLINE)
- antibiotics such as cycloserine (SEROMYCIN), ethionamide (TRECATOR-SC), ciprofloxacin (CIPRO), and metronidazole (FLAGYL)
- diet drugs such as amphetamines (during withdrawal from the drug)
- painkillers or arthritis drugs such as pentazocine (TALWIN), indomethacin (INDOCIN), and ibuprofen (MOTRIN, ADVIL)
- the acne drug isotretinoin (ACCUTANE)
- other drugs including metrizamide (AMIPAQUE), a drug used for diagnosing slipped discs, and disulfiram (ANTABUSE), the alcoholism treatment drug.[21]

The remedy for this kind of depression is to reduce the dose of the drug or stop it altogether if possible. If necessary, switch to another drug that does not cause depression.

Another major cause of drug-induced depression is alcoholism, the treatment of which is difficult.

Situational or reactive depression

Other causes of depression that should not be treated with antidepressant drugs are the "normal" reactions to life problems, such as the loss of a spouse, friend, relative, or job, or other situations that normally make almost anyone sad. If the depression is clearly a response to overwhelming life crises, antidepressants have little value. Other options, such as support from family and friends, psychotherapy with a mental health professional, or a change in your environment, are worth exploring.[27] Doing something nice for yourself, talking with a friend, and exercising every day can help you get through these difficult situations.

Medical conditions that can cause depression

Older adults (or anyone) who appear depressed may have a thyroid disorder, a type of cancer—such as pancreatic, bowel, brain, or lymph node (lymphoma)—viral pneumonia, or hepatitis.[61] In addition, there is evidence that people who have had a stroke or who have Parkinson's disease or Alzheimer's disease may become depressed and, in some cases, may respond to antidepressant drugs.

A major depressive episode: the kind that will usually respond to drugs

If a depressed mood accompanied by several of the following problems has been present for at least several weeks, and a careful history, physical exam, and lab tests have ruled out specific causes of depression, true primary depression is probably the diagnosis. The problems are sadness that impairs normal functioning, difficulty concentrating, low self-esteem, guilt, suicidal thoughts, extreme fatigue, low energy level or agitation, sleep disturbances (increased or decreased), and appetite disturbance (increased or decreased) with associated weight change.[62] Since suicidal thoughts and attempts often characterize depression, the possibility of suicide using antidepressant drugs has to be kept in mind and only a small number of pills (see p. 189) prescribed at one time. Another way of describing the pervasive nature of this kind of severe depression is that the person displays—and relates if asked—a sense of "helplessness, hopelessness, worthlessness and uselessness . . . as well as intense feelings of guilt over real or imagined shortcomings or indiscretions."[63]

Although depression in older adults is usually unipolar (depression alone), occasionally there is a bipolar pattern with alternation of depression and mania. The latter shows up as an elated mood, rapid flow of ideas, and increased "energy." The patient, often seeming hyperactive during this manic phase, can be intrusive, have an infectious sense of humor, and may show poor judgment in business or personal affairs, not infrequently going on spending sprees.[42] Lithium is often used successfully to treat people with bipolar disease (see p. 272). Other drugs approved for treatment of bipolar depression include olanzapine and quetiapine (see pp. 244 and 247).

Serious depressive illness is far less frequent in the elderly. According to data from the National Institute of Mental Health, while nearly 4% of people age 25 to 44 have had a major depression recently, fewer than 1% of people 65 and over have had this misfortune. In spite of this, about one-third of antidepressants are prescribed for people 60 and over even though they make up just one-sixth of the population.

Some of this apparent "overtreatment" may be due to failing to diagnose drug-induced depression and instead using a second drug to treat the depression caused by the first.

Other Uses—Usually Inappropriate— for Antidepressants

In addition to drug-induced depression, medical conditions that can cause depression, and situational or reactive depression—none of which merit treatment with antidepressants— there are other circumstances in which antidepressants are inappropriately dished out. In one community-based study, more than 50% of older people who had been taking antidepressants for a year or more had been started without a clear history of depression. Of these, one-half (or one out of four of all people using antidepressants) were using antidepressants as a sleeping pill, and others were given the drugs as alternatives to tranquilizers.[64] In view of the significant adverse effects of these drugs, their use for such purposes will cause risks that will outweigh the benefits even though, unlike benzodiazepine tranquilizers, they do not cause addiction.

In many countries, including the United States, there has been an extraordinary increase since 1990 in the use of antidepressants, mainly the SSRIs (selective serotonin reuptake inhibitors) such as fluoxetine (PROZAC) and paroxetine (PAXIL). This increase, more than twofold in the 1990s in the United States has been much larger than the smaller decrease in the use of older antidepressants.[65]

A survey in the United States of almost 6,000 people between the ages of 15 and 54 found that primary care physicians were much more likely than psychiatrists to prescribe antidepressants, tranquilizers, or sleeping pills for patients who did not have mood or anxiety disorders. Primary care doctors prescribed antidepressants to 22% of people, tranquilizers to 17% of people, and sleeping pills to 13% of people without mood or anxiety disorders. The author concluded that "primary care physicians are less selective in their use of psychoactive medicines, perhaps because of lower sensitivity and specificity of diagnoses in primary care settings."[4]

What Are the Best and Worst Treatments for Severe Depression?

Everyone with the kind of severe depression described above should be evaluated by a mental health professional to determine what kind of psychotherapy would best supplement the antidepressant drugs that are going to be used.

The decision as to which drug is best will depend largely on which one has the fewest adverse effects, since all antidepressants are equally effective.[42] If depression has occurred previously and responded to one of the drugs without too many adverse effects, that would be the best one to try first. Otherwise, the table on p. 188 compares the 11 tricyclic antidepressants that are listed in this book as well as fluoxetine (PROZAC) and bupropion (WELLBUTRIN).

The Main Risks of Antidepressant Drugs

The four most common groups of adverse effects are anticholinergic, sedative, hypotensive (blood-pressure-lowering), and those effects on heart rate or rhythm. Two serious risks arising from the adverse effects are hip fractures and automobile crashes.

Hip fractures

A study of 1,021 older adults with hip fractures found that 14% of these life-threatening injuries are attributable to the use of mind-affecting drugs, including sleeping pills and minor tranquilizers, antipsychotics, and antidepressants.[11]

There are approximately 227,000 hip fractures each year in the United States, virtually all in older adults.[12] Since the above study found that 14% of hip fractures are drug-induced, this means that if the results of the study are projected nationally, approximately 32,000 hip fractures a year in older adults are caused by the use of mind-affecting drugs. Approximately 60% of these drug-induced hip fractures are caused by antidepressant drugs.

The SSRI antidepressants such as Prozac, Zoloft, and Paxil (see p. 190) are promoted as having fewer adverse effects than the older tricyclic antidepressants such as Elavil (see p. 204) and Tofranil (see p. 196). Canadian researchers recently reported that the SSRIs do not offer any advantage over the older antidepressants with regard to the risk of hip fracture.[66]

Automobile crashes that cause injury

A study involving 495 automobile crashes in older drivers in which an injury occurred found that a significant number of such crashes in older adults aged 65–84 were attributable to the use of benzodiazepine tranquilizers and tricyclic antidepressants. The study was particularly impressive because its findings were strengthened by observing that the rate of

ANTICHOLINERGIC EFFECTS

WARNING: SPECIAL MENTAL AND PHYSICAL ADVERSE EFFECTS

Older adults are especially sensitive to the harmful anticholinergic (see Glossary, p. 889) effects of tricyclic antidepressants. Drugs in this family should not be used unless absolutely necessary.

Mental Effects: confusion, delirium, short-term memory problems, disorientation, and impaired attention.

Physical Effects: dry mouth, constipation, difficulty urinating (especially for a man with an enlarged prostate), blurred vision, decreased sweating with increased body temperature, sexual dysfunction, and worsening of glaucoma.

crashes that caused injury increased in the same group of people when they were using these drugs as opposed to when they were not using the drugs. The majority of the excess number of auto crashes that caused injury were attributable to the benzodiazepines. The authors, stating that the study findings may be generalizable to the population at large, found that if the association is causal, at least 16,000 auto crashes that caused injury each year in older drivers are attributable to psychoactive drug use (specifically benzodiazepines and tricyclic antidepressants), out of the 217,000 crashes that caused injury that occur each year among elderly drivers.[14]

Sedative effects

Most older adults who think they have a sleeping problem do not have the kind of severe depression that justifies the use of these drugs. (See p. 172 for a discussion of nondrug treatments for sleeplessness.) Nevertheless, if the sleep disorder is a consequence of severe depression, the "adverse effect" of sedation may be useful as long as it does not produce too much

sedation, with the risk of falling. This is an important consideration especially in people who already have some impairment of thinking, increased confusion, disorientation, and agitation.[24]

Hypotensive effects: lowering of blood pressure to levels that are too low

Orthostatic (postural) hypotension, or the fall in blood pressure that occurs when someone stands up suddenly, is a common adverse effect of antidepressants, especially in older adults. It can be even more troublesome if the person is already at increased risk for this problem because he or she is taking other drugs to treat high blood pressure. As a result of such a drug-induced drop in blood pressure, falls that result in injury, heart attacks, and strokes can occur. For this reason, before starting treatment with one of these antidepressants, blood pressure should be taken both in the lying position and after standing for two minutes. This should be repeated after using the drug for several weeks.

Drug-induced parkinsonism

Like the antipsychotic drugs, many antidepressants can also cause drug-induced parkinsonism (see p. 30), although this is less common with most antidepressants. Drug-induced parkinsonism involves the following symptoms: difficulty speaking or swallowing; loss of balance; masklike face; muscle spasms; stiffness of arms or legs; trembling and shaking; unusual twisting movements of the body.

Effects on heart rate and rhythm

These drugs can cause the heart to speed up. This is more of a problem with older antidepressants (see table, p. 188). They can also cause a slowing down in the conduction of electricity through the heart, which is especially dangerous if someone already has heart block.[24] For this reason, a baseline electrocardiogram

ADVERSE EFFECTS OF ANTIDEPRESSANTS

Generic/Brand Names	Anticholinergics*	Sedative	Hypotensive Effect	Heart Rate/Rhythm
fluoxetine/PROZAC**	none	none	none	none
paroxetine/PAXIL**	none	none	none	none
sertraline/ZOLOFT**	none	none	none	none
fluvoxamine/LUVOX**	none	none	none	none
bupropion/WELLBUTRIN**	mild	none	none	none
desipramine/NORPRAMIN	mild	mild	mild	mild
nortriptyline/AVENTYL, PAMELOR	moderate	mild	mild	mild
amoxapine/ASENDIN	moderate	mild	moderate	moderate
maprotiline/LUDIOMIL	moderate	moderate	moderate	mild
trazodone/DESYREL	mild	moderate	moderate	moderate
imipramine/TOFRANIL	moderate	moderate	moderate	moderate
doxepin/SINEQUAN	moderate	strong	moderate	moderate
amitriptyline/ELAVIL	strong	strong	moderate	strong

mild = mild adverse effects
moderate = moderate adverse effects
strong = strong adverse effects

*see p. 617
** There is inadequate information for these drugs in older people to ensure that the risk of the adverse effects is as low as it appears; there is more information about nortriptyline and desipramine as far as their reduced amount of adverse effects on older adults in comparison with the drugs listed above them.
These listings are a composite of comparative ratings of 11 of these drugs by four other researchers[70] and information from the references listed for fluoxetine and bupropion on the drug profiles.

should be taken before starting any antidepressant therapy.

Mania induced by selective serotonin reuptake inhibitors (SSRIs)

All currently available antidepressant drugs appear able to induce hypomanic and manic reactions.[67,68] This is a serious concern for people taking the serotonin reuptake inhibitor group of antidepressants, which includes the SSRIs such as fluoxetine[69] but also the antidepressants such as nefazodone that have a combined effect on serotonin and norepinephrine reuptake.[67] This reaction can be severe, having psychotic features or requiring patients to be secluded for extreme agitation.[69]

As can be seen from the table above, the drugs with the fewest overall adverse effects in older adults are desipramine (NORPRAMIN), which has a "mild" for all four kinds of adverse effects,

and nortriptyline (AVENTYL, PAMELOR), which is "mild" for three of the four. Fluoxetine (PROZAC) and bupropion (WELLBUTRIN) may have as few or fewer adverse effects than desipramine and nortriptyline, but adequate comparative studies on older adults have not yet been published. The drug with the worst adverse effects profile in older adults is amitriptyline (ELAVIL), with "strong" adverse effects for three of the four categories. We list this drug as **Do Not Use.**

If the adverse effects of whichever drug is selected are too severe, or if the drug does not seem to be working, talk to your doctor about switching to a drug less likely to cause the troublesome effects.

Increased suicide risk in adults and children

In early 2004, the FDA issued a public health advisory warning, which stated that in studies of depressed adults and children being treated with antidepressants there was an increased risk of suicidal thoughts and actions.[71]

The drugs implicated are bupropion (WELLBUTRIN), citalopram (CELEXA), fluoxetine (PROZAC), fluvoxamine (LUVOX), mirtazapine (REMERON), nefazodone (SERZONE), paroxetine (PAXIL), sertraline (ZOLOFT), escitalopram (LEXAPRO), and venlafaxine (EFFEXOR). It should be noted that the only drug that has received approval for use in children with major depressive disorder is fluoxetine. Several of these drugs are approved for the treatment of obsessive-compulsive disorder in pediatric patients, for example, sertraline, fluoxetine, and fluvoxamine. Fluvoxamine is not approved as an antidepressant in the United States.

The possibility of an increased risk of suicide in patients taking antidepressants is not new. In 1991, Public Citizen's Health Research Group petitioned the FDA to require a black-box warning in the labeling for fluvoxamine about the risk of suicide.[72] Unfortunately, the petition was denied.

How to Reduce the Adverse Effects of Any of These Antidepressants

• Have a baseline electrocardiogram and blood pressure taken before starting.[27]

• Start with a dose of one-third to one-half the usual adult dose, meaning 15–25 milligrams a day, at bedtime. Increase the dose very slowly.[27] It may take three weeks to see an effect. A trial with one of these drugs, should continue until it either works or causes persistent adverse effects.[61]

• Get a prescription for only one week's worth of pills, since more pills increase the chance of a successful suicide attempt by people who are severely depressed.[42] This is much less likely to be a problem with newer antidepressants such as SSRIs or buproprion.

• Lower the dose gradually, as symptoms dic-

tate, after successful treatment for several months.[24]

It is important to realize that long-term treatment with antidepressants is not always necessary even when the drug is being used to treat the kind of serious depression for which its use is proper. In one study, after patients had been successfully treated for four months with antidepressants, half were continued on their drugs and the other half were switched to a placebo. After an additional two months, most of the patients—on either the actual drug or the placebo—were still doing well; only about one-fourth, the same in both groups, had relapsed.[73]

Other recommendations for more effective and safer use of these drugs include:[64]

1. When starting a drug for a specific depressive illness, the doctor should monitor your response carefully to see if a different dose (or drug) should be used.

2. It should be made clear to you that depression can be an episodic illness, that recovery is expected, and that the treatment will probably eventually be stopped.

3. If treatment with drugs is started as a trial in possible depression, you should be informed that it is a trial and that treatment will continue for a specified time, depending on the response of key symptoms.

4. The possibility of adverse effects should be evaluated carefully before these drugs are used primarily as sleeping pills or as an alternative to tranquilizers in the elderly.

DRUG PROFILES

Depression

Selective Serotonin Reuptake Inhibitors (SSRIs)

 Do Not Use

Escitalopram (ess si *tal* oh pram)
LEXAPRO (Forest)

FAMILY: Selective Serotonin Reuptake Inhibitors (SSRIs)
(See p. 184 for discussion of depression.)

We have listed escitalopram (LEXAPRO) as a **Do Not Use** drug rather than as a Do Not Use Until Seven Years After Release drug not because of safety and effectiveness concerns but because there is no significant difference between this drug and citalopram (CELEXA). Switching from citalopram, which is about to become available generically, to escitalopram will cause the health care system economic harm. Patients with poor or nonexistent drug coverage will foot the bill that ensues from doctors being conned into prescribing escitalopram. However, we acknowledge that particular health insurance plans may reimburse for escitalopram and not some other SSRIs that have longer track records.

Escitalopram was approved by the FDA in August 2002, bringing to six the number of selective serotonin reuptake inhibitor (SSRI) antidepressants now on the U.S. market. It is the most recent member of the mirror-image marketing rage, being one-half of the mixture that constitutes citalopram. The other SSRIs currently available are fluoxetine (PROZAC, SARAFEM), fluvoxamine (LUVOX), paroxetine (PAXIL), and sertraline (ZOLOFT).

Both escitalopram and citalopram are pro-

duced by Forest Laboratories, Inc., of St. Louis.

The editors of *The Medical Letter on Drugs and Therapeutics* concluded in their September 30, 2002, review of the drug that: *"Escitalopram (LEXAPRO), the active enantiomer [one of the two mirror images] of citalopram (CELEXA), is effective for treatment of depression, but it has not been shown to be more effective, more rapid-acting or less likely to cause adverse effects, including sexual dysfunction, than citalopram or any other SSRI."* [127]

Limited Use

Citalopram (si *tal* oh pram)
CELEXA (Forest)

Fluoxetine (floo *ox* e teen)
PROZAC, SARAFEM (Lilly)

Fluvoxamine (floo *vox* a meen)
LUVOX (Solvay)

Paroxetine (pa *rox* uh teen)
PAXIL (GlaxoSmithKline)

Sertraline (*ser* tra leen)
ZOLOFT (Pfizer)

GENERIC: not available
FAMILY: Selective Serotonin Reuptake Inhibitors (SSRIs)
(See p. 184 for discussion of depression.)

PREGNANCY WARNING

These drugs caused harm to developing fetuses in animal studies, including decreased growth and survival and malformations of heart and bones. There was, also, an increase in pup deaths and delays in growth. There is new evidence that when women take these drugs in the third trimester of pregnancy, serious complications can arise in their infants' health immediately after delivery. These complications require prolonged hospitalization, respiratory support, and tube feeding.

BREAST-FEEDING WARNING

Because the selective serotonin reuptake inhibitors are excreted in human milk and have been shown to have adverse effects in nursing infants, you should not nurse while taking these drugs.

In addition to being approved by the FDA for major depressive disorder, or MDD, various SSRIs are also approved to treat obsessive-complusive disorder, bulimia, panic disorder, social anxiety disorder, and posttraumatic stress disorder. Fluoxetine, better known as Prozac, is also sold as Sarafem to treat a condition known as premenstrual dysphoric disorder. Women taking Prozac should not be taking Sarafem.

The SSRIs may reduce the risk of suicide in depressed adult patients. However, there have been a few reports that fluoxetine may actually induce suicidal thoughts in selected patients, although this has not been confirmed.[76] Public Citizen's Health Research Group petitioned the FDA in 1991 to require a box warning in the professional product labeling for fluoxetine warning doctors that a small minority of persons taking the drug have experienced intense, violent, suicidal thoughts; agitation; and impul-

All of the SSRI antidepressants have been shown to commonly cause sexual dysfunction in both men and women. In a large prospective study of over 6,000 men and women, sexual dysfunction occurred from 36 to 43% of the time, depending on the drug.[74] Types of sexual dysfunction include problems of desire (libido: sexual interest or drive), arousal (erectile function in men, lubrication in women), and release (ejaculation/orgasm in men and orgasm in women). Strategies to cope with this problem include decreasing the dosage to the lowest effective level; a drug holiday for patients in whom compliance is not a problem; if acceptable to the patient and partner, seeing if the sexual dysfunction resolves without further intervention.[75]

sivity after starting treatment with the drug. You should not take this drug for mild depression or anxiety, or as a sleeping pill.

The FDA-approved professional product labeling for antidepressant drugs sold in the United States carries the following statement:

Suicide: The possibility of a suicide attempt is inherent in major depressive disorder and may persist until significant remission occurs. Close supervision of high-risk patients should accompany initial drug therapy. Prescriptions for Drug X should be written for the smallest quantity of tablets consistent with good patient management, in order to reduce the risk of overdose.

Only fluoxetine is approved for use in children less than 18 years of age for major depressive disorder.

A review of 64 randomized controlled trials comparing SSRIs to the older tricyclic antidepressants such as imipramine (TOFRANIL) found similar benefit from the new and older drugs. When the results of many clinical trials were pooled, called a meta-analysis, no clear benefit was found for the new drugs over the

WARNING: WITHDRAWAL REACTIONS WITH SELECTIVE SEROTONIN REUPTAKE INHIBITOR (SSRI) ANTIDEPRESSANTS

A withdrawal reaction has been reported with all SSRI antidepressants: citalopram (CELEXA); escitalopram (LEXAPRO), fluoxetine (PROZAC, SARAFEM); fluvoxamine (LUVOX); paroxetine (PAXIL); and sertraline (ZOLOFT). The symptoms generally start within one to three days after stopping the drug and generally resolve within one to two weeks after the drug has been discontinued. Withdrawal symptoms may occur even when the dosage of the drug is gradually decreased. The main symptoms of this reaction are dizziness, vertigo, incoordination, nausea and vomiting, and flulike symptoms that include fatigue, lethargy, muscle pain, and chills.

> **WARNING**
>
> A small number of people taking fluoxetine have experienced intense, violent, suicidal thoughts; agitation; and impulsivity. Whether their symptoms were induced by fluoxetine or were related to their underlying psychological problems is unclear. As with any other antidepressant, fluoxetine should only be used under close medical supervision. Patients are advised to consider telling relatives and friends about their use of this drug and the risk of suicidal depression and self-injurious behavior.

> Do not take citalopram, escitalopram, fluoxetine, fluvoxamine, paroxetine, or sertraline with monoamine oxidase (MAO) inhibitors (see Interactions with Other Drugs) because the combinations may produce a syndrome of rising temperature, tremor, and seizures.

older antidepressants. The adverse effects of the new and old antidepressants have little in common except for withdrawal symptoms. For example, SSRIs are less likely than the tricyclic drugs to cause sedation, anticholinergic effects (see p. 181), and heart rhythm disturbances. On the other hand, SSRIs' adverse effects commonly affect the gastrointestinal tract, especially causing nausea and diarrhea, and may also cause insomnia, agitation, extrapyramidal symptoms (drug-induced parkinsonism), and withdrawal effects.

One group of adverse effects is traded for another between the SSRIs and tricyclic antidepressants, and there does not appear to be any difference in the proportion of people who can tolerate these two groups of antidepressants. When the number of people who stopped taking an antidepressant in 58 clinical trials were studied, there was no clinically significant difference between the SSRIs and the tricyclic and related antidepressants.[80]

A large meta-analysis commissioned by the U.S. Department of Health and Human Services through the Agency for Health Care Policy and Research in 1999 found that in general there were no significant differences in the effectiveness of the newer antidepressants such as the SSRIs and the older agents such as the tricyclic antidepressants (see p. 196). In terms of adverse drug reactions, there was no significant difference between the new and old antidepressants in overall discontinuation rates of use of these drugs by patients.[81] Drug discontinuation rates can be used to compare adverse reactions between drugs.

When you take these medicines you may experience some adverse effects. The most frequently reported include nausea, anxiety, headache, and insomnia. These adverse effects tend to be worst at the start of treatment and improve over a few weeks. Akathisia—symptoms of restlessness, constant pacing, and purposeless movements of the feet and legs—may also

> **WARNING:**
> **NEWER ANTIDEPRESSANTS AND THE RISK OF SUICIDE IN CHILDREN LESS THAN 18 YEARS OF AGE**
>
> The FDA and the drug regulatory authorities in Canada and the UK have warned about the possibility of both suicidal ideation and suicide attempts seen in clinical trials of the newer antidepressant drugs, including the selective serotonin reuptake inhibitors (SSRIs), mirtazapine (REMERON), and venlafaxine (EFFEXOR), in children less than 18 years of age.[77-79]
>
> Only fluoxetine is approved for use in children less than 18 years of age for major depressive disorder.

occur. Dry mouth, sweating, diarrhea, tremor, loss of appetite, and dizziness are also common adverse effects.

The length of time it takes an antidepressant to work can overlap with the time of spontaneous recovery, especially if the depression is situational—caused by a death or other external circumstances. The majority of people lift themselves out of depression with friends, spiritual resources, or activities such as exercise, work, reading, play, art, and travel. If depression is not overcome by these measures, seek help from mental health professionals, such as therapists or psychiatrists. Antidepressant drugs should be reserved for depression that is major and does not respond to psychotherapy alone.

Before You Use This Drug

Tell your doctor if you have or have had:

- allergies to drugs
- suicidal thoughts or actions
- kidney or liver problems
- diabetes
- epilepsy or seizures
- history of mania
- Parkinson's disease
- weight loss
- brain disease or damage
- pregnancy or are breast-feeding
- a history of drug abuse or dependence

Tell your doctor about any other drugs you take, including aspirin, herbs, vitamins, and other nonprescription products.

When You Use This Drug

- Until you know how you react to these drugs, do not drive or perform other activities requiring alertness. These drugs may cause drowsiness.
- Do not drink alcohol or take other drugs that can cause drowsiness.

- You may feel dizzy when rising from a lying or sitting position. When getting out of bed, hang your legs over the side of the bed for a few minutes, then get up slowly. When getting up from a chair, stay by the chair until you are sure that you are not dizzy. (See p. 13.)
- Stop taking these drugs and check with your doctor as soon as possible if you develop a skin rash or hives.
- If you develop dryness of the mouth, take sips of water. If dry mouth persists for more than two weeks, check with your doctor.
- Check with your doctor before you take any other drugs, prescription or nonprescription. These drugs frequently interact with other drugs.
- The effects of these drugs may last for several weeks after you stop taking them. Do not drink alcohol and heed all other warnings for this time period.
- Visit your doctor regularly to check on your progess with therapy.

How to Use This Drug

- If you miss a dose, skip the missed dose and continue with your next scheduled dose. **Do not take double doses.**
- **Do not stop taking drug abruptly.**
- Do not share your medication with others.
- Take the drug at the same time(s) each day.
- Take with or without food.
- Measure liquid with a calibrated teaspoon.
- Capsules may be opened and the contents mixed with applesauce, jelly, or ketchup, then swallowed without chewing.
- If you are taking other drugs, take them one to two hours before taking one of these drugs.
- Store at room temperature with cap on tightly. Do not store in the bathroom. Do not expose to heat, moisture, or strong light. Keep out of reach of children.
- Note that it may require four weeks or longer to obtain the desired effects.

Interactions with Other Drugs

The following drugs, biologics (e.g., vaccines, therapeutic antibodies), or foods are listed in *Evaluations of Drug Interactions* 2003 as causing "highly clinically significant" or "clinically significant" interactions when used together with any of the drugs in this section. In some sections with multiple drugs, the interaction may have been reported for one but not all drugs in this section, but we include the interaction because the drugs in this section are similar to one another. We have also included potentially serious interactions listed in the drug's FDA-approved professional package insert or in published medical journal articles. There may be other drugs, especially those in the families of drugs listed below, that also will react with this drug to cause severe adverse effects. Make sure to tell your doctor and pharmacist the drugs you are taking and tell them if you are taking any of these interacting drugs:

At least two weeks should elapse between stopping a monoamine oxidase (MAO) inhibitor and starting one of these drugs. You should wait at least five weeks after stopping one of these drugs and starting one of these MAO inhibitors: deprenyl, ELDEPRYL, furazolidone, FUROXONE, isocarboxazid, MARPLAN, MATULANE, NARDIL, PARNATE, phenelzine, procarbazine, selegiline, tranylcypromine.

Other interacting drugs for the group are: alcohol, alprazolam, amoxapine, ANAFRANIL, ARICEPT, AVENTYL, ayahuasca, carbamazepine, CELEXA, cilostazol, cimetidine, citalopram, clomipramine, clozapine, CLOZARIL, COGNEX, cyclosporine, cyproheptadine, delavirdine, desipramine, DESYREL, dextromethorphan, DIFLUCAN, digoxin, DILANTIN, donepezil, doxepin, DURAGESIC, ERYTHROCIN, erythromycin, escitalopram, ESKALITH, fentanyl, fluconazole, imipramine, IMITREX, INDERAL, IONAMIN, ketorolac, LANOXIN, LEXAPRO, linezolid, lithium, LITHOBID, LITHONATE, marijuana, MAXALT, MERIDIA, moclobemide, NORPRAMIN, nortriptyline, NORVIR, PERIACTIN, phentermine, phenytoin, PLETAL, propranolol, protriptyline, quinidine, RESCRIPTOR, ritonavir, rizatriptan, SANDIMMUNE, sibutramine, SINEQUAN, sumatriptan, SURMONTIL, tacrine, TAGAMET, TEGRETOL, thioridazine, TOFRANIL, tolbutamide, TORADOL, tramadol, trazodone, trimipramine, tryptophan, ULTRACET, ULTRAM, VIVACTIL, XANAX, zotepine, ZYVOX.

Central nervous system (CNS) depressant drugs including alcohol, antidepressants, antihistamines, antipsychotics, some blood pressure medications (reserpine, methyldopa, beta-blockers), motion sickness medications, muscle relaxants, narcotics, sedatives, sleeping pills, and tranquilizers.

Adverse Effects

Call your doctor immediately if you experience:

Signs of allergic reaction or serum sickness–like syndrome:

- skin rash or hives associated with burning or tingling in fingers, hands, or arms
- chills or fever
- swollen glands
- joint or muscle pain
- swelling of feet or lower legs, trouble breathing

Signs of hypoglycemia:

- anxiety
- chills, cold sweats, confusion, cool, pale skin
- difficulty concentrating
- drowsiness
- excessive hunger
- fast heartbeat

- headache
- nervousness, shakiness, unsteady walk
- unusual tiredness or weakness

*Call your doctor immediately if you experi-
ence:*

- suicidal thoughts or behavior
- abnormal bleeding
- breast tenderness or secretion of milk in females
- dizziness or fainting
- slow, fast, or irregular heartbeat
- anxiety
- trouble with urination
- mood changes
- trembling or shaking
- chills, fever, or sore throat
- joint or muscle pain
- skin rash, hives, itching, or peeling of skin
- red, irritated eyes
- difficulty breathing
- cold sweats
- confusion, poor coordination
- excessive hunger
- unusual excitement
- swollen glands
- swelling of feet or lower legs
- difficulty speaking
- dry mouth
- decreased sexual drive, abnormal ejaculation, or impotence
- stomach or abdominal cramps
- black, tarry stools
- gas
- diarrhea
- tiredness or weakness
- trouble sleeping
- mania
- difficult or fast breathing
- unusual facial or body movements

*Call your doctor if these symptoms con-
tinue:*

- anxiety and nervousness
- nausea or vomiting

- diarrhea
- increased or decreased appetite, or weight
  gain or loss
- constipation
- gas
- watering of mouth
- frequent urination
- change in sense of taste
- heartbum
- drowsiness
- dry mouth
- trouble sleeping
- pain in muscles or joints
- menstrual pain
- dizziness or fainting, especially when getting up
- headache (severe and throbbing)
- unusual tiredness
- increased yawning
- increased sweating
- tingling, burning, or prickly feelings on skin
- tooth grinding
- trembling or shaking
- disturbing dreams
- changes in vision
- chest pain
- irregular or fast heartbeat
- stuffy or runny nose
- cough
- impaired concentration
- trembling or quivering
- feeling of warmth or heat
- flushing or redness of skin, especially on
  face and neck
- decreased libido

*Call your doctor if these symptoms occur
after you stop taking the drug:*

- agitation
- anxiety
- dizziness
- fatigue
- headache
- vision changes
- nausea

- sweating
- general feeling of discomfort or illness
- trouble walking
- trouble sleeping
- confusion
- restlessness
- muscle pain
- trembling or shaking

Signs of overdose:

- agitation and restlessness
- dizziness, convulsions
- seizures
- unusual excitement
- severe nausea and vomiting
- severe drowsiness
- dry mouth
- irritability
- large pupils
- fast heartbeat
- sweating
- diarrhea

If you suspect an overdose, call this number to contact your poison control center: (800) 222-1222.

Periodic Tests

Ask your doctor which of these tests should be done periodically while you are taking this drug:

- supervision of depression with suicidal tendencies
- blood count
- liver function tests
- lipid levels in blood

Tricyclics

Limited Use

Amoxapine (a *mox* a peen)
ASENDIN (Lederle)

Doxepin (*dox* e pin)
SINEQUAN (Pfizer)

Imipramine (im *ip* ra meen)
TOFRANIL (Novartis)

GENERIC: available

FAMILY: Tricyclic Antidepressants
(See p. 184 for discussion of depression.)

PREGNANCY WARNING

There have been clinical reports of congenital malformations associated with the use of imipramine. Do not use during pregnancy. Amoxapine and doxepin have not been adequately tested but can be assumed to pose similar risks.

BREAST-FEEDING WARNING

Data suggest that imipramine is excreted in milk. There is a report of trouble breathing and drowsiness in a nursing infant whose mother is taking doxepin, another drug in this group. Because the possibility exists that the drugs can harm the child, mothers taking these drugs should not nurse.

These tricyclic antidepressants are used to treat severe depression that is not caused by other drugs, by alcohol, or by emotional losses (such as a death in the family). You should not be taking them for anxiety or mild depression, or as a sleeping pill. Because these drugs have more harmful adverse effects (see table, p. 188) than the two antidepressants desipramine and nortriptyline (see p. 200), we consider them to be of limited use to older adults.

If you are over 60, you will generally need to take one-third to one-half the dose used by younger adults. If the initial dose is not enough and needs to be increased, this should be done very slowly.

Amoxapine can cause tardive dyskinesia—uncontrolled movements of the jaws, tongue,

ANTICHOLINERGIC EFFECTS

WARNING: SPECIAL MENTAL AND PHYSICAL ADVERSE EFFECTS

Older adults are especially sensitive to the harmful anticholinergic (see Glossary, p. 889) effects of these drugs. Drugs in this family should not be used unless absolutely necessary.

Mental Effects: confusion, delirium, short-term memory problems, disorientation, and impaired attention.

Physical Effects: dry mouth, constipation, difficulty urinating (especially for a man with an enlarged prostate), blurred vision, decreased sweating with increased body temperature, sexual dysfunction, and worsening of glaucoma.

and lips—an affect also seen with antipsychotic drugs (see p. 176). Doxepin has especially strong sedative effects.

A large statistical summary known as a meta-analysis commissioned by the U.S. Department of Health and Human Services through the Agency for Health Care Policy and Research found that in general there were no significant differences in the effectiveness of the newer antidepressants such as the SSRIs (see p. 188) and the older agents such as the tricyclic antidepressants. In terms of adverse drug reactions, there was no significant difference between the new and old antidepressants in overall discontinuation rates of use of these drugs by patients.[81] Drug discontinuation rates can be used to compare adverse reactions between drugs.

The FDA-approved professional product labeling for antidepressant drugs sold in the United States carries the following statement:

Suicide: The possibility of a suicide attempt is inherent in major depressive disorder and may persist until significant remission occurs. Close supervision of high-risk patients should accompany initial drug ther-

apy. Prescriptions for Drug X should be written for the smallest quantity of tablets consistent with good patient management, in order to reduce the risk of overdose.

The length of time it takes an antidepressant to work can overlap with the time of spontaneous recovery, especially if the depression is situational—caused by a death or other external circumstances. The majority of people lift themselves out of depression with friends, spiritual resources, or activities such as exercise, work, reading, play, art, and travel. If depression is not overcome by these measures, seek help from mental health professionals, such as therapists or psychiatrists. Antidepressant drugs should be reserved for depression that is major and does not respond to psychotherapy alone.

Before You Use This Drug

Tell your doctor if you have or have had:

- allergies to drugs
- alcohol dependence
- asthma
- bipolar disorder (manic-depressive illness) or schizophrenia
- blood disorders
- convulsions (seizures)
- difficulty urinating or enlarged prostate
- glaucoma
- heart or blood vessel disease
- high blood pressure
- kidney or liver problems
- overactive thyroid
- stomach or intestinal disorders
- pregnancy or are breast-feeding

Tell your doctor about any other drugs you take, including aspirin, herbs, vitamins, and other nonprescription products.

Ask your doctor to check your blood pressure, once while you are lying down and once after you have been standing up for at least two minutes, and to do an electrocardiogram.

When You Use This Drug

• **Do not stop taking this drug suddenly. Your doctor must give you a schedule to lower your dose gradually, to prevent withdrawal symptoms** such as headache, mood change, nausea, vomiting, diarrhea, and trouble sleeping and vivid dreams.

• Until you know how you react to this drug, do not drive or perform other activities requiring alertness. These drugs may cause blurred vision and drowsiness.

• It may take several weeks before you can tell that these drugs are working. Do not take more drug than prescribed. If the drug works, talk with your doctor about gradually lowering the dose.

• Do not smoke. Smoking may increase the drug's effects on your heart.

• Do not drink alcohol or use other drugs that can cause drowsiness.

• You may feel dizzy when rising from a lying or sitting position. When getting out of bed, hang your legs over the side of the bed for a few minutes, then get up slowly.

• When getting up from a chair, stay beside the chair until you are sure that you are not dizzy. (See p. 13.)

• Check with your doctor before taking any other drugs, prescription or nonprescription. These drugs frequently interact with other drugs.

• The effects of these drugs may last for up to a week after you stop taking them. Avoid alcohol and heed all other warnings for this time period.

• If you plan to have any surgery, including dental, tell your doctor that you take one of these drugs.

• Avoid unprotected exposure to sun.

How to Use This Drug

• *If you miss a dose, use the following guidelines:* If you are taking more than one dose a day of one of these drugs, take the missed dose as soon as you remember, but skip it if it is almost time for the next dose. If you are taking your drug only once a day at bedtime, and you go to sleep without taking that dose, do not take it in the morning. Instead, call your doctor. **Do not take double doses.**

• Do not share your medication with others.

• Take the drug at the same time(s) each day.

• Take with food.

• If you are taking any other drugs, take them one to two hours before you take your antidepressant.

• Capsules may be opened and the contents mixed with applesauce, jelly, or ketchup, then swallowed without chewing.

• Store at room temperature. Do not store in the bathroom. Do not expose to heat, moisture, or strong light. Keep out of reach of children.

Interactions with Other Drugs

The following drugs, biologics (e.g., vaccines, therapeutic antibodies), or foods are listed in *Evaluations of Drug Interactions* 2003 as causing "highly clinically significant" or "clinically significant" interactions when used together with any of the drugs in this section. In some sections with multiple drugs, the interaction may have been reported for one but not all drugs in this section, but we include the interaction because the drugs in this section are similar to one another. We have also included potentially serious interactions listed in the drug's FDA-approved professional package insert or in published medical journal articles. There may be other drugs, especially those in the families of drugs listed below, that also will react with this drug to cause severe adverse effects. Make sure to tell your doctor and pharmacist the drugs you are taking and tell them if you are taking any of these interacting drugs:

The depressant effects of alcohol, barbiturates, and central nervous system (CNS) depressants may be enhanced with the use of these drugs.

ADRENALIN (also in bee sting kits), arbutamine, CELEXA, cimetidine, citalopram,
COMTAN, CYTOMEL, entacapone, epinephrine, flecainide, fluoxetine, guanethidine,
IMDUR, ISMELIN, ISMO, ISORDIL, isosorbide, liothyronine, MELLARIL, MERIDIA,
nitroglycerin (sublingual), NITROBID,
NITRO-DUR, NITROSTAT, NORVIR,
paroxetine, PAXIL, PRIMATENE MIST,
propafenone, PROZAC, quinidine, ritonavir,
RYTHMOL, sertraline, sibutramine,
SORBITRATE, TAGAMET, TAMBOCOR,
thioridazine, tolazamide, TOLINASE,
tramadol, TRANSDERM-NITRO,
TRIOSTAT, ULTRACET, ULTRAM,
ZOLOFT.

You should wait at least 14 days after stopping one of these drugs and starting one of
these MAO inhibitors: deprenyl, ELDE-
PRYL, furazolidone, FUROXONE, isocarboxazid, MARPLAN, MATULANE, NARDIL,
PARNATE, phenelzine, procarbazine, selegiline, tranylcypromine.

Adverse Effects

*Call your doctor immediately if you experi-
ence:*

- irregular blood pressure
- nervousness or restlessness
- loss of bladder control
- severe muscle stiffness
- pale skin
- blurred vision
- constipation
- confusion, delirium, or hallucinations
- decreased sexual ability
- difficulty in speaking or swallowing
- eye pain
- fainting
- loss of balance control
- masklike face
- difficulty urinating
- shakiness or trembling

- shuffling walk
- slowed movements
- stiffness of arms and legs
- anxiety
- breast enlargement in both males and females
- hair loss
- inappropriate secretion of milk
- increased sensitivity to sunlight
- irritability
- twitching muscle
- red or brownish spots on skin
- ringing or buzzing in the ears
- skin rash and itching
- sore throat and fever
- swelling of face and tongue
- swelling of testicles
- trouble with teeth or gums
- yellow skin or eyes

For tricyclic antidepressants:
**Call your doctor if these symptoms con-
tinue:**

- diarrhea
- dizziness
- dry mouth
- drowsiness
- headache
- heartburn
- insomnia
- nausea or vomiting
- increased appetite (may include craving for
  sweets)
- unpleasant taste in mouth
- weight gain
- trouble sleeping

For amoxapine only (in addition to above):
Signs of neuroleptic malignant syndrome:

- convulsions
- difficult breathing
- fast heartbeat or irregular pulse
- fever
- irregular blood pressure
- increased sweating

- loss of control of urination
- severe muscle stiffness
- unusual tiredness or weakness

Call your doctor if these symptoms continue after you stop taking the drug:

- headache
- irritability
- nausea and vomiting
- diarrhea
- restlessness or unusual excitement
- insomnia

For amoxapine only (in addition to above):
Signs of tardive dyskinesia:

- lip smacking or puckering, puffing of cheeks
- rapid or wormlike movements of tongue
- uncontrolled movements of arms, legs, or mouth

Signs of overdose:

- confusion
- severe drowsiness
- fever
- hallucinations
- restlessness and agitation
- seizures
- breathing difficulty
- irregular heartbeat
- unusual tiredness
- weakness
- vomiting
- enlarged pupils

If you suspect an overdose call this number to contact your poison control center: (800) 222-1222.

Periodic Tests

Ask your doctor which of these tests should be done periodically while you are taking this drug:

- complete blood count
- blood pressure
- pulse
- glaucoma tests
- liver function tests
- kidney function tests
- heart function tests such as electrocardiogram (ECG, EKG)
- dental exams (at least twice yearly)
- plasma tricyclic determinations

Desipramine (dess *ip* ra meen)
NORPRAMIN (Aventis)

Nortriptyline (nor *trip* ti leen)
AVENTYL (Lilly)
PAMELOR (Tyco)

GENERIC: available
FAMILY: Tricyclic Antidepressants
(See p. 184 for discussion of depression.)

PREGNANCY AND BREAST-FEEDING WARNING
There are no data available from either animal or human studies. Use during pregnancy only for clear medical reasons. Tell your doctor if you are pregnant or thinking of becoming pregnant before you take this drug.

Desipramine and nortriptyline are tricyclic antidepressants used to treat severe depression that is not caused by other drugs, by alcohol, or by emotional losses (such as a death in the family). These two drugs produce fewer sedative effects and fewer harmful anticholinergic adverse effects (see box) than some other antidepressants, and some clinicians suggest trying one of these two drugs before other drugs in their family (see p. 188 for comparison with other antidepressants). You should not be taking these drugs for mild depression or anxiety, or as a sleeping pill.

If you are over 60, you will generally need to take one-third to one-half the dose used for younger adults. If the initial dose is not enough and must be increased, this should be done very slowly under the guidance of your doctor. Your doctor should monitor the level of

ANTICHOLINERGIC EFFECTS

WARNING: SPECIAL MENTAL AND PHYSICAL ADVERSE EFFECTS

Older adults are especially sensitive to the harmful anticholinergic (see Glossary, p. 889) effects of these drugs. Drugs in this family should not be used unless absolutely necessary.

Mental Effects: confusion, delirium, short-term memory problems, disorientation, and impaired attention.

Physical Effects: dry mouth, constipation, difficulty urinating (especially for a man with an enlarged prostate), blurred vision, decreased sweating with increased body temperature, sexual dysfunction, and worsening of glaucoma.

the drug in your bloodstream, because there is a point at which a higher drug level produces less benefit.

A large statistical summary known as a meta-analysis commissioned by the U.S. Department of Health and Human Services through the Agency for Health Care Policy and Research found that in general there were no significant differences in the effectiveness of the newer antidepressants such as the SSRIs (see p. 188) and the older agents such as the tricyclic antidepressants. In terms of adverse drug reactions, there was no significant difference between the new and old antidepressants in overall discontinuation rates of use of these drugs by patients.[81] Drug discontinuation rates can be used to compare adverse reactions between drugs.

The FDA-approved professional product labeling for antidepressant drugs sold in the United States carries the following statement:

Suicide: The possibility of a suicide attempt is inherent in major depressive disorder and may persist until significant remission occurs. Close supervision of high-risk patients should accompany initial drug therapy. Prescriptions for Drug X should be written for the smallest quantity of tablets consistent with good patient management, in order to reduce the risk of overdose.

The length of time it takes an antidepressant to work can overlap with the time of spontaneous recovery, especially if the depression is situational—caused by a death or other external circumstances. The majority of people lift themselves out of depression with friends, spiritual resources, or activities such as exercise, work, reading, play, art, and travel. If depression is not overcome by these measures, seek help from mental health professionals, such as therapists or psychiatrists. Antidepressant drugs should be reserved for depression that is major and does not respond to psychotherapy alone.

Before You Use This Drug

Tell your doctor if you have or have had:

- allergies to drugs
- alcohol dependence
- asthma
- blood disorders
- heart or blood vessel disease
- epilepsy, seizures
- stomach or intestinal disease
- glaucoma
- kidney, liver, or thyroid problems
- manic-depressive illness, schizophrenia, or paranoia
- retention of urine or enlarged prostate
- pregnancy or are breast-feeding

Tell your doctor about any other drugs you take, including aspirin, herbs, vitamins, and other nonprescription products.

Ask your doctor to check your blood pressure, once while you are lying down and once after you have been standing up for at least two minutes, and to do an electrocardiogram.

When You Use This Drug

- **Do not stop taking this drug suddenly. Your doctor must give you a schedule to lower your dose gradually, to prevent withdrawal symptoms** such as headache, mood change, nausea, vomiting, diarrhea, and trouble sleeping and vivid dreams.
- Do not smoke. Smoking may increase the drug's effects on your heart.
- Until you know how you react to this drug, do not drive or perform other activities requiring alertness. These drugs may cause blurred vision and drowsiness.
- It may take several weeks before you can tell that these drugs are working. If the drug works, talk with your doctor about lowering the dose gradually.
- Do not drink alcohol or use other drugs that can cause drowsiness.
- You may feel dizzy when rising from a lying or sitting position. When getting out of bed, hang your legs over the side of the bed for a few minutes, then get up slowly. When getting up from a chair, stay by the chair until you are sure that you are not dizzy. (See p. 13.)
- Check with your doctor before taking any other drugs, prescription or nonprescription. These drugs frequently interact with other drugs.
- The effects of these drugs may last for up to a week after you stop taking them. Avoid alcohol and heed all other warnings for this time period.
- If you plan to have any surgery, including dental, tell your doctor that you take this drug.

How to Use This Drug

- *If you miss a dose, use the following guidelines:* If you are taking your drug more than once a day, take the missed dose as soon as you remember, but skip it if it is almost time for your next scheduled dose. If you are taking your drug only once a day at bedtime and you go to sleep without taking that dose, do not take it in the morning. Instead, call your doctor. **Do not take double doses.**
- Do not share your medication with others.
- Take the drug at the same time(s) each day.
- Take with food.
- If you are taking other drugs, take them one to two hours before taking your antidepressant.
- Capsules may be opened and the contents mixed with applesauce, jelly, or ketchup, then swallowed without chewing.
- Do not store in the bathroom. Do not expose to heat, moisture, or strong light.

Interactions with Other Drugs

The following drugs, biologics (e.g., vaccines, therapeutic antibodies), or foods are listed in *Evaluations of Drug Interactions* 2003 as causing "highly clinically significant" or "clinically significant" interactions when used together with any of the drugs in this section. In some sections with multiple drugs, the interaction may have been reported for one but not all drugs in this section, but we include the interaction because the drugs in this section are similar to one another. We have also included potentially serious interactions listed in the drug's FDA-approved professional package insert or in published medical journal articles. There may be other drugs, especially those in the families of drugs listed below, that also will react with this drug to cause severe adverse effects. Make sure to tell your doctor and pharmacist the drugs you are taking and tell them if you are taking any of these interacting drugs:

ADRENALIN (also in bee sting kits), arbutamine, CELEXA, chlordiazepoxide, cimetidine, citalopram, COMTAN, CYTOMEL, diazepam, entacapone, epinephrine, flecainide, fluoxetine, guanethidine, halofantrine, IMDUR, INDERAL, INDERAL

LA, ISMELIN, ISMO, ISORDIL, isosorbide, LIBRIUM, liothyronine, marijuana, MEL-LARIL, MERIDIA, nitroglycerin (sublin-gual), NITRO-BID, NITROSTAT, NORVIR, ORAP, paroxetine, PAXIL, phenothiazines, pirnozide, PRIFTIN, PRIMATENE MIST, propafenone, propranolol, PROZAC, quini-dine, rifapentine, ritonavir, RYTHMOL, sertraline, sibutramine, SORBITRATE, TAGAMET, TAMBOCOR, thioridazine, to-lazamide, TOLINASE, tramadol, TRANS-DERM-NITRO, TRIOSTAT, ULTRACET, ULTRAM, VALIUM, ZOLOFT.

You should wait at least 14 days after stop-ping one of these drugs and starting one of these MAO inhibitors: deprenyl, ELDE-PRYL, furazolidone, FUROXONE, isocarbox-azid, MARPLAN, MATULANE, NARDIL, PARNATE, phenelzine, procarbazine, selegiline, tranylcypromine.

Adverse Effects

Call your doctor immediately if you experience:
- signs of parkinsonism: difficulty speaking or swallowing, loss of balance, masklike face, muscle spasms, stiffness of arms or legs, trembling and shaking, unusual twisting movements of body
- irregular blood pressure
- loss of bladder control
- severe muscle stiffness
- pale skin
- blurred vision
- constipation
- confusion, delirium, or hallucinations
- decreased sexual ability
- difficulty in speaking or swallowing
- eye pain
- fainting
- loss of balance control
- difficulty urinating
- shuffling walk

- slowed movements
- anxiety
- breast enlargement in both males and females
- hair loss
- unusual secretion of milk
- increased sensitivity to sunlight
- irritability
- muscle twitching
- red or brownish spots on skin
- ringing or buzzing in the ears
- skin rash and itching
- sore throat and fever
- swelling of face and tongue
- swelling of testicles
- trouble with teeth or gums
- yellow skin or eyes

Call your doctor if these symptoms continue:
- diarrhea
- dizziness
- dry mouth
- headache
- heartburn
- insomnia
- nausea or vomiting
- increased appetite for sweets
- unpleasant taste in mouth
- weight gain
- trouble sleeping

Call your doctor if these symptoms continue after you have stopped taking the drug:
- headache
- irritability
- nausea and vomiting
- diarrhea
- restlessness or unusual excitement
- insomnia

Signs of overdose:
- confusion
- severe drowsiness

- fever
- hallucinations
- restlessness and agitation
- seizures
- shortness of breath, trouble breathing
- unusually fast, slow, or irregular heartbeat
- unusual tiredness
- weakness
- vomiting
- enlarged pupils

If you suspect an overdose, call this number to contact your poison control center: (800) 222-1222.

Periodic Tests

Ask your doctor which of these tests should be done periodically while you are taking this drug:

- complete blood count
- pulse
- blood pressure
- glaucoma tests
- desipramine blood levels
- liver function tests
- kidney function tests
- heart function tests such as electrocardiogram (ECG, EKG)
- dental exams, at least twice yearly

Do Not Use

ALTERNATIVE TREATMENT:
For Depression, see Desipramine and Nortriptyline, p. 200.

Amitriptyline (a mee *trip* ti leen)
ELAVIL (AstraZeneca)

FAMILY: Tricyclic Antidepressants
(See p. 184 for discussion of depression.)

Amitriptyline, a tricyclic antidepressant, is used to treat depression, but we do not recommend its use because it has more harmful adverse effects than any other drug in its family (see table, p. 188). For years these drugs have been on a list of drugs that are inappropriate for use in older adults.[82] If you need an antidepressant drug, either nortriptyline or desipramine is a better choice (see p. 200).

The FDA-approved professional product labeling for antidepressant drugs sold in the United States carries the following statement:

Suicide: The possibility of a suicide attempt is inherent in major depressive disorder and may persist until significant remission occurs. Close supervision of high-risk patients should accompany initial drug therapy. Prescriptions for Drug X should be written for the smallest quantity of tablets consistent with good patient management, in order to reduce the risk of overdose.

The length of time it takes an antidepressant to work can overlap with the time of sponta-

---

ANTICHOLINERGIC EFFECTS

WARNING: SPECIAL MENTAL AND PHYSICAL ADVERSE EFFECTS

Older adults are especially sensitive to the harmful anticholinergic (see Glossary, p. 889) effects of these drugs. Drugs in this family should not be used unless absolutely necessary.

Mental Effects: confusion, delirium, short-term memory problems, disorientation, and impaired attention.

Physical Effects: dry mouth, constipation, difficulty urinating (especially for a man with an enlarged prostate), blurred vision, decreased sweating with increased body temperature, sexual dysfunction, and worsening of glaucoma.

If you use this drug, ask your doctor about switching to another antidepressant. **Do not stop taking this drug suddenly. Your doctor must give you a schedule to lower your dose gradually, to prevent withdrawal symptoms** such as headache, mood change, nausea, vomiting, diarrhea, or trouble sleeping and vivid dreams.

neous recovery, especially if the depression is situational—caused by a death or other external circumstances. The majority of people lift themselves out of depression with friends, spiritual resources, or activities such as exercise, work, reading, play, art, and travel. If depression is not overcome by these measures, seek help from mental health professionals, such as therapists or psychiatrists. Antidepressant drugs should be reserved for depression that is major and does not respond to psychotherapy alone.

 Do Not Use

ALTERNATIVE TREATMENT:
For Depression, see Desipramine and Nortriptyline, p. 200.

Amitriptyline and Chlordiazepoxide
(a mee *trip* ti leen and klor dye az e *pox* ide)
LIMBITROL (Valeant)

FAMILY: Tricyclic Antidepressants
(See p. 184 for discussion of depression.)
Benzodiazepines
(See p. 166 for discussion of sleeping pills and tranquilizers.)

The brand-name drug Limbitrol contains a fixed combination of the tricyclic antidepressant amitriptyline (see p. 204) and a benzodiazepine (tranquilizer or antianxiety drug), chlordiazepoxide (see p. 223). It is used to treat moderate to severe depression associated with

moderate to severe anxiety. We do not recommend that you use it, for several reasons.

This irrational combination product has for years remained on a list of drugs that are inappropriate for use in older adults.[82]

First, combining an antidepressant with a benzodiazepine has not been shown to produce a more effective drug.[83] Second, taking these two drugs together raises the risk of harmful adverse effects. Chlordiazepoxide might increase the harmful anticholinergic effects of amitriptyline (see box), and amitriptyline could increase the drowsiness caused by chlordiazepoxide. Third, the antidepressant in this combination, amitriptyline, has more adverse effects than any other drug in its family (see table, p. 188) and should not be used by older adults, either alone or in a combination such as this one.

If you use Limbitrol, ask your doctor if your treatment can be changed. Do not stop taking this drug suddenly. Your doctor may want to reduce your dose gradually over one or two months before you completely stop taking Limbitrol.

The length of time it takes an antidepressant

ANTICHOLINERGIC EFFECTS

WARNING: SPECIAL MENTAL AND PHYSICAL ADVERSE EFFECTS

Older adults are especially sensitive to the harmful anticholinergic (see Glossary, p. 889) effects of this drug. Drugs in this family should not be used unless absolutely necessary.

Mental Effects: confusion, delirium, short-term memory problems, disorientation, and impaired attention.

Physical Effects: dry mouth, constipation, difficulty urinating (especially for a man with an enlarged prostate), blurred vision, decreased sweating with increased body temperature, sexual dysfunction, and worsening of glaucoma.

to work can overlap with the time of spontaneous recovery, especially if the depression is situational—caused by a death or other external circumstances. The majority of people lift themselves out of depression with friends, spiritual resources, or activities such as exercise, work, reading, play, art, and travel. If depression is not overcome by these measures, seek help from mental health professionals, such as therapists or psychiatrists. Antidepressant drugs should be reserved for depression that is major and does not respond to psychotherapy alone.

 Do Not Use

ALTERNATIVE TREATMENT:
For Depression, see Desipramine and Nortriptyline, p. 200.

Amitriptyline and Perphenazine
TRIAVIL (New River)

FAMILY: Tricyclic Antidepressants
(See p. 184 for discussion of depression.)
Traditional or Typical Antipsychotics (See p. 258.)

The brand-name product Triavil contains a fixed combination of an antidepressant, amitriptyline (see p. 204), and an antipsychotic, perphenazine. It is used to treat moderate to severe anxiety, agitation, and depression. We do not recommend that you use it, for several reasons.

If you use this drug, talk to your doctor about changing your treatment. **Do not stop taking this drug suddenly.** Your doctor may want to give you a schedule to lower your dose gradually to prevent withdrawal symptoms, such as headache, mood change, nausea, vomiting, diarrhea, and trouble sleeping and vivid dreams.

ANTICHOLINERGIC EFFECTS

WARNING: SPECIAL MENTAL AND PHYSICAL ADVERSE EFFECTS

Older adults are especially sensitive to the harmful anticholinergic (see Glossary, p. 889) effects of this drug. Drugs in this family should not be used unless absolutely necessary.

Mental Effects: confusion, delirium, short-term memory problems, disorientation, and impaired attention.

Physical Effects: dry mouth, constipation, difficulty urinating (especially for a man with an enlarged prostate), blurred vision, decreased sweating with increased body temperature, sexual dysfunction, and worsening of glaucoma.

This irrational combination product has for years remained on a list of drugs that are inappropriate for use in older adults.[82]

First, although Triavil is available in different strengths, the dose of each of its two ingredients is fixed and may not exactly fit your needs. Second, combining an antipsychotic with an antidepressant has not been shown to produce a more effective drug.[83] Third, using this combination raises the risk of harmful adverse effects, since it may cause any of the adverse effects of either of its ingredients, including severe drowsiness and other anticholinergic effects (see box). And fourth, the antidepressant ingredient in this combination, amitriptyline, has more adverse effects than any other drug in its family (see table, p. 188) and should not be used by older adults either alone or in combinations such as this one.

Other Drugs for Depression

Limited Use

Bupropion (byu *pro* pee on)
WELLBUTRIN (Glaxo Wellcome)

GENERIC: not available

FAMILY: Other Drugs for Depression
(See p. 184 for a discussion of depression.)

PREGNANCY WARNING

There is concern about the safety of bupropion use in pregnant women: the drug is both genotoxic (damages DNA) and carcinogenic in animal studies. Use in pregnancy only if clearly needed. GlaxoSmithKline maintains a pregnancy registry for which health care providers are encouraged to register their patients.

BREAST-FEEDING WARNING

Bupropion and its metabolites are excreted in human milk. Because of the potential for serious adverse effects in nursing infants, you should not take this drug while nursing.

Bupropion is used to treat severe depression that is not caused by other drugs, alcohol, or emotional losses (such as death in the family). It can take four weeks to be effective. Bupropion controls but does not cure depression. Bupropion is related to amphetamines and diethylpropion (TENUATE, TEPANIL) but purportedly is not habit-forming. Although bupropion is preferred for the elderly by some doctors,[84] it has not been studied much in older people.

Weight loss is a common adverse effect. A

EXTREME CAUTION

Bupropion has been approved by the FDA for smoking cessation for people 18 years of age and older under the brand name Zyban (see p. 786). Zyban and Wellbutrin are exactly the same drug. Taking Zyban and Wellbutrin together will increase the risk of seizure. See the warning about bupropion-induced seizure below.

ANTICHOLINERGIC EFFECTS

WARNING: SPECIAL MENTAL AND PHYSICAL ADVERSE EFFECTS

Older adults are especially sensitive to the harmful anticholinergic (see Glossary, p. 889) effects of this drug. Drugs in this family should not be used unless absolutely necessary.

Mental Effects: confusion, delirium, short-term memory problems, disorientation, and impaired attention.

Physical Effects: dry mouth, constipation, difficulty urinating (especially for a man with an enlarged prostate), blurred vision, decreased sweating with increased body temperature, sexual dysfunction, and worsening of glaucoma.

---

number of people become restless when taking bupropion.

A large statistical summary known as a meta-analysis commissioned by the U.S. Department of Health and Human Services through the Agency for Health Care Policy and Research found that in general there were no significant differences in the effectiveness of the newer antidepressants such as the SSRIs (see p. 190) and the older antidepressants. In terms of adverse drug reactions, there was no significant difference between the new and old antidepressants in overall discontinuation rates of use of these drugs by patients.[81] Drug discontinuation rates can be used to compare adverse reactions between drugs.

Higher doses increase likelihood of harmful effects. With doses more than 450 milligrams per day the risk of seizures increases tenfold.[85] According to the drug's labeling, even doses more than 300 milligrams but less than 450 milligrams per day have been associated with seizures. These doses should be limited to no more than 300 milligrams per day. Bupropion

was temporarily banned in the United States for that reason. People age 60 and over are more likely to experience adverse effects, such as heart complications. Due to age-related decrease in kidney and liver function, the lowest effective dose should be used.

The FDA-approved professional product labeling for antidepressant drugs sold in the United States carries the following statement:

Suicide: The possibility of a suicide attempt is inherent in major depressive disorder and may persist until significant remission occurs. Close supervision of high-risk patients should accompany initial drug therapy. Prescriptions for Drug X should be written for the smallest quantity of tablets consistent with good patient management, in order to reduce the risk of overdose.

The length of time it takes an antidepressant to work can overlap with the time of spontaneous recovery, especially if the depression is situational—caused by a death or other external circumstances. The majority of people lift themselves out of depression with friends, spiritual resources, or activities such as exercise, work, reading, play, art, and travel. If depression is not overcome by these measures, seek help from mental health professionals, such as therapists or psychiatrists. Antidepressant drugs should be reserved for depression that is major and does not respond to psychotherapy alone.

Before You Use This Drug

Do not use if you have or have had:

- eating disorders, such as anorexia or bulimia
- seizures
- pregnancy or are breast-feeding (drug crosses placenta and accumulates in breast milk)

Tell your doctor if you have or have had:

- allergies to drugs
- bipolar disorder (manic depression)
- drug abuse
- electroshock therapy [86]
- head injury
- heart, kidney, or liver problems
- heart attack
- psychosis
- tumor of the central nervous system
- brain tumor
- seizures

Tell your doctor about any other drugs you take, including aspirin, herbs, vitamins, and other nonprescription products.

When You Use This Drug

- Until you know how you react to this drug, do not drive or perform other activities requiring alertness.
- Do not drink alcohol.

How to Use This Drug

- If you miss a dose, take it as soon as you remember, but skip it if it is within four hours of the next dose. **Do not take double doses.**
- Do not share your medication with others.
- Take the drug at the same time(s) each day.
- Take with food.
- Swallow extended-release tablets whole.
- Space doses evenly apart during the day, but avoid taking at bedtime.
- Store tablets at room temperature with lid on tightly. Do not store in the bathroom. Do not expose to heat, moisture, or strong light. Keep out of reach of children.

Interactions with Other Drugs

The following drugs, biologics (e.g., vaccines, therapeutic antibodies), or foods are listed in

Evaluations of Drug Interactions 2003 as causing "highly clinically significant" or "clinically significant" interactions when used together with any of the drugs in this section. In some sections with multiple drugs, the interaction may have been reported for one but not all drugs in this section, but we include the interaction because the drugs in this section are similar to one another. We have also included potentially serious interactions listed in the drug's FDA-approved professional package insert or in published medical journal articles. There may be other drugs, especially those in the families of drugs listed below, that also will react with this drug to cause severe adverse effects. Make sure to tell your doctor and pharmacist the drugs you are taking and tell them if you are taking any of these interacting drugs:

> Do not take bupropion within 14 days of starting or stopping these monoamine oxidase (MAO) inhibitors: deprenyl, ELDEPRYL, furazolidone, FUROXONE, isocarboxazid, MARPLAN, MATULANE, NARDIL, PARNATE, phenelzine, procarbazine, selegiline, tranylcypromine.

> The beta-blocker drugs such as metoprolol (LOPRESSOR). A list of beta blockers can be found on page 52 of Chapter 4, Drugs for Heart Conditions chapter.

> These drugs also can interact with bupropion: alcohol, amitriptyline, AVENTYL, chlorpromazine, clozapine, CLOZARIL, desipramine, DESYREL, ELAVIL, fluoxetine, HALDOL, haloperidol, imipramine, lithium, LITHOBID, LITHONATE, loxapine, LOXITANE, LUDIOMIL, maprotiline, MOBAN, moclobemide, molindone, NAVANE, NORPRAMIN, nortriptyline, NORVIR, pargyline, paroxetine, PAXIL, PROZAC, RISPERDAL, risperidone, ritonavir, sertraline, thioridazine, thiothixene, THORAZINE, TOFRANIL, trazodone, ZOLOFT.

Adverse Effects

Call your doctor immediately if you experience:

- agitation, anxiety, confusion
- seizures
- convulsions
- fainting
- hallucinations
- delusions
- trouble concentrating
- severe headache
- skin rash, itching, hives
- tinnitus (buzzing or ringing in ears)[87]

Call your doctor if these symptoms continue:

- anger, hostility
- low or high blood pressure
- constipation
- diarrhea
- dizziness
- drowsiness
- dry mouth
- increased saliva
- fever
- chills
- sore throat
- impotence
- incoordination
- inflammation of the mouth
- loss of appetite, weight loss
- muscle spasms, tremor, twitching
- muscle pain
- nausea or vomiting
- abdominal pain
- tinnitus (buzzing or ringing in cars)[87]
- increased sweating
- weight change
- unusual tiredness, sleep disturbance
- tremor
- difficulty concentrating
- increase in frequency of urination, especially at night, or difficult urination

- blurred vision
- fast or irregular heartbeat
- change in sense of taste

Periodic Tests

Ask your doctor which of these tests should be done periodically while you are taking this drug:

- kidney function tests
- liver function tests
- supervision for suicidal tendencies

Limited Use

Maprotiline (ma *proe* ti leen)
LUDIOMIL (Novartis)

GENERIC: available

FAMILY: Other Drugs for Depression
(See p. 184 for discussion of depression.)

PREGNANCY WARNING

Maprotiline was not tested adequately in animals to know what the potential risk might be to humans.

BREAST-FEEDING WARNING

Maprotiline is secreted into breast milk. The concentration of maprotiline in breast milk is about the same as that in the mother's blood. Thus, there is a risk of serious adverse effects in nursing infants.

Maprotiline is used to treat severe depression that is not caused by other drugs, by alcohol, or by emotional losses (such as a death in the family). You should not be taking it for anxiety or mild depression, or as a sleeping pill. Because maprotiline has more harmful adverse effects (see table, p.188) than the two antidepressants desipramine and nortriptyline (see p. 200), we consider it to be of limited use to older adults.

If you are over 60, you will generally need to take one-third to one-half the dose used by younger adults. If the initial dose

---

ANTICHOLINERGIC EFFECTS

WARNING: SPECIAL MENTAL AND PHYSICAL ADVERSE EFFECTS

Older adults are especially sensitive to the harmful anticholinergic (see Glossary, p. 889) effects of this drug. Drugs in this family should not be used unless absolutely necessary.

Mental Effects: confusion, delirium, short-term memory problems, disorientation, and impaired attention.

Physical Effects: dry mouth, constipation, difficulty urinating (especially for a man with an enlarged prostate), blurred vision, decreased sweating with increased body temperature, sexual dysfunction, and worsening of glaucoma.

---

is not enough and needs to be increased, this should be done very slowly.

A large statistical summary known as a meta-analysis commissioned by the U.S. Department of Health and Human Services through the Agency for Health Care Policy and Research found that in general there were no significant differences in the effectiveness of the newer antidepressants such as the SSRIs (see p. 188) and the older antidepressants. In terms of adverse drug reactions, there was no significant difference between the new and old antidepressants in overall discontinuation rates of use of these drugs by patients.[81] Drug discontinuation rates can be used to compare adverse reactions between drugs.

The FDA-approved professional product labeling for antidepressant drugs sold in the United States carries the following statement:

Suicide: The possibility of a suicide attempt is inherent in major depressive disorder and may persist until significant remission occurs. Close supervision of high-risk patients should accompany initial drug therapy. Prescriptions for Drug X should be written for the smallest quantity of tablets consistent with good patient management, in order to reduce the risk of overdose.

The length of time it takes an antidepressant to work can overlap with the time of spontaneous recovery, especially if the depression is situational—caused by a death or other external circumstances. The majority of people lift themselves out of depression with friends, spiritual resources, or activities such as exercise, work, reading, play, art, and travel. If depression is not overcome by these measures, seek help from mental health professionals, such as therapists or psychiatrists. Antidepressant drugs should be reserved for depression that is major and does not respond to psychotherapy alone.

Before You Use This Drug

Do not use if you have or have had:

- heart attack
- seizure

Tell your doctor if you have or have had:

- allergies to drugs
- alcohol dependence
- asthma
- difficulty urinating or enlarged prostate
- glaucoma
- severe mental illness (bipolar disorder, schizophrenia)
- stomach or intestinal problems
- heart attack
- heart or blood vessel disease, including stroke
- blood disorders
- thyroid disease
- epilepsy or seizures
- liver problems
- pregnancy or are breast-feeding (level in milk is the same as in blood)

Tell your doctor about any other drugs you take, including aspirin, herbs, vitamins, and other nonprescription products.

Ask your doctor to check your blood pressure, once while you are lying down and once after you have been standing up for at least two minutes, and to do an electrocardiogram.

When You Use This Drug

- **Do not stop taking this drug suddenly. Your doctor must give you a schedule to lower your dose gradually, to prevent withdrawal symptoms** such as headache, mood change, nausea, vomiting, diarrhea, and trouble sleeping and vivid dreams.
- Until you know how you react to this drug, do not drive or perform other activities requiring alertness. This drug may cause blurred vision and drowsiness.
- It may take several weeks before you can tell that this drug is working. If the drug works, talk with your doctor about lowering the dose gradually.
- Do not smoke. Smoking may increase the drug's effects on your heart.
- Do not drink alcohol or use other drugs that can cause drowsiness.
- You may feel dizzy when rising from a lying or sitting position. When getting out of bed, hang your legs over the side of the bed for a few minutes, then get up slowly. When getting up from a chair, stay beside the chair until you are sure that you are not dizzy. (See p. 13).
- Check with your doctor before taking any other drugs, prescription or nonprescription. This drug frequently interacts with other drugs.
- The effects of these drugs may last for up to a week after you stop taking them. Avoid alcohol and heed all other warnings for this time period.
- If you plan to have any surgery, including dental, tell your doctor that you take this drug.

How to Use This Drug

- *If you miss a dose, use the following guidelines:* If you are taking more than one dose a day, take the missed dose as soon as you re-member, but skip it if it is almost time for the next dose. If you are taking your drug only once a day at bedtime, and you go to sleep without taking that dose, do not take it in the morning. Instead, call your doctor. **Do not take double doses.**

- Do not share your medication with others.
- Take the drug at the same time(s) each day.
- Take with food.
- If you are taking any other drugs, take them one to two hours before you take your antidepressant.
- Store at room temperature with lid on tightly. Do not store in the bathroom. Do not expose to heat, moisture, or strong light. Keep out of reach of children.

Interactions with Other Drugs

The following drugs, biologics (e.g., vaccines, therapeutic antibodies), or foods are listed in *Evaluations of Drug Interactions* 2003 as causing "highly clinically significant" or "clinically significant" interactions when used together with any of the drugs in this section. In some sections with multiple drugs, the interaction may have been reported for one but not all drugs in this section, but we include the interaction because the drugs in this section are similar to one another. We have also included potentially serious interactions listed in the drug's FDA-approved professional package insert or in published medical journal articles. There may be other drugs, especially those in the families of drugs listed below, that also will react with this drug to cause severe adverse effects. Make sure to tell your doctor and pharmacist the drugs you are taking and tell them if you are taking any of these interacting drugs:

ADRENALIN (also in bee sting kits), alcohol, cimetidine, COMTAN, CYTOMEL, DILANTIN, entacapone, epinephrine, fluoxetine, guanethidine, IMDUR, ISMELIN, ISMO, ISORDIL, isosorbide, liothyronine, MELLARIL, NITRO-BID, nitroglycerin (sublingual), NITROSTAT, NORVIR, PAR-NATE, paroxetine, PAXIL, phenytoin, PRIMATENE MIST, PROZAC, ritonavir, sertraline, SORBITRATE, TAGAMET, thioridazine, tolazamide, TOLINASE, tramadol, TRANSDERM-NITRO, tranyl-cypromine, TRIOSTAT, ULTRACET, ULTRAM, ZOLOFT.

You should wait at least 14 days after stopping one of these drugs and starting one of these monoamine oxidase (MAO) inhibitors: deprenyl, ELDEPRYL, furazolidone, FUROXONE, isocarboxazid, MARPLAN, MATULANE, NARDIL, PARNATE, phenelzine, procarbazine, selegiline, tranylcypromine.

Adverse Effects

Call your doctor immediately if you experience:

- skin rash, redness, swelling, or itching
- nausea or vomiting
- weight loss
- breast enlargement in both males and females
- delirium
- unusual secretion of milk
- constipation (severe)
- fainting
- shakiness or trembling
- difficulty urinating
- sore throat and fever
- unusual excitement
- yellow eyes or skin
- swelling of testicles

Call your doctor if these symptoms continue:

- blurred vision
- decreased sexual ability or interest

- dizziness or lightheadedness
- drowsiness
- tiredness or weakness
- dry mouth
- headache
- constipation (mild)
- diarrhea
- heartburn
- increased appetite and weight gain
- increased sensitivity to sunlight
- increased sweating
- trouble sleeping

Signs of overdose:

- confusion
- severe drowsiness
- fever
- hallucinations
- muscle stiffness or weakness
- restlessness and agitation
- seizures
- shakiness or trembling
- trouble breathing
- irregular heartbeat
- unusual tiredness
- vomiting

If you suspect an overdose, call this number to contact your poison control center: (800) 222-1222.

Periodic Tests

Ask your doctor which of these tests should be done periodically while you are taking this drug:

- complete blood count
- blood pressure
- heart function tests
- liver function tests
- dental exams (at least twice yearly)

Limited Use

Mirtazapine (mir *taz* a peen)
REMERON (Organon)

GENERIC: not available

FAMILY: Other Drugs for Depression
(See p. 184 for discussion of depression.)

PREGNANCY WARNING

This drug caused harm to developing fetuses in animal studies, including fetal and neonatal deaths and decreased birth weights. Use during pregnancy only for clear medical reasons. Tell your doctor if you are pregnant or thinking of becoming pregnant before you take this drug.

BREAST-FEEDING WARNING

No information is available from either human or animal studies. Since it is likely that this drug, like many others, is excreted in human milk, you should consult with your doctor if you are planning to nurse.

Mirtazapine is used to treat major depression. Mirtazapine resembles a hybrid of other types of antidepressants, namely both tricyclic antidepressants and selective serotonin reuptake inhibitors (SSRIs). Mirtazapine blocks recep-

---

**WARNING:
NEWER ANTIDEPRESSANTS
AND THE RISK OF SUICIDE
IN CHILDREN LESS THAN
18 YEARS OF AGE**

The FDA and the drug regulatory authorities in Canada and the UK have warned about the possibility of both suicidal ideation and suicide attempts seen in clinical trials of the newer antidepressant drugs, including the selective serotonin reuptake inhibitors (SSRIs), mirtazapine (REMERON), and venlafaxine (EFFEXOR) in children less than 18 years of age.

Only fluoxetine is approved for use in children less than 18 years of age for major depressive disorder.

All of the SSRI antidepressants have been shown to commonly cause sexual dysfunction in both men and women. In a large prospective study of over 6,000 men and women, sexual dysfunction occurred from 36 to 43% of the time, depending on the drug.[74] Types of sexual dysfunction include problems of desire (libido: sexual interest or drive), arousal (erectile function in men, lubrication in women), and release (ejaculation/orgasm in men and orgasm in women). Strategies to cope with this problem include decreasing the dosage to the lowest effective level; a drug holiday for patients in whom compliance is not a problem; if acceptable to the patient and partner, seeing if the sexual dysfunction resolves without further intervention.[75]

tors of the neurotransmitters serotonin and norepinephrine.

Older people and those with liver or kidney problems may need a lower dose of mirtazapine. Over half the people who take mirtazapine experience prolonged and often severe drowsiness. Mirtazapine can cause a blood disorder that lowers the number of white blood cells. Called agranulocytosis, it is a serious, sometimes fatal, adverse effect. Another potential life-threatening effect is serotonin syndrome. Symptoms include sweating, shivering, and incoordination. Mirtazapine is not recommended for women who are pregnant or for children under 18.

Published information about this drug is sparse. With so many other antidepressants available, it is wiser to use an antidepressant with better-known safety and effectiveness.

The FDA-approved professional product labeling for antidepressant drugs sold in the United States carries the following statement:

Suicide: The possibility of a suicide attempt is inherent in major depressive disorder and may persist until significant remission occurs. Close supervision of high-risk patients should accompany initial drug therapy. Prescriptions for Drug X should be written for the smallest quantity of tablets consistent with good patient management, in order to reduce the risk of overdose.

The length of time it takes an antidepressant to work can overlap with the time of spontaneous recovery, especially if the depression is situational—caused by a death or other external circumstances. The majority of people lift themselves out of depression with friends, spiritual resources, or activities such as exercise, work, reading, play, art, and travel. If depression is not overcome by these measures, seek help from mental health professionals, such as therapists or psychiatrists. Antidepressant drugs should be reserved for depression that is major and does not respond to psychotherapy alone.

Before You Use This Drug

Tell your doctor if you have or have had:

- allergies to drugs
- heart, kidney, or liver problems
- seizures
- pregnancy or are breast-feeding
- phenylketonuria (some brands contain aspartame)

Tell your doctor about any other drugs you take, including aspirin, herbs, vitamins, and other nonprescription products.

When You Use This Drug

- Do not drink alcohol or use other drugs that can cause drowsiness.
- Until you know how you react to this drug, do not drive or perform other activities that require alertness.
- You may feel dizzy when rising from a lying or sitting position. When getting out of bed, hang your legs over the side of the bed for a few minutes, then get up slowly. When getting up

from a chair, stay beside the chair until you are sure that you are not dizzy. (See p. 13.)

• Have your doctor reassess your need to continue taking mirtazapine periodically.

• If you plan to have any surgery, including dental, tell your doctor that you take this drug.

• Tell your doctor immediately if you have fever, chills, sore throat, or ulcers on mucous membranes.

How to Use This Drug

• If you miss a dose, take it as soon as you remember, but skip it if it is almost time for the next dose. **Do not take double doses.**

• Do not share your medication with others.

• Take the drug at the same time(s) each day.

• Take with or without food.

• Swallow half or whole tablets, according to dose. Take at bedtime.

• **Do not suddenly stop taking this drug.** Check with your doctor.

• Store at room temperature with lid on tightly. Do not store in the bathroom. Do not expose to heat, moisture, or strong light. Keep out of reach of children.

Interactions with Other Drugs

The following drugs, biologics (e.g., vaccines, therapeutic antibodies), or foods are listed in *Evaluations of Drug Interactions* 2003 as causing "highly clinically significant" or "clinically significant" interactions when used together with any of the drugs in this section. In some sections with multiple drugs, the interaction may have been reported for one but not all drugs in this section, but we include the interaction because the drugs in this section are similar to one another. We have also included potentially serious interactions listed in the drug's FDA-approved professional package insert or in published medical journal articles. There may be other drugs, especially those in the families of drugs listed below, that also will react with this drug to cause severe adverse effects. Make sure to tell your doctor and pharmacist the drugs you are taking and tell them if you are taking any of these interacting drugs:

Central nervous system (CNS) depressant drugs, including alcohol, antidepressants, antihistamines, antipsychotics, some blood pressure medications (reserpine, methyldopa, beta-blockers), motion sickness medications, muscle relaxants, narcotics, sedatives, sleeping pills, and tranquilizers.

CATAPRES, Clonidine, diazepam, moclobemide, pargyline, VALIUM.

Do not take mirtazapine within 14 days after stopping or starting any of these monoamine oxidase (MAO) inhibitors: deprenyl, ELDEPRYL, furazolidone, FUROXONE, isocarboxazid, MARPLAN, MATULANE, NARDIL, PARNATE, phenelzine, procarbazine, selegiline, tranylcypromine.

Adverse Effects

Call your doctor immediately if you experience:

• agitation or anxiety
• chills, shivering
• excitement or increased or decreased movement
• apathy
• confusion or abnormal thinking
• dizziness
• fever
• incoordination
• inflammation or sores in mouth
• seizures
• sore throat
• suicidal thoughts
• sweating
• twitching
• menstrual pain or missed periods
• decreased sexual ability
• mood or mental changes
• shortness of breath

- swelling of face
- skin rash
- decreased movement

Call your doctor if these symptoms continue:

- constipation
- drowsiness
- dry mouth
- dizziness
- weakness
- increased appetite, weight gain
- abdominal pain
- abnormal dreams
- back pain
- frequent urge to urinate
- increased sensitivity to touch and pain
- increased thirst
- low blood pressure
- muscle pain
- nausea, vomiting
- trembling, shaking

Ask your doctor which of these tests should be done periodically while you are taking this drug:

- blood tests

Do Not Use

ALTERNATIVE TREATMENT:
See Desipramine and Nortriptyline, p. 200.

Nefazodone (ne *faz* ah done)
SERZONE (Bristol-Myers Squibb)

FAMILY: Other Drugs for Depression
           (See p. 184 for discussion of depression.)

PREGNANCY WARNING

Nefazodone caused harm in animal studies, including decreased pup weights and deaths in pups after birth. Because of the potential for serious adverse effects to the fetus, this drug should not be used by pregnant women.

BREAST-FEEDING WARNING

No information is available from either human or animal studies. However, it is likely that this drug, like many others, is excreted in human milk, and because of the potential for serious adverse effects in nursing infants, you should not take this drug while nursing.

FDA BLACK BOX WARNING

Cases of life-threatening hepatic failure have been reported in patients treated with SERZONE. The reported rate in the United States is about 1 case of liver failure resulting in death or transplant per 250,000–300,000 patient-years of Serzone treatment. The total patient-years is a summation of each patient's duration of exposure expressed in years. For example, 1 patient-year is equal to 2 patients each treated for 6 months, 3 patients each treated for 4 months, etc.

Ordinarily, treatment with SERZONE should not be initiated in individuals with active liver disease or with elevated baseline serum transaminases. There is no evidence that pre-existing liver disease increases the likelihood of developing liver failure, however, baseline abnormalities can complicate patient monitoring.

Patients should be advised to be alert for signs and symptoms of liver dysfunction (jaundice, anorexia, gastrointestinal complaints, malaise, etc.) and to report them to their doctor immediately if they occur.

SERZONE should be discontinued if clinical signs or symptoms suggest liver failure. Patients who develop evidence of hepatocellular injury such as increased serum AST or serum ALT levels >= (greater than or equal to) 3 times the upper limit of NORMAL, while on SERZONE should be withdrawn from the drug. These patients should be presumed to be at increased risk for liver injury if SERZONE is reintroduced. Accordingly, such patients should not be considered for re-treatment.[88]

Nefazodone was cleared for marketing by the FDA in December 1994. On December 10, 2001, the FDA informed nefazodone's manufacturer that it must add a black-box warning to the professional product lable, or "package insert," for the drug, informing doctors and pharmacists that life-threatening liver damage can occur with the use of nefazodone. A black-box warning is the strongest type of warning that the FDA can require on a drug's label. This action followed a warning issued by Canadian government authorities earlier in 2001.

Nefazodone's manufacturer announced on January 8, 2003, that it was pulling the drug in all European countries where it was marketed. Nefazodone was withdrawn from the Swedish market in early 2002 and from Denmark in December 2002 after concerns about liver toxicity. Nefazodone had been linked to liver failure and/or death in 26 patients worldwide.

Public Citizen's Health Research Group has petitioned the FDA on two occasions in 2003 to remove this dangerous drug from the market.[89,90]

———

Limited Use

Trazodone (*traz* oh done)
DESYREL (Apothecon)

GENERIC: available

FAMILY: Other Drugs for Depression
(See p. 184 for discussion of depression.)

PREGNANCY WARNING

This drug caused harm to developing fetuses in animal studies, including death and birth defects. Use during pregnancy only for clear medical reasons. Tell your doctor if you are pregnant or thinking of becoming pregnant before you take this drug.

BREAST-FEEDING WARNING

Trazodone is excreted in rat milk, suggesting that it is likely to be secreted in human milk. There is a risk of serious adverse effects to your infants if you nurse.

Trazodone is used to treat severe depression that is not caused by other drugs, by alcohol, or by emotional losses (such as a death in the family). You should not be taking this drug for anxiety or mild depression, or as a sleeping pill. Because trazodone has more harmful adverse effects (see table, p. 188) than the two antidepressants desipramine and nortriptyline (see p. 200), we consider it to be of limited use to older adults.

If you are over 60, you will generally need to take one-third to one-half the dose used by younger adults. If the initial dose is not enough and needs to be increased, this should be done very slowly.

Trazodone can cause painful, prolonged penile erections (priapism) in men. If you suffer this reaction, stop taking the drug and notify your doctor.

A large statistical summary known as a meta-analysis commissioned by the U.S. Department of Health and Human Services through the Agency for Health Care Policy and Research found that in general there were no significant differences in the effectiveness of the newer antidepressants such as the SSRIs (see p. 188) and the older antidepressants. In terms of ad-

---

ANTICHOLINERGIC EFFECTS

WARNING: SPECIAL MENTAL AND PHYSICAL ADVERSE EFFECTS

Older adults are especially sensitive to the harmful anticholinergic (see Glossary, p. 889) effects of this drug. Drugs in this family should not be used unless absolutely necessary.

Mental Effects: confusion, delirium, short-term memory problems, disorientation, and impaired attention.

Physical Effects: dry mouth, constipation, difficulty urinating (especially for a man with an enlarged prostate), blurred vision, decreased sweating with increased body temperature, sexual dysfunction, and worsening of glaucoma.

verse drug reactions, there was no significant difference between the new and old antidepressants in overall discontinuation rates of use of these drugs by patients.[81] Drug discontinuation rates can be used to compare adverse reactions between drugs.

The FDA-approved professional product labeling for antidepressant drugs sold in the United States carries the following statement:

Suicide: The possibility of a suicide attempt is inherent in major depressive disorder and may persist until significant remission occurs. Close supervision of high-risk patients should accompany initial drug therapy. Prescriptions for Drug X should be written for the smallest quantity of tablets consistent with good patient management, in order to reduce the risk of overdose.

The length of time it takes an antidepressant to work can overlap with the time of spontaneous recovery, especially if the depression is situational—caused by a death or other external circumstances. The majority of people lift themselves out of depression with friends, spiritual resources, or activities such as exercise, work, reading, play, art, and travel. If depression is not overcome by these measures, seek help from mental health professionals, such as therapists or psychiatrists. Antidepressant drugs should be reserved for depression that is major and does not respond to psychotherapy alone.

Do not use if you are recovering from a heart attack.

Before You Use This Drug

Tell your doctor if you have or have had:

- allergies to drugs
- alcohol dependence
- kidney or liver problems
- retention of urine or enlarged prostate
- heart rhythm disturbance

- fever or sore throat
- pregnancy or are breast-feeding

Tell your doctor about any other drugs you take, including aspirin, herbs, vitamins, and other nonprescription products.

Ask your doctor to check your blood pressure, once while you are lying down and once after you have been standing up for at least two minutes, and to do an electrocardiogram.

When You Use This Drug

- **Do not stop taking this drug suddenly. Your doctor must give you a schedule to lower your dose gradually, to prevent withdrawal symptoms** such as headache, mood change, nausea, vomiting, diarrhea, and trouble sleeping and vivid dreams.
- Until you know how you react to this drug, do not drive or perform other activities requiring alertness. This drug may cause blurred vision and drowsiness.
- It may take several weeks before you can tell that this drug is working. If the drug works, talk with your doctor about gradually lowering the dose.
- Do not smoke. Smoking may increase the drug's effects on your heart.
- Do not drink alcohol or use other drugs that can cause drowsiness.
- You may feel dizzy when rising from a lying or sitting position. When getting out of bed, hang your legs over the side of the bed for a few minutes, then get up slowly. When getting up from a chair, stay beside the chair until you are sure that you are not dizzy. (See p. 13.)
- Check with your doctor before taking any other drugs, prescription or nonprescription. This drug frequently interacts with other drugs.
- The effects of this drug may last for up to a week after you stop taking it. Avoid alcohol and heed all other warnings for this time period.
- If you plan to have any surgery, including dental, tell your doctor that you take this drug.

- Check with your doctor if dry mouth continues for more than two weeks.

How to Use This Drug

- If you miss a dose, take it as soon as you remember, but skip it if it is less than four hours until your next scheduled dose. **Do not take double doses.**
- Do not share your medication with others.
- Take the drug at the same time(s) each day.
- Take with food.
- If you are taking any other drugs, take them one to two hours before you take your antidepressant.
- Use sugarless gum, ice, or saliva substitute if you develop a dry mouth.
- Store at room temperature with lid on tightly. Do not store in the bathroom. Do not expose to heat, moisture, or strong light. Keep out of reach of children.

Interactions with Other Drugs

The following drugs, biologics (e.g., vaccines, therapeutic antibodies), or foods are listed in *Evaluations of Drug Interactions* 2003 as causing "highly clinically significant" or "clinically significant" interactions when used together with any of the drugs in this section. In some sections with multiple drugs, the interaction may have been reported for one but not all drugs in this section, but we include the interaction because the drugs in this section are similar to one another. We have also included potentially serious interactions listed in the drug's FDA-approved professional package insert or in published medical journal articles. There may be other drugs, especially those in the families of drugs listed below, that also will react with this drug to cause severe adverse effects. Make sure to tell your doctor and pharmacist the drugs you are taking and tell them if you are taking any of these interacting drugs:

Central nervous system (CNS) depressant drugs, including alcohol, antidepressants, antihistamines, antipsychotics, some blood pressure medications (reserpine, methyldopa, beta-blockers), motion sickness medications, muscle relaxants, narcotics, sedatives, sleeping pills, and tranquilizers.

Other interacting drugs are: digoxin, LANOXIN, ritonavir (NORVIR).

Adverse Effects

Call your doctor immediately if you experience:

- painful, inappropriate erection of the penis
- muscle tremors
- fainting
- skin rash
- unusual excitement

Call your doctor if these symptoms continue:

- dizziness
- dry mouth
- headache
- unpleasant taste in mouth
- blurred vision
- constipation
- nausea and vomiting
- diarrhea
- muscle aches or pains
- unusual tiredness or weakness

Signs of overdose:

- confusion
- severe drowsiness
- fever
- hallucinations
- restlessness and agitation
- seizures
- shortness of breath
- trouble breathing
- irregular heartbeat
- unusual tiredness

- weakness
- nausea and vomiting

If you suspect an overdose, call this number to contact your poison control center: (800) 222-1222.

Periodic Tests

Ask your doctor which of these tests should be done periodically while you are taking this drug:

- complete blood count
- blood pressure
- heart function tests, such as electrocardiogram (ECG, EKG)
- leukocyte and neutrophil counts

Limited Use

Venlafaxine (ven la *fax* een)
EFFEXOR (Wyeth)

GENERIC: not available

FAMILY: Other Drugs for Depression
(See p. 184 for discussion of depression.)

PREGNANCY WARNING

This drug caused harm to developing fetuses in animal studies, including a decrease in birth weight, an increase in still births, and an increase in pup deaths after birth. There is new evidence that when women take this drug in the third trimester of pregnancy, serious complications can arise in their infants' health immediately after delivery. These complications require prolonged hospitalization, respiratory support, and tube feeding.

BREAST-FEEDING WARNING

Venlafaxine and its metabolite are excreted in human milk. Because of the potential for serious adverse reactions in the nursing infant, you should not take this drug while nursing.

Venlafaxine is used to treat major depression. Antidepressants improve symptoms of depression but do not cure depression. Venlafaxine

---

> ## WARNING:
> ## NEWER ANTIDEPRESSANTS AND THE RISK OF SUICIDE IN CHILDREN LESS THAN 18 YEARS OF AGE
>
> The FDA and the drug regulatory authorities in Canada and the UK have warned about the possibility of both suicidal ideation and suicide attempts seen in clinical trials of the newer antidepressant drugs, including the selective serotonin reuptake inhibitors (SSRIs), mirtazapine (REMERON), and venlafaxine (EFFEXOR) in children less than 18 years of age.
>
> Only fluoxetine is approved for use in children less than 18 years of age for major depressive disorder.

blocks the neurotransmitters serotonin and norepinephrine. Adverse effects can be minimized by starting with low doses of 25 milligrams a day.[91] It takes about two weeks for improvement, several weeks for the full effect. If improvement is inadequate, the dose can be increased at intervals of no less than four days up to 150 milligrams a day. The maximum total daily dose is 375 milligrams. People with kidney or liver problems or older adults should take a lower dose. Because of frequently occurring hypertension, blood pressure should be monitored.

Some adverse effects are more likely to occur with higher doses. With prolonged use, a decrease in saliva can cause cavities and other dental problems. A serious, sometimes fatal, effect is called serotonin syndrome. Symptoms include restlessness, shivering, lack of coordination, and profuse sweating. Venlafaxine is not recommended for women who are pregnant or breast-feeding, or children under age 18.

The FDA-approved professional product labeling for antidepressant drugs sold in the United States carries the following statement:

Suicide: The possibility of a suicide attempt is inherent in major depressive disorder and may persist until significant remission occurs. Close supervision of high-risk patients should accompany initial drug therapy. Prescriptions for Drug X should be written for the smallest quantity of tablets consistent with good patient management, in order to reduce the risk of overdose.

The length of time it takes an antidepressant to work can overlap with the time of spontaneous recovery, especially if the depression is situational—caused by a death or other external circumstances. The majority of people lift themselves out of depression with friends, spiritual resources, or activities such as exercise, work, reading, play, art, and travel. If depression is not overcome by these measures, seek help from mental health professionals, such as therapists or psychiatrists. Antidepressant drugs should be reserved for depression that is major and does not respond to psychotherapy alone.

All of the SSRI antidepressants have been shown to commonly cause sexual dysfunction in both men and women. In a large prospective study of over 6,000 men and women, sexual dysfunction occurred from 36 to 43% of the time, depending on the drug.[74] Types of sexual dysfunction include problems of desire (libido: sexual interest or drive), arousal (erectile function in men, lubrication in women), and release (ejaculation/orgasm in men and orgasm in women). Strategies to cope with this problem include decreasing the dosage to the lowest effective level; a drug holiday for patients in whom compliance is not a problem; if acceptable to the patient and partner, seeing if the sexual dysfunction resolves without further intervention.[75]

Before You Use This Drug

Tell your doctor if you have or have had:

- allergies
- blood pressure problems
- heart, kidney, or liver problems
- pregnancy or are breast-feeding
- seizures
- history of mania

Tell your doctor about any other drugs you take, including aspirin, herbs, vitamins, and other nonprescription products.

When You Use This Drug

- Do not drink alcohol or use other drugs that can cause drowsiness.
- Until you know how you react to this drug, do not drive or perform other activities that require alertness.
- You may feel dizzy when rising from a lying or sitting position. When getting out of bed, hang your legs over the side of the bed for a few minutes, then get up slowly. When getting up from a chair, stay beside the chair until you are sure that you are not dizzy. (See p. 13).
- Use sugarless gum, ice, or saliva substitute if you develop a dry mouth.
- Have your doctor assess your need to continue taking this drug periodically.
- If you plan to have any surgery, including dental, tell your doctor that you take this drug.

How to Use This Drug

- If you miss a dose and if it is a prompt-release tablet, take it as soon as you remember, unless it is within two hours of the next dose. **Do not take double doses.** For extended-release tablets, take as soon as possible if remembered the same day. Continue on regular schedule for next dose.
- Do not share your medications with anyone.

- Take your drug at the same time(s) each day.
  - Take at regular intervals with food.
  - Swallow extended-release tablets whole.
  - **Do not stop taking this drug suddenly,** since you could develop signs of withdrawal, such as dizziness, headache, and nausea. Check with your doctor about tapering your dose.
  - Store tablets at room temperature with lid on tightly. Do not store in the bathroom. Do not expose to heat, moisture, or strong light. Keep out of reach of children.
  - Tell your doctor immediately if you have skin rash or hives.

Interactions with Other Drugs

The following drugs, biologics (e.g., vaccines, therapeutic antibodies), or foods are listed in *Evaluations of Drug Interactions* 2003 as causing "highly clinically significant" or "clinically significant" interactions when used together with any of the drugs in this section. In some sections with multiple drugs, the interaction may have been reported for one but not all drugs in this section, but we include the interaction because the drugs in this section are similar to one another. We have also included potentially serious interactions listed in the drug's FDA-approved professional package insert or in published medical journal articles. There may be other drugs, especially those in the families of drugs listed below, that also will react with this drug to cause severe adverse effects. Make sure to tell your doctor and pharmacist the drugs you are taking and tell them if you are taking any of these interacting drugs:

Do not take venlafaxine within 14 days of stopping or starting these monoamine oxidase (MAO) inhibitors: deprenyl, ELDEPRYL, furazolidone, FUROXONE, isocarboxazid, MARPLAN, MATULANE, NARDIL, PARNATE, pheneizine, procarbazine, selegiline, tranylcypromine.

Central nervous system (CNS) depressant drugs, including alcohol, antidepressants, antihistamines, antipsychotics, some blood pressure medications (reserpine, methyldopa, beta-blockers), motion sickness medications, muscle relaxants, narcotics, sedatives, sleeping pills, and tranquilizers.

Other interacting drugs are: cimetidine, COMTAN, entacapone, HALDOL, haloperidol, metoclopramide, MERIDIA, NORVIR, REGLAN, ritonavir, sibutramine, TAGAMET.

Adverse Effects

Call your doctor immediately if you experience:

- agitation
- blood pressure increase
- breathing difficulty
- chest pain
- confusion
- seizures
- decreased sexual desire or ability
- depression
- diarrhea
- dizziness
- extreme drowsiness, tiredness, or weakness
- uncontrolled excitement and activity
- fainting or lightheadedness
- fever
- headache
- more rapid or pounding heartbeat
- incoordination
- itching or skin rash
- lockjaw
- menstrual changes
- mood or mental changes
- restlessness
- ringing or buzzing in ears
- swelling of legs or feet
- twitching
- difficulty urinating

- vision changes
- abnormal thinking

Call your doctor if these symptoms continue:

- abnormal dreams
- anxiety, nervousness
- constipation
- diarrhea
- dry mouth
- insomnia (trouble sleeping)
- loss of appetite
- nausea or vomiting
- runny or stuffed nose
- stomach pain
- taste changes
- tingling sensation
- tiredness, weakness, frequent yawning
- weight loss
- chills
- trembling or shaking
- dizziness
- heartburn
- sweating
- drowsiness

Call your doctor if these symptoms continue after you stop taking the drug:

- nausea
- nervousness
- tiredness or weakness
- abnormal dreams
- dizziness
- dry mouth
- increased sweating
- trouble sleeping
- headache

Periodic Tests

Ask your doctor which of these tests should be done periodically while you are taking this drug:

- blood pressure

Sleeping Pills and Tranquilizers

Benzodiazepines

 Do Not Use

ALTERNATIVE TREATMENT:
*See Nondrug Approaches, p. 172,
Buspirone, p. 232, and Oxazepam, p. 225.*

Chlordiazepoxide (klor dye az e *pox* ide)
LIBRIUM (Valeant)

Clorazepate (klor *az* e pate)
TRANXENE (Ovation)

Diazepam (dye *az* e pam)
VALIUM (Roche)

Estazolam (est *az* oh lam)
PROSOM (Abbott)

Flurazepam (flure *az* e pam)
DALMANE (Valeant)

Halazepam (hal *az* e pam)
PAXIPAM (Schering)

Lorazepam (lor *az* e pam)
ATIVAN (Biovail)

Prazepam (*praz* e pam)
CENTRAX (Parke-Davis)

Quazepam (*kwayz* e pam)
DORAL (Medpointe)

Temazepam (tem *az* e pam)
RESTORIL (Tyco)

Triazolam (trye *ay* zoe lam)
HALCION (Pharmacia and Upjohn)

Do Not Use
Except for Panic Disorder

Alprazolam (al *praz* oh lam)
XANAX (Pharmacia and Upjohn)

FAMILY: Benzodiazepines

PREGNANCY WARNING

An increased risk of congenital malformations associated with the use of minor tranquilizers (diazepam, meprobamate, and chlordiazepoxide) during the first trimester of pregnancy has been suggested in several studies. Because use of these drugs is rarely a matter of urgency, their use during this period should almost always be avoided. The possibility that a woman of childbearing potential may be pregnant when beginning therapy should be considered. Patients should be advised that if they become pregnant during therapy or intend to become pregnant, they should communicate with their physicians about the desirability of discontinuing the drug.

BREAST-FEEDING WARNING

Benzodiazepines are excreted in breast milk. Taking a benzodiazepine (diazepam) caused nursing infants to become lethargic and lose weight. As a general rule, mothers taking benzodiazepines, including Xanax, should not nurse.

These 12 sleeping pills and tranquilizers all belong to the benzodiazepine family. Although they are widely used for older adults, they present significantly higher risks to people over 60 and lack proven long-term benefits. These drugs can cause unsteady gait, dizziness, falling—with an increased risk of hip fractures—automobile accidents that cause injury, impairment of thinking and memory loss, and addiction. While some of these sleeping pills stay in the body so long you can still be sedated during the daytime, other drugs in this family stay in the body such a short time you can get rebound insomnia and become confused the following day. **Many older people who use these drugs should not be taking them. They have significant risks and are often prescribed unnecessarily.**

The available evidence strongly suggests that

---

the use of benzodiazepines by older people increases their risk of hip fracture by at least 50%. Because of the high morbidity and mortality of hip fracture, it can be concluded that older people should rarely be prescribed benzodiazepines and that many older people already taking these drugs should have them withdrawn under appropriate medical supervision.[92]

Based on our review of the benzodiazepine drugs, which are all effective but differ in their degree of safety, we recommend **(for limited use only)** oxazepam (see p. 225) as the safest drug in this family for older adults who truly need a tranquilizer or sleeping pill. The nonbenzodiazepine buspirone (BUSPAR) (see p. 232) is also suggested for limited use.

These 13 benzodiazepine drugs (oxazepam and the 12 listed above) are different from one another, and the difference has to do with the different ways in which they are dangerous for older adults.

The World Health Organization specifically

The best way to reduce the risks from sleeping pills and tranquilizers is to avoid them if at all possible. Before taking one of these powerful medications, see p. 172 for nondrug alternatives to try before using either sleeping pills or tranquilizers.

> One hazard of taking this drug continuously for longer than several weeks is drug-induced dependence. Do not stop taking your drug suddenly. With the help of your doctor, work out a schedule for slowly lowering the amount of the drug you take by about 5 to 10% each day. Keep a written record of the dosage reduction schedule with you. These steps will make it much easier to become drug free without developing distressing symptoms of drug withdrawal.

recommends that older adults should not use the most widely prescribed sleeping pill, flurazepam (DALMANE), "owing to a high incidence of adverse effects."[1] Seven other benzodiazepines are also cleared out of the body more slowly, especially in older adults, and can therefore accumulate, leading to increased risks. These drugs, which also should be avoided by older adults, include diazepam (VALIUM), chlordiazepoxide (LIBRIUM), clorazepate (TRAXENE), prazepam (CENTRAX), halazepam (PAXIPAM), quazepam (DORAL), and estazolam (PROSOM).

Another widely used sleeping pill, triazolam (HALCION), should also be avoided by older adults because it is so short-acting that it can cause rebound insomnia (increased sleeping problems when the drug effect has worn off), anxiety, serious amnesia (forgetfulness or memory loss), and violent, aggressive behavior. In 1992, Public Citizen's Health Research Group petitioned the FDA to ban Halcion. The sleeping pill estazolam (PROSOM) is in the same chemical subclass as Halcion and, according to *The Medical Letter*, there is no reason to use it.[26] It also has the disadvantage of slow clearance from the body.

In a discussion of which of these drugs are best for older adults, it was stated that oxazepam (SERAX) and temazepam (RESTORIL) were the drugs of choice.[27] But it has also been stated that "oxazepam (SERAX) may be the safest benzodiazepine for the older patient" because **"oxazepam may offer the advantages of a short half-life and the absence of active metabolites"** (that is, chemicals into which the body converts the drug that can also have adverse effects).[24] In addition, studies have shown that oxazepam has much less of a "street" drug abuse potential than, for example, diazepam (VALIUM).[28,29]

If you are taking a tranquilizer or sleeping pill other than buspirone or oxazepam, ask your doctor to reevaluate your need for this drug. If you do need such a drug, you should be taking one of these two.

Limited Use

Oxazepam (ox *az* e pam)
SERAX (Alpharma)

GENERIC: available
FAMILY: Benzodiazepines

PREGNANCY WARNING

Several of the benzodiazepines have been associated with an increased risk of congenital malformations when used during the first trimester of pregnancy. Oxazepam has not been studied adequately to know whether it, too, behaves this way, but since the use of these drugs is rarely a matter of urgency, their use should be avoided by pregnant women.

BREAST-FEEDING WARNING

Benzodiazepines are excreted in human milk and have caused adverse effects, including lethargy and weight loss, in nursing infants. Because of the potential for serious adverse effects in nursing infants, you should not take this drug while nursing.

Oxazepam is used to treat anxiety and is the only sleeping pill or tranquilizer in its family that we recommend for older adults. Because oxazepam, like all the drugs in its family, is addictive, you should not be taking it to relieve the stress of daily life (see informa-

---

RULES FOR SAFER USE OF OXAZEPAM

(This is the only benzodiazepine we believe should be prescribed for older adults.)

1. The dose should be one-third to one-half the dose for younger people. This means that the highest starting dose for older adults should be 7.5 milligrams, one to three times a day, if used as a tranquilizer, or 7.5 milligrams at bedtime, if used as a sleeping pill. (This is half of a 15 milligram tablet, generically available.)

2. Ask your doctor to limit the size of the prescription to seven days' worth of pills.

3. Ask your doctor to write NO REFILL on the prescription so that you will not be inclined (because of the "good chemical feelings" these pills may provide) to refill the prescription five times without seeing the doctor again. This dangerously lax refill policy is perfectly legal because oxazepam and other similar drugs are not very carefully controlled by the government. By urging your doctor to write NO REFILL, you are making sure that he or she will reevaluate your condition after you use oxazepam for a short time. You want to discuss how you are doing with your anxiety or sleeping problem, rather than continuing to take the drug without a reevaluation. Continuing to take oxazepam without talking to your doctor could be the first step to addiction or other drug-induced problems.

4. At the end of the first day, and every day you use oxazepam, evaluate what you have done, on your own or by talking to others, to find out what is making you anxious. This includes evaluation of what you have done to alter the internal or external circumstances causing your anxiety. Keep a record of these evaluations. As soon as possible, try reducing the dose, in consultation with your doctor. Since you only have enough medication for one week, it is unlikely you will have become addicted this quickly.

5. Do not drive a car or operate dangerous machinery while using oxazepam.

6. Do not drink alcohol. The combination of this drug with alcohol dangerously increases the effects of both. An overdose of oxazepam in combination with alcohol can be fatal.

Before using oxazepam, make sure that your doctor knows if you are taking other drugs with a sedative or "downer" effect, such as antidepressants, antipsychotics, antihistamines, narcotic painkillers, epilepsy medications, barbiturates, or other sleeping medications. Oxazepam taken with other drugs with sedative effects dangerously increases the risks of both.

---

tion in the box above). There are safer ways to deal with occasional and short-term tension, nervousness, and sleeplessness (see p. 172). Only in a very limited number of circumstances is a sleeping pill or tranquilizer really necessary.

Oxazepam, like Valium, Dalmane, and Librium (see p. 223) belongs to a family of drugs called benzodiazepines. It is safer than these other drugs, and may be the safest benzodiazepine for older adults, because it is short-acting rather than long-acting, meaning that it is eliminated more quickly from your body. This reduces the risk that it will accumulate in your bloodstream and reach dangerously high levels, causing harmful adverse effects. Another reason that oxazepam is safer than other drugs in its family is that your body does not convert it into chemicals called active metabolites that can produce adverse effects.[24]

Studies show that there is much less potential for abusing oxazepam than for abusing diazepam (VALIUM).[28,29] Oxazepam also may have a lower risk of addiction than benzodiazepines that act over a shorter period of time, such as lorazepam (ATIVAN), alprazolam (XANAX), and triazolam (HALCION).[93]

One hazard of taking this drug continuously for longer than several weeks is drug-induced dependence. **Do not stop taking this drug suddenly**. With the help of your doctor, work out a schedule for slowly lowering the amount of the drug you take by about 5 to 10% each day. Keep a written record of the dosage reduction schedule with you. These steps will make it much easier to become drug free without developing distressing symptoms of drug withdrawal.

Oxazepam can cause adverse effects common to all benzodiazepines, and older adults are more likely to experience certain ones: confusion, drowsiness, and incoordination that can result in falls and hip fractures. The available evidence strongly suggests that the use of benzodiazepines by older people increases their risk of hip fracture by at least 50%. Because of the high morbidity and mortality of hip fracture, it can be concluded that older people should rarely be prescribed benzodiazepines and that many older people already taking these drugs should have them withdrawn under appropriate medical supervision.[92]

Before You Use This Drug

Tell your doctor if you have or have had:

- allergies to drugs
- kidney or liver problems
- brief periods of not breathing during sleep (sleep apnea)
- lung disease or breathing problems
- alcohol or drug dependence
- mental depression or illness
- myasthenia gravis
- glaucoma
- epilepsy, seizures
- porphyria
- brain disease
- difficulty swallowing

- hyperactivity
- pregnancy or are breast-feeding

Tell your doctor about any other drugs you take, including aspirin, herbs, vitamins, and other nonprescription products.

When You Use This Drug

- Do not take more than prescribed. Oxazepam is addictive.
- Do not drink alcohol or use other drugs that can cause drowsiness.
- Until you know how you react to this drug, do not drive or perform other activities requiring alertness. Oxazepam may cause drowsiness. **People who take drugs in this family may be more likely to have traffic accidents.**
- If you plan to have any surgery, including dental, tell your doctor that you take this drug.

How to Use This Drug

- If you miss a dose, take it as soon as you remember, but skip it if it is almost time for the next dose. **Do not take double doses.**
- Do not share your medication with others.
- Take the drug at the same time(s) each day.
- Take with food or milk.
- Crush tablet and mix with food (applesauce, jelly, or ketchup) or water, or swallow whole.
- Store at room temperature with lid on tightly. Do not store in the bathroom. Do not expose to heat, moisture, or strong light. Keep out of reach of children.

The best way to reduce the risks from sleeping pills and tranquilizers is to avoid them if at all possible. Before taking one of these powerful medications, see p. 172 for nondrug alternatives to try before using either sleeping pills or tranquilizers.

Interactions with Other Drugs

The following drugs, biologics (e.g., vaccines, therapeutic antibodies), or foods are listed in *Evaluations of Drug Interactions* 2003 as causing "highly clinically significant" or "clinically significant" interactions when used together with any of the drugs in this section. In some sections with multiple drugs, the interaction may have been reported for one but not all drugs in this section, but we include the interaction because the drugs in this section are similar to one another. We have also included potentially serious interactions listed in the drug's FDA-approved professional package insert or in published medical journal articles. There may be other drugs, especially those in the families of drugs listed below, that also will react with this drug to cause severe adverse effects. Make sure to tell your doctor and pharmacist the drugs you are taking and tell them if you are taking any of these interacting drugs:

Alcohol and other central nervous system (CNS) depressant drugs may have an additive effect with oxazepam.

Adverse Effects

Call your doctor immediately if you experience:

- confusion, hallucinations
- trouble sleeping
- unusual excitement, irritability
- mental depression
- skin rash, itching
- sore throat and fever
- yellow eyes or skin
- ulcers or sores in mouth or throat that do not go away
- unusual bleeding or bruising
- clumsiness, unsteadiness, or falling
- seizures
- low blood pressure
- unusual tiredness or weakness
- impaired memory
- muscle weakness
- uncontrolled movements

Call your doctor if these symptoms continue:

- blurred or changed vision
- clumsiness
- dizziness, lightheadedness
- constipation
- diarrhea
- drowsiness
- difficulty urinating
- headache
- dry mouth or increased thirst
- unusual mouth watering
- nausea or vomiting
- slurred speech
- joint or chest pain
- fast heartbeat
- nasal congestion
- abdominal or stomach cramps
- muscle spasms
- change in sex drive or performance

Call your doctor if these symptoms continue after you stop taking this drug:

- irritability, nervousness
- trouble sleeping
- abdominal or stomach cramps
- confusion
- irregular heartbeat
- increased sense of hearing
- increased sensitivity to touch and pain
- sweating
- loss of reality, feelings of distrust or depression
- muscle cramps
- nausea or vomiting
- sensitivity to light
- tingling, burning, or prickly sensation
- trembling
- confusion
- seizures
- hallucinations

Signs of overdose:

- prolonged confusion
- slow reflexes
- severe drowsiness
- slurred speech
- shakiness
- staggering
- slow heartbeat
- shortness of breath
- trouble breathing
- extreme weakness
- seizures

If you suspect an overdose, call this number to contact your poison control center: (800) 222-1222.

Periodic Tests

Ask your doctor which of these tests should be done periodically while you are taking this drug:

- checkups during long-term use to see if the amount and frequency of drug use is right for you
- tests to evaluate how well drug is working

Other Sleeping Pills and Tranquilizers

 Do Not Use

ALTERNATIVE TREATMENT:
See Nondrug Approaches, p. 172, and Zolpidem, p. 230, and Oxazepam, p. 225.

Zaleplon *(zal* e plon)
SONATA (Jones)

FAMILY: Other Sleeping Pills and Tranquilizers

Zaleplon works the same way as the benzodiazepine sleeping pills such as triazolam

> One hazard of taking this drug continuously for longer than several weeks is drug-induced dependence. **Do not stop taking this drug suddenly.** With the help of your doctor, work out a schedule for slowly lowering the amount of the drug you take by about 5 to 10% each day. Keep a written record of the dosage reduction schedule with you. These steps will make it much easier to become drug free without developing distressing symptoms of drug withdrawal.

(HALCION), temazepam (RESTORIL), and flurazepam (DALMANE).[94] Like the benzodiazepines, this drug is regulated as a controlled substance because of its potential to cause dependence.

The editors of *The Medical Letter on Drugs and Therapeutics,* a highly regarded independent source of drug information written for physicians and pharmacists, found that zaleplon is "less potent and has a shorter duration of action than zolpidem (AMBIEN)."[95]

An FDA medical officer's review of zaleplon found the effects of this drug to be "mild to modest at best, yet they are comparable to active comparitors [other sleeping pills]." In the five clinical trials submitted by Wyeth-Ayerst in support of zaleplon's approval, compared to those using an inactive placebo, the median decrease in time to sleep onset ranged from only 8 to 20 minutes in patients taking zaleplon. Zaleplon was not consistently more effective than a placebo in the total time slept or the number of awakenings experienced by patients during the night.[96]

The following drugs, biologics (e.g., vaccines, therapeutic antibodies), or foods are listed in *Evaluations of Drug Interactions* 2003 as causing "highly clinically significant" or "clinically significant" interactions when used together with any of the drugs in this section. In some sections with multiple drugs, the interaction may have been reported for one but not all

> The best way to reduce the risks from sleeping pills and tranquilizers is to avoid them if at all possible. Before taking one of these powerful medications, see p. 172 for nondrug alternatives to try before using either sleeping pills or tranquilizers.

drugs in this section, but we include the interaction because the drugs in this section are similar to one another. We have also included potentially serious interactions listed in the drug's FDA-approved professional package insert or in published medical journal articles. There may be other drugs, especially those in the families of drugs listed below, that also will react with this drug to cause severe adverse effects. Make sure to tell your doctor and pharmacist the drugs you are taking and tell them if you are taking any of these interacting drugs:

alcohol, BENADRYL, carbamazepine, cimetidine, DILANTIN, diphenhydramine, imipramine, LUMINAL, MELLARIL, phenobarbital, phenytoin, RIMACTANE, RIFADIN, rifampin, SOLFOTON, SOMINEX FORMULA, TAGAMET, TEGRETOL, thioridazine, TOFRANIL.

A recently published study compared the effectiveness of drug treatment to behavioral therapy in the management of persistent insomnia. The study is a meta-analysis, or statistical summary of clinical trials involving both types of treatments. The authors of the study concluded: "Overall, behavior therapy and pharmacotherapy produce similar short-term treatment outcomes in primary insomnia."[97] Nondrug treatment is a viable option for the management of insomnia.

Limited Use

Zolpidem (*zole* pi dem)
AMBIEN (Sanofi-Synthelabo)

GENERIC: not available
FAMILY: Other Sleeping Pills and Tranquilizers

PREGNANCY WARNING

This drug caused harm to developing fetuses in animal studies, including incomplete formation of the bones in the back and skull as well as fetal death. Children born of mothers who took sedative/hypnotic drugs are at some risk for withdrawal symptoms as well as lacking muscle strength. Use during pregnancy only if clearly needed. Tell your doctor if you are pregnant or thinking of becoming pregnant before you take this drug.

BREAST-FEEDING WARNING

Zolpidem inhibits milk secretion and is secreted into milk. It should not be used by nursing mothers.

Zolpidem is used for short-term relief of insomnia. Although not classified as a benzodiazepine (related to Valium), zolpidem shares many similarities with that family of drugs.[98] Like the benzodiazepine family of drugs, zolpidem can cause drowsiness. Since it can be habit-forming, zolpidem is a controlled substance.

Interactions with Other Drugs

The following drugs, biologics (e.g., vaccines, therapeutic antibodies), or foods are listed in *Evaluations of Drug Interactions* 2003 as causing "highly clinically significant" or "clinically significant" interactions when used together with any of the drugs in this section. In some sections with multiple drugs, the interaction may have been reported for one but not all

> The best way to reduce the risks from sleeping pills and tranquilizers is to avoid them if at all possible. Before taking one of these powerful medications, see p. 172 for nondrug alternatives to try before using either sleeping pills or tranquilizers.

One hazard of taking this drug continuously for longer than several weeks is drug-induced dependence. **Do not stop taking this drug suddenly.** With the help of your doctor, work out a schedule for slowly lowering the amount of the drug you take by about 5 to 10% each day. Keep a written record of the dosage reduction schedule with you. These steps will make it much easier to become drug free without developing distressing symptoms of drug withdrawal.

drugs in this section, but we include the interaction because the drugs in this section are similar to one another. We have also included potentially serious interactions listed in the drug's FDA-approved professional package insert or in published medical journal articles. There may be other drugs, especially those in the families of drugs listed below, that also will react with this drug to cause severe adverse effects. Make sure to tell your doctor and pharmacist the drugs you are taking and tell them if you are taking any of these interacting drugs:

Central nervous system (CNS) depressant drugs, including alcohol, antidepressants, antihistamines, antipsychotics, some blood pressure medications (reserpine, methyldopa, beta-blockers), motion sickness medications, muscle relaxants, narcotics, sedatives, sleeping pills, and tranquilizers.

Another interacting drug is: rifampin (RIFADIN).

Adverse Effects

Call your doctor immediately if you experience:

- wheezing or difficulty breathing
- irregular or fast heartbeat
- clumsiness or unsteadiness
- swelling of face
- rash

- confusion
- dizziness, lightheadedness, or fainting
- falling
- depression
- unusual excitement, nervousness, or irritability
- hallucinations
- insomnia

Call your doctor if these symptoms continue:

- abnormal dreams, nightmares
- memory problems
- dizziness
- lightheadedness
- abdominal pain
- dry mouth
- back pain or muscle aches
- nausea or vomiting
- diarrhea
- drowsiness during the day
- drugged feelings
- general feeling of discomfort
- headache
- sleepwalking[99]
- problems with vision, including double vision

Call your doctor if these symptoms continue after you stop taking the drug:

- abdominal or stomach cramps
- agitation, nervousness, or feelings of panic
- flushing
- lightheadedness
- muscle cramps
- nausea or vomiting
- worsening of mental or emotional problems
- seizures
- sweating, tremors
- unusual tiredness or weakness
- uncontrolled crying

Signs of overdose:

- severe unsteadiness
- slow heartbeat

- double vision
- severe dizziness
- severe drowsiness
- severe nausea
- trouble breathing
- unconsciousness
- severe vomiting

If you suspect an overdose, call this number to contact your poison control center: (800) 222-1222.

Limited Use

Buspirone (bu *spire* own)
BUSPAR (Bristol-Myers Squibb)

GENERIC: not available
FAMILY: Other Sleeping Pills and Tranquilizers

PREGNANCY WARNING

No valid data are available for buspirone, as it was not tested properly in animal studies. Use during pregnancy only for clear medical reasons. Tell your doctor if you are pregnant or thinking of becoming pregnant before you take this drug.

BREAST-FEEDING WARNING

Buspirone and its metabolites are excreted in milk. Buspirone should not be given to nursing women.

Buspirone is an antianxiety agent, which differs chemically from the benzodiazepine drugs (see p. 223), and appears to lack the potential for addiction common to this family of drugs, such as Xanax and Valium. While buspirone is less apt than the benzodiazepines to cause drowsiness, drowsiness remains a common side

> The best way to reduce the risks from sleeping pills and tranquilizers is to avoid them if at all possible. Before taking one of these powerful medications, see p. 172 for nondrug alternatives to try before using either sleeping pills or tranquilizers.

effect. Although buspirone is preferred for older adults, compared to other drugs available,[100] information about buspirone is limited, and much is still unknown, including its long-term safety and effectiveness.[21,101] Adverse effects are often paradoxical (drowsiness or insomnia, anorexia or weight gain). While buspirone is used for short-term anxiety, it takes a few weeks to work. In some people buspirone may increase anxiety, rather than alleviate it.[102] A decision to use buspirone should be reviewed periodically.

Anxiety is a universal emotion closely allied with appropriate fears.[103] No drug is useful for the stress of everyday living. Try nondrug therapies for anxiety first. Explore preventable causes of anxiety, such as overuse of caffeine, as well as medical/physical causes. Drugs may control but do not cure anxiety.

If you already take a benzodiazepine (see p. 223) or antidepressant (see p. 190), your doctor should taper you off those drugs before trying buspirone. However, if you have already taken a benzodiazepine, the buspirone is less likely to be effective.[104]

Before You Use This Drug

Tell your doctor if you have or have had:

- allergies to drugs
- alcohol or drug dependence
- kidney or liver problems
- pregnancy or are breast-feeding

Tell your doctor about any other drugs you take, including aspirin, herbs, vitamins, and other nonprescription products.

When You Use This Drug

- Do not drink alcohol or use other drugs that can cause drowsiness.
- Until you know how you react to this drug, do not drive or perform other activities that require alertness. Buspirone may cause blurred vision and drowsiness.

• If you plan to have any surgery, including dental, tell your doctor that you take this drug.

• Do not take other drugs without checking with your doctor first—especially nonprescription drugs for appetite control, colds, coughs, hay fever, sinus problems, or sleep.

How to Use This Drug

• If you miss a dose, take it as soon as you remember, but skip it if it is almost time for the next dose. **Do not take double doses.**

• Do not share your medication with others.

• Take the drug at the same time(s) each day.

• Take the drug the same way each time, either with or without food.

• Tablet may be broken in two but not chewed or crushed.

• Do not store in the bathroom. Do not expose to heat, moisture, or strong light.

Interactions with Other Drugs

The following drugs, biologics (e.g., vaccines, therapeutic antibodies), or foods are listed in *Evaluations of Drug Interactions* 2003 as causing "highly clinically significant" or "clinically significant" interactions when used together with any of the drugs in this section. In some sections with multiple drugs, the interaction may have been reported for one but not all drugs in this section, but we include the interaction because the drugs in this section are similar to one another. We have also included potentially serious interactions listed in the drug's FDA-approved professional package insert or in published medical journal articles. There may be other drugs, especially those in the families of drugs listed below, that also will react with this drug to cause severe adverse effects. Make sure to tell your doctor and pharmacist the drugs you are taking and tell them if you are taking any of these interacting drugs:

Taking buspirone with any MAO (monoamine oxidase) inhibitors may increase your blood pressure. Do not take buspirone for at least 10 days after stopping any of these MAO inhibitors: deprenyl, ELDEPRYL, furazolidone, FUROXONE, isocarboxazid, MARPLAN, MATULANE, NARDIL, PARNATE, phenelzine, procarbazine, selegiline, tranylcypromine.

Other interacting drugs are: CALAN SR, carbamazepine, CARDIZEM CD, COVERA-HS, DECADRON, dexamethasone, DILACOR XR, DILANTIN, diltiazem, EES, ERYTHROCIN, erythromycin, itraconazole, ketoconazole, nefazodone, NIZORAL, NORVIR, phenobarbital, phenytoin, RIFADIN, rifampin, RIMACTANE, ritonavir, SERZONE, SPORANOX, TEGRETOL, verapamil.

Adverse Effects

Call your doctor immediately if you experience:

• chest pain
• confusion or depression
• fast or pounding heartbeat
• sore throat or fever
• skin rash or hives
• muscle weakness
• numbness, tingling, pain, or weakness in hands or feet
• uncontrolled movements of the body
• stiffness of arms or legs

Call your doctor if these symptoms continue:

• anger, hostility
• blurred vision
• dizziness, lightheadedness
• constipation
• diarrhea
• sleep or dream disturbance [105]
• drowsiness

- headache
- dry mouth
- involuntary movements
- muscle pain, spasms, cramps, stiffness
- nasal congestion
- numbness
- restlessness, nervousness, insomnia, nightmares
- ringing isn ears
- sweating
- unusual weakness, tiredness
- nausea

Signs of overdose:

- dizziness
- severe drowsiness
- unusually small pupils
- loss of consciousness
- stomach upset including nausea or vomiting

If you suspect an overdose, call this number to contact your poison control center: (800) 222-1222.

Periodic Tests

Ask your doctor which of these tests should be done periodically while you are taking this drug:

- kidney function tests
- liver function tests

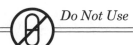

Do Not Use

ALTERNATIVE TREATMENT:
See Nondrug Approaches, p. 172, Oxazepam, p. 225 and Buspirone, p. 232. See also Sleeping Pills and Tranquilizers, p. 166.

Meprobamate (me *proe* ba mate)
EQUANIL (Wyeth-Ayerst)
MILTOWN (Medpointe)

FAMILY: Other Sleeping Pills and Tranquilizers

PREGNANCY WARNING

An increased risk of congenital malformations associated with the use of minor tranquilizers (diazepam, meprobamate, and chlordiazepoxide) during the first trimester of pregnancy has been suggested in several studies. Because use of these drugs is rarely a matter of urgency, their use during this period should almost always be avoided. The possibility that a woman of childbearing potential may be pregnant at the time of institution of therapy should be considered. Patients should be advised that if they become pregnant during therapy or intend to become pregnant, they should communicate with their physicians about the desirability of discontinuing the drug.

Meprobamate is a tranquilizer. It is commonly misused to relieve occasional, short-term anxiety. If you are suffering anxiety and tension from the stress of everyday life, you usually do not need an antianxiety drug. There are safer ways to relieve such anxiety. If you do need a drug for anxiety, oxazepam (see p. 225) or buspirone (see p. 232) is a better choice than meprobamate.

Meprobamate has been included on a list of drugs that are inappropriate for use in older adults.[82,105]

Long-term treatment (longer than four months) of anxiety with meprobamate is rarely effective. It also puts you at risk of developing harmful adverse effects such as drowsiness, dizziness, unsteady gait—with an increased risk of falls and hip fractures—impairment of thinking, memory loss, and addiction.

One hazard of taking this drug continuously for longer than several weeks is drug-induced dependence. **Do not stop taking this drug suddenly.** With the help of your doctor, work out a schedule for slowly lowering the amount of the drug you take by about 5 to 10% each day. Keep a written record of the dosage reduction schedule with you. These steps will make it much easier to become drug free without developing distressing symptoms of drug withdrawal.

Schizophrenia

Atypical Antipsychotics

Do Not Use Until Seven Years After Release

Aripiprazole (ar ee *pip* ra zole)
(Do Not Use Until 2010)
ABILIFY (Bristol-Myers Squibb/
Otsuka America)

GENERIC: not available

FAMILY: Atypical antipsychotics

PREGNANCY WARNING

This drug caused harm to developing fetuses in animal studies, including undescended testicles, delayed bone formation, decreased weight and survival, and increased stillbirths. Do not use during pregnancy. Tell your doctor if you are pregnant or thinking of becoming pregnant before you take this drug.

BREAST-FEEDING WARNING

Aripiprazole is excreted in the milk of rats. It is likely that this drug, like many others, is also excreted in human milk, and because of the potential for serious adverse effects in nursing infants, you should not take this drug while nursing.

Aripiprazole was approved by the FDA for the treatment of schizophrenia in November 2002.

Aripiprazole is a member of a relatively new family of drugs known as atypical antipsychotics. These drugs are also being referred to as second-generation antipsychotics. All antipsychotic drugs usually improve symptoms such as agitation, delusions, hallucinations, and suspiciousness. Atypical antipsychotics additionally tend, more than the older antipsychotics, to improve negative symptoms such as apathy, disorientation, emotional withdrawal, and lack of pleasure. However, there is no clear evidence that atypical antipsychotics are more effective or are better tolerated than the older conventional antipsychotics such as haloperidol (see p. 258).[106]

WARNING: BLOOD SUGAR ELEVATION AND DIABETES MELLITUS

Elevations in blood sugar (glucose),[56-58] in some cases extreme and associated with ketoacidosis or hyperosmolar coma or death, has been reported in patients treated with atypical antipsychotics that include aripiprazole (ABILIFY), clozapine (CLOZARIL), olanzapine (ZYPREXA), quetiapine (SEROQUEL), risperidone (RISPERDAL), and ziprasidone (GEODON).

The relationship between atypical antipsychotic use and glucose abnormalities is complicated by the possibility of an increased background risk of diabetes mellitus in patients with schizophrenia and the increasing incidence of diabetes mellitus in the general population. Given these confounders, the relationship between atypical antipsychotic use and hyperglycemia-related adverse events is not completely understood. Precise risk estimates for hyperglycemia-related adverse events in patients treated with atypical antipsychotics are not available.

Patients with an established diagnosis of diabetes mellitus who are started on atypical antipsychotics should be monitored regularly for worsening of glucose control. Patients with risk factors for diabetes mellitus (e.g., obesity, family history of diabetes) who are starting treatment with atypical antipsychotics should undergo fasting blood glucose testing at the beginning of treatment and periodically during treatment. Any patient treated with atypical antipsychotics should be monitored for symptoms of hyperglycemia, including polydipsia (excessive thirst/drinking of liquids), polyuria (excessive urination), polyphagia (excessive eating), and weakness. Patients who develop symptoms of hyperglycemia during treatment with atypical antipsychotics should undergo fasting blood glucose testing. In some cases, hyperglycemia resolved when the atypical antipsychotic was discontinued; however, some patients required continuation of antidiabetic treatment despite discontinuation of the suspect drug.

WARNING: CEREBROVASCULAR ADVERSE EVENTS, INCLUDING STROKE, IN ELDERLY PATIENTS WITH DEMENTIA

Cerebrovascular adverse events (e.g., stroke, transient ischemic attack), including fatalities, were reported in patients in clinical trials of the atypical antipsychotics in elderly patients with dementia-related psychosis.[59] In placebo-controlled trials, there was a significantly higher incidence of cerebrovascular adverse events in patients treated with these drugs compared to patients treated with placebo. The atypical antipsychotics are not approved for the treatment of patients with dementia-related psychosis.

Three of the five short-term trials submitted to the FDA for aripiprazole's approval showed the efficacy of the drug in doses ranging from 10 milligrams to 30 milligrams per day. There appeared to be no therapeutic advantage of the 30 milligram dose over the lower doses. The FDA-approved dose for the drug ranges from 10 milligrams to 15 milligrams per day. Of the two remaining studies, aripiprazole could not be differentiated from placebo in one, and the other trial failed.[107] One of our reviewers suggests starting with the new 5 milligram dose to minimize the risk of adverse effects.

These trials were not conducted in a way to make direct comparisons between aripiprazole and haloperidol or risperidone, which were used as comparator drugs. And nothing in these five trials can lead one to believe that aripiprazole is a meaningful advancement in the treatment of schizophrenia.

The editors of the highly respected *Medical Letter on Drugs and Therapeutics* concluded in their evaluation of aripiprazole that "published comparisons with other atypical antipsychotics are needed to determine its relative efficacy and safety."[108]

We are concerned about the possibility of eye toxicity with the use of aripiprazole. The studies done in rats before the drug was approved clearly showed degeneration of the retina in animals receiving aripiprazole. The studies done in mice and monkeys found no retinal degeneration, but they were invalid studies. The company committed to doing additional postmarketing research on retinal degeneration in animals as a condition for the approval of aripiprazole. These are studies that clearly should have been completed before the drug was approved.[107]

There are additional findings from the FDA's safety review of aripiprazole that are important. An alteration in the electrical conduction of the heart known as QT prolongation is an important safety issue with both old and new antipsychotic drugs. QT prolongation can lead to life-threatening heart rhythm disturbance.

There was no evidence of QT prolongation with aripiprazole at doses up to 30 milligrams per day. However, in a special study that explored doses of the drug up to 90 milligrams per

---

THE HEALTH RESEARCH GROUP'S SEVEN-YEAR RULE

You should wait at least seven years from the date of release to take any new drug unless it is one of those rare "breakthrough" drugs that offers you a documented therapeutic advantage over older proven drugs. New drugs are tested in a relatively small number of people before being released, and serious adverse effects or life-threatening drug interactions may not be detected until the new drug has been taken by hundreds of thousands of people. A number of new drugs have been withdrawn within their first seven years after release. Also, warnings about serious new adverse reactions have been added to the labeling of a number of drugs, or new drug interactions have been detected, usually within the first seven years after a drug's release.

ANTICHOLINERGIC EFFECTS

WARNING: SPECIAL MENTAL AND PHYSICAL ADVERSE EFFECTS

Older adults are especially sensitive to the harmful anticholinergic (see Glossary, p. 889) effects of this drug. Drugs in this family should not be used unless absolutely necessary.

Mental Effects: confusion, delirium, short-term memory problems, disorientation, and impaired attention.

Physical Effects: dry mouth, constipation, difficulty urinating (especially for a man with an enlarged prostate), blurred vision, decreased sweating with increased body temperature, sexual dysfunction, and worsening of glaucoma.

day, there was substantial prolongation of the QT interval at doses of 75 milligrams and 90 milligrams per day.[107]

Weight gain has also been a problem with the antipsychotic drugs, particularly with the atypical antipsychotics. In the short-term trials, there was a small difference in average weight gain between aripiprazole and placebo patients. The patients given aripiprazole gained on average 1.5 pounds, while the placebo patients lost 0.1 pounds on average. The number of patients gaining more than 7% of their body weight who were taking aripiprazole was equal to 8%, compared to 3% of the placebo patients.[107]

Before You Use This Drug

Tell your doctor if you have or have had:

- allergies to drugs
- Alzheimer's disease
- abuse of drugs or alcohol
- heart problems, such as cerebrovascular disease, conduction abnormalities, ischemic heart disease, heart failure, and heart attack

- blood vessel disease
- high blood pressure
- pneumonia (aspiration)
- pregnancy or are breast-feeding
- seizures
- history of neuroleptic malignant syndrome (NMS)

Tell your doctor about any other drugs you take, including aspirin, blood pressure pills, other drugs for schizophrenia, herbs, vitamins, and other nonprescription products.

When You Use This Drug

- Avoid alcohol.
- Avoid dehydration and overheating, especially during extremely hot weather.
- Do not drive or operate hazardous equipment until you know whether this drug impairs your judgment, thinking, or motor skills.
- Exercise, but avoid overexertion that leads to dehydration.
- Change positions from lying down to sitting, and sitting to standing, gradually.
- Try relaxation to reduce anxiety.
- Check with your doctor or pharmacist before using over-the-counter medications.
- Tell any doctor, dentist, emergency help, or pharmacist you see that you take aripiprazole.
- Tell your doctor if you become pregnant or plan to become pregnant.
- If you take this drug for a long time, have regular visits with your doctor.

How to Use This Drug

- If you miss a dose, take it as soon as possible, unless it is almost time for the next dose. **Do not take double doses.**
- Do not share your medication with others.
- Take at the same time(s) each day
- Swallow tablets with or without food. However, it is advisable to be consistent about whether or not you take with food.

• Store tablets at room temperature with lid on tightly. Do not store in the bathroom. Do not expose to heat, moisture, or strong light. Keep out of reach of children.

Interactions With Other Drugs

The following drugs, biologics (e.g., vaccines, therapeutic antibodies), or foods are listed in *Evaluations of Drug Interactions* 2003 as causing "highly clinically significant" or "clinically significant" interactions when used together with any of the drugs in this section. In some sections with multiple drugs, the interaction may have been reported for one but not all drugs in this section, but we include the interaction because the drugs in this section are similar to one another. We have also included potentially serious interactions listed in the drug's FDA-approved professional package insert or in published medical journal articles. There may be other drugs, especially those in the families of drugs listed below, that also will react with this drug to cause severe adverse effects. Make sure to tell your doctor and pharmacist the drugs you are taking and tell them if you are taking any of these interacting drugs:

Interactions with aripiprazole depend on the enzyme system that breaks down both drugs.

The dose of aripiprazole should be half the normal dose when also taking: amiodarone, CARDIOQUIN, CORDARONE, DIFLUCAN, fluconazole, fluoxetine, itraconazole, ketoconazole, NIZORAL, paroxetine, PAXIL, propafenone, PROZAC, QUINAGLUTE, QUINIDEX, quinidine, QUIN-RELEASE, RYTHMOL, SPORANOX.

The dose of aripiprazole should be doubled up to 30 milligrams if taken with these drugs: carbamazepine, TEGRETOL.

The dose of aripiprazole should be lowered to 10 or 15 milligrams if this drug is stopped: carbamazpeine, TEGRETOL.

When aripiprazole is taken with drugs that have anticholinergic effects, risk of dehydration and disruption of temperature control increases. A partial list includes: amitriptyline, ARTANE, atropine, belladonna, benztropine, COGENTIN, cyclobenzaprine, desipramine, ELAVIL, FLEXERIL, hyoscyamine, meclizine, NORPRAMIN, ORAP, oxybutin, pimozide, scopolamine, TRANS-DERM SCOP, tricyclic antidepressants, trihexyphenidyl.

Adverse Effects

Call your doctor immediately if you experience:

• anxiety or nervousness
• blood pressure increases or decreases
• difficult breathing
• increased sweating
• loss of bladder control
• chest pain
• confusion
• convulsions
• sudden loss of consciousness
• tiredness
• unusually pale skin
• lip smacking
• puffing of cheeks
• uncontrolled chewing movements
• uncontrolled movements of arms and legs
• dizziness, fainting, lightheadedness
• facial grimace
• feelings of depression, euphoria, or suicide
• fever
• flulike symptoms
• faster or slower heartbeats
• hostility
• involuntary movements of all extremities, twisting, snakelike movements
• twitching muscles
• severe muscle stiffness
• pneumonia

- restlessness that is extreme, urgent need of movement
- blue-black, greenish-brown, or yellow patches on skin
- difficulty swallowing
- swelling of ankles or feet
- thirst
- tremor
- blurred vision
- difficulty walking

Call your doctor if you continue to experience:

- appetite decrease
- constipation
- fear
- inability to sit still
- lack of or loss of strength
- lightheadedness
- nervousness
- rash
- trouble sleeping
- blurred vision
- coughing
- fever
- runny nose
- prolonged drowsiness
- inflamed or irritated eyes
- headache
- muscle cramps
- nausea or vomiting
- dry or itchy skin
- profuse sweating
- undesired weight gain

Other adverse effects are possible. Check with your doctor about any concerns.

Signs of overdose:

- sleepiness or unusual drowsiness
- vomiting

If you suspect an overdose, call this number to contact your poison control center: (800) 222-1222.

Periodic Tests

Ask your doctor which of these tests should be done periodically while you are taking this drug:

- AIMS or other rating scale for involuntary movements
- creatinine phosphokinase (CPK)
- kidney function tests
- other evaluations

Last-Choice

Clozapine (*kloe* za peen)
CLOZARIL (Novartis)

GENERIC: not available
FAMILY: Atypical Antipsychotics

PREGNANCY WARNING

Clozapine was not tested adequately to know what the potential effects might be on the fetus. Because of the desirability of keeping all drugs to a minimum during pregnancy, this drug should be used only if clearly needed.

BREAST-FEEDING WARNING

Clozapine appears to be excreted in breast milk and to have an effect on the nursing infant. Women receiving clozapine should not breast-feed their infants.

Clozapine is a drug used to treat schizophrenia. Clozapine is the first atypical antipsychotic, in the same family with olanzapine and the other newer antipsychotics. While all antipsychotics usually improve symptoms such as agitation, delusions, hallucinations, and suspiciousness, atypical antipsychotics tend to improve "negative" symptoms such as apathy, disorientation, emotional withdrawal, and lack of pleasure, more than older antipsychotics. Although the risk of movement disorders is not eliminated with atypical antipsychotics, these drugs have a lower risk of these types of disorders, especially at higher doses. However, there is no clear evi-

FDA BLACK BOX WARNING

1. Agranulocytosis [a serious blood disorder]

Because of a significant risk of agranulocytosis, a potentially life-threatening adverse event, clozapine should be reserved for use in the treatment of severely ill schizophrenic patients who fail to show an acceptable response to adequate courses of standard antipsychotic drug treatment.

Patients being treated with clozapine must have a baseline white blood cell (WBC) and differential count before initiation of treatment as well as regular WBC counts during treatment and for 4 weeks after discontinuation of treatment.

Clozapine is available only through a distribution system that ensures monitoring of WBC counts according to the schedule described below prior to delivery of the next supply of medication.

2. Seizures

Seizures have been associated with the use of clozapine. Dose appears to be an important predictor of seizure, with a greater likelihood at higher clozapine doses. Caution should be used when administering clozapine to patients having a history of seizures or other predisposing factors. Patients should be advised not to engage in any activity where sudden loss of consciousness could cause serious risk to themselves or others.

3. Myocarditis [inflammation of the heart]

Analyses of postmarketing safety databases suggest that clozapine is associated with an increased risk of fatal myocarditis, especially during, but not limited to, the first month of therapy. In patients in whom myocarditis is suspected, clozapine treatment should be promptly discontinued.

4. Other Adverse Cardiovascular and Respiratory Effects

Orthostatic hypotension, with or without syncope, can occur with clozapine treatment. Rarely, collapse can be profound and be accompanied by respiratory and/or cardiac arrest. Orthostatic hypotension is more likely to occur during initial titration in association with rapid dose escalation. In patients who have had even a brief interval off clozapine, i.e., 2 or more days since the last dose, treatment should be started with 12.5 mg once or twice daily.

Since collapse, respiratory arrest and cardiac arrest during initial treatment have occurred in patients who were being administered benzodiazepines or other psychotropic drugs, caution is advised when clozapine is initiated in patients taking a benzodiazepine or any other psychotropic drug.[109]

dence that atypical antipsychotics are more effective or are better tolerated than the older conventional antipsychotics such as haloperidol (see p. 258).[106]

The most serious risk of this drug is a lowering of the number of white blood cells, called agranulocytosis. Clozapine is dispensed only in one-week supplies to assure that monitoring of white blood cells is done, and the dose is ad-justed if necessary. Dry mouth or excess saliva can cause dental problems. Older people are more apt to develop dizziness. Rare, sometimes fatal effects include neuroleptic malignant syndrome (NMS). Symptoms are fever, profuse sweating, and rigid muscles.

Clozapine is not recommended for women who are pregnant or breast-feeding, or for children under age 16.

WARNING: BLOOD SUGAR ELEVATION AND DIABETES MELLITUS

Elevations in blood sugar (glucose),[56-50] in some cases extreme and associated with ketoacidosis or hyperosmolar coma or death, have been reported in patients treated with atypical antipsychotics that include aripiprazole (ABILIFY), clozapine (CLOZARIL), olanzapine (ZYPREXA), quetiapine (SEROQUEL), risperidone (RISPERDAL), and ziprasidone (GEODON).

The relationship between atypical antipsychotic use and glucose abnormalities is complicated by the possibility of an increased background risk of diabetes mellitus in patients with schizophrenia and the increasing incidence of diabetes mellitus in the general population. Given these confounders, the relationship between atypical antipsychotic use and hyperglycemia-related adverse events is not completely understood. Precise risk estimates for hyperglycemia-related adverse events in patients treated with atypical antipsychotics are not available.

Patients with an established diagnosis of diabetes mellitus who are started on atypical antipsychotics should be monitored regularly for worsening of glucose control. Patients with risk factors for diabetes mellitus (e.g., obesity, family history of diabetes) who are starting treatment with atypical antipsychotics should undergo fasting blood glucose testing at the beginning of treatment and periodically during treatment. Any patient treated with atypical antipsychotics should be monitored for symptoms of hyperglycemia including polydipsia (excessive thirst/drinking of liquids), polyuria (excessive urination), polyphagia (excessive eating), and weakness. Patients who develop symptoms of hyperglycemia during treatment with atypical antipsychotics should undergo fasting blood glucose testing. In some cases, hyperglycemia resolved when the atypical antipsychotic was discontinued; however, some patients required continuation of antidiabetic treatment despite discontinuation of the suspect drug.

Before You Use This Drug

Do not use if you have or have had:

- severe central nervous system depression
- history of bone marrow depression
- blood disease
- are breast-feeding

Tell your doctor if you have or have had:

- allergies, including to lactose and iodine
- glaucoma (narrow-angle)
- gastrointestinal problems
- enlarged prostate or difficulty urinating
- heart, kidney, or liver problems
- pregnancy
- seizures

Tell your doctor about any other drugs you take, including aspirin, herbs, vitamins, and other nonprescription products.

When You Use This Drug

- Do not drink alcohol or use other drugs that can cause drowsiness.
- Visit your doctor regularly to check progress and have blood tests.
- Until you know how you react to this drug, do not drive or perform other activities that require alertness.
- You may feel dizzy when rising from a lying or sitting position. When getting out of bed, hang your legs over the side of the bed for a few minutes, then get up slowly. When getting up from a chair, stay beside the chair until you are sure that you are not dizzy. (See p. 13.)
- Use sugarless gum, ice, or saliva substitutes to relieve dry mouth. Check with your doctor or dentist if dryness continues for more than two weeks.
- Check with your doctor before stopping

WARNING: CEREBROVASCULAR ADVERSE EVENTS, INCLUDING STROKE, IN ELDERLY PATIENTS WITH DEMENTIA

Cerebrovascular adverse events (e.g., stroke, transient ischemic attack), including fatalities, were reported in patients in clinical trials of the atypical antipsychotics in elderly patients with dementia-related psychosis.[59] In placebo-controlled trials, there was a significantly higher incidence of cerebrovascular adverse events in patients treated with these drugs compared to patients treated with placebo. The atypical antipsychotics are not approved for the treatment of patients with dementia-related psychosis.

WARNING: LIFE-THREATENING INTERACTION BETWEEN CLOZAPINE AND BENZODIAZEPINES

Public Citizen's Health Research Group petitioned the FDA to require a box warning on the professional product information (package insert), which warns of a potential life-threatening drug interaction between clozapine and drugs like diazepam (VALIUM) or other benzodiazepines (see p. 223). This warning now appears in the clozapine labeling.

clozapine. Ask for a schedule to taper off this drug.

• Tell your doctor immediately if you have any unexplained fatigue, lethargy, weakness, fever, chest pain.

• If you have not taken the drug for two or more days, check with your doctor before restarting clozapine.

• Tell your doctor immediately if you have yellow eyes or skin.

• If you plan to have any surgery, including dental, tell your doctor that you take this drug.

How to Use This Drug

• If you miss a dose, take it as soon as you remember, but skip it if it is almost time for the next dose. **Do not take double doses.**
• Do not share your medication with others.
• Take the drug at the same time(s) each day.
• Take with or without food.
• Do not break, chew, or crush this drug.
• Store at room temperature with lid on tightly. Do not store in the bathroom. Do not expose to heat, moisture, or strong light. Keep out of reach of children.

Interactions with Other Drugs

The following drugs, biologics (e.g., vaccines, therapeutic antibodies), or foods are listed in *Evaluations of Drug Interactions* 2003 as causing "highly clinically significant" or "clinically significant" interactions when used together with any of the drugs in this section. In some sections with multiple drugs, the interaction may have been reported for one but not all

For a variety of reasons, including increased appetite, the newer, so-called atypical antipsychotic drugs commonly cause a significant increase in weight that can be troublesome to and dangerous for patients using these drugs. For various drugs in this group, the usual range of weight gain is from 5 to 20 pounds, but there are a large number of reports of people gaining much more than 20 pounds, especially with longer-term use of the drugs. In addition to and related to weight gain are metabolic disorders including elevated blood sugar, the onset of diabetes, and abnormalities of fat metabolism such as elevated triglyceride levels. Patients should be informed of these effects to help prevent excessive body weight gain.[110]

drugs in this section, but we include the interaction because the drugs in this section are similar to one another. We have also included potentially serious interactions listed in the drug's FDA-approved professional package insert or in published medical journal articles. There may be other drugs, especially those in the families of drugs listed below, that also will react with this drug to cause severe adverse effects. Make sure to tell your doctor and pharmacist the drugs you are taking and tell them if you are taking any of these interacting drugs:

Central nervous system (CNS) depressant drugs, including alcohol, antidepressants, antihistamines, some blood pressure medications (reserpine, methyldopa, beta-blockers), motion sickness medications, muscle relaxants, narcotics, sedatives, sleeping pills, and tranquilizers.

Other drugs that can interact with clozapine are: AGENERASE, amprenavir, bone marrow depressants, carbamazepine, cimetidine, diazepam, EES, ERYTHROCIN, erythromycin, fluvoxamine, lithium, LITHOBID, LITHONATE, LUVOX, NORVIR, RIFADIN, rifampin, ritonavir, TAGAMET, TEGRETOL, VALIUM.

Adverse Effects

Call your doctor immediately if you experience:

- unusual anxiety, nervousness
- bleeding, bruising
- blurred vision
- severe or continuing headaches
- blood pressure decreases or increases
- difficulty breathing
- chills
- sore throat
- confusion
- dizziness or fainting
- fever, sweating

- fast or irregular heartbeat
- severe or continuing headaches
- lip smacking
- muscle stiffness
- restlessness
- seizures
- pale skin
- tremor
- uncontrollable movements of arms, legs, or tongue
- unusual tiredness, weakness
- difficulty urinating
- vision changes
- sores, ulcers, or white spots on lips or mouth
- yellowing of skin or eyes [111]
- puffiness of cheeks
- watering of the mouth
- decreased sexual ability
- depression
- severe drowsiness
- trouble sleeping

Call your doctor if these symptoms continue:

- abdominal discomfort
- heartburn
- constipation
- nausea or vomiting
- weight gain
- dizziness or lightheadedness
- drowsiness
- headache
- too much saliva
- dry mouth
- increased sweating

Signs of overdose:

- fast, slow or irregular heartbeat
- unusual excitement or nervousness
- severe drowsiness or coma
- increased watering of mouth
- dizziness or fainting
- slow, irregular or troubled breathing
- seizures

If you suspect an overdose, call this number to contact your poison control center: (800) 222-1222.

Periodic Tests

Ask your doctor which of these tests should be done periodically while you are taking this drug:

- white blood cell and differential counts
- EKG (ECG) for myocarditis

Limited Use

Olanzapine (oh *lan* za peen)
ZYPREXA (Lilly)

GENERIC: not available
FAMILY: Atypical Antipsychotics

Olanzapine is an antipsychotic used to treat schizophrenia and related psychoses. This drug is chemically similar to clozapine and may work in a similar way to clozapine.[112] All antipsychotics tend to improve symptoms, such as hallucinations, agitation, delusions, suspiciousness, and disorganized thinking. Atypical an-

---

WARNING: BLOOD SUGAR ELEVATION AND DIABETES MELLITUS

Elevations in blood sugar (glucose),[56-58] in some cases extreme and associated with ketoacidosis or hyperosmolar coma or death, have been reported in patients treated with atypical antipsychotics that include aripiprazole (ABILIFY), clozapine (CLOZARIL), olanzapine (ZYPREXA), quetiapine (SEROQUEL), risperidone (RISPERDAL), and ziprasidone (GEODON).

The relationship between atypical antipsychotic use and glucose abnormalities is complicated by the possibility of an increased background risk of diabetes mellitus in patients with schizophrenia and the increasing incidence of diabetes mellitus in the general population. Given these confounders, the relationship between atypical antipsychotic use and hyperglycemia-related adverse events is not completely understood. Precise risk estimates for hyperglycemia-related adverse events in patients treated with atypical antipsychotics are not available.

Patients with an established diagnosis of diabetes mellitus who are started on atypical antipsychotics should be monitored regularly for worsening of glucose control. Patients with risk factors for diabetes mellitus (e.g., obesity, family history of diabetes) who are starting treatment with atypical antipsychotics should undergo fasting blood glucose testing at the beginning of treatment and periodically during treatment. Any patient treated with atypical antipsychotics should be monitored for symptoms of hyperglycemia, including polydipsia (excessive thirst/drinking of liquids), polyuria (excessive urination), polyphagia (excessive eating), and weakness. Patients who develop symptoms of hyperglycemia during treatment with atypical antipsychotics should undergo fasting blood glucose testing. In some cases, hyperglycemia resolved when the atypical antipsychotic was discontinued; however, some patients required continuation of antidiabetic treatment despite discontinuation of the suspect drug.

> ## WARNING: CEREBROVASCULAR ADVERSE EVENTS, INCLUDING STROKE, IN ELDERLY PATIENTS WITH DEMENTIA
>
> Cerebrovascular adverse events (e.g., stroke, transient ischemic attack), including fatalities, were reported in patients in clinical trials of the atypical antipsychotics in elderly patients with dementia-related psychosis.[59] In placebo-controlled trials, there was a significantly higher incidence of cerebrovascular adverse events in patients treated with these drugs compared to patients treated with placebo. The atypical antipsychotics are not approved for the treatment of patients with dementia-related psychosis.

> ## DECREASED SWEATING
>
> This drug may make you sweat less, causing your body temperature to increase. Use extra care not to become overheated during exercise or in hot weather while you are taking this medication, since overheating may result in heatstroke. Also, hot baths or saunas may make you feel dizzy or faint when you are taking this medication.

tipsychotics better improve the "negative" symptoms of schizophrenia, such as apathy, emotional withdrawal, lack of pleasure, and disorientation, than do older antipsychotics. However, there is no clear evidence that atypical antipsychotics are more effective or are better tolerated than the older conventional antipsychotics such as haloperidol (see p. 258).[106]

A randomized controlled clinical trial compared olanzapine to the much older antipsychotic agent haloperidol (HALDOL; see p. 258) and concluded that this trial "found no statistically or clinically significant advantages of olanzapine for schizophrenia on measures of compliance, symptoms, or overall quality of life, nor did it find evidence of reduced inpatient use or total cost."[113]

The results of this trial were considerably less favorable than previously published studies comparing olanzapine with haloperidol. The authors of the study offered two possibilities for the dissimilar results of this and the previous studies. First, haloperidol patients were initially given benztropine (see p. 625) to prevent the development of extrapyramidal symptoms (EPS). Second, in the comparative studies with haloperidol that were favorable to olanzapine, drugs like benztropine were not given until after the development of EPS.

Drowsiness and weight gain are the most common adverse effects with olanzapine. Women, the elderly, and Asians are more prone to adverse effects. A rare but potentially fatal effect is neuroleptic malignant syndrome (NMS). Symptoms of NMS are fever, profuse sweating, rigid muscles, fast or irregular heartbeat, and kidney failure.

Olanzapine has not been studied in children under age 18. Women who are breast-feeding should not take olanzapine. Long-term effects are not yet known. Many studies are as yet unpublished.[114]

Before You Use This Drug

Do not use if you have or have had:

- hypersensitivity to olanzapine
- are breast-feeding

Tell your doctor if you have or have had:

- allergies to drugs
- Alzheimer's disease
- breast cancer
- low blood pressure
- heart or liver problems
- pregnancy
- seizures or stroke

For a variety of reasons, including increased appetite, the newer, so-called atypical antipsychotic drugs commonly cause a significant increase in weight that can be troublesome to and dangerous for patients using these drugs. For various drugs in this group, the usual range of weight gain is from 5 to 20 pounds, but there are a large number of reports of people gaining much more than 20 pounds, especially with longer-term use of the drugs. In addition to and related to weight gain are metabolic disorders including elevated blood sugar, the onset of diabetes, and abnormalities of fat metabolism such as elevated triglyceride levels. Patients should be informed of these effects to help prevent excessive body weight gain.[110]

- drug abuse or dependence
- glaucoma (narrow-angle)
- enlarged prostate
- gastrointestinal obstruction
- dehydration
- dizziness

Tell your doctor about any other drugs you take, including aspirin, herbs, vitamins, and other nonprescription products.

When You Use This Drug

- Have someone stay with you or contact you after you take the first dose, in case you become dizzy or faint.
- Do not drink alcohol or use other drugs that can cause drowsiness.
- Until you know how you react to this drug, do not drive or perform other activities that require alertness.
- You may feel dizzy when rising from a lying or sitting position. When getting out of bed, hang your legs over the side of the bed for a few minutes, then get up slowly. When getting up from a chair, stay beside the chair until you are sure that you are not dizzy. (See p. 13)

- Avoid dehydration. Drink plenty of fluids, especially during hot weather, or if you have nausea, vomiting, or diarrhea.
- Chew sugarless gum, ice, or use saliva substitutes if you develop a dry mouth.
- Have your doctor reassess your need to continue taking this drug periodically.
- If you plan to have any surgery, including dental, tell your doctor that you take this drug.

How to Use This Drug

- If you miss a dose, take it as soon as you remember, but skip it if it is almost time for the next dose. **Do not take double doses.**
- Do not share your medication with others.
- Take the drug at the same time(s) each day.
- Take with or without food.
- Tablet may be broken in two but not chewed or crushed.
- Store at room temperature. Do not store in the bathroom. Do not expose to heat, moisture, or strong light. Keep out of reach of children.

Interactions with Other Drugs

The following drugs, biologics (e.g., vaccines, therapeutic antibodies), or foods are listed in *Evaluations of Drug Interactions* 2003 as causing "highly clinically significant" or "clinically significant" interactions when used together with any of the drugs in this section. In some sections with multiple drugs, the interaction may have been reported for one but not all drugs in this section, but we include the interaction because the drugs in this section are similar to one another. We have also included potentially serious interactions listed in the drug's FDA-approved professional package insert or in published medical journal articles. There may be other drugs, especially those in the families of drugs listed below, that also will react with this drug to cause severe adverse effects. Make sure to tell your doctor and pharmacist the drugs you are taking and tell them if you are taking any of these interacting drugs:

Central nervous system depressant (CNS) drugs, including alcohol, antidepressants, antihistamines, antipsychotics, some blood pressure medications (reserpine, methyldopa, beta-blockers), motion sickness medications, muscle relaxants, narcotics, sedatives, sleeping pills, and tranquilizers.

Other drugs that can interact with olanzapine include: carbamazepine, charcoal, fluvoxamine, LUVOX, NORVIR, RIFADIN, rifampin, RIMACTANE, ritonavir, TEGRETOL.

Adverse Effects

Call your doctor immediately if you experience:

- difficulty in speaking or swallowing
- chest pain
- agitation, hostility
- anxiety
- stiff arms or legs
- dizziness
- excess saliva
- fever
- fast or irregular heartbeat
- trouble breathing
- involuntary movements of hands and fingers or arms and legs
- lip smacking
- muscle spasms in face, neck, and back
- restlessness or nervousness
- confusion
- amnesia
- euphoria
- swelling of face, feet, or ankles
- skin rash
- tremor
- nonaggressive objectionable behavior
- flulike symptoms
- menstrual changes

Call your doctor if these symptoms continue:

- constipation
- drowsiness
- dizziness
- weakness
- dry mouth
- nasal congestion
- nausea or vomiting
- headache
- sleep disturbances
- sweating, increased perspiration
- vision changes
- weight gain or loss
- tremor
- abdominal pain
- joint pain
- stuttering or trouble speaking clearly
- increased salivation
- fast heartbeat
- trouble controlling urine

Signs of overdose:

- drowsiness
- slurred speech

If you suspect an overdose, call this number to contact your poison control center: (800) 222-1222.

Periodic Tests

Ask your doctor which of these tests should be done periodically while you are taking this drug:

- liver function tests

Limited Use

Quetiapine (kwe *tye* a peen)
SEROQUEL (AstraZeneca)

GENERIC: not available
FAMILY: Atypical Antipsychotics

PREGNANCY WARNING

This drug caused harm to developing fetuses in animal studies, including fetal and pup death. Use during pregnancy only for clear medical reasons. Tell your doctor if you are pregnant or thinking of becoming pregnant before you take this drug.

BREAST-FEEDING WARNING

Quetiapine was excreted in the breast milk of treated rats. It is very likely that women taking quetiapine would also excrete the drug into their milk. Because of the potential for serious adverse effects, women taking quetiapine should not breast-feed their infants.

Quetiapine is approved to treat psychotic disorders such as schizophrenia. It belongs to a class of drugs called atypical or second-generation antipsychotics. While all antipsychotics usually improve symptoms such as agitation, delusions, hallucinations, and suspiciousness, atypical antipsychotics claim to improve "negative" symptoms such as apathy, disorientation, emotional withdrawal, and lack of pleasure more than older antipsychotics. However, there is no clear evidence that atypical antipsychotics are more effective or are better tolerated than the older conventional antipsychotics such as haloperidol (see p. 258).[106]

Reports have suggested that the newer atypical antipsyhcotic drugs are associated with the

For a variety of reasons, including increased appetite, the newer, so-called atypical antipsychotic drugs commonly cause a significant increase in weight that can be troublesome to and dangerous for patients using these drugs. For various drugs in this group, the usual range of weight gain is from 5 to 20 pounds, but there are a large number of reports of people gaining much more than 20 pounds, especially with longer-term use of the drugs. In addition to and related to weight gain are metabolic disorders including elevated blood sugar, the onset of diabetes, and abnormalities of fat metabolism such as elevated triglyceride levels. Patients should be informed of these effects to help prevent excessive body weight gain.[110]

ANTICHOLINERGIC EFFECTS

WARNING: SPECIAL MENTAL AND PHYSICAL ADVERSE EFFECTS

Older adults are especially sensitive to the harmful anticholinergic (see Glossary, p. 889) effects of this drug. Drugs in this family should not be used unless absolutely necessary.

Mental Effects: confusion, delirium, short-term memory problems, disorientation, and impaired attention.

Physical Effects: dry mouth, constipation, difficulty urinating (especially for a man with an enlarged prostate), blurred vision, decreased sweating with increased body temperature, sexual dysfunction, and worsening of glaucoma.

development of drug-induced elevations in blood sugar that has led to the development of diabetes.[56–58]

In September 2003, the FDA ordered that the professional product labeling for these drugs warn that patients should be monitored for the symptoms of diabetes mellitus.[115] The drugs requiring the new warning are aripiprazole (ABILIFY), clozapine (CLOZARIL), olanzapine (ZYPREXA), quetiapine (SEROQUEL), risperidone (RISPERDAL), and ziprasidone (GEODON).

Quetiapine can have serious adverse effects. These include neuroleptic malignant syndrome (NMS), a condition that includes a dangerously high fever, muscle rigidity, and altered mental states, heatstroke that can be fatal, and tardive dyskinesia, a serious adverse effect that may be reversible in its early stages. Early signs of tardive dyskinesia include unusual movements of the tongue or mouth, or tremor. If progressive, it may lead to uncontrollable movements of the arms, legs, and tongue, for which there is no known effective treatment. Women and older people are more prone to tardive dyskine-

---

HEAT STRESS ALERT

This drug can affect your body's ability to adjust to heat, putting you at risk of "heat stress." If you live alone, ask a friend to check on you several times during the day. Early signs of heat stress are dizziness, lightheadedness, faintness, and slightly high temperature. Call your doctor if you have any of these signs. Drink more fluids (water, fruit and vegetable juices) than usual—even if you're not thirsty—unless your doctor has told you otherwise. Do not drink alcohol.

---

sia. Extrapyramidal effects, such as drug-induced parkinsonism, may cause a shuffle when walking.

Quetiapine can cause dizziness and low blood pressure. Common anticholinergic effects are drowsiness and dry mouth (see box, p. 181). More than 20% of people taking quetiapine gained weight, sometimes accompanied by an increase in cholesterol level. A common adverse effect is drowsiness. Generally, older people develop adverse effects more often.

In one species of animal (beagles) but not in any other animals, quetiapine caused cataracts. Until the effect of quetiapine on the eyes of humans is determined, you should have eye exams at initiation of treatment and every six months, such as slit lamp exams, to detect the formation of cataracts.

Before You Use This Drug

Do not use if you have or have had:

- hypersensitivity to quetiapine
- are breast-feeding

Tell your doctor if you have or have had:

- allergies, including to iodine or lactose
- Alzheimer's disease
- low blood pressure
- blood problems, such as low white count or increase in blood volume
- breast cancer
- dehydration
- drug abuse or dependence
- epilepsy, seizures, stroke
- heart, kidney, or liver problems
- pregnancy or are breast-feeding
- thyroid problems

Tell your doctor about any other drugs you take, including aspirin, herbs, vitamins, and other nonprescription products.

When You Use This Drug

- Until you know how you react to this drug, do not drive or perform other activities requiring alertness. This drug may cause drowsiness.
- Do not drink alcohol or use other drugs that can cause drowsiness.
- Avoid getting overheated.
- Do not drink grapefruit juice, as quetiapine interacts with it.
- You may feel dizzy when rising from a lying or sitting position. When getting out of bed, hang your feet over the side of the bed for a few minutes, then get up slowly. When getting up from a chair, stay by the chair until you are sure that you are not dizzy. (See p. 13.)
- Chew sugarless gum, candy, or ice or use a saliva substitute if you develop dryness in your mouth. If dryness continues more than two weeks, check with your doctor or dentist.
- Contact your doctor or pharmacist before taking any nonprescription drugs or herbs, especially medicines for colds or allergies.
- Drink plenty of fluids. Avoid dehydration, especially during exercise and hot weather.
- Do not stop taking quetiapine without contacting your doctor.
- Tell any doctor, dentist, emergency medical technician, pharmacist, or surgeon you see that you take quetiapine.

How to Use This Drug

• If you miss a dose, take it as soon as you remember, but skip it if it is almost time for the next dose. **Do not take double doses.**

• Do not share your medication with others.

• Take the drug at the same time(s) each day.

• Take with or without food.

• Do not break, chew, or crush this drug.

• Store quetiapine at room temperature with lid on tightly. Do not store in the bathroom. Do not expose to heat, moisture, or strong light. Keep out of reach of children.

Interactions with Other Drugs

The following drugs, biologics (e.g., vaccines, therapeutic antibodies), or foods are listed in *Evaluations of Drug Interactions* 2003 as causing "highly clinically significant" or "clinically significant" interactions when used together with any of the drugs in this section. In some sections with multiple drugs, the interaction may have been reported for one but not all drugs in this section, but we include the interaction because the drugs in this section are similar to one another. We have also included potentially serious interactions listed in the drug's FDA-approved professional package insert or in published medical journal articles. There may be other drugs, especially those in the families of drugs listed below, that also will react with this drug to cause severe adverse effects. Make sure to tell your doctor and pharmacist the drugs you are taking and tell them if you are taking any of these interacting drugs:

Central nervous system depressant (CNS) drugs, including alcohol, antidepressants, antihistamines, antipsychotics, some blood pressure medications (reserpine, methyldopa, beta-blockers), motion sickness medications, muscle relaxants, narcotics, sedatives, sleeping pills, and tranquilizers.

amiodarone, ATIVAN, BIAXIN, carbamazepine, cimetidine, clarithromycin, CORDARONE, CRIXIVAN, DELTASONE, DIFLUCAN, DILANTIN, EES, ERYTHROCIN, erythromycin, fluconazole, fluoxetine, fluvoxamine, FORTOVASE, indinavir, INVIRASE, itraconazole, ketoconazole, LARODOPA, levodopa, lorazepam, LUMINAL, LUVOX, MELLARIL, METICORTEN, METRETON, nefazodone, nelfinavir, NIZORAL, NORVIR, phenobarbital, phenytoin, prednisolone, prednisone, PROZAC, RIFADIN, rifampin, RIMACTANE, ritonavir, saquinavir, SERZONE, SOLFOTON, sparfloxacin, SPORANOX, TAGAMET, TAO, TEGRETOL, thioridazine, troleandomycin, VIRACEPT, ZAGAM.

Because of its potential for causing low blood pressure, quetiapine may enhance the effects of blood-pressure-lowering drugs.

Adverse Effects

Call your doctor immediately if you experience:

• **signs of tardive dyskinesia:** lip smacking, chewing movements, puffing of cheeks, rapid, darting tongue movements, uncontrolled movements of arms or legs

• **signs of neuroleptic malignant syndrome:** (NMS) troubled or fast breathing, high or low blood pressure, increased sweating, loss of bladder control, muscle stiffness, seizures, unusual tiredness, weakness, fast heartbeat, irregular pulse, pale skin

• **signs of underactive thyroid:** dry, puffy skin, loss of appetite, tiredness, weight gain

• **signs of parkinsonism:** trouble speaking or swallowing, loss of balance, masklike face, shuffling walk, slowed movements, stiffness of arms or legs, trembling and shaking of hands and fingers

• unusual secretion of breast milk in females

- dizziness, fainting, lightheadedness
- fever
- chills
- loss of balance
- menstrual cycle changes
- muscle aches
- dry skin, rash
- sore throat
- difficulty swallowing
- swelling of feet or lower legs
- difficulty speaking
- trouble breathing
- fast, pounding, or irregular heartbeat
- seizures

Call your doctor if these symptoms continue:

- constipation
- dizziness
- drowsiness
- dry mouth
- decreased energy and strength
- headache
- indigestion
- increased muscle tone
- pain in stomach or abdomen (may indicate need for lower dose)
- nasal congestion or runny nose
- profuse sweating
- vision changes
- weight gain (usually related to dose)
- decrease in appetite
- fast or irregular heartbeat

Signs of overdose:

- drowsiness
- fast, slow, or irregular heartbeat
- low blood pressure
- weakness

If you suspect an overdose, call this number to contact your poison control center: (800) 222-1222.

Periodic Tests

Ask your doctor which of these tests should be done periodically while you are taking this drug:

- careful supervision (for patients with suicidal tendencies)
- eye exams
- liver function tests

―――――

Limited Use

Risperidone (ris *per* i done)
RISPERDAL (Janssen)

GENERIC: not available
FAMILY: Atypical Antipsychotics

PREGNANCY WARNING

Risperidone caused harm to developing fetuses in animal studies, including an increase in pup deaths even at drug exposures below those in humans. There is also one report of improper brain formation in an infant exposed to risperidone in the womb. Use during pregnancy only for clear medical reasons. Tell your doctor if you are pregnant or thinking of becoming pregnant before you take this drug.

BREAST-FEEDING WARNING

Risperidone is excreted in human milk. Because of the potential for serious adverse effects, women taking risperidone should not breast-feed their infants.

Risperidone is approved to treat psychotic disorders such as schizophrenia. It belongs to a class of drugs called atypical or second-generation antipsychotics. While all antipsychotics usually improve symptoms such as agitation, delusions, hallucinations, and suspiciousness, atypical antipsychotics claim to improve "negative" symptoms such as apathy, disorientation, emotional withdrawal, and lack of pleasure more than older antipsychotics. However, there is no clear evidence that atypical antipsychotics are more effective or are better tolerated than the older

---

WARNING: BLOOD SUGAR ELEVATION AND DIABETES MELLITUS

Elevations in blood sugar (glucose),[56-58] in some cases extreme and associated with ketoacidosis or hyperosmolar coma or death, have been reported in patients treated with atypical antipsychotics that include aripiprazole (ABILIFY), clozapine (CLOZARIL), olanzapine (ZYPREXA), quetiapine (SEROQUEL), risperidone (RISPERDAL), and ziprasidone (GEODON).

The relationship between atypical antipsychotic use and glucose abnormalities is complicated by the possibility of an increased background risk of diabetes mellitus in patients with schizophrenia and the increasing incidence of diabetes mellitus in the general population. Given these confounders, the relationship between atypical antipsychotic use and hyperglycemia-related adverse events is not completely understood. Precise risk estimates for hyperglycemia-related adverse events in patients treated with atypical antipsychotics are not available.

Patients with an established diagnosis of diabetes mellitus who are started on atypical antipsychotics should be monitored regularly for worsening of glucose control. Patients with risk factors for diabetes mellitus (e.g., obesity, family history of diabetes) who are starting treatment with atypical antipsychotics should undergo fasting blood glucose testing at the beginning of treatment and periodically during treatment. Any patient treated with atypical antipsychotics should be monitored for symptoms of hyperglycemia, including polydipsia (excessive thirst/drinking of liquids), polyuria (excessive urination), polyphagia (excessive eating), and weakness. Patients who develop symptoms of hyperglycemia during treatment with atypical antipsychotics should undergo fasting blood glucose testing. In some cases, hyperglycemia resolved when the atypical antipsychotic was discontinued; however, some patients required continuation of antidiabetic treatment despite discontinuation of the suspect drug.

---

conventional antipsychotics such as haloperidol (see p. 258).[106]

Reports have suggested that the newer atypical antipsychotic drugs are associated with the development of drug-induced elevations in blood sugar that has led to the development of diabetes.[56-58]

Older people are at increased risk for adverse effects. These include neuroleptic malignant syndrome (NMS) characterized by fever, profuse sweating, rigid muscles, fast or irregular heartbeat, and kidney failure. Risperidone can also cause you to sunburn more readily, gain weight, and change the amount of saliva in your mouth, causing cavities. Some adverse effects can be averted by lowering doses. Information about long-term effects of risperidone is still sparse. Continued use should be reassessed periodically. The cost of risperidone is high compared to generic haloperidol. If you switch from other drugs to risperidone, the time the drugs overlap should be minimal.

Before You Use This Drug

Tell your doctor if you have or have had:

- low blood pressure
- breast cancer
- dehydration
- heart, kidney, or liver problems
- hypovolemia
- Parkinson's disease
- seizures or stroke
- brain tumor
- medication overdose
- drug abuse or dependence
- intestinal obstruction
- Reye's syndrome
- slow heartbeat
- pregnancy or are breast-feeding

WARNING: CEREBROVASCULAR ADVERSE EVENTS, INCLUDING STROKE, IN ELDERLY PATIENTS WITH DEMENTIA

Cerebrovascular adverse events (e.g., stroke, transient ischemic attack), including fatalities, were reported in patients in clinical trials of the atypical antipsychotics in elderly patients with dementia-related psychosis.[59] In placebo-controlled trials, there was a significantly higher incidence of cerebrovascular adverse events in patients treated with these drugs compared to patients treated with placebo. The atypical antipsychotics are not approved for the treatment of patients with dementia-related psychosis.

DECREASED SWEATING

This drug may make you sweat less, causing your body temperature to increase. Use extra care not to become overheated during exercise or in hot weather while you are taking this medication, since overheating may result in heat stroke. Also, hot baths or saunas may make you feel dizzy or faint when you are taking this medication.

Tell your doctor about any other drugs you take, including aspirin, herbs, vitamins, and other nonprescription products.

When You Use This Drug

• Until you know how you react to this drug, do not drive or perform other activities that require alertness. Risperidone can cause drowsiness, dizziness, and blurred vision.

• When you first take risperidone, try to have someone stay with you in case you become very weak from the lowering of your blood pressure.

• Do not drink alcohol or use other central nervous system (CNS) depressants, including antidepressants, antihistamines, antipsychotics, some blood pressure medications (reserpine, methyldopa, beta-blockers), motion sickness medications, muscle relaxants, narcotics, sedatives, sleeping pills, and tranquilizers.

• You may feel dizzy when rising from a lying or sitting position. When getting out of bed, hang your legs over the side of the bed for a few minutes, then get up slowly. When getting up from a chair, stay beside the chair until you are sure that you are not dizzy. (See p. 13.)

• Protect yourself from sun. Use sunblock that protects against both UVA and UVB rays and/or wear wide-brim hats, sunglasses, long sleeves, and long slacks. Avoid sunlamps, tanning beds, and tanning booths.

• Avoid heatstroke from exercise, hot baths, or hot weather. Drink adequate fluids during hot weather.

• Chew sugarless gum, candy, or ice or use a saliva substitute if you develop dryness in your mouth. If dryness continues more than two weeks, check with your doctor or dentist.

• Keep regular appointments with your doctor.

• If you plan to have any surgery, including dental, tell your doctor that you take this drug.

How to Use This Drug

• If you miss a dose, take it as soon as you remember, but skip it if it is almost time for the next dose. **Do not take double doses.**

• Do not share your medication with others.

Death has resulted when risperidone has been used to treat dementia in the elderly.

Risperidone is not approved by the FDA to treat patients with dementia, such as Alzheimer's dementia in elderly patients.

For a variety of reasons, including increased appetite, the newer, so-called atypical antipsychotic drugs commonly cause a significant increase in weight that can be troublesome to and dangerous for patients using these drugs. For various drugs in this group, the usual range of weight gain is from 5 to 20 pounds, but there are a large number of reports of people gaining much more than 20 pounds, especially with longer-term use of the drugs. In addition to and related to weight gain are metabolic disorders including elevated blood sugar, the onset of diabetes, and abnormalities of fat metabolism such as elevated triglyceride levels. Patients should be informed of these effects to help prevent excessive body weight gain.[110]

- Take the drug at the same time(s) each day.
- Take with or without food.
- Stir measured dose of oral solution into water, coffee, orange juice, or low-fat milk; do not use cola or tea.
- Store both tablets and oral solution at room temperature with lid on tightly. Do not store in the bathroom. Do not expose to heat, moisture, or strong light. Keep out of reach of children.
- **Do not suddenly stop taking this drug.** Check with your doctor to find out if you need to taper off this drug.

Interactions with Other Drugs

The following drugs, biologics (e.g., vaccines, therapeutic antibodies), or foods are listed in *Evaluations of Drug Interactions* 2003 as causing "highly clinically significant" or "clinically significant" interactions when used together with any of the drugs in this section. In some sections with multiple drugs, the interaction may have been reported for one but not all drugs in this section, but we include the interaction because the drugs in this section are similar to one another. We have also included potentially serious interactions listed in the drug's FDA-approved professional package insert or in published medical journal articles. There may be other drugs, especially those in the families of drugs listed below, that also will react with this drug to cause severe adverse effects. Make sure to tell your doctor and pharmacist the drugs you are taking and tell them if you are taking any of these interacting drugs:

AVELOX, bromocriptine, carbamazepine, clozapine, CLOZARIL, DILANTIN, fluoxetine, LARODOPA, levodopa, moxifloxacin, NORVIR, PARLODEL, phenobarbital, phenytoin, PROZAC, RIFADIN, rifampin, RIMACTANE, ritonavir, TEGRETOL.

Because risperidone may cause low blood pressure (hypotension), it may enhance the blood-pressure-lowering effects of drugs used to treat high blood pressure.

Adverse Effects

Call your doctor immediately if you experience:

- **signs of parkinsonism:** trouble speaking or swallowing, loss of balance, masklike face, shuffling walk, slowed movements, stiffness of arms or legs, trembling and shaking of hands and fingers
  - muscle spasms in face, neck, and back
  - restlessness
  - anxiety, nervousness
  - trouble sleeping
  - decrease in sexual function
  - decrease in appetite
  - weakness or stiffness in arms or legs
  - back pain
  - bleeding
  - irregular blood pressure
  - unusual secretion of milk
  - difficulty breathing
  - puffy cheeks
  - chest pain

- dandruff
- difficulty concentrating or remembering
- dizziness
- drowsiness
- unusual facial expression
- fever
- trembling or shaking of hands or fingers
- irregular heartbeat
- lip smacking or puckering
- menstrual changes
- mood changes, including aggressive behavior or uncontrolled excitement
- stiff muscles
- painful or prolonged penis erection
- restlessness, need to keep moving
- seizures
- decline in sexual desire
- shuffling walk or loss of balance
- itching, oily, or pale skin
- bruises or rash
- difficulty sleeping
- uncontrolled movements of arms, back, face, legs, neck, or trunk
- difficulty swallowing or speaking
- extreme thirst
- ticlike, twisting, or twitching movements of body
- rapid or darting movement of tongue
- difficulty urinating
- blurred or changed vision
- uncontrolled tiredness or weakness

Call your doctor if these symptoms continue:

- tiredness or weakness
- abdominal pain
- constipation
- cough
- diarrhea
- dry mouth
- headache
- heartburn
- joint pain
- nausea
- runny nose

- increase or decrease in saliva (watering of mouth)
- dry or darkened skin
- increased sleep and dreams
- drowsiness
- sore throat
- sunburn
- undesired weight gain or loss
- vomiting

Periodic Tests

Ask your doctor which of these tests should be done periodically while you are taking this drug:

- abnormal movement determinations

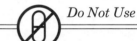 *Do Not Use*

ALTERNATIVE TREATMENT:
See Antipsychotics, p. 176.

Ziprasidone (zi *pras* uh done)
GEODON (Pfizer)

FAMILY: Atypical Antipsychotics

Ziprasidone was approved by the FDA for the treatment of schizophrenia in February 2001. It belongs to a class of drugs called atypical or second-generation antipsychotics. While all antipsychotics usually improve symptoms such as agitation, delusions, hallucinations, and suspiciousness, atypical antipsychotics claim to improve "negative" symptoms such as apathy, disorientation, emotional withdrawal, and lack of pleasure more than older antipsychotics. However, there is no clear evidence that atypical antipsychotics are more effective or are better tolerated than the older conventional antipsychotics such as haloperidol (see p. 258).[106]

Pfizer submitted a New Drug Application (NDA) to the FDA for ziprasidone on March 18,

SELECTED PORTIONS OF THE ZIPRASIDONE WARNING AS IT APPEARS IN THE FDA-APPROVED PROFESSIONAL LABELING

QT PROLONGATION AND RISK OF SUDDEN DEATH

As with other antipsychotic drugs and placebo, sudden unexplained deaths have been reported in patients taking ziprasidone at recommended doses. The premarketing experience for ziprasidone did not reveal an excess risk of mortality for ziprasidone compared to other antipsychotic drugs or placebo, but the extent of exposure was limited, especially for the drugs used as active controls and placebo. Nevertheless, ziprasidone's larger prolongation of QTc length compared to several other antipsychotic drugs raises the possibility that the risk of sudden death may be greater for ziprasidone than for other available drugs for treating schizophrenia. This possibility needs to be considered in deciding among alternative drug products.

Certain circumstances may increase the risk of the occurrence of torsades de pointes and/or sudden death in association with the use of drugs that prolong the QTc interval, including (1) bradycardia [slow heart rate]; (2) hypokalemia [low potassium blood levels] or hypomagnesemia [low magnesium blood levels]; (3) concomitant use of other drugs that prolong the QTc interval; and (4) presence of congenital prolongation of the QT interval.

Ziprasidone use should be avoided in combination with other drugs that are known to prolong the QTc interval. Ziprasidone should also be avoided in patients with congenital long QT syndrome and in patients with a history of cardiac arrhythmias. It is recommended that patients being considered for ziprasidone treatment who are at risk for significant electrolyte disturbances, hypokalemia in particular, have baseline serum potassium and magnesium measurements. Hypokalemia (and/or hypomagnesemia) may increase the risk of QT prolongation and arrhythmia. Hypokalemia may result from diuretic therapy, diarrhea, and other causes. Patients with low serum potassium and/or magnesium should be repleted with those electrolytes before proceeding with treatment. It is essential to periodically monitor serum electrolytes in patients for whom diuretic therapy is introduced during ziprasidone treatment. Persistently prolonged QTc intervals may also increase the risk of further prolongation and arrhythmia, but it is not clear that routine screening ECG measures are effective in detecting such patients. Rather, ziprasidone should be avoided in patients with histories of significant cardiovascular illness, e.g., QT prolongation, recent acute myocardial infarction, uncompensated heart failure, or cardiac arrhythmia. Ziprasidone should be discontinued in patients who are found to have persistent QTc measurements > [greater than] 500 msec [milliseconds].

1998. Three months later, on June 17, the agency sent the company a not-approvable letter based on "the judgment that ziprasidone prolongs the QTc and that this represents a risk of potentially fatal ventricular arrhythmias [heart rhythm disturbances] that is not outweighed by a demonstrated and sufficient advantage of ziprasidone over already marketed antipsychotic drug products."[116]

Ziprasidone causes an adverse effect known as QTc interval prolongation. The QTc interval is the length of time it takes the large chambers of the heart (ventricles) to electrically discharge and recharge. A prolongation of the QTc interval can lead to a type of heart rhythm disturbance, or cardiac arrhythmia, known as torsades de pointes, and sudden death. The QTc interval is measured by an electrocardiogram (EKG or ECG) in milliseconds (msec). The lowercase "c" indicates that the QT interval has been corrected for the patient's heart rate. *Torsades de pointes* is a French phrase that

---

WARNING: BLOOD SUGAR ELEVATION AND DIABETES MELLITUS

Elevations in blood sugar (glucose),[56-58] in some cases extreme and associated with ketoacidosis or hyperosmolar coma or death, have (as elsewhere) been reported in patients treated with atypical antipsychotics that include aripiprazole (ABILIFY), clozapine (CLOZARIL), olanzapine (ZYPREXA), quetiapine (SEROQUEL), risperidone (RISPERDAL), and ziprasidone (GEODON).

The relationship between atypical antipsychotic use and glucose abnormalities is complicated by the possibility of an increased background risk of diabetes mellitus in patients with schizophrenia and the increasing incidence of diabetes mellitus in the general population. Given these confounders, the relationship between atypical antipsychotic use and hyperglycemia-related adverse events is not completely understood. Precise risk estimates for hyperglycemia-related adverse events in patients treated with atypical antipsychotics are not available.

Patients with an established diagnosis of diabetes mellitus who are started on atypical antipsychotics should be monitored regularly for worsening of glucose control. Patients with risk factors for diabetes mellitus (e.g., obesity, family history of diabetes) who are starting treatment with atypical antipsychotics should undergo fasting blood glucose testing at the beginning of treatment and periodically during treatment. Any patient treated with atypical antipsychotics should be monitored for symptoms of hyperglycemia, including polydipsia (excessive thirst/drinking of liquids), polyuria (excessive urination), polyphagia (excessive eating), and weakness. Patients who develop symptoms of hyperglycemia during treatment with atypical antipsychotics should undergo fasting blood glucose testing. In some cases, hyperglycemia resolved when the atypical antipsychotic was discontinued; however, some patients required continuation of antidiabetic treatment despite discontinuation of the suspect drug.

---

means "twisted point," which describes the appearance of this rhythm disturbance on the EKG tracing.

The experience with thioridazine (MELLARIL) (see p. 263) and mesoridazine (SERENTIL) (see p. 261) and another antipsychotic drug, sertindole (SERLECT), places ziprasidone's effect on QTc interval prolongation in some perspective. Sertindole was recommended for approval by an FDA advisory committee and approved on October 2, 1996, but the drug was never marketed in this country. Before sertindole's approval, it was known to increase QTc by about 21 milliseconds, a duration similar to that of ziprasidone. However, sertindole was marketed in the UK but was withdrawn by the company on December 2, 1998, following reports of cardiac arrhythmias and sudden death associated with its use.[117]

Ziprasidone should not be used with any drug that prolongs the QT interval. The only extensive list of drugs that prolong QT intervals is maintained by the University of Arizona Health Sciences Center: http://www.torsades.org.

Pfizer presented the results of five clinical trials to the FDA in support of ziprasidone's approval. Four of these tested the effect of the drug in the management of acute symptoms of schizophrenia. The studies lasted four to six weeks and involved 702 patients who received ziprasidone in doses ranging from 10 milligrams to 200 milligrams, plus 273 patients who received a placebo. One trial included 85 patients who were treated with the old and relatively inexpensive antipsychotic drug haloperidol in a fixed dose of 15 milligrams.

In the single trial in which ziprasidone was compared to 15 milligrams of haloperidol, Pfizer estimated that the treatment effect for haloperidol was greater on the four rating scales used in the study compared to all dosages of ziprasidone tested.[118] Pfizer did not determine if

WARNING: CEREBROVASCULAR ADVERSE EVENTS, INCLUDING STROKE, IN ELDERLY PATIENTS WITH DEMENTIA

Cerebrovascular adverse events (e.g., stroke, transient ischemic attack), including fatalities, were reported in patients in clinical trials of the atypical antipsychotics in elderly patients with dementia-related psychosis.[59] In placebo-controlled trials, there was a significantly higher incidence of cerebrovascular adverse events in patients treated with these drugs compared to patients treated with placebo. The atypical antipsychotics are not approved for the treatment of patients with dementia-related psychosis.

the difference between the drugs was statistically significant and the company did not provide sufficient information to make this determination.

Ziprasidone should be used with caution when it is taken in combination with other drugs that work on the central nervous system. Because of its potential for inducing low blood pressure, ziprasidone may enhance the effects of blood-pressure-lowering drugs. Ziprasidone may antagonize the effects of levodopa (LARO-DOPA). It also interacts with carbamazepine (TEGRETOL) and ketoconazole (NIZORAL).

Traditional or Typical Antipsychotics

Limited Use

Haloperidol (ha loe *per* i dole)
HALDOL (Ortho-McNeil)

GENERIC: available
FAMILY: Traditional or Typical Antipsychotics

Haloperidol is effective for treating mental illnesses called psychoses, including schizophrenia. It should not be used to treat anxiety, to treat the loss of mental abilities (for example, due to Alzheimer's disease) in nonpsychotic people, to sedate, or to control restless behavior or other problems in nonpsychotic people. Haloperidol should also be used sparingly, if at all, for treating depression in older people, since the incidence of tardive dyskinesia (involuntary movements of parts of the body), an often disabling adverse effect of this drug, is 60% in older adults with depression who are given antipsychotic drugs.[46] Most studies find that in-

ANTICHOLINERGIC EFFECTS

WARNING: SPECIAL MENTAL AND PHYSICAL ADVERSE EFFECTS

Older adults are especially sensitive to the harmful anticholinergic (see Glossary, p. 889) effects of this drug. Drugs in this family should not be used unless absolutely necessary.

Mental Effects: confusion, delirium, short-term memory problems, disorientation, and impaired attention.

Physical Effects: dry mouth, constipation, difficulty urinating (especially for a man with an enlarged prostate), blurred vision, decreased sweating with increased body temperature, sexual dysfunction, and worsening of glaucoma.

DECREASED SWEATING

This drug may make you sweat less, causing your body temperature to increase. Use extra care not to become overheated during exercise or in hot weather while you are taking one of these medications, since overheating may result in heatstroke. Also, hot baths or saunas may make you feel dizzy or faint when you are taking this medication.

---

creased age and long duration of therapy are important predictors of increased rates of tardive dyskinesia. Another variable between studies is the differing definitions of tardive dyskinesia.

There is no clear evidence that the newer atypical antipsychotics such as olanzapine (ZYPREXA) (see p. 244) are more effective or are better tolerated than the older conventional antipsychotics such as haloperidol.[106]

A randomized controlled clinical trial compared olanzapine to haloperidol and concluded that this trial "found no statistically or clinically significant advantages of olanzapine for schizophrenia on measures of compliance, symptoms, or overall quality of life, nor did it find evidence of reduced inpatient use or total cost."[113]

The antipsychotics can cause serious adverse effects, including tardive dyskinesia, drug-induced parkinsonism (see p. 30, Chapter 3), the "jitters," and weakness and muscle fatigue (see Adverse Effects).

The table on p. 181 shows the major differences among the various antipsychotic drugs. If your doctor has prescribed one of these drugs and it is causing an unwanted side effect, use this table to find alternative drugs that cause less of that particular effect.

Whichever of these drugs you use, you should be taking between one-tenth and one-fifth of the dose used for younger adults.

Before You Use This Drug

Do not use if you have or have had:

- severe central nervous system depression from drugs
- are breast-feeding

Tell your doctor if you have or have had:

- allergies to drugs
- alcohol dependence
- glaucoma
- heart or blood vessel disease
- Parkinson's disease
- epilepsy, seizures
- kidney or liver problems
- overactive thyroid
- difficulty urinating
- lung disease
- pregnancy or are breast-feeding
- severe drug-induced depression

Tell your doctor about any other drugs you take, including aspirin, herbs, vitamins, and other nonprescription products.

When You Use This Drug

- It may take two to three weeks before you can tell that your drug is working.
- **Do not stop taking this drug suddenly. Your doctor must give your a schedule to lower your dose gradually, to prevent withdrawal symptoms** such as nausea, vomiting, and stomach upset.
- Until you know how you react to this drug, do not drive or perform other activities requiring alertness. These drugs may cause blurred vision, drowsiness, and fainting.
- Do not drink alcohol or use other drugs that can cause drowsiness.
- You may feel dizzy when rising from a lying or sitting position. When getting out of bed, hang your feet over the side of the bed for a few minutes, then get up slowly. When getting out of a chair, stay by the chair until you are sure that you are not dizzy. (See p. 13.)

• Avoid getting overheated. Use caution in hot weather, during exercise, or in hot baths.

• Avoid unprotected exposure to the sun. Use a sunblock that protects against both UVA and UVB rays. Don't use sunlamps or tanning booths.

• If you plan to have any surgery, including dental, tell your doctor that you take this drug.

How to Use This Drug

• If you miss a dose, take it as soon as you remember, but skip it if it is almost time for the next dose. **Do not take double doses.**

• Do not share your medication with others.

• Take the drug at the same time(s) each day.

• Mix liquid dosage form with water, orange juice, apple juice, tomato juice, or cola; do not mix with tea or coffee.

• Avoid skin contact with oral solution.

• Store at room temperature with lid on tightly. Do not store in the bathroom. Do not expose to heat, moisture, or strong light. Do not refrigerate or freeze.

• If you take antacids or diarrhea drugs, take them at least two hours before taking your antipsychotic drug.

Interactions with Other Drugs

The following drugs, biologics (e.g., vaccines, therapeutic antibodies), or foods are listed in *Evaluations of Drug Interactions* 2003 as causing "highly clinically significant" or "clinically significant" interactions when used together with any of the drugs in this section. In some sections with multiple drugs, the interaction may have been reported for one but not all drugs in this section, but we include the interaction because the drugs in this section are similar to one another. We have also included potentially serious interactions listed in the drug's FDA-approved professional package insert or in published medical journal articles.

There may be other drugs, especially those in the families of drugs listed below, that also will react with this drug to cause severe adverse effects. Make sure to tell your doctor and pharmacist the drugs you are taking and tell them if you are taking any of these interacting drugs.

alcohol, AVELOX, carbamazepine, cabergoline, COGNEX, DOSTINEX, ESKALITH, LARODOPA, levodopa, lithium, LITHOBID, LITHONATE, moxifloxacin, NORVIR, pergolide, PERMAX, PRIFTIN, RIFADIN, rifampin, rifapentine, ritonavir, tacrine, TEGRETOL.

Central nervous system (CNS) depressant drugs, including alcohol, antidepressants, antihistamines, antipsychotics, some blood pressure medications (reserpine, methyldopa, beta-blockers), motion sickness medications, muscle relaxants, narcotics, sedatives, sleeping pills, and tranquilizers.

Adverse Effects

Call your doctor immediately if you experience:

• **signs of tardive dyskinesia** (can also occur after stopping the drug): lip smacking, uncontrolled chewing movements, puffing of cheeks, rapid, darting tongue movements, uncontrolled movements of arms or legs

• **signs of parkinsonism:** difficulty speaking or swallowing, loss of balance control, mask-like face, shuffling walk, stiffness of arms or legs, trembling and shaking of hands and fingers

• muscle spasms of face, neck, and back

• ticlike or twitching movements

• inability to move eyes

• weakness of arms and legs

• red and raised or acne-like skin

• **signs of akinesia:** weakness, muscular fatigue, listlessness, depression. Although often confused with true depression, akinesia is actually the most common of a group of adverse effects called extrapyramidal effects.

- changed or blurred vision
- difficulty urinating
- **signs of neuroleptic malignant syndrome:** troubled or fast breathing, high or low blood pressure, increased sweating, loss of bladder control, muscle stiffness, seizures, unusual tiredness, weakness, fast heartbeat, irregular pulse, pale skin
- fever and sore throat
- yellow eyes or skin
- skin rash
- fainting
- hives or itching
- hallucinations
- restlessness and the need to keep moving
- decreased thirst
- unusual bleeding or bruising
- hot, dry skin or lack of sweating
- blinking or spasms of eyelids

Call your doctor if these symptoms continue:

- changes in menstrual period
- constipation
- dry mouth
- swelling or pain in breasts in females
- unusual secretion of milk
- decreased sexual ability
- decreased sweating
- drowsiness
- weight gain
- increased skin sensitivity to sun
- nausea or vomiting
- blurred vision

Signs of overdose:

- severe breathing problems
- dizziness
- severe drowsiness
- severe muscle trembling
- stiffness, jerking or uncontrolled movements
- severe tiredness or weakness

If you suspect an overdose, call this number to contact your poison control center: (800) 222-1222.

Periodic Tests

Ask your doctor which of these tests should be done periodically while you are taking this drug:

- liver function tests
- observation for early signs of tardive dyskinesia
- reevaluation of need for the drug
- observation for the early signs of dehydration
- complete blood count

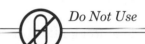 *Do Not Use*

ALTERNATIVE TREATMENT:
Antipsychotics, see p. 176.

Mesoridazine (mez oh *rid* a zeen)
SERENTIL (Novartis)

FAMILY: Traditional or Typical Antipsychotics

FDA BLACK BOX WARNING

SERENTIL (mesoridazine besylate) has been shown to prolong the QTc interval in a dose-related manner, and drugs with this potential, including serentil, have been associated with torsades de pointes–type arrhythmias and sudden death. Due to its potential for significant, possibly life-threatening, proarrhythmic effects, Serentil should be reserved for use in the treatment of schizophrenic patients who fail to show an acceptable response to adequate courses of treatment with other antipsychotic drugs, either because of insufficient effectiveness or the inability to achieve an effective dose due to intolerable adverse effects from those drugs.

ANTICHOLINERGIC EFFECTS

WARNING: SPECIAL MENTAL AND PHYSICAL ADVERSE EFFECTS

Older adults are especially sensitive to the harmful anticholinergic (see Glossary, p. 889) effects of this drug. Drugs in this family should not be used unless absolutely necessary.

Mental Effects: confusion, delirium, short-term memory problems, disorientation, and impaired attention.

Physical Effects: dry mouth, constipation, difficulty urinating (especially for a man with an enlarged prostate), blurred vision, decreased sweating with increased body temperature, sexual dysfunction, and worsening of glaucoma.

Mesoridazine is the active breakdown product of the antipsychotic drug thioridazine (MELLARIL), which we have also listed as a **Do Not Use** drug (see p. 263). Mesoridazine, like thioridazine, required extensive new safety warnings, including a boxed warning, in its professional product labeling or package insert in September 2000 because of life-threatening heart rhythm disturbances and death associated with the use of the drug. The only FDA-approved use for mesoridazine is now "the management of schizophrenic patients who fail to respond adequately to treatment with other antipsychotic drugs."[119]

We have listed mesoridazine as a **Do Not Use** drug because there are a number of safer antipsychotic drugs available on the market. There is simply no longer any reason to expose patients to the risks of mesoridazine.

Mesoridazine causes an adverse effect known as QTc interval prolongation. The QTc interval is the length of time it takes the large chambers of the heart (ventricles) to electrically discharge and recharge. A prolongation of the QTc interval can lead to a type of heart rhythm disturbance, or cardiac arrhythmia, known as torsades de pointes, and sudden death. The QTc interval is measured by an electrocardiogram (EKG or ECG) in milliseconds (msec). The lowercase "c" indicates that the QT interval has been corrected for the patient's heart rate. The QTc prolongation seen with mesoridazine increases with increasing doses of the drug. The new labeling also warns that mesoridazine should not be started if the QTc is greater than 450 milliseconds. In patients already taking the drug, if the QTc is found to be over 500 milliseconds the drug should be stopped. *Torsades de pointes* is a French phrase that means "twisted point," which describes the appearance of this rhythm disturbance on the EKG tracing.

Mesoridazine is now contraindicated in combination with other drugs that can prolong the QTc interval, and in patients who naturally have a long QT interval. The only extensive list of drugs that prolong QT intervals is maintained by the University of Arizona Health Sciences Center: http://www.torsades.org. A naturally long QT interval called "congenital long QT syndrome" and can be detected only by an EKG. Furthermore, mesoridazine is contraindicated in patients with a history of heart rhythm disturbances.

The new warnings in mesoridazine's labeling are based primarily on the FDA's review of a published study involving nine schizophrenic patients who had normal EKG tracings at baseline and no significant heart, kidney, or liver disease.[120] EKG tracings were obtained at baseline, during weeks two, three, and four, and two weeks after the drug's discontinuation. At the lowest dose of mesoridazine, four of nine patients displayed mild to moderate prolongation of the QT interval. At the highest dose, all nine patients had moderate prolongation of the QT interval. Two weeks after discontinuation, EKGs for eight of the nine patients had normalized.

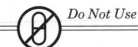

Do Not Use

ALTERNATIVE TREATMENT:
See Antipsychotics, p. 176.

Thioridazine (Thye oh *rid* a zeen)
MELLARIL (Novartis)

FAMILY: Traditional or Typical Antipsychotics

FDA BLACK BOX WARNING

MELLARIL (thioridazine HCl) has been shown to prolong the QTc interval in a dose-related manner, and drugs with this potential, including Mellaril, have been associated with torsades de pointes–type arrhythmias and sudden death. Due to its potential for significant, possibly life-threatening, proarrhythmic effects, Mellaril should be reserved for use in the treatment of schizophrenic patients who fail to show an acceptable response to adequate courses of treatment with other antipsychotic drugs, either because of insufficient effectiveness or the inability to achieve an effective dose due to intolerable adverse effects from those drugs.

Thioridazine required extensive new safety warnings, including a boxed warning, in its professional product labeling or package insert in July 2000 because of life-threatening heart rhythm disturbances and death associated with the use of the drug. The only FDA-approved use for thioridazine is now "the management of schizophrenic patients who fail to respond adequately to treatment with other antipsychotic drugs."[121]

We have listed thioridazine as a **Do Not Use** drug because there are a number of safer antipsychotic drugs available on the market.

ANTICHOLINERGIC EFFECTS

WARNING: SPECIAL MENTAL AND PHYSICAL ADVERSE EFFECTS

Older adults are especially sensitive to the harmful anticholinergic (see Glossary, p. 889) effects of this drug. Drugs in this family should not be used unless absolutely necessary.

Mental Effects: confusion, delirium, short-term memory problems, disorientation, and impaired attention.

Physical Effects: dry mouth, constipation, difficulty urinating (especially for a man with an enlarged prostate), blurred vision, decreased sweating with increased body temperature, sexual dysfunction, and worsening of glaucoma.

There is simply no longer any reason to expose patients to the risk of thioridazine.

Thioridazine causes an adverse effect known as QTc interval prolongation. The QTc interval is the length of time it takes the large chambers of the heart (ventricles) to electrically discharge and recharge. A prolongation of the QTc interval can lead to a type of heart rhythm disturbance, or cardiac arrhythmia, known as torsades de pointes, and sudden death. The QTc interval is measured by an electrocardiogram (EKG or ECG) in milliseconds (msec). The lowercase "c" indicates that the QT interval has been corrected for the patient's heart rate. The QTc prolongation seen with thioridazine increases with increasing doses of the drug. The new labeling also warns that thioridazine should not be started if the QTc is greater that 450 milliseconds. In patients already taking the drug, if the QTc is found to be over 500 milliseconds, the drug should be stopped. Torsades de pointes is a French phrase that means "twisted point," which describes the appearance of this rhythm disturbance on the EKG tracing.

Thioridazine is now contraindicated in combination with other drugs that can prolong the QTc interval and in patients who naturally have a long QT interval. The only extensive list of drugs that prolong QT intervals is maintained by the University of Arizona Health Sciences Center: http://www.torsades.org. This is called "congenital long QT syndrome" and can only be detected by an EKG. Furthermore, thioridazine is also contraindicated in patients with a history of heart rhythm disturbances.

A number of drugs are now contraindicated with the use of thioridazine because they can inhibit one of a group of liver enzymes known as cytochrome P450 that metabolize, or break down, thioridazine. The enzyme that metabolizes thioridazine is cytochrome P450 2D6. If this enzyme is inhibited, increased blood levels of thioridazine can result, leading to a greater risk of a heart rhythm disturbance. The drugs that are listed in the new labeling as not appropriate to use with thioridazine are:

fluoxetine, fluvoxamine, INDERAL, LUVOX, paroxetine, PAXIL, pindolol, propranolol, PROZAC, VISKEN.

Other drugs known to inhibit cytochrome P450 2D6 are: ALERMINE, amiodarone, ANAFRANIL, CARDIOQUIN, CHLOR-TRIMETON, chlorpheniramine, cimetidine, clomipramine, CORDARONE, DOLOPHINE, DURAQUIN, HALDOL, haloperidol, methadone, METHADOSE, mibefradil, NORVIR, POSICOR, QUINAGLUTE DURA-TABS, QUINIDEX, quinidine, ritonavir, TAGAMET.

The new labeling changes were based primarily on the FDA's review of three published studies. The first of these appeared in the journal *Clinical Pharmacology and Therapeutics* in 1996.[122] This study found a dose-related prolongation of the QTc interval between two and eight hours after thioridazine was given. Following a 50 milligram dose of thioridazine, the average QTc increased from 388 (range: 370 to 406) to 411 (range: 397 to 425) milliseconds four hours after the dose. The average maximal increase was 23 milliseconds. This change was statistically greater than that for either an inactive placebo or a 10 milligram dose of thioridazine.

The second study was published in 1991, also in *Clinical Pharmacology and Therapeutics*.[123] This study showed increased blood levels of thioridazine in patients with a genetic defect resulting in the slow inactivation of a research chemical known as debrisoquin. This type of genetic defect is present in about 7% of the Caucasian population. In this study, 19 healthy subjects, 6 slow and 13 rapid inactivators of debrisoquin, received a single 25 milligram oral dose of thioridazine. The slow inactivators reached higher blood levels of thioridazine by 2.4 times, and there was a 4.5-fold increase in the absorption of the drug associated with a two-fold longer half-life compared with that of the rapid inactivators of debrisoquin.

The third study reviewed by the FDA was published in 1999 in the *Journal of Clinical Psychopharmacology*.[124] This study evaluated the effect of the selective serotonin reuptake inhibiting (SSRI) antidepressant fluvoxamine, given in a dose of 25 milligrams twice daily for one week, on thioridazine blood levels in 10 hospitalized male patients with schizophrenia. The levels of thioridazine and its two active breakdown products, mesoridazine (SERENTIL) and sulforidazine, increased threefold following the administration of fluvoxamine.

Limited Use

Thiothixene (thye oh *thix* een)
NAVANE (Pfizer)

GENERIC: available
FAMILY: Traditional or Typical Antipsychotics

This drug caused harm to developing fetuses in animal studies. Use during pregnancy only for clear medical reasons. Tell your doctor if you are pregnant or thinking of becoming pregnant before you take this drug.

There are no data on the transfer of thiothixene to breast milk. However, many drugs are excreted in breast milk. Chlorpromazine, another drug in this class, has a warning not to nurse because of the potential for serious adverse effects on the nursing infant.

Thiothixene is effective for treating mental illnesses called psychoses, including schizophrenia. It should not be used to treat anxiety, to treat the loss of mental abilities (for example, due to Alzheimer's disease) in nonpsychotic people, to sedate, or to control restless behavior or other problems in nonpsychotic people. Thiothixene should also be used sparingly, if at all, for treating depression in older people, since the incidence of tardive dyskinesia (involuntary movements of parts of the body), an often disabling adverse effect of this drug, is 60% in older adults with depression who are given antipsychotic drugs.[46] Most studies find that in-

---

DECREASED SWEATING

This drug may make you sweat less, causing your body temperature to increase. Use extra care not to become overheated during exercise or in hot weather while you are taking one of these medications, since overheating may result in heatstroke. Also, hot baths or saunas may make you feel dizzy or faint when you are taking this medication.

---

creased age and long duration of therapy are important predictors for increased rates of tardive dyskinesia. Another variable between studies is the differing definitions of tardive dyskinesia.

The antipsychotics can cause serious adverse effects, including tardive dyskinesia, drug-induced parkinsonism (see p. 30); the "jitters," and weakness and muscle fatigue (see Adverse Effects).

The table on p. 181 shows the major differences among the various antipsychotic drugs. If your doctor has prescribed one of these drugs and it is causing an unwanted side effect, use this table to find alternative drugs that cause less of that particular effect.

Whichever of these drugs you use, you should be taking between one-tenth and one-fifth of the dose used for younger adults.

ANTICHOLINERGIC EFFECTS

WARNING: SPECIAL MENTAL AND PHYSICAL ADVERSE EFFECTS

Older adults are especially sensitive to the harmful anticholinergic (see Glossary, p. 889) effects of this drug. Drugs in this family should not be used unless absolutely necessary.

Mental Effects: confusion, delirium, short-term memory problems, disorientation, and impaired attention.

Physical Effects: dry mouth, constipation, difficulty urinating (especially for a man with an enlarged prostate), blurred vision, decreased sweating with increased body temperature, sexual dysfunction, and worsening of glaucoma.

Before You Use This Drug

Do not use if you have or have had:

- blood diseases
- bone marrow depression
- central nervous system depression
- drug-induced coma
- collapse of blood vessels

Tell your doctor if you have or have had:

- allergies to drugs
- alcohol dependence

- peptic ulcer
- enlarged prostate or difficulty urinating
- glaucoma
- heart or blood vessel disease
- lung disease or breathing problems
- Parkinson's disease
- epilepsy, seizures
- liver disease
- Reye's syndrome
- pregnancy or are breast-feeding

Tell your doctor about any other drugs you take, including aspirin, herbs, vitamins, and other nonprescription products.

When You Use This Drug

- It may take two to three weeks before you can tell that the drug is working.
- **Do not stop taking this drug suddenly. Your doctor must give you a schedule to lower your dose gradually, to prevent withdrawal symptoms** such as nausea, vomiting, and stomach upset.
- Until you know how you react to this drug, do not drive or perform other activities requiring alertness. This drug may cause blurred vision, drowsiness, and fainting.
- Do not drink alcohol or use other drugs that can cause drowsiness.
- You may feel dizzy when rising from a lying or sitting position. When getting out of bed, hang your feet over the side of the bed for a few minutes, then get up slowly. When getting out of a chair, stay by the chair until you are sure that you are not dizzy. (See p. 13.)
- If you plan to have any surgery, including dental, tell your doctor that you take this drug.
- Take caution during exercise or in hot weather or when taking hot baths to avoid heatstroke.
- Avoid unprotected skin exposure to the sun. Use sunblock products that protect against both UVA and UVB rays. Don't use sunlamps or tanning booths.
- Avoid spilling liquid medication on skin or clothing; it can cause irritation.
- Try sugarless gum or candy, ice, or a saliva substitute for dry mouth.

How to Use This Drug

- If you miss a dose, take it as soon as you remember, but skip it if it is almost time for the next dose. **Do not take double doses.**
- Do not share your medication with others.
- Take the drug at the same time(s) each day.
- Take with food or milk.
- Do not break, chew, or crush this drug.
- Store at room temperature with lid on tightly. Do not store in the bathroom. Do not expose to heat, moisture, or strong light. Do not freeze the liquid form. Keep out of reach of children.
- If you take antacids or diarrhea drugs, wait for two hours before taking your antipsychotic drug.

Interactions with Other Drugs

The following drugs, biologics (e.g., vaccines, therapeutic antibodies), or foods are listed in *Evaluations of Drug Interactions* 2003 as causing "highly clinically significant" or "clinically significant" interactions when used together with any of the drugs in this section. In some sections with multiple drugs, the interaction may have been reported for one but not all drugs in this section, but we include the interaction because the drugs in this section are similar to one another. We have also included potentially serious interactions listed in the drug's FDA-approved professional package insert or in published medical journal articles. There may be other drugs, especially those in the families of drugs listed below, that also will react with this drug to cause severe adverse effects. Make sure to tell your doctor and pharmacist the drugs you are taking and tell them if you are taking any of these interacting drugs:

ADRENALIN (also in bee sting kits), alcohol, cabergoline, DOSTINEX, DURAQUIN, epinephrine, ketorolac, LARODOPA, levodopa, pergolide, PERMAX, PRIMATENE MIST, QUINAGLUTE DURA-TABS, QUINIDEX, quinidine, SINEMET, TORADOL.

Central nervous system (CNS) depressant drugs, including alcohol, antidepressants, antihistamines, antipsychotics, some blood pressure medications (reserpine, methyldopa, beta-blockers), motion sickness medications, muscle relaxants, narcotics, sedatives, sleeping pills, and tranquilizers.

Adverse Effects

Call your doctor immediately if you experience:

- **signs of tardive dyskinesia** (can also occur after discontinuing the drug): lip smacking, chewing movements, puffing of cheeks, rapid, darting tongue movements, uncontrolled movements of arms or legs
- **signs of parkinsonism:** difficulty speaking or swallowing, loss of balance, masklike face, muscle spasms, stiffness of arms or legs, trembling and shaking, unusual twisting movements of body
- **signs of dystonia:** difficulty swallowing, cannot move eyes, twisting and spasms of body
- **signs of restless leg (akathisia):** restless pacing, a feeling of the "jitters"
- **signs of akinesia:** weakness, muscular fatigue, listlessness, depression. Although often confused with true depression, akinesia is actually the most common of a group of adverse effects called extrapyramidal effects.

- **signs of neuroleptic malignant syndrome (NMS):** troubled or fast breathing, high or low blood pressure, increased sweating, loss of bladder control, muscle stiffness, seizures, unusual tiredness, weakness, fast heartbeat, irregular pulse, pale skin
- fever and sore throat
- yellow eyes or skin
- skin rash
- fainting
- changed or blurred vision
- difficulty urinating

Call your doctor if these symptoms continue:

- constipation
- decreased sweating
- dry mouth
- increased appetite and weight
- increased skin sensitivity to sun
- stuffy nose
- changes in menstrual period
- decreased sexual ability
- swelling or pain in breasts in males and females
- unusual secretion of milk
- mild drowsiness
- dizziness or fainting

Signs of overdose:

- convulsions
- severe tiredness or weakness
- coma
- severe breathing problems
- severe dizziness
- severe drowsiness
- fever
- severe muscle trembling
- stiffness
- jerking or uncontrolled movements
- seizures
- unusual excitement
- unusually fast heartbeat
- tiny pupils

If you suspect an overdose, call this number to contact your poison control center: (800) 222-1222.

Periodic Tests

Ask your doctor which of these tests should be done periodically while you are taking this drug:

- complete blood count
- eye examinations
- liver function tests
- observation for early signs of tardive dyskinesia
- reevaluation of need for the drug
- urine tests for bile and bilirubin

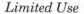

Limited Use

Chlorpromazine (klor *proe* ma zeen)
THORAZINE (GlaxoSmithKline)

Fluphenazine (floo *fen* a zeen)
PROLIXIN (Apothecon)

Trifluoperazine (trye floo oh *pair* a zeen)
STELAZINE (GlaxoSmithKline)

GENERIC: available
FAMILY: Traditional or Typical Antipsychotics

PREGNANCY WARNING

There are reported cases of prolonged jaundice, overactivity or underactivity (hyperreflexia or hyporeflexia), and extrapyramidal signs in infants born to women who were taking these drugs. Studies in rats demonstrated decreased performance with the possibility of permanent neurological damage. Tell your doctor if you are pregnant or thinking of becoming pregnant before you take this drug.

BREAST-FEEDING WARNING

These drugs are excreted in the breast milk of nursing mothers. Because of the potential for serious adverse effects, you should not take these drugs while nursing.

These drugs are in a group called phenothiazines, which are effective for treating mental illnesses called psychoses, including schizophrenia. They should not be used to treat anxiety, to treat the loss of mental abilities (for example, due to Alzheimer's disease) in nonpsychotic people, to sedate, or to control restless behavior or other problems in nonpsychotic people. They should also be used sparingly, if at all, for treating depression in older people, since the incidence of tardive dyskinesia (involuntary movements of parts of the body), an often disabling

ANTICHOLINERGIC EFFECTS

WARNING: SPECIAL MENTAL AND PHYSICAL ADVERSE EFFECTS

Older adults are especially sensitive to the harmful anticholinergic (see Glossary, p. 889) effects of this drug. Drugs in this family should not be used unless absolutely necessary.

Mental Effects: confusion, delirium, short-term memory problems, disorientation, and impaired attention.

Physical Effects: dry mouth, constipation, difficulty urinating (especially for a man with an enlarged prostate), blurred vision, decreased sweating with increased body temperature, sexual dysfunction, and worsening of glaucoma.

DECREASED SWEATING

This drug may make you sweat less, causing your body temperature to increase. Use extra care not to become overheated during exercise or in hot weather while you are taking one of these medications, since overheating may result in heatstroke. Also, hot baths or saunas may make you feel dizzy or faint when you are taking this medication.

SENSITIVITY TO COLD

Drugs such as chlorpromazine (THORAZINE), fluphenazine (PROLIXIN), prochlorperazine (COMPAZINE), thioridazine (Mellaril), and trifluoperazine (STELAZINE) may make you more sensitive to cold temperatures. Dress warmly during cold weather. Be careful during prolonged exposure to cold, such as in winter sports or swimming in cold water.

---

adverse effect of these drugs, is 60% in older adults with depression who are given antipsychotic drugs.[46] Most studies find that increased age and long duration of therapy are important indicators of increased rates of tardive dyskinesia. Another variable between studies is the differing definitions of tardive dyskinesia.

These antipsychotics can cause serious adverse effects, including tardive dyskinesia, drug-induced parkinsonism (see p. 30), the "jitters," and weakness and muscle fatigue (see Adverse Effects).

The table on p. 181 shows the major differences among these drugs. If your doctor has prescribed one of these drugs and it is causing an unwanted side effect, use this table to find alternative drugs that cause less of that particular effect.

Whichever of these drugs you use, you should be taking between one-tenth and one-fifth of the dose used for younger adults.

Before You Use These Drugs

Do not use if you have or have had:

- cardiovascular disease
- severe high or low blood pressure
- comatose states
- history of heart arrhythmias
- genetic defect in drug metabolizing enzyme (2D6)

- severe central nervous system depression
- pregnancy or are breast-feeding

Tell your doctor if you have or have had:

- allergies to phenothiazines, parabans, sulfites, FD&C Yellow No. 5
- alcohol dependence
- blood disease
- breast cancer
- enlarged prostate or difficulty urinating
- heart or blood vessel disease
- Parkinson's disease
- lung disease
- epilepsy, seizures
- glaucoma
- liver disease
- kidney disease
- stomach ulcer
- Reye's syndrome
- severe lethargy
- previous brain damage

Tell your doctor about any other drugs you take, including aspirin, herbs, vitamins, and other nonprescription products.

When You Use This Drug

- It may take two to three weeks before you can tell that the drug is working.
- **Do not stop taking this drug suddenly. Your doctor must give you a schedule to lower your dose gradually, to prevent withdrawal symptoms** such as nausea, vomiting, and stomach upset.
- Until you know how you react to this drug, do not drive or perform other activities requiring alertness. These drugs may cause blurred vision, drowsiness, and fainting.
- Do not drink alcohol or use other drugs that can cause drowsiness.
- You may feel dizzy when rising from a lying or sitting position. When getting out of bed, hang your feet over the side of the bed for a few minutes, then get up slowly. When getting out

of a chair, stay by the chair until you are sure that you are not dizzy. (See p. 13).

- If you plan to have any surgery, including dental, tell your doctor that you take this drug.
- Take caution during exercise or in hot weather or when taking hot baths to avoid heatstroke.
- Avoid unprotected skin exposure to the sun. Use sunblock products that protect against both UVA and UVB rays. Don't use sunlamps or tanning booths.
- Wear sunglasses outdoors.
- Avoid spilling liquid medication on skin or clothing; it can cause irritation.
- Avoid use of over-the-counter medications for colds or allergies.
- Try sugarless gum, candy, or ice or a saliva substitute for dry mouth.
- Long-acting injected liquid form requires precautions for 6 to 12 weeks after stopping the drug.

How to Use This Drug

- If you miss a dose, take it as soon as you remember, but skip it if it is almost time for the next dose. **Do not take double doses.**
- Do not share your medication with others.
- Take the drug at the same time(s) each day.
- Take tablet with food or milk.
- The liquid dosage form should be diluted just before use in tomato or fruit juice, milk, syrup, carbonated beverages, coffee, tea, water, applesauce, jelly, or ketchup.
- Do not break, chew, or crush the tablet.
- Extended-release tablet should be swallowed whole.
- Store at room temperature with lid on tightly. Do not store in the bathroom. Do not expose to heat, moisture, or strong light. Do not freeze the liquid form. Keep out of reach of children.
- If you take antacids or diarrhea drugs, take them at least two hours before taking your antipsychotic drug.

Interactions with Other Drugs

The following drugs, biologics (e.g., vaccines, therapeutic antibodies), or foods are listed in *Evaluations of Drug Interactions* 2003 as causing "highly clinically significant" or "clinically significant" interactions when used together with any of the drugs in this section. In some sections with multiple drugs, the interaction may have been reported for one but not all drugs in this section, but we include the interaction because the drugs in this section are similar to one another. We have also included potentially serious interactions listed in the drug's FDA-approved professional package insert or in published medical journal articles. There may be other drugs, especially those in the families of drugs listed below, that also will react with this drug to cause severe adverse effects. Make sure to tell your doctor and pharmacist the drugs you are taking and tell them if you are taking any of these interacting drugs:

alcohol, amphetamines, ANECTINE, benztropine, bromocriptine, cabergoline, CAPOTEN, captopril, carbamazepine, COGENTIN, COUMADIN, DEMEROL, desipramine, DEXEDRINE, diazoxide, DILANTIN, DOSTINEX, ESKALITH, GLUCOPHAGE, GLUCOVANCE, guanethidine, halofantrine, INDERAL, INDERAL LA, ISMELIN, lithium, LITHOBID, LITHONATE, meperidine, METAGLIP, metformin, NORPRAMIN, NORVIR, ORAP, PARLODEL, PERMAX, pergolide, phenytoin, pimozide, polymyxin B, POLY-RX, PROGLYCEM, propranolol, RIFADIN, rifampin, RIMACTANE, ritonavir, TEGRETOL, tramadol, ULTRACET, ULTRAM, warfarin.

Adverse Effects

Call your doctor immediately if you experience:

- **signs of tardive dyskinesia** (can also occur after drug is discontinued): lip smacking, chewing movements, puffing of cheeks, rapid, darting tongue movements, uncontrolled movements of arms or legs

• **signs of parkinsonism:** difficulty speaking or swallowing, loss of balance, masklike face, muscle spasms, stiffness of arms or legs, trembling and shaking, unusual twisting movements of body

• **signs of restless leg (akathisia):** restless pacing, a feeling of the "jitters"

• **signs of akinesia:** weakness, muscular fatigue, listlessness, depression. Although often confused with true depression, akinesia is actually the most common of a group of adverse effects called extrapyramidal effects.

• **signs of dystonia** (can also occur after drug is discontinued): spasms of face and body; uncontrolled twisting movements; increased blinking or spasms of eyelid

• **signs of neuroleptic malignant syndrome (NMS):** troubled or fast breathing, high or low blood pressure, increased sweating, loss of bladder control, muscle stiffness, seizures, unusual tiredness, weakness, fast heartbeat, irregular pulse, pale skin

• changed or blurred vision; difficulty seeing at night
• difficulty urinating
• dark urine
• fever and sore throat
• yellow eyes or skin
• abdominal or stomach pains
• skin rash or severe sunburn
• fainting or low blood pressure
• abnormal bleeding or bruising
• sore mouth or gums
• nightmares
• nausea or vomiting
• diarrhea
• irregular or slow heart rate

Call your doctor if these symptoms continue:

• blurred vision
• stuffy nose

• constipation
• decreased sweating
• dizziness
• drowsiness
• changes in menstrual period
• decreased sexual ability
• rough or fuzzy tongue
• watering of mouth
• increased sensitivity of eyes to light
• unusual secretion of milk
• swelling or pain in breasts
• unusual weight gain

Call your doctor if these symptoms continue after you stop taking the drug:

• persistent tardive dyskinesia (see adverse effects above)
• persistent tardive dystonia (see adverse effects above)
• dizziness
• nausea, vomiting, stomach pain
• trembling of hands and fingers

Periodic Tests

Ask your doctor which of these tests should be done periodically while you are taking this drug:

• complete blood count
• blood pressure
• electrocardiogram (ECG, EKG)
• blood potassium level
• eye tests
• urine tests
• liver function tests
• levels of medication in blood
• observation for early signs of tardive dyskinesia
• determination of abnormal movement
• urine tests for bile and bilirubin

Mania

Limited Use

Lithium (*lith* ee um)
ESKALITH (SmithKline Beecham)
LITHOBID (Solvay)
LITHONATE (Solvay)

GENERIC: available
FAMILY: Drugs for Mania
(See p. 184 for discussion of depression.)

PREGNANCY WARNING

There are reported cases of heart problems in infants born to women taking lithium. Use during pregnancy only for clear medical reasons. Tell your doctor if you are pregnant or thinking of becoming pregnant before you take this drug.

BREAST-FEEDING WARNING

Lithium is excreted in human breast milk. Infants should not be nursed during drug treatment with lithium.

FDA BLACK BOX WARNING

Lithium toxicity is closely related to serum lithium levels, and can occur at doses close to therapeutic levels. Facilities for prompt and accurate serum lithium determinations should be available before initiating therapy.

Lithium is used to treat manic episodes of manic depression, a condition in which a person's mood swings severely from normal to elated to depressed. It is also used to prevent or decrease the intensity of future manic episodes.

If you are over 60, you generally need to take less than the usual adult dose. Your doctor should frequently measure the levels of lithium in your blood.

Even when the amount of lithium in an older person's body is no more than is needed for

---

HEAT STRESS ALERT

This drug can affect your body's ability to adjust to heat, putting you at risk of "heat stress." If you live alone, ask a friend to check on you several times during the day. Early signs of heat stress are dizziness, lightheadedness, faintness, and slightly high temperature. Call your doctor if you have any of these signs. Drink more fluids (water, fruit and vegetable juices) than usual—even if you're not thirsty—unless your doctor has told you otherwise. Do not drink alcohol.

---

it to work, the drug may cause harm to the central nervous system. Ideally, you should only use lithium if you have a normal salt (sodium) intake and normal heart and kidney function.[103]

Before You Use This Drug

Do not use if you have or have had:

- history of leukemia
- are breast-feeding

Tell your doctor if you have or have had:

- allergies to drugs
- pregnancy
- heart or blood vessel disease
- Parkinson's disease
- epilepsy, seizures
- severe dehydration from vomiting, diarrhea, or profuse sweating
- enlarged prostate or difficulty urinating
- kidney disease
- diabetes
- goiter or thyroid disease
- overactive parathyroid glands
- recent severe infection
- organic brain disease
- schizophrenia

- psoriasis
- a current low-salt diet
- leukemia

Tell your doctor about any other drugs you take, including aspirin, herbs, vitamins, and other nonprescription products.

When You Use This Drug

- It may take one to three weeks before you can tell that this drug is working.
- **Do not stop taking this drug suddenly. Your doctor must give you a schedule to lower your dose gradually, to prevent withdrawal symptoms such as nausea, vomiting, and stomach upset.**
- See your doctor regularly to make sure that the drug is working and that you are not developing adverse effects. Your doctor should regularly measure the amount of drug in your body.
- Follow the diet recommended by your doctor to avoid weight gain, but use caution in dieting.
- Drink plenty of fluids and use an average amount of salt.
- Until you know how you react to this drug, do not drive or perform other activities requiring alertness. Lithium may cause blurred vision, drowsiness, fainting, or slow your reaction time.
- If you plan to have any surgery, including dental, tell your doctor that you take this drug.
- Use caution during exercise, saunas, and hot weather so you don't become dehydrated. The same is true during illness if high fever occurs.
- Be sure your family knows the early symptoms of overdose.
- Use caution in drinking large amounts of caffeinated tea, coffee, or colas because of diuretic effect.

How to Use This Drug

- If you miss a dose, take it as soon as you remember, but skip it if it is less than four hours until your next scheduled dose. If you are taking extended-release tablets, skip the missed dose if it is less than six hours until your next scheduled dose. **Do not take double doses.**
- Do not share your medication with others.
- Take the drug at the same time(s) each day.
- Take with food, juice, or milk.
- Do not break, chew, or crush long-acting forms of this drug.
- Store at room temperature with lid on tightly. Do not store in the bathroom. Do not expose to heat, moisture, or strong light. Do not freeze the liquid form. Keep out of reach of children.

Interactions with Other Drugs

The following drugs, biologics (e.g., vaccines, therapeutic antibodies), or foods are listed in *Evaluations of Drug Interactions* 2003 as causing "highly clinically significant" or "clinically significant" interactions when used together with any of the drugs in this section. In some sections with multiple drugs, the interaction may have been reported for one but not all drugs in this section, but we include the interaction because the drugs in this section are similar to one another. We have also included potentially serious interactions listed in the drug's FDA-approved professional package insert or in published medical journal articles. There may be other drugs, especially those in the families of drugs listed below, that also will react with this drug to cause severe adverse effects. Make sure to tell your doctor and pharmacist the drugs you are taking and tell them if you are taking any of these interacting drugs:

acetazolamide, ACHROMYCIN, ADVIL, ALDOMET, ALEVE, ANAPROX, CALAN SR, carbamazepine, CELEBREX, celecoxib, chlorothiazide, chlorpromazine, COVERA-HS, DIAMOX, DIURIL, ELIXOPHYLLIN, enalapril, FLAGYL, fluoxetine, HALDOL, haloperidol, ibuprofen, imipramine, IMITREX, INDOCIN, indomethacin, ISOPTIN SR, LOPRESSOR, MAZANOR, mazindol, MELLARIL, MERIDIA, metoprolol, methyldopa, metronidazole, MOTRIN, NAPROSYN, naproxen, ORAP, PANMYCIN, PIMA, pimozide, potassium iodide, PROZAC, rofecoxib, SANOREX, sertraline, sibutramine, SLO-BID, sumatriptan, SUMYCIN, TEGRETOL, TERRAMYCIN, tetracycline, THEO-24, THEOLAIR, theophylline, thioridazine, THORAZINE, TOFRANIL, VASOTEC, verapamil, VERELAN, VIOXX, ZOLOFT.

Adverse Effects

Call your doctor immediately if you experience:

- **signs of parkinsonism:** difficulty speaking or swallowing, loss of balance, mask-like face
- face or other muscle spasms, stiffness of arms or legs, trembling and shaking, unusual twisting movements of body
- **signs of low thyroid hormone levels:** dry, rough skin, hair loss, hoarseness, swelling of feet or lower legs, swelling of neck (goiter), increased sensitivity to cold, fatigue, depression, unusual excitement
- increased urination
- increased thirst
- confusion, poor memory
- dizziness
- fainting
- difficulty breathing on exertion
- fast or slow heartbeat, irregular pulse
- weight gain
- blue color and pain in fingers or toes
- cold limbs
- headache
- eye pain, visual problems
- nausea, vomiting
- unusual tiredness or weakness
- noises in ear

Call your doctor if these symptoms continue:

- diarrhea
- increased thirst
- mild nausea
- slight trembling of hands
- slight muscle twitching
- skin rash, acne
- bloated feeling
- fatigue
- loss of bladder control or increased urination

Signs of overdose (early signs):

- diarrhea
- drowsiness
- loss of appetite
- muscle weakness
- nausea or vomiting
- slurred speech
- trembling

Signs of overdose (late signs):

- blurred vision
- ringing in the ears
- clumsiness
- confusion
- dizziness
- seizures
- trembling
- increased amount of urine

If you suspect an overdose, call this number to contact your poison control center: (800) 222-1222.

Periodic Tests

Ask your doctor which of these tests should be done periodically while you are taking this drug:

- white blood cell counts
- blood levels of lithium (more often if taking other drugs)
- blood levels of calcium and phosphate
- electrocardiogram (ECG, EKG)
- kidney function tests
- thyroid function tests
- height and weight evaluation

REFERENCES

1. *Drugs for the Elderly* 2nd ed. Copenhagen, Denmark: World Health Organization, 1997:119–20.

2. Preville M, Hebert R, Boyer R, et al. Correlates of psychotropic drug use in the elderly compared to adults aged 18–64: Results from the Quebec Health Survey. *Aging and Mental Health* 2001; 5:216–24.

3. Harman JS, Rollman BL, Hanusa BH, et al. Physician office visits of adults for anxiety disorders in the United States, 1985–1998. *Journal of General Internal Medicine* 2002; 17:165–72.

4. Mojtabai R. Datapoints: Prescription patterns for mood and anxiety disorders in a community sample. *Psychiatric Services* 1999; 50:1557.

5. Hoffman-LaRoche. "The later years . . . an optimistic outlook." Mailing to physicians, 1979.

6. Catalan J, Gath D, Edmonds G, et al. The effects of non-prescribing of anxiolytics in general practice. I. Controlled evaluation of psychiatric and social outcome. *British Journal of Psychiatry* 1984; 144:593–602.

7. Zung WW, Daniel JT Jr., King RE, et al. A comparison of prazepam, diazepam, lorazepam and placebo in anxious outpatients in non-psychiatric private practices. *Journal of Clinical Psychiatry* 1981; 42:280–4.

8. Institute of Medicine, National Academy of Sciences. Sleeping Pills, Insomnia, and Medical Practice, 1979.

9. Solomon F, White CC, Parron DL, et al. Sleeping pills, insomnia and medical practice. *New England Journal of Medicine* 1979; 300:803–8.

10. Kolata G. Elderly become addicts to drug-induced sleep. *New York Times,* February 1, 1992:5.

11. Ray WA, Griffin MR, Schaffner W, et al. Psychotropic drug use and the risk of hip fracture. *New England Journal of Medicine* 1987; 316:363–9.

12. Riggs BL, Melton LJ III. Involutional osteoporosis. *New England Journal of Medicine* 1986; 314:1676–86.

13. Stenbacka M, Jansson B, Leifman A, et al. Association between use of sedatives or hypnotics, alcohol consumption, or other risk factors and a single injurious fall or multiple injurious falls: A longitudinal general population study. *Alcohol* 2002; 28:9–16.

14. Ray WA, Fought RL, Decker MD. Psychoactive drugs and the risk of injurious motor vehicle crashes in elderly drivers. *American Journal of Epidemiology* 1992; 136:873–83.

15. Beck JC, Benson DF, Scheibel AB, et al. Dementia in the elderly: The silent epidemic. *Annals of Internal Medicine* 1982; 97:231–41.

16. Larson EB, Kukull WA, Buchner D, et al. Adverse drug reactions associated with global cognitive impairment in elderly persons. *Annals of Internal Medicine* 1987; 107:169–73.

17. Use and Misuse of Benzodiazepines. Hearing before the the Subcommittee on Health and Scientific Research of the Committee on Labor and Human Resources, United States Senate, September 10, 1979.

18. Busto U, Sellers EM, Naranjo CA, et al. Withdrawal reaction after long-term therapeutic use of benzodiazepines. *New England Journal of Medicine* 1986; 315:854–9.

19. Dement W. Presentation before the Health, Education and Welfare Joint Coordinating Council for Project Sleep, July 28, 1980.

20. Lakshminarayan S, Sahn SA, Hudson LD, et al. Effect of diazepam on ventilatory responses. *Clinical Pharmacology and Therapeutics* 1976; 20:178–83.

21. Drugs for psychiatric disorders. *Medical Letter on Drugs and Therapeutics* 1986; 28:99–106.

22. Lader M. Anxiety and its treatment. *Scrip* 1992:46–8.

23. Petit L, Azad N, Byszewski A, et al. Non-pharmacological management of primary and secondary insomnia among older people: Review of assessment tools and treatments. *Age and Ageing* 2003; 32:19–25.

24. Vestal RE. ed. *Drug Treatment in the Elderly.* Sydney, Australia: ADIS Health Science Press, 1984:317–37.

25. Choice of benzodiazepines. *Medical Letter on Drugs and Therapeutics* 1981; 23:41–3.

26. Estazolam—a new benzodiazepine hypnotic. *Medical Letter on Drugs and Therapeutics* 1991; 33:91–2.

27. Avorn JL, Lamy PP, Vestal RE. Prescribing for the elderly—safely. *Patient Care* 1982:14–62.

28. Bergman U, Griffiths RR. Relative abuse of diazepam and oxazepam: Prescription forgeries and theft/loss reports in Sweden. *Drug and Alcohol Dependence* 1986; 16:293–301.

29. Griffiths RR, McLeod DR, Bigelow GE, et al. Comparison of diazepam and oxazepam: Preference, liking and extent of abuse. *Journal of Pharmacology and Experimental Therapeutics* 1984; 229:501–8.

30. Lamy PP. Pharmacological considerations in the treatment of Alzheimer's disease. *Geriatric Medicine Today* 1987:29–53.

31. National Institute of Mental Health. Epidemiological Catchment Area Data from 1981–1982, 2004.

32. Hermann RC, Yang D, Ettner SL, et al. Prescription of antipsychotic drugs by office-based physicians in the United States, 1989–1997. *Psychiatric Services* 2002; 53:425–30.

33. Gurwitz JH, Field TS, Avorn J, et al. Incidence and preventability of adverse drug events in nursing homes. *American Journal of Medicine* 2000; 109:87–94.

34. Oborne CA, Hopper R, Li KC, et al. An indicator of appropriate neuroleptic prescribing in nursing homes. *Age and Ageing* 2002; 31:435–9.

35. Beers M, Avorn J, Soumerai SB, et al. Psychoactive medication use in intermediate-care facility residents. *Journal of the American Medical Association* 1988; 260:3016–20.

36. Ray WA, Federspiel CF, Schaffner W. A study of antipsychotic drug use in nursing homes: Epidemiologic evidence suggesting misuse. *American Journal of Public Health* 1980; 70:485–91.

37. Barnes R, Veith R, Okimoto J, et al. Efficacy of antipsychotic medications in behaviorally disturbed dementia patients. *American Journal of Psychiatry* 1982; 139:1170–4.

38. Grimes JD. Drug-induced parkinsonism and tardive dyskinesia in nonpsychiatric patients. *Canadian Medical Association Journal* 1982; 126:468.

39. Cooper JW Jr., Francisco GE Jr. Psychotropic usage in long-term care facility geriatric patients. *Hospital Formulary* 1981; 16:407–13, 417.

40. Ingman SR, Lawson IR, Pierpaoli PG, et al. A survey of the prescribing and administration of drugs in a long-term care institution for the elderly. *Journal of the American Geriatric Society* 1975; 23:309–16.

41. Barton R, Hurst L. Unnecessary use of tranquilizers in elderly patients. *British Journal of Psychiatry* 1966; 112:989–90.

42. Shamoian CA. Psychogeriatrics. *Medical Clinics of North America* 1983; 67:361–78.

43. Peabody CA, Warner MD, Whiteford HA, et al. Neuroleptics and the elderly. *Journal of the American Geriatric Society* 1987; 35:233–8.

44. Llorente MD, Olsen EJ, Leyva O, et al. Use of antipsychotic

drugs in nursing homes: Current compliance with OBRA regulations. *Journal of the American Geriatric Society* 1998; 46:198–201.

45. Evans LK. Sundown syndrome in institutionalized elderly. *Journal of the American Geriatric Society* 1987; 35:101–8.

46. Yassa R, Nastase C, Dupont D, et al. Tardive dyskinesia in elderly psychiatric patients: A 5-year study. *American Journal of Psychiatry* 1992; 149:1206–11.

47. Stephen PJ, Williamson J. Drug-induced parkinsonism in the elderly. *The Lancet* 1984; 2:1082–3.

48. Donlon PT, Stenson RL. Neuroleptic induced extrapyramidal symptoms. *Diseases of the Nervous System* 1976; 37:629–35.

49. Ayd FJ. A survey of drug-induced extrapyramidal reactions. *Journal of the American Medical Association* 1961; 175:102–8.

50. Avorn J, Gurwitz JH, Bohn RL, et al. Increased incidence of levodopa therapy following metoclopramide use. *Journal of the American Medical Association* 1995; 274:1780–2.

51. Gilman AG, Goodman LS, Rall TW, Murad F, eds. *The Pharmacological Basis of Therapeutics*. 7th ed. New York: Macmillan, 1985.

52. Everitt DE, Avorn J. Drug prescribing for the elderly. *Archives of Internal Medicine* 1986; 146:2393–6.

53. Carter CS, Mulsant BH, Sweet RA, et al. Risperidone use in a teaching hospital during its first year after market approval: Economic and clinical implications. *Psychopharmacology Bulletin* 1995; 31:719–25.

54. Young LY, Koda-Kimble MA, eds. *Applied Therapeutics: The Clinical Use of Drugs*. 6th ed. Vancouver, Wash. Applied Therapeutics, Inc., 1995.

55. Knable MB, Heinz A, Raedler T, et al. Extrapyramidal side effects with risperidone and haloperidol at comparable D2 receptor occupancy levels. *Psychiatry Research* 1997; 75:91–101.

56. Olanzapine (Zyprexa) and diabetes. *Current Problems in Pharmacovigilance* 2002; 28:3.

57. Koller E, Schneider B, Bennett K, et al. Clozapine-associated diabetes. *American Journal of Medicine* 2001; 111:716–23.

58. Koller E, Malozowski S, Doraiswamy PM. Atypical antipsychotic drugs and hyperglycemia in adolescents. *Journal of the American Medical Association* 2001; 286:2547–8.

59. *Physicians' Desk Reference*. 58th ed. Montvale, N.J.: Thomson PDR, 2004:1764–8.

60. Salzman C. A primer on geriatric psychopharmacology. *American Journal of Psychiatry* 1982; 139:67–74.

61. Thompson TL, Moran MG, Nies AS. Psychotropic drug use in the elderly [second of two parts]. *New England Journal of Medicine* 1983; 308:194–9.

62. American Psychiatric Association. *Diagnostic and Statistical Manual of Mental Disorders*. 4th ed. Washington, D.C.: American Psychiatric Association, 1994.

63. Salzman C. Clinical guidelines for the use of antidepressant drugs in geriatric patients. *Journal of Clinical Psychiatry* 1985; 46:38–45.

64. Duncan AJ, Campbell AJ. Antidepressant drugs in the elderly: Are the indications as long term as the treatment? *British Medical Journal* 1988; 296:1230–2.

65. McManus P, Mant A, Mitchell PB, et al. Recent trends in the use of antidepressant drugs in Australia, 1990–1998. *Medical Journal of Australia* 2000; 173:458–61.

66. Liu B, Anderson G, Mittmann N, et al. Use of selective serotonin-reuptake inhibitors of tricyclic antidepressants and risk of hip fractures in elderly people. *The Lancet* 1998; 351:1303–7.

67. Dubin H, Spier S, Giannandrea P. Nefazodone-induced mania. *American Journal of Psychiatry* 1997; 154:578–9.

68. Wehr TA, Goodwin FK. Can antidepressants cause mania and worsen the course of affective illness? *American Journal of Psychiatry* 1987; 144:1403–11.

69. Howland RH. Induction of mania with serotonin reuptake inhibitors. *Journal of Clinical Psychopharmacology* 1996; 16:425–7.

70. Rankings of adverse effects are the averages of rankings from Vestal (reference 24), Everitt, et al (reference 52), Salzman (reference 60), and Thompson, et al (reference 61).

71. Food and Drug Administration. FDA Issues Public Health Advisory on Cautions for Use of Antidepressants in Adults and Children, March 22, 2004.

72. Wolfe SM, Hellander I. Citizen's Petition for Revision of Fluoxetine (Prozac) Labeling, May 23, 1991.

73. Georgotas A, McCue RE. Relapse of depressed patients after effective continuation therapy. *Journal of Affective Disorders* 1989; 17:159–64.

74. Clayton AH, Pradko JF, Croft HA, et al. Prevalence of sexual dysfunction among newer antidepressants. *Journal of Clinical Psychiatry* 2002; 63:357–66.

75. Woodrum ST, Brown CS. Management of SSRI-induced sexual dysfunction. *Annals of Pharmacotherapy* 1998; 32:1209–15.

76. Teicher MH, Glod C, Cole JO. Emergence of intense suicidal preoccupation during fluoxetine treatment. *American Journal of Psychiatry* 1990; 147:207–10.

77. Committee on Safety of Medicine, United Kingdom. Selective Serotonin Reuptake Inhibitors—Use in Children and Adolescents with Major Depressive Disorder, December 10, 2003.

78. Health Canada. Health Canada advises Canadians under the age of 18 to consult physicians if they are being treated with newer antidepressants, February 3, 2004. Available at http://www.hc-sc.gc.ca/english/protection/warnings/2004/2004_02.htm

79. Food and Drug Administration. Reports of Suicidality in Pediatric Patients Being Treated with Antidepressant Medications for Major Depressive Disorder (MDD), October 27, 2003.

80. Owens D. New or old antidepressants? Benefits of new drugs are exaggerated. *British Medical Journal* 1994; 309:1281–2.

81. Mulrow CD, Agency for Health Care Policy and Research. Treatment of Depression: Newer Pharmacotherapies, 1999.

82. Fick DM, Cooper JW, Wade WE, et al. Updating the Beers criteria for potentially inappropriate medication use in older adults: Results of a US consensus panel of experts. *Archives of Internal Medicine* 2003; 163:2716–24.

83. Choosing an antidepressive. *Drug and Therapeutics Bulletin* 1984; 22:61–4.

84. Gelenberg AJ. Imperfect drugs in an imperfect world. *Journal of Clinical Psychiatry* 1992; 53:39–40.

85. Davidson J. Seizures and bupropion: A review. *Journal of Clinical Psychiatry* 1989; 50:256–61.

86. Rudorfer MV, Manji HK, Potter WZ. Bupropion, ECT, and dopaminergic overdrive. *American Journal of Psychiatry* 1991; 148:1101–2.

87. Settle EC Jr. Tinnitus related to bupropion treatment. *Journal of Clinical Psychiatry* 1991; 52:352.

88. *Physicians' Desk Reference* 57th ed. Montvale, N.J.: Thomson PDR, 2003:1106–11.

89. Public Citizen's Health Research Group. Petition to the Food and Drug Administration to Ban Nefazodone (Serzone) from the Market, March 6, 2003. Available at: http://www.citizen.org/publications/release.cfm?ID=7233. Accessed February 13, 2004.

90. Public Citizen's Health Research Group. Supplement Petition to the Food and Drug Administration to Ban Nefazodone (Serzone) from the Market, October 29, 2003. Available at: http://www.citizen.org/publications/release.cfm?ID=7288. Accessed February 13, 2004.

91. Cohen LJ. Rational drug use in the treatment of depression. *Pharmacotherapy* 1997; 17:45–61.

92. Cumming RG, Le Couteur DG. Benzodiazepines and risk of hip fractures in older people: a review of the evidence. *CNS Drugs* 2003; 17:825–37.

93. Tyrer P, Murphy S. The place of benzodiazepines in psychiatric practice. *British Journal of Psychiatry* 1987; 151:719–23.

94. Hypnotic drugs. *Medical Letter on Drugs and Therapeutics* 2000; 42:71–2.

95. Zaleplon for insomnia. *The Medical Letter on Drugs and Therapeutics* 1999; 41:93–4.

96. Andreason PJ. FDA Medical Officer Review of Zaleplon (Sonata), July 14, 1998.

97. Smith MT, Perlis ML, Park A, et al. Comparative meta-analysis of pharmacotherapy and behavior therapy for persistent insomnia. *American Journal of Psychiatry* 2002; 159:5–11.

98. *American Hospital Formulary Service Drug Information.* Bethesda, Md.: American Society of Health System Pharmacists, 1996:1744–7.

99. Hypnotic drugs. *Medical Letter on Drugs and Therapeutics* 1996; 38:59–61.

100. *Drugs of Choice.* New Rochelle, N.Y.: Medical Letter, Inc., 1991:29–39.

101. Buspirone—a radical advance in the treatment of anxiety? *The Lancet* 1988; 1:804–6.

102. *American Hospital Formulary Service Drug Information.* Bethesda, Md.: American Society of Hospital Pharmacists, 1992: 1355–61.

103. Gilman AG, Rall TW, Nies AS, Taylor P, eds. *The Pharmacological Basis of Therapeutics.* 8th ed. New York: Pergamon Press, 1990:428–9.

104. Dukes MNG, Beeley L, eds. *Side Effects of Drugs Annual 12* Amsterdam: Elsevier, 1988:45–6.

105. Manfredi RL, Kales A, Vgontzas AN, et al. Buspirone: Sedative or stimulant effect? *American Journal of Psychiatry* 1991; 148:1213–7.

106. Geddes J, Freemantle N, Harrison P, et al. Atypical antipsychotics in the treatment of schizophrenia: Systematic overview and meta-regression analysis. *British Medical Journal* 2000; 321:1371–6.

107. Aripiprazole (Abilify)—FDA Medical Officer Review, 2003. Available at: http://www.fda.gov/cder/foi/nda/2002/21-436_Abilify.htm. Accessed February 12, 2004.

108. Aripiprazole (Abilify) for schizophrenia. *Medical Letter on Drugs and Therapeutics* 2003; 45:15–6.

109. *Physicians' Desk Reference.* 58th ed. Montvale, N.J.: Thomson PDR, 2004:2228–33.

110. Baptista T, Kin NM, Beaulieu S, et al. Obesity and related metabolic abnormalities during antipsychotic drug administration: Mechanisms, management and research perspectives. *Pharmacopsychiatry* 2002; 35:205–19.

111. Macfarlane B, Davies S, Mannan K, et al. Fatal acute fulminant liver failure due to clozapine: A case report and review of clozapine-induced hepatotoxicity. *Gastroenterology* 1997; 112:1707–9.

112. Olanzapine for schizophrenia. *Medical Letter on Drugs and Therapeutics* 1997; 39:5–6.

113. Rosenheck R, Perlick D, Bingham S, et al. Effectiveness and cost of olanzapine and haloperidol in the treatment of schizophrenia: A randomized controlled trial. *Journal of the American Medical Association* 2003; 290:2693–702.

114. Fulton B, Goa KL. Olanzapine: A review of its pharmacological properties and therapeutic efficacy in the management of schizophrenia and related psychoses. *Drugs* 1997; 53:281–98.

115. FDA Orders New Class Warning on Antipsychotics. *Dickinson's FDA Webview,* September 17 2003. Available at http://www.fdaweb.com.

116. Laughren TP. Memo: Team Leader, Psychiatric Drug Products Division of Neuropharmacological Drug Products to the Psychopharmacological Drugs Advisory Committee of Ziprasidone (Geodon), July 19, 2000.

117. Suspension of availability of sertindole (Serolect). *Current Problems in Pharmacovigilance* 1999; 25:1.

118. Pfizer. Briefing Document for Zeldox Capsules (ziprasidone) before the Food and Drug Administration Psychopharmacological Drugs Advisory Committee, July 19, 2000:40.

119. *Physicians' Desk Reference.* 56th ed. Montvale, N.J.: Medical Economics Company, 2002:1057–9.

120. Dillenkoffer RL, Gallant DM, Phillips JH. Electrocardiographic evaluation of mesoridazine (Serentil). *Current Therapeutic Research, Clinical and Experimental* 1972; 14:71–2.

121. *Physicians' Desk Reference.* 57th ed. Montvale, N.J.: Thomson PDR, 2003:2204–6.

122. Hartigan-Go K, Bateman DN, Nyberg G, et al. Concentration-related pharmacodynamic effects of thioridazine and its metabolites in humans. *Clinical Pharmacology and Therapeutics* 1996; 60:543–53.

123. von Bahr C, Movin G, Nordin C, et al. Plasma levels of thioridazine and metabolites are influenced by the debrisoquin hydroxylation phenotype. *Clinical Pharmacology and Therapeutics* 1991; 49:234–40.

124. Carrillo JA, Ramos SI, Herraiz AG, et al. Pharmacokinetic interaction of fluvoxamine and thioridazine in schizophrenic patients. *Journal of Clinical Psychopharmacology* 1999; 19:494–9.

125. *Physicians' Desk Reference.* 41st ed. Oradell, N.J.: Medical Economics Company, 1987.

126. The FDA-approved labeling for all benzodiazepine tranquilizers states that there is no evidence of effectiveness for more than four months.

127. Escitalopram (lexapro) for depression. *Medical Letter on Drugs and Therapeutics* 2002; 44:83–4.

6

DRUGS FOR PAIN AND ARTHRITIS

SALICYLATES

The salicylates are used to relieve pain and to reduce fever and inflammation. Aspirin, a non-steroidal anti-inflammatory drug (NSAID), is the most well-known and frequently used salicylate. Other salicylates discussed in this book are salsalate and choline and magnesium salicylates.

Aspirin

Aspirin is the common name for a chemical called acetylsalicylic acid, or ASA (as it is still known in Canada and some other countries). Aspirin, used as directed, is perhaps the most effective non-narcotic remedy, prescription or nonprescription, for pain, fever, and inflammation. Unfortunately, certain people should not use aspirin.

Aspirin Allergies

Some people are allergic to aspirin and may experience a wide variety of reactions, including hives, rash, swollen lymph nodes, generalized swelling, severe breathing difficulties, or a drop in blood pressure. Simple stomach discomfort following the use of aspirin or any other medication, however, does not indicate that you have an allergy.

Asthmatics seem to be particularly prone to aspirin allergies, as well as allergies to calcium carbaspirin, another member of the salicylate family.

If you have ever had an allergic reaction to aspirin or any other drug, be sure to tell your doctor. This kind of reaction can also occur in response to other related medications, which include prescription drugs containing salicylates or similar ingredients.

Aspirin and the Digestive Tract

Aspirin is a locally irritating, corrosive substance, which when used for a long time or in high doses can increase the likelihood of developing peptic ulcers (in the lower part of the esophagus, the stomach, or the beginning of the small intestine). If you have ulcers, inflammation of the stomach (gastritis), or any form of stomach discomfort, you should not be taking even small quantities of aspirin, in any form.

Aspirin and Bleeding

Aspirin causes bleeding in the stomach; over time, it can weaken the body's ability to slow and contain bleeding. Taking aspirin for a few days can increase the amount of bleeding during childbirth, after tooth extraction, and during surgery. Aspirin should not be taken for at least five days before surgery, even in small doses. Persons with serious liver disease, vitamin K deficiency, or blood clotting disorders, or persons already taking blood thinners (anticoagulants, such as warfarin and heparin) or other drugs, should not take aspirin without strict supervision of a doctor or other health professional.

Aspirin should not be taken in very large doses (more than 12 regular-strength 325 milligram or five-grain tablets per day) or for more than a few days without the supervision of a doctor. Even small doses used over a long period of time may leave certain predisposed individuals at an increased risk of serious bleeding after wounds or cuts.

Aspirin Preparations and Use

Aspirin is highly advertised, and there are many different brands from which to choose. We recommend plain generic aspirin for intermittent use, such as for an occasional headache.

In previous editions of *Worst Pills, Best Pills,* we recommended enteric-coated aspirin (coated so that it does not dissolve in the stomach) because it was thought to cause much less blood loss than regular or buffered aspirin. The weight of the evidence now shows that the risk of GI bleeding is similar among plain, enteric-coated, and buffered aspirin.[19, 51–53]

Enteric-coated aspirin should not be used for occasional problems, such as headaches, because it is absorbed more slowly than regular aspirin and takes more time to relieve pain.

Alka-Seltzer contains aspirin and buffering agents and is much less irritating to the stomach than regular or buffered aspirin, but it is quite expensive and contains a great deal of salt (sodium).[2] If you have to restrict your intake of salt or take a salicylate for a long time, do not use Alka-Seltzer. Since this drug contains aspirin, do not use it as an antacid.

Taking aspirin with food or after meals can decrease stomach upset. If you are on a high-dose salicylate treatment together with antacids, do not suddenly change (start or stop) the way that you take antacids without talking to your doctor first.

If you take aspirin or another salicylate regularly, the level of drug in your blood may have to be checked to make sure that you are taking the best dose. You should also have regular checkups and ask your doctor about the necessity of certain tests including hematocrit (a blood test), kidney and liver function tests, and hearing tests. Also ask if you should take vitamin C or vitamin K.

Salicylates should not be used by anyone with acute liver or kidney failure. They should be discontinued by anyone who has chronic liver or kidney disease if there is any sign of a worsening condition.[3] If you develop ringing in your ears or persistent stomach pain after using aspirin for a long time, call your doctor.

When you buy aspirin, make sure it is pure white and does not contain broken tablets. If it smells like vinegar, do not use it. Do not store your drug in the bathroom medicine cabinet because the heat or moisture might cause it to deteriorate and lose its effectiveness. Keep it away from heat and direct light.

ASPIRIN/REYE'S SYNDROME ALERT

Do not use this product for treating chicken pox, flu, or flulike illness if you are under 40. It will increase the risk of contracting Reye's syndrome, a rare but often fatal disease.

This warning appears in this book in the profiles of drugs that contain aspirin and other salicylates. Although most cases of Reye's syndrome are in children, some occur up to age 40. People under 40 who have chicken pox, flu, or flulike illness and need a drug simply to relieve pain or reduce fever should use acetaminophen (TYLENOL, for example) rather than aspirin.

NONSTEROIDAL ANTI-INFLAMMATORY DRUGS (NSAIDS)

Gastrointestinal (GI) bleeding and perforation are common and serious adverse effects of NSAIDs. These adverse reactions can lead to hospitalization and potentially death. About one-third of all bleeding ulcers in older adults are linked with this family of drugs. The most important factors predisposing people to GI toxicity from NSAIDs are the type and dose of drug (and use of two NSAIDs together), which can increase the risk up to 20-fold. Other risk factors include a history of ulcer, anticoagulants (blood thinners), steroid drugs, smoking, alcohol use, and older age.[4]

An ingenious study published in 1996 involving patients who had bled while taking an NSAID supports a principle long held by Public Citizen's Health Research Group: patients who are informed about the risks of their drugs and instructed what to do if an adverse reaction should occur can avoid serious drug-induced injury.[5]

In the study, patients who had experienced GI bleeding and were subsequently hospitalized knew less about the adverse effects of NSAIDs or what to do when they occurred than those using these drugs that did not have GI bleeding. Fewer patients who bled (16%) than those that did not (41%) remembered having been told of the potential adverse effects of NSAIDs or about what steps to take if they developed an adverse effect (4% versus 21%). Faithful obedience (compliance) in taking an NSAID was more common in patients who bled

---

WARNING

NONSTEROIDAL ANTI-INFLAMMATORY DRUG (NSAID)–INDUCED GASTROINTESTINAL TOXICITY

All members of the NSAID family of drugs can cause gastrointestinal toxicity that can lead to gastrointestinal bleeding and hospitalization or death. The risk of gastrointestinal toxicity from these drugs increases with increasing doses and the length of treatment.

If any of the following symptoms develop while you are taking an NSAID, stop taking the drug immediately and contact your doctor: severe abdominal or stomach pain, cramping, or burning; severe and continuing nausea, heartburn, or indigestion; bloody or black, tarry stools; vomiting blood or material that looks like coffee grounds; or spitting up blood.

(96%) than in those who did not (70%). In addition, 18 (36%) of those who bled had experienced stomach pain before bleeding and all but two had continued to take the drug, while only 15 (15%) of those who did not bleed had stomach pain, of whom 10 had subsequently reduced their intake of the NSAID.

NARCOTICS

Narcotic drugs are prescribed to relieve pain and cough, to treat diarrhea not caused by poisoning, and to cause drowsiness before an operation. These drugs are addictive and have many adverse effects, and their use should be limited to the lowest dose for the shortest period of time except in the case of terminally ill people with extraordinary pain.

Use of Narcotics

Pain relief is the primary legitimate use of narcotics, which are effective for moderate to severe pain that has not responded to nonnarcotic painkillers such as aspirin and other salicylates, acetaminophen, or nonsteroidal anti-inflammatory drugs (NSAIDs). Narcotics can be used alone or in combination with these drugs.

Most of the time when someone is able to swallow, they should first try a nonnarcotic drug such as aspirin taken by mouth. If aspirin alone is not effective, it can be combined with a narcotic, such as codeine. These two drugs work in different ways, and when they are used together, they generally relieve pain that would otherwise require a higher dose of narcotic, while causing fewer adverse effects.[6] A sedative or antianxiety drug is just as effective as a narcotic, without causing vomiting like narcotics can.

Because narcotics are addictive and have many adverse effects, many doctors do not prescribe them freely. This reserve is not always appropriate. In the case of severe pain from late-stage cancer that has spread throughout the body, the pain is often undertreated as far as the use of narcotics is concerned. In an editorial in the *New England Journal of Medicine*, Dr. Marcia Angell wrote: *"Pain is soul destroying. No patient should have to endure intense pain unnecessarily. The quality of mercy is essential to the practice of medicine; here, of all places, it should not be strained."*[7]

Wanted and Unwanted Effects of Narcotics

Narcotics affect the central nervous system, producing pain relief and drowsiness as well as less desirable effects. Older adults may require less than the usual adult dose to produce desired effects because of their bodies' greater sensitivity to the drugs. Some of the adverse effects frequently seen in older adults are slow or troubled breathing (narcotics should never be given to anyone with depressed breathing), stimulation or confusion,[8] and hallucinations and unpleasant dreams (seen more in people using pentazocine).[9]

Other adverse effects are dizziness; drowsiness; feeling faint or lightheaded; nausea or vomiting (which might go away if you lie down for a while); blurry vision or change in vision (double vision); constipation (more often seen with long-term use and with codeine); difficult or painful urination; or need to urinate often; general feeling of discomfort or illness; headache; dry mouth; loss of appetite; bad or unusual dreams; red or flushed face (more often with meperidine or methadone); redness, swelling, pain, or burning at place of injection; stomach pain or cramps; trouble sleeping; abnormal decrease in amount of urine; abnormal increase in sweating (more often with meperidine and methadone); abnormal nervousness, restlessness, tiredness, or weakness; and sexual problems.

Narcotics will add to the effects of alcohol and other drugs that slow down the nervous system: antidepressants, antihistamines, antipsychotics, some blood pressure medications (reserpine, methyldopa, beta-blockers), motion sickness medications, muscle relaxants, narcotics, sedatives, sleeping pills, and tranquilizers. Do not take any of these drugs or drink alcohol when you are taking a narcotic, unless your doctor has told you otherwise.

One hazard of taking narcotics continuously for longer than several weeks is drug-induced dependence. **Do not stop taking your drug suddenly.** With the help of your doctor, work out a schedule for slowly decreasing the amount of the drug you take by about 5 to 10% each day. Keep a written record of the dosage reduction schedule with you. These steps will make it much easier to become drug free without developing distressing symptoms of drug withdrawal. Common withdrawal symptoms include body aches, diarrhea, goosebumps, loss of appetite, nausea or vomiting, nervousness or restlessness, runny nose, shivering or trembling, sneezing, cramps, trouble sleeping, unexplained fever, abnormal increase in sweating or yawning, abnormal irritability, abnormally fast heartbeat, and weakness.

Taking Narcotics

Taking narcotics by mouth is preferred and is usually effective unless the pain is very severe.[10] The drugs can also be given in injections into the muscle or under the skin, intravenously into the bloodstream, alone or mixed with a solution, or into the spinal cord.

Morphine sulfate is available as extended-release tablets, which must be swallowed whole, but tablets of the other narcotics can be crushed. Meperidine sulfate oral solution should be mixed with a half glass of water before you drink it to decrease possible numbness of your mouth and throat.

If you are on a regular dosing schedule and you miss a dose, take it as soon as possible. But if it is almost time for the next dose, skip the missed dose and go back to the regular schedule. **Do not take double doses.** Drink plenty of liquids, as this may help decrease constipation. Call your doctor if you do not have a bowel movement for several days and feel uncomfortable. If you have diarrhea, do not take a drug to stop it. Instead, ask your doctor what to do.

ARTHRITIS AND INFLAMMATION

Arthritis literally means an inflammation of a joint and is a blanket term for a number of ailments with differing significance, various causes, and diverse symptoms. Such conditions are usually characterized by pain when moving or putting weight on the joint. Inflammation (pain, heat, redness, and swelling) may or may not be present.

Pain, stiffness, swelling, or tenderness in any joint, or in the neck or lower back, that lasts longer than six weeks warrants a trip to the doctor to determine the cause of the problem. A long delay in seeking help may result in irreversible damage to joints.

You should seek medical attention for pain in a joint immediately if:

- joint pain or swelling is very sudden and intense;
- joint pain follows an injury (you may have a fracture near the joint); or
- joint problems are accompanied by a fever above 100°F (38°C).

At least 31.6 million Americans suffer from some form of arthritis. The three most common types are rheumatoid arthritis, osteoarthritis, and gout. Each has a different cause, treatment, and probable outcome.

ANTI-INFLAMMATORY DRUGS

1. Nonsteroids

salicylates
  aspirin
  salsalate
nonsalicylates
  celecoxib
  choline and magnesium salicylates
  diclofenac
  diflunisal
  etodolac
  fenoprofen
  flurbiprofen
  ibuprofen
  indomethacin
  ketoprofen
  ketorolac
  meclofenamate
  meloxicam
  nabumetone
  naproxen
  oxaprozin
  piroxicam
  rofecoxib
  salsalate
  sulindac
  tolmetin
  valdecoxib

2. Steroids
  cortisone
  prednisone

ANTIRHEUMATIC DRUGS

1. Gold salts
  auranofin
  aurothioglucose
  gold sodium thiomalate

2. Antimalarial drugs
  chloroquine
  hydroxychloroquine

3. Sulfasalazine

4. Penicillamine

5. Cytotoxic drugs
  azathioprine
  cyclophosphamide
  leflunomide
  methotrexate

6. Immune Response Modifiers
  adalimumab
  anakinra
  etanercept
  infliximab

Rheumatoid Arthritis

Rheumatoid arthritis is an inflammation of the joints caused by disturbances in the body's immune system (which defends it against disease) and can occur at any age. Its victims are more likely to be female and include infants, teenagers, and middle-aged and older adults. It is often characterized by morning stiffness, along with pain and swelling in the joints of fingers, ankles, knees, wrists, and elbows, which improves as the day goes on. The distribution of affected joints is usually symmetrical; that is, if your right wrist is afflicted, your left wrist will probably be afflicted as well.

Treatment

There is no cure for rheumatoid arthritis, but the inflammation may be controlled under medical supervision. Drug therapy draws from two broad categories: the anti-inflammatory drugs and the antirheumatic drugs.

Anti-inflammatory Drugs

Anti-inflammatory drugs can be further divided into nonsteroidal and steroidal drugs. Nonsteroidal anti-inflammatory drugs (NSAIDs) work by inhibiting formation of chemicals in the body that cause pain, fever, and inflammation. NSAIDs can be either salicylate, such as aspirin, or nonsalicylate, such as ibuprofen (MOTRIN, ADVIL, NUPRIN, MEDIPRIN).

The amount of aspirin required to reduce the inflammation of arthritis, however, approaches levels at which a small proportion of people may experience undesirable adverse effects. (High-dose aspirin therapy should never be started without medical supervision to determine the correct dose and to achieve the most therapeutic effect with the fewest adverse effects.)

Aspirin works when it is present in the bloodstream at a certain level, which varies among users. Effective blood levels of aspirin range between 15 and 30 milligrams per deciliter (tenth of a liter of blood). To achieve this level, between 9 and 23 regular aspirin tablets (325 milligrams) must be taken daily (3.0 to 7.5 grams of aspirin).[11] If you are taking aspirin, the level of the drug in your blood should be monitored periodically to prevent toxicity (poisoning). Signs of aspirin toxicity include ringing in the ears, rapid breathing (hyperventilation), mental confusion, shortness of breath, swelling of feet or lower legs (edema), dizziness, headache, nausea or vomiting, sweating, and thirst. These symptoms should be reported to your doctor immediately.

All prescription NSAIDs for rheumatoid arthritis are much more expensive than aspirin, have significant adverse effects, and are no more effective than aspirin. Like aspirin, other NSAIDs may also cause gastrointestinal bleeding or impair kidney function. If you have had an allergic reaction or stomach problems after taking aspirin, however, another NSAID may be better tolerated. Read the information on individual NSAIDs for recommendations and adverse effects. Then discuss these choices with your doctor.

Selective COX-2 inhibitor NSAID drugs

Even before the FDA approved the first two of these drugs, celecoxib (CELEBREX) and rofecoxib (VIOXX), they were widely touted and promoted as the saviors for people who had developed ulcers and other serious gastrointestinal complications from the older NSAIDs. However, two large clinical studies of approximately one-year duration did not support removal of the standard NSAID warning of the risk of serious gastrointestinal events from the Celebrex and Vioxx labels. (see p. 299). These large studies did not show an advantage in overall safety (as measured by the total number of deaths, serious adverse events, and discontinuations and hospitalizations due to adverse events) favoring the selective COX-2 inhibitors compared to the other, older NSAIDs tested.

Further, one large study found a four- to five-fold increase in heart attacks in people using rofecoxib (VIOXX) compared to people using the older NSAID naproxen. The increase in heart attacks was also accompanied by an increase in other thrombotic (blood-clotting) adverse effects such as strokes and clots in the legs as well as problems with high blood pressure in the rofecoxib group compared to those taking naproxen.[12]

A cardiovascular risk warning has been added to the professional product labeling for rofecoxib (VIOXX) (see p. 299) and should also be added to celecoxib's labeling, since there is some concern from a recent review that this risk may be a property of other COX-2 inhibitors such as celexocib in addition to rofecoxib. The authors of this study concluded that "the use of selective COX-2 inhibitors might lead to increased cardiovascular events."[13]

In addition to the concern for increased cardiovascular risk with the COX-2 inhibitors, studies have been published concerning other adverse effects of these drugs, which can inhibit the body's ability to acutely respond to stress. Examples include the heart's ability to respond to heat stress[14] and the healing of a surgical wound,[15] an ulcer,[16] or a ligament injury.[17]

The other type of anti-inflammatory drugs, steroids, are very important hormones that have two functions: controlling inflammation and regulating vital body functions. They are not generally recommended first for treatment of rheumatoid arthritis. Steroids may be useful, however, for older adults who cannot take or do not respond to an NSAID. They can be locally injected into a joint if a specific joint is causing considerable pain. Whenever possible, steroids are to be avoided because they are associated with numerous adverse effects, including an increased risk of developing the bone-weakening disease osteoporosis (which is more likely to affect thin, small-boned white women).

Disease-Modifying Anti-Rheumatic Drugs (DMARDs)

In contrast to the anti-inflammatory drugs just described, the DMARDs not only relieve symptoms but may also slow or even modify the rheumatic disease process itself.

Until recently, most doctors reserved the use of DMARDs for patients who failed to respond to other therapies. Now, many physicians use DMARDs earlier and more aggressively in the hope of slowing disease progression and damage to joints. One of the first, still widely prescribed DMARDs, methotrexate (see p. 342), is often recommended as the first drug to be used in this category for patients with moderate to severe rheumatoid arthritis. There are four newer DMARDs, all of which are biologically based immune response modifiers: adalimumab (HUMIRA), anakinra (KINERET), etanercept (ENBREL), and infliximab (REMICADE) (see p. 327). In many patients, three of these drugs can cause a dramatic improvement in symptoms by blocking the action of a naturally occurring protein called tumor necrosis factor (TNF), believed to play a role in joint inflammation and damage. Elevated levels of TNF are found in the joint fluid of rheumatoid arthritis patients. The drug anakinra apparently works by blocking the receptor for interleukin-1 (IL-1), another naturally occurring protein that has a role in increasing joint inflammation and damage.

As with many drugs with dramatic benefits, these drugs can also pose serious risks by interfering with the body's immune mechanisms for fighting infectious diseases. Thus, it is required that information about increased risks of such diseases are tuberculosis (especially with infliximab) and other infections are included in the warnings for these drugs. As discussed in the monographs for these drugs (see p. 327), if you think you are getting any infection, notify your doctor immediately. For three of the four drugs (etanercept, infliximab, and adalimumab), if you experience the symptoms of heart failure, fatigue, difficulty breathing, swelling (especially in the legs and ankles), or rapid or "galloping" heartbeats, immediately notify your doctor.

Regardless of the drug therapy chosen by you and your doctor, an exercise program and physical therapy should be designed within the limits of pain. This will help to strengthen muscular action and maintain or improve range of motion in the joints. Inflammation also occurs in other rheumatologic diseases such as ankylosing spondylitis, scleroderma, temporal arteritis, and polymalgia rheumatica. Therapy follows the same general anti-inflammatory guidelines that are used to treat rheumatoid arthritis.

Osteoarthritis

Osteoarthritis is the most common type of arthritis and is usually related to the aging of the joint or prior injury. Often a mild condition, it may cause no symptoms or only occasional joint pain and stiffness. Most of the time osteoarthritis is not crippling, although a few people experience considerable pain and disability. It occasionally progresses to a point at which walking is difficult. Osteoarthritis frequently occurs in the finger joints, where it causes knobby bumps, and the spine, where it induces bone-like growths. These, however, do not commonly cause serious problems.

Osteoarthritis can often be treated without medical supervision.

Unlike rheumatoid arthritis, osteoarthritis is a degenerative joint disease that does not always have inflammation as a symptom. Obesity (being excessively overweight) aggravates the wear and tear on the inside surface of the joint. Not surprisingly, the most severe form of osteoarthritis is the type that affects the joints that bear the body's weight, such as the hips and the knees. A marked improvement is often seen after weight loss and an exercise program that helps to preserve full range of movement in the affected joints.

Treatment

Unlike rheumatoid arthritis, which requires high doses of aspirin to reduce inflammation, two 325 milligram tablets four times a day is often sufficient to control osteoarthritic pain in adults. Other pain relievers, including acetaminophen, are recommended for the person who cannot take aspirin. Be aware that in contrast to aspirin, acetaminophen relieves pain, but it is not effective in reducing inflammation. Therefore, we do not recommend the use of acetaminophen for the treatment of arthritis unless it is clear that you have osteoarthritis, which does not have a significant amount of inflammation.

Topical (skin) preparations marketed for treating arthritis (external salicylate-containing painkillers, such as Aspercreme and Myoflex) have no place in arthritis treatment. Salicylates (including aspirin) exert their effect on joints by absorption into the bloodstream. This is best done by swallowing tablets, not by applying cream.

Exercise should put an affected joint through its full range of motion. Swimming and walking are particularly good for this. You can start immediately and gradually improve your strength and flexibility. Under medical supervision, severe osteoarthritis is sometimes treated with physical therapy, orthopedic devices, and, in extreme cases, surgery.

Gout

Gout is related to the formation of uric acid crystals in the joints. White blood cells respond to the crystals by releasing certain enzymes into the joint space. The release of these enzymes causes the intense pain and inflammation of an acute attack of gout. The big toe is a common location of gouty pain. Medical treatment by a professional is required, and is usually sought, as the pain typically comes on suddenly and is often severe.

Treatment

Gout therapy can be divided into treatment of acute (sudden) attacks and prevention of uric acid crystal formation. Colchicine relieves an acute attack by inhibiting the white blood cell response. NSAIDs are also effective for treating an acute attack but require 12 to 24 hours before their onset of action. If you suffer from frequent attacks, or if your uric acid blood levels remain high between attacks, your doctor may prescribe either allopurinol or probenecid to reduce the uric acid in your body. Allopurinol decreases the amount of uric acid produced by the body. Probenecid increases the amount of uric acid that is eliminated by the body.

People who have gout should not use aspirin and other salicylates. Be aware that over-the-counter (nonprescription) products that contain aspirin cause retention of uric acid and may result in a worsening of gouty arthritis. Aspirin also reduces the effectiveness of several anti-gout medications, for example, probenecid.

Infectious Arthritis

Infectious arthritis occurs when a joint is invaded by bacteria, causing it to become red, hot, and swollen. It may be difficult to distinguish this type of arthritis from other types, as it frequently occurs in patients with other kinds of arthritis.

Treatment

This type of infection is almost always accompanied by fever and requires antibiotics, as directed by a physician, as soon as possible; otherwise the joint may be destroyed by the infectious process. No nonprescription preparations are appropriate as the sole treatment for infectious arthritis.

ALCOHOL WARNINGS ON ALL NONPRESCRIPTION PAIN RELIEVERS

The FDA has proposed regulations requiring alcohol warnings for all over-the-counter (OTC) pain relievers, which include aspirin, other salicylates, acetaminophen, ibuprofen, ketoprofen, and naproxen sodium. The proposal includes the following warning statements:

For Acetaminophen-Containing Products
"Alcohol Warning: If you drink three or more alcoholic beverages daily, you should ask your doctor whether you should take [the product name] or other pain relievers. [Product name] may increase your risk of liver damage."

For Aspirin, Carbaspirin Calcium, Choline Salicylate, Ibuprofen, Ketoprofen, Magnesium Salicylate, Naproxen Sodium, and Sodium Salicylate–Containing Products
"Alcohol Warning: If you drink three or more alcoholic beverages daily, ask your doctor whether you should take [the product name] or other pain relievers. [Product name] may increase your risk of stomach bleeding."

Some OTC pain relievers already carry an alcohol warning. This regulation is long overdue.

DRUG PROFILES

Nonsteroidal Anti-inflammatory Drugs (NSAIDs)

(Includes Acetic Acids, Fenamates, Naphthyalkanones, Oxicams, Propionic Acids, COX-2 Inhibitors)

Ibuprofen (eye byou *pro* fen)
Prescription:
MOTRIN (Wyeth)
Nonprescription:
ADVIL (Wyeth)
MEDIPREN (McNeil Consumer Products)

GENERIC: available
FAMILY: Nonsteroidal Anti-inflammatory Drugs (NSAIDs) (see p. 281)

PREGNANCY WARNING
NSAIDs have caused serious harm to human infants born to mothers taking these drugs during pregnancy, particularly in late pregnancy. Such infants have been born with damage to the heart, blood vessels, kidneys, and gastrointestinal tract. Tell your doctor if you are pregnant or thinking of becoming pregnant before you take these drugs.

BREAST-FEEDING WARNING
No information is available from either human or animal studies. Since it is likely that this drug, like many others, is excreted in human milk, you should consult with your doctor if you are planning to nurse.

Ibuprofen belongs to the family of drugs called nonsteroidal anti-inflammatory drugs, shortened to NSAIDs (*n* sayds), often used to treat arthritis in older adults. NSAIDs can cause serious harm, even fatalities, from bleeding in the stomach or intestines. Bleeding can occur at any time and without warning, and older people are more likely to experience adverse effects from bleeding. Older adults are also more likely to have reduced liver and kidney function. Some doctors believe people over age 70 should be

---

WARNING

NONSTEROIDAL ANTI-INFLAMMATORY DRUG (NSAID)–INDUCED GASTROINTESTINAL TOXICITY

All members of the NSAID family of drugs can cause gastrointestinal toxicity that can lead to gastrointestinal bleeding and hospitalization or death. The risk of gastrointestinal toxicity from these drugs increases with increasing doses and the length of treatment. If any of the following symptoms develop while you are taking an NSAID, stop taking the drug immediately and contact your doctor: severe abdominal or stomach pain, cramping, or burning, severe, and continuing nausea; heartburn or indigestion; bloody or black, tarry stools; vomiting blood or material that looks like coffee grounds; or spitting up blood.

---

started with half the usual dose of drugs in this group.[18]

Ibuprofen is used to treat fever and pain, including pain caused by two kinds of arthritis, osteoarthritis and rheumatoid arthritis. **In general, if you are over 60, you should take less than the usual adult dose, especially if you have decreased kidney function.**

Among the NSAIDs, the weight of the evidence is that ibuprofen is less toxic to the gastrointestinal tract, the main safety concern with NSAIDs, than other drugs in this family.[19–23]

Aspirin (see p. 304) is just as effective and less costly than other NSAIDs and is the drug of choice for treating pain, fever, and inflammation in people who do not have ulcers, gastritis (inflammation of the stomach), or an allergy to aspirin. Some rheumatologists (arthritis specialists) prefer aspirin to other NSAIDs for treating rheumatoid arthritis.[24]

Before You Use This Drug

Do not use if you have or have had:

- a severe allergic reaction to aspirin or any other NSAID
- peptic ulcers
- nasal polyps

Tell your doctor if you have or have had:

- a mild allergic reaction to aspirin or other NSAIDs (runny nose, hives, skin rash)
- heart, kidney, or liver problems
- hemophilia or other bleeding problems
- high blood pressure
- anemia
- asthma
- active alcohol dependence
- edema
- diabetes
- pregnancy or are breast-feeding
- stomach or intestinal problems, including Crohn's disease, peptic ulcer, and diverticulitis
- tobacco use
- inflammation of the mouth

Tell your doctor about any other drugs you take, including aspirin, herbs, vitamins, and other nonprescription products.

When You Use This Drug

- Get regular checkups when you take the drug for a long time.
- Do not drink alcohol. It irritates the stomach lining and increases the risk of stomach bleeding.
- Do not take two or more NSAID drugs at the same time.
- Protect yourself from the sun.
- Call your doctor immediately if you have flulike symptoms (chills, fever, muscle aches or pains) shortly before or at the same time as a skin rash. This may be a sign of a serious reaction to ibuprofen.

• You may feel dizzy when rising from a lying or sitting position. If you are lying down, hang your legs over the side of the bed for a few minutes, then get up slowly. When getting up from a chair, stay by the chair until you are sure that you are not dizzy.

• If you plan to have any surgery, including dental, tell your doctor that you take this drug.

How to Use This Drug

• If you miss a dose, take it as soon as possible, but skip it if it is almost time for the next dose. **Do not take double doses.**

• Do not share your medication with others.

• Take the drug at the same time(s) each day.

• Take with food or antacids to reduce stomach irritation.

• Take wih **a full glass (eight ounces) of water.** Do not lie down for 15 to 30 minutes afterward.

• Read patient information provided if you buy ibuprofen without a prescription.

• Store at room temperature, with lid on tightly. Do not store in the bathroom. Do not expose to heat, moisture, or strong light. Keep out of reach of children.

Interactions with Other Drugs

The following drugs, biologics (e.g., vaccines, therapeutic antibodies), or foods are listed in *Evaluations of Drug Interactions* 2003 as causing "highly clinically significant" or "clinically significant" interactions when used together with any of the drugs in this section. In some sections with multiple drugs, the interaction may have been reported for one but not all drugs in this section, but we include the interaction because the drugs in this section are similar to one another. We have also included potentially serious interactions listed in the drug's FDA-approved professional package insert or in published medical journal articles. There may be other drugs, especially those in the families of drugs listed below, that also will react with this drug to cause severe adverse effects. Make sure to tell your doctor and pharmacist the drugs you are taking and tell them if you are taking any of these interacting drugs:

abciximab, ardeparin, bendroflumethiazide, BENEMID, CAPOTEN, captopril, certoparin, clopidogrel, COUMADIN, cyclosporine, digoxin, DILANTIN, enoxaparin, eptifibatide, GARAMYCIN, gentamicin, INDERAL, INDERAL LA, INTEGRILIN, ketorolac, labetalol, LANOXICAPS, LANOXIN, lithium, LITHOBID, LITHONATE, LOVENOX, methotrexate, MINIPRESS, nadroparin, NATURETIN, NEORAL, NORMODYNE, NORVIR, phenytoin, PLAVIX, prazosin, probenecid, propranolol, TREXALL DOSE PACK, ritonavir, SANDIMMUNE, TORADOL, TRANDATE, warfarin.

The NSAIDs may diminish the blood-pressure-lowering effect of the angiotensin converting enzyme (ACE) inhibitors. See page 91 in chapter 4, Drugs for Heart Conditions, for a listing of ACE inhibitors.

The NSAIDs may reduce the effect of furosemide (LASIX).

The NSAIDs may reduce the effect of the thiazide diuretics (water pills). See page 60 in chapter 4, Drugs for Heart Conditions, for a listing of thiazide diuretics.

Adverse Effects

Call your doctor immediately if you experience:

• abdominal pain or swelling
• appetite loss
• bloody or black, tarry stools
• increase or decrease in blood pressure
• difficulty breathing
• unusual bruising

- chest pain
- chills
- confusion
- cough or hoarseness
- depression
- drowsiness
- pain, dryness, redness, irritation, or swelling of the eyes
- facial skin color changes
- fever
- gastrointestinal pain, cramping, or burning
- swollen glands
- hallucinations
- headache
- hearing change or ringing or buzzing in the ears
- heartburn
- hives on face, eyelids, or tongue
- indigestion
- lower back, neck, or side pain
- unusually heavy menstrual bleeding
- muscle cramps or pain
- nausea, vomiting
- nosebleeds, runny nose, or sneezing
- numbness, tingling, pain, or weakness in hands or feet
- pinpoint red spots on skin
- skin rash, blisters, hives, itching, scaling
- sore throat
- sores, ulcers, or white spots on lips or in mouth
- swelling of face, lips, tongue, fingers, lower legs, or feet
- unusual tiredness or weakness
- difficulty urinating
- bloody or cloudy urine
- vision change
- vomiting blood or material that looks like coffee grounds
- rapid weight gain
- yellow eyes or skin

Call your doctor if these symptoms continue:

- dizziness
- drowsiness
- mild to moderate headache
- pounding heartbeat
- trouble sleeping
- abdominal cramps, pain, or discomfort
- bloated feeling or gas
- constipation
- decrease or loss of appetite
- diarrhea
- stomach pain or discomfort
- heartburn
- indigestion
- nausea or vomiting
- irritation, dryness, or soreness of mouth
- nervousness or irritability
- sunburn

Periodic Tests

Ask your doctor which of these tests should be done periodically while you are taking this drug:

- kidney function tests
- liver function tests
- stool tests for possible blood loss
- hematocrit and/or hemoglobin test
- blood concentrations of creatinine, potassium, and urea nitrogen
- white blood cell count
- upper GI diagnostic tests
- ophthalmologic exams

———————

Flurbiprofen (flure *by* proe fen)
ANSAID (Pharmacia & Upjohn)
OCUFEN (Allergan)

Ketoprofen (kee toe *proe* fen)
ORUDIS (Wyeth-Ayerst)

Naproxen (na *prox* en)
ANAPROX (Roche Palo)
NAPROSYN (Roche Palo)

Limited Use

Diclofenac (dye *kloe* fen ak)
VOLTAREN (Novartis)

Etodolac (ee *toe* doe lak)
LODINE (Wyeth)

Fenoprofen (fen oh *proe* fen)
NALFON (Ranbaxy)

Meclofenamate (me kloe *fen* am ate)
(Mylan)

Mefenamic Acid (me fe *nam* ik)
PONSTEL (First Horizon)

Nabumetone (na *byoo* me tone)
RELAFEN (GlaxoSmithKline)

Oxaprozin (ox a *pro* zin)
DAYPRO (Searle)

Sulindac (syl *in* dak)
CLINORIL (Merck)

Tolmetin (*tole* me tin)
TOLECTIN (Ortho-McNeil)

GENERIC: available

FAMILY: Nonsteroidal Anti-inflammatory Drugs (NSAIDs)
(see p. 281)

PREGNANCY WARNING

NSAIDs have caused serious harm to infants born to mothers taking these drugs during pregnancy, particularly in late pregnancy. Such infants have been born with damage to the heart, blood vessels, kidneys, and gastrointestinal tract. Tell your doctor if you are pregnant or thinking of becoming pregnant before you take these drugs.

BREAST-FEEDING WARNING

Many NSAIDs are excreted in human milk. Because of the potential for adverse effects in nursing infants, you should not take these drugs while nursing.

These drugs belong to the family of drugs called nonsteroidal anti-inflammatory drugs, short-

---

> ## WARNING
>
> ### NONSTEROIDAL ANTI-INFLAMMATORY DRUG (NSAID)–INDUCED GASTROINTESTINAL TOXICITY
>
> All members of the NSAID family of drugs can cause gastrointestinal toxicity that can lead to gastrointestinal bleeding and hospitalization or death. The risk of gastrointestinal toxicity from these drugs increases with increasing doses and the length of treatment. If any of the following symptoms develop while you are taking an NSAID, stop taking the drug immediately and contact your doctor: severe abdominal or stomach pain, cramping, or burning; severe, and continuing nausea; heartburn or indigestion; bloody or black, tarry stools; vomiting blood or material that looks like coffee grounds; or spitting up blood.

ened to NSAIDs (*n* sayds), often used to treat arthritis in older adults. NSAIDs can cause serious harm, even fatalities, from bleeding in the stomach or intestines. Bleeding can occur at any time and without warning and older people are more likely to experience adverse effects from bleeding. Older adults are also more likely to have reduced liver and kidney function. Some doctors believe people over age 70 should be started with half the usual dose of drugs in this group.[18]

These drugs are used to treat mild to moderate pain and symptoms of rheumatoid arthritis, osteoarthritis, and spondylitis. **In general, if you are over 60, you should take less than the usual adult dose, especially if you have decreased kidney function.**

Among the NSAIDs, the weight of the evidence is that ibuprofen (see p. 288) is less toxic to the gastrointestinal tract, the main safety concern with NSAIDs, than other drugs in this family.[19–23]

Aspirin (see p. 279) is just as effective and

less costly than other NSAIDs and is the drug of choice to treat pain, fever, and inflammation in people who do not have ulcers, gastritis (inflammation of the stomach), or an allergy to aspirin. Some rheumatologists (arthritis specialists) prefer aspirin to other NSAIDs for rheumatoid arthritis.[24]

Before You Use This Drug

Do not use if you have or have had:

- a severe allergic reaction to aspirin or any other NSAID
- peptic ulcers
- nasal polyps
- bone marrow depression (diclofenac)
- blood diseases (diclofenac)
- are breast-feeding

Tell your doctor if you have or have had:

- a mild allergic reaction to aspirin or any other NSAIDs
- heart, kidney, or liver problems
- hemophilia or other bleeding problems
- high blood pressure
- blood transfusion[25]
- hemorrhoids[26]
- active alcohol dependence
- occupational exposure to chemicals[25]
- psoriasis[27]
- salt-restricted diet[18]
- seizures[28]
- anemia
- asthma
- diabetes
- pregnancy
- stomach or intestinal problems, including Crohn's disease, peptic ulcer, and diverticulitis
- inflammation of the mouth
- tobacco use

Tell your doctor about any other drugs you take, including aspirin, herbs, vitamins, and other nonprescription products.

When You Use This Drug

- Get regular checkups when you take the drug for a long time.
- Do not take two or more NSAID drugs at the same time.
- Protect yourself from the sun.
- Do not drink alcohol. It irritates the stomach lining and increases the risk of stomach bleeding.
- Call your doctor immediately if you have flulike symptoms (chills, fever, muscle aches or pains) shortly before or with a skin rash. This may indicate a serious reaction to diclofenac.
- You may feel dizzy when rising from a lying or sitting position. If you are lying down, hang your legs over the side of the bed for a few minutes, then get up slowly. When getting up from a chair, stay by the chair until you are sure that you are not dizzy. (See p. 13.)
- Do not drive or perform other activities that require alertness, because this drug may make you drowsy, dizzy, or lightheaded.
- If you plan to have any surgery, including dental, tell your doctor that you take this drug.

How to Use This Drug

- If you miss a dose, take it as soon as possible, but skip it if it is almost time for the next dose. **Do not take double doses.**
- Do not share your medication with others.
- Take the drug at the same time(s) each day.
- Take with food or antacids to reduce stomach irritation.
- Take with a full glass (eight ounces) of water. Do not lie down for 15 to 30 minutes afterward.
- Store at room temperature with lid on tightly. Do not store in the bathroom. Do not expose to heat, moisture, or strong light. Keep out of reach of children.

Interactions with Other Drugs

The following drugs, biologics (e.g., vaccines, therapeutic antibodies), or foods are listed in *Evaluations of Drug Interactions* 2003 as causing "highly clinically significant" or "clinically significant" interactions when used together with any of the drugs in this section. In some sections with multiple drugs, the interaction may have been reported for one but not all drugs in this section, but we include the interaction because the drugs in this section are similar to one another. We have also included potentially serious interactions listed in the drug's FDA-approved professional package insert or in published medical journal articles. There may be other drugs, especially those in the families of drugs listed below, that also will react with this drug to cause severe adverse effects. Make sure to tell your doctor and pharmacist the drugs you are taking and tell them if you are taking any of these interacting drugs:

abciximab, alendronate, ardeparin, bendroflumethiazide, CAPOTEN, captopril, certoparin, clopidogrel, COUMADIN, cyclosporine, digoxin, DILANTIN, DYAZIDE, DYRENIUM, enoxaparin, eptifibatide, FOLEX, FOSAMAX, GARAMYCIN, gentamicin, gold sodium thiomalate, INDERAL, INDERAL LA, INTEGRILIN, ketorolac, LANOXICAPS, LANOXIN, lithium, LITHOBID, LITHONATE, LOVENOX, MAXZIDE, methotrexate, MEXATE, MINIPRESS, MYOCHRYSINE, nadroparin, NATURETIN, NEORAL, NORVIR, phenytoin, PLAVIX, prazosin, propranolol, ritonavir, SANDIMMUNE, TORADOL, TREXALL DOSE PACK, triamterene, triamterene and hydrocholorothiazide, warfarin.

The NSAIDs may diminish the blood-pressure-lowering effect of the angiotensin converting enzyme (ACE) inhibitors. See page 91 in chapter 4, Drugs for Heart Conditions, for a listing of ACE inhibitors.

The NSAIDs may reduce the effect of furosemide (LASIX).

The NSAIDs may reduce the effect of the thiazide diuretics (water pills). See page 60 in chapter 4, Drugs for Heart Conditions, for a listing of thiazide diuretics.

Adverse Effects

Call your doctor immediately if you experience:

- abdominal pain or swelling
- appetite loss
- bloody or black, tarry stools
- increase or decrease in blood pressure
- difficulty breathing
- unusual bruising
- chest pains
- chills
- confusion
- convulsions
- cough or hoarseness
- depression
- drowsiness
- color changes in facial skin
- fever
- forgetfulness
- gastrointestinal pain, cramping, or burning
- swollen glands
- headache
- hearing change or ringing or buzzing in the ears
- heartburn
- hives on face, eyelids, or tongue
- indigestion
- lower back, neck, or side pain
- unusually heavy menstrual bleeding
- muscle cramps or pain
- nausea, vomiting
- nosebleeds

- numbness, tingling, pain, or weakness in hands or feet
- pinpoint red spots on skin
- psychotic reaction
- rectal bleeding
- skin rash, blisters, hives, itching, scaling
- sore throat
- sores, ulcers, or white spots on lips or in mouth
- swelling of face, lips, tongue, fingers, lower legs, or feet
- unusual tiredness or weakness
- difficulty urinating
- bloody or cloudy urine
- vision change
- vomiting blood or material that looks like coffee grounds
- rapid weight gain
- yellow eyes or skin

Call your doctor if these symptoms continue:

- constipation
- diarrhea
- bloated feeling or gas
- heartburn
- indigestion
- nausea, vomiting
- decreased appetite
- general feeling of discomfort or illness
- irritation, dryness, or soreness of mouth
- muscle weakness
- abdominal cramps, pain, or discomfort (mild to moderate)
- dizziness
- flushing or hot flashes
- fast or pounding heartbeat
- dizziness
- drowsiness
- mild to moderate headache
- trouble sleeping
- nervousness, irritability
- sunburn
- sweating

- bitter taste
- trembling or twitching
- unusual weakness with no other symptoms
- hair loss or changes in nails[29]

Periodic Tests

Ask your doctor which of these tests should be done periodically while you are taking this drug:

- kidney function tests
- liver function tests
- stool tests for possible blood loss
- hematocrit and/or hemoglobin test
- blood concentrations of creatinine, potassium, and urea nitrogen
- white blood cell count
- upper GI diagnostic tests
- ophthalmologic exams

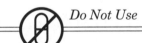

Do Not Use

ALTERNATIVE TREATMENT:
See Aspirin, p. 279, or Ibuprofen, p. 288.

Indomethacin (in doe *meth* a sin)
INDOCIN (Merck)

FAMILY: Nonsteroidal Anti-inflammatory Drugs (NSAIDs)
(see p. 281)

Indomethacin belongs to the family of drugs called nonsteroidal anti-inflammatory drugs, shortened to NSAIDs, often used to treat arthritis in older adults. NSAIDs can cause serious harm, even fatalities, from bleeding in the stomach or intestines. Bleeding can occur at any time and without warning and older people are more likely to experience adverse effects from bleeding. Older adults are also more likely to have reduced liver and kidney function. Some doctors believe people over age 70 should be

WARNING

NONSTEROIDAL ANTI-INFLAMMATORY DRUG (NSAID)–INDUCED GASTROINTESTINAL TOXICITY

All members of the NSAID family of drugs can cause gastrointestinal toxicity that can lead to gastrointestinal bleeding and hospitalization or death. The risk of gastrointestinal toxicity from these drugs increases with increasing doses and the length of treatment. If any of the following symptoms develop while you are taking an NSAID, stop taking the drug immediately and contact your doctor: severe abdominal or stomach pain, cramping, or burning; severe and continuing nausea, heartburn, or indigestion; bloody or black, tarry stools; vomiting blood or material that looks like coffee grounds; or spitting up blood.

started with half the usual dose of drugs in this group.[18]

Indomethacin relieves the pain and inflammation of rheumatoid arthritis and acute gout, and reduces fever. This drug is not recommended for older adults.[30] It can cause depression, mood changes, and confusion. Indomethacin may also make epilepsy or Parkinson's disease worse, cause more stomach and intestinal bleeding than aspirin, and hide the signs of any infection you might have.

Among the NSAIDs, the weight of the evidence is that ibuprofen (see p. 288) is less toxic to the gastrointestinal tract, the main safety concern with NSAIDs, than other drugs in this family.[19–23]

Indomethicin is included on a well-recognized list of drugs that are inappropriate for use in older adults because of all of the available NSAIDs; this drug produces the most central nervous system adverse effects.[30]

Aspirin (see p. 279) is just as effective and less costly than other NSAIDs and is the drug of choice for treating pain, fever, and inflammation in people who do not have ulcers, gastritis (inflammation of the stomach), or an allergy to aspirin. Some rheumatologists (arthritis specialists) prefer aspirin to other NSAIDs for treating rheumatoid arthritis.[24]

Do Not Use

ALTERNATIVE TREATMENT:
See Narcotics, p. 282.

Ketorolac (kee *toe* role ak)
TORADOL (Roche)

FAMILY: Nonsteroidal Anti-inflammatory Drugs (NSAIDs)
(see p. 281)

The following is an excerpt from the black-box warning required on the professional product label or package insert for this drug.[31]

Ketorolac belongs to the family of drugs called nonsteroidal anti-inflammatory drugs, shortened to NSAIDs, often used to treat arthritis in older adults. NSAIDs can cause serious harm, even fatalities, from bleeding in the stomach or intestines. Bleeding can occur at any time and without warning and older people are more likely to experience adverse effects from bleeding. Older adults are also more likely to have reduced liver and kidney function. Some doctors believe people over age 70 should be started with half the usual dose of drugs in this group.[18]

Ketorolac is only approved for short-term use, five days or less, in the treatment of acute pain. This drug is available in both oral (by mouth) and injectable forms.

The professional product labeling or package insert for ketorolac warns about the risks of gastrointestinal bleeding and kidney and liver damage, warns against the use of the drug in

FDA BLACK BOX WARNING

TORADOL, a nonsteroidal anti-inflammatory drug (NSAID), is indicated for the short-term (up to 5 days in adults) management of moderately severe acute pain that requires analgesia at the opioid level. It is NOT indicated for minor or chronic painful conditions. TORADOL is a potent NSAID analgesic, and its administration carries many risks. The resulting NSAID-related adverse events can be serious in certain patients for whom TORADOL is indicated, especially when the drug is used inappropriately. Increasing the dose of TORADOL beyond the label recommendations will not provide better efficacy but will result in increasing the risk of developing serious adverse events.

GASTROINTESTINAL EFFECTS

TORADOL can cause peptic ulcers, gastrointestinal bleeding, and/or perforation. Therefore, TORADOL is contraindicated in patients with active peptic ulcer disease, in patients with recent gastrointestinal bleeding or perforation, and in patients with a history of peptic ulcer disease or gastrointestinal bleeding.

RENAL [KIDNEY] EFFECTS

TORADOL is contraindicated in patients with advanced renal impairment and in patients at risk for renal failure due to volume depletion.

RISK OF BLEEDING

TORADOL inhibits platelet function and is, therefore, contraindicated in patients with suspected or confirmed cerebrovascular bleeding, patients with hemorrhagic diathesis, incomplete hemostatis and those at high risk of bleeding.

TORADOL is contraindicated as a prophylactic analgesic before any major surgery and is contraindicated intraoperatively when hemostatis is critical because of the increased risk of bleeding.

HYPERSENSITIVITY

Hypersensitivity reactions, ranging from bronchospasm to anaphylactic shock, have occurred and appropriate counteractive measures must be available when administering the first dose of TORADOL IM/IV. TORADOL is contraindicated in patients with previously demonstrated hypersensitivity to ketorolac tromethamine or allergic manifestations to aspirin or other nonsteroidal anti-inflammatory drugs (NSAIDs).

INTRATHECAL OR EPIDURAL ADMINISTRATION [SPINAL ADMINISTRATION]

TORADOL is contraindicated in intrathecal or epidural administration due to its alcohol content.

LABOR, DELIVERY AND NURSING

The use of TORADOL in labor and delivery is contraindicated because it may adversely affect fetal circulation and inhibit uterine contractions.

The use of TORADOL is contraindicated in nursing mothers because of the potential adverse effects of prostaglandin-inhibiting drugs on neonates.

CONCOMITANT USE WITH NSAIDS

TORADOL is contraindicated in patients currently receiving ASA [aspirin] or NSAIDs because of the cumulative risk of inducing serious NSAID-related side effects.

WARNING

NONSTEROIDAL
ANTI-INFLAMMATORY
DRUG (NSAID)–INDUCED
GASTROINTESTINAL TOXICITY

All members of the NSAID family of drugs can cause gastrointestinal toxicity that can lead to gastrointestinal bleeding and hospitalization or death. The risk of gastrointestinal toxicity from these drugs increases with increasing doses and the length of treatment. If any of the following symptoms develop while you are taking an NSAID, stop taking the drug immediately and contact your doctor: severe abdominal or stomach pain, cramping, or burning; severe and continuing nausea, heartburn, or indigestion; bloody or black, tarry stools; vomiting blood or material that looks like coffee grounds; or spitting up blood.

---

labor and delivery, against the drug being used by nursing mothers, that it should not be used before or during surgery, and using anything but the lowest dose in small or older adults.

Among the NSAIDs, the weight of the evidence is that ibuprofen (see p. 288) is less toxic to the gastrointestinal tract, the main safety concern with NSAIDs, than other drugs in this family.[19–23]

Ketorolac remains on a well-recognized list of drugs that are inappropriate for use in older adults.[30]

Aspirin (see p. 304) is just as effective as and less costly than other NSAIDs and is the drug of choice for treating pain, fever, and inflammation in people who do not have ulcers, gastritis (inflammation of the stomach), or an allergy to aspirin. Some rheumatologists (arthritis specialists) prefer aspirin to other NSAIDs for treating rheumatoid arthritis.[24]

 Do Not Use

ALTERNATIVE TREATMENT:
See Aspirin, p. 304, or Ibuprofen, p. 288.

Piroxicam (peer *ox* i cam)
FELDENE (Pfizer)

FAMILY: Nonsteroidal Anti-inflammatory Drugs (NSAIDs)
(see p. 281)

WARNING

NONSTEROIDAL
ANTI-INFLAMMATORY
DRUG (NSAID)–INDUCED
GASTROINTESTINAL TOXICITY

All members of the NSAID family of drugs can cause gastrointestinal toxicity that can lead to gastrointestinal bleeding and hospitalization or death. The risk of gastrointestinal toxicity from these drugs increases with increasing doses and the length of treatment. If any of the following symptoms develop while you are taking an NSAID, stop taking the drug immediately and contact your doctor: severe abdominal or stomach pain, cramping, or burning; severe and continuing nausea, heartburn, or indigestion; bloody or black, tarry stools; vomiting blood or material that looks like coffee grounds; or spitting up blood.

Piroxicam belongs to the family of drugs called nonsteroidal anti-inflammatory drugs, shortened to NSAIDs, often used to treat arthritis in older adults. NSAIDs can cause serious harm, even fatalities, from bleeding in the stomach or intestines. Bleeding can occur at any time and without warning and older people are more likely to experience adverse effects from bleeding. Older adults are also more likely to have reduced liver and kidney function. Some doctors believe people over age 70 should be started with half the usual dose of drugs in this group.[18]

Public Citizen's Health Research Group unsuccessfully petitioned the Food and Drug Administration (FDA) to remove piroxicam from the market in 1994 because of its toxicity.[32]

Piroxicam relieves pain and inflammation caused by two kinds of arthritis, rheumatoid arthritis and osteoarthritis. **It has caused serious adverse effects and numerous deaths,** especially in oder adults.[33],[34] **People over 60 are more likely than other users of this drug to suffer stomach and intestinal bleeding, ulcers, and perforations.** These adverse effects have occurred even when patients were taking only the recommended dose. People in all age groups have had **serious skin reactions, some of which have been fatal, while taking piroxicam.**

Piroxicam remains on a list of drugs that are inappropriate for use in older adults because of its toxicity.[30]

Among the NSAIDs, the weight of the evidence is that ibuprofen (see p. 288) is less toxic to the gastrointestinal tract, the main safety concern with NSAIDs, than other drugs in this family.[19–23]

Aspirin is just as effective and less costly than other NSAIDs and is the drug of choice for treating pain, fever, and inflammation in people who do not have ulcers, gastritis (inflammation of the stomach), or an allergy to aspirin. Some rheumatologists (arthritis specialists) still prefer aspirin to other NSAIDs for treating rheumatoid arthritis.[24]

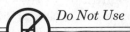 *Do Not Use*

ALTERNATIVE TREATMENT:
See Aspirin, p. 304, or Ibuprofen, p. 288.

Celecoxib (sell a *kox* ib)
CELEBREX (Pfizer, Pharmacia & Upjohn)

Meloxicam (mel *ox* i cam)
MOBIC (Boehringer Ingelheim)

Rofecoxib (roe fe *kox* ib)
VIOXX (Merck)

Valdecoxib (val de *kox* ib)
BEXTRA (Pfizer)

GENERIC: not available

FAMILY: Nonsteroidal Anti-inflammatory Drugs (NSAIDs) (see p. 281)

PREGNANCY WARNING

These drugs caused fetal harm in animal studies including an increase in skeletal malformations, heart defects, and fetal death. Because of the potential for serious adverse effects to the fetus, these drugs should not be used by pregnant women.

BREAST-FEEDING WARNING

These drugs are excreted in animal milk at concentrations equal to that in the mother's plasma; it is likely that this also occurs in humans. Because of the potential for serious adverse effects in nursing infants, you should not take these drugs while nursing.

WARNING

NONSTEROIDAL ANTI-INFLAMMATORY DRUG (NSAID)–INDUCED GASTROINTESTINAL TOXICITY

All members of the NSAID family of drugs can cause gastrointestinal toxicity that can lead to gastrointestinal bleeding and hospitalization or death. The risk of gastrointestinal toxicity from these drugs increases with increasing doses and the length of treatment. If any of the following symptoms develop while you are taking an NSAID, stop taking the drug immediately and contact your doctor: severe abdominal or stomach pain, cramping, or burning; severe and continuing nausea, heartburn, or indigestion; bloody or black, tarry stools; vomiting blood or material that looks like coffee grounds; or spitting up blood.

One large study found a four- to-fivefold increase in heart attacks in people using rofecoxib (VIOXX) compared to people using the older NSAID naproxen. The increase in heart attacks was also accompanied by an increase in other thrombotic (blood-clotting) adverse effects such as strokes and clots in the legs as well as problems with high blood pressure.[12] This risk may be a property of other COX-2 inhibitors such as celecoxib in addition to rofecoxib.[13]

In addition to the concern for increased cardiovascular risk with the COX-2 inhibitors, studies have been published concerning other adverse effects of these drugs that can inhibit the body's ability to acutely respond to stress. Examples include the heart's ability to respond to heat stress[14] and the healing of a surgical wound,[15] an ulcer,[16] or a ligament injury.[17]

Celecoxib

This drug exploded onto the market in early 1999 with a successfully managed media campaign as "super-aspirin," a "breakthrough" drug that is as effective as the older nonsteroidal anti-inflammatory drugs (NSAIDs) and supposedly without the same risk of gastrointestinal (GI) toxicity, the adverse effect that is the most serious concern with the use of NSAIDs.

Overlooked by uncritical journalists, too many health care professionals, and a duped public was the fact that celecoxib was approved by the FDA with exactly the same warnings about risk of GI bleeding and death as the other 19 NSAIDs that were on the market at that time.[35] Celecoxib's manufacturer could not, and has not, proved to the FDA that their drug was any safer as far as GI toxicity is concerned than the legion of other NSAIDs already available at much lower cost.

Celecoxib is remarkable in one respect. Despite the fact that it is an unremarkable treatment for arthritis and pain, it racked up $1 billion in sales before a single clinical trial was published comparing it to an existing drug for the treatment of arthritis.[36] In recent years, the core business of the pharmaceutical industry has been marketing, not research, and celecoxib is the icon of how successful marketing can be, even for a drug that is no better or safer (just more expensive) than drugs already on the market.

Celecoxib's image was fashioned around the theory that it is a specific inhibitor of cyclooxygenase-2—COX-2 for short. All NSAIDs, including celecoxib, work by inhibiting the COX enzymes. Two forms of this enzyme are known to exist, COX-1 and COX-2. In theory, both COX-1 and COX-2 reduce the symptoms of arthritis but also lead to the adverse effects associated with NSAIDs. If COX-2 were selectively blocked, the reasoning goes, arthritis pain would be relieved, without the serious GI and other adverse effects seen with the use of NSAIDs.

In December 1998, the Public Citizen's Health Research Group testified before the FDA's Arthritis Drug Advisory Committee reviewing celecoxib. We cautioned that the COX-2 enzyme may have other important physiological functions. These include GI tract tissue repair, cell integrity, kidney function, kidney development in the fetus during pregnancy, ovarian function and fertility, and cartilage repair. New classes of drugs such as celecoxib, and other COX-2 drugs in the pipeline, offer not only new mechanisms of action but also new mechanisms of potential toxicity and the possibility of a new spectrum of adverse effects.[37]

The manufacturer scored an egregious advertising coup with the publication of the CLASS study (Celecoxib Long-term Arthritis Safety Study) in the September 13, 2000, issue of the *Journal of the American Medical Association (JAMA)*.[38] The results of this six-month-long study were "spun" to say that celecoxib was safer on the GI tract than other NSAIDs. A cautiously optimistic editorial about the therapeutic benefits of celecoxib accompanied the publication of the CLASS study.[39]

The FDA's Arthritis Advisory Committee met on February 7, 2001, to review a request by celecoxib's manufacturer to change the drug's labeling to indicate that it is a GI-safe NSAID, based on the results of the CLASS study. A company must first prove to the FDA any claim of superiority for its drug over other drugs before the claim can legally be made. At this meeting it was revealed that the company actually had data on the safety of celecoxib for as long as 16 months, rather than just the six months of results published in *JAMA*.

The FDA medical officer who reviewed the CLASS study for the February advisory committee meeting concluded that the company had failed to show a statistically significant lower rate of serious GI adverse reactions compared to the other drugs included in the study. The other NSAIDs were usual doses of ibuprofen (MOTRIN) and diclofenac (VOLTAREN).[39]

We mentioned earlier our concern about the possibility of new adverse reactions when drugs work in new ways, such as the selective inhibition of the COX-2 enzyme. A recent reanalysis of the CLASS study indicated the possibility of an increased risk of cardiovascular adverse events with COX-2 drugs.[13] A cardiovascular risk warning has been added to the professional product labeling for rofecoxib (VIOXX), another COX-2 NSAID (see p. 299), and should also be added to celecoxib's labeling.

Because celecoxib is chemically related to the sulfonamides (sulfa drugs), it must not be taken by those who have had an allergic reaction to a sulfa drug.

Meloxicam

This NSAID was approved in April 2000 by the FDA, making it the 23rd nonsteroidal anti-inflammatory drug on the United States market. We have listed meloxicam as **Do Not Use** because there is no evidence that it is safer or

more effective than some of the older NSAIDs such as ibuprofen (MOTRIN), and because of its excessive cost compared to the older generic NSAIDs.

Meloxicam is approved only for the relief of the signs and symptoms of osteoarthritis, not for acute pain or for the treatment of rheumatoid arthritis.

Meloxicam is by no means a new drug and it joins the list of old drugs first marketed in other countries that have been recycled in the United States. Meloxicam has been available in the UK since September 1996 and has been promoted there as a selective and thus supposedly safer NSAID for the GI tract. GI adverse effects are the most serious reactions seen with the NSAIDs.

All NSAIDs, including meloxicam, work by inhibiting the enzyme cyclooxygenase, or COX for short. Two forms of COX are known to exist, COX-1 and COX-2. In theory, blocking both of these enzymes reduces the symptoms of arthritis but also leads to the adverse GI effects associated with NSAIDs. It is thought, in theory, that if COX-2 is selectively blocked, arthritis pain would be relieved without the serious GI adverse effects seen with other NSAIDs.

In the August 1998 issue of *Current Problems in Pharmacovigilance*, a newsletter published by the British Medicines Control Agency and the Committee on Safety of Medicines, it was reported that in the first year and nine months of marketing experience with meloxicam in that country, there had been a total of 1,339 adverse reactions reported to the government for the drug. Of these, 41 percent, or 549, were GI adverse effects, 99 being reports of perforations, ulcers, or bleeding, including five deaths. The British drug regulatory authorities required a major revision in the warnings for meloxicam because of these severe GI adverse effects.[40]

The internationally respected *Drug and Therapeutics Bulletin*, the UK's equivalent of our *Medical Letter on Drugs and Therapeutics*, said in its August 1998 issue: *"There is no convincing evidence that the risk of the severest gastrointestinal events, namely peptic ulceration, perforation and bleeding, is lower with meloxicam than with other NSAIDs when given at equi-effective doses. Meloxicam has not been compared with ibuprofen [MOTRIN] which comes out best in most safety assessments."* [41]

If you require treatment with an NSAID, you should not be taking meloxicam. There are more effective, safer, and less expensive drugs on the market such as ibuprofen.

Rofecoxib

This is another heavily promoted, overpriced nonsteroidal anti-inflammatory drug (NSAID) that now carries a new warning in its professional product labeling or package insert about its use by people with a history of heart disease. The drug is approved by the FDA for the management of osteo- and rheumatoid arthritis, acute pain, and painful menstrual periods.

Rofecoxib's image was fashioned around the theory that it is a specific inhibitor of cyclooxygenase-2—COX-2 for short. All NSAIDs, including rofecoxib, work by inhibiting the COX enzymes. Two forms of this enzyme are known to exist, COX-1 and COX-2. In theory, both COX-1 and COX-2 reduce the symptoms of arthritis but also lead to the adverse effects associated with NSAIDs. If COX-2 were selectively blocked, the reasoning goes, arthritis pain would be relieved, without the serious GI and other adverse effects seen with the use of NSAIDs.

The heart disease warning is based on results of a study called VIGOR, short for Vioxx GI Clinical Research study.[42] VIGOR was submitted to the FDA by Merck in a request to change rofecoxib's professional product labeling or package insert to say that it is a safer NSAID in regards to GI toxicity compared to the numerous other drugs in its family. This is important for drug companies because they cannot legally make superiority claims for either safety or effectiveness for their products unless they first submit proof for such claims to the FDA.

The VIGOR study was discussed at an FDA Arthritis Advisory Committee meeting held on February 8, 2001, at which time it was revealed that patients taking rofecoxib who should have been taking aspirin had a statistically significant, fivefold increase in heart attacks compared to patients taking naproxen (NAPROSYN), another NSAID. This amounted to 20 heart attacks with rofecoxib (out of 4,047 patients) compared to four with naproxen (out of 4,029 patients). The increase in heart attacks was also accompanied by an increase in other thrombotic (blood-clotting) adverse effects such as strokes and clots in the legs as well as problems with high blood pressure in the rofecoxib group compared to those taking naproxen.[12]

Rofecoxib was found to cause fewer serious adverse GI reactions compared to naproxen in the VIGOR study in those patients who were not taking rofecoxib and aspirin together. At this time, it is not known if adding aspirin to rofecoxib will abolish the GI protective effect seen with rofecoxib alone compared to naproxen.[43] Rofecoxib can be promoted as safer than naproxen on the GI tract, but not as the safest NSAID, for two reasons. First, to make the claim as the safest NSAID the VIGOR study would need to be repeated, comparing rofecoxib directly to ibuprofen. Second, adding up rofecoxib's GI toxicity with its cardiovascular toxicity, it is clearly not the safest NSAID.

The FDA did not allow Merck to remove the GI toxicity warning (see our boxed warning above) from the drug's label that is the same for all NSAIDs on the market. Aspirin and naproxen inhibit the clumping together of elements in the blood called platelets; rofecoxib does not. Platelets are one of the body's first defenses against bleeding, but they are also involved early in the development of heart attack and stroke. This is why aspirin is prescribed to prevent heart attack and stroke in those at high risk of developing these serious cardiovascular events.

The text of the new warning contains the information we discussed above in dense technical jargon:

"Because of its lack of platelet effects, VIOXX is not a substitute for aspirin for cardiovascular prophylaxis. Therefore, in patients taking VIOXX, antiplatelet therapies should not be discontinued and should be considered in patients with an indication for cardiovascular prophylaxis. Prospective, long-term studies on concomitant administration of VIOXX and aspirin evaluating cardiovascular outcomes have not been conducted."[44]

Merck argued at the February 8, 2001, Arthritis Advisory Committee meeting that the increased number of serious cardiovascular events seen compared to naproxen in the VIGOR study was solely due to the "protective" effect of naproxen on platelets. The FDA medical officer who reviewed the VIGOR study agreed that Merck's explanation could not be totally discarded, but he found several lines of evidence against the theory that the effect of naproxen on platelets is the only explanation for the VIGOR results.

There are no studies with naproxen to support the assumption that it is effective in decreasing the risk of cardiovascular events. The effect of naproxen on platelets is short-lived, while that of aspirin is irreversible. The effect of naproxen in reducing cardiovascular events relative to rofecoxib in the VIGOR study was 58%. This effect exceeds that of aspirin compared to placebo in reducing cardiovascular risks in other trials, which is 25 to 30%. The medical officer also commented that the absence of cardiovascular problems in the original review of rofecoxib may be explained by the short duration and low doses of rofecoxib used in the majority of the studies submitted to the FDA by Merck.[43]

The most likely explanation, in our view, is that the VIGOR results are a combination of naproxen's ability to inhibit platelets and rofecoxib's new way of working (selective inhibition of the COX-2 enzyme) to directly increase the risk of cardiovascular adverse events.

Valdecoxib

Valdecoxib is another redundant "me too" drug in the crowded NSAID family of drugs. This drug is chemically similar to celecoxib, and both valdecoxib and celecoxib are produced by the same manufacturer.

Valdecoxib's image was fashioned around the theory that it is a specific inhibitor of cyclooxygenase-2—COX-2 for short. All NSAIDs, including valdecoxib, work by inhibiting the COX enzymes. Two forms of this enzyme are known to exist, COX-1 and COX-2. In theory, both COX-1 and COX-2 reduce the symptoms of arthritis but also lead to the adverse effects associated with NSAIDs. If COX-2 were selectively blocked, the reasoning goes, arthritis pain would be relieved, without the serious GI and other adverse effects seen with the use of NSAIDs.

This NSAID carries the same warning in its professional product labeling or package insert about GI toxicity, as do all of the other drugs in the NSAID family.[45]

Valdexocib was to be the second prong of a two-pronged marketing strategy that would begin with parecoxib, an injectable form of valdecoxib that breaks down in the body to valdecoxib. The plan was to have both an injectable and an oral drug. The manufacturer submitted its application for the approval of parecoxib to the FDA in October 2000 for the management of acute pain.[46] The FDA informed Pharmacia in July 2001 that parecoxib was "not approvable." The company did not reveal why the application for parecoxib was rejected.[47]

The manufacturer filed its application for valdecoxib's FDA marketing clearance in March 2001, asking that it be approved for the treatment of acute pain, painful menstrual periods, and osteo- and rheumatoid arthritis.[48] When valdecoxib was approved in November 2001, the drug had failed to gain FDA approval for acute pain and is still not approved to treat acute pain.[45]

Pfizer did not let the failure to gain FDA approval for acute pain for valdecoxib deter it from making the drug a marketing success. The *New York Times* reported on November 22, 2002, that an article published in the *Journal of the American Dental Association*[49] concluded that valdecoxib was effective for acute pain following dental surgery. This was six months after the FDA rejected the drug for acute pain.[50]

Valdecoxib sold almost $1 billion in 2003.

If you require treatment with an NSAID, you should not be taking valdecoxib. There are more effective, safer, and less expensive drugs on the market, such as ibuprofen.

Salicylates

Aspirin/Acetylsalicylic Acid
GENUINE BAYER ASPIRIN
(Bayer Healthcare)
ECOTRIN ENTERIC-COATED
(GlaxoSmithKline)
EASPRIN 975 MILLIGRAMS
(Parke-Davis)

GENERIC: available
FAMILY: Salicylates
(see p. 279)

PREGNANCY WARNING

NSAIDs have caused serious harm to human infants born to mothers taking these drugs during pregnancy, particularly the third trimester of pregnancy. Such infants have been born with damage to the heart, blood vessels, kidney, and gastrointestinal tract. Tell your doctor if you are pregnant or thinking of becoming pregnant before you take these drugs.

BREAST-FEEDING WARNING

Many NSAIDs are excreted in human milk. Because of the potential for adverse effects in nursing infants, you should not take these drugs while nursing.

ASPIRIN/REYE'S SYNDROME ALERT

Do not use this product for treating chicken pox, flu, or flulike illness if you are under 40. It will increase the risk of contracting Reye's syndrome, a rare but often fatal disease.

WARNING

NONSTEROIDAL ANTI-INFLAMMATORY DRUG (NSAID)–INDUCED GASTROINTESTINAL TOXICITY

All members of the NSAID family of drugs can cause gastrointestinal toxicity that can lead to gastrointestinal bleeding and hospitalization or death. The risk of gastrointestinal toxicity from these drugs increases with increasing doses and the length of treatment.

If any of the following symptoms develop while you are taking an NSAID, stop taking the drug immediately and contact your doctor: severe abdominal or stomach pain, cramping, or burning; severe and continuing nausea, heartburn, or indigestion; bloody or black, tarry stools; vomiting blood or material that looks like coffee grounds; or spitting up blood.

Aspirin belongs to the family of drugs called nonsteroidal anti-inflammatory drugs, shortened to NSAIDs, often used to treat arthritis in older adults. NSAIDs can cause serious harm, even fatalities, from bleeding in the stomach or intestines. Bleeding can occur at any time and without warning, and older people are more likely to experience adverse effects from bleeding. Older adults are also more likely to have reduced liver and kidney function. Some doctors believe people over age 70 should be started with half the usual dose of drugs in this group.[18]

There are several forms of aspirin available. These are plain aspirin, enteric-coated aspirin, and buffered aspirin. In previous editions of *Worst Pills, Best Pills,* we recommended the use of enteric-coated aspirin over plain or buffered aspirin because enteric coating was once thought to reduce the overall risk of GI bleeding, as this form of aspirin does not dissolve in the stomach. The weight of the evidence now indicates that the risk of GI bleeding is similar among plain, enteric-coated, and buffered aspirin,[19,51–53] probably because, in part, once aspirin is absorbed into the blood it can cause GI bleeding not related to local irritation but due to its effects on diminishing the natural protection of the GI tract and blood clotting.

We have listed buffered aspirin as a **Do Not Use** drug (see p. 308) because it is no better than plain aspirin and is more costly.

Aspirin is also prescribed as a preventive measure for illnesses such as heart disease. The FDA has approved the use of aspirin for patients

- who have had a previous heart attack or unstable chest pain (angina) to reduce death and nonfatal heart attacks;
- with chronic stable angina to reduce MI and sudden death;
- who have undergone revascularization procedures, such as the placement of a stent, for a preexisting condition;
- with a suspected acute heart attack to reduce vascular mortality;
- who have had ischemic stroke or transient ischemia of the brain due to fibrin platelet emboli (clot) to reduce death and nonfatal stroke.

The use of aspirin in the above situation is known as *secondary prevention* because the patient already had a preexisting medical cardiovascular condition.

In 2003, Bayer, the producer of Genuine Bayer Aspirin, petitioned the FDA to allow the use of aspirin to reduce the risk of a first heart attack in patients with a coronary heart disease risk of 10% or greater over 10 years. This is known as *primary prevention.*

On December 8, 2003, the FDA's Cardio-Renal Drugs Advisory Committee met to evaluate the results of five published clinical trials[54–58] submitted by Bayer to support their petition. The committee refused to recommend aspirin for primary prevention. Some of the concerns raised by the committee or by FDA staff included:

- In only one[57] of the five studies submitted by Bayer was there a reduction in fatal heart attacks. In this study there was a larger, though not statistically significant, increase in fatal sudden death, strokes, or other fatal cardiovascular events.
- "The lack of efficacy [prevention of cardiovascular events, primarily a first heart attack] in the face of associated morbidity, i.e., bleeding, prevents the recommendation of use of aspirin for the primary prevention of cardiovascular morbidity and mortality."[59]

The lack of evidence of an aspirin benefit in the primary prevention of heart attack is clearly outweighed by the increased risk of bleeding from aspirin, and aspirin should not be used for the primary prevention of heart attacks.

Before You Use This Drug

Do not use if you have or have had:

- bleeding ulcers
- other bleeding problems
- severe sensitivity reaction to aspirin or other NSAIDs (for aspirin only)
- nasal polyps associated with asthma (for aspirin only)
- poor kidney function (for choline and magnesium salicylates)
- are breast-feeding

Tell your doctor if you have or have had:

- mild allergic reaction to aspirin or other NSAIDs
- bleeding problems
- vitamin K deficiency
- ulcer or other stomach problems
- kidney, liver, or heart problems
- asthma (for aspirin only)
- anemia
- glucose-6-phosphate dehydrogenase deficiency
- gout
- overactive thyroid
- high blood pressure
- symptoms of nasal polyps

Tell your doctor about any other drugs you take, including aspirin, herbs, vitamins, and other nonprescription products.

When You Use This Drug

- Get regular checkups when you take the drug for a long time.
- Caution if you take other aspirin or salicylate drugs at the same time to avoid overdose.
- If taking for pain and pain lasts longer than ten days for adults or five days for children, contact your doctor.
- If taking for fever and fever lasts longer than three days or you get worse, new symptoms, redness, or swelling, contact your doctor.
- If taking for sore throat and sore throat is severe, persists longer than two days, or there is fever, headache, rash, nausea, or vomiting, contact your doctor.
- Do not drink alcohol. This combination increases the risk of stomach or intestinal bleeding.
- Never take more than the amount prescribed by your doctor or recommended on the package label.
- **Caution diabetics:** see p. 405.
- If you are treating yourself, call your doctor if your symptoms do not improve or if you have

a fever that lasts more than three days or returns.

- Do not take aspirin for five days before any surgery, unless your doctor tells you otherwise. Aspirin interferes with your body's ability to stop bleeding.
- Never place aspirin directly on teeth or gums because it irritates these tissues.
- Do not chew aspirin within one week after you have had any type of surgery in your mouth.

How to Use This Drug

- If you miss a dose, take it as soon as you remember, but skip it if it is almost time for the next dose. **Do not take double doses.**
- Do not share your medication with others.
- Take the drug at the same time(s) each day.
- Take tablets with food and **a full glass (eight ounces) of water.** Do not break, chew, or crush long-acting forms of this drug. Do not lie down for 30 minutes.
- Store at room temperature with lid on tightly. Do not store in the bathroom. Do not expose to heat, moisture, or strong light. Keep out of reach of children.

Interactions with Other Drugs

The following drugs, biologics (e.g., vaccines, therapeutic antibodies), or foods are listed in *Evaluations of Drug Interactions* 2003 as causing "highly clinically significant" or "clinically significant" interactions when used together with any of the drugs in this section. In some sections with multiple drugs, the interaction may have been reported for one but not all drugs in this section, but we include the interaction because the drugs in this section are similar to one another. We have also included potentially serious interactions listed in the drug's FDA-approved professional package insert or in published medical journal articles. There may be other drugs, especially those in the families of drugs listed below, that also will react with this drug to cause severe adverse effects. Make sure to tell your doctor and pharmacist the drugs you are taking and tell them if you are taking any of these interacting drugs:

acetazolamide, AGGRASTAT, alcohol, aluminum hydroxide/magnesium hydroxide, AMARYL, CAPOTEN, captopril, chlorpropamide, COUMADIN, danaparoid, DEPAKEN/DEPAKOTE, DIABINESE, DIAMOX, GARAMYCIN, gentamicin, glimepiride, heparin, ketorolac, MAALOX, MAALOX TC, MEDROL, methotrexate, methylprednisolone, MEXATE, nadroparin, reteplase, TREXALL DOSE PACK, TICLID, ticlopidine, tirofiban, TORADOL, valproic acid, warfarin.

Adverse Effects

Call your doctor immediately if you experience:

- **an allergic reaction:** bluish discoloration or flushing or redness of skin, coughing, difficulty swallowing, dizziness or lightheadedness, skin rash, hives, or itching, stuffy nose, swelling of eyelids, face, or lips, tightness in chest, trouble breathing and/or wheezing
  - vomiting material that looks bloody or like coffee grounds
  - unusual tiredness or weakness (aspirin only)
  - skin rash, hives, or itching
  - bloody or black, tarry stools
  - severe stomach pain
  - wheezing, tightness in chest, or trouble breathing
  - fainting or dizzy spells

Call your doctor if these symptoms continue:

- heartburn, indigestion, nausea with or without vomiting, or mild stomach pain
- abnormal weakness or fatigue

Signs of overdose (mild):

- continued ringing or buzzing in ears or hearing loss
- confusion
- extreme drowsiness
- nausea or vomiting
- stomach pain and/or headache
- dizziness or lightheadedness
- abnormally fast or deep breathing, or trouble breathing
- abnormal or uncontrolled flapping of hands
- nervousness or excitement

Signs of overdose (severe):

- bloody urine
- convulsions
- hallucinations
- severe nervousness, excitement, or confusion
- shortness of breath or troubled breathing
- unexplained fever

If you suspect an overdose, call this number to contact your poison control center: (800) 222-1222.

Periodic Tests

Ask your doctor which of these tests should be done periodically while you are taking this drug:

- liver function tests
- hematocrit determinations
- salicylate concentrations
- serum magnesium levels (for choline and magnesium salicylates)

Do Not Use

ALTERNATIVE TREATMENT:
See Aspirin, p. 279.

Buffered Aspirin
BUFFERIN (Bristol-Myers)
ASCRIPTIN, ASCRIPTIN A/D (Rorer)

Diflunisal (dye *floo* ni sal)
DOLOBID

Salsalate (*sal* sa late)
DISALCID

FAMILY: Nonsteroidal Anti-inflammatory Drugs (NSAIDs)
(see p. 281)
Salicylates (see p. 279)

ASPIRIN/REYE'S SYNDROME ALERT

Do not use this product for treating chicken pox, flu, or flulike illness if you are under 40. It will increase the risk of contracting Reye's syndrome, a rare but often fatal disease.

Buffered aspirin is aspirin with a "buffer" or "acid neutralizer" added. Advertisements for buffered aspirin claim that it relieves pain faster than plain aspirin because it is absorbed better and also that it is less irritating to the stomach and intestines than plain aspirin. These claims cannot be justified.

The amount of buffer in buffered aspirin is very small, only a fraction of the amount found in even one teaspoon of many antacids. An FDA advisory committee found that although buffered aspirin may be absorbed more quickly than plain aspirin, it does not provide much faster pain relief. The committee also found no evidence that buffered aspirin is any gentler to the stomach than plain aspirin. Alka-

---

WARNING

NONSTEROIDAL ANTI-INFLAMMATORY DRUG (NSAID)–INDUCED GASTROINTESTINAL TOXICITY

All members of the NSAID family of drugs can cause gastrointestinal toxicity that can lead to gastrointestinal bleeding and hospitalization or death. The risk of gastrointestinal toxicity from these drugs increases with increasing doses and the length of treatment.

If any of the following symptoms develop while you are taking an NSAID, stop taking the drug immediately and contact your doctor: severe abdominal or stomach pain, cramping, or burning; severe and continuing nausea, heartburn, or indigestion; bloody or black, tarry stools; vomiting blood or material that looks like coffee grounds; or spitting up blood.

Seltzer, a brand of buffered aspirin, should not be taken by anyone whose salt (sodium) intake has been limited.

If you take aspirin only occasionally, plain generic aspirin (see p. 279) is better than buffered, because it is much less expensive and relieves pain just as quickly.

Diflunisal and salsalate should not be used because they have no advantage over plain aspirin (see p. 279).

Nonnarcotic Painkillers

Acetaminophen (a seat a *mee* noe fen)
TYLENOL (Ortho-McNeil Consumer Products)

GENERIC: available
FAMILY: Nonnarcotic Painkillers (see p. 308)

PREGNANCY WARNING

Acetominophen crosses the placenta and exposes the fetus to the drug. Tell your doctor if you are pregnant or thinking of becoming pregnant before you take this drug.

BREAST-FEEDING WARNING

Acetaminophen is excreted in human milk. You should consult with your doctor if you are planning to nurse.

WARNING

There have been a number of case reports of liver damage involving a possible drug interaction between isoniazid, a medication used to prevent and treat tuberculosis (TB), and acetaminophen, an over-the-counter painkiller and the active ingredient in Tylenol. Isoniazid alone, especially as people get older, has been documented to cause liver damage. Acetaminophen, alone in large doses or probably in combination with alcohol, also increases the risk of liver damage. The combination of acetaminophen with isoniazid, according to the authors of these case reports, may also be dangerous.

If you are taking isoniazid for tuberculosis or have a positive TB skin test and are using the drug, consult your physician before using acetaminophen or any combination product containing acetaminophen. Discuss alternatives to acetaminophen with your physician.

DRUG INTERACTION WARNING

INCREASED RISK OF BLEEDING WHEN ACETAMINOPHEN AND WARFARIN (COUMADIN) ARE TAKEN TOGETHER

Acetaminophen may interact with warfarin to increase the risk of bleeding. This risk increases with increasing doses of acetaminophen. The risk of bleeding has been found to increase tenfold in people who were taking 28 or more regular-strength acetaminophen tablets per week, or the equivalent of 18 or more extra-strength tablets per week, compared to those taking warfarin and no acetaminophen.[60] A regular-strength tablet contains 325 milligrams of acetaminophen, and an extra-strength tablet contains 500 milligrams of the drug.

Warfarin is a drug of considerable benefit after heart valve replacement and in preventing blood clots from a type of heart rhythm disturbance known as atrial fibrillation. It also reduces the risk of death, recurrent heart attacks, and stroke after a heart attack.

Based on this new evidence, if you are taking warfarin, you should notify your doctor before taking any product containing acetaminophen.

Acetaminophen, like aspirin, kills pain and reduces fever, but unlike aspirin, it does not help the redness, stiffness, or swelling of inflammation. Because of this, aspirin (see p. 304) is much more effective for treating the inflammation of arthritis.[2]

In general, you should not take anything to reduce a fever until the cause of the fever is known. It is rarely necessary to treat a fever. However, if a fever is having damaging effects or is making you extremely uncomfortable, it can be reduced with acetaminophen. When you are taking acetaminophen to reduce a fever, you should take it regularly every three or four hours, and stop taking it when the underlying problem is gone or has been controlled through other treatment.

One advantage of acetaminophen over aspirin is that acetaminophen does not cause the stomach bleeding that aspirin can cause. For this reason, doctors often prescribe or recommend acetaminophen to people who are likely to suffer from bleeding when they take aspirin. This includes most people taking blood-thinning drugs like warfarin or heparin and people who have ulcers, gout, or bleeding problems such as hemophilia. Also, people who are allergic to aspirin can often take acetaminophen.

Acetaminophen has its own harmful effects—

it can cause liver damage, sometimes fatal, especially in older adults. Acetaminophen overdose and idiosyncratic adverse drug reactions involving the liver have replaced viral hepatitis (inflammation of the liver) as the most frequent apparent causes of acute liver failure in the United States.[61,62]

Before You Use This Drug

Tell your doctor if you have or have had:

- allergies to acetaminophen or aspirin
- pregnancy or are breast-feeding
- alcohol dependence
- liver problems
- viral hepatitis
- kidney problems
- phenylketonuria
- diabetes (drug can interfere with blood glucose tests)

Tell your doctor about any other drugs you take, including aspirin, herbs, vitamins, and other nonprescription products.

When You Use This Drug

- If taking for pain, including arthritic pain, and pain persists for longer than 10 days or condition becomes worse, or new symptoms occur, or the painful area is red or swollen, contact your doctor.
- If taking for fever, and fever persists for longer than three days, condition becomes worse, or new symptoms occur, contact your doctor.
- If taking for sore throat, and sore throat is severe, persists for longer than two days, or occurs together with or is followed by fever, headache, rash, nausea, or vomiting, contact your doctor.
- Avoid use of alcohol if taking more than an occasional one to two doses.
- Get emergency help if you suspect an overdose, even if no symptoms have appeared. Treatment started 24 hours following overdose may not work in prevent liver damage or death.

If you suspect an overdose, call this number to contact your poison control center: (800) 222-1222.

How to Use This Drug

- If you miss a dose, take it as soon as you remember, but skip it if it is almost time for the next dose. **Do not take double doses.**
- Do not share your medication with others.
- Take the drug at the same time(s) each day.
- Store at room temperature with lid on tightly. Do not store in the bathroom. Do not expose to heat, moisture, or strong light. Keep out of reach of children.

Interactions with Other Drugs

The following drugs, biologics (e.g., vaccines, therapeutic antibodies), or foods are listed in *Evaluations of Drug Interactions* 2003 as causing "highly clinically significant" or "clinically significant" interactions when used together with any of the drugs in this section. In some sections with multiple drugs, the interaction may have been reported for one but not all drugs in this section, but we include the interaction because the drugs in this section are similar to one another. We have also included potentially serious interactions listed in the drug's FDA-approved professional package insert or in published medical journal articles. There may be other drugs, especially those in the families of drugs listed below, that also will react with this drug to cause severe adverse effects. Make sure to tell your doctor and pharmacist the drugs you are taking and tell them if you are taking any of these interacting drugs:

INH, isoniazid.

Adverse Effects

Call your doctor immediately if you experience:

- yellow eyes or skin
- bloody or cloudy urine
- fever with or without chills
- trouble urinating, painful urination, or sudden decrease in amount of urine
- skin rash, hives, or itching
- unexplained fever or sore throat
- unusual bleeding or bruising
- unusual tiredness or weakness
- bloody or black, tarry stools
- severe lower back or side pain
- pinpoint red spots on skin
- sores, ulcers, or white spots on lips or in mouth

Signs of overdose:

- diarrhea
- loss of appetite
- nausea or vomiting
- pain or cramps in stomach
- pain, tenderness, and/or swollen upper abdomen
- abnormal increase in sweating

If you suspect an overdose, call the following number to contact your poison control center: (800) 222-1222.

Periodic Tests

Ask your doctor which of these tests should be done periodically while you are taking this drug:

- liver function tests, for long-term or high-dose therapy

Opiate-Containing Painkillers

Codeine (*koe* deen)
CODEINE SULFATE TABLETS USP (Roxane)

Codeine and Acetaminophen
(*koe* deen and a seat a *mee* noe fen)
TYLENOL WITH CODEINE (Ortho-McNeil)

Hydrocodone and Acetaminophen
(hye droe *koe* done and a seat a *mee* noe fen)
LORTAB (UCB)
VICODIN (Abbott)

Hydrocodone and Ibuprofen
(hye droe *koe* done and eye byoo *proe* fen)
VICOPROFEN (Abbott)

Hydromorphone (hye dro *mor* fone)
DILAUDID (Abbott)

Morphine (*mor* feen)
MS CONTIN (Purdue Frederick)

Limited Use

Meperidine (me *per* i deen)
DEMEROL (Sanofi-Synthelabo)

Oxycodone (ox ee *koe* done)
OXYCONTIN (Purdue Frederick)

Oxycodone and Acetaminophen
(ox ee *koe* done and a seat a *mee* noe fen)
PERCOCET (Endo)
ROXICET (Roxane)

Oxycodone and Aspirin
(ox ee *koe* done and *as* pir in)
PERCODAN (Endo)

GENERIC: available

FAMILY: Narcotics (see p. 287)
Nonnarcotic Painkillers
Salicylates (see p. 279)

PREGNANCY WARNING

Some opioids caused fetal harm in animal studies including neurological, soft tissue, and skeletal abnormalities; exposure during pregnancy was also associated with reduction in growth and a number of behavioral abnormalities. In humans, infants born to mothers who have taken opioids chronically may exhibit withdrawal symptoms (irritability and excessive crying, tremors, hyperactive reflexes, diarrhea, sneezing, yawning, vomiting, and fever), reversible reduction in brain volume, small size, and increased risk of sudden infant death syndrome. These drugs should be used by a pregnant woman only if the need for opioid analgesia clearly outweighs the potential risks to the fetus.

BREAST-FEEDING WARNING

It is known that some of these drugs are excreted in human milk. Because of the potential for serious adverse effects in nursing infants, you should not take these drugs while nursing.

FDA BLACK BOX WARNING

OxyContin is an opioid agonist and a Schedule II controlled substance with an abuse liability similar to morphine.

Oxycodone can be abused in a manner similar to other opioid agonists, legal or illicit. This should be considered when prescribing or dispensing OxyContin in situations where the physician or pharmacist is concerned about an increased risk of misuse, abuse, or diversion.

OxyContin Tablets are a controlled-release oral formulation of oxycodone hydrochloride indicated for the management of moderate to severe pain when a continuous, around-the-clock analgesic is needed for an extended period of time.

OxyContin Tablets are NOT intended for use as a prn [as needed] analgesic.

OxyContin 80 mg and 160 mg Tablets ARE FOR USE IN OPIOID-TOLERANT PATIENTS ONLY. These tablet strengths may cause fatal respiratory depression when administered to patients not previously exposed to opioids.

OxyContin Tablets are to be swallowed whole and are not to be broken, chewed, or crushed. Taking broken, chewed, or crushed OxyContin Tablets leads to rapid release and absorption of a potentially fatal dose of Oxycodone.

One hazard of taking these drugs continuously for longer than several weeks is drug-induced dependence. **Do not stop taking your drug suddenly.** With the help of your doctor, work out a schedule for slowly lowering the amount of the drug you take by about 5 to 10% each day. Keep a written record of the dosage reduction schedule with you. These steps will make it much easier to become drug free without developing distressing symptoms of drug withdrawal.

These drugs can increase the risk of hip fracture.

Codeine, hydrocodone, hydromorphone, morphine, meperidine, and oxycodone are narcotics basically derived from morphine. They are prescribed to relieve pain and cough, to treat diarrhea not caused by poisoning, and to cause drowsiness before an operation. These drugs can cause dependence and have many adverse effects, and their use should be limited to the lowest dose for the shortest period of time except in the case of terminally ill people with extraordinary pain.

If you are taking any of the combination drugs listed above, you should also read the information about acetaminophen (see p. 308), ibuprofen (see p. 288), or aspirin (see p. 304).

Narcotic drugs affect the central nervous system, producing pain relief and drowsiness as well as less desirable effects. Older adults may require less than the usual adult dose to produce desired effects because of their bodies' greater sensitivity to the drugs. Some of the adverse effects frequently seen in older adults are slow or troubled breathing (narcotics should never be given to anyone with depressed breathing), stimulation or confusion,[8] and hallucinations and unpleasant dreams.[9]

Other adverse effects seen with the narcotics

are dizziness, drowsiness, feeling faint or light-headed, nausea or vomiting (which might go away if you lie down for a while), blurry vision or change in vision (double vision), constipation (more often seen with long-term use and with codeine), difficult or painful urination, or needed to urinate often, general feeling of discomfort or illness, headache, dry mouth, loss of appetite, bad or unusual dreams, red or flushed face (more often with meperidine or methadone), redness, swelling, pain, or burning at place of injection, stomach pains or cramps, trouble sleeping, abnormal decrease in amount of urine, abnormal increase in sweating (more often with meperidine and methadone), abnormal nervousness, restlessness, tiredness or weakness, and sexual problems.

Meperidine

Meperidine is on a list of drugs that are inappropriate for use in older adults because the drug is not particularly effective in the oral doses commonly prescribed. It may also cause confusion and has many disadvantages over other narcotic drugs.[30]

Before You Use This Drug

Do not use if you have or have had:

- respiratory depression
- diarrhea caused by antibiotics or poisoning
- are breast-feeding

Tell your doctor if you have or have had:

- an unusual reaction to any narcotics
- brain disease or head injury
- recent surgery in gastrointestinal tract
- colitis (inflammation of the colon)
- emphysema, asthma, or other lung disease
- enlarged prostate or trouble urinating
- gallbladder disease or gallstones
- heart, kidney, or liver problems
- seizures

- underactive thyroid gland
- alcohol or drug abuse
- emotional problems
- pregnancy or are breast-feeding

Tell your doctor about any other drugs you take, including aspirin, herbs, vitamins, and other nonprescription products.

When You Use This Drug

- Do not drink alcohol or take any drugs that make you drowsy unless you have checked with your doctor first. When codeine is combined with these substances, it will make you even more drowsy, which puts you at risk of having accidents.
- Do not drive or perform other activities that require alertness, because this drug may make you drowsy, dizzy, or lightheaded.
- If this drug seems less effective after a few weeks of use, do not increase the dose. Call your doctor instead.
- Lie down if you have nausea, vomiting, dizziness, or lightheadedness.
- If you use this drug for a long time, have regular checkups.
- You may feel dizzy when rising from a lying or sitting position. If you are lying down, hang your legs over the side of the bed for a few minutes, then get up slowly. When getting up from a chair, stay by the chair until you are sure that you are not dizzy. (See p. 13.)
- If you plan to have any surgery, including dental, tell your doctor that you take this drug.
- Check with your doctor before discontinuing medication after prolonged use or high doses.
- Use sugarless gum or candy, ice, or a saliva substitute for dry mouth.
- Get emergency help at once if you suspect an overdose.

If you suspect an overdose, call this number to contact your poison control center: (800) 222-1222.

How to Use This Drug

• If you miss a dose, take it as soon as you remember, but skip it if it is almost time for the next dose. **Do not take double doses.**
• Do not share your medication with others.
• Take the drug at the same time(s) each day.
• Meperidine syrup: mix with one half glass (four ounces) of water.
• Morphine oral liquid: may be mixed with fruit juice to improve taste.
• Morphine and oxycodone extended-release tablets: swallow whole; do not break, crush, or chew.
• Store at room temperature with lid on tightly. Do not store in the bathroom. Do not expose to heat, moisture, or strong light. Keep out of reach of children. Protect liquid form from freezing.

Interactions with Other Drugs

The following drugs, biologics (e.g., vaccines, therapeutic antibodies), or foods are listed in *Evaluations of Drug Interactions* 2003 as causing "highly clinically significant" or "clinically significant" interactions when used together with any of the drugs in this section. In some sections with multiple drugs, the interaction may have been reported for one but not all drugs in this section, but we include the interaction because the drugs in this section are similar to one another. We have also included potentially serious interactions listed in the drug's FDA-approved professional package insert or in published medical journal articles. There may be other drugs, especially those in the families of drugs listed below, that also will react with this drug to cause severe adverse effects. Make sure to tell your doctor and pharmacist the drugs you are taking and tell them if you are taking any of these interacting drugs:

abciximab, acetazolamide, AGGRASTAT, alcohol, aluminum/magnesium antacids, AMARYL, ANTURANE, ardeparin, CAPOTEN, captopril, carbamazepine, certoparin, chlorpromazine, chlorpropamide, cimetidine, clopidogrel, COUMADIN, danaparoid, DEPAKENE, DIABINESE, DIAMOX, digoxin, DILANTIN, enoxaparin, eptifibatide, glimepiride, GLUCHOPHAGE, GLUCOVANCE, heparin, INTEGRILIN, ketorolac, LANOXIN, LOVENOX, methotrexate, MEDROL, MERIDIA, METAGLIP, metformin, MEXATE, methylprednisolone, nadroparin, naltrexone, NARDIL, NORVIR, PENTOTHAL, phenelzine, phenytoin, PLAVIX, quinidine, reteplase, REVIA, ritonavir, sibutramine, sulfinpyrazone, TAGAMET, TEGRETOL, thiopental, THORAZINE, TICLID, ticlopidine, tirofiban, TORADOL, tramadol, trovafloxacin, TROVAN, TUBARINE, tubocrarine, ULTRAM, valproic acid, warfarin.

These drugs will increase the effects of other drugs that cause dizziness or drowsiness.

Adverse Effects

Call your doctor immediately if you experience:

• feelings of unreality
• hallucinations
• unusual excitement or restlessness
• skin rash, hives, or itching
• depression or other mood or mental change
• ringing or buzzing sound in ears
• slow, irregular, or troubled breathing
• swollen, red, or flushed face
• trembling or uncontrolled or rigid muscle movements
• abnormal (slow, fast, or pounding) heartbeat
• increased sweating

Call your doctor if these symptoms continue:

- dizziness
- drowsiness
- confusion
- headache
- feeling faint or lightheaded
- nausea or vomiting
- loss of appetite
- stomach cramps or pain
- constipation
- dry mouth
- false sense of well-being
- general feeling of discomfort
- nervousness or restlessness
- unusual tiredness or weakness
- nightmares or insomnia
- difficult or painful urination, frequent urge to urinate
- vision changes

Call your doctor if these symptoms continue after you stop taking this drug:

- shivering or trembling
- stomach cramps
- body aches
- diarrhea
- fast heartbeat
- fever, runny nose, or sneezing
- increased yawning
- loss of appetite
- nausea or vomiting
- unusual excitement, nervousness, or restlessness
- trouble sleeping
- unusually large pupils
- weakness

Signs of overdose:

- cold, clammy skin
- seizures
- severe dizziness or drowsiness
- severe nervousness or restlessness
- confusion
- convulsions
- pinpoint pupils
- unconsciousness

- abnormally low blood pressure
- slow heartbeat
- slow or troubled breathing
- severe weakness

If you suspect an overdose, call this number to contact your poison control center: (800) 222-1222.

Periodic Tests

Ask your doctor which of these tests should be done periodically while you are taking this drug:

- respiratory function tests

Limited Use

Fentanyl Patches (*fen* ta nil)
DURAGESIC TRANSDERMAL THERAPEUTIC SYSTEM (Janssen)

GENERIC: not available

FAMILY: Opiate-containing Painkillers

PREGNANCY WARNING

Fentanyl caused fetal death in animal studies. Because of the potential for serious adverse effects to the fetus, this drug should not be used by pregnant women.

BREAST-FEEDING WARNING

Fentanyl is excreted in human milk. Because of the potential for adverse effects in nursing infants, you should not take this drug while nursing.

Fentanyl is a synthetic narcotic that relieves pain. Most studies about fentanyl focus on the injectable form used during surgery. Fewer studies have been done on the transdermal (patch) form, and even fewer studies have been done on older people using fentanyl patches.

Fentanyl patches, which slowly release medication over three days, are used for chronic pain, such as cancer pain. Pain relief usually

FDA BLACK BOX WARNING

Because serious or life-threatening hypoventilation [respiratory depression] could occur, Duragesic (fentanyl transdermal system) is contraindicated:

- In the management of acute or postoperative pain, including use in outpatient surgeries
- In the management of mild or intermittent pain responsive to PRN (as needed) for non-opioid therapy
- In doses exceeding 25 ug/h at the initiation of opioid therapy

Safety of Duragesic has not been established under 2 years of age. Duragesic should be administered to children only if they are opioid-tolerant and age 2 years or older.

One hazard of taking this drug continuously for longer than several weeks is drug-induced dependence. **Do not stop taking your drug suddenly.** With the help of your doctor, work out a schedule for slowly lowering the amount of the drug you take by about 5 to 10% each day. Keep a written record of the dosage reduction schedule with you. These steps will make it much easier to become drug free without developing distressing symptoms of drug withdrawal.

---

improves sleep. People with swallowing difficulties or poor veins benefit from the topical application. Others find the patch convenient. However, fentanyl is not a Band-Aid for mild or intermittent pain, and is not usually used until doses of oral morphine have become high and frequent. The first dose of fentanyl is usually 25 micrograms (this refers to the number of micrograms released each hour). Doses must be estimated according to prior use of other analgesics. Older people usually need less fentanyl than younger people. It may take a few days until adequate pain relief is achieved. During the transition, other shorter-acting analgesics relieve breakthrough pain. One drawback of the patches is less flexibility in doses, which are currently limited to four sizes and their combinations. People who lose weight may need to have their dose lowered, since fentanyl is stored in fat tissue.

Fentanyl is not recommended for those weighing less than 110 pounds. Common adverse effects of fentanyl are nausea, vomiting, constipation, and skin irritation from the adhesive on the patch. Fentanyl patches are not recommended after surgery due to risk of severe respiratory problems. Like morphine, fentanyl is a controlled substance and could be habit-forming. The cost of fentanyl patches is more than short-acting oral morphine, similar to long-acting oral morphine, and usually less than injectable morphine, which involves costs for supplies and equipment.

Before You Use This Drug

Do not use if you have or have had:

- diarrhea
- respiratory depression
- are breast-feeding

Tell your doctor if you have or have had:

- allergies to medications or adhesives
- emphysema, asthma, or other lung problems
- colitis or inflammatory bowel disease
- alcohol or drug abuse
- gallbladder problems
- head injuries or brain tumor
- kidney or liver problems
- gastrointestinal problems
- thyroid problems
- slow heartbeat
- emotional problems
- enlarged prostate or difficulty urinating
- recent urinary tract surgery
- pregnancy or are breast-feeding

Tell your doctor about any other drugs you take, including aspirin, herbs, vitamins, and other nonprescription products.

When You Use This Drug

• Read the patient instructions carefully before using.

• To avoid constipation, drink plenty of water or fluids. Eat fiber. Take a stool softener. If constipation develops, you may need a laxative or enema.

• Do not use more than directed by your doctor; it may take 24 hours before effects are felt.

• Until you know how you react to fentanyl, avoid driving or performing other activities requiring alertness, as fentanyl can cause drowsiness.

• Avoid drinking alcohol, which adds to central nervous system (CNS) effects of fentanyl.

• Until your dose of fentanyl stabilizes, you may need another short-acting pain reliever for breakthrough pain.

• If you plan to have any surgery, including dental, tell your doctor that you take this drug.

• Do not use heating pads, electric blankets, heated water beds, hot tubs, saunas, or heat lamps. These could cause fentanyl to be too rapidly absorbed, especially if devices slip onto the patch while you sleep.

• You may feel dizzy when rising from a lying or sitting position. When getting out of bed, hang your legs over the side of the bed for a few minutes, then get up slowly. When getting up from a chair, stay beside the chair until you are sure that you are not dizzy.

• If nausea develops, try lying down until it subsides.

• You may wear fentanyl patches while bathing, showering, or swimming, but do not rub the patch vigorously or stay for a prolonged time in hot water. If the patch loosens or dislodges, discard it and apply new patch on a dry area.

• If you sleep or nap near someone else, cover the area of the patch with clothing. Otherwise, the patch could transfer to the other person. This has caused children to receive overdoses.

How to Use This Drug

• If you miss a dose, take it as soon as possible, but skip it if it is almost time for the next dose. **Do not take double doses.**

• Do not share your medication with others.

• Take the drug at the same time(s) each day.

• Prepare the site with water. Do not shave the site or use soap, alcohol, or lotions. Do not apply to areas that are burned, cut, or irritated. Clip hair if necessary.

• Remove liner just before using. Take care not to touch the adhesive surface. Wash with clean water any area the medication unintentionally touches.

• Do not use if seal is broken or patch is otherwise damaged or cut.

• Apply entire patch to dry skin above the waist. Press firmly with palm of hand for at least 30 seconds, especially around the edges.

• If applying more than one patch, do not let edges overlap or touch.[63] Rotate site of application, preferably alternating sides of the body.

• Change patch every three days, unless your doctor tells you to change at a different frequency.

• Do not apply more than the prescribed dose.

• Fold used patches in half with adhesive layer inside the fold. Flush down toilet or otherwise dispose of in secure manner.

• Wash hands.

• Do not stop using abruptly. A gradual reduction prevents withdrawal symptoms. Even if you stop using fentanyl patches, some of the drug can remain in older people for a few days.

• Store at room temperature. Do not expose to heat, moisture, or strong light. Keep out of reach of children.

Interactions with Other Drugs

The following drugs are listed in the *Evaluations of Drug Interactions* 2003 as causing "highly clinically significant" or "clinically significant" interactions when used together with this drug. We have also included potentially serious interactions listed in the drug's FDA-approved professional product labeling or package insert. New scientific techniques have allowed researchers to predict some drug interactions before they have been documented in people. There may be other drugs, especially those in the families of drugs listed below, that also will react with this drug to cause severe adverse effects. The number of new drugs approved for marketing increases the chance of drug interactions, and new drug interactions are being identified with old drugs. Be vigilant. Make sure to tell your doctor and pharmacist the drugs you are taking and tell your doctor if you are taking any of these interacting drugs:

People who take monoamine oxidase inhibitors should be off these drugs for 14 days before starting fentanyl.[64] These include: deprenyl, ELDEPRYL, furazolidone, FUROXONE, isocarboxazid, MARPLAN, MATULANE, NARDIL, PARNATE, phenelzine, procarbazine, selegiline, tranylcypromine.

Central nervous system (CNS) depressant drugs, including alcohol, antidepressants, antihistamines, antipsychotics, some blood pressure medications (reserpine, methyldopa, beta-blockers), motion sickness medications, muscle relaxants, narcotics sedatives, sleeping pills, and tranquilizers. Doses of fentanyl and any of these drugs may need to be lowered by 50%. If any of these drugs are discontinued while you use fentanyl, adjustments in doses may be required.

Other drugs that can interact with fentanyl are: carbamazepine, DILANTIN, EES, erythromycin, ketoconazole, MERIDIA, naltrexone, NIZORAL, NORVIR, phenytoin, REVIA, RIFADIN, rifampin, ritonavir, sibutramine, TEGRETOL.

Adverse Effects

Call your doctor immediately if you experience:

- abdominal swelling
- **difficulty breathing** (If you care for a person who uses fentanyl patches and their breathing slows while sleeping, try to waken them. If breathing does not improve once awake, call their doctor.)[63]
- fainting
- problems speaking
- chest pain
- slow, fast, pounding, or irregular heartbeat
- confusion
- dizziness, incoordination, or fainting
- fever with or without chills (your dose may be lowered temporarily)[63]
- hallucinations
- restlessness or nervousness
- cold, red, swollen, or blistered skin with or without itching at patch
- thickened or scaly skin
- fluid-filled blisters
- spitting blood
- combative and/or suspicious thoughts
- difficulty urinating (decreased frequency and/or volume)
- mental or mood changes
- unusual bruising
- swollen glands
- any change in vision
- bladder pain

Call your doctor if these symptoms continue:

- decreased appetite
- anxiety, confusion
- constipation
- diarrhea

- dizziness
- unusual dreams
- memory loss
- drowsiness
- dry mouth
- headache
- blurred vision
- nausea or vomiting
- red or itchy skin, sweating, tingling or burning sensation
- weakness
- abdominal or stomach pain
- indigestion, gas
- weight loss
- sweating

Call your doctor if these symptoms continue after you stop taking this drug:

- diarrhea
- body aches
- increased heartbeat
- nervousness, restlessness, or irritability
- nausea or vomiting
- unusually enlarged pupils
- shivering or trembling
- increased sweating
- fever, runny nose, or sneezing
- stomach cramps
- trouble sleeping
- weakness
- increased yawning
- loss of appetite

Periodic Tests

Ask your doctor which of these tests should be done periodically while you are taking this drug:

- blood pressure
- heart rate
- respiratory rate
- degree of sedation

Limited Use

Methadone (*meth* a done)
DOLOPHINE (Roxane)

GENERIC: available for oral forms
FAMILY: Opiate-containing Painkillers

PREGNANCY WARNING

Opioids have been associated with a variety of effects on growth and development including abnormal behavior. Safe use in pregnancy has not been established. Infants born to mothers who have taken opioids regularly will exhibit withdrawal symptoms (including excessive crying, tremors, increased rate of breathing, diarrhea, vomiting, and fever) and are at increased risk for sudden death syndrome. Consult with your doctor if you are pregnant or thinking of becoming pregnant before you take this drug.

BREAST-FEEDING WARNING

Methadone is excreted in human milk. Because of the potential for serious adverse effects in nursing infants, you should not take methadone while nursing. If you are already on high-dose methadone maintenance and are already breast-feeding, you need to wean your infant gradually to prevent withdrawal symptoms.

FDA BLACK BOX WARNING

Laboratory studies, both *in vivo* and *in vitro*, have demonstrated that methadone inhibits cardiac potassium channels and prolongs the QT interval. (See below for further information about QT prolongation.) Cases of QT interval prolongation and serious arrhythmia (torsades de pointes) have been observed during treatment with methadone. These cases appear to be more commonly associated with, but not limited to, higher dose treatment (> 200 mg/day). Most cases involve patients being treated for pain with large, multiple daily doses of methadone, although cases have been reported in patients receiving doses commonly used for maintenance treatment of opioid addiction.

Methadone is a synthetic opiate belonging to the same family as morphine. Methadone is approved by the FDA to treat severe pain and detoxify addiction to other narcotics,[65] and for maintenance in opiate-dependent drug users.

In opiate-dependent individuals, methadone, which is long-acting, is given to replace the shorter-acting drugs of abuse such as heroin. It is also given by mouth instead of intravenously, like heroin. This reduces harm caused by drug abuse. It prevents withdrawal, suppresses craving for heroin, and avoids unsafe injections[66] and death from overdose.[67] Methadone also reduces harm because pharmaceutical-grade methadone is formulated consistently, unlike street heroin, which can have variable doses and be contaminated. Methadone maintenance also reduces, but does not necessarily eliminate, illicit drug use, crime, risk of HIV infection, and unemployment, and it helps to stabilize social relations.[68] However, methadone can be habit-forming.[69]

The prescription of methadone for opiate indications such as methadone maintenance is limited to registered drug treatment facilities and certain pharmacies. When patients who have been receiving morphine (see p. 311), hydromorphone (see p. 311), or fentanyl (see p. 315) experience intolerable adverse effects, or pain is not well controlled, a switch to methadone may be considered. Several protocols determine the amount of methadone to use when switching, to avoid withdrawal. The amount depends on the dose of the other narcotic and the degree of tolerance developed, if any. Switches typically require several days.[70–72]

QT Prolongation

The QT interval is the length of time it takes the large chambers of the heart (ventricles) to electrically discharge and recharge. A prolongation of the QT interval can lead to a type of heart rhythm disturbance, or cardiac arrythmia, known as torsades de pointes, and sudden death. The QT interval is measured by an electrocardiogram (EKG or ECG) in milliseconds

(msec). *Torsades de pointes* is a French phrase that means "twisted point," describing the appearance of this rhythm disturbance on the EKG tracing.

Substantial risk exists when methadone is given in combination with other drugs known to prolong the QT interval. The only extensive list of drugs that prolong QT intervals is maintained by the University of Arizona Health Sciences Center, at http://www.torsades.org.

The most frequent and persistent adverse effect of opioids such as methadone is constipation. The other adverse effects of methadone are similar to those of morphine. The risk of respiratory depression rises when used with alcohol, benzodiazepines such as diazepam (Valium) (see p. 223) and illicit narcotics such as heroin. To avoid respiratory depression, the dose is increased slowly.[73] Gradually, the interval between doses can be lengthened.[74] The toxic dose of methadone is much lower in people who have not used it or other narcotics before.[73]

Before You Use This Drug

Do not use if you have or have had:

- diarrhea from pseudomembranous colitis caused by certain antibiotics (cephalosporins, clindamycin topical, lincomycin, or penicillin)
- diarrhea caused by poisoning
- respiratory disease or impairment

Tell your doctor if you have or have had:

- allergy to methadone
- pregnancy or are breast-feeding
- abdominal problems
- asthma
- respiratory problems
- heart problems
- convulsions
- drug abuse
- alcohol abuse
- emotional problems

- suicide attempts or suicidal thoughts
- gallbladder problems
- recent gastrointestinal surgery
- head injury
- liver problems
- low thyroid activity
- bowel disease
- enlarge prostate
- kidney or urinary problems or recent urinary tract surgery

Tell your doctor about any other drugs you take, including aspirin, herbs, vitamins, and other nonprescription products.

When You Use This Drug

- Visit your doctor regularly to check your progress during long-term therapy.
- Avoid alcohol and other central nervous system drugs, such as alprazolam (XANAX) and diazepam (VALIUM), unless approved by your doctor.
- Do not drive or operate hazardous equipment until you know whether you become dizzy or drowsy or have a false sense of well-being when taking methadone.
- When you change position from lying down to sitting to standing, do so gradually.
- Lie down if you become dizzy, drowsy, lightheaded, or nauseous.
- If you plan to have any surgery, including dental, tell your doctor that you take this drug.
- If you have dry mouth, use sugarless gum, hard candy, or a saliva substitute to prevent cavities. Check with your dentist if dry mouth continues for more than two weeks.

How to Use This Drug

- If you miss a dose, take it as soon as you remember, but skip the dose if it is almost time for the next dose. **Do not take double doses.**
- Do not share your medication with others.
- Take the drug at the same time(s) each day.

- Dissolve dispersible tablets in water or fruit juice.
- Dilute oral concentrate with at least one ounce of water, unless prediluted by your provider.
- Do not suddenly stop taking this drug without checking with your doctor to find out if you need to taper off.
- If you stop taking this medication, remember that adverse effects can still occur even after drug is discontinued.
- Store at room temperature with lid on tightly. Do not store in the bathroom. Do not expose to heat, moisture, or strong light. Keep out of reach of children.

Interactions with Other Drugs

The following drugs, biologics (e.g., vaccines, therapeutic antibodies), or foods are listed in *Evaluations of Drug Interactions* 2003 as causing "highly clinically significant" or "clinically significant" interactions when used together with any of the drugs in this section. In some sections with multiple drugs, the interaction may have been reported for one but not all drugs in this section, but we include the interaction because the drugs in this section are similar to one another. We have also included potentially serious interactions listed in the drug's FDA-approved professional package insert or in published medical journal articles. There may be other drugs, especially those in the families of drugs listed below, that also will react with this drug to cause severe adverse effects. Make sure to tell your doctor and pharmacist the drugs you are taking and tell them if you are taking any of these interacting drugs:

Methadone taken with these drugs may increase the methadone level in the blood and could lead to overdose of methadone: KALETRA, lopinavir, naltrexone, nelfinavir, nevirapine, REVIA, RIFAMATE, rifampin, RIFATER, RIMACTANE, TRAMADOL, ULTRAM, VIRACEPT, VIRAMUNE.

Methadone with other drugs that also depress the central nervous system or have anticholinergic effects could add to adverse effects, such as drowsiness and constipation. Doses may need adjusting. These include: alcohol, antidepressants (for example, imipramine [TOFRANIL]), antihistamines (for example, diphenhydramine [BENADRYL]), antinausea agents (for example, prochlorperazine [COMPAZINE]), antipsychotic agents (for example, chlorpromazine [THORAZINE]), motion sickness pills (for example, meclizine [ANTIVERT]), other narcotics (for example, morphine), sedatives (for example, oxazepam [SERAX]), tranquilizers (for example, diazepam [VALIUM]).

Adverse Effects

Call your doctor immediately if you experience:

- difficult, irregular, or slow breathing; wheezing
- facial swelling
- unusual excitement or restlessness
- confusion
- pounding, rapid, or slow heartbeat
- hallucinations
- blood pressure decrease
- profuse sweating
- flushed or red face
- mental depression
- bloating
- constipation that is severe
- nausea or vomiting
- stomach cramps or pain

Contact your doctor if these symptoms continue:

- more frequent, difficult, or painful urination, or decrease in the amount of urine
- stomach cramps or pain
- skin rash, hives, and/or itching
- vision changes
- constipation

- nausea or vomiting
- dizziness, fainting, lightheadedness
- drowsiness
- general feeling of discomfort or illness
- dry mouth
- appetite decrease
- false sense of well-being
- headache
- nervousness
- trouble sleeping
- tiredness or weakness that is unusual

Call your doctor if these symptoms continue after you stop taking this drug:

- sweating
- yawning
- appetite loss
- gooseflesh
- fast heartbeat
- irritability, nervousness, restlessness
- dilated pupils
- tremor, twitching, shivering
- body aches
- abdominal cramps
- diarrhea
- fever, runny nose, or sneezing
- insomnia
- weakness

Signs of overdose:

- blood pressure drop
- difficult breathing
- cold, clammy skin
- confusion
- convulsions
- severe dizziness
- severe drowsiness
- slow heartbeat
- nervousness or restlessness
- pinpoint pupils
- severe weakness
- unconsciousness

If you suspect an overdose, call this number to contact your poison control center: (800) 222-1222.

Periodic Tests

Ask your doctor which of these tests should be done periodically while you are taking this drug:

- drug, blood, or urine tests
- respiratory function tests

 Do Not Use

ALTERNATIVE TREATMENT:
See Narcotics, p. 282.

Butorphanol (byoo *tor* fa nole)
STADOL, STADOL NS
(Bristol-Myers Squibb)

FAMILY: Opiate-containing Painkillers

One hazard of taking this drug continuously for longer than several weeks is drug-induced dependence. **Do not stop taking your drug suddenly.** With the help of your doctor, work out a schedule for slowly lowering the amount of the drug you take by about 5 to 10% each day. Keep a written record of the dosage reduction schedule with you. These steps will make it much easier to become drug free without developing distressing symptoms of drug withdrawal.

Butorphanol is a strong pain reliever chemically related to morphine, and milligram for milligram, it is about 25 to 50 times more potent. In 1978, the FDA ignored the advice of its own advisory committee, which had voted 12 to 2 to classify the injectable form of butorphanol as a controlled substance, and allowed the drug to be marketed as a nonnarcotic.

The scope of distribution of butorphanol changed dramatically when, in 1992, Bristol-Myers Squibb sought and received approval for butorphanol nasal spray. Once this dosage form was approved, the company embarked on a major promotional campaign for butorphanol nasal spray. Advertising to doctors minimized the drug's adverse effects and addictive potential. During the first three years after the appearance of butorphanol nasal spray, the number of adverse drug reaction reports to the FDA increased from 60 to about 400 per year. Dependence and/or addiction was by far the most common adverse reaction.[75]

After 19 years on the market with countless unsuspecting consumers having become addicted to butorphanol, the Drug Enforcement Administration finally decided—in July 1997—to classify this drug as a controlled substance.

Though more potent, butorphanol is no more effective a pain reliever than morphine or other morphine-like drugs and is more expensive, particularly the nasal spray. There is no medical reason why you should be using butorphanol rather than morphine or other morphine-like drugs to control severe pain.

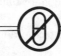 *Do Not Use*

ALTERNATIVE TREATMENT:
See Narcotics, p. 282.

Pentazocine (pen *taz* oh seen)
TALWIN (Sanofi)

Pentazocine and Naloxone
(pen *taz* oh seen and nal *ox* one)
TALWIN-NX (Sanofi)

FAMILY: Opiate-containing Painkillers

Pentazocine relieves moderate to severe pain. Older adults should not use this drug, either alone or in combination with naloxone, because of the high risk of adverse effects, especially confusion. The risk is so high that the World

One hazard of taking this drug continuously for longer than several weeks is drug-induced dependence. **Do not stop taking your drug suddenly.** With the help of your doctor, work out a schedule for slowly lowering the amount of the drug you take by about 5 to 10% each day. Keep a written record of the dosage reduction schedule with you. These steps will make it much easier to become drug free without developing distressing symptoms of drug withdrawal.

Health Organization recommends that this drug not be used if possible.[76]

This drug remains on a well-recognized list of drugs that are inappropriate for use in older adults. Pentazocine causes more central nervous system adverse effects, including confusion and hallucination, more often than other narcotic drugs.[30]

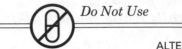

Do Not Use

ALTERNATIVE TREATMENT:
See Narcotics, p. 282.

Propoxyphene (proe *pox* i feen)
DARVON, DARVON-N (aaiPHARMA)

Propoxyphene and Acetaminophen
(proe *pox* i feen and a seat a *mee* noe fen)
DARVOCET-N (aaiPHARMA)
WYGESIC (Women First)

Propoxyphene, Aspirin, and Caffeine
(proe *pox* i feen, *as* pir in, and kaf *een*)
DARVON COMPOUND (aaiPHARMA)
DARVON COMPOUND-65 (aaiPHARMA)

FAMILY: Opiate-containing Painkillers
Nonnarcotic Painkillers

FDA BLACK BOX WARNING

- Do not prescribe propoxyphene for patients who are suicidal or addiction-prone.
- Prescribe propoxyphene with caution for patients taking tranquilizers or antidepressant drugs and patients who use alcohol in excess.
- Tell your patients not to exceed the recommended dose and to limit their intake of alcohol.

Propoxyphene products, in excessive doses, either alone or in combination with other CNS depressants, including alcohol, are a major cause of drug related deaths. Fatalities within the first hour of overdosage are not uncommon. In a survey of deaths due to overdosage conducted in 1975, in approximately 20% of the fatal cases, death occurred within the first hour (5% occurred within 15 minutes). Propoxyphene should not be taken in doses higher than those recommended by the physician. The judicious prescribing of propoxyphene is essential to the safe use of this drug. With patients who are depressed or suicidal, consideration should be given to the use of nonnarcotic analgesics. Patients should be cautioned about the concomitant use of propoxyphene products and alcohol because of potentially serious CNS-additive effects of these agents. Because of its added depressant effects, propoxyphene should be prescribed with caution for those patients whose medical condition requires the concomitant administration of sedatives, tranquilizers, muscle relaxants, antidepressants, or other CNS-depressant drugs. Patients should be advised of the additive depressant effects of these combinations. Many of the propoxyphene-related deaths have occurred in patients with previous histories of emotional disturbances or suicidal ideation or attempts, as well as histories of misuse of tranquilizers, alcohol, and other CNS-active drugs. Some deaths have occurred as a consequence of the accidental ingestion of excessive quantities of propoxyphene alone or in combination with other drugs. Patients taking propoxyphene should be warned not to exceed the dosage recommended by the physician.

These drugs can increase the risk of hip fracture.

WARNING

There have been a number of case reports of liver damage involving a possible drug interaction between isoniazid, a medication used to prevent and treat tuberculosis (TB), and acetaminophen, an over-the-counter painkiller and the active ingredient in Tylenol. Isoniazid alone, especially as people get older, has been documented to cause liver damage. Acetaminophen, alone in large doses or probably in combination with alcohol, also increases the risk of liver damage. The combination of acetaminophen with isoniazid, according to the authors of these case reports, may also be dangerous.

If you are taking isoniazid for tuberculosis or have a positive TB skin test and are using the drug, consult your physician before using acetaminophen or any combination product containing acetaminophen. Discuss alternatives to acetaminophen with your physician.

One hazard of taking these drugs continuously for longer than several weeks is drug-induced dependence. **Do not stop taking your drug suddenly**. With the help of your doctor, work out a schedule for slowly lowering the amount of the drug you take by about 5 to 10% each day. Keep a written record of the dosage reduction schedule with you. These steps will make it much easier to become drug free without developing distressing symptoms of drug withdrawal.

Propoxyphene is a narcotic that relieves mild to moderate pain. For years we have recommended that you do not use it because it is no more effective than aspirin (see p. 304) or codeine (see p. 311) and it is much more dangerous than aspirin. If you have taken aspirin for your pain and it has not worked, propoxyphene will probably not do any better.[77] In fact, some found that propoxyphene by itself is no more effective than a sugar pill (placebo).[78] Most studies show that propoxyphene is less effective than aspirin and that it has a potential for addiction and overdose.

The Public Citizen's Health Research Group petitioned the government in 1978 to remove this dangerous drug from the market.[79]

Propoxyphene has remained on a list of drugs for years that are inappropriate for use in older adults.[30] Unfortunately, it is still being widely prescribed to elderly patients. In 1998, among Medicare beneficiaries, 6.8% of these people living at home were receiving propoxyphene and 15.5% who were institutionalized were prescribed propoxyphene.[80]

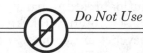 *Do Not Use*

ALTERNATIVE TREATMENT:
See Narcotics, p. 282.

Tramadol (tra *ma* dol)
ULTRAM (Ortho-McNeil)

Tramadol and Acetaminophen
(tra *ma* dol and a seat a *mee* noe fen)
ULTRACET (Ortho-McNeil)

FAMILY: Opiate-containing Painkillers
Nonnarcotic Painkillers

Tramadol is an old German painkiller first marketed in 1977 but not sold in the United States until 1995. It is heavily promoted to doctors as being equivalent to acetaminophen and codeine (TYLENOL WITH CODEINE, see p. 311) and having a low potential to cause addiction. In fact, tramadol appears to be no more and sometimes less effective than combinations of codeine with aspirin or acetaminophen.[81]

Tramadol was approved without being classified as a controlled substance, even though it has many chemical similarities to narcotic drugs like morphine and codeine. After being on the market for only one year in the United States, serious adverse reactions were reported with tramadol, even after the first dose, including seizures, dependence, and severe allergic reactions.

Within the first year of marketing, the FDA had received 83 reports of seizures or convulsions among people using tramadol.[82] During its second year on the market, the FDA received more than 200 reports of seizures. Many of these reports noting seizures occurred within one day of starting tramadol. Most of these people were healthy and between the ages of 20 and 39 years, and most had no previous history of seizures. This adverse reaction can occur at recommended dosages, although an overdose may increase the risk of tramadol-related seizures. Taking tramadol with antidepressant drugs, including the new selective serotonin reuptake inhibitors and older tricyclic antidepressants, increases the risk of seizures.[83] The FDA conservatively estimates that for every report of an adverse drug reaction, 10 go unreported.

Tramadol has effects similar to the narcotic pain relievers morphine and codeine, including the potential to cause addiction, but it was not classified as a controlled substance at the time of its approval. Ortho-McNeil Pharmaceutical of Raritan, New Jersey, the producer of the drug, advertised heavily to doctors that tramadol had a low potential for abuse. Within the drug's first year on the market, the FDA had received 115 reports of adverse events described as drug abuse, dependence, withdrawal, or intentional overdose associated with the use of tramadol.[82] Countless consumers who were not told that tramadol was addicting may have unknowingly become dependent on this drug.

Problems with tramadol are beginning to appear in other countries. For example, in 2002 tramadol was the third most frequently involved drug in withdrawal reactions reported to British drug regulatory authorities.[84]

Barbiturates

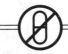 *Do Not Use*

ALTERNATIVE TREATMENT:
See Acetaminophen, p. 308.

Butalbital, Acetaminophen, and Caffeine
(byoo *tal* bi tal, a seat a *mee* noe fen, and kaf *een*)
ESGIC PLUS (Forest)
FIORICET (Watson)

Butalbital, Caffeine, and Aspirin
(byoo *tal* bi tal, kaf *een*, and *as* pir in)
FIORINAL (Watson)

Butalbital, Caffeine, Aspirin, and Codeine
(byoo *tal* bi tal, kaf *een*, *as* pir in and *ko* deen)
FIORINAL WITH CODEINE (Watson)

FAMILY: Barbiturates
Nonnarcotic Painkillers
Opiate-containing Painkillers
Salicylates (see p. 279)

> One hazard of taking butalbital or codeine continuously for longer than several weeks is drug-induced dependence. **Do not stop taking your drug suddenly.** With the help of your doctor, work out a schedule for slowly lowering the amount of the drug you take by about 5 to 10% each day. Keep a written record of the dosage reduction schedule with you. These steps will make it much easier to become drug free without developing distressing symptoms of drug withdrawal.

Like other fixed-combination products, these combinations curtail the ability to vary doses of

WARNING

There have been a number of case reports of liver damage involving a possible drug interaction between isoniazid, a medication used to prevent and treat tuberculosis (TB), and acetaminophen, an over-the-counter painkiller and the active ingredient in Tylenol. Isoniazid alone, especially as people get older, has been documented to cause liver damage. Acetaminophen, alone in large doses or probably in combination with alcohol, also increases the risk of liver damage. The combination of acetaminophen with isoniazid, according to the authors of these case reports, may also be dangerous.

If you are taking isoniazid for tuberculosis or have a positive TB skin test and are using the drug, consult your physician before using acetaminophen or any combination product containing acetaminophen. Discuss alternatives to acetaminophen with your physician.

Fiorinal with Codeine can increase the risk of hip fracture.[85]

ASPIRIN/REYE'S SYNDROME ALERT

Do not use the aspirin-containing products for treating chicken pox, flu, or flulike illness. They will increase the risk of contracting Reye's syndrome, a rare but often fatal disease.

each drug—irrationally combining, in the case of Fioricet, an ineffective drug (caffeine), one effective painkiller (acetaminophen), and one excessively dangerous drug (butalbital).

Caffeine has not proven effective in relieving pain. It can aggravate incontinence, produce insomnia, and lead to dependence-causing withdrawal headaches.

Butalbital is a barbiturate, and because of the serious adverse effects and addictive nature of all barbiturates, older adults should not use it. The barbiturates, other than using phenobarbital for seizure, has been on a list of drugs that are inappropriate for use in older adults.[30]

Acetaminophen is an effective painkiller, available separately without a prescription (see p. 308), as is aspirin (see p. 304).

Drugs for Arthritis and Gout

Limited Use

Adalimumab (ad a *lim* you mab)
HUMIRA (Abbott)

Anakinra (an a *kin* rah)
KINERET (Amgen)

Etanercept (ee tan *ner* cept)
ENBREL (Amgen)

Infliximab (in *flix* i mab)
REMICADE (Centocor)

GENERIC: not available
FAMILY: Drugs for Arthritis and Gout (see pp. 283 and 287)
Tumor Necrosis Factor (TNF) Blockers
Interleukin-1 (IL-1) Blockers

PREGNANCY WARNING
There is only limited data from animal studies. Use during pregnancy only for clear medical reasons. Tell your doctor if you are pregnant or thinking of becoming pregnant before you take these drugs.

BREAST-FEEDING WARNING
Although they have not been tested, it is likely that these drugs are excreted in human milk. Because of the potential for serious adverse effects in nursing infants, you should not take these drugs while nursing.

FDA BLACK BOX WARNING

HUMIRA
RISK OF INFECTIONS

Cases of tuberculosis (frequently disseminated or extrapulmonary at clinical presentation) have been observed in patients receiving HUMIRA.

Patients should be evaluated for latent tuberculosis infection with a tuberculin skin test. Treatment of latent tuberculosis infection should be initiated prior to therapy with HUMIRA.

FDA BLACK BOX WARNING

REMICADE
RISK OF INFECTIONS

Tuberculosis (frequently disseminated or extrapulmonary at clinical presentation), invasive fungal infections, and other opportunistic infections have been observed in patients receiving Remicade; some of these infections have been fatal.

Patients should be evaluated for latent tuberculosis infection with a tuberculin skin test. Treatment of latent tuberculosis infection should be initiated prior to therapy with Remicade.

Adalimumab

This genetically engineered drug is a monoclonal antibody that blocks the interaction of tumor necrosis factor (TNF) with TNF receptors. TNF plays an important role in the inflammatory processes of rheumatoid arthritis.

Adalimumab is approved by the FDA to treat moderate to severe rheumatoid arthritis. This drug is intended for adults who have failed at least one disease-modifying antirheumatic drug (DMARD) and for use with other DMARDs such as methotrexate (see p. 342).[86] It is injected every other week.[87]

The major serious adverse drug reactions associated with the use of adalimumab are serious infections (see the Humira black-box warning above); nervous system diseases that have been seen with the TNF blockers; certain types of cancers reportedly associated with TNF blocker use; lupuslike symptoms such as chest pains, shortness of breath, joint pain or rash, and sun sensitivity; and severe allergic reactions.[88]

Anakinra

This drug is an interleukin-1 (IL-1) receptor blocker. It is approved by the FDA for the treatment of moderate to severe rheumatoid arthritis in adults who have failed at least one disease-modifying antirheumatic drug (DMARD), such as methotrexate (see p. 342). IL-1 may play a role in the inflammation and local bone degradation seen with rheumatoid arthritis.[89]

Anakinra has been associated with an increased incidence of serious infections. This drug should be discontinued if you develop an infection and should not be started if you have an active infection. Other serious adverse reactions seen with anakinra are an effect on blood

---

WARNINGS

Kineret has been associated with an increased incidence of serious infections (2%) vs. placebo (> 1%). Administration of Kineret should be discontinued if a patient develops a serious infection. Treatment with Kineret should not be initiated in patients with active infections. The safety and efficacy of Kineret in immunosuppressed patients or in patients with chronic infections have not been evaluated. In a 24-week study of concurrent Kineret and etanercept therapy, the rate of serious infections in the combination arm (7%) was higher than with etanercept alone (0%). The combination of Kineret and etanercept did not result in higher ACR response rates compared to etanercept alone.

cells and the appearance of certain types of malignancies.[90]

Etanercept

This drug blocks and inactivates TNF. It is approved by the FDA for rheumatoid arthritis, psoriatic arthritis, juvenile rheumatoid arthritis, and ankylosing spondylitis,[91] but is not indicated for Crohn's disease.[92,93]

Serious adverse drug reactions associated with the use of etanercept include serious infections; nervous system diseases that have been seen with the TNF blockers; blood cell problems that have been seen with the use of this drug; heart problems; and severe allergic reactions.[91]

Infliximab

This drug is also a TNF blocker. It was approved by the FDA for rheumatoid arthritis and Crohn's disease, including fistulizing Crohn's disease.[94] Infliximab is not effective in treating ulcerative colitis.[95]

Serious adverse drug reactions associated with the use of infliximab include serious infections that have sometimes been fatal, a lupus-like syndrome, heart problems, and the appearance of certain types of malignancies.[94]

Some physicians advise women of childbearing age to use birth control when using etanercept or infliximab.[96]

ETANERCEPT WARNING

INFECTIONS

In post-marketing reports, serious infections and sepsis, including fatalities, have been reported with the use of Enbrel. Many of the serious infections have occurred in patients on concomitant immunosuppressive therapy that, in addition to their underlying disease, could predispose them to infections. Rare cases of tuberculosis (TB) have been observed in patients with TNF antagonists, including Enbrel. Patients who develop a new infection while undergoing treatment with Enbrel should be monitored closely. Administration of Enbrel should be discontinued if a patient develops a serious infection or sepsis. Treatment with Enbrel should not be initiated in patients with active infections including chronic or localized infections. Physicians should exercise caution when considering the use of Enbrel in patients with a history of recurring infections or with underlying conditions which may predispose patients to infections, such as advanced or poorly controlled diabetes.

In a 24-week study of concurrent Enbrel and anakinra therapy, the rate of serious infections in the combination arm (7%) was higher than with Enbrel alone (0%). The combination of Enbrel and anakinra did not result in higher ACR response rates compared to Enbrel alone.

Before You Use This Drug

Do not use if you have or have had:

- allergy to E. coli proteins, rubber, latex, or mouse proteins
- allergy to etanercept, infliximab, or adalimumab
- diabetes
- heart problems, such as congestive heart failure
- active infections, including chronic or localized
- problems with your immune system
- diseases of the nervous system
- history of blood problems
- sepsis
- tuberculosis
- cancer
- are breast-feeding

Tell your doctor if you have or have had:

- pregnancy or are breast-feeding
- rheumatoid arthritis

Tell your doctor about any other drugs you take, including immunosuppressants, herbs, vitamins, and other nonprescription products.

When You Use This Drug

• Update your vaccinations before starting therapy.

• Visit your doctor regularly to check progress.

• If you experience the symptoms of heart failure—fatigue, difficulty breathing, swelling (especially in the legs and ankles), or rapid or "galloping" heartbeats—notify the prescribing physician immediately.

• Tell your doctor immediately if you have chest pain, fever, chills, facial flushing, itching, hives, or troubled breathing within a few hours of receiving.

• After you start therapy, avoid vaccination with live viruses.

• Use caution driving or performing tasks requiring alertness or coordination, since this drug may cause dizziness.

• Follow good food safety. Avoid foods that could be contaminated with Listeria monocytogenes, such as soft cheese and unpasteurized milk. Reheat ready-to-eat foods until steaming, such as cold cuts and hot dogs.[97]

• Avoid exposure to histoplasmosis, such as cleaning chicken coops or bird-roosting sites.[98]

• Exercise.

• Stop smoking.[99]

• If you have psoriatic arthritis, see a dermatologist, as well as your rheumatologist.

• Tell any doctor, dentist, emergency help, pharmacist, or surgeon you see that you use an immune modulator.

How to Use This Drug

• If you self-administer these drugs, obtain training and carefully follow accompanying instructions on how to prepare, measure, and inject the drug.

• Wash your hands thoroughly and prepare in a clean area.

• Do not add other medications to the solution.

• Inspect solution to be sure it is not discolored and has no particles floating in it.

• Rotate sites of injection, moving at least one inch from last site. Do not rub the injection site.

• Adalimumab and etanercept can be self-injected subcutaneously (SC) just under the skin at home. Do not handle the needle cover of adalimumab if you are allergic to latex (rubber).

• Anakinra is usually administered by a health professional. It should be injected at the same time each day.

• Infliximab is injected intravenously with an in-line filter over at least two hours, and started within three hours of preparation. It should be administered where emergency assistance is available in case of allergic reactions.

• If you miss a dose of etanercept, contact your doctor about when to inject the next dose.

• If you miss a dose of adalimumab, inject the next dose right away, then inject the following dose at the next scheduled time.

• **Do not take double doses.**

• Do not reuse needles or syringes.

• Do not share these drugs with others.

• Store injection solution in refrigerator, protected from light. Do not freeze or shake. Keep out of reach of children.

• Do not use beyond the expiration date. Discard needles and syringes in a puncture-resistant container.

Interactions with Other Drugs

The following drugs, biologics (e.g., vaccines, therapeutic antibodies), or foods are listed in *Evaluations of Drug Interactions* 2003 as causing "highly clinically significant" or "clinically significant" interactions when used together with any of the drugs in this section. In some sections with multiple drugs, the interaction may have been reported for one but not all drugs in this section, but we include the interaction because the drugs in this section are similar to one another. We have also included potentially serious interactions listed in the drug's FDA-approved professional package insert or in published medical journal articles. There may be other drugs, especially those in the families of drugs listed below, that also will react with this drug to cause severe adverse effects. Make sure to tell your doctor and pharmacist the drugs you are taking and tell them if you are taking any of these interacting drugs:

> TNF blockers with live virus vaccinations may be less effective and could induce infection. Do not use: adenovirus, BCG, influenza intranasal virus, measles, mumps, polio (Sabin), rotovirus, rubella, typhoid, varicella, or yellow fever vaccines.

> Avoid using anakinra (KINERET) with: ENBREL, etanercept, infliximab, REMICADE.

Adverse Effects

Call your doctor immediately if you experience:

- abdomen wall bulges (hernia)
- body aches or pains
- bleeding or bruising
- blood pressure increase or decrease
- breathing problems
- tightness in chest
- painful or tender cheekbones
- chills
- constipation
- cough
- diarrhea
- dizziness, fainting
- painful, tender, or yellow eyes
- facial flushing
- falls
- feeling of fullness
- fever
- general feeling of illness
- swollen glands
- headache
- irregular or pounding heartbeat
- infection
- bleeding, itching, swelling, or rash or pain at injection site
- irritated or white patches on mouth or tongue
- nasal congestion
- nausea or vomiting
- numbness or tingling
- pain in abdomen, back, bone, joints, muscles, rectum, side, stomach (severe), or pain that spreads to left shoulder
- redness around fingernails or toenails
- runny nose
- cracks at corners of mouth, hives, itching, pus, rash, pinpoint red spots on skin, or tender, red, or yellow skin
- sneezing
- sore throat
- black, bloody, or tarry stools
- unusual tiredness or weakness
- difficult, frequent, or painful urination or urine appears bloody or cloudy
- vision changes
- weight loss
- wheezing

Periodic Tests

Ask your doctor which of these tests should will be done periodically while you are taking this drug:

- blood counts
- computed tomography (CT) scan for tuberculosis
- heart status
- infectious disease testing
- neutrophil counts

Limited Use

Allopurinol (al oh *pure* i nole)
ZYLOPRIM (Prometheus)

GENERIC: available

FAMILY: Drugs for Arthritis and Gout (see pp. 283 and 287)

PREGNANCY WARNING

There is a published report of allopurinol causing deaths and malformations in an animal study. Because of the potential for serious adverse effects to the fetus, this drug should not be used by pregnant women.

BREAST-FEEDING WARNING

Allopurinol is excreted in human milk. Because of the potential for adverse effects in nursing infants, you should not take this drug while nursing.

Allopurinol helps to prevent gout attacks. Gout occurs when you have a high level of uric acid in your body, and an attack occurs when crystals of uric acid form in your joints and your body releases chemicals in response to the crystals. This causes pain and inflammation. Allopurinol works by decreasing your body's production of uric acid, thereby lowering the level of uric acid in your blood.[100]

Allopurinol will not relieve a gout attack that has already started. If you are taking allopurinol, keep taking it during an attack, even if another drug is prescribed to treat the attack.

After you start using allopurinol, your gout attacks may become more frequent for a while. Keep taking the drug. If you take it regularly, the attacks gradually will become less frequent and less painful, and they may stop completely after several months.

Allopurinol can cause skin rashes, allergic reactions, and kidney stones. Stop taking allopurinol and call your doctor at the first sign of skin rash or allergic reaction. To help prevent kidney stones while taking allopurinol, drink at least 10 to 12 full glasses (eight ounces each) of fluid each day, unless your doctor tells you otherwise. Too much vitamin C (see p. 809) also increases your risk of forming kidney stones, so do not take vitamin C supplements while you are taking allopurinol unless you have checked with your doctor first.

Before You Use This Drug

Tell your doctor if you have or have had:

- history of allergy to allopurinol
- kidney function impairment
- diabetes
- heart disease or high blood pressure
- pregnancy or are breast-feeding

Tell your doctor about any other drugs you take, including aspirin, herbs, vitamins, and other nonprescription products.

When You Use This Drug

- Do not drink alcohol. Alcohol increases the amount of uric acid in your blood and may make your gout attacks more frequent and more difficult to control. It also increases your risk of stomach problems.
- Discontinue immediately if a skin rash develops.
- Drink large amounts of fluids.
- Until you know how you react to this drug, do not drive or perform other activities requiring alertness. Allopurinol can cause drowsiness.

How to Use This Drug

- If you miss a dose, take it as soon as you remember, but skip it if it is almost time for the next dose. **Do not take double doses.**
- Do not share your medication with others.
- Take the drug at the same time(s) each day.
- Take after meals to decrease stomach upset. If this does not work and your stomach continues to be upset, check with your doctor.
- Store at room temperature with lid on tightly. Do not store in the bathroom. Do not expose to heat, moisture, or strong light. Keep out of reach of children.

Interactions with Other Drugs

The following drugs, biologics (e.g., vaccines, therapeutic antibodies), or foods are listed in *Evaluations of Drug Interactions* 2003 as causing "highly clinically significant" or "clinically significant" interactions when used together with any of the drugs in this section. In some sections with multiple drugs, the interaction may have been reported for one but not all drugs in this section, but we include the interaction because the drugs in this section are similar to one another. We have also included potentially serious interactions listed in the drug's FDA-approved professional package insert or in published medical journal articles. There may be other drugs, especially those in the families of drugs listed below, that also will react with this drug to cause severe adverse effects. Make sure to tell your doctor and pharmacist the drugs you are taking and tell them if you are taking any of these interacting drugs:

AMOXIL, ampicillin, amoxicillin, ARA-A, ARABINOSIDE, azathioprine, chlorpropamide, cyclophosphamide, cyclosporine, CYTOXAN, DIABINESE, dicumarol, DILANTIN, ELIXOPHYLLIN, IMURAN, mercaptopurine, OMNIPEN, phenytoin, PURINETHOL, SANDIMMUNE, SLO-BID, THEO-24, theophylline, vidarabine, VIRA-A.

Adverse Effects

Call your doctor immediately if you experience:

- skin rash, hives, or itching
- bloody or cloudy urine
- difficult or painful urination
- lower back or side pain
- chills, fever, or muscle aches
- nausea or vomiting along with chills or fever
- numbness or tingling of hands or feet
- red, thick, tender, burning, or peeling skin
- chill, sore throat, and fever
- unusual bleeding or bruising
- unusual tiredness or weakness
- sudden decrease in amount of urine
- yellow eyes or skin
- loosening of fingernails
- rapid weight gain
- difficulty breathing
- tightness in chest or wheezing
- unexplained nosebleeds
- bloody or black, tarry stools
- bleeding sores on lips
- pinpoint red spots on skin
- sores, ulcers, or white spots in mouth or on lips
- swelling in stomach area
- nausea or vomiting
- swelling of face, fingers, feet, or lower legs
- swollen glands

Call your doctor if these symptoms continue:

- diarrhea
- drowsiness
- nausea or vomiting without symptoms of skin rash
- stomach pain
- headache
- chills or fever
- muscle aches or pains
- unusual hair loss

Periodic Tests

Ask your doctor which of these tests should be done periodically while you are taking this drug:

- complete blood count
- liver function tests
- kidney function tests
- blood levels of uric acid

Limited Use

Azathioprine (aze *thy* o prin)
IMURAN (Prometheus)

GENERIC: not available for tablets

FAMILY: Drugs for Arthritis and Gout (see pp. 283 and 287)
Immunosuppressants

PREGNANCY WARNING

Immune system and skeletal abnormalities have occurred in infants of women taking azathioprine during pregnancy. This drug should not be used by pregnant women.

BREAST-FEEDING WARNING

Azathioprine is excreted in human milk. Because of the potential for adverse effects in nursing infants, including the possibility of tumors, you should not take this drug while nursing.

FDA BLACK BOX WARNING

Chronic immunosuppression with this purine antimetabolite increases risk of neoplasia [cancer] in humans. Physicians using this drug should be very familiar with this risk as well as with the mutagenic potential to both men and women and with possible hematologic [blood cell] toxicities.[101]

Azathioprine is a potent drug reserved for severe conditions. It prevents rejection of transplanted organs, particularly kidneys, by suppressing the immune system. When all other treatments (rest, anti-inflammatory drugs, gold compounds) fail to relieve rheumatoid arthritis, azathioprine may slow damage to the joints and control symptoms but does not cure any condition. It is an alternative when surgery for some disabling arthritis cannot be done, and is used to lower the dose of steroids, often given along with azathioprine. It may take several weeks or even a few months for improvement to show.

Older people with age-related decrease in kidney function are more likely to need a low dose. In all ages, the lowest effective dose should be used.

During the first couple of weeks of therapy with azathioprine, nausea is common. Since azathioprine affects your immune system, you may get infections, which can more easily become fatal. Azathioprine increases the risk of skin cancer, cervical cancer, Kaposi's sarcoma, and leukemia.[102] These risks increase when the drug is used for transplants and after the drug has been used for five years.[103] Azathioprine can also irritate your pancreas, damage your bone marrow, and harm your liver enough to be life-threatening. This liver damage is more apt to happen to men.[64] Lowering the dose may reverse some of these problems.

Before You Use This Drug

Because your risk of developing cancer would rise, discuss the benefit/risk balance of using azathioprine with your doctor if you are taking or have previously taken: ALKERAN, chlorambucil, cyclophosphamide, CYTOXAN, LEUKERAN, melphalan.

Do not use if you are:

- pregnant or breast-feeding

Tell your doctor if you have or have had:

- allergy to azathioprine
- chicken pox
- gout
- hepatitis zoster
- herpes
- infection
- kidney or liver problems
- pancreatitis

- radiation therapy
- severe xanthine oxidase deficiency
- previous exposure to cytotoxic drugs or radiation

Tell your doctor about any other drugs you take, including aspirin, herbs, vitamins, and other nonprescription products.

When You Use This Drug

- Keep your appointments for lab work. For the first two months blood tests should be done at least weekly, and at least monthly thereafter.
- Your doctor should be experienced in immunosuppressive therapy.
- Avoid places and people that expose you to bacterial or viral infections. Avoid crowds during flu seasons. Report the first sign of any infection to your doctor: cough, hoarseness, fever, chills, lower back or side pain, or painful or difficult urination.
- Avoid immunizations unless approved by your doctor. Others in patient's household should avoid oral polio vaccine.
- Check with your doctor immediately if you have unusual bleeding or bruising, black, tarry stools, blood in urine or stools, or pinpoint red spots on skin.
- Practice good hygiene. Wash your hands before touching your eyes or the inside of your nose.
- Check with your dentist about teeth-cleaning methods suited to your condition. Check with your physician before having dental work done.
- Be cautious using knives, razors, nail clippers, and other sharp objects.
- Avoid engaging in contact sports, moving heavy objects, and activities where you might get bruised.
- Continue to rest, get physical therapy, and use anti-inflammatory drugs if you have rheumatoid arthritis.
- If you undergo emergency care, or surgery, including dental, tell your doctor that you take azathioprine.

- If you must take allopurinol, your dose of azathioprine should be reduced to one-fourth the usual dose.

How to Use This Drug

- *If you miss a dose, use the following guidelines:* If you take the drug once a day, do not take the missed dose nor double the next dose. If you take the drug several times a day, then take it as soon as you remember or double the next dose only. Check with your doctor if you miss more than one dose.
- Do not share your medication with others.
- Take the drug at the same time(s) each day.
- Swallow tablet whole or break in half. If you take azathioprine once a day, take it at bedtime to reduce stomach upset. Otherwise, take it after a meal.
- If your doctor prescribes a suspension, shake it well before measuring.
- Store tablets at room temperature with lid on firmly. Do not expose to light and heat. Store other forms according to the prescription label. Keep out of reach of children.

Interactions with Other Drugs

The following drugs, biologics (e.g., vaccines, therapeutic antibodies), or foods are listed in *Evaluations of Drug Interactions* 2003 as causing "highly clinically significant" or "clinically significant" interactions when used together with any of the drugs in this section. In some sections with multiple drugs, the interaction may have been reported for one but not all drugs in this section, but we include the interaction because the drugs in this section are similar to one another. We have also included potentially serious interactions listed in the drug's FDA-approved professional package insert or in published medical journal articles. There may be other drugs, especially those in the families of drugs listed below, that also will react with this drug to cause severe adverse effects. Make sure to tell your doctor and pharmacist the drugs you are taking and tell them if you are taking any of these interacting drugs:

allopurinol, BACTRIM, co-trimoxazole, COUMADIN, warfarin (do not suddenly stop taking azathioprine or warfarin; check with your doctor), ZYLOPRIM.

The use of angiotensin converting enzyme (ACE) inhibitors to lower blood pressure together with azathioprine has been reported to cause a severe decrease in white blood cells.

Avoid live virus vaccines, such as polio vaccines, for at least three months after stopping azathioprine. Not only might the vaccine be ineffective, but you may be more apt to have adverse reactions to the vaccine. It is very important that you not come in close contact with anyone else, such as your grandchildren, getting live virus vaccines. If you must come in contact, especially with infants, wear a mask over your mouth and nose. Let someone else change and dispose of their diapers.

Adverse Effects

Call your doctor immediately if you experience:

- bloody or black, tarry, or pale stools
- unusual bleeding or bruising
- difficulty breathing
- chills
- cough, hoarseness
- severe diarrhea
- dizziness
- sudden fever
- rapid heartbeat
- severe nausea or vomiting
- pain in lower back, muscles, joints, side, or stomach
- pinpoint red spots, redness, blisters on skin
- sores in mouth or lips

- swelling of feet or legs
- unusual tiredness or weakness
- painful or difficult urination
- dark or bloody urine
- yellowing of eyes or skin
- unusual feeling of discomfort or illness

Call your doctor if these symptoms continue:

- abdominal pain
- constipation
- depression[104]
- hair loss
- headache
- heartburn
- loss of appetite
- low blood pressure
- nausea or vomiting
- skin rash, itching
- unusually deep suntan[105]
- blurred vision[104]

Call your doctor if these symptoms continue after you stop taking this drug:

- black, tarry stools
- blood in urine
- cough or hoarseness
- fever or chills
- lower back or side pain
- painful or difficult urination
- pinpoint red spots on skin
- unusual bleeding or bruising

Signs of overdose:

- pinpoint red spots on skin
- unusual bleeding or bruising
- diarrhea
- fever or chills
- cough or hoarseness
- lower back or side pain
- painful or difficult urination
- nausea or vomiting

If you suspect an overdose, call this number to contact your poison control center: (800) 222-1222.

Periodic Tests

Ask your doctor which of these tests should be done periodically while you are taking this drug:

- complete blood count
- liver function tests

Colchicine (*kol* chi seen)

GENERIC: available

FAMILY: Drugs for Arthritis and Gout (see pp. 283 and 287)

PREGNANCY WARNING

Colchicine caused fetal malformations in animal studies. Because of the potential for serious adverse effects, this drug should not be used by pregnant women.

BREAST-FEEDING WARNING

No information is available from either human or animal studies. However, it is likely that this drug, like many others, is excreted in human milk and, because of the potential for adverse effects in nursing infants, you should not take this drug while nursing.

Colchicine prevents and treats gout attacks, and reduces inflammation and relieves pain from acute gouty arthritis.

Gout occurs in people who have high levels of uric acid in their body, and an attack occurs when crystals of uric acid form in the joints and the body responds by releasing harmful chemicals. This causes pain and inflammation.

Colchicine prevents and treats attacks by decreasing the amount of chemicals that your body releases into the joints. It does not lower the level of uric acid in your body, which is the root cause of the problem. Colchicine has several harmful adverse effects (see Adverse Effects) and you may be better off taking large doses of an anti-inflammatory drug such as naproxen (a nonsteroidal anti-inflammatory drug, see p. 281), which has fewer harmful effects. Stop taking colchicine and call your doctor immediately if you have diarrhea, nausea, vomiting, or stomach pain. Older adults are more susceptible to colchicine's adverse effects. If you have decreased kidney function, you should be on a low dose of colchicine in order to reduce adverse effects such as muscle and nerve damage.

Before You Use This Drug

Do not use if you have or have had:

- liver or kidney disease
- pregnancy or are breast-feeding

Tell your doctor if you have or have had:

- allergy to colchicine
- alcohol abuse
- bone marrow depression, or blood cell diseases
- heart, kidney, or liver problems
- severe intestinal disease
- ulcer or other stomach problem

Tell your doctor about any other drugs you take, including aspirin, herbs, vitamins, and other nonprescription products.

When You Use This Drug

- Do not take more than prescribed, even if the pain is not relieved or if you do not experience adverse effects.
- Do not drink alcohol. Alcohol increases the amount of uric acid in your blood and may make your gout attacks more frequent or more difficult to control. It also increases the likelihood of stomach problems.

How to Use This Drug

- If you miss a dose, take it as soon as you remember, but skip it if it is almost time for the next dose. **Do not take double doses.**
- Do not share your medication with others.
- Take the drug at the same time(s) each day.
- If you take other drugs to prevent gout attacks and your doctor prescribes colchicine

when you have an attack, keep taking the other drugs as directed by your doctor.

• If you take colchicine only when you have an attack, take it at the first sign of attack. Stop taking it as soon as pain is relieved or at first sign of diarrhea, nausea, vomiting, or stomach pain. Do not take it more often than every three days, unless your doctor tells you otherwise.

• If you take colchicine regularly to prevent attacks, do not increase your dose during an acute attack unless directed by your doctor. If your doctor increases your dose during an attack, return to your regular dose after the attack is over.

• Store at room temperature with lid on tightly. Do not store in the bathroom. Do not expose to heat, moisture, or strong light. Keep out of reach of children.

Interactions with Other Drugs

Some other drugs that you may be taking (either over-the-counter or prescription) can interact with this one, causing adverse effects. Ask your doctor what these drugs are and let him or her know if you are taking any of them.

Such interacting drugs are: cyclosporine, grapefruit juice, SANDIMMUNE.

Adverse Effects

Call your doctor immediately if you experience:

- numbness or tingling in fingers or toes
- skin rash or hives
- huge, hive-like swellings on face, eyelids, mouth, lips, and/or tongue
- sore throat
- fever with or without chills
- sores, ulcers, white spots on lips or in mouth
- headache
- difficulty breathing
- tarry stools

- blood in urine
- pinpoint red spots on skin
- muscle weakness
- unusual bleeding or bruising
- unusual tiredness or weakness

Call your doctor if these symptoms continue:

- loss of appetite
- diarrhea
- nausea or vomiting
- stomach pain
- unusual hair loss

Signs of overdose:

- bloody urine
- burning feeling in stomach throat, or skin
- seizures
- bloody diarrhea
- fever
- mood or mental changes
- severe muscle weakness
- sudden decrease in amount of urine
- difficulty breathing
- severe vomiting
- hair loss
- sores, ulcers, or white spots on lips or in mouth

If you suspect an overdose, call this number to contact your poison control center: (800) 222-1222.

Periodic Tests

Ask your doctor which of these tests should be done periodically while you are taking this drug:

- complete blood count

Limited Use

Hydroxychloroquine (hye drox ee *klor* oh kwin)
PLAQUENIL (Sanofi)

GENERIC: available

FAMILY: Drugs for Arthritis and Gout (see pp. 283 and 287)

PREGNANCY WARNING

Hydroxychlorquine rapidly crossed the placenta in an animal study and accumulated in fetal eyes; it remained there for five months after it had been removed from the rest of the body. Irreversible retinal damage has occurred in some patients taking this drug. Because of the potential for serious adverse effects to the fetus, this drug should not be used by pregnant women except for the treatment of malaria.

BREAST-FEEDING WARNING

There is no information on excretion of hydroxychloroquine in milk. However, because of the potential for serious adverse effects in nursing infants, you should not take this drug while nursing.

Hydroxychloroquine is used to treat malaria, rheumatoid arthritis, and lupus erythematosus. Like other antiarthritis drugs, it reduces symptoms caused by inflammation. Because hydroxychloroquine has serious adverse effects, you should not be taking it for rheumatoid arthritis unless you have already tried other drugs that reduce inflammation and they have not worked.

Hydroxychloroquine takes time to produce results, and you may not notice improvement in your condition for weeks or months. Continue to take the drug as directed by your doctor, and use a nonsteroidal anti-inflammatory drug such as aspirin at the same time to relieve your symptoms until the hydroxychloroquine works. If the drug doesn't begin to work after six months, it should be discontinued.

Hydroxychloroquine can cause serious adverse effects, some of which may occur months after you have stopped using it. The drug can collect in your eyes and cause vision problems, so an eye specialist should check your eyes before and during your treatment with hydroxychloroquine. If you develop blurred vision, difficulty reading, or any other change in your vision, stop taking the drug and call your doctor.

Hydroxychloroquine has also caused some cases of rash, hearing loss, muscle weakness, and blood disorders. You should not take a dose greater than 400 milligrams per day, since taking such a large dose for a long time increases your risk of adverse effects.

Keep this drug out of the reach of children. Children are especially sensitive to the effects of hydroxychloroquine, and some have died after taking as few as three or four tablets.

Before You Use This Drug

Tell your doctor if you have or have had:

- allergies to drugs
- alcohol dependence
- liver or kidney problems
- severe blood disorders
- gastrointestinal disease
- glucose-6-phosphate dehydrogenase deficiency
- disorders of the nervous system or seizures
- psoriasis
- eye disease
- porphyria
- pregnancy or are breast-feeding

Tell your doctor about any other drugs you take, including aspirin, herbs, vitamins, and other nonprescription products.

When You Use This Drug

- Do not drink alcohol.
- Be alert to changes in vision and stop drug immediately. Hydroxychloroquine can cause irreversible damage to the eyes.
- Have regular eye exams during and after long-term use.
- Check with your doctor if there is no improvement in your arthritis after a few weeks or months. If there is no improvement in rheuma-

toid arthritis joint swelling or mobility after six months, the drug should be discontinued.

• Until you know how you react to this drug, do not drive or perform other activities requiring alertness. Hydroxychloroquine causes lightheadedness and drowsiness.

How to Use This Drug

• *If you miss a dose, use the following guidelines:* If you take the drug once a week, take the missed dose as soon as you remember and resume your regular schedule. If you take the drug once a day, take the missed dose as soon as you remember, but skip it if you don't remember until the next day. If you take the drug more than once a day, take the missed dose if you remember less than an hour after you were supposed to take it. If more than an hour has passed since you were supposed to take it, skip it. Continue to follow your regular schedule. **Do not take double doses.**

• Take with food or milk to reduce stomach upset.

• Store at room temperature with lid on tightly. Do not store in the bathroom. Do not expose to heat, moisture, or strong light. Keep out of reach of children.

Interactions with Other Drugs

The following drugs, biologics (e.g., vaccines, therapeutic antibodies), or foods are listed in *Evaluations of Drug Interactions* 2003 as causing "highly clinically significant" or "clinically significant" interactions when used together with any of the drugs in this section. In some sections with multiple drugs, the interaction may have been reported for one but not all drugs in this section, but we include the interaction because the drugs in this section are similar to one another. We have also included potentially serious interactions listed in the drug's FDA-approved professional package insert or in published medical journal articles. There may be other drugs, especially those in the families of drugs listed below, that also will react with this drug to cause severe adverse effects. Make sure to tell your doctor and pharmacist the drugs you are taking and tell them if you are taking any of these interacting drugs:

digoxin, FLAGYL, LANOXICAPS, LANOXIN, metronidazole.

Adverse Effects

Call your doctor immediately if you experience:

• changes of vision
• seizures
• mood or mental changes
• hearing loss; ringing or buzzing in ears
• unusual bleeding or bruising
• unusual muscle weakness
• sore throat and fever
• fatigue, weakness

Call your doctor if these symptoms continue:

• vision changes
• diarrhea
• loss of appetite
• nausea, stomach cramps or pain
• headache
• itching
• bleaching of hair or increased hair loss
• blue-black discoloration of skin, fingernails, or inside mouth
• dizziness or lightheadedness
• nervousness or restlessness
• skin rash

Call your doctor if this symptom continues after you stop taking this drug:

• blurred vision or any change in vision

Signs of overdose:

• difficulty breathing
• drowsiness
• fainting

- seizure
- coma
- headache
- very excitable

If you suspect an overdose, call this number to contact your poison control center: (800) 222-1222.

Periodic Tests

Ask your doctor which of these tests should be done periodically while you are taking this drug:

- eye exams (before use, and at least every six months during long-term use)
- complete blood count
- neuromusclar exams

 Do Not Use

ALTERNATIVE TREATMENT:
See Methotrexate (TREXALL), p. 342.

Leflunomide (le *flun* o mide)
ARAVA (Aventis)

FAMILY: Drugs for Arthritis and Gout (see pp. 283 and 287)

FDA BLACK BOX WARNING

CONTRAINDICATIONS AND WARNINGS

Pregnancy must be excluded before the start of treatment with Arava. Arava is contraindicated in pregnant women, or women of childbearing potential who are not using reliable contraception. Pregnancy must be avoided during Arava treatment or prior to the completion of the drug elimination procedure after Arava treatment.

Leflunomide was approved by the FDA in September 1998 for the treatment of active rheumatoid arthritis in adults. On March 28, 2002, Public Citizen's Health Research Group petitioned the Department of Health and Human Services to remove leflunomide immediately from the market.[106] Through the end of September 2001 leflunomide had been associated with at least 130 severe liver reactions, including 56 hospitalizations and 22 deaths. Two of these reactions were in patients in their 20s. In 12 of these deaths, leflunomide-induced liver toxicity appears to be the most plausible explanation.

Leflunomide is much more toxic to the liver than methothrexate (TREXALL), the alternative arthritis drug mentioned below (see p. 342).

The European Agency for the Evaluation of Medicinal Products (EMEA) issued a warning in March 2001 to patients and physicians concerning the potential link of leflunomide to severe liver injury, including death.[107] The highly regarded French source of independent drug information, *Prescrire International,* reviewed leflunomide and other drugs for rheumatoid arthritis and concluded "leflunomide appears to be less effective than methotrexate; and it has been associated with more severe adverse events than methotrexate or sulfasalazine [AZULFIDINE]." Furthermore, *Prescrire* added, "Leflunomide provides no clinically tangible advantage in the management of patients with rheumatoid arthritis who require treatment with a disease modifying drug. When long-term treatment with such a drug is warranted, methotrexate remains the first-choice option if maximal efficacy is sought, while antimalarials and oral suflasalazine have fewer adverse effects."[108] Antimalarial drugs include products such as hydroxychloroquine (PLAQUENIL) (see p. 339).

The United States perspective on the therapeutic value of leflunomide echoed the European view. The editors of *The Medical Letter on Drugs and Therapeutics,* a U.S. source of high-quality drug information, concluded their 1998 review of leflunomide by saying it "offers no clear advantage over better established and less expensive drugs such as methotrexate."[109]

Clinical trials submitted to the FDA by Aventis demonstrated that the effectiveness of leflunomide was likely inferior to methotrexate. In one trial, leflunomide and methotrexate were considered equally effective, with 41% of patients on leflunomide, 35% on methotrexate, and 19% on placebo responding to treatment.[110] But, in a much larger trial comparing methotrexate to leflunomide, methotrexate was significantly superior, with a 57% response rate compared to a 43% rate for those on leflunomide.[111]

Evidence of leflunomide's liver toxicity appeared during the clinical trials submitted to the FDA, with four cases of extremely elevated abnormal liver function test (LFT) enzymes and two patients requiring liver biopsies. Elevated LFTs of greater than three times the upper limit of what is considered normal is an early indicator of possible liver toxicity. One patient in these trials had elevations of 39 times and another 80 times the upper limit of normal. In the most carefully conducted study comparing leflunomide with methotrexate, 7.1% of patients on leflunomide had abnormal LFTs compared to 3.3% of patients on methotrexate 1.7% of those on placebo. Patients on leflunomide were also more likely to withdraw from the trial due to adverse events: 22% of patients on leflunomide versus 10% on methotrexate and 9% on placebo.[112]

In randomized controlled trials, there were more than three times as many cases of hypertension caused by leflunomide than by methotrexate. Since the drug came on the market, there have been 38 reports of hypertension with leflunomide but only one with methotrexate, even though there were more than five times as many prescriptions filled for methotrexate than for leflunomide.

Leflunomide offers no therapeutic advantage to patients over other drugs approved for rheumatoid arthritis. It poses an increased likelihood of serious adverse reactions such as liver toxicity and hypertension when compared to methotrexate, the current gold standard. With a variety of better drug treatments available, there is no reason to subject patients to an accumulating list of added risks; leflunomide should be promptly removed from the market.

───────

Limited Use

Methotrexate (meth oh *trex* ate)
TREXALL (Barr)

GENERIC: available

FAMILY: Drugs for Arthritis and Gout (see pp. 283 and 287)

┌─────────────────────────────────────┐
| **PREGNANCY WARNING** |
| |
| Methotrexate can cause fetal death and malformations when given to pregnant women. Because of the potential for serious adverse effects to the fetus, methotrexate should not be used by pregnant women. |
└─────────────────────────────────────┘

┌─────────────────────────────────────┐
| **BREAST-FEEDING WARNING** |
| |
| Because of the potential for serious adverse effects in nursing infants, you should not take this drug while nursing. |
└─────────────────────────────────────┘

Immediately below are excerpts from the methotrexate black-box warning required by the FDA. The entire warning can be found in the drug's professional product labeling or package insert. The package insert can be obtained from a pharmacist.

Methotrexate is used to treat rheumatoid arthritis and a few types of cancer.

FDA BLACK BOX WARNING

Methotrexate should be used only by physicians whose knowledge and experience include the use of antimetabolite therapy.

Because of the possibility of serious toxic reactions (which can be fatal):

Methotrexate should be used only in life threatening neoplastic diseases, or in patients with psoriasis or rheumatoid arthritis with severe, recalcitrant, disabling disease which is not adequately responsive to other forms of therapy.

Deaths have been reported with the use of methotrexate in the treatment of malignancy, psoriasis, and rheumatoid arthritis.

Patients should be closely monitored for bone marrow, liver, lung, and kidney toxicities.

Patients should be informed by their physician of the risks involved and be under a physician's care throughout therapy.

1. Methotrexate has been reported to cause fetal death and/or congenital anomalies. Therefore, it is not recommended for women of childbearing potential unless there is clear medical evidence that benefits can be expected to ourweigh the considered risks. Pregnant women with psoriasis or rheumatoid arthritis should not receive methotrexate.

2. Unexpectedly severe (sometimes fatal) bone marrow suppression, aplastic anemia and gastrointestinal toxicity have been reported with concomitant administration of methotrexate (usually in high dosage) along with some nonsteroidal anti-inflammatory drugs (NSAIDs). [See p. 281 for a list of NSAIDs.]

3. Methotrexate causes hepatotoxicity [liver toxicity], fibrosis and cirrhosis, but generally only after prolonged use.

4. Methotrexate-induced lung disease is a potentially dangerous lesion, which may occur acutely at any time during therapy and which has been reported at doses as low as 7.7 mg/week. It is not always fully reversible. Pulmonary symptoms (especially a dry, nonproductive cough) may require interruption of treatment and careful investigation.

5. Malignant lymphomas, which may regress following withdrawal of methotrexate, may occur in patients receiving low-dose methotrexate and, thus may not require cytotoxic treatment.

6. Severe, occasionally fatal, skin reactions have been reported following single or multiple doses of methotrexate.

7. Potentially fatal opportunistic infections, especially *Pneumocystis carinii* pneumonia, may occur with methotrexate therapy.

For rheumatoid arthritis, methotrexate is used in severe cases that have not responded to treatment with other drugs. Before prescribing methotrexate, your doctor should try anti-inflammatory drugs such as aspirin (see p. 304) or ibuprofen (see p. 288) and other antiarthritis drugs such as gold salts or penicillamine. You should only use methotrexate if these other drugs are not effective.

Methotrexate takes time to relieve the symptoms of arthritis, and you may not see improvement for weeks or months. Continue to take the drug as directed by your doctor, and also use a nonsteroidal anti-inflammatory drug other than aspirin until the methotrexate begins to work.

If you are using methotrexate for cancer, you may have to take it despite adverse effects such

Drugs used to treat cancer often cause severe nausea and vomiting, either immediately after the drug is taken or several hours later. You can treat this kind of nausea and vomiting by changing your diet or by taking an antinausea drug. You should always try dietary changes first.

• Eat small, frequent meals so that your stomach is never empty.

• When you get up from sleeping or resting, eat some dry crackers or toast before you start being active.

• Drink carbonated drinks or other clear liquids such as soups and gelatin.

• Eat tart foods such as lemons and pickles.

• Do not eat foods with strong smells.

as sore mouth, stomach upset, nausea, vomiting, and loss of appetite. If an adverse effect is causing you problems, ask your doctor or other health professional to suggest ways to avoid or decrease the problem.

Before You Use This Drug

Do not use if you have or have had:

• pregnancy or are breast-feeding
• bone marrow depression
• severe liver or kidney disease

Tell your doctor if you have or have had:

• allergy to methotrexate
• alcohol dependence
• bone marrow depression
• recent infection
• kidney or liver problems
• colitis
• stomach ulcers
• intestinal obstruction
• cytotoxic drugs or radiation
• chicken pox exposure or infection
• shingles (herpes zoster)
• mouth sores or inflammation

Tell your doctor about any other drugs you take, including aspirin, herbs, vitamins, and other nonprescription products.

When You Use This Drug

• Schedule regular visits with your doctor to check your blood counts, liver function, and progress on the drug.
• Use a doctor who is experienced in antimetabolite drug use.
• Do not use more or less often or in a higher or lower dose than prescribed.
• Check with your doctor before you stop using this drug.
• Do not drink alcohol. It increases your chances of liver damage.
• Avoid salicylate-containing products or NSAIDs.
• Notify your doctor at once if adverse events occur.
• Try to stay out of the sun. Methotrexate makes your skin more sensitive to sunlight.
• Do not get immunizations without your doctor's approval, and avoid exposure to people who have colds or other infections or who have recently been immunized. Because methotrexate decreases the number of white blood cells, which fight infection, you are more likely to get an infection while you are taking it.
• If you plan to have any surgery, including dental, tell your doctor that you take this drug.

How to Use This Drug

• If you miss a dose, take it as soon as you remember, but skip it if it is almost time for the next dose. **Do not take double doses.**
• Do not share your medication with others.
• Take the drug at the same time(s) each day.
• Store at room temperature with lid on tightly. Do not store in the bathroom. Do not expose to heat, moisture, or strong light. Keep out of reach of children.
• Call your doctor if you miss a dose or vomit shortly after taking the drug.

Interactions with Other Drugs

The following drugs, biologics (e.g., vaccines, therapeutic antibodies), or foods are listed in *Evaluations of Drug Interactions* 2003 as causing "highly clinically significant" or "clinically significant" interactions when used together with any of the drugs in this section. In some sections with multiple drugs, the interaction may have been reported for one but not all drugs in this section, but we include the interaction because the drugs in this section are similar to one another. We have also included potentially serious interactions listed in the drug's FDA-approved professional package insert or in published medical journal articles. There may be other drugs, especially those in the families of drugs listed below, that also will react with this drug to cause severe adverse effects. Make sure to tell your doctor and pharmacist the drugs you are taking and tell them if you are taking any of these interacting drugs:

ARAVA, asparaginase, aspirin, azapropazone, BACTRIM, BENEMID, chloramphenicol, cisplatin, COTRIM, DILANTIN, ECOTRIN, EMPIRIN, etretinate, GENUINE BAYER ASPIRIN, ketoprofen, leflunomide, leucovorin, MATULANE, neomycin, NEO-RX, ORUDIS, ORUVAIL, phenytoin, piperacillin, PLATINOL, PROBALAN, probenecid, procarbazine, rofecoxib, SEPTRA, SUMYCIN, TEGISON, tetracycline, trimethoprim/sulfamethoxazole, VIOXX, WELLCOVORIN, ZOSYN.

Adverse Effects

Call your doctor immediately if you experience:

- black, tarry stools
- stomach pain
- diarrhea
- bloody vomit
- fever, chills, or sore throat
- unusual bleeding or bruising
- lower back or side pain
- sores in mouth or on lips
- blood in urine
- painful or difficult urination
- swelling of feet or lower legs
- joint pain
- cough, shortness of breath
- dark urine
- yellow eyes or skin
- pinpoint red spots on skin
- blurred vision
- convulsions
- dizziness

Call your doctor if these symptoms continue:

- nausea, vomiting, loss of appetite
- hair loss
- skin rash, hives, or itching
- acne or boils
- pale or reddened skin

Periodic Tests

Ask your doctor which of these tests should be done periodically while you are taking this drug:

- kidney function tests
- monthly liver function tests
- monthly complete blood tests (including hematocrit, platelet count, white blood cell count)
- examination for mouth ulcers

Limited Use

Probenecid (proe *ben* e sid)
PROBALAN (Lannett)

GENERIC: available

FAMILY: Drugs for Arthritis and Gout (see pp. 283 and 287)
Antibiotic Therapy Aid

Probenacid crosses the placenta exposing the fetus to the drug. Use during pregnancy only for clear medical reasons. Tell your doctor if you are pregnant or thinking of becoming pregnant before you take this drug.

No information is available from either human or animal studies. Since it is likely that this drug, like many others, is excreted in human milk, you should consult with your doctor if you are planning to nurse.

Probenecid helps to prevent gout attacks. Gout occurs when you have high levels of uric acid in your body, and an attack occurs when crystals of uric acid form in your joints and your body releases chemicals in response to the crystals. This causes pain and inflammation. Probenecid works by causing more uric acid to leave your body through the kidneys, thereby lowering the level of uric acid in your blood.

Probenecid will not relieve a gout attack that has already started. If you are taking probenecid, keep taking it during an attack, even if another drug is prescribed to treat the attack.

After you start using probenecid, you may still have gout attacks for a while. Keep taking the drug. If you take it regularly, the attacks gradually will become less frequent and less painful, and they may stop completely after several months.

Probenecid can increase your risk of getting kidney stones. To help prevent kidney stones while using probenecid, drink at least 10 to 12 full glasses (eight ounces each) of fluid each day, unless your doctor tells you otherwise. Too much vitamin C (see p. 809) also increases your risk of kidney stones, so do not take vitamin C supplements while taking probenecid unless you have checked with your doctor.

Before You Use This Drug

Tell your doctor if you have or have had:

- allergies to drugs
- kidney problems
- kidney stones
- blood disease
- stomach ulcer
- cancer treated by antineoplastics or radiation
- pregnancy or breast-feeding

Tell your doctor about any other drugs you take, including aspirin, herbs, vitamins, and other nonprescription products.

When You Use This Drug

- Do not take aspirin and other drugs in its family (salicylates, see p. 304) because they may make probenecid less effective.
- Do not drink alcohol. Alcohol increases the amount of uric acid in your blood and it may make your gout attacks more frequent and more difficult to control. It also increases the likelihood of stomach problems.
- **Caution diabetics:** Probenecid may cause false results in copper sulfate urine sugar tests (Clinitest). It will not interfere with glucose enzymatic urine sugar tests (Clinistix).

How to Use This Drug

- If you miss a dose, take it as soon as you remember, but skip it if it's almost time for your next dose. **Do not take double doses.**
- Do not share your medication with others.
- Take the drug at the same time(s) each day.
- Take with food to decrease stomach upset. If this does not work and your stomach continues to be upset, check with your doctor.
- Store at room temperature with lid on tightly. Do not store in the bathroom. Do not expose to heat, moisture, or strong light. Keep out of reach of children.

Interactions with Other Drugs

The following drugs, biologics (e.g., vaccines, therapeutic antibodies), or foods are listed in

Evaluations of Drug Interactions 2003 as causing "highly clinically significant" or "clinically significant" interactions when used together with any of the drugs in this section. In some sections with multiple drugs, the interaction may have been reported for one but not all drugs in this section, but we include the interaction because the drugs in this section are similar to one another. We have also included potentially serious interactions listed in the drug's FDA-approved professional package insert or in published medical journal articles. There may be other drugs, especially those in the families of drugs listed below, that also will react with this drug to cause severe adverse effects. Make sure to tell your doctor and pharmacist the drugs you are taking and tell them if you are taking any of these interacting drugs:

aspirin, cephalothin, CYTOVENE, DILOR, dyphylline, ECOTRIN, ganciclovir, GENUINE BAYER ASPIRIN, INDOCIN, indomethacin, KEFLIN, ketorolac, LUFYLLIN, meropenem, MERREM, methotrexate, RETROVIR, TORADOL, TREXALL DOSE PACK, zidovudine (AZT).

Probenecid will increase the blood levels of certain antibiotics. Sometimes this is done therapeutically but it can also increase the risk of adverse drug reactions.

Adverse Effects

Call your doctor immediately if you experience:

- bloody or cloudy urine
- difficult or painful urination
- back or rib pain
- difficulty breathing

- unusual weight gain
- swelling of feet, legs, fingers, or face
- sore throat and fever
- unusual bleeding or bruising
- unusual tiredness or weakness
- decrease in amount of urine
- yellow eyes or skin
- cough or hoarseness
- sores, ulcers, or white spots on lips or mouth
- swollen and/or painful glands

Call your doctor if these symptoms continue:

- headache
- joint pain, redness, or swelling
- loss of appetite
- nausea or vomiting
- dizziness
- flushing or redness of face
- frequent urge to urinate
- sore gums

Signs of overdose:

- convulsions
- severe vomiting
- trouble breathing
- puffiness or swelling of eyelids
- changes in facial skin color, skin rash, hives, or itching

If you suspect an overdose, call this number to contact your poison control center: (800) 222-1222.

Periodic Tests

Ask your doctor which of these tests should be done periodically while you are taking this drug:

- blood and urine levels of uric acid

REFERENCES

1. Drugs for rheumatoid arthritis. *Medical Letter on Drugs and Therapeutics* 1991; 33:65–70.

2. Arthropan liquid and other salicylates for arthritis. *Medical Letter on Drugs and Therapeutics* 1976; 18:119.

3. Orland MJ, Saltman RJ, eds. *Manual of Medical Therapeutics.* 25th ed. Boston: Little, Brown and Company, 1986:373.

4. Herxheimer A. Many NSAID users who bleed don't know when to stop. *British Medical Journal* 1998; 316:492.

5. Wynne HA, Long A. Patient awareness of the adverse effects of non-steroidal anti-inflammatory drugs (NSAIDs). *British Journal of Clinical Pharmacology* 1996; 42:253–6.

6. Gilman AG, Goodman LS, Rall TW, Murad F, eds. *The Pharmacological Basis of Theapeutics.* 7th ed. New York: Macmillan, 1985.

7. Angell M. The quality of mercy. *New England Journal of Medicine* 1982; 306:98–9.

8. Simonson W. *Medications and the Elderly.* Rockville, Md.: Aspen Systems Corporation, 1984:116.

9. Drug treatment of cancer pain. *Medical Letter on Drugs and Therapeutics* 1982; 24:95–6.

10. AMA Department of Drugs. *AMA Drug Evaluations.* 5th ed. Chicago: American Medical Association, 1983.

11. Vestal RE. ed. *Drug Treatment in the Elderly.* Sydney, Australia: ADIS Health Science Press, 1984:179.

12. Targum SL. Food and Drug Administration Review of Cardiovascular Safety for Vioxx (rofecoxib), February 1, 2001:18.

13. Mukherjee D, Nissen SE, Topol EJ. Risk of cardiovascular events associated with selective COX-2 inhibitors. *Journal of the American Medical Association* 2001; 286:954–9.

14. Arnaud C, Joyeux-Faure M, Godin-Ribuot D, et al. COX-2: An in vivo evidence of its participation in heat stress–induced myocardial preconditioning. *Cardiovascular Research* 2003; 58:582–8.

15. Ott E, Nussmeier NA, Duke PC, et al. Efficacy and safety of the cyclooxygenase 2 inhibitors parecoxib and valdecoxib in patients undergoing coronary artery bypass surgery. *Journal of Thoracic and Cardiovascular Surgery* 2003; 125:1481–92.

16. Halter F, Tarnawski AS, Schmassmann A, et al. Cyclooxygenase-2 implications on maintenance of gastric mucosal integrity and ulcer healing: Controversial issues and perspectives. *Gut* 2001; 49:443–53.

17. Ekman EF. A cyclooxegenase-2 inhibitor impairs ligament healing in the rat. *American Journal of Sports Medicine* 2002; 30:457.

18. *USP DI, Drug Information for the Health Care Professional.* 12th ed. Rockville, Md.: United States Pharmacopeial Convention, 1992:460–70.

19. Garcia Rodriguez LA, Jick H. Risk of upper gastrointestinal bleeding and perforation associated with individual non-steroidal anti-inflammatory drugs. *The Lancet* 1994; 343:769–72.

20. Henry D, Dobson A, Turner C. Variability in the risk of major gastrointestinal complications from nonaspirin nonsteroidal anti-inflammatory drugs. *Gastroenterology* 1993; 105:1078–88.

21. Kaufman DW, Kelly JP, Sheehan JE, et al. Nonsteroidal anti-inflammatory drug use in relation to major upper gastrointestinal bleeding. *Clinical Pharmacology and Therapeutics* 1993; 53:485–94.

22. Langman MJ, Weil J, Wainwright P, et al. Risks of bleeding peptic ulcer associated with individual non-steroidal anti-inflammatory drugs. *The Lancet* 1994; 343:1075–8.

23. Savage RL, Moller PW, Ballantyne CL, et al. Variation in the risk of peptic ulcer complications with nonsteroidal anti-inflammatory drug therapy. *Arthritis and Rheumatism* 1993; 36:84–90.

24. Nonsteroidal anti-inflammatory drugs for rheumatoid arthritis. *Medical Letter on Drugs and Therapeutics* 1980; 22:29–31.

25. Gay GR. Another side effect of NSAIDs. *Journal of the American Medical Association* 1990; 264:2677–8.

26. Stadler P, Armstrong D, Margalith D, et al. Diclofenac delays healing of gastroduodenal mucosal lesions: Double-blind, placebo-controlled endoscopic study in healthy volunteers. *Digestive Diseases and Science* 1991; 36:594–600.

27. Dukes MNG, ed. *Side Effects of Drugs Annual* 13. Amsterdam: Elsevier, 1989:80.

28. Heim M, Nadvorna H, Azaria M. Grand mal seizures following treatment with diclofenac and pentazocine. *South African Medical Journal* 1990; 78:700–1.

29. Dukes MNG, ed. *Side Effects of Drugs Annual* 13. Amsterdam: Elsevier, 1989:74.

30. Fick DM, Cooper JW, Wade WE, et al. Updating the Beers criteria for potentially inappropriate medication use in older adults: results of a US consensus panel of experts. *Archives of Internal Medicine* 2003; 163:2716–24.

31. Toradol (ketorolac) Professional Product Labeling, September 1, 2002. Available at: http://www.rocheusa.com/products/toradol/pi.pdf. Accessed March 17, 2004.

32. Ahmad SR, Wolfe SM. Citizen's Petition to Withdraw Approval of Piroxicam (Feldene) from the Market, December 5, 1994.

33. Wolfe SM. Safety of piroxicam. *The Lancet* 1986; 2:808–9.

34. Armstrong CP, Blower AL. Ulcerogenicity of piroxicam: an analysis of spontaneously reported data. *British Medical Journal* 1987; 294:772.

35. *Physicians' Desk Reference.* 56th ed. Montvale, N.J.: Medical Economics Company, Inc., 2002:2676–80.

36. Lieberman T. Health Matters: When Hype Stands in for Solid Science. *Los Angeles Times,* June 18, 2001:S1.

37. Wolfe SM, Sasich LD. Public Citizen's Health Research Group—Statement Before the Arthritis Drugs Advisory Committee on Celecoxib (Celebrex), December 1, 1998.

38. Silverstein FE, Faich G, Goldstein JL, et al. Gastrointestinal toxicity with celecoxib vs nonsteroidal anti-inflammatory drugs for osteoarthritis and rheumatoid arthritis: the CLASS study: A randomized controlled trial. Celecoxib Long-term Arthritis Safety Study. *Journal of the American Medical Association* 2000; 284:1247–55.

39. Lichtenstein DR, Wolfe MM. COX-2-Selective NSAIDs: New and improved? *Journal of the American Medical Association* 2000; 284:1297–9.

40. Meloxicam (Mobic): Gastrointestinal and skin reactions. *Current Problems in Pharmacovigilance* 1998; 24:11–14.

41. Meloxicam—a safer NSAID? *Drug and Therapeutics Bulletin* 1998; 24:62–4.

42. Bombardier C, Laine L, Reicin A, et al. Comparison of upper gastrointestinal toxicity of rofecoxib and naproxen in patients with rheumatoid arthritis. VIGOR Study Group. *New England Journal of Medicine* 2000; 343:1520–8.

43. Villalba ML, Goldkind L. Food and Drug Administration Advisory Committee Briefing Document: Overall Safety, Rofecoxib (Vioxx), February 8, 2001:12.

44. *Physicians' Desk Reference.* 58th ed. Montvale, N.J.: Thomson PDR, 2004:2108–13.

45. *Physicians' Desk Reference.* 58th ed. Montvale, N.J.: Thomson PDR, 2004:2709–13.

46. Pharmacia submits NDA for "first" COX-2 injectable for acute pain. *Dickinson's FDA Webview,* July 16, 2001. Available at: http://www.fdaweb.com. Accessed March 17, 2004.

47. NDA deficiencies bring Pharmacia a "not approvable" letter for paracoxib. *Dickinson's FDA Webview,* July 16, 2001. Available at: http://www.fdaweb.com. Accessed March 16, 2004.

48. PR Newswire. Pharmacia submits new drug application for valdecoxib, March 23, 2001.

49. Daniels SE, Desjardins PJ, Talwalker S, et al. The analgesic efficacy of valdecoxib vs. oxycodone/acetaminophen after oral surgery. *Journal of the American Dental Association* 2002; 133:611–21.

50. Petersen, M. Madison Ave. Has Growing Role in the Business of Drug Research. *New York Times,* November 22, 2002.

51. Weil J, Colin-Jones D, Langman M, et al. Prophylactic aspirin and risk of peptic ulcer bleeding. *British Medical Journal* 1995; 310:827–30.

52. Kelly JP, Kaufman DW, Jurgelon JM, et al. Risk of aspirin-associated major upper-gastrointestinal bleeding with enteric-coated or buffered product. *The Lancet* 1996; 348:1413–6.

53. Derry S, Loke YK. Risk of gastrointestinal haemorrhage with long term use of aspirin: meta-analysis. *British Medical Journal* 2000; 321:1183–7.

54. de Gaetano G. Low-dose aspirin and vitamin E in people at cardiovascular risk: A randomised trial in general practice. Primary Prevention Project. *The Lancet* 2001; 357:89–95.

55. Hansson L, Zanchetti A, Carruthers SG, et al. Effects of intensive blood-pressure lowering and low-dose aspirin in patients with hypertension: Principal results of the Hypertension Optimal Treatment (HOT) randomised trial. HOT Study Group. *The Lancet* 1998; 351:1755–62.

56. Thrombosis prevention trial: Randomised trial of low-intensity oral anticoagulation with warfarin and low-dose aspirin in the primary prevention of ischaemic heart disease in men at increased risk. The Medical Research Council's General Practice Research Framework. *The Lancet* 1998; 351:233–41.

57. Steering Committee of the Physicians' Health Study Research Group. Final report on the aspirin component of the ongoing Physicians' Health Study. *New England Journal of Medicine* 1989; 321:129–35.

58. Peto R, Gray R, Collins R, et al. Randomised trial of prophylactic daily aspirin in British male doctors. *British Medical Journal* 1988; 296:313–6.

59. Pelayo, JC. Citizen's Petition Requesting the Commissioner of Food and Drug Administration to Amend the Final Rule for Professional Labeling for Aspirin. Docket: 77N-0094, September 2, 2003:26–7.

60. Hylek EM, Heiman H, Skates SJ, et al. Acetaminophen and other risk factors for excessive warfarin anticoagulation. *Journal of the American Medical Association* 1998; 279:657–62.

61. Ostapowicz G, Fontana RJ, Schiodt FV, et al. Results of a prospective study of acute liver failure at 17 tertiary care centers in the United States. *Annals of Internal Medicine* 2002; 137:947–54.

62. Lee WM. Acute liver failure in the United States. *Seminars in Liver Disease* 2003; 23:217–26.

63. *USP DI, Drug Information for the Health Care Professional.* 16th ed. Rockville, Md.: United States Pharmacopeial Convention, Inc., 1996:1448–54.

64. *American Hospital Formulary Service Drug Information.* Bethesda, Md.: American Society of Health System Pharmacists, 1996.

65. Professional Product Labeling for Methadone Hydrochloride Injection, USP, February 14, 2004. Available at: http://www.fda.gov/cder/foi/label/2004/21624slr001_methadone_hcl_lbl.pdf. Accessed March 12, 2004.

66. Cone EJ, Preston KL. Toxicologic aspects of heroin substitution treatment. *Therapeutic Drug Monitoring* 2002; 24:193–8.

67. Acute reactions to drugs of abuse. *Medical Letter on Drugs and Therapeutics* 2002; 44:21–4.

68. Ward J, Hall W, Mattick RP. Role of maintenance treatment in opioid dependence. *The Lancet* 1999; 353:221–6.

69. *USP-DI, Drug Information for the Health Care Professional.* 23rd ed. Greenwood Village, Col.: Micromedex, 2003.

70. Mercadante S, Casuccio A, Calderone L, et al. Switching from morphine to methadone in cancer patients with poor response to morphine. *Journal of Clinical Oncology* 1999; 17:3307–12.

71. Ripamonti C, Groff L, Brunelli C, et al. Switching from morphine to oral methadone in treating cancer pain: What is the equianalgesic dose ratio? *Journal of Clinical Oncology* 1998; 16:3216–21.

72. Tse DM, Sham MM, Ng DK, et al. An ad libitum schedule for conversion of morphine to methadone in advanced cancer patients: an open uncontrolled prospective study in a Chinese population. *Palliative Medicine* 2003; 17:206–11.

73. Eap CB, Buclin T, Baumann P. Interindividual variability of the clinical pharmacokinetics of methadone: implications for the treatment of opioid dependence. *Clinical Pharmacokinetics* 2002; 41:1153–93.

74. Shir Y, Rosen G, Zeldin A, et al. Methadone is safe for treating hospitalized patients with severe pain. *Canadian Journal of Anaesthesia* 2001; 48:1109–13.

75. Fisher MA, Glass S. Butorphanol (Stadol): a study in problems of current drug information and control. *Neurology* 1997; 48:1156–60.

76. *Drugs for the Elderly.* 2nd ed. Copenhagen, Denmark: World Health Organization, 1997:95.

77. Miller RR, Feingold A, Paxinos J. Propoxyphene hydrochloride: A critical review. *Journal of the American Medical Association* 1970; 213:996–1006.

78. Moertel CG, Ahmann DL, Taylor WF, et al. A comparative evaluation of marketed analgesic drugs. *New England Journal of Medicine* 1972; 286:813–5.

79. Public Citizen's Health Research Group. Letter to Joseph Califano, Secretary, Department of Health, Education, and Welfare, to Withdraw Propoxyphene (Darvon) from the Market, November 21, 1978.

80. Kamal-Bahl SJ, Doshi JA, Stuart BC, et al. Propoxyphene use by community-dwelling and institutionalized elderly Medicare beneficiaries. *Journal of the American Geriatrics Society* 2003; 51:1099–1104.

81. Tramadol—a new oral analgesic. *Medical Letter on Drugs and Therapeutics* 1995; 37:59–62.

82. Gibson T. Dear Health Care Professional Letter—Ultram (tramadol), March 20, 1996.

83. Kahn LH, Alderfer RJ, Graham DJ. Seizures reported with tramadol. *Journal of the American Medical Association* 1997; 278:1661.

84. Withdrawal syndrome and dependence: Tramadol too. *Prescrire International* 2003; 12:99–100.

85. Shorr RI, Griffin MR, Daugherty JR, et al. Opioid analgesics and the risk of hip fracture in the elderly: codeine and propoxyphene. *Journal of Gerontology* 1992; 47:M111–5.

86. Adalimumab (humira) for rheumatoid arthritis. *Medical Letter on Drugs and Therapeutics* 2003; 45:25–7.

87. Furst DE, Schiff MH, Fleischmann RM, et al. Adalimumab, a fully human anti tumor necrosis factor-alpha monoclonal antibody, and concomitant standard antirheumatic therapy for the treatment of rheumatoid arthritis: Results of STAR (Safety Trial of Adalimumab in Rheumatoid Arthritis). *Journal of Rheumatology* 2003; 30:2563–71.

88. Humira (adalimumab) Professional Product Labeling, January 1, 2003. Available at: http://www.rxabbott.com/pdf/humira.pdf. Accessed March 15, 2004.

89. Anakinra (Kineret) for rheumatoid arthritis. *Medical Letter on Drugs and Therapeutics* 2002; 44:18–9.

90. *Physicians' Desk Reference.* 58th ed. Montvale, N.J.: Thomson PDR, 2004:587–9.

91. *Physicians' Desk Reference.* 58th ed. Montvale, N.J.: Thomson PDR, 2004:573–8.

92. Marzo-Ortega H, McGonagle D, O'Connor P, et al. Efficacy of etanercept for treatment of Crohn's related spondyloarthritis but not colitis. *Annals of Rheumatologic Disease* 2003; 62:74–6.

93. Van den Brande JM, Braat H, van den Brink GR, et al. Infliximab but not etanercept induces apoptosis in lamina propria T-lymphocytes from patients with Crohn's disease. *Gastroenterology* 2003; 124:1774–85.

94. *Physicians' Desk Reference.* 58th ed. Montvale, N.J.: Thomson PDR, 2004:1145–8.

95. Probert CS, Hearing SD, Schreiber S, et al. Infliximab in moderately severe glucocorticoid resistant ulcerative colitis: a randomised controlled trial. *Gut* 2003; 52:998–1002.

96. Chakravarty EF, Sanchez-Yamamoto D, Bush TM. The use of disease modifying antirheumatic drugs in women with rheumatoid arthritis of childbearing age: a survey of practice patterns and pregnancy outcomes. *Journal Rheumatology* 2003; 30:241–6.

97. Slifman NR, Gershon SK, Lee JH, et al. Listeria monocytogenes infection as a complication of treatment with tumor necrosis factor alpha-neutralizing agents. *Arthritis and Rheumatism* 2003; 48:319–24.

98. Lee JH, Slifman NR, Gershon SK, et al. Life-threatening histoplasmosis complicating immunotherapy with tumor necrosis factor alpha antagonists infliximab and etanercept. *Arthritis and Rheumatism* 2002; 46:2565–70.

99. Bieber J, Kavanaugh A. Cigarette smoking, TB, and TNF inhibitors. *Annals of Rheumatic Disease* 2003; 62:1118–9.

100. Terkeltaub RA. Clinical practice. Gout. *New England Journal of Medicine* 2003; 349:1647–55.

101. *Physicians' Desk Reference.* 58th ed. Montvale, N.J.: Thomson PDR, 2004:402–3.

102. Younger IR, Harris DW, Colver GB. Azathioprine in dermatology. *Journal of the American Academy of Dermatology* 1991; 25:281–6.

103. Yudkin PL, Ellison GW, Ghezzi A, et al. Overview of azathioprine treatment in multiple sclerosis. *The Lancet* 1991; 338:1051–5.

104. Singh G, Fries JF, Williams CA, et al. Toxicity profiles of disease modifying antirheumatic drugs in rheumatoid arthritis. *Journal of Rheumatology* 1991; 18:188–94.

105. Callen JP, Spencer LV, Burruss JB, et al. Azathioprine: An effective, corticosteroid-sparing therapy for patients with recalcitrant cutaneous lupus erythematosus or with recalcitrant cutaneous leukocytoclastic vasculitis. *Archives of Dermatology* 1991; 127:515–22.

106. Barbehenn E, Lurie P, and Wolfe SM. Citizen's Petition to Remove Leflunomide (Arava) from the Market, March 28, 2002.

107. European Agency for the Evaluation of Medicinal Products. EMEA Public Statement on Leflunomide (Arava)—Severe and Serious Hepatic Reactions, March 12, 2001.

108. Leflunomide and rheumatoid arthritis: new preparation. Neither the safest nor the most effective slow-acting antirheumatic drug. *Prescrire International* 2001; 10:36–9.

109. New drugs for rheumatoid arthritis. *Medical Letter on Drugs and Therapeutics* 1998; 40:110–2.

110. Hyde J. Food and Drug Administration Medical Officer Review of Arava (leflunomide), September 3, 1998:21.

111. Hyde J. Food and Drug Administration Medical Officer Review of Arava (leflunomide), September 3, 1998:33.

112. Strand V, Cohen S, Schiff M, et al. Treatment of active rheumatoid arthritis with leflunomide compared with placebo and methotrexate. Leflunomide Rheumatoid Arthritis Investigators Group. *Archives of Internal Medicine* 1999; 159:2542–50.

7

DRUGS FOR COLD, COUGH, ALLERGY, AND ASTHMA

COUGH AND COLD

Combination Drugs for Cold, Cough, or Allergy

Many prescription or over-the-counter drug combinations of two or more ingredients should not be used because they are irrational combinations of single ingredients, some of which are safe and effective and sensible to use alone if treating the symptom for which they are intended. The combinations, however, present extra risks for extra ingredients that will usually not add any benefit (possibly a risk) to the first ingredient and will invariably cost much more than the single ingredient alone. They represent a "shotgun" approach to multiple symptoms of colds, coughs, and allergies that rarely occur in force in the combination that is suggested by the two ingredients in these products. (See p. 378 for details of these drugs.)

The viral infection we call "the common cold" can usually be treated without any professional help by rest and plenty of liquids, occasionally aided by the use of simple over-the-counter (nonprescription) remedies for relief of certain symptoms. There are no drugs that can kill the viruses that cause colds.

A cold cannot be "cured," except by time, but you are less likely to catch a cold if you do not smoke, since smoking paralyzes the hairlike cells (cilia) that clean out the body's airways. Colds are usually spread by hand more often than they are spread through the air. It's a good idea to prevent the spread of viruses by trying not to touch your eyes, mouth, or nose, and by washing your hands frequently when you are ill or with an ill person.

Certain other illnesses appear similar to colds but warrant medical advice. If you have a high fever (above 101°F, or 38.3°C) accompanied by chills and you are coughing up thick phlegm, or if coughing or breathing deeply causes sharp chest pain, you may have pneumonia. You should call your doctor for diagnosis and appropriate treatment.

The safest, best, and least expensive way to care for a cold is to not take anything at all and let the illness run its short, usually self-limiting course. If necessary, purchase single-ingredient products to treat the individual symptoms that you have.

What Is the Common Cold?

The common cold is a viral infection of the upper respiratory tract (nose, throat, and upper airways), resulting in inflammation of the mucous membrane lining of those areas. The most common symptoms are runny nose, sneezing, and a sore throat. The sore throat accompanying a cold is the most common kind of sore throat.

How to Treat a Cold

Nondrug Measures

A cold is best treated without drugs by drinking plenty—at least 8 to 10 full (eight-ounce) glasses per day—of nonalcoholic liquids (especially warm or hot liquids), getting enough rest, and not smoking.

Drugs to Use

If symptoms do not respond to these nondrug measures and interfere with normal activities, the following products are safe and effective. Please note that all of the drug products we recommend for treating various cold symptoms— stuffy nose, fever, nonproductive cough—are available without a prescription (over-the-counter [OTC]). None of the prescription cough or cold drugs is recommended; they are classified as **Do Not Use.**

For a runny nose: No OTC or prescription drug is appropriate. A runny nose promotes drainage and should not be treated with medication. If it lasts longer than a week, call your doctor.

For a stuffy nose: If your nose is blocked, especially if you can't breathe through it, use nose drops or spray containing oxymetazoline hydrochloride (AFRIN, for example), xylometazoline hydrochloride (OTRIVIN NASAL SPRAY, for example), or phenylephrine hydrochloride (NEO-SYNEPHRINE nose drops and nasal spray, for example). Buy a less expensive generic or store brand product of any of these if it is available. Do not use these drugs for more than three days because they can cause local irritation and then promote congestion.

For fever, headaches, and body aches: Use aspirin or acetaminophen, if needed (see pp. 304 and 308). (Also see Reye's Syndrome Warning, p. 281.) *For a cough:* A productive cough (when you are coughing something up) should not be treated. An unproductive (dry) cough associated with a cold also does not require treatment (see p. 354).

Cold Remedies (Not to Use)

Oral nasal decongestants (pills or syrup): We do not recommend the use of any nasal decongestants that are taken by mouth for treatment of a cold, although an FDA panel has found two ingredients, pseudoephedrine and phenylephrine, safe and effective. These decongestant ingredients are in the OTC drugs Actifed and Sudafed and others of the prescription cough and cold drugs presented in this book. The reason we do not recommend them is that they all contain large amounts of amphetamine-like drugs that can increase your heart rate and blood pressure. In addition, they can make you jittery and keep you awake. By using nose drops or spray, for one to three days (no more), you get less than ⅕₅ as much of these drugs—and just in your nose where they are needed, instead of throughout your system as you do when you take these drugs by mouth.

Antihistamines: Although the FDA has tentatively approved these drugs for colds, we do not recommend the use of the following for treatment of a cold, largely because they are ineffective for this purpose: Chlor-Trimeton and Dimetane (OTC) or any of the prescription antihistamines (see p. 363).

The most widely read book on drugs, a standard reference for doctors called *The Pharmacological Basis of Therapeutics,* says this about the use of antihistamines for treating the common cold: "Despite early claims and persistent popular belief, histamine-blocking drugs [antihistamines] are without value in combating the common cold." Antihistamines also have a sedative effect.

Another reason to avoid unnecessary use of antihistamines is that older adults are more sensitive to their adverse effects. (See Chapter 2, Adverse Drug Reactions, p. 10.)

Sore Throat

Sore throats are one of the leading causes of visits to doctors, with more than 10 million such visits a year. The only kind of sore throat that merits treatment with an antibiotic is a bacterial sore throat caused by group A beta-hemolytic streptococci, the so-called strep throat. Although only approximately 10% of adults seen by a doctor for a sore throat actually have strep throat, 75% of patients with sore throats seen by doctors are prescribed an antibiotic.[1] Though the likelihood that a sore throat in a child is a strep throat is somewhat higher, perhaps 25%, the majority of children are also treated with antibiotics. The risks of unnecessary antibiotic prescribing, discussed further in chapter 24, Drugs for Infections, include the adverse reactions, sometimes quite serious, to a drug that should have not been prescribed in the first place as well as unnecessary worsening of the already serious problem of antibiotic resistance.

As discussed in the section above about colds, a viral infection such as a cold is by far the most common cause of a sore throat. Although it is possible to have both a cold and a strep throat as the cause of your sore throat, most of the time it is one or the other, usually a viral infection. Among the clinical findings that make it more likely that you have a strep throat, rather than a viral sore throat, are the absence of a cough, the presence of not only a fever but chills and the presence of exudate (pus) on your tonsils. The most sensitive and specific test for a strep throat is the old-fashioned throat culture. Then, your doctor can write a prescription for an antibiotic, but it can be filled only if the throat culture turns out to be positive. The newer rapid diagnostic tests for strep are not quite as accurate but are in widespread use.

Cough: A Necessary Evil

Your lungs clean themselves constantly in order to maintain efficient breathing. Mucus normally lines the walls of the lungs and captures foreign particles, such as inhaled smoke and infecting virus particles. Hairlike cells (cilia) push this out of the lungs. Coughing adds an additional, rapid-fire means of removing unwanted material from the lungs.

A cough is beneficial as long as it is bringing up material, such as sputum (phlegm), from your airways and lungs. This is called a productive cough and is often seen with colds, bronchitis, and pneumonia. A dry, hacking, non-productive cough, on the other hand, can be irritating and keep you awake at night. Cough can also be part of a chronic condition, such as asthma or emphysema, or it may be caused by cigarette smoking.

Cough resulting from a chronic condition should be evaluated by your doctor. You should also seek medical advice if your sputum (phlegm) becomes greenish, yellowish, or foul-smelling, if your cough is accompanied by a high fever lasting several days, if coughing or breathing deeply causes sharp chest pain, or if you develop shortness of breath. Any of the symptoms may indicate pneumonia. Anyone who coughs up blood should call a doctor.

Types of Coughs

A *productive cough* is useful in helping you to recover from a cold or flu. You should do what you can to encourage the clearance of material from your lungs by "loosening up" the mucus. This is the purpose of an expectorant, which thins secretions so that they can be removed more easily by coughing (or "expectoration"). The best expectorant is water, especially in warm liquids such as soup, which thins the mucus and increases the amount of fluid in the respiratory tract. A moist environment also helps this effort. You should drink plenty of liquids and, if you can, moisten the air in your home with a humidifier or plain water steamed by a vaporizer. A pan of water on the radiator can help in the winter.

A *nonproductive cough,* a dry cough bringing up no mucus, should not be treated with a cough suppressant, also called an antitussive, if it is only associated with a cold. A nonproductive cough associated with cancer, for example, that keeps you up at night or is extremely exhausting may call for the use of benzonatate (TESSALON). Cough suppressants should be used only in a single-ingredient product. Rest and plenty of fluids are also in order.

Cough Remedies (Not to Use)

Acute cough due to an upper respiratory tract infection is mild and self-limiting. Two of the most popular cough suppressants, dextromethorphan (see p. 375) and diphenhydramine (see p. 363) have not been shown to be effective for this type of cough in children and adults and should not be used.

Another ingredient in prescription (and OTC) cough products that we recommend against using is the expectorant guaifenesin (in all Robitussin products). We believe guaifenesin lacks evidence of effectiveness in loosening secretions (see Robitussin and Mucinex, p. 377).

Fever, Headache, and Muscle Aches

Fever, headache, and muscle aches are sometimes companions of the common cold. They are best treated without drugs, with rest and adequate fluids, or with plain aspirin or acetaminophen. (A generic or store brand is as effective as heavily advertised brand names such as Genuine Bayer or Tylenol and generally costs less.)

Never give aspirin to a feverish person under 40 years old: he or she may have influenza rather than a cold. There is strong evidence that young people who take aspirin when they have flu (or chicken pox) have a greatly increased risk of later getting Reye's syndrome. This is a rather rare but potentially fatal disease that often leaves its victims mentally impaired for life, if they survive.

Call your doctor if a fever climbs above 103°F (39.4°C), or if a fever at or above 100°F (38°C) lasts for more than four days. Under either of these circumstances, the patient probably does not have a cold.

When to Seek Medical Help

Seek Medical Help When Any of the Following Occur:

- a fever greater than 101°F (38.3°C) accompanied by chills and coughing up thick phlegm (especially if greenish or foul-smelling)
- sharp chest pain when taking a deep breath
- coldlike symptoms that do not improve after seven days
- any fever greater than 103°F (39.4°C)
- coughing up blood
- a painful throat with any of the following
  1. pus (yellowish-white spots) on the tonsils or the throat
  2. fever greater than 101°F (38.3°C)
  3. swollen or tender glands or bumps in the front of the neck
  4. exposure to someone who has a documented case of strep throat
  5. a rash that came during or after a sore throat
  6. a history of rheumatic fever, rheumatic heart disease, kidney disease, or chronic lung disease such as emphysema or chronic bronchitis

ALLERGY AND HAY FEVER

If you suffer from an itchy and runny nose, watery eyes, sneezing, and a tickle in the back of your throat, then you probably have an allergy. An allergy means a hypersensitivity to a particular substance called an allergen. Hypersensitivity means that the body's immune system, which defends against infection, disease, and foreign bodies, reacts inappropriately to the allergen. Examples of common allergens are pollen, mold, ragweed, dust, feathers, cat hair, makeup, walnuts, aspirin, shellfish, poison ivy, and chocolate.

There are four common types of allergic responses, although many substances can cause more than one type of response in a given person:

- Itchy and runny nose, watery eyes, sneezing, and a tickle in the back of your throat. This type of allergy is sometimes called allergic rhinitis and is commonly caused by exposure to allergens in the air, such as pollen, dust, and animal feathers or hair. It is called hay fever when it occurs seasonally, in response to ragweed in the fall.
- Hives or other skin reactions. These commonly result from something you eat or from skin exposure to an allergenic substance, such as poison ivy or chemicals. Allergic skin reactions may also follow insect bites or an emotional disturbance.
- Asthma (see p. 358).
- Sudden, generalized itching, rapidly followed by difficulty breathing, and possible shock (extremely low blood pressure) or death. This rare and serious allergic response, called anaphylaxis, usually occurs as a response to certain injections (including allergy shots), drugs (including antibiotics such as penicillin and many arthritis drugs such as celecoxib [CELEBREX]), and insect bites as from a bee or wasp. This reaction may become increasingly severe with repeated exposures. Anaphylaxis is a medical emergency requiring an immediate trip to an emergency room, clinic, or doctor's office. If you are likely to have an anaphylactic response to an allergen, such as a bee sting, in a locale where medical attention may be out of reach, you should obtain a prescription from a doctor for an emergency kit containing injectable epinephrine to keep with you, and learn how to use it.

How to Treat Allergic Symptoms

The best way to treat an allergy is to discover its cause and, if possible, to avoid the substance. Sometimes this is easy, but in many cases it is not. If, for example, your eyes swell, your nose runs, and you break out in hives each time you are around cats, avoid cats and you have solved your problem.

If, however, you sneeze during one particular season (typically, late spring, summer, or fall) each year or all year round, there is not too much you can do to avoid the pollens, dust, or grass particles in the air. Some people find relief in an indoor retreat where it is cooler, closed, and less dusty, but this is not always possible.

If you can't seem to figure out the cause of your allergy, have tried eliminating most of the common allergens from your environment, and are still suffering significant discomfort, you may have to see your doctor or another health professional. It is possible that you may be an appropriate candidate for skin testing and may be referred to a doctor specializing in allergies.

Beware of the allergist who sends you home with a long list of substances to avoid because they gave positive patch tests. Even if you avoid all of them, you may be left with your allergy if none of the substances on the list is the particular one responsible for your symptoms.

When identifying the cause of your allergy is not possible, you may choose to treat the symptoms. Allergy symptoms are caused primarily by the release of a chemical in your body called histamine, and a class of drugs known as the antihistamines is the most effective initial treatment available. We recommend that you use antihistamines in a single-ingredient preparation to treat your symptoms. Another choice are the steroid-containing nasal sprays (see p. 379).

Allergic rhinitis should not be treated with topical nasal decongestants (drops, sprays, and inhalers) that are recommended for treating the temporary stuffy nose of a cold. Allergies are long-term conditions, lasting for weeks, months, or years, and use of these topical decongestants for more than a few days can lead to rebound congestion (an increase in nasal stuffiness after the medication wears off) and sometimes permanent damage to the membranes lining the nose. If you think your congestion is caused by allergies, don't use an OTC nasal spray, or you may eventually find that you cannot breathe through your nose without it.

Drugs for Allergy

Antihistamines: Of all the products sold for allergy, we recommend that you use a single-ingredient product containing only an antihistamine. Antihistamines are the most effective ingredients you can buy for treating an allergy, and you will minimize the adverse effects by buying the single-ingredient formulation.

A major adverse effect of antihistamines is drowsiness. If they make you drowsy, you should avoid driving a motor vehicle or operating heavy machinery while taking these drugs. Even if they don't make you drowsy, they may still slow your reaction time. Additionally, keep in mind that drowsiness is increased dramatically by adding other sedatives, including alcoholic beverages.

The amount of drowsiness produced by an antihistamine differs depending on the person who takes it and the antihistamine that is used. Of antihistamines classified by the FDA as safe and effective for OTC use, those causing the least drowsiness are chlorpheniramine maleate, brompheniramine maleate, pheniramine maleate, and clemastine. For daytime use, we urge you to use one of these.

Other FDA-approved antihistamines causing a great deal of drowsiness include diphenhydramine hydrochloride and doxylamine succinate, which are the ingredients in some currently available OTC sleep aids.

The advent of the less sedating but dangerous prescription antihistamines, the first of which were astemizole and terfenadine, now banned, has lessened the tendency of physicians and patients to use the lowest possible dose of the older, less expensive, and safer antihistamines such as chlorpheniramine maleate, the active ingredient in Chlor-Trimeton and dozens of other prescription and over-the-counter allergy medicines. By trying a lower dose, you may find that you significantly reduce the sedating effects. There are now other, less dangerous nonsedating antihistamines on the market (see p. 369).

Another common adverse effect of antihistamines is dryness of the mouth, nose, and throat. Other less common adverse effects include blurred vision, dizziness, loss of appetite, nausea, upset stomach, low blood pressure, headache, and loss of coordination. Difficulty in urinating is often a problem in older men with enlarged prostate glands. Antihistamines occasionally cause nervousness, restlessness, or insomnia, especially in children.

For antihistamine treatment of allergies, your first choice should be a low dose of chlorpheniramine in an OTC single-ingredient product such as Chlor-Trimeton. Check the label and be sure that nothing else is in the product. Chlor-Trimeton Decongestant and Dimetapp both contain an additional ingredient that is not necessary for the treatment of allergy. Less expensive store brand or generic equivalents are often available and should be purchased if possible. If you can't find them, ask the pharmacist.

You should not use antihistamines for self-medication if you have asthma, glaucoma, or difficulty urinating due to enlargement of the prostate gland.

Nasal decongestants: Many over-the-counter products sold for allergies contain amphetamine-like nasal decongestants, such as pseudoephedrine hydrochloride or ingredients found in many oral cold preparations (see earlier discussion on oral decongestants for colds). Some of these adverse effects and adverse reactions (such as jitteriness, sleeplessness, and potential heart problems) occur even more frequently when they are used to treat allergies, because allergy medication is usually taken for a longer period of time than a cold remedy is.

More to the point, nasal decongestants do not treat the symptoms most frequently experienced by allergy sufferers: the runny nose, itchy and watery eyes, sneezing, cough, and the tickle in the back of the throat. They treat only a stuffy nose, which is not the major problem for most allergy sufferers.

Examples of OTC nasal decongestants that are labeled to treat symptoms "without drowsiness" (since they do not contain antihistamines) include Afrinol and Sudafed. We do not recommend the use of these products for allergies.

Combination allergy products: As usual in the OTC market (particularly in the cold and allergy area), most products available are fixed-combination products using a "shotgun" approach to your ailment. The majority of allergy combination products contain antihistamines and nasal decongestants; some also contain pain relievers. We do not recommend any of these for self-treatment.

It is our opinion that nasal decongestants should not be used for allergy symptoms that are appropriate for self-treatment. The likelihood of adverse effects is increased by taking a combination product, and decongestants are seldom useful for allergy symptoms.

Examples of OTC combination drugs for allergy, which we cannot recommend, are Actifed Cold & Allergy Tablets, Chlor-Trimeton Allergy-D 12 Hour Tablets, and Drixoral Cold & Allergy Tablets. Many of the combination cold products that we urge you not to use are also marketed for allergic symptoms and hay fever. We do not recommend using any of these products for allergies either.

ASTHMA, CHRONIC BRONCHITIS, AND EMPHYSEMA

Asthma, chronic bronchitis, and emphysema all occur commonly, may occur together, and may have similar treatments.

Asthma is a disease in which the smaller air passages in the lungs are hyperirritable. Attacks, which may be initiated by various influences, lead to narrowing of the airways and difficulty breathing. Wheezing, chest tightness, and an unproductive cough usually accompany the sensation of shortness of breath. Most asthmatics have only occasional trouble breathing.

Asthma attacks are commonly caused by exposure to specific allergens, air pollutants, industrial chemicals, or infection. They can be caused by exercise (especially in cold air). Asthma can be worsened by emotional factors, and the disease often runs in families. Other ailments common to many asthma sufferers, or their family members, are hay fever and an allergic skin condition called eczema.

Chronic bronchitis is a disease in which the cells lining the lungs secrete excess mucus, leading to a chronic cough, usually accompanied by phlegm.

Emphysema is due to destruction of the walls of lung air sacs and is characterized by shortness of breath, with or without a cough. There is a fair degree of overlap between chronic bronchitis and emphysema, and the two are sometimes lumped together into "chronic obstructive pulmonary disease," or COPD. Wheezing may occur with chronic bronchitis or emphysema.

Chronic bronchitis or emphysema is most commonly the end result of many years of cigarette smoking. Other causes include occupational or environmental air pollution, chronic lung infections, and hereditary factors.

Asthma, chronic bronchitis, and emphysema may be occupational illnesses (a problem related to the workplace). Asthma frequently occurs among meat wrappers, bakers, woodworkers, and farmers, and among workers exposed to specific chemicals. Chronic bronchitis frequently is the result of exposure to dusts and noxious gases.

Asthma, bronchitis, and emphysema may be mild. For some people, however, these diseases can become life-threatening or can cause restriction in lifestyle. For all people afflicted with these problems, the types of drugs prescribed to treat or prevent the attacks are quite strong. If used incorrectly, they may have an immediate and dangerous effect on the health of the user.

Do not try to diagnose or treat yourself. Asthma, chronic bronchitis, and emphysema must be diagnosed and treated by a doctor or other health professional. Two other common conditions that cause breathing difficulties, congestive heart failure and pneumonia, have similar symptoms, and many of the drugs used to treat asthma or COPD may worsen these conditions. Therefore, it is extremely important that you have your condition properly diagnosed before starting any medication.

Treatment

Like its diagnosis, the treatment of asthma or COPD should be determined by a doctor. Attacks of asthma can be very frightening, and sufferers often overtreat themselves, especially when the desired relief has not been provided by the recommended dosage. Do not use more or less than the prescribed dose of any asthma or bronchitis medication without first consulting your doctor.

All medications for the treatment of these disorders, including those available without a prescription, should be chosen by you and your doctor together. A doctor is likely to prescribe one or more prescription drugs for the asthmatic. The currently available nonprescription (over-the-counter) drugs should not be used even for the treatment of minor or infrequent asthmatic episodes. The drug of choice for treatment of occasional acute symptoms of asthma is an inhaled short-acting beta2-agonist, such as albuterol (PROVENTIL, VENTOLIN), or pirbuterol (MAXAIR).[2] These drugs are also commonly used for chronic bronchitis or emphysema.

Corticosteroids such as oral prednisone (DELTASONE, METICORTEN), or inhaled beclomethasone (BECLOVENT, VANCERIL), flunisolide (AEROBID), and triamcinolone (AZMACORT) are commonly used when severe acute symptoms of asthma do not improve after treatment with inhaled albuterol.[2] These are not used in COPD unless there is a component of asthma on top of the COPD.

Theophylline and aminophylline are commonly used for suppressing the symptoms of chronic asthma, bronchitis, or emphysema. Aminophylline is identical to theophylline except that aminophylline contains a salt called ethylenediamine, which has caused rashes and hives in some people. Oxtriphylline (CHOLEDYL) is not recommended because it is no more effective than theophylline and costs more. These drugs must be taken exactly as prescribed, and the level of drug in the bloodstream must be monitored by a doctor. These measures will prevent adverse effects and ensure the optimal dose.

Montelukast (SINGULAIR) and zafirlukast (ACCOLATE) are members of a family of asthma drugs called leukotriene antagonists. Both of these drugs are approved only to prevent asthma attacks in people with chronic asthma, not to treat acute attacks of asthma. Montelukast is also approved for seasonal allergy.[3] Montelukast is associated with liver toxicity. Production of the third leukotriene antagonist zileutin (ZYFLOW) was halted in December 2003. The manufacturer cited poor sales as the reasons; however, zileutin was also associated with liver toxicity.

The National Institutes of Health's 1997 *Guidelines for the Diagnosis and Management of Asthma* said of the leukotriene inhibitors that "further clinical experience and study are needed to establish their roles in therapy." At this time, the role of the leukotriene inhibitors in the management of asthma is still far from established.[4]

The leukotriene inhibitors are promoted as useful in helping patients reduce their dosages of steroid drugs, for example triamcinolone (AZMACORT). The *Cochrane Database of Systematic Reviews* published in 2002 found, in comparing leukotriene inhibitors to placebo in people also using steroids, that the dosage of inhaled steroids can be safely reduced without requiring the use of leukotriene inhibitors. Furthermore, the dose of leukotriene inhibitors required to achieve a significant reduction in steroid dosage is several times the currently approved maximum dosage.

Proper Use of Inhalers

To receive the most benefit from your inhaler, follow the directions below,[5] even though they may not agree with the directions on the drug manufacturer's packaging. Always shake well before taking each dose. Remove the plastic cap that covers the mouthpiece. Hold the inhaler upright, approximately 1 to 1½ inches from your lips. Open your mouth widely. Breathe out as fully as you comfortably can. Breathe in deeply as you press down on the can with your index finger. When you have finished breathing in, hold your breath as long as you comfortably can (try to hold it for 10 seconds). This allows time for the medication to treat your lungs before you breathe it out. If you have difficulty with hand-breath coordination, as many people do, ask your doctor for an "add-on" device that attaches to your inhaler. It allows you to close your lips around the inhaler, yet still receive the full therapeutic benefit from that dose.

If your doctor has told you to take more than one puff at each treatment, wait one minute, shake the can again, and repeat. If you also take a bronchodilator in addition to the corticosteroids, you should inhale the bronchodilator first. Wait 15 minutes before inhaling the corticosteroids. This allows more corticosteroid to be absorbed into the lungs.

Your inhaler should be cleaned every day. To do this properly, remove the can from the plastic case. Rinse the plastic case and cap under warm running water. Dry thoroughly. Using a gentle, twisting motion, replace the metal can into the case. Put the cap on the mouthpiece.

> Inhaled steroids for asthma have been available in the United States mainly in pressurized metered-dose inhalers, which require a propellant. The chlorofluorocarbon (CFC) propellants in these formulations are being changed for environmental reasons. Dry-powder inhalers, which are activated by inhalation, do not require a propellant, and people who have difficulty with hand-breath coordination find them easier to use.
>
> If you have difficulty with hand-breath coordination, talk to your doctor about a dry-powder inhaler.

DRUG PROFILES

Cough, Cold, and Allergy

Antihistamines

 Do Not Use

ALTERNATIVE TREATMENT:
See Chlorpheniramine, p. 363.

Azelastin (a *zel* as teen)
AZTELIN (Wallace)

FAMILY: Antihistamines (see p. 356)

Azelastine is an antihistamine nasal spray. About 40% of each dose of the drug is absorbed into the bloodstream. This may explain why in clinical trials 11.5% of patients using azelastine experienced drowsiness compared to 5.4% of those using a placebo.[6] Also, between 9 and 12% of azelastine users complain of a bitter taste in the mouth.[7]

The editors of *The Medical Letter on Drugs and Therapeutics,* an independent source of drug information written for pharmacists and physicians, concluded their review of the drug by saying that oral antihistamines (see p. 353) or corticosteroid nasal sprays are preferred to azelastine.[7]

We can think of no reason why you should be paying almost $70 (price on the Internet from a national chain pharmacy, April 12, 2004) per bottle for a prescription antihistamine nasal spray when there is no evidence that it is any safer or more effective than oral nonprescription antihistamines.

Hydroxyzine (hy *drox* i zeen)
ATARAX (Pfizer)
VISTARIL (Pfizer)

GENERIC: available
FAMILY: Antihistamines (see p. 356)

Limited Use

Cetirizine (se *ti* ra zeen)
ZYRTEC (Pfizer)

GENERIC: not available
FAMILY: Antihistamines (see p. 356)

BREAST-FEEDING WARNING

Cetirizine was excreted in breast milk in animal studies and caused retarded weight gain in nursing pups. There is no information on hydroxyzine from either human or animal studies. However, since it is likely that this drug, like many others, is excreted in human milk, there is the potential for serious adverse events in nursing infants, if you take either of these drugs.

PREGNANCY WARNING

Hydroxyzine caused fetal abnormalities in animal studies and is contraindicated in early pregnancy. There is limited data on effects of cetirizine in pregnant animals. Use during pregnancy only for clear medical reasons. Tell your doctor if you are pregnant or thinking of becoming pregnant before you take this drug.

ADDITIONAL PRECAUTIONS

Avoid exposure to things that trigger your allergies or asthma, such as animals, bedding, chemicals, cosmetics, drugs, dust, mold, foods, pollens, and smoke. Wearing a mask reduces inhalation of drugs, pollens, and smoke. Many people with mildly red, itching eyes require no treatment. Cold compresses to the eyes may prove helpful. Using eye drops with vasoconstrictors whitens eyes for a while, but rebound redness can occur. Misuse of vasoconstrictors sets up a vicious cycle.

Cetirizine is an antihistamine. Antihistamines relieve symptoms of seasonal allergies due to pollens, reduce sneezing, and tearing due to dust mites, dander, and molds, chronic hives and itching, but do not cure any condition.

Cetirizine is the metabolic breakdown product of the older antihistamine hydroxyzine (ATARAX, VISTARIL). Although cetirizine does not cause as much drowsiness as hydroxyzine, it may cause more drowsiness than newer "nonsedating" antihistamines. Small studies suggest cetirizine does not slow the heart, but studies on drug interactions are limited. People with kidney and liver impairment, and older adults, should take five milligrams a day. Older people are more apt to develop dry mouth, which can increase dental problems. Men are more apt to experience urinary retention. Cetirizine is not recommended in early pregnancy or during nursing.

Hydroxyzine is used to treat itching and hives caused by allergic reactions and to relieve drug withdrawal symptoms, nausea, and anxiety. It also promotes sleep. If you need a sleeping pill, an antihistamine such as hydroxyzine is preferable to the overprescribed and addictive benzodiazepine sleeping pills and tranquilizers such as Valium, Librium, and Dalmane (see p. 223).

Do not use these drugs to treat a cold. Colds and allergies have different causes, and these drugs are not effective against either the cause of a cold or its symptoms. In fact, they can make a cold or cough worse by thickening nasal secretions and drying mucous membranes.

These drugs can cause harmful adverse effects, most commonly in people over 60. These effects include confusion, dizziness, fainting, difficult or painful urination, dry mouth, nose, or throat, nightmares, unusual excitement, nervousness, restlessness, and irritability.

Before You Use This Drug

Tell your doctor if you have or have had:

- allergies to drugs
- glaucoma
- kidney problems
- pregnancy or are breast-feeding
- prostate problems
- urinary retention

Tell your doctor about any other drugs you take, including aspirin, herbs, vitamins, and other nonprescription products.

When You Use This Drug

- Do not drink alcohol or use other drugs that can cause drowsiness.
- Until you know how you react to this drug, do not drive or perform other activities that require alertness.

ANTICHOLINERGIC EFFECTS

WARNING: SPECIAL MENTAL AND PHYSICAL ADVERSE EFFECTS

Older adults are especially sensitive to the harmful anticholinergic (see Glossary, p. 889) effects of this drug. Drugs in this family should not be used unless absolutely necessary.

Mental Effects: confusion, delirium, short-term memory problems, disorientation, and impaired attention.

Physical Effects: dry mouth, constipation, difficulty urinating (especially for a man with an enlarged prostate), blurred vision, decreased sweating with increased body temperature, sexual dysfunction, and worsening of glaucoma.

• Protect yourself from sunburn, using a sunscreen or wearing protective clothing (cetirizine).
• Do not breast-feed.
• Use sugarless gum, ice, or saliva substitutes if dry mouth develops.
• If you plan to have any surgery, including dental surgery, tell your doctor that you take this drug.

How to Use This Drug

• If you miss a dose, take it as soon as you remember, but skip it if it is almost time for the next dose. **Do not take double doses.**
• Do not share your medication with others.
• Take the drug at the same time(s) each day.
• Take with food, water, or milk.
• Swallow tablets whole. If you become drowsy, take at bedtime.
• Store at room temperature with lid on tightly. Do not store in the bathroom. Do not expose to heat, moisture, or strong light. Keep out of reach of children.

Interactions with Other Drugs

The following drugs, biologics (e.g., vaccines, therapeutic antibodies), or foods are listed in *Evaluations of Drug Interactions* 2003 as causing "highly clinically significant" or "clinically significant" interactions when used together with any of the drugs in this section. In some sections with multiple drugs, the interaction may have been reported for one but not all drugs in this section, but we include the interaction because the drugs in this section are similar to one another. We have also included potentially serious interactions listed in the drug's FDA-approved professional package insert or in published medical journal articles. There may be other drugs, especially those in the families of drugs listed below, that also will react with this drug to cause severe adverse effects. Make sure to tell your doctor and pharmacist the drugs you are taking and tell them if you are taking any of these interacting drugs:

Central nervous system (CNS) depressant drugs, including alcohol, antidepressants, antihistamines, antipsychotics, some blood pressure medications (reserpine, methyldopa, beta-blockers), motion sickness medications, muscle relaxants, narcotics, sedatives, sleeping pills, and tranquilizers.

Adverse Effects

Call your doctor immediately if you experience:

• unusual bleeding or bruising
• cough
• difficulty swallowing
• dizziness
• fast or irregular heartbeat (cetirizine)
• chills
• convulsions or seizures
• tightness in chest
• puffiness or swelling of eyelids or around eyes, face, lips, or tongue

- shortness of breath
- skin rash, hives, or itching
- unusual tiredness or weakness
- wheezing
- abdominal or stomach pain
- clay-colored stools or dark urine
- diarrhea
- fever
- headache

Call your doctor if these symptoms continue:

- confusion (cetirizine)
- dizziness
- headache
- dryness of mouth, nose, or throat (cetirizine)
- increased sweating (cetirizine)
- loss of appetite (cetirizine)
- nightmares (cetirizine)
- unusual excitement, nervousness, or irritability (cetirizine)
- ringing or buzzing in ears (cetirizine)
- skin rash (cetirizine)
- upset or painful stomach or nausea (cetirizine)
- constipation
- diarrhea
- change in menstrual cycle
- tremor
- drowsiness
- fast heartbeat (cetirizine)
- clumsiness or unsteadiness
- sunburn (cetirizine)
- tiredness
- difficult or painful urination (cetirizine)
- changes in vision (cetirizine)
- increased appetite or weight gain (cetirizine)

Signs of overdose:

- clumsiness or unsteadiness
- severe dry mouth, nose, or throat
- flushed or red face
- shortness of breath

- trouble breathing
- fast or irregular heartbeat
- severe drowsiness
- seizures
- hallucinations
- trouble sleeping
- faintness or lightheadedness

If you suspect an overdose, call this number to contact your poison control center: (800) 222-1222.

_____

Chlorpheniramine (klor fen *eer* a meen)
CHLOR-TRIMETON (Schering-Plough)

Diphenhydramine (di fen *hye* dra meen)
BENADRYL (Parke-Davis)
SOMINEX FORMULA (GlaxoSmithKline)

GENERIC: available

FAMILY: Antihistamines (see p. 356)

PREGNANCY AND BREAST-FEEDING WARNINGS

There is no information in the labels for these drugs. Consult with your doctor or pharmacist if you already are or are planning to become pregnant or to breast-feed.

ANTICHOLINERGIC EFFECTS

WARNING: SPECIAL MENTAL AND PHYSICAL ADVERSE EFFECTS

Older adults are especially sensitive to the harmful anticholinergic (see Glossary, p. 889) effects of this drug. Drugs in this family should not be used unless absolutely necessary.

Mental Effects: confusion, delirium, short-term memory problems, disorientation, and impaired attention.

Physical Effects: dry mouth, constipation, difficulty urinating (especially for a man with an enlarged prostate), blurred vision, decreased sweating with increased body temperature, sexual dysfunction, and worsening of glaucoma.

ADDITIONAL PRECAUTIONS

Avoid exposure to things that trigger your allergies or asthma, such as animals, bedding, chemicals, cosmetics, drugs, dust, mold, foods, pollens, or smoke. Wearing a mask reduces inhalation of drugs, pollens, and smoke. Many people with mildly red, itching eyes require no treatment. Cold compresses to the eyes may prove helpful. Using eye drops with vasoconstrictors whitens eyes for a while, but rebound redness can occur. Misuse of vasoconstrictors sets up a vicious cycle.

Chlorpheniramine relieves the symptoms of hay fever and other allergic reactions. Diphenhydramine is used to treat allergic reactions, coughing, insomnia, motion sickness, and Parkinson's disease.

Do not use these drugs to treat a cold. Colds and allergies have different causes, and chlorpheniramine is not effective against either the cause of a cold or its symptoms. In fact, these drugs can make a cold or cough worse by thickening nasal secretions and drying mucous membranes.

These drugs can cause harmful adverse effects, most commonly in people over 60. These effects include confusion, dizziness, fainting, difficult or painful urination, dry mouth, nose, or throat, nightmares, unusual excitement, nervousness, restlessness, and irritability. If you have any of these symptoms while taking chlorpheniramine, ask your doctor about changing or discontinuing this drug. Since older people can be more sensitive to the usual adult dose, start with a low dose. This may decrease adverse effects.

Before You Use This Drug

Tell your doctor if you have or have had:

- allergies to drugs
- problems with urination
- glaucoma
- enlarged prostate
- kidney problems
- pregnancy or are breast-feeding

Tell your doctor about any other drugs you take, including aspirin, herbs, vitamins, and other nonprescription products.

When You Use This Drug

- Do not drink alcohol or use other drugs that can cause drowsiness.
- Until you know how you react to this drug, do not drive or perform other activities requiring alertness.
- If you plan to have any surgery, including dental surgery, tell your doctor that you take this drug.
- Use sugarless gum, ice, or saliva substitutes if dry mouth develops.

How to Use This Drug

- If you miss a dose, take it as soon as you remember, but skip it if it is almost time for the next dose. **Do not take double doses.**
- Do not share your medication with others.
- Swallow tablets whole. Take at about the same time(s) each day.
- Take with food, water, or milk.
- Store at room temperature with lid on tightly. Do not store in the bathroom. Do not expose to heat, moisture, or strong light. Do not allow liquid form to freeze. Keep out of reach of children.

Interactions with Other Drugs

The following drugs, biologics (e.g., vaccines, therapeutic antibodies), or foods are listed in *Evaluations of Drug Interactions* 2003 as causing "highly clinically significant" or "clinically significant" interactions when used together with any of the drugs in this section. In some sections with multiple drugs, the interaction may have been reported for one but not all drugs in this section, but we include the interaction because the drugs in this section are similar to one another. We have also included potentially serious interactions listed in the drug's FDA-approved professional package insert or in published medical journal articles. There may be other drugs, especially those in the families of drugs listed below, that also will react with this drug to cause severe adverse effects. Make sure to tell your doctor and pharmacist the drugs you are taking and tell them if you are taking any of these interacting drugs:

alcohol, DILANTIN, phenytoin, RESTORIL, temazepam.

Antihistamines, when taken together with other drugs that affect the central nervous system (CNS), will cause additional drowsiness.

Adverse Effects

Call your doctor immediately if you experience:

- cough
- difficulty swallowing
- dizziness
- hives
- itching
- puffiness or swelling of the eyelids or around the eyes, face, lips, or tongue
- shortness of breath
- skin rash
- tightness in chest
- unusual tiredness or weakness
- wheezing
- abdominal or stomach pain
- chills
- clay-colored stools or dark urine
- fever
- headache
- fast or irregular heartbeat

Call your doctor if these symptoms continue:

- gastrotintestinal upset (diphenhydramine)
- clumsiness or unsteadiness
- stomach pain or nausea (diphenhydramine)
- blurred or any change in vision (diphenhydramine)
- drowsiness
- constipation
- increased sweating (chlorpheniramine)
- diarrhea
- loss of appetite (chlorpheniramine)
- dizziness
- nightmares (diphenhydramine)
- unusual excitement (both)
- painful or difficult urination (chlorpheniramine)
- nervousness or restlessness (both)
- change in menstrual cycle
- thickening of mucus (diphenhydramine)
- confusion (diphenhydramine)

Signs of overdose:

- clumsiness or unsteadiness
- severe dry mouth, nose, or throat
- flushed or red face
- shortness of breath
- trouble breathing
- fast or irregular heartbeat
- severe drowsiness
- seizures
- hallucinations
- trouble sleeping
- faintness or lightheadedness

If you suspect an overdose, call this number to contact your poison control center: (800) 222-1222.

Cyproheptadine (si proe *hep* ta deen)
PERIACTIN (Merck)

GENERIC: available
FAMILY: Antihistamines

PREGNANCY WARNING

Cyproheptadine caused fetal harm in an animal study. Because of the potential for serious adverse effects to the fetus, this drug should not be used by pregnant women.

BREAST-FEEDING WARNING

Cyproheptadine should not be used by nursing women.

Cyproheptadine was approved by the FDA in 1961. At one time the drug was heavily promoted as an appetite stimulant for children.[8] Appetite stimulation is not an FDA-approved use for this drug and it should not be used for this purpose.

Cyproheptadine should not be used to treat a cold. Colds and allergies have different causes, and cyproheptadine is not effective against either the cause of a cold or its symptoms. In fact, the drug can make a cold or cough worse by thickening nasal secretions and drying mucous membranes. It also causes drowsiness.

Cyproheptadine can cause harmful adverse effects, most commonly in people over 60. These effects include confusion, dizziness, fainting, difficult or painful urination, dry mouth, nose, or throat, nightmares, unusual excitement, nervousness, restlessness, and irritability. If you have any of these while taking cyproheptadine, ask your doctor about changing or discontinuing this drug.

Before You Use This Drug

Tell your doctor if you have or have had:

- allergies to drugs
- peptic ulcer

ADDITIONAL PRECAUTIONS

Avoid exposure to things that trigger your allergies or asthma, such as animals, bedding, chemicals, cosmetics, drugs, dust, mold, foods, pollens, or smoke. Wearing a mask reduces inhalation of drugs, pollens, and smoke. Many people with mildly red, itching eyes require no treatment. Cold compresses to the eyes may prove helpful. Using eye drops with vasoconstrictors whitens eyes for a while, but rebound redness can occur. Misuse of vasoconstrictors sets up a vicious cycle.

ANTICHOLINERGIC EFFECTS

WARNING: SPECIAL MENTAL AND PHYSICAL ADVERSE EFFECTS

Older adults are especially sensitive to the harmful anticholinergic (see Glossary, p. 889) effects of this drug. Drugs in this family should not be used unless absolutely necessary.

Mental Effects: confusion, delirium, short-term memory problems, disorientation, and impaired attention.

Physical Effects: dry mouth, constipation, difficulty urinating (especially for a man with an enlarged prostate), blurred vision, decreased sweating with increased body temperature, sexual dysfunction, and worsening of glaucoma.

- problems with urination
- gastrointestinal obstruction
- glaucoma
- kidney problems
- enlarged prostate
- pregnancy or are breast-feeding

Tell your doctor about any other drugs you take, including aspirin, herbs, vitamins, and other nonprescription products.

When You Use This Drug

• Do not drink alcohol or use other drugs that can cause drowsiness.

• Until you know how you react to this drug, do not drive or perform other activities requiring alertness.

• If you plan to have any surgery, including dental surgery, tell your doctor that you take this drug.

• Protect yourself from sunburn, using a sunscreen or wearing protective clothing.

• Use sugarless gum, ice, or saliva substitutes if dry mouth develops.

How to Use This Drug

• If you miss a dose, take it as soon as you remember, but skip it if it is almost time for the next dose. **Do not take double doses.**

• Do not share your medication with others.

• Take the drug at the same time(s) each day.

• Take with food, water, or milk to avoid stomach upset.

• Swallow extended-release forms whole.

• Do not store in the bathroom. Do not expose to heat, moisture, or strong light. Do not allow liquid form to freeze. Keep out of reach of children.

Interactions with Other Drugs

The following drugs, biologics (e.g., vaccines, therapeutic antibodies), or foods are listed in *Evaluations of Drug Interactions* 2003 as causing "highly clinically significant" or "clinically significant" interactions when used together with any of the drugs in this section. In some sections with multiple drugs, the interaction may have been reported for one but not all drugs in this section, but we include the interaction because the drugs in this section are similar to one another. We have also included potentially serious interactions listed in the drug's FDA-approved professional package insert or in published medical journal articles.

There may be other drugs, especially those in the families of drugs listed below, that also will react with this drug to cause severe adverse effects. Make sure to tell your doctor and pharmacist the drugs you are taking and tell them if you are taking any of these interacting drugs:

DILANTIN, EFFEXOR, fluoxetine, fluvoxamine, LUVOX, nefazodone, paroxetine, PAXIL, phenytoin, PROZAC, SERZONE, venlafaxine.

Adverse Effects

Call your doctor immediately if you experience:

• sore throat
• cough
• difficulty swallowing
• dizziness
• hives
• itching
• puffiness or swelling of the eyelids or around the eyes, face, lips, or tongue
• shortness of breath
• skin rash
• unusual bleeding or bruising
• tightness in chest
• unusual tiredness or weakness
• wheezing
• abdominal or stomach pain
• diarrhea
• chills
• clay-colored stools or dark urine
• fever
• headache
• convulsions or seizures
• burning, prickly, tingling sensations
• fast or irregular heartbeat
• tingling

Call your doctor if these symptoms continue:

• increased appetite or weight gain
• thickening of mucus

- blurred vision or any change in vision
- confusion
- difficult or painful urination
- dizziness
- increased sweating
- increased appetite or weight gain
- nightmares
- loss of appetite
- ringing or buzzing in ears
- skin rash
- stomach upset or pain
- nausea or vomiting
- unusually fast heartbeat
- increased sensitivity to the sun
- clumsiness or unsteadiness
- constipation
- menstrual cycle changes
- tremor
- diarrhea
- fatigue
- tremor

Signs of overdose:

- clumsiness or unsteadiness
- severe dry mouth, nose, or throat
- flushed or red face
- shortness of breath
- trouble breathing
- fast or irregular heartbeat
- severe drowsiness
- seizures
- hallucinations
- trouble sleeping
- faintness or lightheadedness

If you suspect an overdose, call this number to contact your poison control center: (800) 222-1222.

 Do Not Use

ALTERNATIVE TREATMENT:
See Chlorpheniramine, p. 363.

Desloratadine (des lor *at* a dine)
CLARINEX (Schering-Plough)

FAMILY: Antihistamines (see p. 356)

Desloratadine is Schering-Plough's replacement for its $3 billion a year antihistamine loratadine (CLARITIN, see p. 369). Desloratadine is only technically a new drug. Patients who have been taking the older loratadine since it was approved in 1994 have been producing desloratadine with each dose of loratadine. Loratadine is broken down, or metabolized, in the body to desloratadine.[9] Thus, desloratadine is referred to as an active metabolite of loratadine.

Desloratadine's manufacturer abused the basic intent of our patent law (which is to reward ingenuity and originality) and managed

---

ANTICHOLINERGIC EFFECTS

WARNING: SPECIAL MENTAL AND PHYSICAL ADVERSE EFFECTS

Older adults are especially sensitive to the harmful anticholinergic (see Glossary, p. 889) effects of this drug. Drugs in this family should not be used unless absolutely necessary.

Mental Effects: confusion, delirium, short-term memory problems, disorientation, and impaired attention.

Physical Effects: dry mouth, constipation, difficulty urinating (especially for a man with an enlarged prostate), blurred vision, decreased sweating with increased body temperature, sexual dysfunction, and worsening of glaucoma.

ADDITIONAL PRECAUTIONS

Avoid exposure to things that trigger your allergies or asthma, such as animals, bedding, chemicals, cosmetics, drugs, dust, mold, foods, pollens, or smoke. Wearing a mask reduces inhalation of drugs, pollens, and smoke. Many people with mildly red, itching eyes require no treatment. Cold compresses to the eyes may prove helpful. Using eye drops with vasoconstrictors whitens eyes for a while, but rebound redness can occur. Misuse of vasoconstrictors sets up a vicious cycle.

---

to get a patent for desloratadine, an active metabolite of loratadine. Then they got desloratadine through the FDA's 40-year-old legal standard for approving new drugs, which does not require new drugs to be better than older ones.

There are no studies or data to show that loratadine and desloratadine are clinically different. The company submitted four clinical trials to the FDA comparing various doses of desloratadine to a placebo for support of the drug's approval. Only in two of these studies was the approved five-milligram-per-day dose found to be effective.[10] However, this was sufficient under current law to justify the drug's approval.

The FDA medical officer's review indicates that Schering-Plough was trying to convince the agency that desloratadine's onset of effect was between one and two hours. The medical officer concluded, "There is adequate data to support a claim for effectiveness of 5 mg of DCL [desloratadine] beginning within two days of initiating treatment."[10]

In December 2002, the European Medicines Evaluation Agency added a warning to the professional product labeling of drugs containing desloratadine indicating that they should not be used during pregnancy. Desloratadine and

loratadine have been linked to a fetal malformation known as hypospadias (penile malformation).[11]

Overall, desloratadine is an unremarkable antihistamine, as is loratadine. The nonprescription antihistamines such as generic chlorpheniramine (CHLOR-TRIMETON) are effective, perhaps equally or more so than desloratadine. The drowsiness that may be experienced by some people using generic chlorpheniramine can be avoided by starting with a low dose and slowly working up to a dose that relieves symptoms without sedation. This can save a substantial amount of money.

Limited Use

Fexofenadine (fex o *fen* a deen)
ALLEGRA (Aventis)

GENERIC: not available

Loratadine (lor *at* a deen)
CLARITIN (Schering)

GENERIC: available
FAMILY: Antihistamines (see p. 356)

PREGNANCY WARNING

Fexofenadine caused decreased weight gain and survival in developing fetuses in animal studies. Use during pregnancy only for clear medical reasons. Tell your doctor if you are pregnant or thinking of becoming pregnant before you take these drugs.

BREAST-FEEDING WARNING

No information is available from either human or animal studies. It is likely that these drugs are excreted in human milk, and because of the potential for adverse effects in nursing infants, you should avoid these drugs while nursing.

Fexofenadine is an antihistamine that is the metabolic breakdown product of the antihistamine terfenadine (SELDANE), which was re-

---

ADDITIONAL PRECAUTIONS

Avoid exposure to things that trigger your allergies or asthma, such as animals, bedding, chemicals, cosmetics, drugs, dust, mold, foods, pollens, or smoke. Wearing a mask reduces inhalation of drugs, pollens, and smoke. Many people with mildly red, itching eyes require no treatment. Cold compresses to the eyes may prove helpful. Using eye drops with vasoconstrictors whitens eyes for a while, but rebound redness can occur. Misuse of vasoconstrictors sets up a vicious cycle.

ANTICHOLINERGIC EFFECTS

WARNING: SPECIAL MENTAL AND PHYSICAL ADVERSE EFFECTS

Older adults are especially sensitive to the harmful anticholinergic (see Glossary, p. 889) effects of this drug. Drugs in this family should not be used unless absolutely necessary.

Mental Effects: confusion, delirium, short-term memory problems, disorientation, and impaired attention.

Physical Effects: dry mouth, constipation, difficulty urinating (especially for a man with an enlarged prostate), blurred vision, decreased sweating with increased body temperature, sexual dysfunction, and worsening of glaucoma.

---

moved from the market because it caused fatal heart rhythm disturbances. Fexofenadine does not appear to cause the fatal heart rhythm disturbances seen with terfenadine.[12]

Fexofenadine relieves symptoms of seasonal allergies such as sneezing, itchy, watery eyes, and red eyes but does not cure allergies. How this antihistamine compares with other antihistamines remains to be determined.[12]

Loratadine is now sold both as an over-the-counter and as a prescription drug. Loratadine is broken down in the body to desloratadine (CLARINEX) (see p. 368). It relieves the symptoms of seasonal allergies and chronic itching but does not cure any condition. High doses increase the risk of adverse effects with loratadine. People with impaired kidney or liver function should only take 10 milligrams of the drug every other day. Older people may be more prone to adverse effects, such as dizziness and dry mouth. A dry mouth for a prolonged time can lead to dental problems.

Loratadine passes into the breast milk and should not be used when nursing. Do not use in the third trimester of pregnancy.

Before You Use This Drug

Tell your doctor if you have or have had:

- allergies to drugs
- problems with urination
- kidney problems
- glaucoma
- enlarged prostate
- pregnancy or are breast-feeding

Tell your doctor about any other drugs you take, including aspirin, herbs, vitamins, and other nonprescription products.

When You Use This Drug

- Do not drink alcohol or use other drugs that can cause drowsiness.
- Until you know how you react to this drug, do not drive or perform other activities requiring alertness.
- If you plan to have any surgery, including dental surgery, tell your doctor that you take this drug.
- Protect yourself from sunburn, using a sunscreen or wearing protective clothing (loratadine).

- Use sugarless gum, ice, or saliva substitutes if dry mouth develops.

How to Use This Drug

- If you miss a dose, take it as soon as you remember, but skip it if it is almost time for the next dose. **Do not take double doses.**
- Do not share your medication with others.
- Take the drug at the same time(s) each day.
- Take with food, water, or milk to avoid stomach upset.
- Swallow extended-release forms whole.
- Do not store in the bathroom. Do not expose to heat, moisture, or strong light. Do not allow liquid form to freeze. Keep out of reach of children.

Interactions with Other Drugs

The following drugs, biologics (e.g., vaccines, therapeutic antibodies), or foods are listed in *Evaluations of Drug Interactions* 2003 as causing "highly clinically significant" or "clinically significant" interactions when used together with any of the drugs in this section. In some sections with multiple drugs, the interaction may have been reported for one but not all drugs in this section, but we include the interaction because the drugs in this section are similar to one another. We have also included potentially serious interactions listed in the drug's FDA-approved professional package insert or in published medical journal articles. There may be other drugs, especially those in the families of drugs listed below, that also will react with this drug to cause severe adverse effects. Make sure to tell your doctor and pharmacist the drugs you are taking and tell them if you are taking any of these interacting drugs:

AGENERASE, aluminum/magnesium antacids, amprenavir, NORVIR, ritonavir.

Adverse Effects

Call your doctor immediately if you experience:

- unusual bleeding or bruising
- unusual tiredness or weakness
- cough
- difficulty swallowing
- dizziness
- fast or irregular heartbeat
- puffiness or swelling of eyelids or around eyes, face, lips, or tongue
- shortness of breath
- skin rash, hives, or itching
- tightness in chest
- wheezing
- abdominal or stomach pain
- clay-colored stools or dark urine
- chills
- diarrhea
- headache
- convulsions or seizures

Call your doctor if these symptoms continue:

- confusion (loratadine)
- dizziness
- any change in vision (loratadine)
- constipation
- diarrhea
- headache
- dryness of mouth, nose, or throat (loratadine)
- difficult or painful urination (loratadine)
- nightmares (fexofenadine)
- loss of appetite (loratadine)
- increased appetite or weight gain (loratadine)
- unusual excitement, nervousness, restlessness, or irritability
- ringing or buzzing in ears (loratadine)
- skin rash
- stomach upset or pain
- nausea (loratadine)

- increased sweating (loratadine)
- unusually fast heartbeat (loratadine)
- increased sensitivity to the sun (loratadine)
- drowsiness (loratadine)
- clumsiness or unsteadiness
- tremor
- menstrual cycle change

Signs of overdose:

- clumsiness or unsteadiness
- severe dry mouth, nose, or throat
- flushed or red face
- shortness of breath
- trouble breathing
- fast or irregular heartbeat
- severe drowsiness
- seizures
- hallucinations
- trouble sleeping
- faintness or lightheadedness

If you suspect an overdose, call this number to contact your poison control center: (800) 222-1222.

Decongestants

Saline Nasal Spray/Mist/Wash (*say* leen)
AYR (Ascher)
BREATHE RIGHT (CNS)
ENTSOL (Kenwood Therapeutics)
LITTLE NOSES (Vetco)
OCEAN (Fleming)
SEA MIST (Thames)
SIMPLY SALINE (Blairex)

GENERIC: available

FAMILY: Decongestants (see p. 357)

Saline nasal sprays/mists/washes are a safe, simple combination of salt and water that can be extremely helpful in relieving nasal stuffiness, congestion, and dryness. Normal (isotonic) saline has the same concentration of salt that is normally found in the body and is therefore very gentle. Saline can even be made at home: mix one-half teaspoon uniodized salt (the iodine can be irritating) with eight ounces (one cup) of water that has been boiled and is still warm. You may add one small pinch of baking soda to decrease stinging. Allow the mixture to cool to body temperature before using. You can use an ear-bulb syringe to squirt the saline up your nostrils.

Before You Use This Drug

Tell your doctor if you have or have had:

- allergies to drugs
- pregnancy or are breast-feeding

Tell your doctor about any other drugs you take, including aspirin, herbs, vitamins, and other nonprescription products.

When You Use This Drug

- There is no limit to how often you can use normal saline to irrigate your nose. A minimum of four times per day until symptoms resolve is generally recommended.
- Commercial saline products may contain preservatives that can be irritating. If you experience irritation, you may want to switch to homemade saline.

How to Use This Drug

- Store commercial saline at room temperature with lid on tightly. Keep homemade saline in the refrigerator for up to 24 hours and then throw it out and make a new batch if needed. Do not freeze. Do not store in the bathroom. Do not expose to heat, moisture, or strong light. Keep out of reach of children.
- Wipe the tip of the applicator with a clean, damp tissue and replace the cap right after use.
- Do not share your saline with others.

Interactions with Other Drugs

Since saline does not contain any medication, it is unlikely to cause any drug interactions.

Adverse Effects

Call your doctor immediately if you experience:

- severe stinging or burning in your nose

———————

Oxymetazoline (ox ee met *ah* zoh leen)
AFRIN (Schering-Plough)
DRISTAN NASAL SPRAY/MIST (Whitehall-Robins)
DRIXORAL NASAL SOLUTION (Schering-Plough)
DURAMIST NASAL DECONGESTANT SPRAY (Pfeiffer Pharmaceuticals)
NEO-SYNEPHRINE DROPS/SPRAY (Bayer Healthcare)
NOSTRILLA NASAL DECONGESTANT (Insight Pharmaceuticals)
VICKS SINEX NASAL SPRAY/MIST (Procter & Gamble)

GENERIC: available

FAMILY: Decongestants (see p. 357)

PREGNANCY AND BREAST-FEEDING WARNINGS
There is no information in the labels for these drugs. Consult with your doctor or pharmacist if you already are or are planning to become pregnant or to breast-feed.

Oxymetazoline is the active ingredient in over-the-counter nasal drops, mists, and sprays used for temporary relief of nasal congestion from the common cold, sinusitis, hay fever, or allergies. The medication lasts up to 12 hours. Nasal decongestants are useful because they treat congested noses topically, as discussed in the introduction to this section (see p. 357). Treatment should be limited to a stuffed-up nose, since a runny nose promotes drainage. Minimal medication gets into the rest of your body, thereby avoiding the need for an oral decongestant medicine that treats your symptoms indirectly and requires over 25 times more medication, therefore causing more adverse effects. Nasal decongestant sprays should not be used for more than three days in a row, however, because they can cause "rebound congestion," in which the lining of the nose becomes more swollen.

Before You Use This Drug

Tell your doctor if you have or have had:

- pregnancy or are breast-feeding
- allergies or sensitivity to oxymetazoline or other nasal decongestants
- coronary artery disease
- heart disease, including angina
- hypertension
- enlarged prostate
- diabetes
- glaucoma
- hyperthyroidism
- dry mucous membranes

Tell your doctor about any other drugs you take, including aspirin, herbs, vitamins, and other nonprescription products.

When You Use This Drug

- Do not use this drug for more than three days without checking with your doctor.

How to Use This Drug

- If you miss a dose, take it as soon as you remember, but skip it if it is almost time for the next dose. **Do not take double doses.**
- Do not share your medication with others.
- Take the drug at the same time(s) each day.
- Store at room temperature with lid on tightly. Do not store in the bathroom. Do not ex-

pose to heat, moisture, or strong light. Keep out of reach of children.

• Wipe the tip of the applicator with a clean, damp tissue and replace the cap right after use.

Interactions with Other Drugs

Some other drugs that you may be taking (either over-the-counter or prescription) can interact with this one, causing adverse effects. Ask your doctor what these drugs are and let him or her know if you are taking any of them.

Adverse Effects

Call your doctor immediately if you experience:

• rebound congestion (increased runny or stuffy nose)

Call your doctor immediately if you experience symptoms of systemic absorption:

• blurred vision
• fast, irregular, or pounding heartbeat
• headache, dizziness, drowsiness, lightheadedness
• high blood pressure
• nervousness
• trembling
• trouble sleeping
• weakness

Call your doctor if these symptoms continue:

• burning, dryness, or stinging of nasal mucosa
• increase in nasal discharge
• sneezing

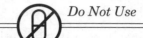

Do Not Use

ALTERNATIVE TREATMENT:
See Saline Nasal Spray/Mist/Wash, p. 372, or Oxymetazoline, p. 373.

Pseudoephedrine (soo doe e *fed* rin)
SUDAFED (Warner Lambert)

FAMILY: Decongestants (see p. 357)

Pseudoephedrine is related both chemically and pharmacologically to the group of "speedlike" drugs that include the amphetamines, the dangerous dietary supplement ephedra (see p. 835 in chapter twenty-eight, Dietary Supplements), ephedrine, which is a constituent of ephedra, and the banned nasal decongestant phenylpropanolamine (PPA). All of these drugs can raise heart rate and blood pressure that can lead to serious cardiovascular consequences.

PPA was banned by the FDA because of an increased risk of hemorrhagic stroke in women.[13]

In addition to the possibility of raising heart rate and blood pressure, there have been reports in the medical literature of a serious gastrointestinal (GI) adverse effect known as ischemic colitis. In this condition, the blood supply to a section of the GI tract can be compromised.[14,15] Ischemic colitis led to the original market withdrawal of alosetron (LOTRONEX) (see p. 555) and a new warning on the drug tegaserod (ZELNORM) (see p. 557).

Normal saline nasal wash or oxymetazoline nasal spray offer safer and equally effective alternatives to pseudoephedrine.

Cough Suppressants

 Do Not Use

ALTERNATIVE TREATMENT:
Acute cough due to an upper respiratory tract infection (URI) is mild and self-limiting and does not require treatment (see Cough, p. 353).

Dextromethorphan
DELSYM (Celltech)

FAMILY: Cough Suppressants

Dextromethorphan is an over-the-counter drug that is sold alone and in combination with other products as a cough suppressant for children and adults. We have previously recommended dextromethorphan as a safe and effective cough suppressant for both children and adults. However, the weight of the evidence now suggests that dextromethorphan is no more effective than an inactive placebo syrup in suppressing a nighttime cough in children.

The study tipping the balance for us to a **DO NOT USE** classification for dextromethorphan was published in the July 2004 issue of the journal *Pediatrics* and was conducted by researchers from the Pennsylvania State College of Medicine, Hershey, Pennsylvania.[88]

Sleep quality was used as the measure of effectiveness in the study of the two drugs and the placebo. The study involved 100 children with coughs and their parents and used a five-question questionnaire to access sleep quality both children and their parents. The median age of the children was 4.5 years and their ages ranged from 2.0 years to 16.5 years. To be eligible to participate in the study, the children had to have an acute cough as a result of an upper respiratory tract infection.

The questionnaire was administered on two consecutive days. No medication was given the night before the first day; on the second day, the questionnaire was administered after the drug or the placebo had been given the previous night.

The study concluded that dextromethorphan was not superior to the placebo in providing nighttime symptomatic relief for children with a cough and sleep difficulty as a result of an upper respiratory tract infection. In addition, the use of dextromethorphan did not result in improved sleep quality for the children's parents. In other words, neither drug had any effect on the natural course of cough improvement over a 24-hour period.

Older research on the value of these drugs as cough suppressants was conflicting. Recently, a type of statistical summary of multiple studies known as a meta-analysis published in the February 9, 2002, *British Medical Journal* concluded, "Over the counter cough medicines for acute cough cannot be recommended because there is no good evidence for their effectiveness."[89]

The American Academy of Pediatrics' Committee on Drugs has not supported the use of dextromethorphan primarily because there is a lack of proven benefit and some potential for toxicity and overdose.

Even ineffective drugs have the potential to cause adverse effects. In usual doses, dextromethorphan has been associated with loss of muscle tone, severe allergic reactions, and the proliferation of a type of cell called mast cells that may appear as a blister. Overdose of dextromethorphan may result in psychosis, mania, or hallucinations. Deaths have been reported from an overdose of this drug.

Parents and health professionals have a strong urge to "do something" to ease symptoms in children, even in a mild, self-limiting illness like an upper respiratory tract infection. The lesson from this study is that it is sometimes better to do nothing because the medications have no therapeutic benefit but do carry a known risk of potentially serious adverse reactions.

—————

Limited Use

Benzonatate (ben *zone* a tate)
TESSALON (Forest)

GENERIC: not available
FAMILY: Cough Suppressants

PREGNANCY WARNING

No animal studies were done. Thus, it is not known whether this drug would cause harm to developing fetuses. Use during pregnancy only for clear medical reasons. Tell your doctor if you are pregnant or thinking of becoming pregnant before you take this drug.

BREAST-FEEDING WARNING

No information is available from either human or animal studies. It is likely that this drug is excreted in human milk. You should consult with your doctor if you are planning to nurse.

Benzonatate was first marketed in this country in 1958 and is approved by the FDA for the symptomatic relief of cough. It is chemically related to anesthetic agents such as procaine and tetracaine.[16]

In the absence of convincing published research on the value of benzonatate in the management of cough due to upper respiratory tract infection (URI) we do not recommend it for this use. The best therapeutic role for this drug may be in the management of cough due to pulmonary cancers.[63]

Severe hypersensitivity reactions that include cardiovascular collapse have been reported when the benzonatate capsule is sucked or chewed instead of swallowed. Also, because of the drug's local anesthetic effect, choking can occur when the capsule is sucked or chewed.[16]

You should not use benzonatate or any other drug to treat a cough that is producing mucus, because this is the body's way of ridding itself of secretions and decreasing infection. If you have this kind of cough, drinking lots of liquids, especially soup and other hot drinks, and inhaling steam from hot showers and warm baths will help to loosen secretions and clean and soothe mucous membranes. For more information on treating coughs, see Cough, p. 353, and Allergy and Hay Fever, p. 355.

Before You Use This Drug

Tell your doctor if you have or have had:

- productive cough
- allergy to benzonatate or topical anesthetics

Tell your doctor about any other drugs you take, including aspirin, herbs, vitamins, and other nonprescription products.

When You Use This Drug

- Check with doctor if still coughing after seven days or if high fever, skin rash, or continuing headache is present.

How to Use This Drug

- If you miss a dose, take it as soon as you remember, but skip it if it is almost time for the next dose. **Do not take double doses.**
- Do not share your medication with others.
- Do not chew or suck on capsules. Swallow whole.
- Store at room temperature. Do not store in the bathroom. Do not expose to heat, moisture, or strong light. Keep out of reach of children.

Interactions with Other Drugs

Some other drugs that you may be taking (either over-the-counter or prescription) can interact with this one, causing adverse effects. Ask your doctor what these drugs are and let him or her know if you are taking any of them.

Adverse Effects

Call your doctor immediately if you experience:

- shortness of breath
- trouble breathing
- skin rash, itching
- tightness in chest
- wheezing
- difficulty speaking
- hallucinations
- confusion

Call your doctor if these symptoms continue:

- mild drowsiness
- mild dizziness
- nausea or vomiting
- stuffy nose
- nasal congestion
- constipation
- headache
- skin rash
- itching
- burning eyes

Signs of overdose:

- convulsions
- restlessness
- trembling
- loss of feeling in mouth and throat if capsules are chewed or dissolved in mouth

If you suspect an overdose, call this number to contact your poison control center: (800) 222-1222.

 Do Not Use

ALTERNATIVE TREATMENT:
See Cold, p. 351, and Allergy and Hay Fever, p. 355.

Guaifenesin (gwye *fen* e sin)
ROBITUSSIN (Whitehall-Robins)
MUCINEX (Adams)

FAMILY: Expectorants

Guaifenesin was first marketed in the United States in 1951. It is currently approved by the FDA to help loosen phlegm (mucus) and thin bronchial secretions to make coughs more productive. Doubts about the effectiveness of guaifenesin stretch back to the early 1970s.[17]

Our suggestion is to drink lots of liquids, especially soup and other hot drinks, and inhale steam from hot showers and warm baths to help to loosen secretions rather than take guaifenesin.

If you have a cough, it is not necessarily a good idea to take a cough suppressant. Coughing clears mucous plugs and thick secretions from your airways and opens collapsed segments of your lungs.

Even a dry, irritating cough associated with an upper respiratory infection that is not producing mucus is best not treated with a drug. If

WARNING

Beware of physicians prescribing and pharmacists compounding guaifenesin to treat fibromyalgia. Our search of the medical literature (April 26, 2004) found no published studies documenting the use of guaifenesin for this use. Drugs compounded by pharmacists are not approved by the FDA and are not produced in facilities meeting Good Manufacturing Practice guidelines.

your cough persists, you should see a doctor or other health professional, especially if you are a smoker.

Combination Antihistamines, Decongestants, and/or Cough Preparations

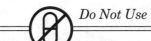 *Do Not Use*

ALTERNATIVE TREATMENT:
See individual drug families in this chapter.

All of the following prescription or over-the-counter drug combinations of two or more ingredients should not be used because they are irrational combinations of single ingredients, some of which are safe and effective and sensible to use alone if treating the symptom for which they are intended. The combinations, however, present extra risks for extra ingredients that will usually not add any benefit (possibly a risk) to the first ingredient and will invariably cost much more than the single ingredient alone. They represent a "shotgun" approach to multiple symptoms of colds, coughs, and allergies that rarely occur in the combination that is suggested by the ingredients in these products.

Alternative treatments include nose spray or drops for a stuffed nose from a cold (see AFRIN p. 373), and a single-ingredient oral antihistamine for allergies (see chlorpheniramine, p. 363). Coughs associated with upper respiratory infections are best not treated with drugs.

The various categories of combinations, the products in each category, and the main reasons we recommend against their use are as follows:

Antihistamines and decongestants

Loratadine and Pseudoephedrine
(lor *at* a deen and soo doe e *fed* rin)
CLARITIN D (Schering)

Triprolidine and Pseudoephedrine
(trye *proe* li deen and soo doe e *fed* rin)
ACTIFED (GlaxoSmithKline)

Promethazine and Phenylephrine
(proe *meth* a zeen and fen ill *ef* rin)
PROMETHAZINE VC (Cenci, Morton Grove)

Fexofenadine/Pseudoephedrine
(fex o *fen* a deen/soo doe e *fed* rin)
ALLEGRA D (Aventis)

There are two reasons why we oppose these combinations for colds:

1. There is no adequate evidence that the use of an antihistamine for a cold, which is an infectious, not an allergic, phenomenon, will help treat the cold. However, the mucous membrane drying effect of the antihistamine may actually impair the healing of the cold.

2. We have consistently opposed the use of systemic (oral) decongestants—all of which are stimulants—for treating the nasal congestion of a cold because they involve using 25 to 50 times more of the drug than would be used in the form of nose drops or nasal spray, the preferred treatments if your nose is really stopped up. (See AFRIN, p. 373.)

Our opposition to these combinations for the treatment of allergies is based on the fact that there is no satisfactory evidence that people with allergies will benefit from a nasal decongestant.

Cough suppressants and antihistamines

Hydrocodone and Chlorpheniramine
(hye dro *koe* done and klor fen *eer* a mine)
TUSSIONEX (Celltech)

Promethazine and Codeine
(proe *meth* a zeen)
PHENERGAN WITH CODEINE
(Wyeth-Ayerst)

Promethazine and Dextromethorphan
(proe *meth* a zeen/dex tro me *thor* fan)
PHENERGAN DM (Wyeth-Ayerst)

If you have a cold and a cough, the use of an antihistamine can impair the healing of your cold. Coughs associated with upper respiratory infections are best not treated with drugs.

Cough suppressants and decongestants

Pseudoephedrine and Codeine
(soo doe e *feh* drin and *koe* deen)

Coughs associated with upper respiratory infection are best not treated with drugs. As stated above, for the stuffed nose of a cold, nose sprays or drops are much safer than systemic (oral) drugs because the dose is much lower.

Expectorants and cough suppressants

Guaifenesin and Dextromethorphan
(gwye *fen* e sin and dex tro meth *or* fan)
ROBITUSSIN DM

Guaifenesin and Codeine
(gwye *fen* e sin and *koe* deen)

Both guaifenesin and dextromethorphan lack adequate evidence of effectiveness to be recommended as part of treatment for coughs or colds (see pp. 375–7).[17,88] Coughs associated with upper respiratory infections are best not treated with drugs.

Expectorants and decongestants

Guaifenesin and Pseudoephedrine
(gwye *fen* e sin and soo doe e *feh* drin)
GUIFENEX PSE (Ethex)

We oppose this combination because of the lack of effectiveness of guaifenesin and our opposition to the large systemic doses of the decongestant pseudoephedrine as a decongestant.

Anticholinergics and cough suppressants

Hydrocodone and Homatropine
(hye dro *koe* done and hom a *troe* peen)
HYCODAN (Endo)

The inclusion of an anticholinergic drug such as homatropine in a cough medicine adds considerable risk (see anticholinergic box, p. 362) without any significant benefit.

Nasal Steroids

Beclomethasone (bek low *meth* a sone)
BECONASE AQ (GlaxoSmithKline)
VANCENASE AQ (Schering)

Budesonide (byoo *des* o nyde)
RHINOCORT AQUA (AstraZeneca)

Fluticasone (*flew* ti cas sone)
FLONASE (GlaxoSmithKline)

Mometasone (mow *met* a sone)
NASONEX (Schering)

Triamcinolone (try am *sin* o lone)
NASACORT AQ (Aventis)

GENERIC: not available
FAMILY: Allergy Drugs (see p. 356)
Nasal Steroids (Sprays)

PREGNANCY WARNING

Corticosteroids caused fetal death and fetal malformations in animal studies. Because of the potential for serious adverse effects to the fetus, these drugs should not be used by pregnant women.

BREAST-FEEDING WARNING

Corticosteroids are excreted in human milk. Because of the potential for adverse effects in nursing infants, you should not take these drugs while nursing.

Nasal sprays of steroids primarily reduce inflammation in the nose due to allergies or unidentifiable causes.[18–20] The condition, called rhinitis, may be seasonal or continuous. Nasal steroids also reduce inflammation of the lower airway in rhinitis in people with or without asthma.[21]

The first step to control rhinitis is to eliminate or avoid as much as possible any cause of allergies. If this is insufficient, drugs may be tried. Antihistamines such as chlorpheniramine (see p. 363) relieve most symptoms, except nasal congestion. Antihistamines work just as well as nasal steroids to relieve eye symptoms.[22]

The effectiveness of beclomethasone, budesomide, fluticasone, mometasone, and triamcinolone nasal sprays are similar.[23–28] Nasal steroids are not intended for the common cold.[29] These drugs control, but do not cure, rhinitis. Beclomethasone is also approved for prevention of nasal polyp regrowth after surgical removal.[30]

Some of the nasal steroid is absorbed systemically and can cause supression of adrenal gland function.[31–33] Suppression of adrenal glands can cause low blood sugar, unconsciousness, convulsions, coma, or death. Onset in adults may start with drowsiness and nausea. This can occur during fasting or if steroids are stopped abruptly.

Steroids can suppress growth in children and adolescents, especially if high doses are used for long periods. Although effect based on short-term studies shows minimal effect on growth and development, long-term studies are needed to determine effect on final adult height.[34]

Steroids can reduce immunity, making you more prone to infections, and prolong healing of wounds. Avoid exposure to chicken pox or measles. A fungus, aspergillus, can develop and spread, leading to loss of vision or death.[35]

Sometimes, perforation of the nasal septum occurs, more so in women during the first few months of use. Avoid trauma with tip of nozzle on the septum. Some people develop cataracts.

Before You Use This Drug

Do not use if you are:

* pregnant or breastfeeding

Tell your doctor if you have or have had:

* allergies, including to lactose
* asthma
* diabetes
* glaucoma
* herpes in the eye
* infection (bacterial, fungal, parasitic, or viral)
* liver problems
* myocardial infarction (heart attack) or other heart problems
* pregnancy or are breast-feeding
* surgery, trauma, or ulcers of nose that are not yet healed, including nosebleeds
* low thyroid (hypothyroidism)
* tuberculosis
* recent nasal ulcers, surgery, or trauma

Tell your doctor about any other drugs you take, including aspirin, herbs, vitamins, and other nonprescription products.

When You Use This Drug

* Request training on use of this drug from your doctor and read patient instructions carefully before use.
* Avoid allergens that trigger your rhinitis.
* Check with your doctor before getting any immunizations.

- If you have excess nasal mucus or swelling of nose, use a vasoconstrictor for two to three days to enable the steroid to reach site of action.
- It may take up to three weeks for full benefit.
- Tell any doctor, dentist, emergency help, or pharmacist you see that you use a nasal steroid.

How to Use This Drug

- Follow specific use and cleaning instructions accompanying your device.
- Shake well before each use.
- Hold head in a neutral upright position.
- Gently blow nose to clear of any thick or excessive mucus, if present.
- Insert spray nozzle into the nose and toward the outer portion of the eye or the top of the ear on that side. If possible, use the right hand to spray the left nostril and left hand to spray the right nostril, to direct spray away from the septum.
- Activate the device as recommended by the manufacturer and with the number of sprays recommended by your doctor.
- Gently breathe in or sniff during the spraying.
- Breathe out through the nose.
- Avoid swallowing.
- Do not spray in eyes.
- Use drug at same time(s) each day. If you use more than once a day, schedule doses 12 hours apart.
- If you miss a dose, take it if you remember it within an hour. Otherwise, wait until next regular dose. **Do not take double doses.**
- Do not share your medication with others.
- Store device at room temperature (canister does not work well if cold). Protect from light. Do not freeze. Keep out of reach of children for whom not prescribed.
- Store budesonide with valve up; do not store in damp places.
- Discard after the labeled number of actuations has been reached. Discard beclometh-asone solution three months after opening package.
- Do not transfer any remaining amount to another container. Any residual amount may not deliver the full dose.

Interactions with Other Drugs

Evaluations of Drug Interactions 2003 lists no drugs, biologics (e.g., vaccines, therapeutic antibodies), or foods as causing "highly clinically significant" or "clinically significant" interactions when used together with the drugs in this section. We also found no interactions in the drug's FDA-approved professional package inserts. However, as the number of new drugs approved for marketing increases and as more experience is gained with these drugs over time, new interactions may be discovered.

No studies have been done on interactions with fluticasone nasal spray. Manufacturers advise caution when budesomide or fluticasone is used with: ketoconazole, NIZORAL, NORVIR, ritonavir.

Manufacturers also advise caution when budesmoide is used with: AZITHROMYCIN, clarithromycin, E-MYCIN, ERYBID, ERYTHROCIN, ERYC, ERY-TABS, erythromycin, ILOSONE, PCE.

Adverse Effects

Call your doctor immediately if you experience:

- breathing difficulty
- tightness in chest
- cough
- dizziness or lightheadedness
- ringing in ears
- dry, irritated, painful, red, swollen, or watery eyes or eyelid, or discharge from eye
- fever
- flulike symptoms

- headache
- hoarseness
- muscle pain
- nausea or vomiting
- nosebleed, blood in mucus, nasal burning, stinging, crusting, or dryness, irritation inside nose or stuffy nose, or sores or white patches inside nose
- hives, itching, or rash
- sore throat or white patches in throat
- stomach pain
- swelling of face, lips, or eyelids
- unusual tiredness or weakness
- vision blurs or blindness
- wheezing

Call your doctor if these symptoms continue:

- burning, dryness, or other irritation inside the nose (mild and transient)
- sneezing attacks
- stuffy nose or headache; throat discomfort

Signs of overdose:

- acne
- blurred vision
- blood pressure increase
- bone fracture
- excess facial hair in women
- impotence in men
- menstruation changes
- muscle wasting and weakness
- excess fullness or rounding of face, neck, and trunk
- thirst increase
- urination increase

If you suspect an overdose, call this number to contact your poison control center: (800) 222-1222.

Periodic Tests

Ask your doctor which of these tests should be done periodically while you are taking this drug:

- adrenal function test
- eye, ear, nose, and throat exam

Asthma

Beta Agonists

Albuterol (al *byoo* ter ol)
PROVENTIL (Schering)
VENTOLIN (GlaxoSmithKline)

Pirbuterol (per *butte* er all)
MAXAIR (3M)

GENERIC: available
FAMILY: Beta Agonists

PREGNANCY WARNING

Albuterol caused malformations in human infants including cleft palate and limb defects. There is no human data for pirbuterol, but it caused abortions and fetal death in animal studies. Because of the potential for serious adverse effects to the fetus, these drugs should not be used by pregnant women.

BREAST-FEEDING WARNING

No information is available from either human or animal studies. However, it is likely that these drugs, like many others, are excreted in human milk, and because of the potential for adverse effects in nursing infants, including the potential for cancer with albuterol, you should not take these drugs while nursing.

Inhaled albuterol is used to treat asthma, as well as chronic bronchitis and emphysema. Within five minutes it begins to subdue wheezing and improve breathing.

It belongs to the same family as pirbuterol (MAXAIR). According to Goodman and Gilman's *The Pharmacological Basis of Therapeutics,* there is little basis to choose one of this drug family over another.[36]

Albuterol can cause tremors, jitters, and nervousness, especially in older adults.[37] Albuterol has also been found to cause benign tumors in the ligament surrounding the ovaries in rats.[38]

If you are taking one of these drugs and are suffering from adverse effects, ask your doctor to change your prescription to the other one. **If you are over 60, you will generally need to**

Do not stop any asthma medication without first consulting your physician. Abruptly stopping a medication may result in acutely deteriorating asthma control.

This drug can cause or worsen high blood pressure. It is especially dangerous for people who have high blood pressure, heart disease, diabetes, or thyroid disease. People over 60 are more likely than younger people to experience effects on the heart and blood pressure, restlessness, nervousness, and confusion.

---

take less than the usual adult dose of these drugs, especially if you have heart disease.

Whichever of these drugs you take, use only the inhaled form. Do not take the tablets, capsules, or liquids. Because these forms are swallowed, the drug is distributed throughout your body, increasing the risk of adverse effects. An inhaler deposits most of the drug in the lungs, where it is needed.

Before You Use This Drug

Tell your doctor if you have or have had:

- allergies to drugs
- an allergy to other sympathomimetic drugs such as the decongestants pseudoephedrine and phenylpropanolamine (PPA)
- heart or blood vessel disease
- pheochromocytoma

ADDITIONAL PRECAUTIONS

Avoid exposure to things that trigger your allergies or asthma, such as animals, bedding, chemicals, cosmetics, drugs, dust, mold, foods, pollens, or smoke. Wearing a mask reduces inhalation of drugs, pollens, and smoke.

Aspirin can trigger asthma in people who are aspirin-allergic, as can beta-blockers. Infections aggravate lung problems. During epidemics of respiratory illnesses, avoid crowded places and wash your hands frequently to help prevent infection. If you have asthma, get a flu vaccination.

Note: The information in this profile addresses the care of asthma that is not serious enough to need emergency treatment.

- high blood pressure
- heart rhythm problems
- pregnancy or are breast-feeding
- enlarged thyroid

Tell your doctor about any other drugs you take, including aspirin, herbs, vitamins, and other nonprescription products.

When You Use This Drug

- Check with your doctor immediately if breathing problem persists or if condition becomes worse. Call your doctor if you do not feel better after taking the usual dose, if you still have trouble breathing one hour after a dose, if symptoms return within four hours, or if your condition worsens.
- Check with your doctor immediately if more than your usual inhalations are needed to relieve an acute attack.
- If you plan to have any surgery, including dental surgery, tell your doctor that you take an asthma drug.
- Check with your doctor about anti-inflammatory drug use.

• Do not take other drugs without talking to your doctor first, especially nonprescription drugs for appetite control, asthma, colds, coughs, hay fever, or sinus problems.

How to Use This Drug

• Read patient instructions first.
• If you miss a dose, take it as soon as you remember, then space remaining doses for the day at regular intervals. Do not take more often than prescribed.
• Do not share your medication with others.
• Be careful not to get medicine in your eyes.
• If using an anti-inflammatory drug, check with your doctor before stopping or reducing amount.
• Do not store in the bathroom. Do not expose to heat, moisture, or strong light. Do not allow inhaled form to freeze. Keep out of reach of children.

For the aerosol for oral inhalation:

• Invert the can, then shake well.
• Exhale as completely as possible.
• Place mouthpiece into the mouth. Close lips loosely around it. Tilt inhaler upward and head backward, then inhale slowly and deeply while actuating the inhaler. (Some physicians recommend placing inhaler about two inches from the front of the open mouth.) Remove inhaler from mouth. Hold breath a few seconds, then exhale slowly.
• Avoid contact with the eyes. If you do get drug in your eyes, flush immediately with cool water.
• Clean the inhaler and plastic mouthpiece with warm water. Save inhaler, as refill canister may be available.
• Do not puncture, burn, or incinerate the container.

Interactions with Other Drugs

The following drugs, biologics (e.g., vaccines, therapeutic antibodies), or foods are listed in *Evaluations of Drug Interactions* 2003 as causing "highly clinically significant" or "clinically significant" interactions when used together with any of the drugs in this section. In some sections with multiple drugs, the interaction may have been reported for one but not all drugs in this section, but we include the interaction because the drugs in this section are similar to one another. We have also included potentially serious interactions listed in the drug's FDA-approved professional package insert or in published medical journal articles. There may be other drugs, especially those in the families of drugs listed below, that also will react with this drug to cause severe adverse effects. Make sure to tell your doctor and pharmacist the drugs you are taking and tell them if you are taking any of these interacting drugs:

flecainide, FLUOTHANE, GLUCOPHAGE, GLUCOVANCE, halothane, imipramine, INDERAL, INDERAL LA, METAGLIP, metformin, propranolol, TAMBOCOR, TOFRANIL.

Adverse Effects

Call your doctor immediately if you experience:

• hives
• increased shortness of breath
• skin rash
• swelling of face, lips, or eyelids
• tightness in chest or wheezing
• trouble breathing

Call your doctor if these symptoms continue:

• irregular heartbeat
• headache
• nervousness
• trembling
• coughing or other bronchial irritation
• dizziness or lightheadedness

- dryness or irritation of mouth or throat
- low potassium
- chest discomfort or pain
- drowsiness or weakness
- muscle cramps or twitching
- nausea and/or vomiting
- restlessness
- trouble sleeping

Signs of overdose:

- dizziness or lightheadedness
- continuing trembling
- vomiting
- agitation
- hallucinations or paranoia with nebulized albuterol
- seizures
- fast and irregular heartbeat

If you suspect an overdose, call this number to contact your poison control center: (800) 222-1222.

Fluticasone and Salmeterol inhalation powders
(*flew* ti cas sone and sall *met* er all)
ADVAIR DISKUS (GlaxoSmithKline)

GENERIC: not available for combination
FAMILY: Inhalation Steroids with Beta Agonists

PREGNANCY WARNING

Fluticasone and salmeterol caused fetal harm in animal studies, including delayed bone formation, malformations, and fetal death. Because of the potential for serious adverse effects to the fetus, this drug should not be used by pregnant women.

BREAST-FEEDING WARNING

Fluticasone is excreted in animal milk, and it is likely that this occurs in humans. Although fluticasone was not tested, other corticosteroids have been detected in human milk. Because of the potential for serious adverse effects in nursing infants, you should not take fluticasone and salmeterol while nursing.

Advair combines powders that are inhaled by mouth of both a steroid (fluticasone) and a long-acting beta-blocker (salmeterol). The combination allows for lower dose of fluticasone.[39] It is approved by the FDA for the treatment of chronic asthma but is not intended for treatment of acute episodes, or if asthma is rapidly deteriorating.

FDA BLACK BOX WARNING

Data from a large placebo-controlled US study that compared the safety of salmeterol (SEREVENT Inhalation Aerosol) or placebo added to usual asthma therapy showed a small but significant increase in asthma-related deaths in patients receiving salmeterol (13 deaths out of 13,174 patients treated for 28 weeks) versus those on placebo (4 of 13,179).

Subgroup analyses suggest the risk may be greater in African-American patients compared to Caucasians.

Do not stop any asthma medication without first consulting your physician. Abruptly stopping a medication may result in acutely deteriorating asthma control.

Advair decreases constriction of bronchial smooth muscle and inflammation of the airway. This may reduce need of rescue medications, such as albuterol, reduce severity of shortness of breath, reduce mortality, improve lung function, improve ability to endure strenuous activity, and increase number of symptom-free days.[40–42]

While inhaled steroids reduce likelihood of systemic effects, the risks are not eliminated. Steroids can damage adrenal glands and potentially change bone mineral density.[43–45] High-dose steroids used over six months are more associated with adrenal crisis.[46] Suppression of adrenal glands can cause low blood sugar, unconsciousness, convulsions, coma, or death. Onset in adults may start with drowsiness and nausea.

A detachment of the retina called chorioretinopathy has been associated with steroid inhalers, especially in women.[47]

Before You Use This Drug

Do not use if you have or have had:

- tuberculosis
- herpes simplex (eye)
- untreated infections (bacterial, fungal, parasitic, or viral)
- allergy to fluticasone or salmeterol
- asthma called status asthmaticus
- pregnancy

Tell your doctor if you have or have had:

- heart problems
- high blood pressure
- breast-feeding
- seizures
- thyrotoxicosis

Tell your doctor about any other drugs you take, including aspirin, herbs, vitamins, and other nonprescription products.

When You Use This Drug

- Request training for self-management of asthma.[48,49]
- Always have a short-acting rescue medication available.
- Limit exposure to allergens that trigger asthma. Stop smoking.
- Avoid exposure to chicken pox or measles.
- Contact your doctor if symptoms do not improve, or if you increase use of short-acting beta-blockers.
- If bronchospasm occurs shortly after using, use a short-acting beta-blocker for immediate relief, then call your doctor about discontinuing this combination product.
- If you are being transferred from systemic oral tablets of steroids to inhaled steroids, carry a warning card that you may need systemic steroids during stress or severe asthma attacks.
- Tell any doctor, dentist, emergency help, or pharmacist you see that you use ADVAIR.

How to Use This Drug

- Do not use combination for acute attacks of asthma, including asthma induced by exercise.
- Carefully follow instructions accompanying the device.
- Activate device in a level, horizontal position. Inhale through the mouth. Never use with a spacer. Do not exhale into the device.
- Rinse mouth with water after inhalation, but do not swallow.
- Schedule doses 12 hours apart.
- If you miss a dose, take it as soon as you remember, but skip it if it is almost time for the next dose. **Do not take double doses.**
- Keep the device dry. Do not wash the device or take it apart.
- Store device at room temperature. Do not store in the bathroom. Do not expose to heat, moisture, or sunlight. Keep out of reach of children. Discard one month after removing moisture-protective foil, or after each blister has been used (dose indicator reads zero). Do not take the device apart.

Interactions with Other Drugs

Evaluations of Drug Interactions 2003 lists no drugs, biologics (e.g., vaccines, therapeutic antibodies), or foods as causing "highly clinically significant" or "clinically significant" interactions when used together with the drugs in this section. We also found no interactions in the drug's FDA-approved professional package inserts. However, as the number of new drugs approved for marketing increases and as more experience is gained with these drugs over time, new interactions may be discovered.

The manufacturer carries a reminder not to use Advair with other inhaled long-acting beta-blockers for asthmas: formoterol, FORADIL.

The USP (United States Pharmacopeia) ranks as a major interaction use of Advair within two weeks of: amitriptyline, amoxapine, ANAFRANIL, ASENDIN, AVENTYL, clomipramine, desipramine, doxepin, ELAVIL, imipramine, isocarboxazid, MARPLAN, monoamine oxidase (MAO) inhibitor, NARDIL, NORPRAMIN, nortriptyline, PAMELOR, PARNATE, phenelzine, protriptyline, SINEQUAN, SURMONTIL, TOFRANIL, tranylcypromine, tricyclic antidepressant, trimipramine, VIVACTIL.

USP also states severe bronchospasm could result from using ADVAIR with nonselective systemic beta-blockers: acebutolol, BETAPACE, carteolol, CARTROL, CORGARD, CORZIDE, INDERAL, labetalol, LEVATOL, nadolol, OCUPRESS, oxprenolol, penbutolol, pindolol, propranolol, SECTRAL, sotalol, TRANDATE, TRASICOR, VISKAZIDE, VISKEN.

Adverse Effects

Call your doctor immediately if you experience:

- unusual bleeding or bruising
- difficult or noisy breathing
- chest pain or tightness
- chills
- cough
- fever
- swollen glands
- sores, ulcers, or white spots on lips or mouth
- rash
- numbness, tingling, pain, or burning sensation in arms, feet, hands, or legs
- sensation of pins and needles
- spasm of bronchials
- black or tarry stools
- sore or dry throat
- unusual tiredness or weakness
- difficult or painful urination
- wheezing

Call your doctor if these symptoms continue:

- body aches
- abdominal pain
- appetite loss
- breathing that produces high-pitched noise
- tender cheekbones
- choking
- cough with mucus
- diarrhea
- irritated or inflamed, painful, or tender eyes
- flulike symptoms
- tender or swollen glands in neck
- headache
- fast, irregular, or pounding heartbeat or pulse
- hoarseness
- irritated, swollen, or spasmodic larynx
- white patches in mouth, tongue, or throat
- muscle pain
- nausea
- nervousness
- nosebleed, inflamed sinuses, runny or stuffy nose
- sleep problems
- sneezing
- stomach upset or pain
- difficulty swallowing
- tremors
- voice changes

Other adverse effects are possible. Contact your doctor with any concerns.

Signs of overdose:

- appetite loss
- difficult breathing or breath that has fruit-like odor
- chest pain or tightness
- confusion
- convulsions
- diarrhea
- dizziness
- dry mouth
- fainting
- fatigue, general feeling of discomfort or illness
- headaches
- fast, irregular, or pounding heartbeat or pulse
- hunger increases
- lightheadedness when changing position
- mental depression, mood changes
- muscle cramps or pain
- nausea or vomiting
- nervousness
- numbness or tingling in hands, feet, or lips
- darkened or dry skin, rash
- sleeping problems
- sudden sweating, thirst increase
- unusual tiredness or weakness
- tremors
- urine decrease
- blurred vision

If you suspect an overdose, call this number to contact your poison control center: (800) 222-1222.

Periodic Tests

Ask your doctor which of these tests should be done periodically while you are taking this drug:

- adrenal function test, such as low-dose Synathen stimulation test
- asthma quality-of-life questionnaire
- growth and development (children)
- lung function tests
- skin testing for allergens

Do Not Use

ALTERNATIVE TREATMENT:
See Asthma: Inhaled Steroids, p. 394, and Asthma: Short-Acting Beta Agonists, p. 382.

Salmeterol (sal *met* er all)
SEREVENT (GlaxoSmithKline)

FAMILY: Long-Acting Beta Agonists

FDA BLACK BOX WARNING

Data from a large placebo-controlled US study that compared the safety of salmeterol (SEREVENT Inhalation Aerosol) or placebo added to usual asthma therapy showed a small but significant increase in asthma-related deaths in patients receiving salmeterol (13 deaths out of 13,174 patients treated for 28 weeks) versus those on placebo (4 of 13,179).

Subgroup analyses suggest the risk may be greater in African-American patients compared to Caucasians and that people using salmeterol were more likely to die than those using salmeterol combined with a steroid.

Salmeterol belongs to a family of asthma medications known as long-acting beta2-receptor agonists, or just beta agonists. In contrast, drugs such as albuterol (PROVENTIL, VENTOLIN), metaproterenol (ALUPENT), and pirbuterol (MAXAIR) are short-acting beta agonists. Salmeterol and formoterol (FORADIL) are the only long-acting beta agonists marketed in the United States.

In August 2003, the FDA announced that a black-box warning (see above) is required on the

> Do not stop any asthma medication without first consulting your physician. Abruptly stopping a medication may result in acutely deteriorating asthma control.

professional product labeling or package inserts for drug products containing salmeterol. This requirement applies to both SEREVENT and the combination of salmeterol with the steroid fluticasone sold as ADVAIR (see p. 385). The FDA has the regulatory authority to require box warnings for drugs that have been associated with the deaths or serious injuries of patients and may also require them if there is strong evidence from animal experiments that they may be dangerous. A black-box warning is the strongest type of safety warning that the FDA can mandate in a drug's professional product labeling.

The black-box warning was promoted by a study known as the Salmeterol Multicenter Asthma Research Trial, or SMART for short, that was terminated early. This study was initiated by GlaxoSmithKline in 1996 and was designed to assess the safety of salmeterol because of concerns regarding the safety of regular use of the combination of short- and long-acting beta agonists in the management of asthma after reports of death had been submitted to the FDA.

Unfortunately, information about the SMART study is only fragmentary. GlaxoSmithKline has not published a full description of the study and its outcomes in a medical journal. What is known about the SMART study is contained in an FDA January 23, 2003, announcement and the new additions to salmeterol's professional product labeling.

A very troubling aspect of the FDA's announcement was the number of patients in the trial not using an inhaled steroid as the foundation of their asthma treatment. The National Asthma Education and Prevention Program (NAEPP) guidelines published in 1997 recommend that patients requiring more medicine than needed for simply treating an acute attack with short-acting beta agonists should be using regular and adequate doses of an inhaled steroid for optimal management of their asthma. There are a number of inhaled steroids on the market in the United States, including beclomethasone (BECLOVENT, VANCERIL), budesonide (PULMICORT), flunisolide (AEROBID), fluticasone (FLOVENT), and triamcinolone (AZMACORT).

Historically, worldwide, there have been two beta agonist–induced epidemics of increased deaths in asthmatics. In the 1960s, an isoproterenol (ISUPREL) inhaler containing five times the usual concentration of the drug was marketed in the UK. Isoproterenol is a short-acting beta agonist. While this product was being prescribed in the UK, there was a significant increase in asthma deaths. A parallel increase was not seen in other countries in which the high-concentration preparation was not available.[50]

Fenoterol, a long-acting beta agonist that was never marketed in the United States, was shown to be associated with an epidemic of asthma deaths in New Zealand starting in 1976. This epidemic ended abruptly after New Zealand authorities warned of the possible link between the drug and deaths.[51]

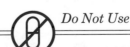

Do Not Use

ALTERNATIVE TREATMENT:
See Asthma: Inhaled Steroids (p. 394) and Asthma: Short-Acting Beta Agonists (p. 382).

Isoetharine (eye soe *eth* a reen)
BETA-2 (Nephron)

FAMILY: Short-Acting Beta Agonists

ADDITIONAL PRECAUTIONS

Avoid exposure to things that trigger your allergies or asthma, such as animals, bedding, chemicals, cosmetics, drugs, dust, mold, foods, pollens, or smoke. Wearing a mask reduces inhalation of drugs, pollens, and smoke.

Aspirin can trigger asthma in people who are aspirin-allergic, as can beta-blockers. Infections aggravate lung problems. During epidemics of respiratory illnesses, avoid crowded places and wash your hands frequently to help prevent infection. If you have asthma, get a flu vaccination.

Note: The information in this profile addresses the care of asthma that is not serious enough to need emergency treatment.

Isoetharine is used to treat mild asthma, chronic bronchitis, emphysema, or occasional acute spasms of the airways called bronchospasm. If you have any of these conditions, the best drug to use is either albuterol or pirbuterol (see p. 382), rather than isoetharine.

Isoetharine is an older inhaled drug that lasts for a shorter time than albuterol.[52] It is more likely to cause high blood pressure and an increase in your heart rate than the similar drugs albuterol, metaproterenol, and terbutaline.[53,54] If you are using isoetharine and have adverse effects, ask your doctor to change your inhalant to albuterol or pirbuterol.

Whichever drug you take, use only the inhaled forms. Do not use the tablets, capsules, or liquids. Because these forms are swallowed, the drug is distributed throughout the body, increasing the risk of adverse effects. An inhaler deposits most of the drug in the lungs, where it is needed.

Xanthines

Limited Use

Aminophylline (am in *off* a lin)

Theophylline (thee *off* a lin)
ELIXOPHYLLIN (Forest)
QUIBRON-T-SR (Monarch)
THEOLAIR (3M)
THEOLAIR-SR (3M)
THEO-24 (UCB)
UNIPHYL (Purdue Frederick)

GENERIC: available
FAMILY: Xanthines

PREGNANCY WARNING

Theophylline caused malformations and death in developing fetuses in animal studies. Because of the potential for serious adverse effects to the fetus, these drugs should not be used by pregnant women.

BREAST-FEEDING WARNING

Theophylline is excreted in human milk. The concentration of theophylline in breast milk is the same as the serum concentration of the mother. Newborns and children under one year are at increased risk. Because of the potential for serious adverse effects in nursing infants, you should not take these drugs while nursing.

These drugs are used to treat symptoms of chronic asthma, bronchitis, and emphysema, including trouble breathing, wheezing, chest tightness, or shortness of breath.

Aminophylline is identical to theophylline, except that aminophylline contains a salt called ethylenediamine, which has caused rashes and hives in some people.[55] For this reason, theophylline is preferable to aminophylline if you need to take a drug in this family by mouth. (Both drugs are also available in an intravenous form for hospital use.)

You must take these drugs exactly as prescribed. Because there is a narrow range between a helpful and harmful amount of this drug in your body, your doctor must monitor

---

ADDITIONAL PRECAUTIONS

Avoid exposure to things that trigger your allergies or asthma, such as animals, bedding, chemicals, cosmetics, drugs, dust, mold, foods, pollens, or smoke. Wearing a mask reduces inhalation of drugs, pollens and smoke. Aspirin can trigger asthma in people who are aspirin-allergic, as can beta-blockers. Infections aggravate lung problems. During epidemics of respiratory illnesses, avoid crowded places and wash your hands frequently to help prevent infection. If you have asthma, get a flu vaccination.

Note: The information in this profile addresses the care of asthma that is not serious enough to need emergency treatment.

WARNING

Extreme caution should be used when fluoroquinolones such as ciprofloxacin (CILOXAN, CIPRO), enoxacin (PENETREX), lomefloxacin (MAXAQUIN), norfloxacin (CHIBROXIN, NOROXIN), and ofloxacin (FLOXIN, OCUFLOX) are to be prescribed in conjunction with aminophylline or theophylline, particularly in elderly patients. Aminophylline doses should be adjusted, perhaps reduced by 30 to 50% at the start of fluoroquinolone therapy. The reduction in dose must be guided by the clinical conditions of the patient, the use of other medications, and the baseline level of the aminophylline in the blood. In addition, blood aminophylline levels should be obtained following the initiation of a fluoroquinolone no later than two days into therapy.

---

your dose and the level of the drug in your bloodstream. Too little drug may bring on an asthma attack; too much can lead to an overdose. The more serious signs of an overdose include seizures, irregular heart rhythms, and pounding heartbeat. Less severe signs may or may not appear before the serious ones.[56]

These drugs interact with a wide variety of other drugs. Most frequently, the interactions result in increased or decreased blood levels of these drugs or of the other drugs.

Before You Use This Drug

Tell your doctor if you have or have had:

- an allergy to caffeine or any other xanthine, such as theobromine (found in chocolate or theophylline)
- rapid heartbeat
- heart failure
- pregnancy or are breast-feeding
- stomach inflammation
- ulcers
- gastroesophageal reflux
- prolonged fever

- respiratory infections
- seizures
- liver problems
- underactive thyroid

Tell your doctor about any other drugs you take, including aspirin, herbs, vitamins, and other nonprescription products.

When You Use This Drug

- Do not use more often or in a higher dose than prescribed by your doctor. Do not change brands or dosage forms without checking with your doctor or pharmacist first.
- See your doctor regularly to check on progress.
- Reduce your intake of charcoal-broiled foods and foods that contain caffeine, such as chocolate, cocoa, tea, coffee, and colas.
- Call your doctor immediately if you get a fever because this increases your chance of developing adverse effects from the drug.
- Notify your doctor if you have started or stopped other medicines, started or stopped

smoking, or made an extended change in your diet.

• If you plan to have any surgery, including dental surgery, tell your doctor that you take this drug.

How to Use This Drug

• If you miss a dose, take it as soon as you remember, but skip it if it is almost time for the next dose. **Do not take double doses.**
• Do not share your medication with others.
• Take the drug at the same time(s) each day.
• *For liquids and immediate-release capsules or tablets:* Take on an empty stomach with a glass of water. If the drug upsets your stomach, take with food instead.
• *For once-a-day dosage forms:* Take either in the morning at least one hour before eating or in the evening without food. Be consistent as to whether you take with or without food.
• *For enteric-coated tablets or delayed-release tablets:* Swallow whole.
• *For extended-release forms:* Capsules may be opened and the contents mixed with applesauce, jelly, or ketchup, then swallowed without chewing.
• Do not store in the bathroom. Do not expose to heat, moisture, or strong light. Keep out of reach of children.

Interactions with Other Drugs

The following drugs, biologics (e.g., vaccines, therapeutic antibodies), or foods are listed in *Evaluations of Drug Interactions* 2003 as causing "highly clinically significant" or "clinically significant" interactions when used together with any of the drugs in this section. In some sections with multiple drugs, the interaction may have been reported for one but not all drugs in this section, but we include the interaction because the drugs in this section are similar to one another. We have also included potentially serious interactions listed in the drug's FDA-approved professional package insert or in published medical journal articles. There may be other drugs, especially those in the families of drugs listed below, that also will react with this drug to cause severe adverse effects. Make sure to tell your doctor and pharmacist the drugs you are taking and tell them if you are taking any of these interacting drugs:

adenosine, alcohol, allopurinol, aminoglutethimide, ANTABUSE, ANTURANE, ATAVAN, BIAXIN, caffeine, CALAN, carbamazepine, charcoal, CIPRO, ciprofloxacin, clarithromycin, COGNEX, CYTADREN, DALMANE, diazepam, DILANTIN, dipyridamole, disulfiram, EES, enoxacin, erythromycin, estrogen-containing oral contraceptives, ETHOZINE, FLUOTHANE, flurazepam, fluvoxamine, halothane, *Hypericum perforatum,* INDERAL, interferon alpha, INTRON A, KETALAR, ketamine, lithium, LITHOBID, lorazepam, LUMINAL, LUVOX, methotrexate, mexiletine, MEXITIL, MINTEZOL, modafinil, moricizine, NORVIR, pancuronium, PAVULON, PENETREX, pentoxifylline, PERSANTINE, phenobarbital, phenytoin, propafenone, propranolol, PROVIGIL, RIFADIN, rifampin, ritonavir, ROFERON-A, RYTHMOL, St. John's wort, sulfinpyrazone, tacrine, TAO, TEGRETOL, thiabendazole, TICLID, ticlopidine, TRENTAL, troleandomycin, VALIUM, verapamil, VERELAN, ZYLOPRIM.

Adverse Effects

Call your doctor immediately if you experience:

• heartburn and/or vomiting
• skin rash or hives (aminophylline)

Call your doctor if these symptoms continue:

- headache
- fast heartbeat
- trouble sleeping
- increased urination
- anxiety
- nausea, vomiting
- nervousness
- trembling

Signs of overdose:

- dark or bloody vomit, continuing vomiting
- severe or continuing abdominal pain
- continuing nervousness or restlessness
- confusion or change in behavior
- diarrhea
- dizziness or lightheadedness
- convulsions
- fast and irregular heartbeat
- trembling

If you suspect an overdose, call this number to contact your poison control center: (800) 222-1222.

Periodic Tests

Ask your doctor which of these tests should be done periodically while you are taking this drug:

- blood levels of aminophylline or theophylline
- lung function tests
- caffeine concentrations

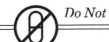 *Do Not Use*

ALTERNATIVE TREATMENT:
See Theophylline, p. 390.

Oxtriphylline (ox *trye* fi lin)
CHOLEDYL SA (Warner-Chilcott)

FAMILY: Xanthines

ADDITIONAL PRECAUTIONS

Avoid exposure to things that trigger your allergies or asthma, such as animals, bedding, chemicals, cosmetics, drugs, dust, mold, foods, pollens, or smoke. Wearing a mask reduces inhalation of drugs, pollens, and smoke. Aspirin can trigger asthma in people who are aspirin-allergic, as can beta-blockers. Infections aggravate lung problems. During epidemics of respiratory illnesses, avoid crowded places and wash your hands frequently to help prevent infection. If you have asthma, get a flu vaccination.

Note: The information in this profile addresses the care of asthma that is not serious enough to need emergency treatment.

Oxtriphylline is used to treat symptoms of chronic asthma, bronchitis, and emphysema. It opens airways in the lungs and increases the flow of air through them, making breathing easier. Oxtriphylline is identical to theophylline, except that it contains a salt not found in theophylline. It is no more effective than theophylline (see p. 390), yet it costs more.[57] If you take oxtriphylline, ask your doctor to change your prescription to theophylline.

If you continue to use oxtriphylline, take it exactly as prescribed. Because there is a narrow range between a helpful and a harmful amount of this drug in your body, your doctor must monitor your dose and the level of the drug in your bloodstream. Too little oxtriphylline may bring on an asthma attack; too much can lead to an overdose. The more serious signs of an overdose include seizures, irregular heart rhythms, and pounding heartbeat. Less severe signs may or may not appear before the serious ones.[56]

Inhaled Steroids

Beclomethasone (beh kloe *meth* a sone)
QVAR AEROSOL (Ivax)

Fluticasone (flue *tik* a sone)
FLOVENT (GlaxoSmithKline)
FLOVENT DISKUS (GlaxoSmithKline)
FLOVENT ROTADISK (GlaxoSmithKline)

Triamcinolone Inhalation
(trye am *sin* oh lone)
AZMACORT AEROSOL CANISTER
(Aventis)

GENERIC: not available
FAMILY: Inhaled Steroids

PREGNANCY WARNING
Corticosteroids cause death and malformations in fetuses, including cleft palate, skeletal defects, and central nervous system and/or brain malformations. Because of the potential for serious adverse effects to the fetus, these drugs should not be used by pregnant women.

BREAST-FEEDING WARNING
Corticosteroids are excreted in human milk. Because of the potential for adverse effects in nursing infants, you should not take these drugs while nursing.

Steroids inhaled by mouth prevent or reduce inflammation due to asthma when used routinely. These drugs are not bronchodilators that open airways, and are not intended for treatment of acute asthma attacks or status asthmaticus.[58]

Asthma is a progressive disease that can develop at any age. Lung function declines and irreversible obstruction of the airways can occur. Diseases of the nose or sinuses and viral infections may worsen asthma.[59] Drugs control symptoms of shortness of breath, chest tightness, wheezing, and coughing but do not cure asthma.

The steroids beclomethasone, fluticasone, and triamcinolone have similar efficacy when inhaled.[60,61] In addition to reducing inflammation, these drugs improve lung function and reduce the number of acute asthma attacks.[61]

FDA BLACK BOX WARNING

TRIAMCINOLONE

Particular care is needed in patients who are transferred from systemically active corticosteroids to Azmacort Inhalation Aerosol because deaths due to adrenal insufficiency have occurred in asthmatic patients during and after transfer from systemic corticosteroids to aerosolized steroids in recommended doses. After withdrawal from systemic corticosteroids, a number of months are usually required for recovery of hypothalamic-pituitary-adrenal (HPA) function (i.e., start producing your own corticosteroids after suppression by systemic corticosteroids). For some patients who have received large doses of oral steroids for long periods of time before therapy with Azmacort Inhalation Aerosol is initiated, recovery may be delayed for one year or longer. During this period of HPA suppression, patients may exhibit signs and symptoms of adrenal insufficiency when exposed to trauma, surgery, or infections, particularly gastroenteritis or other conditions with acute electrolyte loss. Although Azmacort Inhalation Aerosol may provide control of asthmatic symptoms during these episodes, in recommended doses it supplies only normal physiological amounts of corticosteroid systemically and does NOT provide the increased systemic steroid which is necessary for coping with these emergencies.

During periods of stress or a severe asthmatic attack, patients who have been recently withdrawn from systemic corticosteroids should be instructed to resume systemic steroids (in large doses) immediately and to contact their physician for further instruction. These patients should also be instructed to carry a warning card indicating that they may need supplementary systemic steroids during periods of stress or a severe asthma attack.

Important to the effectiveness of inhalers is proper technique in using the device delivering the steroid.[62]

Steroids inhaled by mouth are available as an aerosol or as dry powder to be inhaled through an accompanying device. Doses are measured in micrograms, abbreviated as mcg. Time for initial improvement varies from 1 to 14 days; full benefits take several weeks to months.

If you take systemic steroids, the dose needs to be tapered down slowly and carefully, since it takes several months for adrenal function to recover. Deaths from adrenal insufficiency have occurred during this process. Trauma, surgery, infections, or gastroenteritis are times to be especially watchful.

While inhaled steroids reduce likelihood of systemic effects, the risks are not eliminated. Steroids can damage adrenal glands and potentially change bone mineral density.[44–45] Suppression of adrenal glands can cause low blood sugar, unconsciousness, convulsions, coma, or death. This can also occur during fasting or if steroids are stopped abruptly.[44]

A detachment of the retina called chorioretinopathy has been associated with steroid inhalers, especially in women.[47]

A rare disease called Churg-Strauss syndrome has been associated with both systemic and inhaled steroids.[64]

Steroids, both systemic and inhaled, can slow growth and development in children. Safety and effectiveness in children under three months of age has not been established.

Steroids also can make you more susceptible to infections. These can lead to fungal infection of the mouth, throat, and voice box called candidiasis or aspergillosis. Risk increases with higher doses. Risk may be higher with fluticasone.[65,66] Avoiding swallowing after rinsing your mouth helps reduce risk. Children or adults who have not had chicken pox or measles should avoid exposure to these diseases.

Before You Use This Drug

Do not use if you are:

- pregnant or breast-feeding
- allergic to lactose (fluticasone)

Tell your doctor if you have or have had:

- glaucoma
- infections (bacterial, fungal, parasitic, or viral)
- liver problems, such as cirrhosis
- osteoporosis
- hypothyroidism
- tuberculosis

Tell your doctor about any other drugs you take, including aspirin, herbs, vitamins, and other nonprescription products.

When You Use This Drug

- Request training for self-management of asthma.[67]
- Read patient instructions carefully.
- Limit exposure to triggers of asthma. Wear protective devices or masks. Stop smoking.
- Avoid exposure to chicken pox or measles.
- Contact your doctor if symptoms do not improve, or if you increase use of short-acting beta agonists.
- If you are being transferred from systemic oral tablets of steroids to inhaled steroids, carry identification with you stating that supplemental systemic steroid therapy may be required in emergencies, periods of unusual stress, or acute asthma attack.
- Use every day in regularly spaced doses.
- Tell any doctor, dentist, emergency help, pharmacist, or surgeon you see that you use a steroid inhaler.

How to Use This Drug

- Do not use for acute attacks of asthma.
- Success depends on technique. Follow printed instructions that accompany the partic-

ular inhaler device carefully about when and how to prime the container, inhalation technique by mouth, and disposal precautions.

• Children should use a spacer device.

• Do not spray in eyes or nose.

• Gargle and rinse mouth with water after use. Spit out. Do not swallow. This reduces dry mouth, hoarseness, and risk of systemic absorption.

• Schedule doses at even intervals.

• If you miss a dose, take it as soon as you remember, but skip it if it is almost time for the next dose. Space any remaining doses of the day at regular intervals. **Do not take double doses.**

• **Do not stop taking this drug suddenly.** Contact your doctor.

• Do not share your medication with others.

• Do not use actuator for other inhalation drugs.

• Store inhalers in dry place at room temperature. Coldness can reduce the amount of drug inhaled. Do not freeze. Protect from sunlight. Do not use or store near heat or open flame. High temperatures may cause bursting. Keep out of reach of children for whom not prescribed.

• Store fluticasone with nozzle end down.

• Dispose after full number of actuations used or indicator reads zero. Follow accompanying instructions precisely. Do not throw into fire or incinerator. Do not reuse Diskus device.

• The triamcinolone canister contains chlorofluorocarbon (CFC) as a propellant.

Interactions with Other Drugs

Evaluations of Drug Interactions 2003 lists no drugs, biologics (e.g., vaccines, therapeutic antibodies), or foods as causing "highly clinically significant" or "clinically significant" interactions when used together with the drugs in this section. We also found no interactions in the drug's FDA-approved professional package inserts. However, as the number of new drugs approved for marketing increases and as more experience is gained with these drugs over time, new interactions may be discovered.

Adverse Effects

Call your doctor immediately if you experience:

• aggressive behavior
• anxiety
• bleeding from rectum
• blood pressure increase
• difficult breathing
• bruises
• chest pain or burning
• diarrhea
• dizziness, fainting
• fat deposits in face, neck, or trunk
• fever
• general feeling of discomfort or illness
• slowed growth (children)
• fast or irregular heartbeat
• menstruation change
• vaginal infection
• mood or mental change
• creamy-white patches in mouth or throat
• nausea or vomiting
• numbness
• pain in abdomen, arms, back, chest, legs, ribs, or stomach
• sense of constant movement of self or surroundings
• diminished or lost senses of smell and taste
• sinus problems
• skin itching, hives, rash
• bloody stools
• painful swallowing or eating
• swelling of ankles, eyelids, face, feet, fingers, lips, lower legs
• unusual thirst
• unusual tiredness or weakness
• frequent, bloody, burning, or painful urination
• blurred or changed vision

- weight gain
- severe wheezing
- osteoporosis (occurs with long-term use; pain in back, ribs, arms, or legs)

Call your doctor if these symptoms continue:

- sinus problems
- cough
- dry mouth or throat
- headache
- sore throat, hoarseness, or voice change
- throat irritation
- constipation
- diarrhea
- trouble sleeping
- nausea or vomiting
- unpleasant taste in mouth
- nosebleeds or other nasal problems
- general aches

Other adverse effects are possible. Contact your doctor with any concerns.

Periodic Tests

Ask your doctor which of these tests should be done periodically while you are taking this drug:

- adrenal function test
- eye test
- growth and development (in children)
- lung function test
- signs of bruising
- test of technique in using inhaler
- weight

Leukotriene Inhibitors

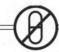 *Do Not Use*

ALTERNATIVE TREATMENT:
See Asthma: Short-Acting Beta Agonsists, p. 382, and Asthma: Single-Agent Inhaled Steroids, p. 394.

Montelukast (mon te *loo* kast)
SINGULAIR (Merck)

Zafirlukast (az fer *loo* kast)
ACCOLATE (Astra Zeneca)

FAMILY: Leukotriene Inhibitors

Montelukast and zafirlukast are members of the leukotriene inhibitor family of asthma drugs. These drugs work by blocking the function or preventing the production of chemicals called leukotrienes, which are thought to play a role in asthma.

The leukotriene inhibitors are the first new family of asthma drugs to be introduced in 20 years. However, they are not as effective or as

---

ADDITIONAL PRECAUTIONS

Avoid exposure to things that trigger your allergies or asthma, such as animals, bedding, chemicals, cosmetics, drugs, dust, mold, foods, pollens, or smoke. Wearing a mask reduces inhalation of drugs, pollens, and smoke.

Aspirin can trigger asthma in people who are aspirin-allergic, as can beta-blockers. Infections aggravate lung problems. During epidemics of respiratory illnesses, avoid crowded places and wash your hands frequently to help prevent infection. If you have asthma, get a flu vaccination.

Note: The information in this profile addresses the care of asthma that is not serious enough to need emergency treatment.

safe as the currently recommended drugs for treatment and prevention of asthma, which are inhaled steroids,[68] for example, beclomethasone (VANCERIL). Steroids are also used in combination with an inhaled beta2-agonist such as albuterol (VENTOLIN) for rescue therapy in case of a sudden asthma attack. In addition to being used on their own, leukotriene inhibitors are promoted as useful in helping patients reduce their dosages of steroid drugs. However, studies comparing leukotriene inhibitors to placebo in people using steroids reveal that the dosage of inhaled steroids can be safely reduced without requiring the use of leukotriene inhibitors.[69] Furthermore, the dose of leukotriene inhibitors required to achieve a significant reduction in steroid dosage is several times the currently approved maximum dosage. If you are concerned about the amount of exposure to steroids you are receiving, consult with your doctor to see if lowering your dosage is appropriate.

Montelukast and zafirlukast are associated with an adverse reaction known as Churg-Strauss syndrome, a condition in which blood vessels become inflamed.[70,71] Though some researchers believe that such events are caused by changes in steroid dosage following the use of these drugs, Churg-Strauss has been documented in patients using these drugs but not receiving steroids at the time the syndrome was diagnosed.[72,73] Zafirlukast use has also been linked to drug-induced lupus[74] and a recurrence of ulcerative colitis (inflammation of the colon).[75]

Cases of liver toxicity with zafirlukast have been reported in the medical literature.[76–78]

The liver toxicity warning in zafirlukast's professional product labeling or package insert was strengthened in April 2004 to say that cases of life-threatening liver failure have been reported in patients treated with the drug. In some cases these patients have progressed to liver transplantation and death.

If you are taking zafirlukast and develop the signs and symptoms of liver toxicity, for example, abdominal pain on the upper right side, nausea, fatigue, lethargy, itching, jaundice (yellowing of the skin or eyes), flulike symptoms, or loss of appetite, you should contact your physician immediately.

The FDA approved montelukast for the relief of symptoms of seasonal allergic rhinitis (hay fever) in adults and children two years of age and older in January 2003. The approval was based on five clinical trials, all of which were similar in design. There were a total of 5,029 patients involved, of whom 1,799 were treated with montelukast.

The effectiveness of montelukast in the five trials was assessed using the average change from the beginning of the study in the daytime nasal symptoms score. This score is the average of individual scores of nasal congestion, rhinorrhea (runny nose), nasal itching, and sneezing as assessed by patients in the trial on a 0–3 point scale.

Four of the five trials found montelukast superior to a placebo (an inactive "dummy" drug). In the fifth trial, montelukast was compared to an active antihistamine, loratadine (CLARITIN). In this trial, the score for loratadine was superior to that of montelukast.[3]

The Medical Letter on Drugs and Therapeutics, a highly respected, independent source of drug information written for health professionals, reviewed montelukast and concluded:

"Montelukast (Singulair) might be as effective as an oral antihistamine for treatment of seasonal allergic rhinitis (more data are needed), but it is less effective than an intranasal corticosteroid, and more expensive than either. We agree. Intranasal corticosteroids, or steroids, are also effective for hay fever."[79]

The Medical Letter was referring to studies showing that fluticasone (FLONASE) was better than either montelukast or loratadine for hay fever. Some other intranasal steroids on the market are beclomethasone (BECONASE AQ) and budesonide (RHINOCORT AQUA).

Overall, montelukast is an unremarkable treatment for hay fever, as is loratadine or its close chemical relative desloratadine (CLARINEX), for that matter. Clinical trials of the leukotriene inhibitors have shown that when used alone these drugs are inferior to inhaled steroids in preventing and treating asthma, and their use to help reduce exposure to steroids is questionable. Overall, the lack of a documented therapeutic advantage over current treatment and the chance of some serious adverse reactions should rule out the use of these drugs.

Chronic Obstructive Pulmonary (Lung) Disease (COPD)

Ipratropium (ip ra *trop* ee um)
ATROVENT (Boehringer Ingelheim)

Ipratropium and Albuterol
(ip ra *trop* ee um and al *byoo* ter ol)
COMBIVENT (Boehringer Ingelheim)

GENERIC: not available
FAMILY: Chronic Obstructive Pulmonary Disease (COPD)
Beta Agonists

PREGNANCY WARNING

Albuterol, a component of COMBIVENT, caused malformations in human infants. Because of the potential for serious adverse effects to the fetus, ipratropium with albuterol should not be used by pregnant women. There were no adverse effects seen in animal studies with ipratropium when used alone, and there were no human data.

BREAST-FEEDING WARNING

No information is available from either human or animal studies. However, because many drugs are excreted in human milk, it is likely that these drugs are present in milk. Because of the potential for adverse effects in nursing infants, particularly the potential for cancer with albuterol, you should not take the combination of ipratropium and albuterol while nursing.

Ipratropium is approved by the FDA for the management of chronic obstructive pulmonary disease, known as COPD. It is not approved for the treatment of asthma.[80] It is an anticholinergic drug in the same family as atropine.[81] Ipratropium takes about 15 minutes to work and lasts about three to six hours.

Ipratropium enlarges the bronchial tubes, but may also enlarge the intestines.[82] It does not control symptoms nor reduce inflammation, a drawback for treating asthma according to a report of the International Asthma Management Project.[83] Ipratropium may thicken secretions in the lungs, cause retention of urine, and cause or worsen narrow-angle glaucoma. It does not relieve nasal congestion or sneezing. While ipratropium is often preferred for use in people over age 60, it should be used cautiously in older men with prostate problems.[84]

COMBIVENT is a combination of ipratropium with the beta agonist bronchodilator albuterol. See p. 382 for more information on albuterol.

ANTICHOLINERGIC EFFECTS

WARNING: SPECIAL MENTAL AND PHYSICAL ADVERSE EFFECTS

Older adults are especially sensitive to the harmful anticholinergic (see Glossary, p. 889) effects of this drug. Drugs in this family should not be used unless absolutely necessary.

Mental Effects: confusion, delirium, short-term memory problems, disorientation, and impaired attention.

Physical Effects: dry mouth, constipation, difficulty urinating (especially for a man with an enlarged prostate), blurred vision, decreased sweating with increased body temperature, sexual dysfunction, and worsening of glaucoma.

Before You Use This Drug

Tell your doctor if you have or have had:

- allergies to ipratropium or belladonna alkaloids (ipratropium)
- allergies to ipratropium, atropine, or albuterol (ipratropium and albuterol)
- allergies to soya lecithin, soybean protein, or peanuts (when using metered-dose inhaler)
- narrow-angle glaucoma (ipratropium)
- difficulty urinating (ipratropium)
- heart problems (albuterol)
- high blood pressure (albuterol)
- pregnancy or are breast-feeding

Tell your doctor about any other drugs you take, including aspirin, herbs, vitamins, and other nonprescription products.

When You Use This Drug

- Check with your doctor if symptoms do not improve within 30 minutes of use. Check immediately if using ipratropium with albuterol and breathing difficulty persists or gets worse.
- If you plan to have any surgery, including dental surgery, tell your doctor that you take this drug.

How to Use This Drug

- If you miss a dose, take it as soon as you remember, and evenly space the remaining doses for that day.
- Do not share your medication with others.
- Take the drug at the same time(s) each day.
- Read instructions carefully before using.
- Avoid getting ipratropium in your eyes. Use a well-fitting mask, goggles, or T-piece extension, or at least close your eyes.[85–87] If nasal spray gets in eyes, flush eyes for several minutes with cool tap water. If you get eye pain or blurred vision, check with your doctor immediately.

- Shake canister well before using. Dilute solutions before using, according to instructions.
- If you use a spacer device or nebulizer, be sure you understand the instructions for use. Ask questions and practice until you are comfortable using the device. Ask your doctor if a paper bag can be substituted.
- Discard solutions of ipratropium stored at room temperature without a preservative within 24 hours; discard within 48 hours if refrigerated.
- Do not store in the bathroom. Do not expose to heat, moisture, or strong light. Store metered dose inhaler at room temperature. Store solutions according to instructions on the label. Keep out of reach of children.

Interactions with Other Drugs

The following drugs, biologics (e.g., vaccines, therapeutic antibodies), or foods are listed in *Evaluations of Drug Interactions* 2003 as causing "highly clinically significant" or "clinically significant" interactions when used together with any of the drugs in this section. In some sections with multiple drugs, the interaction may have been reported for one but not all drugs in this section, but we include the interaction because the drugs in this section are similar to one another. We have also included potentially serious interactions listed in the drug's FDA-approved professional package insert or in published medical journal articles. There may be other drugs, especially those in the families of drugs listed below, that also will react with this drug to cause severe adverse effects. Make sure to tell your doctor and pharmacist the drugs you are taking and tell them if you are taking any of these interacting drugs:

cromolyn solution (if mixed with ipratropium a cloudy sludge will form; do not use such mixtures), GASTROCOM, INTAL, NASALCROM.

For albuterol: GLUCOPHAGE, GLUCO-VANCE, METAGLIP, metformin.

Adverse Effects

Call your doctor immediately if you experience:

- constipation, or lower abdominal pain or bloating
- difficulty breathing: shortness of breath or wheezing
- chest discomfort or pain
- severe eye pain
- swelling of face, lips, or eyelids
- swelling of the mouth or throat
- dizziness

- unusually fast heartbeat (ipratropium and albuterol)
- skin rash or hives

Call your doctor if these symptoms continue:

- cough
- dry mouth or throat
- headache
- nausea
- increased nasal congestion
- nasal itching, burning, or irritation
- increased runny nose
- nervousness
- change in sense of taste
- dizziness
- trembling

REFERENCES

1. Neuner JM, Hamel MB, Phillips RS, et al. Diagnosis and management of adults with pharyngitis: A cost-effectiveness analysis. *Annals of Internal Medicine* 2003; 139:113–122.

2. Drugs for asthma. *Medical Letter on Drugs and Therapeutics* 1987; 29:11–16.

3. *Physicians' Desk Reference.* 58th ed. Montvale, N.J.: Thomson PDR, 2004:2076–81.

4. National Heart, Lung, and Blood Institute. National Asthma Education and Prevention Program Expert Panel Report 2: Guidelines for the Diagnosis and Management of Asthma, July 1, 1997. Available at: http://www.nhlbi.nih.gov/guidelines/asthma/asthgdln.htm. Accessed April 27, 2004.

5. Newhouse MT, Dolovich MB. Control of asthma by aerosols. *New England Journal of Medicine* 1986; 315:870–4.

6. *Physicians' Desk Reference.* 58th ed. Montvale, N.J.: Thomson PDR, 2004:1913–5.

7. Azelastine nasal spray for allergic rhinitis. *Medical Letter on Drugs and Therapeutics* 1997; 39:45–7.

8. Cyproheptadine (Periactin). *Medical Letter on Drugs and Therapeutics* 1971; 13:17–8.

9. Desloratadine (Clarinex). *Medical Letter on Drugs and Therapeutics* 2002; 44:27–8.

10. Nicklas R. Food and Drug Administration Medical Officer Review of Desloratadine (Clarinex), September 29, 2000; 3–8.

11. Loratadine, desloratadine and pregnancy: Don't use, risk of hypospadias. *Prescrire International* 2003; 12:183.

12. Fexofenadine. *Medical Letter on Drugs and Therapeutics* 1996; 38:95–6.

13. Kernan WN, Viscoli CM, Brass LM, et al. Phenylpropanolamine and the risk of hemorrhagic stroke. *New England Journal of Medicine* 2000; 343:1826–32.

14. Klestov A, Kubler P, Meulet J. Recurrent ischaemic colitis associated with pseudoephedrine use. *Internal Medicine Journal* 2001; 31:195–6.

15. Ischaemic colitis on pseudoephedrine. *Prescrire International* 2001; 21:117.

16. *Physicians' Desk Reference.* 58th ed. Montvale, N.J.: Thomson PDR, 2004:1308.

17. AMA Department of Drugs. *AMA Drug Evaluations.* 1st ed. Chicago: American Medical Association, 1971:355.

18. Wihl JA, Andersson KE, Johansson SA. Systemic effects of two nasally administered glucocorticosteroids. *Allergy* 1997; 52:620–6.

19. Jeal W, Faulds D. Triamcinolone acetonide: A review of its pharmacological properties and therapeutic efficacy in the management of allergic rhinitis. *Drugs* 1997; 53:257–80.

20. Davies RJ, Nelson HS. Once-daily mometasone furoate nasal spray: efficacy and safety of a new intranasal glucocorticoid for allergic rhinitis. *Clinical Therapeutics* 1997; 19:27–38.

21. Sandrini A, Ferreira IM, Jardim JR, et al. Effect of nasal triamcinolone acetonide on lower airway inflammatory markers in patients with allergic rhinitis. *Journal of Allergy and Clinical Immunology* 2003; 111:313–20.

22. Yanez A, Rodrigo GJ. Intranasal corticosteroids versus topical H1 receptor antagonists for the treatment of allergic rhinitis: a systematic review with meta-analysis. *Annals of Allergy, Asthma and Immunology* 2002; 89:479–84.

23. Mometasone furoate nasal spray for allergic rhinitis. *Medical Letter on Drugs and Therapeutics* 1999; 41:16–7.

24. Mandl M, Nolop K, Lutsky BN. Comparison of once daily mometasone furoate (Nasonex) and fluticasone propionate aqueous nasal sprays for the treatment of perennial rhinitis. *Annals of Allergy, Asthma and Immunology* 1997; 79:370–8.

25. Lee DK, Robb FM, Sims EJ, et al. Systemic bioactivity of intranasal triamcinolone and mometasone in perennial allergic rhinitis. *British Journal of Clinical Pharmacology* 2003; 55:310–3.

26. Ciprandi G, Canonica WG, Grosclaude M, et al. Effects of budesonide and fluticasone propionate in a placebo-controlled study on symptoms and quality of life in seasonal allergic rhinitis. *Allergy* 2002; 57:586–91.

27. Berger WE, Kaiser H, Gawchik SM, et al. Triamcinolone acetonide aqueous nasal spray and fluticasone propionate are equally effective for relief of nasal symptoms in patients with seasonal allergic rhinitis. *Otolaryngology and Head and Neck Surgery* 2003; 129:16–23.

28. Bachert C, El Akkad T. Patient preferences and sensory comparisons of three intranasal corticosteroids for the treatment of allergic rhinitis. *Annals of Allergy, Asthma and Immunology* 2002; 89:292–7.

29. Silverman M, Wang M, Hunter G, et al. Episodic viral wheeze in preschool children; effect of topical nasal corticosteroid prophylaxis. *Thorax* 2003; 58:431–4.

30. *Physicians' Desk Reference.* 58th ed. Montvale, N.J.: Thomson PDR, 2004.

31. Wilson AM, McFarlane LC, Lipworth BJ. Effects of intranasal corticosteroids on adrenal, bone, and blood markers of systemic activity in allergic rhinitis. *Journal of Allergy and Clinical Immunology* 1998; 102:598–603.

32. Wilson AM, Lipworth BJ. 24 hour and fractionated profiles of adrenocortical activity in asthmatic patients receiving inhaled and intranasal corticosteroids. *Thorax* 1999; 54:20–6.

33. Benninger MS, Hadley JA, Osguthorpe JD, et al. Techniques of intranasal steroid use. *Otolaryngology and Head and Neck Surgery* 2004; 130:5–24.

34. Agertoft L, Pedersen S. Short-term lower leg growth rate in children with rhinitis treated with intranasal mometasone furoate and budesonide. *Journal of Allergy and Clinical Immunology* 1999; 104:948–52.

35. Banov CH, Silvers WS, Green AW, et al. Placebo-controlled, double-blind study of the efficacy and safety of triamcinolone acetonide aerosol nasal inhaler in pediatric patients with seasonal allergic rhinitis. *Clinical Therapeutics* 1996; 18:265–72.

36. Gilman AG, Rall TW, Nies AS, Taylor P, eds. *The Pharmacological Basis of Therapeutics.* 8th ed. New York: Pergamon Press, 1990.

37. Drugs for asthma. *Medical Letter on Drugs and Therapeutics* 1982; 24:83–6.

38. *Physicians' Desk Reference.* 41st ed. Oradell, N.J.: Medical Economics Company, 1987:1948.

39. Busse W, Koenig SM, Oppenheimer J, et al. Steroid-sparing effects of fluticasone propionate 100 microg and salmeterol 50 microg administered twice daily in a single product in patients previously controlled with fluticasone propionate 250 microg administered twice daily. *Journal of Allergy and Clinical Immunology* 2003; 111:57–65.

40. Nelson HS, Chapman KR, Pyke SD, et al. Enhanced synergy between fluticasone propionate and salmeterol inhaled from a single inhaler versus separate inhalers. *Journal of Allergy and Clinical Immunology* 2003; 112:29–36.

41. Mahler DA, Wire P, Horstman D, et al. Effectiveness of fluticasone propionate and salmeterol combination delivered via the Diskus device in the treatment of chronic obstructive pulmonary disease. *American Journal of Respiratory and Critical Care Medicine* 2002; 166:1084–91.

42. Calverley P, Pauwels R, Vestbo J, et al. Combined salmeterol and fluticasone in the treatment of chronic obstructive pulmonary disease: A randomised controlled trial. *The Lancet* 2003; 361:449–56.

43. Pescollderungg L, Radetti G, Gottardi E, et al. Systemic activity of inhaled corticosteroid treatment in asthmatic children: Corticotrophin releasing hormone test. *Thorax* 2003; 58:227–30.

44. Todd GR, Acerini CL, Ross-Russell R, et al. Survey of adrenal crisis associated with inhaled corticosteroids in the United Kingdom. *Archives of Diseases in Children* 2002; 87:457–61.

45. Sim D, Griffiths A, Armstrong D, et al. Adrenal suppression from high-dose inhaled fluticasone propionate in children with asthma. *European Respiratory Journal* 2003; 21:633–6.

46. Nguyen KL, Lauver D, Kim I, et al. The effect of a steroid "burst" and long-term, inhaled fluticasone propionate on adrenal reserve. *Annals of Allergy, Asthma and Immunology* 2003; 91:38–43.

47. Haimovici R, Gragoudas ES, Duker JS, et al. Central serous chorioretinopathy associated with inhaled or intranasal corticosteroids. *Ophthalmology* 1997; 104:1653–60.

48. Sheth K, Bernstein JA, Lincourt WR, et al. Patient perceptions of an inhaled asthma medication administered as an inhalation powder via the Diskus or as an inhalation aerosol via a metered-dose inhaler. *Annals of Allergy, Asthma and Immunology* 2003; 91:55–60.

49. Dinakar C, Reddy M. The yellow zone in asthma treatment: is it a gray zone? *Annals of Allergy, Asthma and Immunology* 2004; 92:7–16.

50. Stolley PD. Asthma mortality: Why the United States was spared an epidemic of deaths due to asthma. *American Review of Respiratory Disease* 1972; 105:883–90.

51. Beasley R, Pearce N, Crane J, et al. Withdrawal of fenoterol and the end of the New Zealand asthma mortality epidemic. *International Archives of Allergy and Immunology* 1995; 107:325–7.

52. Kastrup EK, ed. *Facts and Comparisons.* St. Louis: J.B. Lippincott, January 1986.

53. AMA Department of Drugs. *AMA Drug Evaluations.* 5th ed. Chicago: American Medical Association, 1983:580.

54. Shrestha M, Gourlay S, Robertson S, et al. Isoetharine versus albuterol for acute asthma: greater immediate effect, but more side effects. *American Journal of Medicine* 1996; 100:323–7.

55. Dukes MNG, ed. *Side Effects of Drugs Annual* 10. New York: Elsevier, 1986.

56. *USP DI Drug Information for the Health Care Provider.* 7th ed. Rockville, Md.: The United States Pharmacopeial Convention Inc., 1987.

57. Kastrup EK, ed. *Facts and Comparisons.* St. Louis: J.B. Lippincott, July 1987.

58. *Physicians' Desk Reference.* 58th ed. Montvale, N.J.: Thomson PDR, 2004:1461–3.

59. Tosca MA, Cosentino C, Pallestrini E, et al. Improvement of clinical and immunopathologic parameters in asthmatic children treated for concomitant chronic rhinosinusitis. *Annals of Allergy, Asthma and Immunology* 2003; 91:71–8.

60. Fairfax A, Hall I, Spelman R. A randomized, double-blind comparison of beclomethasone dipropionate extrafine aerosol and fluticasone propionate. *Annals of Allergy, Asthma and Immunology* 2001; 86:575–82.

61. Kelly HW. Pharmaceutical characteristics that influence the clinical efficacy of inhaled corticosteroids. *Annals of Allergy, Asthma and Immunology* 2003; 91:326–34.

62. Devadason SG, Huang T, Walker S, et al. Distribution of technetium-99m-labelled QVAR delivered using an Autohaler device in children. *European Respiratory Journal* 2003; 21:1007–11.

63. Homsi J, Walsh D, Nelson KA. Important drugs for cough in advanced cancer. *Supportive Care in Cancer* 2001; 9:565–74.

64. Cooper SM, Libman BS, Lazarovich M. Churg-Strauss syndrome in a group of patients receiving fluticasone for asthma. *Journal of Rheumatology* 2002; 29:2651–2.

65. Kanda N, Yasuba H, Takahashi T, et al. Prevalence of esophageal candidiasis among patients treated with inhaled fluticasone propionate. *American Journal of Gastroenterology* 2003; 98:2146–8.

66. Fukushima C, Matsuse H, Tomari S, et al. Oral candidiasis associated with inhaled corticosteroid use: comparison of fluticasone and beclomethasone. *Annals of Allergy, Asthma and Immunology* 2003; 90:646–51.

67. Gani F, Pozzi E, Crivellaro MA, et al. The role of patient training in the management of seasonal rhinitis and asthma: Clinical implications. *Allergy* 2001; 56:65–8.

68. Ducharme FM, Hicks GC. Anti-leukotriene agents compared to inhaled corticosteroids in the management of recurrent and/or chronic asthma in adults and children. *Cochrane Database of Systematic Reviews* 2002; CD002314.

69. Ducharme F, Hicks G, Kakuma R. Addition of anti-leukotriene agents to inhaled corticosteroids for chronic asthma. *Cochrane Database of Systematic Reviews* 2002; CD003133.

70. Tuggey JM, Hosker HS. Churg-Strauss syndrome associated with montelukast therapy. *Thorax* 2000; 55:805–6.

71. Wechsler ME, Finn D, Gunawardena D, et al. Churg-Strauss syndrome in patients receiving montelukast as treatment for asthma. *Chest* 2000; 117:708–13.

72. Green RL, Vayonis AG. Churg-Strauss syndrome after zafirlukast in two patients not receiving systemic steroid treatment. *The Lancet* 1999; 353:725–6.

73. Katz RS, Papernik M. Zafirlukast and Churg-Strauss syndrome. *Journal of the American Medical Association* 1998; 279:1949.

74. Finkel TH, Hunter DJ, Paisley JE, et al. Drug-induced lupus in a child after treatment with zafirlukast (Accolate). *Journal of Allergy and Clinical Immunology* 1999; 103:533–4.

75. Kroegel C, Reissig A, Hengst U, et al. Ulcerative colitis following introduction of zafirlukast and corticosteroid withdrawal in severe atopic asthma. *European Respiratory Journal* 1999; 14:243.

76. Moles JR, Primo J, Fernandez JM, et al. Acute hepatocellular injury associated with zafirlukast. *Journal of Hepatology* 2001; 35:541–2.

77. Actis GC, Morgando A, Lagget M, et al. Zafirlukast-related hepatitis: Report of a further case. *Journal of Hepatology* 2001; 35:539–41.

78. Torres M, Reddy KR. Severe liver injury. *Annals of Internal Medicine* 2001; 135:550.

79. Montelukast (singulair) for allergic rhinitis. *Medical Letter on Drugs and Therapeutics* 2003; 45:21–2.

80. *Physicians' Desk Reference.* 58th ed. Montvale, N.J.: Thomson PDR, 2004:996–7.

81. Ipratropium. *Medical Letter on Drugs and Therapeutics* 1987; 29:71–2.

82. Dukes MNG, Beeley L, eds. *Side Effects of Drugs Annual* 15. Amsterdam: Elsevier, 1991.

83. Randall T. International consensus report urges sweeping reform in asthma treatment. *Journal of the American Medical Association* 1992; 267:2153–4.

84. Pras E, Stienlauf S, Pinkhas J, et al. Urinary retention associated with ipratropium bromide. *DICP: The Annals of Pharmacotherapy* 1991; 25:939–40.

85. Humphreys DM. Acute angle closure glaucoma associated with

nebulised ipratropium bromide and salbutamol. *British Medical Journal* 1992; 304:320.

86. Shah P, Dhurjon L, Metcalfe T, et al. Acute angle closure glaucoma associated with nebulised ipratropium bromide and salbutamol. *British Medical Journal* 1992; 304:40–1.

87. AMA Department of Drugs. *AMA Drug Evaluations Annual* 1992. Chicago: American Medical Association, 1992.

88. Paul IM, Yoder KE, Crowell KR, et al. Effect of dextromethorphan, diphenhydramine, and placebo on nocturnal cough and sleep quality for coughing children and their parents. *Pediatrics* 2004; 114:e85–90.

89. Schroeder K, Fahey T. Systematic review of randomised controlled trials of over the counter cough medicines for acute cough in adults. *British Medical Journal* 2002; 324:329–31.

8

DRUGS FOR DIABETES

DIABETES PREVENTION AND TREATMENT

What Is Diabetes?

Diabetes (diabetes mellitus) is a malfunction of the body's system that regulates glucose. Normally, sweets and starches (carbohydrates) are broken down in the intestines to simple sugars, mostly glucose. Glucose then circulates in the blood and enters cells all over the body where it is either stored or burned to produce energy. Insulin is a hormone made in the pancreas and released into the bloodstream. It enables some of the body's organs to take sugar from the blood-stream and use it for energy. When there isn't enough insulin, or when cells have too few receptors that recognize insulin, sugar is not removed from the bloodstream and high levels accumulate. High blood sugar arises from a defect in insulin production or a defect in insulin action or both.

Diabetes can lead to kidney disease, damage to the retina leading to blindness, nerve damage, foot ulcers, hardening of the arteries, heart disease, and bacterial or fungal infections. Three out of four diabetics die of cardiovascular (heart and blood vessel) disease related to their diabetes, and two of those three deaths are from heart disease.

Insulin-Dependent Diabetes Mellitus (IDDM, Type-1)

A small fraction of all diabetics have IDDM and require insulin to live. With insulin, many live to an old age. Although this type of diabetes most commonly appears in childhood or adolescence, the term "juvenile-onset" is misleading. IDDM can first occur in much older patients as well. Therefore, physicians often refer to this type of diabetes in non-age-restricted terms as IDDM, or type-1 diabetes.

In type-1 diabetes, the pancreas cannot produce insulin. When diabetics eat carbohydrates, their blood sugar rises sharply. This is because without insulin, glucose moves into the cells very slowly. Therefore, while a diabetic's blood contains concentrations of sugar, the cells are not able to absorb the glucose properly. Deprived of glucose, the cells may be forced to burn fat at an abnormally fast rate, a process that in turn floods the body with substances called ketones. This can lead to a condition known as ketoacidosis. Symptoms of ketoacidosis include vomiting, weakness, stomach pain, dehydration, and very low blood pressure. Untreated, it may even lead to coma and death.

To prevent toxic levels of ketones from accumulating in the blood, a type-1 diabetic needs insulin injections daily. By adhering strictly to the American Diabetes Association's diet, a type-1 diabetic can regulate the amount and type of sugar taken into the body at various times throughout the day. The type-1 diabetic needs both insulin injections and a regimented diet to live.

Non-Insulin-Dependent Diabetes Mellitus (NIDDM, Type-2)

Of the millions of older Americans who have diabetes, 85 to 90% have type-2 diabetes. The vast majority of these people are obese, averaging about 50% over their ideal body weight. Type-2 diabetics have a hereditary tendency toward diabetes, which is magnified when they become overweight. The symptoms of adult-onset diabetes involve, at the worst, increased urination, excessive eating and drinking, and perhaps occasional dizziness. Because of the vagueness of the symptoms, type-2 diabetes can often only be diagnosed with blood tests. The many long-term complications of diabetes, especially heart attacks and strokes, make this disease the sixth leading cause of death in this country.

Like their type-1 counterparts, type-2 diabetics cannot remove sugar from the blood at a normal rate, but partly for a different reason. Type-2 diabetics can make some insulin, but not as much as can nondiabetics. But type-2 diabetics do not respond normally to insulin (this is called "insulin resistance"); they require much larger amounts of insulin than are present in nondiabetics in order to control blood glucose. This resistance to insulin appears to be hereditary. This combination of increased insulin requirements and limited insulin secretion leads to the loss of control of blood glucose.

Obesity itself causes insulin resistance. Thus, type-2 diabetics who are overweight have even higher needs for insulin than do those who are not. Weight loss is the cornerstone of treatment for type-2 diabetics who are overweight: losing the excess weight makes the body more sensitive to insulin, and the amount of insulin naturally produced will have much greater effects. Physically and psychologically, the benefits of a low-calorie diet are achieved early (often within days) when patients are still overweight.[1] This happens when their blood sugar becomes more normal.

Prevention

In a book published 30 years ago, *Off Diabetes Pills,*[2] we reviewed extensive evidence from observational studies in clinics and by physicians who, with proper attention to diet and exercise, had been able to successfully prevent or treat type-2 diabetes without the use of prescription drugs. Only more recently, in the last several years, has this approach to preventing diabetes been subjected to the rigors of randomized studies, wherein a fraction of the people are assigned to the intervention (diet and exercise) and the others to usual medical care.

Preventing Diabetes in People at High Risk

In a landmark study, published in the *New England Journal of Medicine* in 2002, 3,234 nondiabetic people with abnormally high blood sugar levels, placing them at increased risk of developing diabetes, were randomized to get either usual medical care alone (with a placebo drug), a lifestyle modification program of diet and exercise (plus a placebo drug), or a diabetes drug, metformin (GLUCOPHAGE).[3]

After an average follow-up of almost three years, the best result, by far, in preventing people from developing actual diabetes was observed in the group randomized to get the lifestyle modification program, consisting of at least a 7% weight loss (14 pounds out of 200 pounds) and at least 150 minutes of moderate physical activity (such as brisk walking) each week (an average of slightly more than 21 minutes a day). Compared to the group getting usual medical care and a placebo, people in the lifestyle intervention group were 58% less likely to develop diabetes in the 2.8-year average of the follow-up. This result was almost twice as good as was seen in the group taking the diabetes drug metformin (see p. 421), in which the reduction in developing diabetes, compared to the placebo group, was only 31%.

This important intervention was similar in men and women, in all racial and ethnic groups, and was at least as effective in older people as in those who were younger. The intervention was particularly effective, compared to most drug treatments for most diseases, in that one case of diabetes was prevented for every seven persons treated for three years.

In comments on this study, reviewers stated: "Lifestyle modification requires expertise in behavior modification and the effective mobilization of community resources to support the patient. Financial and logistical barriers may limit the implementation of an intensive lifestyle-modification in clinical practice. However, this evidence [the study discussed above] justifies efforts to remove these barriers and, on a broader scale, to promote a healthier lifestyle to control the diabetes epidemic."[4]

Lifestyle Modifications for the Treatment of Diabetes

Recent randomized studies have looked at the effectiveness of lifestyle modifications on di-

abetes control in people already diagnosed with type-2 diabetes. Unfortunately, in contrast to the prevention study described above, at the start of these studies the majority of people were already using oral diabetes drugs and/or insulin, but the important additional role of lifestyle modification in improving diabetes control could still be assessed.

In one such rural community-based study lasting for three months, all participants received basic diabetes education, but half participated in 11 weekly nutritional classes and, if exercise was safe for them, they participated in group walking exercise three times a week for one hour each time. The other half merely got the basic education but no additional dietary or exercise intervention. At the conclusion of the study, those in the lifestyle modification group had significantly lower (better) levels of glycosylated hemoglobin (also known as Hemoglobin A1c) and fasting blood sugar than the group who received only diabetes education.[5]

Treatment

There are three kinds of treatment of type-2 diabetes: diet, oral hypoglycemic pills (antidiabetes drugs taken by mouth), or insulin injections, alone or in combination. Below is a ranking of treatments from most hazardous, diabetes pills, to the safest, diet.

Diabetes pills, although the easiest therapy to follow, actually undermine the purpose of treating diabetes because they may increase your chances of dying from cardiovascular disease. The University Group Diabetes Program (UGDP) study, a study done on insulin and the antidiabetes drugs tolbutamide (a member of the sulfonylurea group of drugs) and phenformin (banned from the market—a biguanide drug and a first cousin to metformin [GLUCOPHAGE]) failed to prove that diabetes pills prevent the long-term complications of diabetes, such as heart disease, kidney disease, and blindness.[1] Moreover, it is probable that these drugs cause premature deaths from cardiovascular disease.[6]

Unlike insulin, oral hypoglycemics are only somewhat effective in lowering blood sugar. They fail to adequately control blood sugar in 20 to 40% of patients. But even if they work at first, they may fail later in as many as 30% of patients per year.[7]

After the UGDP report was released, two clinics that stopped using the sulfonylurea oral hypoglycemics found no change in blood sugar in about one-third to one-half of patients after stopping the drug, indicating that these people did not need to be on the drug in the first place.[6] The remaining patients were able to lower their blood sugar with diet alone or diet plus insulin. These results suggest that a majority of the people who take the sulfonylurea oral hypoglycemics could get along with mild dietary changes and not risk premature cardiovascular death.

Two oral hypoglycemics pose additional problems, especially for older people. Chlorpropamide (DIABINESE) may cause life-threatening, long-lasting periods of low blood sugar. It may also cause difficulty breathing, drowsiness, muscle cramps, seizures, swelling of face, hands, or ankles, and unconsciousness, water retention, or weakness that could be life-threatening to people who have congestive heart failure or cirrhosis of the liver.[8] For these reasons, the World Health Organization recommends that chlorpropamide not be used by people 60 years and older. A second drug, acetohexamide (DYMELOR) is eliminated from the body predominantly by the kidneys. Since kidney function decreases steadily with age, there is a possibility that toxic amounts of this drug may accumulate in older people.

Chlorpropamide and acetohexamide should not be used in older people **and probably should be avoided at any age.** Other diabetes pills should only be used by people whose diabetes is not controlled by diet and who cannot inject insulin. Below is an informed consent statement containing information that Public Citizen's Health Research Group believes all patients should receive and sign before they are prescribed diabetes pills.

INFORMED CONSENT FOR USE OF ORAL DIABETES DRUGS

1. I have participated in a program of dietary control and physical exercise including at least 25 hours of instruction.
2. This program did not succeed in weight reduction or control of blood sugar. Dr. _____ told me that insulin was the preferred drug if one had to be used.
3. I refuse (or am physically unable) to take insulin.

In light of the above, I agree to take

_____ (oral diabetes drug)

_____ Date

_____ Patient's signature

Insulin, like the diabetes pills, alters only the symptoms of the disease without treating the cause. In too large a dose, it may cause trembling, hunger, weakness, and irritability—symptoms of low blood sugar that can progress to insulin shock. Unlike the diabetes pills, however, insulin has not been shown to increase your chance of cardiovascular disease, **but it does carry a risk of severe hypoglycemia (low blood sugar).**

It is very important that you understand the correct use of the needle and syringe and instructions that come in the insulin package. Ask for help if you are not sure about any part of your treatment. Your doctor or the diabetes nurse-educator at your hospital can help you. Improper cleansing or injection technique may cause skin problems or infections. Tell your doctor if you are having skin problems or difficulty injecting insulin. Disposable syringes and needles are meant to be used only once. United States Pharmacopeia medical panels do not recommend reusing them. However, if you do reuse them, the syringe and needle must be used for only one person. After each use, wipe the needle with alcohol and replace the cap. These needles should definitely not be used more than a few times. Glass syringes need to be sterilized each time they are used.

Insulin should be refrigerated but not frozen. It can be kept at room temperature for a month, but it is better to keep it in the refrigerator. Do not expose it to hot temperatures or sunlight.

Insulin is available in a wide variety of preparations. Some last longer than others. Local allergy is more common with the less pure, older insulins and may be recognized by a hard, red, itching area at the injection site. **You should be using a human insulin rather than the older animal insulins.** Some people experience more serious allergic reactions (skin rash, swelling, upset stomach, difficulty breathing, and, very rarely, low blood pressure or even death).[8] Call your doctor immediately if you think you may be experiencing an allergic reaction.

Diet is the safest, most effective treatment available for the vast majority of adult-onset diabetics. More than 90% of type-2 diabetics are overweight. In many cases, blood sugar levels return to normal and symptoms go away when the diabetic loses enough weight.

Since a large proportion of diabetics can be treated by diet alone, why are so many people taking pills? There are three reasons: drug companies, doctors, and patients. When the oral hypoglycemic agents became available, they were intended to serve as substitutes for insulin in the few adult-onset diabetics who needed diet plus insulin to control their diabetes. Instead, the pills became substitutes for the diet. With the availability of oral drugs, experts stopped stressing the role of diet in controlling the disease, mostly in those very people whose diabetes could have been controlled by an appropriate diet.

Doctors find it easier to prescribe a pill than to assertively help patients lose weight. Some assume that older people will not change their diet or lose weight. Many doctors may not even suggest a trial weight-loss period, but simply begin treatment by prescribing an oral hypoglycemic pill. Patients who receive complex diet instructions from their physician and are referred to a dietitian for instructions on weighing food portions and memorizing food choices often find it easier to take a pill than to change eating habits.

However, it is foolhardy to increase the already present risk of heart and blood vessel disease for the convenience of popping a pill, when proper instruction, limited dietary changes, and a little encouragement can help you to reach optimal weight, better health, and improved control of blood sugar. Below are some suggestions for successful weight loss, guidelines for developing a healthier diet, and details of some of the common pitfalls that cause people to become discouraged and discontinue dietary therapy for diabetes.

Diets that are very complicated or very different from what you are used to are hard to follow. The American Diabetes Association (ADA) diet is a highly structured plan based on exchange lists. Although it serves its purpose of regulating calorie and sugar intake quite well, the ADA diet may be difficult for older people to use. Successful use of this diet requires considerable time spent planning meal patterns and food portions. Older people often have trouble with this diet because the food lists are long and complicated and require considerable memorization. The amount of patience and manual dexterity necessary to properly weigh and measure foods may prove difficult, especially for older people. Furthermore, rigid control, such as that provided by the ADA diet, is often not necessary in type-2 diabetics. More gradual dietary change will frequently reduce weight and lower blood sugar. See if your doctor or a dietitian can help you plan an easy-to-follow diet that will help to control your diabetes. The diet for a type-2 diabetic is based on the same nutritional principles as for a nondiabetic. Special foods ("dietetic") and imbalanced fad diets are unnecessary and sometimes dangerous. **The basic plan should be to avoid sugar and instead eat a diet high in starch and fiber.**

Many people are already eating a diet that is partly appropriate for diabetics. Only small changes may be needed. Eat fewer simple sugars. Instead of soft drinks, snack foods, and cookies, substitute sugar-free drinks, graham crackers, or bread sticks. To reduce your risk of atherosclerosis (hardening of the blood vessels), ask your doctor for a list of foods to avoid to reduce your intake of cholesterol and saturated fat. Start by cutting back meals that contain red meat (beef, pork, lamb) to three or fewer per week. These can be replaced with fish, chicken, turkey, or vegetable dishes.

A regular exercise program is recommended for people who have diabetes. Exercise helps to lower blood sugar and to reduce weight. It does not have to be strenuous; walking is often the best form of exercise. Some complications of diabetes can limit your ability to exercise. Make sure your doctor thinks you have picked a form of exercise that is safe for you.

Health Care for Diabetics

Because diabetes is such a complex disease, your overall health and your response to treatment need to be checked periodically. Schedule regular appointments with your doctor.

Most diabetics, even those treated by diet alone, should use one of the many machines currently available to test blood glucose at home at least once a day. This will let you know how well controlled your blood sugar is and will tell you if it is getting out of control. You should rotate the time of measurement (before breakfast one day, before lunch the next day, before supper the next, at bedtime the next, and then back to breakfast); this way you will know what happens to your blood sugar throughout the day. Write down your measurements and show them to your doctor at each visit (your doctor should make a copy for your medical record).

Also, at least two or three times a year your doctor should order a blood test called hemoglobin A1c or glycosylated hemoglobin. This will tell your doctor how well your blood sugar has been controlled during the previous two to three months. If this test indicates that your blood sugar has been more than just slightly elevated, your doctor should consider changes in your treatment.

Foot care is a particular problem for diabetics. Between appointments be sure to check your feet regularly for sores, infections, and ulcers. These need prompt medical attention. Use cotton socks and wear well-fitted shoes.

Diabetic eye disease is one of the major causes of blindness in our country. Schedule an appointment with an ophthalmologist (an eye doctor with an MD degree) at least every 12 months.

A number of drugs may raise blood sugar as an adverse effect. The most common are clonidine, corticosteroids, diuretics, gemfibrozil, narcotics, progesterone, and theophylline. If you are taking one of these drugs, ask your doctor whether you still need the medicine or if there is an alternative. Older people should not use chlorpropamide or acetohexamide.

DRUG PROFILES

Sulfonylureas

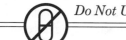 *Do Not Use*

ALTERNATIVE TREATMENT:
See Tolbutamide, Glipizide, and Tolazamide, p. 412.

Acetohexamide (a set oh *hex* a mide)
DYMELOR (Barr)

Chlorpropamide (klor *proe* pa mide)
DIABINESE (Pfizer)

FAMILY: Sulfonylureas

Acetohexamide was approved for use in the United States in 1964. This drug should not be used by people who have impaired kidney function.[9] Since many older adults do have impaired kidney function, even though they have normal kidney function tests, we do not recommend this drug for people over 60. We also strongly recommend that you do not use it because it takes a long time to be eliminated from the body and is more likely than other diabetes pills to cause serious adverse effects associated with low blood sugar.

Chlorpropamide (DIABINESE)

Chlorpropamide is a member of the sulfonylurea family of antidiabetic drugs and has been on the U.S. market since 1959.

Problems were recognized with chlorpropamide at the time of its original FDA approval in this country. *The Medical Letter on Drugs and Therapeutics,* a publication we frequently cite because it is a consistent source of objective drug information, reviewed chlorpropamide in March 1959 and concluded: "Whatever the incidence, the toxicity of Diabi-

nese is clearly much greater than that of Orinase [see p. 412] and it seems highly inadvisable to substitute Diabinese for Orinase. The convenience of taking Diabinese only once daily is hardly worth the added risk."[10]

In 1978, we raised concerns about the safety of chlorpropamide and other diabetes drugs in the book titled *Off Diabetes Pills* published by the Health Research Group.[2] We have listed chlorpropamide as a **Do Not Use** drug ever since publication of the 1988 edition of *Worst Pills, Best Pills* because it was more likely than other diabetic drugs to cause low blood sugar in the elderly. This recommendation was based on a 1985 World Health Organization publication.[11]

A new warning was added in May 2002 to the professional product labeling or package insert for chlorpropamide concerning its use in the elderly. The new warning cites increased risks of low blood sugar (hypoglycemia), low blood sodium levels (hyponatremia), or both in patients aged 65 and over. The text of the warning reads:

Geriatric Use

The safety and effectiveness of Diabinese in patients aged 65 and over has not been properly evaluated in clinical studies. Adverse event reporting suggests that elderly patients may be more prone to developing hypoglycemia and/or hyponatremia when using Diabinese. Although the underlying mechanisms are unknown, abnormal renal (kidney) function, drug interaction, and poor nutrition appear to contribute to these events.

Chlorpropamide remains on a list of drugs that are inappropriate for use in older adults because it can cause prolonged low blood sugar and is the only oral antidiabetes drug that causes an adverse effect known as the syndrome of inappropriate secretion of antidiuretic hormone (SIADH).[12]

Limited Use

Glimepiride (gli *mip* ear ride)
AMARYL (Aventis)

Glipizide (*glip* i zide)
GLUCOTROL (Pfizer)

Glyburide (*glye* byoo ride)
DIABETA (Aventis)
MICRONASE (Pharmacia & Upjohn)

Tolazamide (tole *az* a mide)
TOLINASE (Pharmacia & Upjohn)

Tolbutamide (tole *byoo* ta mide)
ORINASE (Pharmacia & Upjohn)

GENERIC: available except for Glimepiride
FAMILY: Sulfonylureas

PREGNANCY WARNING

These drugs caused fetal death in animal studies. Prolonged severe hypoglycemia (4 to 10 days) has been reported in infants born to mothers who were receiving a sulfonylurea drug at time of delivery. Many experts recommend that insulin be used during pregnancy to maintain blood glucose levels. Tell your doctor if you are pregnant or thinking of becoming pregnant before you take these drugs.

BREAST-FEEDING WARNING

Sulfonylurea drugs are excreted in animal milk and cause skeletal deformities in nursing pups. They are also excreted in human milk. Since nursing infants can also become hypoglycemic, you should not breast-feed while taking these drugs.

These drugs are taken by mouth (orally) to lower high blood sugar levels caused by NIDDM (type-2) diabetes (see p. 406). Most type-2 diabetics can control their disease by following a prescribed diet, or, if diet alone does not work, by following a diet and injecting insulin (see p. 405). The main reason to use these drugs is if diet alone fails to control your diabetes and you cannot inject insulin. These drugs, all known as sulfonylureas, work by stimulating the release

---

HEAT STRESS ALERT

This drug can affect your body's ability to adjust to heat, putting you at risk of "heat stress." If you live alone, ask a friend to check on you several times during the day. Early signs of heat stress are dizziness, lightheadedness, faintness, and slightly high temperature. Call your doctor if you have any of these signs. Drink more fluids (water, fruit and vegetable juices) than usual—even if you're not thirsty—unless your doctor has told you otherwise. Do not drink alcohol.

---

of insulin for cells in the pancreas. If you do use these drugs, it is best to use them temporarily, while losing weight, not permanently.

If you have type-2 diabetes, before taking any of these pills you should try following a prescribed diet to reduce your blood sugar levels and, if you are overweight, to lose weight. If this does not work and you need to take a drug, insulin is a better choice than any of these pills. Although taking these pills is easier and more convenient than injecting insulin, they have significant risks, including an increased risk of death from heart attacks and blood vessel disease.

If you do take a diabetes pill, you should make sure that you are taking the safest possible one. Tolbutamide is less likely than the other diabetes pills to cause low blood sugar (see Adverse Effects on p. 414) and takes less time to be eliminated from your body. It is also available in an inexpensive generic form.

If you are over 60 and you use a diabetes pill, your doctor should start you off at no more than half the usual adult dose.

Before You Use This Drug

Do not use if you have or have had recent:

- severe burns or injuries
- severe infection

RISK OF LOW BLOOD SUGAR (HYPOGLYCEMIA) WITH INDIVIDUAL SULFONYLUREAS IN OLDER PEOPLE

A study has been published assessing the risk of serious hypoglycemia in diabetics over age 65 taking one of the sulfonylurea drugs.[13] The new sulfonylurea drug glimepiride was not included in the study.

Serious hypoglycemia was more than four times more frequent in those using glyburide or chlorpropamide than in users of tolbutamine. Serious hypoglycemia occurred twice as often among users of glyburide compared to those taking glipizide. Compared to tolbutamide, those taking glipizide experienced serious hypoglycemia 2.5 times more often in the study.

Listed below are the drugs taken by diabetics in the study, from glyburide, which caused the most reactions, to tolbutamide, which caused the fewest.

FREQUENCY OF SERIOUS HYPOGLYCEMIC REACTIONS WITH SULFONYLUREAS

1. glyburide
2. chlorpropamide
3. acetohexamide
4. tolzamide
5. glipizide
6. tolbutamide

- major surgery or trauma
- high ketone levels
- acidosis
- diabetic coma or ketoacidosis
- any condition with severe changes in blood glucose levels
- any condition that causes insulin needs to change rapidly
- breast-feeding

Tell your doctor if you have or have had:

- allergies to drugs, particularly to another diabetes drug, a sulfonamide (sulfa) antibiotic, or a thiazide diuretic (water pill)
- adrenal gland disease
- kidney or liver problems
- thyroid disease
- pituitary gland disease
- recent nausea, vomiting, or high fever
- malnutrition
- severe diarrhea
- delayed stomach emptying
- intestinal obstruction
- female hormone changes
- severe infection
- severe mental stress
- heart disease and water retention (for chlorpropamide and tolbutamide)
- pregnancy

Tell your doctor about any other drugs you take, including aspirin, herbs, vitamins, and other nonprescription products.

When You Use This Drug

- Call your doctor immediately and eat or drink something with sugar in it (but low in fat) if you experience symptoms of low blood sugar (see Adverse Effects on p. 414).
- Do not stop taking your drug without talking to your doctor.
- If you have a high fever, nausea and vomiting, severe infection, or any severe injury, tell your doctor. Your treatment may have to be changed.
- Do not drink alcohol. The combination of alcohol and diabetes pills may cause abdominal cramps, nausea, vomiting, headaches, flushing, and low blood sugar.
- If you plan to have any surgery, including dental, tell your doctor that you take an oral hypoglycemic.
- Carry medical history and medication list with you for emergency situations.

• Wear medical identification

• Keep quick-acting sugar and glucagon kit and needles near you.

• Know signs of high blood sugar (see Adverse Effects, below).

• For chlorpropamide only: Someone should check on you regularly for at least three to five days after you experience symptoms of low blood sugar.

How to Use This Drug

• If you miss a dose, take it as soon as you remember, but skip it if it is almost time for the next dose. **Do not take double doses.**

• Do not share your medication with others.

• Take the drug at the same time(s) each day.

• For extended-release glipizide tablets, swallow pills whole.

• Do not store in the bathroom. Store pills at room temperature. Do not expose to heat, moisture, or strong light. Keep out of reach of children.

• Stick to regime of diet, exercise, and glucose monitoring.

Interactions with Other Drugs

The following drugs, biologics (e.g., vaccines, therapeutic antibodies), or foods are listed in *Evaluations of Drug Interactions* 2003 as causing "highly clinically significant" or "clinically significant" interactions when used together with any of the drugs in this section. In some sections with multiple drugs, the interaction may have been reported for one but not all drugs in this section, but we include the interaction because the drugs in this section are similar to one another. We have also included potentially serious interactions listed in the drug's FDA-approved professional package insert or in published medical journal articles. There may be other drugs, especially those in the families of drugs listed below, that also will react with this drug to cause severe adverse effects. Make sure to tell your doctor and pharmacist the drugs you are taking and tell them if you are taking any of these interacting drugs:

The family of drugs known as monoamine oxidase (MAO) inhibitors: deprenyl, ELDEPRYL, furazolidone, FUROXONE, isocarboxazid, MARPLAN, MATULANE, NARDIL, PARNATE, phenelzine, procarbazine, selegiline, tranylcypromine.

The beta-blockers, which include propranolol (INTERAL). A list of beta-blockers can be found on p. 87 of chapter 4, Drugs for Heart Conditions.

Other drugs that can interact are: alcohol, aspirin, ATROMID-S, charcoal, chloramphenicol, CHLOROMYCETIN, cholestyramine, cimetidine, CIPRO, ciprofloxacin, clofibrate, clopidogrel, cortisone, CORTONE, dicumarol, doxepin, ECOTRIN, ESIDRIX, gemfibrozil, GENUINE BAYER ASPIRIN, hydrochlorothiazide, HYDRODIURIL, levothyroxine, LOCHOLEST, LOPID, NORVIR, oxytetracycline, PLAVIX, PRIFTIN, QUESTRAN, rifapentine, ritonavir, sertraline, SINEQUAN, sulfamethizole, SYNTHROID, TAGAMET, TERRAMYCIN, THIOSULFIL, ZOLOFT.

Adverse Effects

Call your doctor immediately if you experience:

• **signs of low blood sugar:** anxiety, blurred vision, cold sweats or cool, pale skin, confusion, difficulty concentrating, drowsiness, increased hunger, headache, nausea, nervousness, nightmares and restless sleep, rapid heartbeat, shakiness, slurred speech, unsteady walk, abnormal tiredness or weakness, behavior change similar to drunkenness, weight gain

- **signs of high blood sugar:** blurred vision, drowsiness, dry, flushed skin, breath smells of fruit, increased urination, loss of appetite, tiredness, abnormal thirst, deep rapid breathing, dizziness, dry mouth, headache, stomachache, nausea, vomiting
- dark urine or pale stools
- itching, peeling, red skin, or rash
- yellow eyes and skin
- sore throat and fever
- unusual bleeding or bruising
- weakness or tiredness
- fainting or unconsciousness
- coma or seizures
- chest pain
- chills
- coughing up blood or increased amount of phlegm
- skin blisters
- sweating
- pale skin
- sensitivity to the sun
- difficulty breathing
- weight gain
- headache

Call your doctor if these symptoms continue:

- diarrhea
- dizziness
- drowsiness
- headache
- heartburn
- nausea, vomiting, loss or increase in appetite
- stomach pain
- skin rash
- change in sense of taste
- constipation
- increased volume and frequency of urination
- blurred vision
- increased sensitivity of skin to sunlight

Periodic Tests

Ask your doctor which of these tests should be done periodically while you are taking this drug:

- complete blood count
- blood levels of sugar and glycosylated hemoglobin
- urine levels of sugar and ketones
- chronic high blood sugar levels
- potassium and sodium serum concentrations

Insulins

Glargine (*glare* jeen) Insulin
LANTUS (Aventis)

Human Insulin
HUMULIN (Lilly)

Lispro (*lye* sproe) Insulin
HUMALOG (Lilly)

GENERIC: not available
FAMILY: Nonanimal insulins

PREGNANCY WARNING

No information is available on the effects of insulin on the developing fetus from either human or animal studies. Insulin does not cross the placenta, and it is thought that the benefits would outweigh any risk to the fetus. Tell your doctor if you are pregnant or thinking of becoming pregnant.

BREAST-FEEDING WARNING

It is likely that this drug, like many others, is excreted in human milk. Because of the potential for adverse effects of insulin on nursing infants, you should consult your physician as to the safety of breast-feeding.

The first insulin came from animal sources, the pancreases of cattle or swine. Today the majority of insulin used in the United States is produced in bacteria using DNA biotechnology. Animal-source insulin differs slightly in chemical structure from that of human insulin. Humulin, produced using DNA technology, is chemically identical to human insulin. Glargine insulin and lispro insulin, also produced by DNA technology, are modifications of human insulin and are referred to as insulin analogs.

Insulin works by regulating the amount of sugar (glucose) in the blood and the speed at which sugar moves into cells. In diabetics, instead of moving into the cells, the sugar accumulates in the blood, resulting in very high blood sugar levels. Your diet affects your cells' need for insulin and the insulin's ability to lower blood sugar when necessary. Therefore, for insulin to work, you must also follow a prescribed diet; insulin is not a replacement for such a diet.

Too much insulin may cause low blood sugar (hypoglycemia). This happens most often in people who are over 60, especially if they have reduced kidney function, and also occurs frequently in young diabetics with type-1, so-called juvenile-onset diabetes. You may be more likely to suffer hypoglycemia if you skip or delay eating meals, exercise more than usual, or drink a significant amount of alcohol.

Properly designed clinical trials have shown that strict control of blood sugar in patients with type-1 diabetes using insulin reduces the risk of the serious complications of diabetes.[14,15]

Although there is an emphasis on stricter glucose control than before, there are still concerns about the hazards of low blood sugar (hypoglycemia) if control is too strict.[16–19] Overly strict glucose control also resulted in more auto accidents for diabetics, due to sudden episodes of hypoglycemia.[17,18] Studies conflict on whether severe and frequent episodes of low blood sugar hasten decline in intellectual ability.[16,20,21] Prior objections to frequent testing centered on making people too preoccupied with being ill. Diabetic therapy must be individualized.

Human Insulin

Human insulin produced by DNA technology is formulated in a number of different forms to alter both its onset and duration of effect. These forms may also be mixed, under the instruction of your physician or diabetes educator, to better individualize blood sugar control.

Glargine Insulin

Glargine insulin is a long-acting insulin analog produced using DNA technology and approved by the FDA in April 2000.

Glargine insulin must not be diluted or mixed with any other insulin or solution.

In one clinical trial submitted to the FDA in support of glargine insulin's approval, one measure of eye damage from diabetes (retinopathy) in patients with type-2 diabetes showed a higher incidence with glargine insulin than with NPH insulin (an older form of long-acting insulin). The difference was 7.5% versus 2.5% respectively.[22]

The FDA medical officer who reviewed glargine insulin prior to its marketing approval recommended that the professional product labeling or package insert for this product say that "no claim of superiority to NPH insulin should be allowed."[23]

Lispro Insulin

Lispro insulin has a more rapid onset of action and shorter duration than human insulin. Clinical trials show that there is no difference in diabetes control according to the type of insulin used, in either type-1 or type-2 diabetes. Some cases of resistance to human insulin have been successfully treated with lispro insulin.[24] According to a meta-analysis, a type of statistical summary, of trials comparing lispro insulin with human insulin, lispro insulin does not alter the risk of hypoglycemia.[25] In practice, lispro insulin can be administered just before meals, which is an advantage over human insulin, which has to be administered 30 to 45 minutes before meals.

Before You Use This Drug

Tell your doctor if you have or have had:

- allergies to insulins
- adrenal or pituitary gland problems[19]
- eating disorders
- kidney or liver problems
- loss of consciousness
- nausea, vomiting, or diarrhea, or other stomach disorders, especially delayed stomach emptying
- severe infections
- severe injuries or surgery
- thyroid problems
- changes in female hormones
- high fever
- psychological stress
- pregnancy or are breast-feeding

Tell your doctor about any other drugs you take, including aspirin, herbs, vitamins, and other nonprescription products.

When You Use This Drug

- Know the warning signs of low blood sugar, high blood sugar, and ketoacidosis (see Adverse Effects on p. 419).
- Keep sugar on hand. Tubes or tablets of glucose, a piece of fruit, pure orange juice, cheese, soda crackers, or one or two cups of milk will suffice. Honey, sugar candy, or syrup can also be used. Carry some with you at all times. Avoid chocolate, which is high in fat.
- Monitor your blood glucose. All diabetics should be using a machine to monitor blood glucose. Be sure you receive adequate instruction.

Do not hesitate to ask or repeat questions until you feel comfortable using the device.

- Eat a diet high in complex carbohydrates and fiber, but low in saturated fats. Avoid sugar, alcohol, and smoking. Distribute your calories over several small meals, or meals and snacks, to prevent low blood sugar. While these general diet guidelines should help, older diabetics should be aware that little information is available on the effect of diets in the elderly.
- Whenever you cannot eat properly due to illness (fever, nausea, vomiting), continue your insulin, but realize your insulin requirements may change. Close medical supervision and hospitalization may be required. Also, not taking enough insulin, skipping a dose, getting less exercise, overeating, or not eating the right foods can affect insulin requirements.
- If you plan to have any surgery, including dental, tell your doctor that you are diabetic and take insulin.
- Carry identification stating your condition and the type of insulin(s) you use.
- When you travel, pack an extra supply of insulin, syringes, glucose and ketone testing materials, snacks, and a prescription. Carry your supplies with you instead of checking them.
- Exercise regularly. Inconsistent exercise risks low blood sugar on days you exert more.
- Keep your feet clean, warm, and dry. If you cannot cut your toenails yourself, find a community group that provides the service. Call your doctor if signs of infection appear.
- Wear well-fitting shoes and break them in gradually. Avoid thongs, chemical corn and callus removers, and hot soaks or pads.
- Be cautious while driving. Do not drive when your glucose levels are unstable.
- Choose nonprescription drugs and vitamins without sugar and alcohol. Lists of acceptable products are generally available from diabetes associations, your doctor, and your pharmacy. Check with your doctor if you have any doubts.

How to Use This Drug

• Select the syringe of proper units of measure for the amount of insulin you need. The syringe should be made to measure insulin in units to facilitate accurate measurement of the dose of insulin. A ³⁄₁₀ cubic centimeter syringe measures up to 30 USP (United States Pharmacopoeia) units of insulin. A ½ cubic centimeter syringe measures up to 50 USP units, and a 1 cubic centimeter syringe measures up to 100 USP units.

• If you cannot see well enough to measure the insulin, contact community agencies to find someone to predraw your insulin.

• Insulin is stable for two weeks in plastic syringes; in glass, it is stable for one week when refrigerated.[26]

• Verify the label on your insulin and examine the appearance of the insulin. Do not use regular insulin if it is cloudy or thick. Other insulins should appear uniformly milky, but not lumpy, grainy, stuck on the bottle, or unable to shake into suspension. Return questionable, unopened vials to your pharmacy.

• Wash your hands. Swab the top of the vial with alcohol.

• Except for regular (short-acting) insulin, roll the vial slowly between the palms of the hands until the insulin is uniformly mixed.

• Do not shake vigorously, or bubbles may interfere with a correct measurement of insulin.

• Draw air into the syringe equal to your insulin dose. Insert needle into the vial, then expel the air. Draw insulin into the syringe; check for air bubbles. Double-check your dose.

• If you use more than one type of insulin, always draw in the same order. Draw regular (short-acting) insulin first. Before injecting, roll the syringe to remix. Several premixed insulins are now available. Do not mix buffered insulins with lente (longer-acting) insulins. Store prefilled syringes of mixtures vertically with the needle upward to avoid plugging the needle.

• Select a site to inject insulin in the abdomen, buttocks, front thigh, or back of the arm. Stick to one area, then rotate sites within that area to prevent breakdown of fat tissue.[27] Maintain the same posture each time you inject. Avoid inflamed or infected sites.

• Clean the site before injecting. Inject needle at a 90-degree angle just under the skin (subcutaneously). Pull back on the plunger. If blood appears, try again. Inject in less than five seconds. Massaging the site after injection may speed absorption of the insulin.[28]

• Insulin comes in a variety of forms with different lengths of action. Do not change brands, strength, or type of insulin without checking with your doctor. Switches may call for a change in your insulin dose. If you use a less common form of insulin, deal with a pharmacy that promises to keep some in stock.

• Refrigeration prolongs stability and prevents contamination of insulin. According to the International Diabetes Institute, unopened insulin, properly stored, loses 5% potency in 10 years.[29] Insulin (even old-style) may be stored at room temperature. Once assembled, Novolin-Pen or PenFill must be stored at room temperature and must not be refrigerated.

Today, at home, most people with diabetes refrigerate insulin vials until opened, then store the vial being used at room temperature. Do not expose to high temperatures or sunlight. Never freeze insulin or warm it in a microwave. Once opened, vials should be discarded after several weeks.[30] Policies for storing insulin in congregate living and institutions may differ from home practices.

• Dispose of your syringes according to local waste disposal regulations.

Interactions with Other Drugs

The following drugs, biologics (e.g., vaccines, therapeutic antibodies), or foods are listed in *Evaluations of Drug Interactions* 2003 as causing "highly clinically significant" or "clinically

significant" interactions when used together with any of the drugs in this section. In some sections with multiple drugs, the interaction may have been reported for one but not all drugs in this section, but we include the interaction because the drugs in this section are similar to one another. We have also included potentially serious interactions listed in the drug's FDA-approved professional package insert or in published medical journal articles. There may be other drugs, especially those in the families of drugs listed below, that also will react with this drug to cause severe adverse effects. Make sure to tell your doctor and pharmacist the drugs you are taking and tell them if you are taking any of these interacting drugs:

alcohol, ARMOUR THYROID, ATROMID-S, clofibrate, fenugreek, guanethidine, INDERAL, INDERAL LA, ISMELIN, LEVOTHROID, levothyroxine, NARDIL, oxytetracycline, phenelzine, propranolol, SYNTHROID, TERRAMYCIN, thyroid, timolol, TIMOPTIC.

In addition, the 2003 edition of the USP's (United States Pharmacopoeia's) *Drug Information for the Health Care Professional* lists these drugs as having interaction of major significance: the family of drugs known as beta-blockers, which includes propranolol (INDERAL). A list of the beta-blockers can be found page 87 of chapter 4, Drugs for Heart Conditions.

Corticosteroids, which include drugs such as prednisone (DELTASONE, METICORTEN).

Adverse Effects

Any insulin may cause allergies in a few individuals.[31,32] Skin cleansers and preservatives in the insulin also can cause local allergic reactions.

Call your doctor immediately if you experience:

- **signs of low blood sugar:** anxiety, blurred vision, cold sweats or cool, pale skin, confusion, difficulty concentrating, drowsiness, increased hunger, headache, nausea, nervousness, numbness, nightmares and restless sleep, rapid heartbeat, shakiness, slurred speech, unsteady walk, abnormal tiredness or weakness, behavior change similar to drunkenness, seizures
- **signs of high blood sugar:** blurred vision, drowsiness, dry, flushed skin, breath smells of fruit, increased urination, loss of appetite, tiredness, abnormal thirst, deep, rapid breathing, dizziness, dry mouth, headache, stomachache, nausea, vomiting
- **allergic reactions:** itching, rapid heartbeat, shortness of breath, swelling at injection site
- out-of-control blood sugar
- weight gain
- severe vomiting
- seizures
- faintness or unconsciousness
- depressed or thickened skin at injection site
- swelling of face, fingers, feet, or ankles

Low blood sugar
- Low blood sugar can be caused by missed meals, increased exercise, consuming alcohol, changes in insulin dose, use of long-acting insulins, use of continuous infusion pumps,[18,32] and certain illnesses.[19] An increase of even one unit of insulin can cause low blood sugar.[33]
- Hunger, sweating, and trembling are signs most diabetics rely on as a warning.[34,35] However, warnings vary with the individual, and whether or not an insulin pump is used. Warning signs may change if low blood sugar occurs often.[16]
- Every instance of these symptoms does not mean you have low blood sugar. Do not rely only on warning signs, but also test your blood sugar to see if it actually is low, if time permits.[19]

• More than half of episodes of low blood sugar happen during the night.[18] Testing blood glucose at bedtime is advisable.[16] So is keeping a source of sugar by your bed. However, you may not always be aware of low blood sugar that happened during the night. Clues on waking up are:[27] morning headaches, night sweats, symptoms of hypothermia (see Glossary, p. 894).

• If you have low blood sugar often, call your doctor.

High blood sugar

• Symptoms of high blood sugar in the elderly may vary but they can include: blurred vision, drowsiness, dry, flushed skin, breath smells of fruit, increased urination, loss of appetite, tiredness, abnormal thirst, deep, rapid breathing, dizziness, dry mouth, headache, stomachache, nausea, vomiting, swelling of feet and legs.[27]

• High blood sugar is often due to severe lack of insulin or infection.

Periodic Tests

Ask your doctor which of these tests should be done periodically while you are taking this drug and how often they should be done:

- blood levels of glucose, ketones, and potassium
- blood pH
- blood pressure
- glycosylated hemoglobin
- urine ketone

Thiazolidinediones (Glitazones)

 Do Not Use

ALTERNATIVE TREATMENT:
See p. 405, Drugs for Diabetes

Pioglitazone (pye oh *gli* ta zone)
ACTOS (Takeda Chemical Industries)

Rosiglitazone (*ros* e glit a zone)
AVANDIA (GlaxoSmithKline)

FAMILY: Thiazolidinediones (glitazones)

PREGNANCY WARNING

These drugs caused harm in animal studies including embryo death and delayed development. Because of the potential for adverse effects to the fetus, these drugs should not be used during pregnancy. Many experts recommend the use of insulin during pregnancy to maintain blood glucose levels.

BREAST-FEEDING WARNING

These drugs are excreted in animal milk. It is likely that these drugs, like many others, are also excreted in human milk, and because of the potential for serious adverse effects in nursing infants, you should not take these drugs while nursing.

Rosiglitazone and pioglitazone are members of the thiazolidinedione (or glitazone) class of antidiabetic drugs, which are thought to work by increasing the body's sensitivity to insulin. The first glitazone to reach the market, troglitazone (REZULIN), was banned in the United States in March 2000 due to liver toxicity and deaths caused by use of this drug.[36]

In research conducted as part of the approval process for rosiglitazone and pioglitazone, a significant number of trial participants experienced elevations in liver enzymes, an early sign of possible liver damage. Furthermore, cases of liver failure associated with both rosiglitazone and pioglitazone have been reported in the medical literature, indicating that these drugs are capable of inflicting clinically significant damage.[37–40]

Public Citizen's Health Research Group has petitioned the FDA to change the professional product labeling or package insert of the glitazones to reflect their therapeutic inferiority to other oral antidiabetic drugs and to better explain the safety problems associated with the use of these drugs, including an increased occurrence of heart failure in people using them.[41]

Clinical trials show that patients who previously had used nonglitazone antidiabetic therapy did not respond to the glitazones as well as they did to nonglitazones. Moreover, in 9 out of the 10 head-to-head trials of glitazone versus other antidiabetic drugs, the glitazone tested was considered the inferior drug.[41]

Weight gain is a consistent finding with all the glitazones. This occurs for two reasons. First, these drugs promote the conversion of sugar to fat, and the production of new fat cells in the body.[42,43]

Second, glitazones have the property of causing fluid accumulation in the legs, ankles, and lungs.[44,45] Fluid accumulation may lead to difficult breathing and heart failure, especially in those patients with a history of cardiovascular disease. It is not known how much weight gain can be expected with long-term use of these drugs, or if the negative effects of weight gain are outbalanced by the decrease in blood sugar.

Anemia is also associated with glitazone use and appears to be more pronounced when the glitazone is used with metformin (GLUCOPHAGE), another antidiabetic drug.[42] Glitazone-induced anemia is thought to be caused by fat cells accumulating in the bone marrow, thus limiting blood cell production.[46]

The FDA professional product labeling or package inserts for these drugs are very clear that they can cause or worsen heart failure.[47,48] Unfortunately, these drugs and another antidiabetes drug that can cause or worsen heart failure, metformin (see p. 421), are being inappropriately prescribed to patients with heart failure. Researchers found that in the group

hospitalized because of heart failure during 1998 to 1999, 7.1% were discharged with a prescription for metformin and 7.2% with a prescription for a glitazone, either pioglitazone or rosiglitazone. In a similar group of 13,158 patients hospitalized between 2000 and 2001, the researchers found that prescriptions for metformin had increased to 11.2 percent and glitazone use had jumped to 16.1 percent. The differences between the two time periods were statistically significant, and similar increases were found when the data was analyzed to take into account age, race, and sex.[49]

The only role for the glitazones in the management of diabetes is their addition to the treatment of the small number of patients in whom blood sugar cannot be adequately controlled with the sulfonylureas and diet, and in whom the use of insulin is too dangerous.

███

Biguanides

Limited Use

Metformin (met *for* min)
GLUCOPHAGE (Bristol-Myers Squibb)

GENERIC: available
FAMILY: Biguanides

PREGNANCY WARNING

No valid data are available for metformin. Many experts recommend that insulin be used during pregnancy to maintain blood glucose levels. Tell your doctor if you are pregnant or thinking of becoming pregnant before you use this drug.

BREAST-FEEDING WARNING

Metformin is excreted in animal milk. It is likely that this drug, like many others, is also excreted in human milk and, because of the potential for serious adverse effects in nursing infants, you should not take this drug while nursing.

Metformin was approved for use in the United States in March 1995 but was available in some

FDA BLACK BOX WARNING

LACTIC ACIDOSIS

Lactic acidosis is a rare, but serious, metabolic complication that can occur due to metformin accumulation during treatment with GLUCOPHAGE or GLUCOPHAGE XR; when it occurs, it is fatal in approximately 50% of cases. Lactic acidosis may also occur in association with a number of pathophysiologic conditions, including diabetes mellitus, and whenever there is significant tissue hypoperfusion and hypoxemia. Lactic acidosis is characterized by elevated blood lactate levels (>5 mmol/L), decreased blood pH, electrolyte disturbances with an increased anion gap, and an increased lactate/pyruvate ratio. When metformin is implicated as the cause of lactic acidosis, metformin plasma levels >5 μg/mL are generally found.

The reported incidence of lactic acidosis in patients receiving metformin hydrochloride is very low (approximately 0.03 cases/1000 patient-years, with approximately 0.015 fatal cases/1000 patient-years). Reported cases have occurred primarily in diabetic patients with significant renal insufficiency, including both intrinsic renal disease and renal hypoperfusion, often in the setting of multiple concomitant medical/surgical problems and multiple concomitant medications. Patients with congestive heart failure requiring pharmacologic management, in particular those with unstable or acute congestive heart failure who are at risk of hypoperfusion and hypoxemia, are at increased risk of lactic acidosis. The risk of lactic acidosis increases with the degree of renal dysfunction and the patient's age. The risk of lactic acidosis may, therefore, be significantly decreased by regular monitoring of renal function in patients taking GLUCOPHAGE or GLUCOPHAGE XR and by use of the minimum effective dose of GLUCOPHAGE or GLUCOPHAGE XR. In particular, treatment of the elderly should be accompanied by careful monitoring of renal function. GLUCOPHAGE or GLUCOPHAGE XR treatment should not be initiated in patients = 80 years of age or older unless measurement of creatinine clearance demonstrates that renal function is not reduced, as these patients are more susceptible to developing lactic acidosis. In addition, GLUCOPHAGE and GLUCOPHAGE XR should be promptly withheld in the presence of any condition associated with hypoxemia, dehydration, or sepsis. Because impaired hepatic function may significantly limit the ability to clear lactate, GLUCOPHAGE and GLUCOPHAGE XR should generally be avoided in patients with clinical or laboratory evidence of hepatic disease. Patients should be cautioned against excessive alcohol intake, either acute or chronic, when taking GLUCOPHAGE or GLUCOPHAGE XR, since alcohol potentiates the effects of metformin hydrochloride on lactate metabolism. In addition, GLUCOPHAGE and GLUCOPHAGE XR should be temporarily discontinued prior to any intravascular radiocontrast study and for any surgical procedure.

The onset of lactic acidosis often is subtle, and accompanied only by nonspecific symptoms such as malaise, myalgias, respiratory distress, increasing somnolence, and nonspecific abdominal distress. There may be associated hypothermia, hypotension, and resistant bradyarrhythmias with more marked acidosis. The patient and the patient's physician must be aware of the possible importance of such symptoms and the patient should be instructed to notify the physician immediately if they occur.

GLUCOPHAGE and GLUCOPHAGE XR should be withdrawn until the situation is clarified. Serum electrolytes, ketones, blood glucose and, if indicated, blood pH, lactate levels, and even blood metformin levels may be useful. Once a patient is stabilized on any dose level of GLUCOPHAGE or GLUCOPHAGE XR, gastrointestinal symptoms, which are common during initiation of therapy, are unlikely to be drug related. Later occurrence of gastrointestinal symptoms could be due to lactic acidosis or other serious disease.

(continued on p. 423)

(FDA Black Box Warning continued from p. 422)

Levels of fasting venous plasma lactate above the upper limit of normal but less than 5 mmol/L in patients taking GLUCOPHAGE or GLUCOPHAGE XR do not necessarily indicate impending lactic acidosis and may be explainable by other mechanisms, such as poorly controlled diabetes or obesity, vigorous physical activity, or technical problems in sample handling.

Lactic acidosis should be suspected in any diabetic patient with metabolic acidosis lacking evidence of ketoacidosis (ketonuria and ketonemia). Lactic acidosis is a medical emergency that must be treated in a hospital setting. In a patient with lactic acidosis who is taking GLUCOPHAGE or GLUCOPHAGE XR, the drug should be discontinued immediately and general supportive measures promptly instituted. Because metformin hydrochloride is dialyzable (with a clearance of up to 170 mL/min under good hemodynamic conditions), prompt hemodialysis is recommended to correct the acidosis and remove the accumulated metformin. Such management often results in prompt reversal of symptoms and recovery.

European countries and Canada for 30 years before it was sold in this country. This drug is a member of the biguanide family of antidiabetes drugs, the same family as phenformin (DBI), which was withdrawn from the market in 1977 because of hundreds of deaths from lactic acidosis, a serious disease—in this case an adverse drug reaction—caused by a buildup of lactic acid in the blood. Metformin also causes lactic acidosis, though to a lesser extent than phenformin. Lactic acidosis is estimated to be fatal about 50% of the time.

Lactic acidosis remains a serious concern with metformin and is the reason that this drug is required to display a black-box warning in its professional product labeling or package insert. Metformin's black-box warning starts on p. 422. A black-box warning is the strongest type of warning that the FDA can require.

The signs of lactic acidosis are:

- feeling very weak, tired, or uncomfortable
- unusual muscle pain
- trouble breathing
- unusual or unexpected stomach discomfort
- feeling cold
- feeling dizzy or lightheaded
- suddenly developing a slow or irregular heartbeat

Metformin is approved by the FDA in addition to diet and exercise to control blood sugar in patients with type-2 diabetes.[50] In common with other oral drugs approved to treat type-2 diabetes, no claim is made in the drug's professional product labeling that it reduces the long-term consequences of this disease, simply that it lowers blood sugar.

Metformin is not to be used in individuals with congestive heart failure that is serious enough to require drug treatment. Unfortunately, metformin and two other antidiabetes drugs known as glitazones (see p. 420) that can also cause or worsen heart failure are being inappropriately prescribed to patients with heart failure. Researchers found that in a group hospitalized because of heart failure in 1998 and 1999, 7.1% were discharged with a prescription for metformin and 7.2% with a prescription for a glitazone, either pioglitazone or rosiglitazone. In a similar group of 13,158 patients hospitalized between 2000 and 2001, the researchers found that prescriptions for metformin had increased to 11.2% and glitazone use had jumped to 16.1%. The differences between the two time periods were statistically significant, and similar increases were found when the data was analyzed to take into account age, race, and sex.[49]

We initially listed metformin as a **Do Not Use** drug when it came on the U.S. market. This recommendation was modified to Limited Use with the publication of the United Kingdom Prospective Diabetes Study. This study was the largest and longest ever conducted in patients with type-2 diabetes with a median follow-up of 10 years. In overweight diabetic patients with stable blood sugar levels taking metformin to reach a target blood sugar concentration of 108 milligrams per deciliter, there was a statistically significant decrease in overall mortality, mortality linked to diabetes, and the incidence of a first clinical complication of diabetes. However, in those obese patients whose blood sugar was difficult to control, there was a statistically significant increase in the number of diabetes-related deaths in those taking older diabetes drugs plus metformin versus those being treated with an older drug alone.[51,52]

Before You Use This Drug

Do not use except in special situations if you have or have had:

- severe burns
- dehydration
- diabetic coma
- diabetic ketoacidosis
- hyperosmolar nonketotic coma
- severe infection
- major surgery
- severe trauma
- cardiorespiratory insufficiency
- cardiovascular collapse
- congestive heart failure
- heart attack
- liver disease
- lactic acidosis
- kidney disease or poor kidney function

- diagnostic or medical procedures using IV contrast media containing iodine

Tell your doctor if you have or have had:

- allergies to drugs
- pregnancy or are breast-feeding
- diarrhea
- gastroparesis
- intestinal blockage
- vomiting
- conditions causing delayed food absorption
- female hormonal changes
- high fever
- high levels of cortisol
- hyperthyroidism
- adrenal insufficiency
- pituitary insufficiency
- hypothyroidism

Tell your doctor about any other drugs you take, including aspirin, herbs, vitamins and other nonprescription drugs.

When You Use This Drug

- Call your doctor immediately and eat or drink something with sugar in it if you experience the symptoms of low blood sugar.
- Call your doctor immediately if you experience the symptoms of lactic acidosis.

How to Use This Drug

- If you miss a dose, take it as soon as you remember, but skip it if it is almost time for the next dose. **Do not take double doses.**
- Store between 59°F and 86°F in a light-resistant container, unless otherwise specified by the manufacturer.

Interactions with Other Drugs

The following drugs, biologics (e.g., vaccines, therapeutic antibodies), or foods are listed in *Evaluations of Drug Interactions* 2003 as causing "highly clinically significant" or "clinically

significant" interactions when used together with any of the drugs in this section. In some sections with multiple drugs, the interaction may have been reported for one but not all drugs in this section, but we include the interaction because the drugs in this section are similar to one another. We have also included potentially serious interactions listed in the drug's FDA-approved professional package insert or in published medical journal articles. There may be other drugs, especially those in the families of drugs listed below, that also will react with this drug to cause severe adverse effects. Make sure to tell your doctor and pharmacist the drugs you are taking and tell them if you are taking any of these interacting drugs:

Metformin should be temporarily discontinued if you are undergoing a radiologic procedure that requires the use of an intravenous contrast product containing iodine.

The thiazide diuretics, or water pills (see p. 60), interact with metformin.

Other drugs that interact with metformin are: acetophenazine, ACTH, ADDERAL, ADVIR, AEROBID, albuterol, ALUPENT, amiloride, amlodipine, ARAMINE, ARMOUR THYROID, BACTRIM, beclomethasone, BECLOVENT, benzphetamine, bepridil, bitolterol, BRONKOSOL, CALAN, CARDENE, CARDIZEM, chloral hydrate, chlorpromazine, CHOLOXIN, cimetidine, COMPAZINE, corticotropin, cortisone, cosyntropin, COTROSYN, COVERA, DECADRON, DEPO-MEDROL, desoxycorticosterone, DEXADRINE, dexamethasone, dextroamphetamine, dextrothyroxine, DIDREX, diethylpropion, digoxin, DILACOR, DILANTIN, diltiazem, DIULO, dobutamine, DOBUTREX, DOCA, dofetilide, dopamine, DYNACIRC, DYRENIUM, ephedrine, epinephrine, ETRAFON, FASTIN, felodipine, flunisolide, fluphenazine, furosemide, hydrocortisone, indapamide, INH, isoetharine, isoniazid, isoproterenol, isradipine, ISUPRIL, LANOXIN, LASIX, levothyroxine, LOZOL, MAXIR, mazindol, MEDROL, mephentermine, mesoridazine, metaproterenol, metaraminol, methamphetamine, methdilazine, methylphenidate, methylprednisolone, metolazone, MIDAMOR, midodrine, morphine, NASALIDE, nicardipine, nimodipine, NIMOTOP, nisoldipine, NOCTEC, norepinephrine, NORVASC, oral contraceptives, orlistat, PERMITIL, perphenazine, PHENERGAN, phenmetrazine, phentermine, phenylephrine, phenytoin, piperacetazine, pirbuterol, PLENDIL, PRELUDIN, PROAMATINE, procainamide, PROCANBID, prochlorperazine, promethazine, PROVENTIL, pseudoephedrine, QUIDE, QUINAGLUTE, QUINIDEX, quinidine, quinine, ranitadine, RITALIN, ritodrine, salmeterol, SANOREX, SEREVENT, SERENTIL, STELAZINE, SUDAFED, SULAR, sulfamethoxazone-trimethoprim, SYNTHROID, TACRYL, TAGAMET, TENUATE, THORAZINE, thyroid, TIAZAC, TIKOSYN, TINDAL, TORNALATE, triamterene, trifluoperazine, VANCENASE, VANCERIL, VASCOR, verapamil, WYAMINE, XENICAL, YUTOPAR, ZANTAC.

Adverse Effects

Call your doctor immediately if you experience:

- tiredness and/or weakness
- **signs of low blood sugar:** anxiety, blurred vision, cold sweats or cool, pale skin, confusion, difficulty concentrating, drowsiness, increased hunger, headache, nausea, nervousness, nightmares and restless sleep, rapid heartbeat, shakiness, slurred speech, unsteady walk, abnormal tiredness or weakness, behavior change similar to drunkenness, weight gain

- **signs of high blood sugar:** blurred vision, drowsiness, dry, flushed skin, breath smells of fruit, increased urination, loss of appetite, tiredness, abnormal thirst, deep, rapid breathing, dizziness, dry mouth, headache, stomachache, nausea, vomiting
  - lactic acidosis

Call your doctor if these symptoms continue:

- loss of appetite
- diarrhea
- upset stomach
- passing of gas
- headache
- metallic taste
- nausea
- vomiting
- weight loss

Periodic Tests

Ask your doctor which of these tests should be done periodically while you are taking this drug and how often they should be done:

- folic acid and vitamin B_{12} levels
- blood sugar levels
- glycosylated hemoglobin (hemoglobin A1c) levels
- routine blood tests
- regular physical examinations
- kidney function tests

Meglitinides

Do Not Use

ALTERNATIVE TREATMENT:
See p. 405, Drugs for Diabetes

Nateglinide (na *teg* li nide)
STARLIX (Novartis)

Repaglinide (re *pag* lin ide)
PRANDIN (Novo Nordisk)

FAMILY: Meglitinides

Repaglinide and nateglinide are the first two members of a new family of antidiabetic drugs known as meglitinides. Repaglinide was approved by the FDA in December 1997 and nateglinide in December 2000.

Both nateglinide and repaglinide work in a manner similar to the oldest class of diabetes drugs, the sulfonylureas—glipizide (GLUCOTROL) is an example—by stimulating the release of insulin from cells in the pancreas.

These two drugs are approved for use only when elevated blood sugar levels cannot be controlled satisfactorily by diet and exercise alone. The approved use of nateglinide is even more restrictive. Patients whose blood sugar has not been controlled with the older sulfonylurea class of drugs should not be switched to nateglinide, nor should nateglinide be added to their treatment. If the older drugs do not help, neither will nateglinide. Both drugs can be used in combination with metformin (GLUCOPHAGE) (see p. 421), a member of the biguanide class of antidiabetic drugs.

In considering the use of oral antidiabetic drugs, it should be recognized that blood sugar control using diet, insulin, or some older drugs in type-2 diabetes has only been shown to delay the long-term complications to the eye, nervous system, and kidney. The picture is not as clear concerning the effect of any oral antidiabetic drugs on controlling blood sugar and the cardiovascular complications of diabetes such as heart attacks and strokes, even though there is some suggestion that coronary heart disease and high blood sugar levels are linked.

The professional product labeling or package insert for nateglinide suggests that this drug is minimally effective in lowering blood sugar and another measure of diabetes control, hemoglobin A1c (HbA1c) blood levels. A study described in the package insert found a negligible effect on blood sugar and HbA1c levels even at the drug's highest recommended dose.[53] These results were statistically significant in favor of nateglinide, but as is often the case with many new drugs, the clinical effect was insignificant.

In another clinical trial summarized in nateglinide's package insert, involving patients whose blood sugar was not controlled after treatment with a sulfonylurea, the effect of nateglinide was compared with the sulfonylurea glyburide (DIABETA). Patients switched to natelinide had significant *increases* in their average blood sugar and HbA1c levels compared to those taking glyburide, thus worsening their diabetes control.

The editors of *The Medical Letter on Drugs and Therapeutics,* a source we often cite because of its reputation for providing independent drug information, reviewed nateglinide in April 2001. Their conclusion was, "Nateglinide is a short-acting hypoglycemic agent that is less convenient and less effective than a sulfonylurea and much more expensive. Its long-term safety remains to be established."[54]

The drug companies are attempting to create a "hook" to sell repaglinide and nateglinide by making it seem that despite their less convenient three times daily dosing requirements, these drugs are a novel advance in the treatment of type-2 diabetes. The spin goes like this: there is a better correlation between the risk of cardiovascular disease from diabetes and blood sugar levels after eating than there is for fasting blood sugar levels (one of the blood tests usually performed to monitor diabetes treatment). It is thus implied that targeting elevated blood sugar levels after eating reduces cardiovascular risk and this can be accomplished by meglitinides because they have a rapid onset of action and must be given three times a day.

A physician who has taken money from Novo Nordisk and Novartis played up the "benefits" of treating post-eating blood sugar levels in the the medical journal *The Lancet.*[55] She was quickly taken to task in a January 12, 2002, letter to *The Lancet*'s editor that emphasized that "no data yet support postprandial glycaemia [elevated blood sugar after eating] as a therapeutic target for cardiovascular risk reduction."[56] The letter pointed out that this is a misleading claim made by manufacturers of the meglitinide diabetes drugs.

REFERENCES

1. Meinert CL, Knatterud GL, Prout TE, et al. A study of the effects of hypoglycemic agents on vascular complications in patients with adult-onset diabetes. II. Mortality results. *Diabetes* 1970; 19(suppl):830.

2. Warner R, Wolfe SM. *Off Diabetes Pills*. Washington, D.C.: Public Citizen's Health Research Group, 1978.

3. Knowler WC, Barrett-Connor E, Fowler SE, et al. Reduction in the incidence of type 2 diabetes with lifestyle intervention or metformin. *New England Journal of Medicine* 2002; 346:393–403.

4. Montori VM. A lifestyle intervention or metformin prevented or delayed the onset of type 2 diabetes in persons at risk. *American College of Physician's Journal Club* 2002; 137:55.

5. Goldhaber-Fiebert JD, Goldhaber-Fiebert SN, Tristan ML, et al. Randomized controlled community-based nutrition and exercise intervention improves glycemia and cardiovascular risk factors in type 2 diabetic patients in rural Costa Rica. *Diabetes Care* 2003; 26:24–9.

6. Chalmers TC. Editorial: Settling the UGDP controversy. *Journal of the American Medical Association* 1975; 231:624–5.

7. Vestal RE. ed. *Drug Treatment in the Elderly*. Sydney, Australia: ADIS Health Science Press, 1984:231.

8. AMA Department of Drugs. *AMA Drug Evaluations*. 5th ed. Chicago: American Medical Association, 1983:1045.

9. Peden N, Newton RW, Feely J. Oral hypoglycaemic agents. *British Medical Journal* 1983; 286:1564–7.

10. Orinase and Diabinese. *Medical Letter on Drugs and Therapeutics* 1959; 1:17–8.

11. *Drugs for the Elderly*. 2nd ed. Copenhagen, Denmark: World Health Organization, 1997:46.

12. Fick DM, Cooper JW, Wade WE, et al. Updating the Beers criteria for potentially inappropriate medication use in older adults: Results of a US consensus panel of experts. *Archives of Internal Medicine* 2003; 163:2716–24.

13. Shorr RI, Ray WA, Daugherty JR, et al. Individual sulfonylureas and serious hypoglycemia in older people. *Journal of the American Geriatrics Society* 1996; 44:751–5.

14. Reichard P, Berglund B, Britz A, et al. Intensified conventional insulin treatment retards the microvascular complications of insulin-dependent diabetes mellitus (IDDM): The Stockholm Diabetes Intervention Study (SDIS) after 5 years. *Journal of Internal Medicine* 1991; 230:101–8.

15. The Diabetes Control and Complications Trial Research Group. The effect of intensive treatment of diabetes on the development and progression of long-term complications in insulin-dependent diabetes mellitus. *New England Journal of Medicine* 1993; 329:977–86.

16. Reichard P, Berglund A, Britz A, et al. Hypoglycaemic episodes during intensified insulin treatment: Increased frequency but no effect on cognitive function. *Journal of Internal Medicine* 1991; 229:9–16.

17. Ratner RE, Whitehouse FW. Motor vehicles, hypoglycemia, and diabetic drivers. *Diabetes Care* 1989; 12:217–22.

18. The DCCT Research Group. Epidemiology of severe hypoglycemia in the diabetes control and complications trial. *American Journal of Medicine* 1991; 90:450–9.

19. Feingold KR. Hypoglycemia—a major risk of insulin therapy. *Western Journal of Medicine* 1991; 154:469–71.

20. Kerr D, Reza M, Smith N et al. Importance of insulin in subjective, cognitive, and hormonal responses to hypoglycemia in patients with IDDM. *Diabetes* 1991; 40:1057–62.

21. Langan SJ, Deary IJ, Hepburn DA, et al. Cumulative cognitive impairment following recurrent severe hypoglycaemia in adult patients with insulin-treated diabetes mellitus. *Diabetologia* 1991; 34:337–44.

22. Insulin glargine (Lantus), a new long-acting insulin. *Medical Letter on Drugs and Therapeutics* 2001; 43:65–6.

23. Misbin, RI. Food and Drug Adminstration (FDA) Medical Officer Review of Lantus (glargine insulin), January 21, 2000.

24. Insulin lispro: New preparation. Faster acting. *Prescrire International* 1998; 7:67–8.

25. Davey P, Grainger D, MacMillan J, et al. Clinical outcomes with insulin lispro compared with human regular insulin: A meta-analysis. *Clinical Therapeutics* 1997; 19:656–74.

26. Olin BR, ed. *Facts and Comparisons*. St. Louis: J.B. Lippincott, 1992:129f–30d.

27. Gilman AG, Rall TW, Nies AS, Taylor P, eds. *The Pharmacological Basis of Therapeutics*. 8th ed. New York: Pergamon Press, 1990:1463.

28. Dunagan WC, Ridner ML, eds. *Manual of Medical Therapeutics*. St. Louis: Washington University, 1989:381.

29. Raab RS. Letter from International Diabetes Institute, May 4, 1990.

30. *American Hospital Formulary Service Drug Information*. Bethesda, Md.: American Society of Hospital Pharmacists, 1992:1883–8.

31. Balsells MC, Corcoy RM, Lleonart RB, et al. Primary allergy to human insulin in patient with gestational diabetes. *Diabetes Care* 1991; 14:423–4.

32. Dukes MNG, Beeley L, eds. *Side Effects of Drugs Annual*. 14 Amsterdam: Elsevier, 1990:372–3.

33. Gin H, Aparicio M, Potaux L, et al. Low-protein, low-phosphorus diet and tissue insulin sensitivity in insulin-dependent diabetic patients with chronic renal failure. *Nephron* 1991; 57:411–5.

34. Egger M, Smith GD, Teuscher AU, et al. Influence of human insulin on symptoms and awareness of hypoglycaemia: A randomised double blind crossover trial. *British Medical Journal* 1991; 303:622–6.

35. Muhlhauser I, Heinemann L, Fritsche E, et al. Hypoglycemic symptoms and frequency of severe hypoglycemia in patients treated with human and animal insulin preparations. *Diabetes Care* 1991; 14:745–9.

36. Gale EA. Lessons from the glitazones: A story of drug development. *The Lancet* 2001; 357:1870–5.

37. Al Salman J, Arjomand H, Kemp DG, et al. Hepatocellular injury in a patient receiving rosiglitazone: A case report. *Annals of Internal Medicine* 2000; 132:121–4.

38. Forman LM, Simmons DA, Diamond RH. Hepatic failure in a patient taking rosiglitazone. *Annals of Internal Medicine* 2000; 132:118–21.

39. May LD, Lefkowitch JH, Kram MT, et al. Mixed hepatocellular-cholestatic liver injury after pioglitazone therapy. *Annals of Internal Medicine* 2002; 136:449–52.

40. Ravinuthala RS, Nori U. Rosiglitazone toxicity. *Annals of Internal Medicine* 2000; 133:658.

41. Public Citizen's Health Research Group. Citizen's Petition to Require Class Labeling for the Diabetes Drugs Troglitazone (Rezulin), Rosiglitazone (Avandia), and Pioglitazone (Actos), March 7, 2000.

42. Food and Drug Administration Medical Officer Review of Rosiglitazone (Avandia), April 16, 1999.

43. Food and Drug Administration Medical Officer Reveiw of Pioglitazone (Actos), June 23, 1999.

44. Phillips LS, Grunberger G, Miller E, et al. Once- and twice-daily

dosing with rosiglitazone improves glycemic control in patients with type 2 diabetes. *Diabetes Care* 2001; 24:308–15.

45. Lebovitz HE, Dole JF, Patwardhan R, et al. Rosiglitazone monotherapy is effective in patients with type 2 diabetes. *Journal of Clinical Endocrinology and Metabolism* 2001; 86:280–8.

46. Gimble JM, Robinson CE, Wu X, et al. Peroxisome proliferator-activated receptor-gamma activation by thiazolidinediones induces adipogenesis in bone marrow stromal cells. *Molecular Pharmacology* 1996; 50:1087–94.

47. *Physicians' Desk Reference.* 58th ed. Montvale, N.J.: Thomson PDR, 2004:1452–6.

48. *Physicians' Desk Reference.* 58th ed. Montvale, N.J.: Thomson PDR, 2004:3186–90.

49. Masoudi FA, Wang Y, Inzucchi SE, et al. Metformin and thiazolidinedione use in Medicare patients with heart failure. *Journal of the American Medical Association* 2003; 290:81–5.

50. *Physicians' Desk Reference.* 57th ed. Montvale, N.J.: Thomson PDR, 2003:1079–85.

51. King P, Peacock I, Donnelly R. The UK prospective diabetes study (UKPDS): Clinical and therapeutic implications for type 2 diabetes. *British Journal of Clinical Pharmacology* 1999; 48:643–8.

52. Reducing long-term complications of type 2 diabetes. *Drug and Therapeutics Bulletin* 1999; 37:84–7.

53. *Physicians' Desk Reference.* 56th ed. Montvale, N.J.: Medical Economics Company, Inc., 2002:2401–4.

54. Nateglinide for type 2 diabetes. *Medical Letter on Drugs and Therapeutics* 2001; 43:29–30.

55. Dornhorst A. Insulinotropic meglitinide analogues. *The Lancet* 2001; 358:1709–16.

56. Yudkin JS. Post-load hyperglycaemia—an inappropriate therapeutic target. *Lancet* 2002; 359:166–7.

9

DIET DRUGS

NO EVIDENCE THAT DIET DRUGS WORK

The subtitle for this chapter on diet drugs could be "Clinically Trivial, Statistically Significant, and Too Often Toxic." This phrase sums up what we know about the effectiveness and safety of the diet drugs.

The FDA has set the bar too low for the approval of diet drugs. In June 1968, FDA Medical Officer Robert O. Knox, MD, refused to approve the New Drug Application (NDA) for a diet drug. This disapproval touched off a dispute between the FDA and the drug's manufacturer, A.H. Robbins, that eventually led to the drug's approval and Dr. Knox's transfer to another area within the FDA. His reason for not approving the drug: obesity is a chronic disease and there is no evidence that these drugs affect the course of the disease over the long term.[1]

The drug Dr. Knox refused to approve was fenfluramine (PONDIMIN), a drug that ultimately became the "fen" portion of the notorious "fenphen" combination of diet drugs, that was removed from the market on September 15, 1997.[2] These drugs caused heart valve damage and a potentially fatal adverse reaction of the lungs known as primary pulmonary hypertension.[3,4]

Thirty years of experience with diet drugs has clearly vindicated Dr. Knox's views. If his recommendation had been heeded in 1968, and the FDA had adopted a standard that required the demonstration of a health benefit from these drugs, the public may have had better drugs, hundreds of millions of dollars would have been saved, and an immeasurable number of patients would have been spared serious harm and even death.

Prevention may be the best treatment for obesity. Our advice about losing weight and diet pills has been the same for 20 years: Eat less, exercise more. This approach to losing weight is slow but effective. The only one who profits from it is you. That's why it isn't sold.

DRUG PROFILES

 Do Not Use

ALTERNATIVE TREATMENT:
Lifestyle changes, diet, and exercise.

Benzphetamine (benz *fet* a meen)
DIDREX (Pharmacia & Upjohn)

Diethylpropion (dye eth il *proe* pee on)
TENUATE, TENUATE DOSPAN (Aventis)

Phendimetrazine (fen dye *met* ra zeen)
BONTRIL (Amarin Pharmaceuticals)

Phentermine (*fen* ter meen)
IONAMIN (Celltech)

FAMILY: Diet Drugs

These four drugs are grouped together because of their chemical and pharmacological similarities to amphetamine, the prototype of "speed"like drugs. All four drugs carry similar information in their FDA-approved professional product labeling or package insert on the substantial toxicity and limited effect on weight of these drugs:[5–8]

- All four raise blood pressure and cause central nervous system stimulation similar to amphetamine.
- All are controlled substances; tolerance and a potential for dependence develops with their use.
- The magnitude of weight loss with these drugs compared to a placebo is only a fraction of a pound per week.
- These drugs are approved by the FDA only for a few weeks' use in combination with a regimen of weight reduction based on caloric restriction.
- None of these drugs should be used in people with arteriosclerosis, cardiovascular disease, moderate or severe high blood pressure, overactive thyroid, glaucoma, agitated states, or in those taking other central nervous system stimulants or the monoamine oxidase (MAO) inhibitor antidepressants.

Phentermine was the "phen" half of the once widely prescribed "fen-phen" diet drug combination. The "fen" portion of this combination, now banned, was fenfluramine (PONDIMIN). Fen-phen was one of the major driving forces behind the lucrative diet clinic industry of the early and mid-1990s. The economic boom for diet clinic doctors abruptly ended in September 1997 when phentermine and its close chemical cousin dexfenfluramine (REDUX) were removed from the market because of life-threatening adverse drug reactions.[2]

Phentermine was not removed from the market, but additional warnings were added to its professional product labeling about the development of heart valve damage, about a severe adverse reaction of the lungs known as primary pulmonary hypertension, and stating that the drug should be used alone only for a short period of time.

No diet drug, including these four, has ever been shown to confer a health benefit in terms of reducing the serious complications associated with long-term obesity.

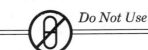

Do Not Use

ALTERNATIVE TREATMENT:
Lifestyle changes, diet, and exercise.

Orlistat (*or* li stat)
XENICAL (Roche)

FAMILY: Diet Drugs

Orlistat, like other diet drugs, is approved by the FDA for use in conjunction with a reduced-calorie diet. Also like other diet drugs, orlistat was approved without scientific evidence showing that there is a health benefit for those who use it. In other words, there is no evidence that orlistat, or any diet drug, will reduce risk of premature death or illness associated with long-term obesity and inactivity.

Unlike other obesity drugs, orlistat prevents enzymes in the gastrointestinal (GI) tract from breaking down dietary fats into smaller molecules that can be absorbed by the body; thus, absorption of fat is decreased by about 30%, leading to orlistat's most common adverse effects: oily spotting, gas with discharge, fecal urgency, fatty/oily stools, and frequent bowel movements. Because orlistat reduces the absorption of some fat-soluble vitamins and beta-carotene, patients must take a supplement that contains fat-soluble vitamins (A, D, E, and K) and beta-carotene.

In May 1997, Public Citizen's Health Research Group appeared before the FDA's advisory committee, which reviews diet drugs, to urge that orlistat not be recommended for approval unless there was evidence that it offers a health benefit by reducing the illness and death associated with obesity.[9] Because this drug has not been shown to confer a health benefit, the FDA-approved professional product labeling or package insert states: "The long-term effects of orlistat on morbidity and mortality associated with obesity have not been established."[10]

An editorial published in the January 1, 1998, *New England Journal of Medicine* sums up how little we know about the effect of weight loss and health:

> Given the enormous social pressure to lose weight, one might suppose there is clear and overwhelming evidence of the risks of obesity and the benefits of weight loss. Unfortunately, the data linking overweight and death, as well as the data showing the beneficial effects of weight loss, are limited, fragmentary, and often ambiguous. Most of the evidence is either indirect or derived from observational epidemiologic studies, many of which have serious methodologic flaws. Many studies fail to consider confounding variables, which are extremely difficult to assess and control for in this type of study. For example, mortality among obese people may be misleadingly high because overweight people are more likely to be sedentary and of low socioeconomic status. Thus, although some claim that every year 300,000 deaths in the United States are caused by obesity, that figure is by no means well established.[11]

 Do Not Use

ALTERNATIVE TREATMENT:
Lifestyle changes, diet, and exercise.

Sibutramine (si *byoo* tra mine)
MERIDIA (Abbott)

FAMILY: Diet Drugs

Sibutramine received marketing approval from the FDA in November 1997 for weight loss and weight maintenance when used with a reduced-calorie diet in those who meet the medical definition of being overweight.

The drug was evaluated at the September 1996 meeting of the FDA Endocrinologic and Metabolic Drugs Advisory Committee. This committee voted five to four against recommending approval of sibutramine on the grounds that the risks of this drug outweighed its benefits. Committee members were concerned about sibutramine's potential to raise blood pressure and increase heart rate.[12] These adverse effects could make this a dangerous drug for people with high blood pressure, heart disease, blood vessel disease, congestive heart failure, stroke, heart rhythm disturbances, and high thyroid hormone levels (hyperthyroidism).

The FDA medical officer who reviewed the drug wrote that "sibutramine has an unsatisfactory risk-benefit ratio and therefore this Reviewer recommends non-approval of the original submission."[13] The concern of both the advisory committee and the FDA medical officer was based on the fact that sibutramine significantly increases blood pressure and heart rate in many people. The FDA, against the advice of the advisory committee, deemed that sibutramine could be approved.[14]

In the April 1998 issue of *Worst Pills, Best Pills News* we listed sibutramine as a **Do Not Use** drug because of its risks and the meager amount of weight loss seen in clinical trials.

On March 19, 2002, Public Citizen's Health Research Group petitioned the FDA to immediately remove sibutramine from the market for safety reasons. Publicly available material obtained from the FDA showed that from the time it was introduced in February 1998 to September 30, 2001, there were almost 400 serious adverse reactions in patients taking sibutramine. This included 19 cardiac deaths, including 10 in people under the age of 50, three of whom were women under 30. The average yearly weight loss for patients taking the usual 10 milligram dose was only six and a half pounds more than the loss of weight in those taking a placebo.[15]

Due to a rising number of severe adverse drug reactions being reported with sibutramine, and the failure of the FDA to take action, the Health Research Group amended the original petition with new information and resubmitted it to the FDA on September 3, 2003. In the 18 months subsequent to the original petition, October 1, 2001, through March 31, 2003, there had been an additional 30 reports of cardiovascular deaths in people using sibutramine, for a total of 49 cardiovascular deaths.[16]

The FDA-approved professional product labeling or package insert for sibutramine mentions that the use of the drug is not recommended during pregnancy and that women of childbearing potential should employ adequate contraception while taking sibutramine.

An analysis of an adverse event not discussed in our original petition, fetal toxicity, was included in the resubmitted petition of September 3, 2003. Our analysis of the FDA Adverse Event Reports (AERS) database, from the original marketing of the drug through March 2003, yielded 54 reports with the term "Complications of maternal exposure" or "Maternal drugs affecting fetus" where sibutramine was listed as the primary suspect drug.

It was surprising to find so many reports, including reports on four babies with cardiovascular birth defects. These defects are: (1) bicuspid aortic valve with cardiac murmur; (2) cardiomegaly (large heart), congenital anomaly; (3) congenital heart disease; (4) ventricular hypoplasia (underdeveloped heart chamber).

In addition to the cardiovascular defects in infants, there are reports of spontaneous abortions, stillbirths, and congenital malformations, including those of the central nervous system (hydrocephalus, Chiari malformation, brain neoplasm, spina bifida).

The FDA-approved professional product information for sibutramine contains a number of important warnings: "The long-term effects of Meridia on the morbidity and mortality associated with obesity have not been established. . . . The safety and effectiveness of Meridia, as demonstrated in double-blind, placebo-controlled trials, have not been determined beyond one year at this time. . . . Meridia is contraindicated in patients taking other centrally acting appetite suppressant drugs." Sibutramine also carries the following warning in bold uppercase letters:

MERIDIA SUBSTANTIALLY INCREASES BLOOD PRESSURE IN SOME PATIENTS. REGULAR MONITORING OF BLOOD PRESSURE IS REQUIRED WHEN PRESCRIBING MERIDIA.[17]

Sibutramine inhibits the reuptake of the brain transmitter serotonin, as do the class of antidepressant drugs known as selective serotonin reuptake inhibitors (SSRIs). These antidepressants include escitalopram (LEXAPRO), fluoxetine (PROZAC), fluvoxamine (LUVOX), paroxetine (PAXIL), and sertraline (ZOLOFT). A rare but serious condition termed serotonin syndrome has been reported with the use of SSRIs, including sibutramine in combination with drugs for migraine headache treatment, such as sumatriptan (IMITREX) and dihydroergotamine (D.H.E. 45); certain opioids, such as dextromethorphan (DELSYM), meperidine (DEMEROL), pentazocine (TALWIN), and fentanyl (DURAGESIC); lithium (LITHOBID,

LITHONATE); and tryptophan. Serotonin syndrome has also been reported when two SSRIs are taken together.

Serotonin syndrome requires immediate medical attention and may include one or more of the following symptoms: excitement, restlessness, loss of consciousness, confusion, disorientation, anxiety, agitation, weakness, tremor, incoordination, shivering, sweating, vomiting, and rapid heartbeat.

Sibutramine is another in the long list of diet drugs that have never been shown they can be taken safely for a long enough period of time to reduce the morbidity and mortality associated with obesity.

REFERENCES

1. Dorsen N, Weiner N, Astin AA, et al. *Investigation of Allegations Relating to the Bureau of Drugs, Food and Drug Administration.* Department of Health, Education, and Welfare, 1977:279–344.

2. Food and Drug Administration. FDA Announces Withdrawal of Fenfluramine and Dexfenfluramine, September 15, 1997.

3. Abenhaim L, Moride Y, Brenot F, et al. Appetite-suppressant drugs and the risk of primary pulmonary hypertension. International Primary Pulmonary Hypertension Study Group. *New England Journal of Medicine* 1996; 335:609–16.

4. Connolly HM, Crary JL, McGoon MD, et al. Valvular heart disease associated with fenfluramine-phentermine. *New England Journal of Medicine* 1997; 337:581–8.

5. *Physicians' Desk Reference.* 50th ed. Montvale, N.J.: Medical Economics Company, Inc., 1996:2607–8.

6. *Physicians' Desk Reference.* 48th ed. Montvale, N.J.: Medical Economics Company, Inc., 1994:1328–9.

7. *Physicians' Desk Reference.* 57th ed. Montvale, N.J.: Thomson PDR, 2003:567.

8. *Physicians' Desk Reference.* 56th ed. Montvale, N.J.: Thomson PDR, 2002:1163–4.

9. Public Citizen's Health Research Group. Comments Before the Food and Drug Administration's Endocrinologic and Metabolic Drugs Advisory Committee on Orlistat (Xenical) for the Long Term Treatment of Obesity, May 14, 1997.

10. *Physicians' Desk Reference.* 57th ed. Montvale, N.J.: Thomson PDR, 2003:2959–63.

11. Kassirer JP, Angell M. Losing weight—an ill-fated New Year's resolution. *New England Journal of Medicine* 1998; 338:52–4.

12. U.S. FDA panel rejects Knoll's sibutramine. *SCRIP* 1996:21.

13. Coleman E. Sibutramine (Meridia). *Medical Officer Review* 1996:162.

14. Knoll Meridia "approvable": Labeling discussion on use by diabetics. *F-D-C Reports* 1996:5–7.

15. Public Citizen's Health Research Group. Petition to ban sibutramine (Meridia), March 19, 2002. Available at: http://www.citizen.org/publications/release.cfm?ID=7160. Accessed Novemver 29, 2003.

16. Public Citizen's Health Research Group. Amended petition to ban sibutramine (Meridia), September 3, 2003. Available at: http://www.citizen.org/publications/release.cfm?ID=7273. Accessed November 29, 2003.

17. *Physicians' Desk Reference.* 57th ed. Montvale, N.J.: Thomson PDR, 2003:475–80.

10

ORAL CONTRACEPTIVES

Some oral contraceptive pills (OCPs), also known as birth control pills (BCPs), can be used as emergency contraception to prevent pregnancy if taken as soon as possible after having unprotected sex. There are also some pills packaged specifically for use as emergency contraception, like PREVEN (levonorgestrel and ethinyl estradiol) and PLAN B (levonorgestrel). If you need emergency contraception, ask a doctor how to use the pill you are taking as emergency contraception, or if a medicine like PREVEN or PLAN B would be right for you.[1]

PREGNANCY PREVENTION

Birth control pills (BCPs) were hailed as women's liberators when first approved in 1960. They are currently used by over 100 million women all over the world and 10 million women in the United States as an effective method for avoiding pregnancy. When used properly without missing any pills, they prevent pregnancy over 98% of the time, though typical failure rates are about 5% per year. However, they do not protect against sexually transmitted diseases such as HIV/AIDS, and they are not safe for every woman.[2]

All birth control pills work by giving your body hormones so that it is fooled into thinking it is pregnant. There are two kinds of hormones in the pill: estrogen and progestin. Combination pills contain both estrogen and progestin. Some pills, known as minipills, have only progestin in them. They are not used as much as combination pills because they are more difficult to take properly and do not work as well. If you are breast-feeding or have had problems with the estrogen in combination pills, though, talk to your doctor about minipills.

The different combinations and strengths in combination pills all have the same efficacy, but they can have different adverse effects. There are three kinds of combination pills: monophasic, biphasic, and triphasic. Monophasic pills have one strength and color of pill, biphasic pills have two, and triphasics have three strengths and colors of pills. Almost all combinations then have one week of pills that do not have any hormone in them, called inert pills. You take the inert pills at the end of the pill pack, and that is when you get your period.

ADVERSE EFFECTS

The pill can cause many adverse effects. Some of them are merely a nuisance, while others can be life-threatening. The pill can cause headaches, bloating, nausea, irregular bleeding and spotting, breast tenderness, weight gain, or vision changes. Other more serious adverse effects that can occur from a few months to a few years after starting oral contraceptives include high blood pressure, gallbladder disease, liver tumors, depression, and metabolic disorders, such as diabetes. Temporary infertility has been associated with the period of time right after pill use is stopped. But the two most dangerous risks associated with taking birth control pills are blood clots and cancer.

Blood clots most commonly form in the veins in your legs. They can then travel to the lungs, where they can cause severe breathing problems and even death. Blood clots can also cause a heart attack or stroke. People with high blood pressure are already at higher risk for heart attacks and strokes, so the pill is probably not right for you if you have high blood pressure. Not moving for long periods of time can increase your likelihood of forming clots, so if you are going to have surgery that requires bed rest, you should talk to your doctor about stopping the pill. Clotting can also cause problems during surgery, so ask your doctor if you need to stop the pill at least four weeks before having surgery.

The estrogen in the pill was formerly the main culprit in causing blood clots, which is why the amount of estrogen in the pill has decreased so dramatically since the pill was first introduced.[3] **Make sure your pill has less than 0.05 milligrams of estradiol, and preferably less than 0.035 milligrams.**

The progestin in the newer third-generation pills can also increase your risk of blood clots (see Desogen, Mircette, and Ortho-Cept, p. 442). Combination pills all have the same kind of estrogen, called estradiol, but there are two main kinds of progestins. The third-generation progestins are desogestrel, gestodene, and norgestimate. Of these, only desogestrel is available in the United States.

The progestin drospirenone, available in Yasmin (see p. 444), presents the unacceptable risk of dangerously increasing potassium blood levels.

Smoking greatly increases your risk of developing blood clots, especially if you smoke 15 or more cigarettes a day. **If you take the pill, you should not smoke. The risk is especially high for smokers over age 35.** For most women, the risks associated with pregnancy are higher than the risk of blood clots, but for smokers over age 35 and even nonsmokers over age 40 the risks are higher from the pill. In fact, if you are over 40 and a smoker, you are four times more likely to die from taking the pill than from getting pregnant.[4]

There has been some controversy about the link between the pill and both breast and cervical cancer. Whereas the evidence for cervical cancer is now strong, for breast cancer some studies show increased risks, while others do not. Until we know more, your best bet is to examine your breasts every month (ask your doctor to show you how), have your doctor check your breasts at least once a year, get a Pap smear once a year, and use a condom to prevent sexually transmitted diseases (cervical cancer is primarily caused by a sexually transmitted virus). You should not take the pill if you have or have had a history of cancer of the breast, cervix, vagina, or endometrium (lining of the uterus).

HEALTH BENEFITS

There are also health benefits associated with oral contraceptives. The pill probably helps to prevent ectopic pregnancies (pregnancies outside of the uterus) and cancers of the ovary and the endometrium (lining of the uterus), and it can decrease cramping associated with your period.[5]

One reason women like the pill is because it is good at controlling when you get your menstrual period. For years gynecologists have recommended skipping that last week of inert pills and starting the next pack right away to change when your period comes. This is easiest and safest to do with monophasic pills, since their hormone levels do not change from week to week. A new pill, Seasonale, was approved by the FDA in September of 2003. It is an extended-cycle monophasic pill that you take for 12 weeks before getting your period during the 13th week. Since it was approved recently, there is no long-term safety data yet, but keep in mind that if you take Seasonale you are getting an extra nine weeks of estrogen and progestin and their adverse effects. Also, since you only get your period four times a year on Seasonale, if you become pregnant while on the pill it may take you longer to realize it, and no birth control pill should be taken while you are pregnant. Seasonale contains estrogen and levonorgestrel, a second-generation progestin.

Is the pill right for you? Only you and your doctor can decide that. However, the pill is *not* right for you if you smoke, have high blood pressure, diabetes, high cholesterol, liver or gallbladder problems, clotting disorders, or have ever had a heart attack, stroke, or cancer of the breast, endometrium, cervix, or vagina. If you do decide to take the pill, choose one containing a low dose of estrogen and a second-generation progestin (see p. 438), and remember also to use condoms to prevent sexually transmitted infections.

DRUG PROFILES

Second-Generation Oral Contraceptives

Levonorgestrel/Ethinyl Estradiol
(*lee* voh nor jes trel and *eth* in il es tra *dye* ole)
ALESSE 28 (Wyeth)

TRIPHASIL (Wyeth)
TRIVORA-28 (Watson)

Norethindrone/Ethinyl Estradiol
(nor eth *in* drone and *eth* in il es tra *dye* ole)
LOESTRIN FE 1/20 (Parke-Davis)
NECON 1/35 (Watson)
ORTHO-NOVUM 7/7/7 (Ortho-McNeil)

Norgestimate/Ethinyl Estradiol
(nor *jes* ti mate and *eth* in il es tra *dye* ole)
ORTHO CYCLEN (Ortho-McNeil)
ORTHO TRI-CYCLEN (Ortho-McNeil)

Norgestrel/Ethinyl Estradiol
(nor *jes* trel and *eth* in il es tra *dye* ole)
LOW-OGESTREL (Watson)
LO/OVRAL 28 (Wyeth)

GENERIC: available

FAMILY: Second Generation Oral Contraceptives

BREAST-FEEDING WARNING

Oral contraceptive steroids are excreted in breast milk and have caused adverse effects in nursing infants, including jaundice and breast enlargement. These drugs may also decrease the amount and quality of breast milk. Use another form of birth control until the infant is completely weaned.

PREGNANCY WARNING

These drugs should not be used if you are pregnant or are thinking of becoming pregnant. The risk of use of this drug in pregnant women clearly outweighs any possible benefit.

Are birth control pills the safest contraceptive option for you? There are many issues to consider, and like every other decision concerning your health, this is a highly individual one. Unfortunately, you will not be able to base your decision on assurances of absolute safety. In fact, even after over 40 years of studying the pill,

---

much about its long-term effect on human physiology is still unknown.

Although the convenience of the pill is obvious from the start, soon its acute problems may become evident. Many women suffer from headaches, bloating, nausea, irregular bleeding, breast tenderness, weight gain, or optical (visual) changes. The use of oral contraceptives is also associated with increased risk of a number of very serious conditions, including heart attack, blood clots, stroke, liver tumors, and gallbladder disease.

We have long been concerned about the pill's relationship to the risk of breast cancer.[3] The best evidence indicates that women who are currently using a combined oral contraceptive or have done so within the last 10 years are at slightly increased risk of being diagnosed with breast cancer.[6]

Oral contraceptives have been suspected of being associated with development of cervical cancer. There is now compelling evidence of this link. Women who have taken oral contraceptives for five to nine years were almost three times more likely than nonusers to develop cervical cancer. Those who used the pill for more than 10 years were four times more likely than nonusers to develop the disease.[7]

True, oral contraceptives have come a long way since the early days—the 1960s and 1970s—when women were first given hormone doses so potent that heart attacks and strokes were not unusual among pill users. With hormone levels in the pill now much lower, the number of women suffering from heart attacks and strokes also appears to have dropped.

Today's pill is clearly safer in many respects. When used properly, it prevents pregnancy more than 98 percent of the time, and its unwanted clotting properties have been significantly reduced.

Ortho Tri-Cyclen, which contains the progestin norgestimate, is included with the second-generation oral contraceptives because it is rapidly converted in the body to norgestrel.[8] Ortho Tri-Cyclen is also approved for the treatment of acne in women over age 15 who have no contraindications to oral contraceptives, who wish to use an oral contraceptive, have achieved menarche, and who are unresponsive to topical antiacne medications.[4]

Before You Use This Drug

Do not use if you have or have had:

- cancer of the breast, known or suspected
- abnormal mammogram (breast X-ray)
- cancer of the cervix or endometrium (lining of the uterus)
- unexplained vaginal bleeding
- jaundice (yellowing of the skin or eyeballs) during previous pregnancy or with prior use of birth control pills
- liver disease, including tumors or cancer of the liver
- pregnancy or are breast-feeding
- blood clots in legs, lungs, or eyes
- heart attack or stroke
- chest pain
- uncontrolled high blood pressure
- plans to have surgery requiring bed rest
- heart valve or heart rhythm disorders
- headaches with neurological symptoms
- heart disease

Tell your doctor if you have or have had:

- migraine headache
- mental depression

- diabetes
- epilepsy
- gallbladder disease
- history of irregular menstrual periods
- high blood pressure
- strong family history of breast cancer
- elevated cholesterol or triglycerides
- liver disease

Tell your doctor about any other drugs you take, including aspirin, herbs (including St. John's wort), vitamins, and nonprescription products, and whether you smoke.

When You Use This Drug

- You should receive regular checkups by your doctor at least every 6 to 12 months.
- You should examine your breasts every month (ask your doctor to show you how), and your doctor should check your breasts at least every year.
- Tell any doctor, dentist, emergency medical technician, pharmacist, or surgeon you see that you take oral contraceptives.
- Use an additional birth control method when you are using ampicillin, penicillin V, ritonavir, tetracyclines, or hepatic enzyme inducers.
- Stop medication immediately and check with your doctor if you think you may be pregnant. Contact your doctor immediately if you miss two periods.
- Call your doctor if vaginal bleeding occurs.
- Have your dentist clean your teeth regularly. Ask about any swelling, tenderness, or bleeding of gums.

How to Use This Drug

- If you miss taking a pill, follow the directions in the FDA-approved patient information leaflet that you should receive from your pharmacist each time you get a prescription for birth control pills. This information will tell you what

to do and when to use a backup method of contraception.
- Do not share your medication with others.
- Take the drug at the same time each day.
- Do not break, chew, or crush this drug.
- Your pharmacist is required to dispense an FDA-approved patient information leaflet each time you receive a prescription for an oral contraceptive. Since the many different brands of oral contraceptives vary in the number of tablets taken per month and the colors of the pills, consult this information for the drug you receive before starting to take your pills. Make sure you are receiving the FDA-approved information for the brand of birth control pills you are taking and not just the printout from the pharmacist's computer system.
- Try to keep an extra month's supply available.
- Store at room temperature. Do not store in the bathroom. Do not expose to heat, moisture, or strong light. Keep out of reach of children.

Interactions with Other Drugs

The following drugs, biologics (e.g., vaccines, therapeutic antibodies), or foods are listed in *Evaluations of Drug Interactions* 2003 as causing "highly clinically significant" or "clinically significant" interactions when used together with any of the drugs in this section. In some sections with multiple drugs, the interaction may have been reported for one but not all drugs in this section, but we include the interaction because the drugs in this section are similar to one another. We have also included potentially serious interactions listed in the drug's FDA-approved professional package insert or in published medical journal articles. There may be other drugs, especially those in the families of drugs listed below, that also will react with this drug to cause severe adverse effects. Make sure to tell your doctor and pharmacist the drugs you are taking and tell them if you are taking any of these interacting drugs:

carbamazepine, DILANTIN, EVISTA, FUL-VICIN, GRIFULVIN V, GRIS-PEG, GRIS-ACTIN, griseofulvin, LUMINAL, nelfinavir, NORVIR, phenobarbital, phenytoin, ralox-ifene, RIFADIN, rifampin, RIMACTANE, ritonavir, SOLFOTON, ST. JOHN'S WORT, TEGRETOL, TOPAMAX, topiramate, VIRACEPT.

Other antibiotics, drugs used for seizures, and drugs used for HIV/AIDS may also interact with birth control pills.

You may need to use additional forms of contraception when you take these drugs.

Adverse Effects

Call your doctor immediately if you experience:

- sharp chest pain
- crushing chest pain or heaviness
- coughing up blood
- sudden loss of coordination
- lumps in breast
- mood changes
- pain in the calf or groin
- sudden partial or complete loss of vision
- severe pain or tenderness in the stomach area
- severe and sudden headache, vomiting, dizziness, fainting
- sudden slurring of speech
- sudden shortness of breath
- weakness, or numbness in arms or legs
- yellowing of the skin or eyeballs, accompanied frequently by fever, fatigue, loss of appetite, dark-colored urine, or light brown–colored bowel movements
- changes in menstrual bleeding
- depression
- fainting, nausea, pale or sweating skin (if you have diabetes)
- increased blood pressure
- insomnia (difficulty sleeping)

- worsening migraines
- vaginal infection such as a yeast infection
- stoppage of menstrual bleeding over several months
- breakthrough bleeding
- prolonged or very light bleeding

Signs of overdose:

- irregular bleeding cycle
- nausea or vomiting
- withdrawal bleeding

If you suspect an overdose, call this number to contact your poison control center: (800) 222-1222.

Call your doctor if these symptoms continue:

- abdominal cramping or bloating
- acne
- breast pain, tenderness, or swelling
- dizziness or fainting
- swelling of ankles or feet
- unusual tiredness or weakness
- nausea or vomiting
- brown, blotchy spots on skin
- gain or loss of body or facial hair
- weight gain or loss
- increased sensitivity to the sun
- sexual interest decrease or increase

Periodic Tests

Ask your doctor which of these tests should be done periodically while you are taking this drug:

- blood pressure
- liver function tests
- Pap smear
- breast exams
- glucose (sugar), lipid (cholesterol), and lipoprotein serum levels
- FSH levels (if you are close to menopause)

Third-Generation Oral Contraceptives

 Do Not Use

ALTERNATIVE TREATMENT:
See Second Generation Oral Contraceptives, p. 438.

Desogestrel/Ethinyl Estradiol
(des oh *jes* trel and *eth* in il es tra *dye* ole)
DESOGEN (Organon)
MIRCETTE (Organon)
ORTHO-CEPT (Ortho-McNeil)

FAMILY: Third Generation Oral Contraceptives

PREGNANCY WARNING

This drug should not be used if you are pregnant or are thinking of becoming pregnant. The risk of use of this drug in pregnant women clearly outweighs any possible benefit.

FDA BLACK BOX WARNING

Cigarette smoking increases the risk of serious cardiovascular adverse effects from oral contraceptive use. This risk increases with age and with heavy smoking (15 or more cigarettes per day) and is quite marked in women over 35 years of age. Women who use oral contraceptives are strongly advised not to smoke.

A bitter scientific debate began raging in late 1995 and early 1996 when four observational studies were published showing that the risk of blood clots, or deep venous thrombosis, with third-generation oral contraceptives is two times higher than with second-generation birth control pills (see p. 438).

Combination oral contraceptives contain the hormones estrogen and progestin. These pills are commonly referred to as second or third generation based on their progestin component. Two third-generation brands are available in the United States, Ortho-Cept, produced by Ortho-McNeil Pharmaceuticals of Raritan, New Jersey, and Desogen, sold by Organon Incorporated of West Orange, New Jersey. Both drugs are exactly the same, containing 0.15 milligrams of the progestin desogestrel and 0.03 milligrams of the estrogen ethinyl estradiol. Second-generation contraceptives contain the progestins norgestrel, levonorgestrel, and norethindrone.

A worldwide study conducted by the World Health Organization (WHO) and published in late 1995 found that the third-generation oral contraceptives containing the progestins desogestrel and gestodene (this progestin is not available in the United States) were associated with an increased risk of blood clots.[9] Shortly thereafter, four more observational studies, published in rapid succession, confirmed that the risk of blood clots with the third-generation pills was two times greater than with the older second-generation contraceptives.[10–13]

In October 1995, the United Kingdom's equivalent of our Food and Drug Administration (FDA), the Committee on Safety of Medicines (CSM), warned the British public that third-generation birth control pills containing the progestins desogestrel or gestodene could double the risk of blood clots compared to older second-generation oral contraceptives containing the progestins norgestrel, levonorgestrel, or norethindrone. British doctors were told that the third-generation products should not be routinely prescribed and that women should be offered the choice to switch to the older, safer second-generation pills. The CSM decided that the increased risk—estimated at 30 cases of blood clots for every 100,000 users of third-generation pills a year, compared with 15 cases for every 100,000 women on second-generation pills a year—was sufficient to warrant an urgent alert to women and their doctors.[14]

Proponents of the third-generation pills maintained that any increase in the risks of blood clots may be offset by a reduced risk of heart attack.[15,16] The key phrase in the last sentence is "may be." The third-generation pill proponents have not been able to produce any convincing evidence that there is any difference in the risk of heart attack between women using second- or third-generation pills.

While the British authorities took the responsible step in 1995 to inform women and their doctors about the risk of blood clots with the third-generation pills, the FDA took no similar action in alerting the public. The action of the British authorities allowed "the user to be the chooser" by providing women with the information to make an informed decision about which contraceptive to use.

The professional product labeling or package insert and the patient labeling for Ortho-Cept now warn doctors and women about the risks of blood clots, but few doctors or pharmacists read the product labeling in detail, and not every woman receives the FDA-approved patient labeling from their pharmacist when Ortho-Cept is dispensed. Unlike the British authorities, who used the news media to warn doctors and women, the FDA relied on the drug's labeling as the only warning. This is the statement contained in the Ortho-Cept professional package insert: "Data from case-control and cohort studies report that oral contraceptives containing desogestrel (ORTHO-CEPT contains desogestrel) are associated with a twofold increase in the risk of venous thromboembolic disease as compared to other low-dose (containing less than 50 micrograms of estrogen) pills containing other progestins. According to these studies, this twofold risk increases the yearly occurrence of venous thromboembolic disease by about 10–15 cases per 100,000 women."

The Ortho-Cept package insert also makes reference to the unsubstantiated theory that third-generation birth control pills protect users from heart attacks. This is the statement, again directly from the Ortho-Cept package insert: "Desogestrel has minimum androgenic activity, and there is some evidence that the risk of myocardial infarction (heart attack) associated with oral contraceptives is lower when the progestogen has minimal androgenic activity."

Organon, the producer of Desogen, makes similar statements about the risks of blood clots and heart attacks in the Desogen professional package insert and the patient labeling for the drug.

To settle questions about oral contraceptives, the World Health Organization convened an international meeting of experts in Switzerland in November 1997 with the overall objective of reviewing the current scientific data on the use of oral contraceptives and the risk of heart attack, stroke, and blood clots. Regarding blood clots and heart attack, the Scientific Group concluded:

• Current users of combined oral contraceptives have a low absolute risk of venous thromboembolism, which is nonetheless three- to sixfold higher than in nonusers. The risk is probably highest in the first year of use and declines thereafter, but persists until discontinuation.

• Combined oral contraceptive preparations containing desogestrel and gestodene probably carry a small risk of venous thromboembolism beyond that attributable to combined oral contraceptives containing levonorgestrel. There are insufficient data to draw conclusions with regard to combined oral contraceptives or combined oral contraceptives containing norgestimate.

• The available data do not allow a conclusion that the risk of myocardial infarction (heart attack) in users of low-dose combined oral contraceptives is related to progestogen type. The suggestion that gestodene- or desogestrel-containing low-dose combined oral contraceptives may carry a lower risk of myocardial infarction compared with low-dose formulations

containing levonorgestrel remains to be sub-
stantiated.[17]

The risk of blood clots with combined oral contraceptives is small, but it is a real risk, and this
risk is greater with the third-generation pills
than with the second-generation oral contraceptives. There is no acceptable scientific evidence
that a woman taking third-generation pills reduces her risk of heart attack over a woman
using the second-generation products, and the
second- and third-generation pills are equally
effective in preventing pregnancy. In summary,
there is no reason why women should be using
third-generation pills when equally effective
and safer oral contraceptives are available.

Other Oral Contraceptives

 Do Not Use

ALTERNATIVE TREATMENT:
See Second Generation Oral Contraceptives, p. 438.

Drospirenone/Ethinyl Estradiol
(draw *speer* a none and *eth* in il es tra *dye* ole)
YASMIN (Berlex)

FAMILY: Other Oral Contraceptives

PREGNANCY WARNING

This drug should not be used if you are pregnant or are thinking of becoming pregnant. The risk of use of this drug in pregnant women clearly outweighs any possible benefit.

The combination birth control pill of ethinyl
estradiol with drospirenone was approved by
the FDA in April 2001. Combination birth control pills containing the hormones estrogen and
progestin are referred to as combined hormonal
oral contraceptives. In the case of Yasmin, the
estrogen is ethinyl estradiol and the progestin
is drospirenone. The difference between Yasmin
and the other birth control pills on the market is

that drospirenone has never before been marketed in the United States and is unlike other
progestins available in this country.

Drospirenone is a close chemical cousin of
spironolactone (ALDACTONE) (see p. 74), a
diuretic (water pill) that causes the body to retain potassium. Spironolactone is known as a
potassium-sparing diuretic and a 3 milligram
dose of drospirenone (the amount in a daily pill)
is equivalent to 25 milligrams of spironolactone.

Two facts form our basis for listing Yasmin as
a **Do Not Use** drug. First, drospirenone causes
elevated blood levels of potassium that may
cause serious heart and other health conditions
such as change in the acid balance of the blood
and muscle weakness. Second, there is no evidence that Yasmin is superior in any way to
older contraceptive products.

It is not known if the risk of developing blood
clots is more or less in women using Yasmin
than it is in women using the second- or third-
generation oral contraceptives (see p. 438 and
p. 442). The Netherlands Pharmacovigilance
Centre has reported five cases of blood clots that
are possibly linked to the use of Yasmin.[18]

The use of Yasmin is contraindicated (should
not be used) in women with the following conditions:

- kidney or liver problems
- adrenal disease
- disorders that lead to formation of blood
  clots or a past history of blood clots

- cerebral-vascular or coronary-artery disease
- known or suspected cancer of the breast
- cancer of the endometrium or other known or suspected estrogen-dependent cancer
- undiagnosed abnormal genital bleeding
- cholestatic jaundice (yellowing of the skin or eyes) during pregnancy or jaundice with prior pill use
- liver tumor (benign or malignant) or active liver disease
- known or suspected pregnancy
- heavy smoking (more than 15 cigarettes per day) and over age 35

A number of prescription and nonprescription drugs can contribute to increased blood levels of potassium. These include:

- nonsteroidal anti-inflammatory drugs (NSAIDs), such as ibuprofen (MOTRIN), naproxyn (ALEVE), phenylbutazone (BUTAZOLIDIN), and celecoxib (CELEBREX), when taken long-term and daily for the treatment of arthritis and other problems
- potassium-sparing diuretics, such as spironolactone (ALDACTONE), triamterene (DYRENIUM), and amiloride (MIDAMOR)
- potassium supplementation that includes the use of unregulated dietary supplements labeled as containing potassium
- angiotensin converting enzyme (ACE) inhibitors, such as captopril (CAPOTEN) and enalapril (VASOTEC)
- angiotensin receptor blockers, also known as angiotensin-II receptor antagonists, such as losartan (COZAAR) and valsartan (DIOVAN)
- heparin, an injectable anticoagulant (blood thinner) that is rarely used outside of the hospital

Yasmin's professional product labeling or package insert requires that a blood test be done during the first month of use to check the potassium level if the above-listed drugs are also being taken. This blood test is not required for any other birth control pill currently on the market.

Yasmin is required to contain the following boldface warning: YASMIN contains 3 mg of the progestin drospirenone that has antimineralocorticoid activity, including the potential for hyperkalemia [elevated blood levels of potassium] in high-risk patients, comparable to a 25 mg dose of spironolactone. YASMIN should not be used in patients with conditions that predispose to hyperkalemia (i.e. renal insufficiency, hepatic dysfunction and adrenal insufficiency). Women receiving daily, long-term treatment for chronic conditions or diseases with medications that may increase serum potassium, should have their serum potassium level checked during the first treatment cycle. Drugs that may increase serum potassium include ACE inhibitors, angiotensin-II receptor antagonists, potassium-sparing diuretics, heparin, aldosterone antagonists, and NSAIDs.[19]

Yasmin and other birth control pills may interact with the following drugs:

- Rifampin (RIMACTANE, RIFADIN), a drug used for tuberculosis. The breakdown (metabolism) of ethinyl estradiol and some progestins is increased by rifampin. A reduction in contraceptive effectiveness and an increase in menstrual irregularities have been associated with concomitant use of rifampin.
- Anticonvulsants such as phenobarbital (LUMINAL, SOLFOTON), phenytoin (DILANTIN), and carbamazepine (TEGRETOL) have been shown to increase the metabolism of ethinyl estradiol and/or some progestins, which could result in a reduction of contraceptive effectiveness.
- Antibiotics. Pregnancy while taking birth control pills has been reported when oral contraceptives were taken with antibiotics such as ampicillin (OMNIPEN, POLYCILLIN), tetracycline (ACHROMYCIN, SUMYCIN), and griseofulvin (FULVICIN, GRIFULVIN V, GRISACTIN, GRIS-PEG).

• Atorvastatin (LIPITOR), a cholesterol-lowering statin drug. Coadministration of atorvastatin and an oral contraceptive increases the absorption of the progestin norethindrone and ethinyl estradiol by approximately 30% and 20%, respectively.

• St. John's wort. Herbal supplement drugs containing St. John's wort *(Hypericum perfora-tum)* may induce liver enzymes that may reduce the effectiveness of oral contraceptives and emergency contraceptive pills. This may also result in breakthrough bleeding.

• Other. Ascorbic acid (vitamin C) and acetaminophen (TYLENOL) may increase plasma levels of some synthetic estrogens, possibly by inhibition of their metabolism.

REFERENCES

1. Westhoff C. Clinical practice: Emergency contraception. *New England Journal of Medicine* 2003; 349:1830–5.

2. Petitti DB. Clinical practice: Combination estrogen-progestin oral contraceptives. *New England Journal of Medicine* 2003; 349:1443–50.

3. Wolfe SM. *Women's Health Alert*. Reading, Mass.: Addison-Wesley, 1991:122–3.

4. *Physicians' Desk Reference*. 58th ed. Montvale, N.J.: Thomson PDR, 2004:2476–84.

5. Burkman RT. Oral contraceptives: Current status. *Clinical Obstetrics and Gynecology* 2001; 44:62–72.

6. Collaborative Group on Hormonal Factors in Breast Cancer. Breast cancer and hormonal contraceptives: Collaborative reanalysis of individual data on 53,297 women with breast cancer and 100,239 women without breast cancer from 54 epidemiological studies. *The Lancet* 1996; 347:1713–27.

7. Moreno V, Bosch FX, Munoz N, et al. Effect of oral contraceptives on risk of cervical cancer in women with human papillomavirus infection: The IARC multicentric case-control study. *The Lancet* 2002; 359:1085–92.

8. Schindler AE, Campagnoli C, Druckmann R, et al. Classification and pharmacology of progestins. *Maturitas* 2003; 46 (suppl 1):S7–16.

9. World Health Organization Collaborative Study of Cardiovascular Disease and Steroid Hormone Contraception. Venous thromboembolic disease and combined oral contraceptives: Results of international multicentre case-control study. *The Lancet* 1995; 346:1575–82.

10. World Health Organization Collaborative Study of Cardiovascular Disease and Steroid Hormone Contraception. Effect of different progestagens in low oestrogen oral contraceptives on venous thromboembolic disease. *The Lancet* 1995; 346:1582–8.

11. Jick H, Jick SS, Gurewich V, et al. Risk of idiopathic cardiovascular death and nonfatal venous thromboembolism in women using oral contraceptives with differing progestagen components. *The Lancet* 1995; 346:1589–93.

12. Bloemenkamp KW, Rosendaal FR, Helmerhorst FM, et al. Enhancement by factor V Leiden mutation of risk of deep-vein thrombosis associated with oral contraceptives containing a third-generation progestagen. *The Lancet* 1995; 346:1593–6.

13. Spitzer WO, Lewis MA, Heinemann LA, et al. Third generation oral contraceptives and risk of venous thromboembolic disorders: An international case-control study. Transnational Research Group on Oral Contraceptives and the Health of Young Women. *British Medical Journal* 1996; 312:83–8.

14. Carnall D. Controversy rages over new contraceptive data. *British Medical Journal* 1995; 311:1117–8.

15. MacRae K, Kay C. Third generation oral contraceptive pills. *British Medical Journal* 1995; 311:1112.

16. Lewis MA, Spitzer WO, Heinemann LA, et al. Third generation oral contraceptives and risk of myocardial infarction: An international case-control study. Transnational Research Group on Oral Contraceptives and the Health of Young Women. *British Medical Journal* 1996; 312:88–90.

17. WHO scientific group meeting on cardiovascular disease and steroid hormone contraceptives. *WHO Weekly Epidemiological Record* 1997; 72:357–64.

18. van Grootheest K, Vrieling T. Thromboembolism associated with the new contraceptive Yasmin. *British Medical Journal* 2003; 326:257.

19. *Physicians' Desk Reference*. 58th ed. Montvale, N.J.: Thomson PDR, 2004:924–32.

11

DRUGS FOR MIGRAINE HEADACHES

TREATING MIGRAINE HEADACHES

Clinical guidelines published by the American College of Physicians—American Society Internal Medicine in 2002 recommend the use of aspirin (see p. 304) or nonsteroidal anti-inflammatory drugs (NSAIDs) such as ibuprofen (MOTRIN) (see p. 288 for the first-line treatment for acute attacks of migraine headache, including those that are severe and that have responded to these drugs during previous attacks.[1] Acetaminophen (TYLENOL) (see p. 308) has also been shown effective in the management of acute migraine attack.[2]

For reasons of both safety and cost, the newer migraine drugs known as triptans, the main topic of this chapter, should be used only after determining that the NSAIDs and acetaminophen fail to work. The triptans can dangerously, even fatally, narrow arteries in the heart.

A number of factors have been reported that trigger the onset of a migraine attack.[1] These factors are listed on the table on this page. Try and identify these triggers and, if you can, learn to avoid them.

SOME TRIGGERS OF MIGRAINE HEADACHE

Food Triggers
alcohol
caffeine
chocolate
monosodium glutamate
nitrate-containing foods

Behavioral-Physiologic Triggers
too much or too little sleep
skipped meals
stress or poststress
menstruation
fatigue
physical activity

Environmental Triggers
loud noises
weather changes
perfumes or fumes
high altitude
exposure to glare or flickering lights

DRUG PROFILES

Serotonin Stimulators

Do Not Use Until Seven Years After Release

Almotriptan (*al* moh trip tan)
(Do Not Use Until 2008)
AXERT (Pharmacia & Upjohn)

Eletriptan (*el* eh trip tan)
(Do Not Use Until 2010)
RELPAX (Pfizer)

Frovatriptan (*fro* vah trip tan)
(Do Not Use Until 2008)
FROVA (Elan)

Limited Use

Naratriptan (*nar* a trip tan)
AMERGE (GlaxoSmithKline)

Rizatriptan (*rye* za trip tan)
MAXALT, MAXALT MLT (Merck)

Sumatriptan (*soo* ma trip tan)
IMITREX (GlaxoSmithKline)

Zolmitriptan (*zoll* ma trip tan)
ZOMIG, ZOMIG ZMT (AstraZeneca)

GENERIC: not available
FAMILY: Serotonin Stimulators (triptans)

PREGNANCY WARNING

The triptans caused harm to developing fetuses in animal studies, including malformations of bone, blood vessels and kidneys as well as fetal death. Use during pregnancy only for clear medical reasons. Tell your doctor if you are pregnant or thinking of becoming pregnant before you take these drugs.

Two pharmaceutical companies have Pregnancy Registries to monitor fetal outcomes of pregnant women who are taking these drugs:

Merck & Co., Inc: (800) 986-8999
GlaxoSmithKline: (800) 336-2176

BREAST-FEEDING WARNING

The triptans have been shown to be excreted in high levels in rat and/or human milk. Because of the potential for serious adverse effects in nursing infants, you should not take these drugs while nursing.

THE HEALTH RESEARCH GROUP'S SEVEN-YEAR RULE

You should wait at least seven years from the date of release to take any new drug unless it is one of those rare "breakthrough" drugs that offer you a documented therapeutic advantage over older proven drugs. New drugs are tested in a relatively small number of people before being released, and serious adverse effects or life-threatening drug interactions may not be detected until the new drug has been taken by hundreds of thousands of people. A number of new drugs have been withdrawn within their first seven years after release. Also, warnings about serious new adverse reactions have been added to the labeling of a number of drugs, or new drug interactions have been detected, usually within the first seven years after a drug's release.

WARNING EFFECTS ON THE HEART

The triptans have caused serious effects on the heart, some of which have been fatal. These drugs can cause the vessels of the heart to contract and should not be taken by people with heart disease, including chest pain (angina) and/or history of heart attack.

The newest family of drugs for migraines is called triptans. These drugs are used to relieve migraine headaches, with or without aura, in adults. Triptans are thought to work by narrowing swollen blood vessels in the brain that, when overdilated, cause migraine pain.

Triptans do not prevent or cure migraines, do not reduce frequency of migraines, and are not recommended for migraines described as basilar or hemiplegic. About 25% of patients do not respond to any of the triptans.[3] Triptans should only be used after determining that acetaminophen (TYLENOL), or nonsteroidal anti-inflammatory drugs (NSAIDs), such as ibuprofen (MOTRIN, ADVIL) fail to work, or cannot be taken due to allergies.

The first triptan to be approved was sumitriptan (IMITREX), first marketed in 1995. As of this writing seven triptans are available on the U.S. market. Triptans are also called serotonin stimulators. Safety, effectiveness, and adverse effects among triptans are similar. Triptan symptoms of tingling, numbness, tightness in the chest and neck, and a sensation of warmth are common adverse effects of this drug family. About 20% of patients treated with triptans experience these chest symptoms.[4] Other common adverse effects include dizziness, dry mouth, fatigue, nausea, and skeletal pain. Generally, higher doses lead to more adverse effects.[5] Long-term use may affect your eyesight. Overuse may lead to withdrawal.[6]

The main differences among triptans include how fast the drug is absorbed and how long it stays in the body. Generally, the faster a triptan is absorbed, the more quickly it may relieve the migraine, but the shorter the time it remains in the body. Rizatriptan acts quickly, but migraines may recur not long after.[5] Frovatriptan and naratriptan do not act as quickly as other triptans, but stay longer in the body, so migraines may be less apt to recur.[5]

Drug interactions may differ among triptans.[4] Only the injectable form of sumatriptan is also approved to treat cluster headaches. An advantage of sumatriptan is longer clinical experience. The amount of published information available also differs among triptans. This prompted *The Lancet,* a leading medical jour-

nal, to comment that what little information was available about frovatriptan suggested it may be less effective than other triptans.[7]

Older people who use frovatriptan may need a lower dose. Other differences among triptans include the routes of administration available. Injections and nasal sprays are more quickly absorbed. Disintegrating tablets and wafers are convenient, dissolving quickly on the tongue, but more expensive. People with phenylketonuria should not take these rapid forms of rizatriptan and zolmitriptan, as these contain aspartame.

If you have severe liver problems, do not take almotriptan, eletriptan, frovatriptan, or naratriptan.[8,9] Even if you have less severe liver problems, be cautious of taking any triptan. People who have severe kidney problems should not take naratriptan. People on dialysis should be cautious of using rizatriptan or sumatriptan. If you have moderate or mild kidney problems, your doctor may prescribe a lower dose of naratriptan.

People whose high blood pressure is not controlled should not take triptans. If your blood pressure is controlled, be aware that triptans may cause your blood pressure to rise.[10] None of the triptans are approved by the FDA for use in children under the age of 18 years.

Before You Use This Drug

Do not use if you have or have had:

- coronary artery disease, especially angina, history of a myocardial infarction (heart attack), or ischemia
- uncontrolled high blood pressure
- basilar or hemiplagic migraines
- breast-feeding

Tell your doctor if you have or have had:

- allergies to other drugs, including aspartame (NutraSweet in zolmitriptan orally disintegrating tablets), or sulfa drugs (al-

motriptan, eletriptan, naratriptan, suma-triptan)[11]
- ischemic bowel disease
- family history of heart disease
- heart problems (especially angina, coronary artery disease, fast heartbeat, ischemia, myocardial infarction [heart attack], or stroke)
- high blood pressure
- kidney problems
- liver problems
- peripheral vascular disease
- phenylketonuria (for zolmitriptan)
- pregnancy
- risk factors for heart disease: diabetes, high blood pressure, high cholesterol, overweight, smoking, past menopause, men over 40 years old

Tell your doctor about any other drugs you take, including aspirin, herbs, vitamins, and other nonprescription products.

When You Use This Drug

- Until you know how you react to this drug, do not drive or perform other activities requiring mental alertness.
- Avoid alcohol, which aggravates headaches.
- Avoid smoking.
- Avoid triggers to your migraine.
- Do not overuse pain relievers to prevent rebound headaches.
- Protect yourself from sunlight (including tanning booths) with sunscreen or protective clothing.
- Tell any doctor, dentist, emergency help, pharmacist, or surgeon you see that you take a triptan.

How to Use This Drug

- If you have risks for heart disease (such as diabetes, high blood pressure, high cholesterol, overweight, smoking, or family history of heart disease), it is advisable to take your first dose under medical supervision.[12]
- Use a triptan at onset of a migraine, with or without aura. Do not take for a headache different from your usual migraines; instead, check with your doctor.
- For regular, oral tablets, swallow dose with a glass of water. If tablets are scored, these may be cut in half. Do not crush or chew tablets. Eating food may delay relief from sumatriptan up to 30 minutes.
- For oral disintegrating tablets, use dry, clean hands to peel back the foil of blister-pack. Place tablet on the tongue, where it dissolves rapidly. Do not eat, drink, smoke, or chew tobacco while this tablet dissolves. Do not remove disintegrating tablets from blister-pack prior to time needed.
- For nasal spray, blow your nose to clear nasal passage. Hold head upright. Close one nostril with an index finger. Breathe through your mouth. Hold spray container with your other hand, using your thumb to support the bottle. Hold your other index and middle fingers on either side of the nozzle. Insert the nozzle into your open nostril about one-half inch. Tilt your head back slightly. Close your mouth while taking a breath through your nose, and press on the plunger to release your dose. Avoid contact with eyes. Remove nozzle from your nose. Hold head back for 10 to 20 seconds while breathing in through your nose and breathing out through your mouth. For large doses, you may spray some in each nostril. Clean nozzle, then recap container.
- For injection, inspect the solution to be sure it is not discolored and has no particles floating in the solution. Wash your hands. Cleanse the injection site. Inject just below the skin (subcutaneously), in the upper thigh or outer upper arm. Do not inject into veins or muscles. An auto-injector syringe is available, which penetrates one-fourth inch below the skin. Be sure to select a site that accommodates this depth.

• After taking your prescribed dose, lie down in a quiet, dark space if possible. Ice packs or massage on your forehead or temples may help alleviate pain. If you get no relief, do not take another dose. Call your doctor.

• If you get partial relief, or symptoms return after two hours, you may repeat an additional dose. For frovatriptan and rizatriptan, you may take a third dose if you have inadequate relief from the second dose after another two hours. Do not exceed a total of 30 milligrams of rizatriptan within 24 hours. If you also take propranolol, do not take more than 15 milligrams of rizatriptan within 24 hours. For zolmitriptan you may take doses at two hour intervals as long as you do not exceed a total of 10 milligrams within 24 hours. Do not exceed more than 200 milligrams of oral sumatriptan within 24 hours. Do not inject more than 12 milligrams of sumatriptan injection within one or two days.

• **Do not take double doses** of any triptan.

• Have your blood pressure checked.

• Generally, if you have more than three migraine headaches within 30 days, avoid using a triptan for additional headaches. For almotriptan, frovatriptan, naratriptan, rizatriptan, or sumatriptan, you may use for up to four migraines within 30 days.

• Store tablets at controlled room temperature, out of the reach of children. Protect from heat, light, and moisture. Protect injection and nasal spray from light and freezing.

Interactions with Other Drugs

The following drugs, biologics (e.g., vaccines, therapeutic antibodies), or foods are listed in *Evaluations of Drug Interactions* 2003 as causing "highly clinically significant" or "clinically significant" interactions when used together with any of the drugs in this section. In some sections with multiple drugs, the interaction may have been reported for one but not all drugs in this section, but we include the inter-

action because the drugs in this section are similar to one another. We have also included potentially serious interactions listed in the drug's FDA-approved professional package insert or in published medical journal articles. There may be other drugs, especially those in the families of drugs listed below, that also will react with this drug to cause severe adverse effects. Make sure to tell your doctor and pharmacist the drugs you are taking and tell them if you are taking any of these interacting drugs:

Do not take these monoamine oxidase (MAO) inhibitors within 14 days of taking a triptan: ELDEPRYL, furazolidone, FUROXONE, isocarboxazid, MARPLAN, MATULANE, moclobemide, NARDIL, PARNATE, phenelzine, PROCARBAZINE, selegiline, tranylcypromine.

Do not take these drugs within 72 hours of almotriptan or eletriptan: BIAXIN, CALAN, clarithromycin, fluconazole, ISOPTIN, ketoconazole, nefazodone, nelfinavir, NIZORAL, NORVIR, ritonavir, SPORANOX, TAO, troleandomycin, verapamil, VIRACEPT.

Do not take any other triptan within 24 hours of the first triptan you use.

Also, do not take these drugs within 24 hours of taking a triptan: BELLERGAL-S, bromcriptine, cabergoline, CAFERFOT, CAFERGOT-PB, DHE-45, dihydroergotamine, DOSTINEX, ERGOMAR, ergonovine, ERGOSTAT, ergotamine, HYDERGINE, methylergonovine, methylsergide, pergolide, PERMAX, SANSERT, WIGRAINE.

The combination of a triptan with these drugs could cause incoordination, increase in reflexes, weakness, a serotonin syndrome, or other complications. Signs of serotonin syndrome include altered consciousness, irritability of the nervous system, shivering, and weakness. Avoid these drugs: CELEXA, citalopram, fluvoxamine, fluoxetine,

LUVOX, MELLARIL (with sumatriptan), MERIDIA, paroxetine, PAXIL, PROZAC, sertraline, sibutramine, thioridazine, ZOLOFT.

If you take this drug while on a triptan, your doctor may adjust your doses or prescribe alternative drugs:[3] cimetidine, INDERAL, oral contraceptives (for frovatriptan), propranolol, TAGAMET.

Doses of zolmitriptan should not exceed 5 milligrams per day if you take cimetidine (TAGAMET).[11]

Adverse Effects

Call your doctor immediately if you experience (for all):

- blood pressure increase or decrease
- difficult, fast, or irregular breathing, or wheezing
- severe chest pain
- heaviness, tightness, or pressure in chest, throat, and/or neck
- sensation of burning, warmth, or heat
- sensation of numbness, tightness, or tingling
- irregular or slow heartbeat

In addition, for zolmotriptan:

- severe abdominal pain, diarrhea
- loss of appetite
- nausea
- fever or chills
- cough or hoarseness
- lower back or side pain
- painful or difficult urination

In addition, for sumatriptan:

- changes in facial skin color, skin rash, hives, itching
- swelling of eyes, face, or lips
- seizures
- difficulty swallowing

In addition, for almotriptan:

- discharge from eye, redness of inner lining of eyelid
- shortness of breath
- tightness in the throat
- skin rash
- difficulty swallowing
- heartburn
- eye pain
- fever
- abdominal pain
- irregular or rapid heartbeat
- rapid breathing
- diarrhea, nausea, vomiting
- loss of vision
- fainting
- earache

Signs of overdose:

- slow heartbeat
- dizziness
- severe and continuing headache
- sleepiness
- fainting
- vomiting
- arms or legs appear red
- blood pressure increases
- tension in neck
- chest pain
- difficult breathing
- subdued or withdrawn behavior
- seizures
- problems with muscle control or coordination
- lightheadedness
- paralysis
- skin appears blue-gray
- skin sheds at site of injection
- tension in neck
- tremors.

If you suspect an overdose, call this number to contact your poison control center: (800) 222-1222.

Call your doctor if these symptoms continue:

- agitation
- anxiety
- unusual tiredness or muscle weakness
- depression
- bleeding from ear, eye, nose, or throat
- clumsiness
- confusion
- constipation
- coughing up mucus
- depression
- discomfort in jaw, mouth, tongue, throat, nasal passages, or sinuses
- dizziness or lightheadedness
- drowsiness
- dry mouth
- buzzing or ringing in ears, hearing loss, or intense sense of hearing
- dry or painful eyes
- facial flushing
- fainting
- hallucinations
- shaking or trembling hands or feet
- headaches other than migraine or aggravation of migraine
- indigestion, heartburn, belching
- irritation at injection site (for those triptans that are injected)
- nasal irritation (for those triptans that are nasal sprays) or discharge
- difficulty swallowing
- painful menstruation
- mood changes
- muscle or joint aches, cramps, pain, spasms, stiffness, or weakness
- nausea or vomiting
- nervousness
- pain in bone or joints
- restlessness, feelings of constant movement
- increase in saliva
- change in sense of smell
- increased sensitivity to light and noise, decreased sensitivity to touch

- burning, painful, or red skin at site of injection
- skin rash, itching
- sleeping problems
- sneezing
- sore throat
- sunburn
- profuse sweating
- swelling of face, fingers, feet, or lower legs
- change in sense of taste
- difficulty talking
- increased thirst
- sudden increase in frequency and quantity of urination
- blurred, doubled, or otherwise changed vision

Periodic Tests

Ask your doctor which of these tests should be done periodically while you are taking this drug:

- electrocardiogram (ECG or EKG)
- blood pressure
- cholesterol
- creatine
- gamma glutamyl transpeptidase (GGT)
- glucose

Other Drugs for
Migraine Headaches

Do Not Use

ALTERNATIVE TREATMENT:
See Aspirin, p. 279, Acetaminophen, p. 308,
or Nonsteroidal Anti-inflammatory Drugs (NSAIDs)
such as Ibuprofen, p. 288.

Isometheptene, Dichloralphenazone, and Acetaminophen (eye soe meth *ep* teen, dye klor al *fen* a zone, and a seat a *min* oh fen)
MIDRIN (Women First Healthcare)

FAMILY: Migraine Headache Drugs
          Nonnarcotic Painkillers

This old three-drug combination of isomethep-tene, dichloralphenazone, and acetaminophen was approved by the FDA before 1962, when amendments to the Food, Drug, and Cosmetic Act were passed that required manufacturers to show "substantial evidence" that their products would do what they claimed. In other words, that their drugs were effective.

The 1962 law required the FDA to review the effectiveness for all prescription drugs approved for marketing between 1938, when safety first became a standard for marketing, and 1962. The FDA entered into a contract with the National Academy of Sciences–National Research Council (NAS-NRC) in 1966 to fulfill its legal requirement. Drug companies were asked to submit data to the NAS-NRC to support their claims of effectiveness.[14] This process was known as the Drug Efficacy Study Implementation (DESI) program.

The FDA was supposed to begin marketing withdrawal procedures if substantial evidence of effectiveness was not presented. Unfortunately, the FDA failed to do its job, and 38 years after the DESI program began, numerous, less-than-effective drugs remain on the market today. The combination of isometheptene, dichloralphenazone, and acetaminophen is one of them.

The FDA-approved professional product labeling or package insert for the drug is required to display the following cryptic statement, in a box:[15]

> Based on a review of this drug (isometheptene mucate) by the National Academy of Sciences–National Research Council and/or other information, FDA has classified the other indication as "possibly" effective in the treatment of migraine headache. Final classification to the less-than-effective indication requires further investigation.

The NAS-NRC translation of "possibly" effective is that substantial research is needed to substantiate effectiveness. According to one former NAS-NRC scientific panelist, "this designation means that in the best judgment of the panel members, if appropriate controlled studies were to be done, the result would be negative."

In August 2001, the Drug Enforcement Administration reclassified Midrin as a controlled substance because the ingredient dichloralphenazone breaks down to chloral hydrate (NOCTEC), a very old sleeping medication that is a controlled substance.[16]

REFERENCES

1. Snow V, Weiss K, Wall EM, et al. Pharmacologic management of acute attacks of migraine and prevention of migraine headache. *Annals of Internal Medicine* 2002; 137:840–9.

2. Lipton RB, Baggish JS, Stewart WF, et al. Efficacy and safety of acetaminophen in the treatment of migraine: Results of a randomized, double-blind, placebo-controlled, population-based study. *Archives of Internal Medicine* 2000; 160:3486–92.

3. Deleu D, Hanssens Y. Current and emerging second-generation triptans in acute migraine therapy: A comparative review. *Journal of Clinical Pharmacology* 2000; 40:687–700.

4. Nappi G, Sandrini G, Sances G. Tolerability of the triptans: Clinical implications. *Drug Safety* 2003; 26:93–107.

5. Jhee SS, Shiovitz T, Crawford AW, et al. Pharmacokinetics and pharmacodynamics of the triptan antimigraine agents: A comparative review. *Clinical Pharmacokinetics* 2001; 40:189–205.

6. Katsarava Z, Fritsche G, Muessig M, et al. Clinical features of withdrawal headache following overuse of triptans and other headache drugs. *Neurology* 2001; 40:189–205.

7. Ferrari MD, Roon KI, Lipton RB, et al. Oral triptans (serotonin 5-HT(1B/1D) agonists) in acute migraine treatment: A meta-analysis of 53 trials. *The Lancet* 2001; 358:1668–75.

8. Keam SJ, Goa KL, Figgitt DP. Almotriptan: A review of its use in migraine. *Drugs* 2002; 62:387–414.

9. *Physicians' Desk Reference.* 58th ed. Montvale, N.J.: Thomson PDR, 2004:2626–30.

10. Fleishaker JC, McEnroe JD, Azie NE, et al. Cardiovascular effect of almotriptan in treated hypertensive patients. *Clinical Pharmacology and Therapeutics* 2002; 71:169–75.

11. Gawel MJ, Worthington I, Maggisano A. A systematic review of the use of triptans in acute migraine. *Canadian Journal of Neurological Sciences* 2001; 28:30–41.

12. Tepper SJ. Safety and rational use of the triptans. *Medical Clinics of North America* 2001; 85:959–70.

13. Goldberg MR, Sciberras D, De Smet M, et al. Influence of beta-adrenoceptor antagonists on the pharmacokinetics of rizatriptan, a 5-HT1B/1D agonist: Differential effects of propranolol, nadolol and metoprolol. *British Journal of Clinical Pharmacology* 2001; 52:69–76.

14. Wofle SM, Coley CM. *Pills That Don't Work.* N.Y.: Farrar Straus Giroux, 1981.193–8.

15. *Physicians' Desk Reference.* 58th ed. Montvale, N.J.: Thomson PDR, 2004:3396.

16. Drug Enforcement Administration. Schedule of Controlled Substances: Placement of Dichloalphenazone into Schedule IV. *Federal Register* 2001; 66:42943–4.

12

THYROID REPLACEMENT DRUGS

THYROID HORMONE

Thyroid hormone is naturally produced by the body. This hormone affects all organ systems principally by increasing the production of energy and heat, especially in tissues such as skeletal muscle, the heart, the kidneys, and the liver. Equally important, thyroid hormone increases the synthesis of proteins in all body tissues. Thyroid hormone is thus essential for growth and development. A normal thyroid state is called euthyroid. During severe illness, such as infection or a heart attack, people who are euthyroid may develop temporary changes in thyroid function.[1,2]

The production of too much thyroid hormone is referred to as hyperthyroidism or thyrotoxicosis. This condition occurs in Grave's disease and during the early stages of thyroiditis (inflammation of the thyroid gland). Hyperthyroidism can also be caused by too high a dose of thyroid hormone replacement products. Common symptoms of hyperthyroidism are warm, moist skin, raised temperature, and rapid heart rate. Untreated, excess thyroid hormone production can lead to heart problems and osteoporosis.

Too little, or a lack of thyroid hormone, is called hypothyroidism. Hypothyroidism can result from the later stages of thyroiditis, from thyroid cancer, thyroid surgery, radioactive iodine, or treatment for hyperthyroidism. Thyroid dysfunction is common in alcoholism.[3] As many as 10% of older women have subclinical hypothyroidism.[4,5] Symptoms of hypothyroidism include low energy, slow heartbeat, weight gain, easily chilled, aching muscles, puffy eyes, brittle nails, hair loss, dry hair and skin, and vitiligo (white patches of skin). Untreated hypothyroidism may lead to atherosclerosis or coronary artery disease.[4]

Levothyroxine and the FDA

In July 2001 the media reported that the FDA was threatening to withdraw levothyroxine (SYNTHROID) from the market. This drug has been sold in the United States since the 1950s and in 2000 Synthroid was the third most frequently prescribed brand name drug in the United States—almost 40 million prescriptions were dispensed, with retail sales approaching $650 million. The implication in the media reports was that the drug is not safe and effective. Needless to say, this alarmed many patients and physicians.

Synthroid was produced by the Knoll Pharmaceutical Company of Mount Olive, New Jersey, from 1995 until the company was purchased in March 2001 by the Illinois-based Abbott Laboratories. Knoll had acquired Synthroid from a British concern, Boots Co. PLC.

Levothyroxine was introduced into the market before there was a requirement that manufacturers submit New Drug Applications (NDAs) to the FDA as part of the drug approval process.[6] An NDA contains the studies submitted by manufacturers to prove to the FDA's satisfaction that a new drug is both safe and effective. In addition, a manufacturer must report in detail exactly how the drug is manufactured. This includes not only the synthesis of the active ingredients but what inactive ingredients are used and, in the case of tablets and capsules, specifications for stability, disintegration, and dissolution. In other words, the FDA approves not only what a drug contains but how it is manufactured. This is crucial, because unless the manufacturing process can be carefully and consistently controlled, a drug may not be fully potent through the labeled expiration date, or be of consistent potency from lot to lot.

Variations in the amount of active levothyroxine available in a tablet can affect both the safety and effectiveness of the drug. Levothyroxine is unstable in the presence of light, temperature, air, and humidity. Patients who receive superpotent tablets (too much levothyroxine) experience chest pain, rapid heart rate, or heart rhythm disturbances. There is also evidence that overtreatment can cause the bone-weakening disease osteoporosis. Subpotent (too little levothyroxine) tablets will not be effective in controlling the symptoms of low thyroid hormone production (hypothyroid).

Because levothyroxine products had been marketed without an approved NDA, manufacturers did not seek FDA approval each time they reformulated their products. In 1982, for example, one manufacturer reformulated its levothyroxine product by removing two inactive ingredients and changing the physical form of the coloring agents. The reformulated product increased potency of the drug significantly. One study found that the reformulated product contained 100% of the stated content of levothyroxine compared to 78% before the reformulation.[7]

Over the years, there has been evidence from product recalls and adverse drug experience reports that even when a physician consistently prescribed the same brand of levothyroxine, patients sometimes received products of variable potency at a given dose. Such variations in drug potency present actual safety and effectiveness concerns.

Because of the accumulation of evidence showing significant stability and potency problems with levothyroxine products, plus the fact that these products fail to maintain potency through their expiration dates, and tablets of the same labeled dosage strength from the same manufacturer vary from lot to lot in the amount of active ingredient present, the FDA took action on August 14, 1997. It announced that manufacturers wishing to continue marketing levothyroxine products must submit NDAs within three years. Manufacturers who contended that their levothyroxine product was not subject to this requirement were given the option of submitting a citizen's petition asking that their drug be "generally recognized" as safe and effective. Companies that did not comply with the FDA's notice would have their drugs removed from the market.[7]

Knoll, then the manufacturer of Synthroid, chose to file a citizen's petition that was submitted December 15, 1997, and managed to delay any final action on levothyroxine products. On April 26, 2000, the FDA issued a second notice extending the deadline for obtaining approved NDAs for one year (until August 14, 2001).[8] The FDA, in a letter dated April 26, 2001, denied Knoll's petition that Synthroid be generally recognized as safe and effective.

In July 2001—by which time Knoll had sold Synthroid to Abbott Laboratories—the FDA issued instructions that manufacturers of levothyroxine products must phase out the distribution of their levothyroxine products unless they submit an NDA and obtain approval for their drug.[9] Abbott filed an NDA for Synthroid on August 1, 2001, which was finally approved by the FDA on July 24, 2002.

The first levothyroxine product with an FDA-approved NDA was Unithroid, which was granted approval on August 22, 2000.[10] Other levothyroxine products are now marketed under FDA-approved NDAs. These are listed in the drug profile for levothyroxine (see p. 461).

T4 Alone or Combined with T3?

The human thyroid gland produces two hormones: tetraiodothyronine (T4 or levothyroxine) and triiodothyronine (T3 or liothyronine). A long-standing controversy spurred more by "natural product" enthusiasts than science is the claim that T4 given in combination with T3 is a superior form of thyroid hormone replacement than T4 given alone. Thyroid Tablets USP (see p. 460), derived from animal sources, contain both T4 and T3, and are touted as being superior by some natural-product advocates. There are still combination products of synthetic T4 and T3 available (see liotrix, p. 461).

In 1970, it was found that T4 was broken down in the body to T3 and that T4 given alone would therefore result in normal levels of both T4 and T3.[11]

Three randomized controlled studies published in late 2003 failed to confirm any benefit of combined T4 and T3 treatment compared to T4 given alone.[12–14] Unfortunately, science frequently fails to dissuade natural-product zealots. However, there may be a role for combined T4 and T3 therapy in the subset of patients that have no thyroid gland.[11] This has yet to be confirmed.

Beware of Doctors Diagnosing "Wilson's Syndrome" and Compounding Pharmacists

The American Thyroid Association (ATA) issued a statement on "Wilson's Syndrome" that was posted on their Web site in November 1999.[15]

"Wilson's Syndrome" refers to a set of common and nonspecific symptoms, relatively low body temperature, and normal levels of thyroid hormones in blood. Dr. E. Denis Wilson, a disciplined Florida physician who named the syndrome after himself, contends that it represents a form of thyroid hormone deficiency responsive to treatment with a special preparation of triiodothyronine (T3 or liothyronine).

The ATA concluded their review of this bogus disorder by saying:

> The American Thyroid Association has found no scientific evidence supporting the existence of "Wilson's syndrome." The theory proposed to explain this condition is at odds with established facts about thyroid hormone. Diagnostic criteria for "Wilson's syndrome" are imprecise and could lead to misdiagnosis of many other conditions. The T3 therapy advocated for "Wilson's syndrome" has never been evaluated objectively in a properly designed scientific study. Furthermore, administration of T3 can produce abnormally high concentrations of T3 in the blood, subjecting patients to new symptoms and potentially harmful effects on the heart and bones.

The "treatment" for "Wilson's Syndrome" is time-released T3 prepared by a compounding pharmacist. Products prepared by compounding pharmacists are not FDA-approved. They have not been tested for safety or effectiveness and are not produced in facilities, or under conditions, meeting the FDA's Good Manufacturing Practice guidelines.

Patients have been needlessly injured by pharmacy-compounded T3 capsules. Three patients suffered severe illness and were hospitalized in Atlanta from T3 prepared to treat "Wilson's Syndrome" in 2001.[16] There is no way to tell how many patients have actually been harmed from compounding pharmacists because they are not required to report problems with the drugs they prepared to either the FDA or state boards of pharmacy.

DRUG PROFILES

 Do Not Use

ALTERNATIVE TREATMENT:
See Levothyroxine, p. 461.

Thyroid Tablets USP
ARMOUR THYROID (Forest)

FAMILY: Hormones (Thyroid)

In the first edition of *Worst Pills, Best Pills,* we wrote that natural or desiccated (dried) thyroid extract products, such as Armour Thyroid, should not be used except by those who have successfully taken it for years to control their symptoms of low thyroid hormone production (hypothyroidism).[17] Remarkably, Armour Thyroid remains among the Top 200 drugs in the United States with almost 2 million prescriptions dispensed in 2002 despite the fact that for decades levothyroxine has been recommended as the better product for the vast majority of pa-

---

Drugs with thyroid hormone activity, alone or together with other therapeutic agents, have been used for the treatment of obesity. In euthyroid (normal thyroid) patients, doses within the range of daily hormonal requirements are ineffective for weight reduction. Larger doses may produce serious or even life-threatening manifestations of toxicity, particularly when given in association with sympathomimetic amines (speedlike drugs) such as those used for their anorectic (weight loss) effects.

---

tients. Yet, the number of Armour Thyroid prescriptions appears to be growing.

Advocates of natural thyroid hormone replacement therapy maintain that products like Armour Thyroid are superior not only because they are from a natural source (feed animals in this case) but because they contain both important thyroid hormones, tetraiodothyronine (T4) and triiodothyronine (T3). However, in 1970 it was found that T4 was broken down to T3 in the body and that T4 given alone would give normal levels of both T4 and T3.[11] Three randomized controlled studies published in late 2003 failed to confirm any benefit of combined T4 and T3 treatment compared to T4 given alone.[12–14]

The Medical Letter on Drugs and Therapeutics, an independent source of drug information written for physicians and pharmacists that we frequently cite, concluded that synthetic levothyroxine is preferred over other forms of thyroid replacement drugs. This recommendation was originally made in 1977.[18]

The fifth edition of the *AMA Drug Evaluations*—an excellent source of drug information before the AMA (American Medical Association) became so tied to the pharmaceutical industry—again made the recommendation in 1983 that synthetic levothyroxine is the preferred thyroid hormone replacement treatment.[19]

The American Thyroid Association clearly stated in 2003 on its Web site: "[T]here is no evidence that desiccated thyroid, a biological preparation, has any advantage over synthetic thyroxine."[20]

The United States Pharmacopoeia (USP) long ago established standards for all thyroid products from animal sources sold in the United States. Active thyroid hormones contain iodine and the USP standards allow that the uniformity of Thyroid Tablets USP, such as Armour Thyroid, is based on iodine content,[21] not on the direct measurement of the amount of T4 and T3 in the tablets. The advantage of synthetic levothyroxine (T4) over natural thyroid hormone is a predictable effect because of standard hormonal content.[22]

Desiccated thyroid remains on a list of drugs that are inappropriate for use in older adults.[23]

Why, after over 25 years of advice to the contrary, is Armour Thyroid in the top 200 most frequently prescribed drugs in the United States? One explanation appears to be that thyroid replacement therapy with natural thyroid appears to have become a niche market for unscrupulous complementary and alternative medicine (CAM) practitioners, some of whom are licensed MDs. Some of these CAM practitioners are also promoting natural thyroid hormone as a part of their weight loss programs. This is a dangerous practice, but it is not new.

The U.S. Senate held hearings on the diet pill industry 36 years ago, in 1968.[24] During these hearings, the dangerous practice of "diet doctors" who prescribed thyroid hormone alone or in combination with the heart drug digitalis or amphetamines (speedlike drugs)—or all three together—came to light. In some cases, these diet doctors were selling these drugs directly to their patients.

Levothyroxine (lee voe thy *rox* een)
(tetraiodothyronine, l-thyroxine, thyroxine, T-4)
LEVO-T (Alara Pharm)
LEVOXYL (Jones Pharma)
NOVOTHYROX (Genpharm)
SYNTHROID (Abbott)
THYRO-TABS (Lloyd)
UNITROID (Jerome Stevens)

Limited Use

Liothyronine (lye oh *thye* roe neen)
(triiodothyronine or T-3)
CYTOMEL (Monarch Pharmaceuticals)

Liotrix (*lye* oh trix)
(pure synthetic triiodothyronine and tetraiodothyronine)
THYROLAR (Forest)

GENERIC: available except for Liothyronine
FAMILY: Hormones (Thyroid)

PREGNANCY WARNING
Thyroid hormones appear to be safe to take during pregnancy.

BREAST-FEEDING WARNING
Adequate replacement doses are generally needed to maintain normal lactation. However, thyroid hromones are excreted in human milk; the infant should be monitored when the mother is using these drugs.

Thyroid hormone replacement therapy is prescribed for patients who do not produce any, or enough, thyroid hormone.

Among the thyroid hormone replacement drugs, levothyroxine has been the preferred product for decades.[18–20] This pure, crystalline, synthetic product produces the same activity as the natural hormone. It has the most reliable and uniform potency and is easier to monitor.[22]

Thyroid hormone replacement drugs come in a wide range of strengths expressed as milligrams (mg) or micrograms (mcg), which can be confusing. Compared to other drugs, prescriptions for thyroid hormone replacement drugs

Drugs with thyroid hormone activity, alone or together with other therapeutic agents, have been used for the treatment of obesity. In euthyroid (normal thyroid) patients, doses within the range of daily hormonal requirements are ineffective for weight reduction. Larger doses may produce serious or even life-threatening manifestations of toxicity, particularly when given in association with sympathomimetic amines (speedlike drugs) such as those used for their anorectic (weight loss) effects.

are prone to errors in filling prescriptions. For example, 125 micrograms is the same as 0.125 milligram. Errors may be made if leading zeroes are missing or decimal points misplaced. Errors may also occur due to handwriting or unclear abbreviations.

Physicians are encouraged to print prescriptions for these drugs and to specify the strength in micrograms or state the strength in both milligrams and micrograms. Pharmacies are encouraged to have computer alerts for doses over 200 micrograms.[25,26]

People who are older, or who have heart problems or myxedema (boggy swelling of the face, hands, and occasionally the legs caused by hypothyroidism) should be started on low doses of thyroid, then increase gradually if necessary.[4]

Thyroid hormone treatment is not approved by the FDA for weight loss. Unscrupulous diet doctors have prescribed thyroid in combination with digitalis, amphetamines, and diuretics, at times with fatal results. Neither is thyroid approved for treating infertility.

Before You Use This Drug

Tell your doctor if you have or have had:

- allergies, including to aspirin, iodine, lactose, pork, or tartrazine
- Addison's disease or adrenal gland problems
- bowel disease
- heart disease, such as angina, arteriosclerosis, coronary artery disease, myocardial infarction (heart attack)
- diabetes
- hyperthyroidism
- hypothyroidism
- malabsorption conditions, such as celiac disease
- myxedema
- pituitary gland problems
- pregnancy or are breast-feeding
- thyrotoxicosis being treated with antithyroid medication

Tell your doctor about any other drugs you take, including aspirin, herbs, vitamins, and other nonprescription products.

When You Use This Drug

- Be vigilant in checking both new and refilled prescriptions. Check for color, shape, correct strength, and manufacturer. If your medication appears to be different, inquire about this from the pharmacist before leaving the pharmacy. It is usually best to stick with a product from the same manufacturer instead of switching brands.
- Tell any doctor, dentist, pharmacist, or surgeon you see that you take thyroid.

How to Use This Drug

- If you miss a dose, take it as soon as you remember, but skip it if it is almost time for the next dose. **Do not take double doses.**
- Do not share your medication with others.
- Take the drug at the same time(s) each day, usually before breakfast.
- Swallow tablet(s) with water. Thyroid is absorbed better without food.
- If tablets are scored, break tablets as appropriate to your dose.
- Levothyroxine tablets may be crushed and placed in baby formula or water, or sprinkled on applesauce or cereal, or given via a nasogastric tube. Preparation of such doses should be fresh and not saved.
- Contact your doctor if you miss two or more doses in a row.
- Store tablets at room temperature with lid on tightly. Do not store in the bathroom. Do not expose to heat, moisture, or strong light. Keep out of reach of children.
- Check with your doctor before you stop taking this drug.

Interactions with Other Drugs

The following drugs, biologics (e.g., vaccines, therapeutic antibodies), or foods are listed in *Evaluations of Drug Interactions* 2003 as causing "highly clinically significant" or "clinically significant" interactions when used together with any of the drugs in this section. In some sections with multiple drugs, the interaction may have been reported for one but not all drugs in this section, but we include the interaction because the drugs in this section are similar to one another. We have also included potentially serious interactions listed in the drugs' FDA-approved professional package insert or in published medical journal articles. There may be other drugs, especially those in the families of drugs listed below, that also will react with this drug to cause severe adverse effects. Make sure to tell your doctor and pharmacist the drugs you are taking and tell them if you are taking any of these interacting drugs:

If you take these drugs with thyroid, risk of heart complications increases: ADRENALIN, amitriptyline, bee-sting kits, ELAVIL, epinephrine, imipramine, KETALAR, ketamine, LUDIOMIL, maprotiline.

If you take anticoagulants or drugs for diabetes, extra monitoring may be required, especially if you stop, start, or change doses of either thyroid or: acarbose, acetohexamide, ACTOS, AMARYL, AVANDIA, chlorpropamide, COUMADIN, DIABINESE, DIAMICRON, DYMELOR, glicaside, glimepiride, glipizide, GLUCOPHAGE, GLUCOTROL, GLUCOVANCE, glyburide, GLYNASE, insulin, metformin, nateglinide, ORINASE, pioglitazone, PRANDIN, PRECOSE, repalginide, rosiglitazone, STARLIX, tolazamide, tolbutamide, TOLINASE, warfarin.

Many other drugs can interact with thyroid products and may require adjustments in doses. These include: carbamazepine, digoxin, DILANTIN, LANOXIN, LUMINAL, oral contraceptives, oral estrogens, phenobarbital, phenytoin, PREMARIN, PREMPRO, RIFADIN, rifampin, rifapentine, RIMACTANE, ROFACT, TEGRETOL.

Some drugs are more apt to interact with thyroid in high doses. Of particular note are: DECADRON (dexamethasone) over 4 milligrams per day, Inderal (propranolol) over 160 milligrams per day, salicylates, such as aspirin or sodium salicyclate, over 2 grams (2,000 milligrams) per day.

The following drugs may prevent absorption of thyroid drugs. If you take these, take four to five hours apart from thyroid: ALUDROX, aluminum, antacids, calcium carbonate, CARAFATE, cholestyramine, COLESTID, colestipol, FEOSOL, ferrous sulfate, iron preparations, KAYEXALATE, MAALOX, magnesium, MYLICON, QUESTRAN, simethicone, sucralfate, TUMS.

If you take these drugs, it could affect results of thyroid monitoring tests: amiodarone, carbamazepine, CORDARONE, iodine, sertraline, TEGRETOL, ZOLOFT.

Adverse Effects

Call your doctor immediately if you experience:

- breathing difficulty
- changes in appetite
- chest pain
- fever
- headache that is severe in children (pseudotumor cerebri)
- heartbeat becomes irregular or fast
- irritability
- leg cramps
- menstrual periods change
- nervousness
- sensitivity to heat
- skin rash or hives

- sleeping problems
- sweating profusely
- vomiting
- weight loss

Signs of overdose:

- change in appetite
- change in menstrual periods
- chest pain
- diarrhea
- fast or irregular heartbeat
- fever
- hand tremors
- headache
- irritability
- jaundice
- leg cramps
- mood swings
- muscle wasting
- nervousness
- psychosis
- restlessness
- sensitivity to heat
- shortness of breath
- sweating
- trouble sleeping
- vomiting
- extreme weakness
- weight loss

If you suspect an overdose, call this number to contact your poison control center: (800) 222-1222.

Call your doctor if you continue to experience:

- clumsiness
- coldness
- constipation
- hair loss
- headaches
- listlessness
- menstrual periods change
- muscle aches
- sleepiness
- tiredness
- skin is dry, puffy
- weakness
- weight gain

Periodic Tests

Ask your doctor which of these tests should be done periodically while you are taking this drug:

- measurement of bone age and density
- measurement of growth
- measurement of psychomotor development
- observation for signs of ischemia or tach-yarrhythmias
- TSH (thyroid-stimulating hormone); T-3 (triiodothyronine); free T-4 (thyroxine); T-4 resin uptake determinations; or total serum T-3 or T-4 (thyroid function tests)

REFERENCES

1. Friberg L, Werner S, Eggertsen G, et al. Rapid down-regulation of thyroid hormones in acute myocardial infarction: Is it cardioprotective in patients with angina? *Archives of Internal Medicine* 2002; 162:1388–94.

2. Langton JE, Brent GA. Nonthyroidal illness syndrome: Evaluation of thyroid function in sick patients. *Endocrinology and Metabolism Clinics of North America* 2002; 31:159–72.

3. Hermann D, Heinz A, Mann K. Dysregulation of the hypothalamic-pituitary-thyroid axis in alcoholism. *Addiction* 2002; 97:1369–81.

4. Klein I, Ojamaa K. Thyroid hormone and the cardiovascular system. *New England Journal of Medicine* 2001; 344:501–9.

5. Redmond GP. Hypothyroidism and women's health. *International Journal of Fertility and Women's Medicine* 2002; 47:123–7.

6. What is going on with levothyroxine. *Medical Letter on Drugs and Therapeutics* 2003; 43:57–8.

7. Food and Drug Administration. Prescription Drug Products; Levothyroxine Sodium. *Federal Register* 1997; 62:43535–8.

8. Food and Drug Administration. Prescription Drug Products; Levothyroxine Sodium; Extension of Compliance Date. *Federal Register* 2000; 65:24488–9.

9. Food and Drug Administration. Guidance for Industry on Levothyroxine Sodium Products—Enforcement of August 14, 2001, Compliance Date and Submission of New Applications. *Federal Register* 2001; 66:36794–5.

10. Food and Drug Administration. FDA Approves First NDA for Levothyroxine Sodium. *FDA Talk Paper* 2000:1–2.

11. Cooper DS. Combined T4 and T3 therapy—back to the drawing board. *Journal of the American Medical Association* 2003; 290:3002–4.

12. Sawka AM, Gerstein HC, Marriott MJ, et al. Does a combination regimen of thyroxine (T4) and 3,5,3'-triiodothyronine improve depressive symptoms better than T4 alone in patients with hypothyroidism? Results of a double-blind, randomized, controlled trial. *Journal of Clinical Endocrinology and Metabolism* 2003; 88:4551–5.

13. Walsh JP, Shiels L, Lim EM, et al. Combined thyroxine/liothyronine treatment does not improve well-being, quality of life, or cognitive function compared to thyroxine alone: A randomized controlled trial in patients with primary hypothyroidism. *Journal of Clinical Endrocrinology and Metabolism* 2003; 88:4543–50.

14. Clyde PW, Harari AE, Getka EJ, et al. Combined levothyroxine plus liothyronine compared with levothyroxine alone in primary hypothyroidism. *Journal of the American Medical Association* 2003; 290:2952–8.

15. American Thyroid Association. American Thyroid Association Statement on "Wilson's Syndrome," 2003. Available at: http://www.thyroid.org/professionals/publications/statements/99_11_16_wilsons.html. Accessed December 12, 2003.

16. Teegardin C. State drug agents looking for link between thyroid capsules, ailments. *Atlanta Journal-Constitution,* March 29, 2001:A1.

17. Wolfe SM, Fugate L, Kamimoto LE. *Worst Pills, Best Pills.* Washington, D.C.: Public Citizen's Health Research Group, 1988:507–8.

18. Thyroid replacement therapy. *Medical Letter on Drugs and Therapeutics* 1977; 19:50–1.

19. AMA Department of Drugs. *AMA Drug Evaluations.* 5th ed. Chicago: American Medical Association, 1983:1056–64.

20. American Thyroid Association. Thyroid hormone treatment, 2003. Available at: http://www.thyroid.org. Accessed December 11, 2003.

21. *The United States Pharmacopoeia USP 26—The National Formulary NF 21.* Rockville, Md.: United States Pharmacopoeial Convention, Inc., 2003:1830–1.

22. *USP DI— Drug Information for the Health Care Professional.* 23rd ed. Greenwood Village, Col.: Thomson Micromedex, 2003:2583–9.

23. Fick DM, Cooper JW, Wade WE, et al. Updating the Beers criteria for potentially inappropriate medication use in older adults: Results of a US consensus panel of experts. *Archives of Internal Medicine* 2003; 163:2716–24.

24. United States Senate Committee on the Judiciary Subcommittee on Antitrust and Monopoly. Diet Pill Industry. 1968.

25. Institute for Safe Medicine Practice. FDA Advise-ERR: Medication errors associated with levothyroxine products, September 6, 2000. Available at: http://www.ismp.org. Accessed December 14, 2003.

26. Institute for Safe Medicine Practice. ISMP Quarterly Action Agenda, 2003. Available at: http://www.ismp.org. Accessed December 14, 2003.

13

DRUGS FOR ATTENTION DEFICIT HYPERACTIVITY DISORDER

> Drug treatment is not suitable for all children with attention deficit hyperactivity disorder (ADHD). Drug treatment is not intended for use in patients who exhibit symptoms of the disorder that result primarily from environmental factors (school, home), learning disabilities, and/or other psychiatric disorders, including psychosis.

DIAGNOSIS AND TREATMENT

The cause of attention deficit hyperactivity disorder (ADHD) is unknown, and there is no single specific diagnostic test to identify this disorder. To correctly establish the diagnosis of ADHD requires the use not only of medical but also of special psychological, educational, and social resources. Many children diagnosed with ADHD actually have problems that are primarily caused or worsened by inadequate teachers, unsuitable educational settings, or by problems with their parents. Similarly, many adults diagnosed with ADHD may have interpersonal problems that need to be dealt with by psychotherapy.

The diagnosis of ADHD in a child must be based on a complete history and evaluation of the patient and not solely on the presence of the required number of characteristics listed in the American Psychiatric Association's *Diagnostic and Statistical Manual of Mental Disorders,* fourth edition (DSM-IV). If you are worried that your child may have ADHD, tell your child's school that you want an evaluation as part of an individualized education program (IEP). The school is required by law to provide a free and timely evaluation and appropriate interventions. Also, talk to your child's doctor about getting ADHD checklist forms for you, other caregivers, and your child's teachers to complete.

The diagnosis of ADHD implies the presence of symptoms of hyperactivity—impulsivity or inattention that cause impairment and that were present before the age of seven. The symptoms must be persistent, must be more severe than is typically observed in individuals at a comparable level of development, must cause clinically significant impairment—for example, in social, academic, or occupational functioning—and must be present in two or more settings, such as school (or work) and home. The symptoms must not be better accounted for by another mental disorder.[1]

About 85% of children with ADHD respond to stimulants. Stimulants have the potential to be abused, and their common street names are "speed" or "uppers." We do not know why, but people with ADHD paradoxically become less hyper when given stimulant medications. Common adverse effects include headache, stomach pain, and decreased appetite. Stimulants are also marketed as appetite suppressants. Some children do not grow well while on ADHD medications because of the decrease in appetite. If that happens with your child, talk to your child's doctor about strategies to help your child eat better, such as timing meals to coincide with when the medication is wearing off or taking drug breaks on weekends and holidays.

The stimulant methylphenidate may assist in focusing, sustaining attention and lessening impulsiveness, reducing aggression, and combating other problems in children with ADHD.[2,3]

ADHD IN ADULTS

In addition to the more well-known occurrence of ADHD in children, the disorder affects an estimated 2% or more of adults. In adults, it can cause educational as well as occupational and interpersonal problems. Although the origin of adult ADHD is in childhood, and many cases are diagnosed then, for many other people the diagnosis is not made until adulthood. It is likely that some physicians taking care only of adults will not be as aware of the problem as pediatricians or family practitioners. The correct diagnosis in adults shares many of the elements of diagnosis in children, including efforts to determine patterns of behavior when the adult was younger, and a psychiatric and developmental history and physical exam to rule out other causes of ADHD such as thyroid disease and other neurological problems. Whereas in children, frequent symptoms are hyperactivity and impulsiveness, in adults the more common findings include procrastination, lack of motivation, mood liability, and low self-esteem, as well as the frequent occurrence of anxiety and depression.[4]

DRUG PROFILES

Central Nervous System Stimulants

Limited Use

Amphetamine mixtures (am *fet* a meen)
ADDERALL (Shire Richwood)

Dextroamphetamine (dex tro am *fet* a meen)
DEXEDRINE (GlaxoSmithKline)

GENERIC: available
FAMILY: Central Nervous System Stimulants

PREGNANCY WARNING

Amphetamines caused malformations and fetal death in animal studies. Infants born to mothers dependent on amphetamines are at increased risk of premature delivery and low birth weight and may experience withdrawal symptoms. Because of the potential for serious adverse effects to the fetus, these drugs should not be used by pregnant women.

BREAST-FEEDING WARNING

Amphetamines are excreted in human milk. Because of the potential for serious adverse effects in nursing infants, you should not take amphetamines if you are nursing.

FDA BLACK BOX WARNING

AMPHETAMINES HAVE A HIGH POTENTIAL FOR ABUSE. ADMINISTRATION OF AMPHETAMINES FOR PROLONGED PERIODS OF TIME MAY LEAD TO DRUG DEPENDENCE. PARTICULAR ATTENTION SHOULD BE PAID TO THE POSSIBILITY OF SUBJECTS OBTAINING AMPHETAMINES FOR NON-THERAPEUTIC USE OR DISTRIBUTION TO OTHERS AND THE DRUGS SHOULD BE PRESCRIBED OR DISPENSED SPARINGLY.

> Drug treatment is not suitable for all children with attention deficit hyperactivity disorder (ADHD). Drug treatment is not intended for use in patients who exhibit symptoms of the disorder that result primarily from environmental factors (school, home), learning disabilities, and/or other psychiatric disorders, including psychosis.

Amphetamine and dextroamphetamine are approved by the FDA to treat symptoms of attention deficit hyperactivity disorder (ADHD), and for narcolepsy, a rare sleep disorder. Amphetamine and dextroamphetamine are for all practical purposes the same drug.

Many drugs, such as amphetamine, exist as mixtures of chemically identical compounds that are mirror images of each other. One of the compounds that make up amphetamine is dextroamphetamine. All of the atoms in the amphetamine mixture are the same, only their spatial orientation is different. Separating these mirror images, or recombining them, and selling the combination as a "new" drug is a successful business scheme to protect patents, not a strategy to improve public health.

Amphetamine and dextroamphetamine belong to a family of central nervous system stimulant drugs sometimes called psychostimulants. Amphetamine and dextroamphetamine affect the neurotransmitters dopamine and norepinephrine.[2] Exactly how these drugs work is not fully known. Amphetamines may control symptoms of some conditions but are not a cure for any condition.[5]

Amphetamine and dextroamphetamine are classified as Schedule-II controlled substances by U.S. federal law. Misuse can result in criminal charges. All children prescribed amphetamine should be cautioned not to share or sell their medication. Each new and refill prescription requires a new, handwritten prescription. If your child is taking more than one dose a day, ask your pharmacist to divide your prescription into two labeled containers, one for home and one for school or work. Check with schools about their security procedures. Be sure requests for refill correspond to the time for the amount prescribed.

If you are subject to urine tests for employment or school, inform them that you take an amphetamine medication.

People with uncontrolled high blood pressure should not take any amphetamine.[6] This includes patients with mild high blood pressure.[7]

Periodically, your doctor should reassess your need to continue taking amphetamines.

Before You Use This Drug

Tell your doctor if you have or have had:

- allergies, including to lactose, tartrazine, or aspirin
- agitation
- anorexia
- arteriosclerosis
- cardiovascular disease
- drug abuse or dependence
- high blood pressure
- glaucoma
- heart problems
- hyperthyroidism (overactive thyroid)
- pregnancy or are breast-feeding
- psychosis
- tics
- Tourette's syndrome

Tell your doctor about any other drugs you take, including aspirin, herbs, vitamins, and other nonprescription products.

When You Use This Drug

- For narcolepsy, avoid drugs that induce sleep. Avoid other stimulants, such as caffeine, methylphenidate (RITALIN), and pseudoephedrine (SUDAFED).
- Do not drive, operate hazardous equipment, or perform dangerous activities if you ex-

perience dizziness or euphoria, or your narcolepsy is not controlled.

• Minimize distractions at school or work. For example, sit toward the front of the classroom. Seek schools and work with structured settings, and establish short-term goals.

• Try scheduling naps if you have narcolepsy.

• Check with your doctor if you think you may have become dependent on amphetamine.

• Augment treatment with biofeedback, cognitive-behavioral therapy, educational skills training, parenting skills, and/or social skills.

How to Use This Drug

• If you miss a dose of a short-acting form, take it within the hour. If remembered later, wait until the next scheduled dose. If you miss a dose of a long-acting form, take it as soon as possible, unless it is too close to bedtime. Otherwise, wait until the following day.

• **Do not take double doses.**

• Do not share your medication with others.

• Take the drug at the same time(s) each day. Swallow capsule or tablet in the morning. Take scheduled doses at specified intervals, taking the last dose of short-acting forms at least six hours before bedtime, of long-acting forms 10 to 14 hours before bedtime. Take with or without food, but it is best to be consistent about which way it is taken.

• For extended-release forms, do not break, chew, or crush this drug. Capsules may be opened and the contents mixed with applesauce, jelly, or ketchup, then swallowed without chewing. Vitamin C (ascorbic acid), present in fruit juice, may reduce absorption.

• Store at room temperature with lid on tightly. Do not store in the bathroom. Do not expose to heat, moisture or strong light.

• Do not discontinue taking medication without checking with your doctor, who will likely put you on a tapering schedule.

Interactions with Other Drugs

The following drugs, biologics (e.g., vaccines, therapeutic antibodies), or foods are listed in *Evaluations of Drug Interactions* 2003 as causing "highly clinically significant" or "clinically significant" interactions when used together with any of the drugs in this section. In some sections with multiple drugs, the interaction may have been reported for one but not all drugs in this section, but we include the interaction because the drugs in this section are similar to one another. We have also included potentially serious interactions listed in the drug's FDA-approved professional package insert or in published medical journal articles. There may be other drugs, especially those in the families of drugs listed below, that also will react with this drug to cause severe adverse effects. Make sure to tell your doctor and pharmacist the drugs you are taking and tell them if you are taking any of these interacting drugs:

acebutolol, acetazolamide, amitriptyline, ammonium chloride, amoxapine, ANAFRANIL, ascorbic acid, ASENDIN, atenolol, AVANDAMET, AVENTYL, BETAGAN, BETAPACE, betaxolol, BETAXON, BETOPTIC, BIOCADREN, bisoprolol, caffeine, cartelol, CARTOL, chlorpromazine, clomipramine, CORGARD, CORZIDE, cyclobenzaprine, DEMEROL, desipramine, DIAMOX, digoxin, doxepin, ELAVIL, ELDEPRYL, FLEXERIL, fruit juices, furazolidone, FUROXONE, GLUCOVANCE, guanethidine, imipramine, INDERAL, INDERIDE, ISMELIN, isocarboxazid, KERLONE, LANOXIN, LEVATOL, LOPRESSOR, LOPRESSOR HTC, MARPLAN, MATULANE, meperidine, METAGLIP, metformin, metipranolol, metoprolol, naldolol, NARDIL, NORPRAMIN, NORTRIPTYLINE, OCUPRESS, OPTIPRANOLOL, orlistat, PAMELOR, PARNATE, penbutolol, PERTOFRANE, phenelzine, pinolol, procarbazine, propranolol, protriptyline, pseudoephedrine (present in numerous cough and cold remedies), SECTRAL, selegiline, SINEQUAN, sotalol, SUDAFED, SURMONTIL, TENORETIC, TENORMIN, THORAZINE, TIMOLIDE, timolol, TIMOPTIC, TOFRANIL, tranylcypromine, trimipramine, VISKAZIDE, VISKEN, vitamin C (especially in high doses),VIVACTIL, XENICAL, ZEBETA, and ZIAC.

Use of amphetamines with monoamine oxidase (MAO) inhibitors can cause dangerous increases in blood pressure, called a hypertensive crisis. Do not take amphetamines within fourteen days of an MAO inhibitor.

Adverse Effects

Call your doctor immediately if you experience:

- blood pressure increase
- breathing difficulty
- chest pain or discomfort
- dizziness or faintness
- pounding or irregular heartbeat
- psychosis (hallucinations)
- mood or mental changes
- uncontrolled movements of head, neck, arms, and legs
- extremely high body temperature
- unusual tiredness or weakness

Signs of overdose:

- agitation
- assaultive behavior
- blood pressure increase or decrease
- rapid breathing
- confusion
- diarrhea
- fast, pounding, or irregular heartbeat
- confusion
- dry mouth
- euphoria
- fever
- hallucinations

- severe headache
- muscle twitch
- nausea
- enlarged pupils
- overactive reflexes
- panic
- restlessness
- shaking
- stomach cramps
- increased sweating
- trembling
- vomiting

These symptoms may be followed by fatigue and depression.

If you suspect an overdose, call this number to contact your poison control center: (800) 222-1222.

Call your doctor if these symptoms continue:

- appetite decrease
- constipation
- diarrhea
- dizziness or lightheadedness
- drowsiness, fatigue
- dry mouth
- false sense of well-being
- headache, migraine headache[8]
- fast or pounding heartbeat
- trouble sleeping
- irritability
- mental depression
- nausea or vomiting
- nervousness, restlessness
- change in sexual desire or ability
- stomach cramps or pain
- increased sweating
- sense of taste becomes unpleasant
- trembling
- blurred vision
- weight loss

Call your doctor if these symptoms continue after you stop taking this drug:

- mental depression
- nausea
- stomach cramps or pain
- vomiting
- trembling
- unusual tiredness or weakness

Periodic Testing

Ask your doctor which of these tests should be done periodically while you are taking this drug:

By your doctor:

- assessment for drug tolerance, blood pressure, electrocardiogram (EKG or ECG), pulse, tics, weight and height, and reassessment for continuing need for therapy, dose of medication, and signs of dependence or abuse
- standard sleepiness scale, Test of Variables of Attention (TOVA)

By your parent(s):

- rating scales, such as Achenbach's Child Behavior Checklist, Conner's Parent Questionnaire

By your teacher(s):

- rating scales, such as Child Attention Problems, Conner's Teacher Rating Scale

Do Not Use Until Seven Years After Release

Atomoxetine (at oh *mox* i teen)
(Do Not Use Until 2010)
STRATTERA (Lilly)

GENERIC: not available

FAMILY: Central Nervous System Stimulants

PREGNANCY WARNING

Atomoxetine caused fetal harm in animal studies, including fetal resorptions, atypical or missing arteries in the heart, in-

complete bone formation of the spine, as well as decreases in pup weight and survival. Because of the potential for serious adverse effects to the fetus, this drug should not be used by pregnant women.

BREAST-FEEDING WARNING

Atomoxetine was excreted in animal milk. It is likely that this drug, like many others, is also excreted in human milk, and because of the potential for serious adverse effects in nursing infants, you should not take this drug while nursing.

Atomoxetine is approved by the FDA to treat attention deficit hyperactivity disorder (ADHD) in children, adolescents, and adults. Atomoxetine increases function of the neurotransmitter norepinephrine. Atomoxetine is intended to be part of a therapy that includes educational, psychological, and social measures.[1] It may control but does not cure ADHD.

Atomoxetine should not be used by people with narrow-angle glaucoma. The drug has not been studied in children under the age of six years or in the elderly. The effectiveness of atomoxetine beyond 9 weeks in children or 10 weeks in adults has not been evaluated. Safety

THE HEALTH RESEARCH GROUP'S SEVEN-YEAR RULE

You should wait at least seven years from the date of release to take any new drug unless it is one of those rare "breakthrough" drugs that offer you a documented therapeutic advantage over older proven drugs. New drugs are tested in a relatively small number of people before being released, and serious adverse effects or life-threatening drug interactions may not be detected until the new drug has been taken by hundreds of thousands of people. A number of new drugs have been withdrawn within their first seven years after release. Also, warnings about serious new adverse reactions have been added to the labeling of a number of drugs, or new drug interactions have been detected, usually within the first seven years after a drug's release.

beyond one year has not been studied in controlled trials. Long-term effects are not known. Short-term studies show children gain less height and weight when using atomoxetine.[1]

Concern exists about long-term use effect on growth of children, and heart and circulation adverse effects in children and adults.[9] If height and weight gain in children are insufficient, consideration should be given to interrupting therapy.

Common adverse effects with atomoxetine include indigestion, fatigue, dizziness, decreased appetite, and mood swings. Adverse effects that have caused adults to discontinue atomoxetine include chest pain, insomnia, and urinary retention, while children and adolescents were more apt to stop due to aggression, drowsiness, irritability, and vomiting.

Before You Use This Drug

Do not use if you have or have had:

- allergy to atomoxetine or any of its components

Tell your doctor if you have or have had:

- high blood pressure
- glaucoma
- heart problems
- liver problems
- pregnancy or are breast-feeding

Tell your doctor about any other drugs you take, including aspirin, herbs, vitamins, and other nonprescription products.

When You Use This Drug

- Do not drive or operate hazardous equipment until you know whether atomoxetine causes you to be dizzy.
- Make regular visits to your doctor to see how you are doing and decide if you should continue using the drug.
- Tell your doctor if you are nursing, pregnant, or thinking of becoming pregnant.

Drug treatment is not suitable for all children with attention deficit hyperactivity disorder (ADHD). Drug treatment is not intended for use in patients who exhibit symptoms of the disorder that result primarily from environmental factors (school, home) learning disabilities and/or other psychiatric disorders, including psychosis (see the introduction to this chapter, p. 466).

- Tell your doctor right away if you get swelling, hives, or any symptoms that concern you.
- Reduce distractions; for example, sit toward the front of classrooms, or make lists of several small deadlines at work.
- Select schools that have structured rules and expectations and that provide regular feedback.
- Seek education about ADHD and counseling for skills development, or join support groups.
- Augment treatment with biofeedback, cognitive-behavioral therapy, educational skills training, parenting skills, and/or social skills.
- Try parent counseling to increase self-confidence and learn to discipline consistently and appropriately, reinforcing good behavior with immediate rewards, reducing disruptive behavior, and decreasing family stress.
- Tell any doctor, dentist, emergency help, or pharmacist you see that you take atomoxetine.
- Use sugarless candy or gum, ice, or a saliva substitute for dry mouth, but check with your doctor if dry mouth continues for more than two weeks.

How to Use This Drug

- If you miss a dose, take it as soon as you remember, but do not take more than your daily dose within 24 hours. **Do not take double doses.**
- Do not share your medication with others.
- Take the drug at the same time(s) each day.
- Swallow capsules whole with water. Take

with or without food, but it is best to be consistent. High-fat meals may slow the rate at which atomoxetine is absorbed.

• If you are prescribed a second dose in a day, take the second dose by late afternoon or early evening.

• Store at room temperature with lid on tightly. Do not store in the bathroom. Do not expose to heat, moisture, or strong light. Keep out of reach of children.

Interactions with Other Drugs

Atomoxetine is a relatively new drug, and information about drug interactions is scant. People in clinical trials are usually on few other drugs and have few other conditions. Listed are potentially serious interactions in FDA-approved labeling and other medical references that are known or suspected to date. New scientific techniques allow researchers to predict some drug interactions before they have been documented in people. There may be other drugs, especially those in the families of drugs listed below, that also will react with this drug to cause severe adverse effects. The number of new drugs approved for marketing increases the chance of drug interactions, and new drug interactions are being identified with old drugs. Be vigilant. Make sure to tell your doctor and pharmacist the drugs you are taking and tell your doctor if you are taking any of these interacting drugs:

Drugs that inhibit monoamine oxidase (MAO inhibitors) may cause serious, at times fatal reactions, such as extreme agitation, rapid fluctuations of mental status, rigid muscles, twitching, or coma. Do not take atomoxetine within two weeks of: deprenyl, ELDEPRYL, furazolidone, FUROXONE, isocarboxazid, MARPLAN, MATULANE, NARDIL, PARNATE, phenelzine, procarbazine, selegiline, tranylcypromine.

Using atomoxetine with asthma drugs called beta agonists may add to adverse effects of the heart and circulation: albuterol, PROVENTIL, VENTOLIN, VOLMAX.

If you use atomoxetine with these drugs, your doctor may adjust your doses: CARDIO-QUIN, fluoxetine, PAXIL, paroxetine, PROZAC, QUINAGLUTE, QUINIDEX, quinidine, quinidine gluconate, quinidine polygalacturonate, quinidine sulfate.

Using atomoxetine with anticholinergic drugs (see p. 617) could add to the adverse effect of urinary retention: amitriptyline, AMOXAPINE, antidepressants (tricyclic), antihistamines, ARTANE, ASENDIN, atropine, AVENTYL, belladonna, benztropine, clidinium, COGENTIN, cyclobenzaprine, desipramine, DETROL, dicyclomine, DITROPAN, doxepin, ELAVIL, FLEXERIL, glycopyrrolate, hyoscyamine, imipramine, LIBRAX, NORPRAMIN, nortriptyline, oxybutin, PROBANTHINE, propantheline, protriptyline, scopolamine, SINEQUAN, SURMONTIL, TOFRANIL, tolterodine, TRANS-DERM SCOP, trihexyphenidyl, trimipramine, VISTARIL, VIVACTIL.

Adverse Effects

Call your doctor immediately if you experience:

• irregular heart rate
• itching or skin rash
• large, hive-like swelling on face, eyelids, lips, tongue, throat, hands, legs, feet, or sex organs

Call your doctor if these symptoms continue:

• appetite decrease
• stomach pain
• coldness of hands or feet
• constipation
• diarrhea

- fatigue
- chills, cold sweats, confusion
- gas
- indigestion
- menstruation changes
- mood swings, irritability
- sinus headache
- joint pain or swollen joints
- muscle aches
- nausea or vomiting
- enlarged pupils
- sleep changes, such as insomnia or early awakening
- tics
- difficult or less frequent urination
- undesirable weight change
- pain, cramps, heavy bleeding
- loss of sexual ability or drive
- unusual tiredness or weakness
- hot flushes
- itching

Periodic Testing

Ask your doctor which of these tests should be done periodically while you are taking this drug:

By your doctor:

- blood pressure
- height and weight (in children)
- pulse
- reevaluation of continued need for therapy, dose of medication, and signs of dependence or abuse
- Test of Variables of Attention (TOVA)

By your parent(s):

- rating scales, such as Achenbach's Child Behavior Checklist, Conner's Parent Questionnaire

By your teacher(s):

- rating scales, such as Child Attention Problems, Conner's Teacher Rating Scale

Do Not Use

ALTERNATIVE TREATMENT:
See Methylphenidate (RITALIN), p. 476.

Dexmethylphenidate (dex meth il *fen* i date)
FOCALIN (Novartis)

FAMILY: Central Nervous System Stimulants

FDA BLACK BOX WARNING: DRUG ABUSE AND DEPENDENCE

Dexmethylphenidate should be given cautiously to emotionally unstable patients, such as those with a history of drug dependence or alcoholism, because such patients may increase dosage on their own initiative.

Chronically abusive use can lead to marked tolerance and psychic dependence with varying degrees of abnormal behavior. Frank psychotic episodes can occur, especially with parenteral abuse. Careful supervision is required during drug withdrawal, since severe depression as well as the effects of chronic overactivity can be unmasked. Long-term follow-up may be required because of the patient's basic personality disturbances.

Dexmethylphenidate was approved by the FDA in November 2001 for the management of attention deficit hyperactivity disorder (ADHD).

Dexmethylphenidate is identical to one-half of the chemical mixture that makes up the 40-year-old drug methylphenidate (see p. 476), a type of compound known as an optical isomer of the older drug. Both drugs are produced by the same company, Novartis Pharmaceuticals of New Jersey, but methylphenidate is also available in generic form.

In studies that Novartis submitted to the FDA in support of the newer drug's approval,

Drug treatment is not suitable for all children with attention deficit hyperactivity disorder (ADHD). Drug treatment is not intended for use in patients who exhibit symptoms of the disorder that result primarily from environmental factors (school, home), learning disabilities, and/or other psychiatric disorders, including psychosis.

several safety risks (similar to those of methylphenidate) were identified. They included loss of appetite that accompanied loss of weight, fluctuations in blood pressure and heart rate, abdominal pain, nausea, vomiting, and headaches. There was one case of convulsion reported, in addition to possible onsets of psychotic and other behavioral disturbances.[10]

In one study there was an average increase in systolic blood pressure (the upper number) of 20 millimeters of mercury (mmHg) and 30 beats per minute in heart rate in 12 children who had received a 10 milligram dose of dexmethylphenidate.[10] This is a significant increase, even in children.

A common strategy of drug companies trying to sell what is essentially an old drug with a new name is simply to "spin"; that is, to suggest that the improvement is more than merely cosmetic. Unfortunately, this strategy works, not only with patients but with many health professionals as well. Novartis tried to claim that "the duration of activity was statistically significantly longer" than with methylphenidate. But the FDA medical officer who reviewed Novartis's data disagreed: "This statement is misleading for several reasons."[10]

A number of possible drug interactions with methylphenidate apply with dexmethylphenidate. Both drugs, because they increase blood pressure, decrease the effectiveness of high blood pressure drugs. Studies have shown that methylphenidate may inhibit the breakdown of anticoagulants (blood thinners) such as warfarin (COUMADIN). In addition, the break-

down of anticonvulsants such as phenobarbital (LUMINAL, SOLFOTON), phenytoin (DILANTIN), and primidone (MYSOLINE) may be inhibited. Also, tricyclic antidepressants—amitriptyline (ELAVIL) and imipramine (TOFRANIL) are examples—and selective serotonin reuptake inhibitor (SSRI) antidepressants such as fluoxetine (PROZAC) and paroxetine (PAXIL) are inhibited in their breakdown.

It may be necessary to adjust the dose and monitor drug concentration in the blood or, in the case of warfarin, the effect on blood clotting when starting or stopping methylphenidate or dexmethylphenidate.[10]

Serious adverse reactions have occurred when methylphenidate has been used in combination with clonidine (CATAPRES). The same may apply to dexmethylphenidate.[10]

Dexmethylphenidate should not be used in combination with a group of antidepressants called monoamine oxidase (MAO) inhibitors or for at least 14 days after an MAO inhibitor because of the risk of an acute elevation in blood pressure. The MAO inhibitor drugs include furazolidone (FUROXONE), isocarboxazid (MARPLAN), phenelzine (NARDIL), procarbazine (MATULANE), selegiline (ELDEPRYL), and tranylcypromine (PARNATE).[10]

The conclusion of the editors of the highly respected *Medical Letter on Drugs and Therapeutics* in their May 13, 2002, review of dexmethylphenidate was: "There is no evidence that dexmethylphenidate (FOCALIN) offers an advantage over any other formulation of methylphenidate (RITALIN and others). Older drugs with better established dosages and longer safety records are preferred."[10]

Limited Use

Methylphenidate (meth ill *fen* i date)
(immediate release)
RITALIN (Novartis)
METHYLIN (Mallinckrodt)

Methylphenidate (meth ill *fen* i date)
(extended release)
CONCERTA (McNeil)
METADATE CD (Celltech)
METADATE ER (Celltech)
METHYLIN ER (Mallinckrodt)
RITALIN LA (Novartis)

Methylphenidate (meth ill *fen* i date)
(sustained release)
RITALIN-SR (Novartis)

GENERIC: not available

FAMILY: Central Nervous System Stimulants

PREGNANCY WARNING

Methylphenidate caused malformations in animal studies. It also caused DNA damage (a precursor to some tumors) as well as a rare liver tumor in mice. Because of the potential for serious adverse effects to the fetus, these drugs should not be used by pregnant women.

BREAST-FEEDING WARNING

No information is available from either human or animal studies. It is likely that this drug, like many drugs, is excreted in human milk, and, because of the potential for adverse effects in nursing infants, you should not take this drug while nursing.

Methylphenidate is approved by the FDA for the treatment of attention deficit hyperactivity disorder (ADHD) and narcolepsy. Methylphenidate increases the neurotransmitters dopamine and norepinephrine.[11] This drug is not a cure for either ADHD or narcolepsy.

The chemical structure of methylphenidate resembles that of amphetamine ("speed"like drugs).[12] U.S. federal law classifies methylphenidate as a Schedule-II controlled substance that requires a new handwritten prescription for each new and refill prescription.

FDA:BLACK BOX WARNING: DRUG ABUSE AND DEPENDENCE

Methylphenidate should be given cautiously to emotionally unstable patients, such as those with a history of drug dependence or alcoholism, because such patients may increase dosage on their own initiative.

Chronically abusive use can lead to marked tolerance and psychic dependence with varying degrees of abnormal behavior. Frank psychotic episodes can occur, especially with parenteral abuse. Careful supervision is required during drug withdrawal, since severe depression as well as the effects of chronic overactivity can be unmasked. Long-term follow-up may be required because of the patient's basic personality disturbances.

Narcolepsy is uncontrolled sleepiness, especially during the day. It is a rare condition. The use of most stimulants for narcolepsy lacks a well-documented benefit-to-risk ratio, since most studies are small.[13]

Little information on long-term safety and effectiveness of methylphenidate is available. The safety and efficacy in children under age six have not been established.

Suppression of growth (weight gain, and/or height) has been reported with the long-term use of stimulants in children.[11]

Nearly one-half of almost 13,000 poisoning exposures to methylphenidate involved children under age 6 who usually swallowed prescriptions belonging to others. From ages 6 to 12, one-third involved the child's own medication.[12] Over age 12, about one-third involved their own prescription and some poisonings were suicide attempts. Many incidents involved unintentionally administering an incorrect dose.[14]

Methylphenidate may induce psychosis with mood changes and hallucinations, especially when used for a long time and in higher doses.

> Drug treatment is not suitable for all children with attention deficit hyperactivity disorder (ADHD). Drug treatment is not intended for use in patients who exhibit symptoms of the disorder that result primarily from environmental factors (school, home), learning disabilities, and/or other psychiatric disorders, including psychosis.

Tics, a condition that waxes and wanes, occur mostly in children ages 7 to 13. There are reports of methylphenidate both decreasing vocal tics and worsening tics.[3]

Common adverse effects are headache, stomachache, and loss of appetite. Short-acting forms are more apt to cause dizziness, long-acting forms to cause insomnia.[2] The shell of the extended-release tablets (Concerta) may be observed in the stool. This does not mean the methylphenidate was not absorbed.

Before You Use This Drug

Do not use if you have or have had:

- agitation, anxiety, or tension
- mental depression
- glaucoma
- motor tics other than Tourette's syndrome

Tell your doctor if you have or have had:

- allergies, including to lactose or aspartame (NutraSweet)
- anorexia, bulimia, or failure to thrive[2]
- dependence on alcohol or drugs
- epilepsy
- gastrointestinal obstructions
- growth retardation[2]
- heart problems
- high blood pressure
- phenylketonuria (PKU)
- pregnancy or are breast-feeding
- psychosis
- seizures
- difficulty swallowing[2]

- Tourette's syndrome, including family history, or other motor tics

Tell your doctor about any other drugs you take, including aspirin, herbs, vitamins, and other nonprescription products.

When You Use This Drug

- Avoid using alcohol and recreational drugs.
- Avoid or limit caffeine.[2]
- Do not take more than the prescribed amount because of possible habituation.
- Do not drive, ride a bicycle, operate hazardous equipment, or perform dangerous activities if you experience dizziness or euphoria or if your narcolepsy is not controlled.

For ADHD:

- Reduce distractions, for example, sit toward the front of classrooms, or make lists of several small deadlines at work.[15]
- Select schools that have structured rules and expectations, and that provide regular feedback.[15]
- Recognize that your appetite may be greatest late in the day as methylphenidate wears off.
- Seek education about ADHD and counseling for skills development, or join support groups.
- Augment treatment with biofeedback, cognitive-behavioral therapy, educational skills training, parenting skills, and/or social skills.
- Try parent counseling to increase self-confidence, and learn to discipline consistently and appropriately, reinforcing good behavior with immediate rewards, reducing disruptive behavior, and decreasing family stress.[15,16]

For narcolepsy:

- Avoid alcohol and drugs that cause drowsiness. These include amitriptyline, benzodiazepines, buspirone, chlorpromazine, diphenhydramine, hydrocodone, meprobamate, methyldopa, phenobarbital, and propranolol.[17]

• Do not drive until sleepiness is controlled. Avoid other dangerous activities.

• Try scheduling naps.

• Tell any doctor, dentist, emergency help, or pharmacist you see that you take methylphenidate.

How to Use This Drug

• If you miss a dose, take it as soon as you remember, but skip it if it is almost time for the next dose or it is after 6 P.M. Then take any remaining doses for that day at regularly spaced intervals. **Do not take double doses.**

• Do not share your medication with others.

• Take the drug at the same time(s) each day.

• The initial dose of methylphenidate is taken in the morning. For immediate-release forms, doses may be repeated once or twice more, at least four hours apart. The last dose usually is taken by late afternoon or at least by 6 P.M. to avoid insomnia. Taking with food may prevent abdominal pain and insomnia. However, avoid high-fat meals, which may delay absorption and cause erratic effects.

• Chew chewable tablets with at least eight ounces of fluid. Fluid is necessary to prevent tablets from swelling in your throat and causing choking.

• Swallow extended-release tablets (Concerta) whole with or without food. It is preferable to be consistent about taking with or without food. Do not chew, crush, or divide.

• Swallow methylphenidate (METADATE CD) capsules whole with fluid, or empty entire capsule contents onto soft food, such as applesauce, jelly, or ketchup. Do not crush or chew. Swallow immediately. Follow with fluids. Do not store mixtures for future use.

• Store at room temperature with lid on tightly. Do not store in the bathroom. Do not expose to heat, moisture, or strong light.

• If you take more than prescribed, call the poison control center (800-222-1222) immediately.

Interactions with Other Drugs

The following drugs, biologics (e.g., vaccines, therapeutic antibodies), or foods are listed in *Evaluations of Drug Interactions* 2003 as causing "highly clinically significant" or "clinically significant" interactions when used together with any of the drugs in this section. In some sections with multiple drugs, the interaction may have been reported for one but not all drugs in this section, but we include the interaction because the drugs in this section are similar to one another. We have also included potentially serious interactions listed in the drug's FDA-approved professional package insert or in published medical journal articles. There may be other drugs, especially those in the families of drugs listed below, that also will react with this drug to cause severe adverse effects. Make sure to tell your doctor and pharmacist the drugs you are taking and tell them if you are taking any of these interacting drugs:

Use of methylphenidate with monoamine oxidase (MAO) inhibitors may cause a dangerous increase in blood pressure called hypertensive crisis. Do not take within two weeks of taking methylphenidate: deprenyl, ELDEPRYL, furazolidone, FUROXONE, isocarboxazid, MARPLAN, MATULANE, NARDIL, PARNATE, phenelzine, procarbazine, selegiline, tranylcypromine.

Methylphenidates may inhibit anticoagulants. Your doctor may do more tests and adjust doses of: COUMADIN, warfarin.

This drug may antagonize the effect of methylphenidate, and your dose may be adjusted: HALDOL, haloperidol.

Methylphenidate may cause tics. If tics are present, methylphenidate should be discontinued to determine if the medication is the cause before using it for tics: ORAP, pimozide.

Although generally classified as less apt to be clinically significant, methylphenidate can affect a number of other drugs that may result in the need for adjustments in doses.

Methylphenidate may increase anticonvulsants, and dose of anticonvulsant may be lowered: DILANTIN, LUMINAL, MYSOLINE, phenobarbital, phenytoin, primidone.

Use of other stimulants may add to the effects of methylphenidate. These include caffeine, ephedrine (in numerous over-the-counter medications, herbs, and club drugs), phenylpropanolamine (removed from market in 2000), pseudoephedrine (present in numerous cough and cold products), SUDAFED.

Methylphenidate may decrease the effectiveness of drugs used for high blood pressure, and doses may be adjusted: all blood pressure pills (see p. 45), ACE inhibitors (see p. 91), beta-blockers (see p. 87), calcium channel blockers (see p. 96), and reserpine.

Methylphenidate with certain antidepressants may require less antidepressant: desipramine, imipramine, NORPRAMIN, PERTOFRANE, SSRIs, TOFRANIL, tricyclics.

Many other drugs may interact with methylphenidate, such as AVANDAMET, GLUCOVANCE, METAGLIP, metformin, orlistat, and XENICAL. Check any concerns with your doctor or pharmacist.

Adverse Effects

Call your doctor immediately if you experience:

- unusual bleeding or bruising
- blood pressure increase
- chest pain
- confusion
- convulsions
- muscle cramps
- delusions
- feelings of estrangement, being automated, or extremities changing size
- hallucinations
- fast or irregular heartbeat
- fever
- mood changes
- uncontrolled movements of body
- pinpoint red spots, hives, or rash on skin
- black, bloody, or tarry stools
- tics
- bloody urine
- blurred or changed vision
- vocal outbursts that are uncontrolled
- weight loss

Signs of overdose:

- agitation
- blood pressure increase
- fast, pounding, or irregular heartbeat
- extreme confusion
- dry mouth
- false sense of well-being
- fever
- hallucination
- severe headache
- muscle twitch
- enlarged pupils
- overactive reflexes
- increased sweating
- shaking or trembling
- vomiting

If you suspect an overdose, call this number to contact your poison control center: (800) 222-1222.

Call your doctor if these symptoms continue:

- appetite decrease
- coughing increase
- dizziness
- drowsiness

- hair pulling, nail biting, or skin picking
- headache
- nausea
- nervousness
- sleeping problems
- stomach pain

Call your doctor immediately if these symptoms occur after you stop taking this drug:

- depression
- unusual behavior
- unusual tiredness or weakness

Periodic Testing

Ask your doctor which of these tests should be done periodically while you are taking this drug:

By your doctor:

- blood pressure and pulse
- complete blood count, differential and platelet counts
- monitoring of growth, both height and weight gain, in children

- reassessment of continued need for therapy, dose of medication, and signs of dependence or abuse
- Test of Variables of Attention

By parent(s):

- rating scales, such as Achenbach's Child Behavior Checklist, Conner's Parent Questionnaire

By teacher(s):

- rating scales, such as Child Attention Problems, Conner's Teacher Rating Scale

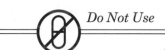

Do Not Use

ALTERNATIVE TREATMENT:
See Methylphenidate (RITALIN), p. 476.

Pemoline (pem *oh* leen)
CYLERT (Abbott)

FAMILY: Central Nervous System Stimulants

FDA BLACK BOX WARNING

Because of its association with life threatening hepatic failure, CYLERT should not ordinarily be considered as first-line drug therapy for ADHD. Because CYLERT provides an observable symptomatic benefit, patients who fail to show substantial clinical benefit within three weeks of completing dose titration, should be withdrawn from CYLERT.

Since CYLERT's marketing in 1975, 15 cases of acute hepatic failure have been reported to the FDA. While the absolute number of reported cases is not large, the rate of reporting ranges from 4 to 17 times the rate expected in the general population. This estimate may be conservative because of under-reporting and because the long latency between initiation of CYLERT treatment and the occurrence of hepatic failure may limit recognition of the association. If only a portion of actual cases were recognized and reported, the risk could be substantially higher.

Of the 15 cases reported as of December 1998, 12 resulted in death or liver transplantation, usually within four weeks of the onset of signs and symptoms of liver failure. The earliest onset of hepatic abnormalities occurred six months after initiation of CYLERT. Although some reports described dark urine and nonspecific prodromal symptoms (e.g., anorexia, malaise, and gastrointestinal symptoms), in other reports it was not clear if any prodromal symptoms preceded the onset of jaundice.

(continued on p. 481)

(continued from p. 480)

Treatment with CYLERT should be initiated only in individuals without liver disease and with normal baseline liver function tests. It is not clear if baseline and periodic liver function testing are predictive of these instances of acute liver failure; however it is generally believed that early detection of drug-induced hepatic injury along with immediate withdrawal of the suspect drug enhances the likelihood for recovery. Accordingly, the following liver monitoring program is recommended: Serum ALT (SGPT) levels should be determined at baseline, and every two weeks thereafter. If CYLERT therapy is discontinued and then restarted, liver function test monitoring should be done at baseline and reinitiated at the frequency above.

CYLERT should be discontinued if serum ALT (SGPT) is increased to a clinically significant level, or any increase ≥ 2 times the upper limit of normal, or if clinical signs and symptoms suggest liver failure.

The physician who elects to use CYLERT should obtain written informed consent from the patient prior to initiation of CYLERT therapy.

Pemoline (CYLERT) was withdrawn from the market in the UK in the fall of 1997 and in Canada in 1999 because of serious liver toxicity.[18]

Pemoline was originally approved for use in the United States in January 1975. The drug was withdrawn from the market in the UK in the fall of 1997 because of cases of serious liver toxicity.[18] The decision by British authorities was based on 33 serious liver reactions reported in the United States that led to liver transplantation in two cases and death in another six patients. In addition, the evidence for pemoline's effectiveness in treating ADHD is limited and there is no good evidence from appropriate clinical trials that it is effective for patients who have failed to respond to alternative drugs.

As of 1996, there had been 193 cases of liver toxicity, including nine deaths in children under age 20.[19]

Extensive safety labeling changes were finally required in this country in June 1999 that included a black-box warning about the drug's liver toxicity and the necessity for the prescribing physician to obtain the patient's written informed consent before prescribing pemoline. A black-box warning is the strongest type of warning that the FDA can require in a drug's professional product labeling or package insert. The text of pemoline's black-box warning appears above.[20]

Drug treatment is not suitable for all children with attention deficit hyperactivity disorder (ADHD). Drug treatment is not intended for use in patients who exhibit symptoms of the disorder that result from environmental factors (school, home) learning disabilities and/or other psychiatric disorders, including psychosis.

REFERENCES

1. *Physicians' Desk Reference.* 58th ed. Montvale, N.J.: Thomson PDR, 2004:1850–4.

2. Greydanus DE, Sloane MA, Rappley MD. Psychopharmacology of ADHD in adolescents. *Adolescent Medicine* 2002; 13:599–624.

3. Pliszka SR. The use of psychostimulants in the pediatric patient. *Pediatric Clinics of North America* 1998; 45:1085–98.

4. Weiss M, Murray C. Assessment and management of attention-deficit hyperactivity disorder in adults. *Canadian Medical Association Journal* 2003; 168:715–22.

5. Carrey NJ, Wiggins DM, Milin RP. Pharmacological treatment of psychiatric disorders in children and adolescents: Focus on guidelines for the primary care practitioner. *Drugs* 1996; 51:750–9.

6. Spencer T, Biederman J, Wilens T, et al. Efficacy of a mixed amphetamine salts compound in adults with attention-deficit/hyperactivity disorder. *Archives of General Psychiatry* 2001; 58:775–82.

7. *Physicians' Desk Reference.* 58th ed. Montvale, N.J.: Thomson PDR, 2004:3143–4.

8. Horrigan JP, Barnhill LJ. Low-dose amphetamine salts and adult attention-deficit/hyperactivity disorder. *Journal of Clinical Psychiatry* 2000; 61:414–7.

9. Wernicke JF, Faries D, Girod D, et al. Cardiovascular effects of atomoxetine in children, adolescents, and adults. *Drug Safety* 2003; 26:729–40.

10. Glass, RL. Food and Drug Administration Medical Officer Review of Dexmethylphenidate (Focalin), August 25, 2001.

11. *Physicians' Desk Reference.* 58th ed. Montvale, N.J.: Thomson PDR, 2004:2297–8.

12. Klein-Schwartz W, McGrath J. Poison centers' experience with methylphenidate abuse in pre-teens and adolescents. *Journal of the American Academy of Child and Adolescent Psychiatry* 2003; 42:288–94.

13. Littner M, Johnson SF, McCall WV, et al. Practice parameters for the treatment of narcolepsy: An update for 2000. *Sleep* 2001; 24:451–66.

14. Klein-Schwartz W. Pediatric methylphenidate exposures: 7-year experience of poison centers in the United States. *Clinical Pediatrics* 2003; 42:159–64.

15. Cyr M, Brown CS. Current drug therapy recommendations for the treatment of attention deficit hyperactivity disorder. *Drugs* 1998; 56:215–23.

16. Monastra VJ, Monastra DM, George S. The effects of stimulant therapy, EEG biofeedback, and parenting style on the primary symptoms of attention-deficit/hyperactivity disorder. *Applied Psychophysiology and Biofeedback* 2002; 27:231–49.

17. Roth T, Roehrs TA. Etiologies and sequelae of excessive daytime sleepiness. *Clinical Therapeutics* 1996; 18:562–76.

18. Volital (Pemoline) has been withdrawn. *Current Problems in Pharmacovigilance* 1997; 23:9–12.

19. Safer DJ, Zito JM, Gardner JE. Pemoline hepatotoxicity and postmarketing surveillance. *Journal of the American Academy of Child and Adolescent Psychiatry* 2001; 40:622–9.

20. *Physicians' Desk Reference.* 54th ed. Montvale, N.J.: Medical Economics Company, Inc., 2000:420–1.

14

MUSCLE RELAXANTS

LACK OF EFFECTIVENESS

Some of the widely prescribed muscle relaxants covered in this chapter have been on the market for more than 40 years. Yet five of these drugs were among the top 200 most frequently prescribed medications in the United States in 2002, with more than 30 million prescriptions dispensed. Of course, there is nothing necessarily wrong with older drugs per se. Many of the proven, safest, and most effective products are older drugs. The problem with this particular group of drugs is that they have not disappeared from the market despite substantial shortcomings, including a lack of effectiveness and some serious adverse effects. Worse yet, some have become "blockbusters."

Since their original marketing, there has been very little reliable evidence that these drugs actually relax muscles. The editors of *The Medical Letter on Drugs and Therapeutics,* a highly respected independent source of drug information written for pharmacists and physicians, wrote in 1961: *"Some oral drugs, whether or not offered as muscle relaxants, do have a relaxing effect, but the evidence indicates that this effect results not from any specific action on the muscles, but rather from their central-nervous-system depressing sedative action."* [1]

In other words, these drugs work by causing drowsiness. In fact, the FDA-approved professional product labeling or package inserts for these drugs indicate that they do not directly relax muscles in people.

In 1961, the *Medical Letter* editors also commented on the therapeutic value of these drugs: "In a few controlled trials placebos have given much better results than some of the drugs."

As with other therapeutic agents, the accumulating evidence of controlled clinical trials with muscle relaxants shows that neither favorable animal experiments, uncontrolled trials, nor wide acceptance by physicians can be relied upon to establish the value of a drug. [1]

The American Medical Association concluded their 1986 review of the muscle relaxants by saying: *"All spasmolytic (muscle-relaxing) drugs are superior to placebo in alleviating the symptoms and signs of localized muscle spasm. However, none of these agents have been shown conclusively to be more effective than analgesic-anti-inflammatory agents in relieving the pain of acute or chronic localized muscle spasm."* [2]

Although these muscle relaxants have been on the market for decades, their effectiveness, compared to that of anti-inflammatory drugs such as aspirin or ibuprofen, is still unknown. A 2003 systematic review of the muscle relaxants in the treatment of nonspecific low back pain found:

"Muscle relaxants are effective in the management of nonspecific low back pain, but the adverse effects require that they be used with caution. Trials are needed that evaluate if muscle relaxants are more effective than analgesics or nonsteroidal anti-inflammatory drugs."[3]

DRUG PROFILES

 Do Not Use

ALTERNATIVE TREATMENT:
Rest, exercise, physical therapy, and an anti-inflammatory drug such as aspirin.

Carisoprodol (kar eye soe *proe* dole)
SOMA (Wallace)

Carisoprodol with Aspirin
(kar eye soe *proe* dole with *as* per in)
SOMA COMPOUND (Wallace)

Carisoprodol, Aspirin, and Codeine
(car eye soe *proe* dole, *as* per in, and *koe* deen)
SOMA COMPOUND WITH CODEINE (Wallace)

FAMILY: Muscle Relaxants

Carisoprodol has been sold in this country since April 1959. The drug is approved by the FDA in addition to rest, physical therapy, and other measures for the relief of discomfort associated with acute, painful muscle conditions. Carisoprodol does not directly relax tense skeletal muscles in humans and the drug's effect may be related to its sedative properties.[4]

The body breaks down carisoprodol to meprobamate (EQUANIL, MILTOWN), an old tranquilizer, which is also listed as a **Do Not Use** drug (see p. 234). Meprobamate is a controlled substance and some feel that carisoprodol should also be listed as a controlled substance. In addition, carisoprodol, like meprobamate, has also been shown to have a potential for abuse.[5]

Carisoprodol has not been shown to be any more effective than painkillers or anti-inflammatory drugs such as aspirin for relieving the pain of local muscle spasm.

Some people taking carisoprodol have experienced drowsiness, lightheadedness, dizziness, nausea, vomiting, heartburn, abdominal distress, constipation, diarrhea, and loss of appetite as adverse effects.[2]

Carisoprodol occasionally causes a reaction within the first few minutes or hours after the first dose. Symptoms of a reaction are agitation, confusion, unsteadiness, disorientation, weakness, speech or vision problems, and temporary inability to move arms or legs.

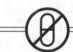 *Do Not Use*

ALTERNATIVE TREATMENT:
Rest, exercise, physical therapy, and an anti-inflammatory drug such as aspirin.

Chlorzoxazone (klor *zox* a zone)
PARAFON FORTE DSC (Ortho-McNeil)

FAMILY: Muscle Relaxants

Chlorzoxazone was first sold in the United States in August 1958. The drug is approved by the FDA in addition to rest, physical therapy, and other measures for the relief of discomfort associated with acute, painful musculoskeletal conditions. The way chlorzoxazone works has not been clearly identified but may be related to its sedative properties. Chlorzoxazone does not directly relax tense skeletal muscles in people.[6]

Chlorzoxazone has not been shown to be any more effective than painkillers or anti-inflammatory drugs such as aspirin for relieving the pain of local muscle spasm.[2]

Some people taking chlorzoxazone have experienced drowsiness, headache, upset stomach, nausea, vomiting, heartburn, constipation, diarrhea, and loss of appetite as adverse effects.

Serious, sometimes fatal, liver toxicity has been reported in patients taking chlorzoxazone. The way chlorzoxazone causes liver toxicity is unknown but appears to be idiosyncratic and unpredictable. You should stop taking chlorzoxazone and contact your physician immediately if you develop the symptoms of liver toxicity, such as fever, rash, loss of appetite, nausea, vomiting, fatigue, abdominal pain, dark urine, or jaundice (yellowing of the skin or eyes).[6]

The use of chlorzoxazone together with alcohol or other central nervous system depressants may have an additive sedative effect.

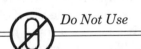

Do Not Use

ALTERNATIVE TREATMENT:
Rest, exercise, physical therapy, and an anti-inflammatory drug such as aspirin.

Cyclobenzaprine (sye kloe *ben* za preen)
FLEXERIL (McNeil Consumer & Specialty Pharmaceuticals)

FAMILY: Muscle Relaxants

Cyclobenzaprine was approved for marketing by the FDA in August 1977. This drug is approved, in addition to rest and physical therapy, for relief of muscle spasm associated with acute, painful musculoskeletal conditions.[7] Cyclobenzaprine is very close in chemical structure to the tricyclic antidepressant amitriptyline (ELAVIL) (see p. 204) and may cause some of the same adverse effects and dangerous drug interactions.

Cyclobenzaprine has not been shown to be any more effective than painkillers or anti-inflammatory drugs such as aspirin for relieving the pain of local muscle spasm.[2]

A systematic analysis of clinical trials in which cyclobenzaprine was used to manage low back pain found that the drug was more effective than a placebo. However, the authors of the analysis commented: "Studies comparing the relative value of acetaminophen, nonsteroidal anti-inflammatory drugs, and cyclobenzaprine individually and in combination for the treatment of back pain are needed."[8]

Cyclobenzaprine must not be used with the family of antidepressants known as monoamine oxidase (MAO) inhibitors or within 14 days after stopping an MAO inhibitor. Seizure resulting from a high fever and deaths have occurred in patients receiving cyclobenzaprine (or structurally similar tricyclic antidepressants) and MAO inhibitor drugs.

The risk of seizure is enhanced when cyclobenzaprine is taken with the pain reliever tramadol (ULTRAM) or tramadol with acetaminophen (ULTRACET). Both Ultram and Ultracet are also listed as **Do Not Use** drugs (see p. 325).

Cyclobenzaprine, especially when used with alcohol or other central nervous system (CNS) depressants, can impair mental or physical abilities, or both, required for the performance of hazardous tasks, such as operating machinery or driving a motor vehicle. In the elderly, the frequency and severity of adverse events associated with the use of cyclobenzaprine, with or without the use of other drugs, are increased.

In 1999 cyclobenzaprine's manufacturer applied to the FDA to market the drug over the counter in a five-milligram strength. The advisory committee reviewing the studies submitted by the company found that "the efficacy of 5-mg Flexeril had not been established . . . and that . . . by day 7 about 70% of back spasm was resolved—including those on placebo."[9]

Remarkably, in 2003 the FDA approved cyclobenzaprine in the 5-milligram strength as a prescription drug. The new strength is being promoted as less sedating. Although this is undoubtedly true, sedation may still be the way this drug works.

Do Not Use

ALTERNATIVE TREATMENT:
*Rest, exercise, physical therapy, and an
anti-inflammatory drug such as aspirin.*

Methocarbamol (meth oh *kar* ba mole)
ROBAXIN (Schwarz)

FAMILY: Muscle Relaxants

Methocarbamol was first sold in the United
States in July 1957. The drug is FDA-approved
to be used with rest, physical therapy, and other
measures for the relief of discomfort associated
with acute, painful musculoskeletal conditions.
The way methocarbamol works has not been
clearly identified but may be related to its sedative properties. Methocarbamol does not directly relax tense skeletal muscles in people.[10]

Methocarbamol has not been shown to be
any more effective than painkillers or anti-
inflammatory drugs such as aspirin for relieving the pain of local muscle spasm.[2]

Methocarbamol's adverse effects include
drowsiness, lightheadedness, dizziness, nausea, vomiting, heartburn, abdominal distress,
constipation, diarrhea, and loss of appetite.

Since methocarbamol possesses a central nervous system (CNS) depressant effect, patients
must be careful about the combined effects
when the drug is used with alcohol and other
CNS depressants.

Do Not Use

ALTERNATIVE TREATMENT:
*Rest, exercise, physical therapy, and an
anti-inflammatory drug such as aspirin.*

Orphenadrine (or *fen* a dreen)
NORFLEX (3M)

Orphenadrine, Aspirin, and Caffeine
NORGESIC FORTE (3M)

FAMILY: Muscle Relaxants
              Painkillers

Orphenadrine was cleared for sale in the
United States in November 1959 and is approved by the FDA in addition to rest, physical
therapy, and other measures for the relief of discomfort associated with acute painful musculoskeletal conditions. The way orphenadrine
works has not been clearly identified. The drug
does not directly relax tense skeletal muscles.[11]

Orphenadrine has not been shown to be

ANTICHOLINERGIC EFFECTS

WARNING: SPECIAL MENTAL AND PHYSICAL ADVERSE EFFECTS

Older adults are especially sensitive to the harmful anticholinergic (see Glossary, p. 889) effects of
orphenadrine because of its similarity to the antihistamines. Drugs in this family should not be used
unless absolutely necessary.

Mental Effects: confusion, delirium, short-term
memory problems, disorientation, and impaired
attention.

Physical Effects: dry mouth, constipation, difficulty urinating (especially for a man with an
enlarged prostate), blurred vision, decreased
sweating with increased body temperature, sexual
dysfunction, and worsening of glaucoma.

any more effective than painkillers or anti-inflammatory drugs, such as aspirin alone, for relieving the pain of local muscle spasm. It has a higher risk of adverse effects than these painkillers. Because orphenadrine is similar to a family of drugs called antihistamines, used to relieve symptoms of hay fever and other allergies, it may cause some of the same adverse effects and dangerous drug interactions as antihistamines. Some people taking orphenadrine experience blurred vision, dry mouth, mild excitement, temporary dizziness, and lightheadedness. Many of these effects occur more often in older adults. Orphenadrine is particularly dangerous for people who have glaucoma, myasthenia gravis, heart problems, or an enlarged prostate.

In the combination product Norgesic Forte, the aspirin by itself may be helpful along with rest, exercise, physical therapy, and/or other treatment recommended by your doctor. When taking this product you are, in fact, taking three drugs, each with its own cautions, adverse effects, and drug interactions. Like other fixed-combination products, this combination curtails the ability to vary doses of each drug.

REFERENCES

1. Muscle Relaxants—I. *Medical Letter on Drugs and Therapeutics* 1961; 3:89–90.

2. AMA Department of Drugs. *AMA Drug Evaluations.* 6th ed. Chicago: American Medical Association, 1986:232–3.

3. Van Tulder MW, Touray T, Furlan AD, et al. Muscle relaxants for nonspecific low back pain: A systematic review within the framework of the Cochrane Collaboration. *Spine* 2003; 28:1978–92.

4. *Physicians' Desk Reference.* 57th ed. Montvale, N.J.: Thomson PDR, 2003:3254–7.

5. Reeves RR, Carter OS, Pinkofsky HB, et al. Carisoprodol (soma): Abuse potential and physician unawareness. *Journal of Addictive Disease* 1999; 18:51–6.

6. *Physicians' Desk Reference.* 56th ed. Montvale, N.J.: Medical Economics, Inc., 2002:2582.

7. *Physicians' Desk Reference.* 57th ed. Montvale, N.J.: Thomson PDR, 2003:1897–8.

8. Browning R, Jackson JL, O'Malley PG. Cyclobenzaprine and back pain: a meta-analysis. *Archives of Internal Medicine* 2001; 161:1613–20.

9. Minutes of the Food and Drug Administration's Nonprescription Drugs and Arthritis Advisory Committees, July 20, 1999.

10. *Physicians' Desk Reference.* 57th ed. Montvale, N.J.: Thomson PDR, 2003:1294–5.

11. *Physicians' Desk Reference.* 57th ed. Montvale, N.J.: Thomson PDR, 2003:1888–9.

15

DRUGS FOR ENLARGED PROSTATE

BENIGN PROSTATIC HYPERTROPHY

The prostate gland becomes enlarged in many men as they age.[1] This condition is known as benign prostatic hyperplasia (BPH), or benign prostatic hypertrophy. BPH rarely causes symptoms before age 40, but more than half of men in their sixties, and as many as 90% in their seventies and eighties, have some symptoms of BPH.[2]

Many of the symptoms of BPH result from the partial obstruction of the urethra, resulting in thickening of the bladder. This thickening causes the bladder to hold less urine, leading to urinary frequency during the day and night. The gradual loss of bladder function may also result in incomplete emptying of the bladder. The symptoms of BPH vary, but the most common ones involve changes or problems with urination, such as

- a hesitant, interrupted, weak stream
- urgency and leaking or dribbling
- more frequent urination, especially at night

The symptoms of BPH arise from both prostate enlargement leading to mechanical obstruction and increased tone of the smooth muscle in the prostate. The size of the prostate does not always determine how severe the obstruction or the symptoms will be. Some men with greatly enlarged glands have little obstruction and few symptoms while others, whose glands are less enlarged, have more blockage and greater problems.[2]

The alpha-blocker family, which acts to relax the smooth muscle of the prostate, includes five drugs: alfuzosin (UROXATRAL), doxazosin (CARDURA), prazosin (MINIPRESS), tamsulosin (FLOMAX), and terazosin (HYTRIN). Three of these drugs—doxazosin, prazosin, and terazosin—are approved by the FDA to treat high blood pressure. Alfuzosin and tamsulosin are FDA-approved to treat BPH, or enlarged prostate gland. Terazosin and doxazosin are approved for both high blood pressure and enlarged prostate. Prazosin is not approved for the treatment of BPH. We have listed the alpha-blockers as **Do Not Use** drugs for the treatment of high blood pressure (see p. 102 in Chapter 4, Drugs for Heart Conditions).

Another type of drug for the treatment of BPH is the 5-alpha reductase inhibitor finasteride (PROSCAR), which acts to shrink the prostate and was approved by the FDA in June 1992 (see p. 494). Finasteride was also marketed in December 1997 as PROPECIA for hair regrowth. A second drug in this category, dutasteride (AVODART), has recently been approved, but there is no study that compares its usefulness to finasteride, itself a last-choice drug for treating BPH (see below).

A large clinical trial published in 1996 compared the effect of the 5-alpha reductase inhibitor finasteride with the alpha-blocker terazosin in more than 1,000 men with BPH. This study lasted one year. Overall, it was found that terazosin was effective therapy, finasteride was not, and the combination of terazosin and finasteride was not more effective than terazosin alone. However, the researchers did find that finasteride was effective in a group of men with very large glands, while terazosin was effective in men with a very large or smaller prostate gland.[3]

A different conclusion was reached in a clinical trial published in 2003 that involved over 3,000 men and lasted 4.5 years. This trial is known as the Medical Therapy of Prostatic Symptoms Study, or MTOPS. It concluded that the combination of finasteride and terazosin was superior to either of the drugs used alone.[4] There are several possible reasons for these divergent results.

First, the MTOPS trial lasted much longer than the trial published in 1996, 4.5 years versus one year. This is important because finasteride does not act rapidly and often requires six months to a year to work.[5] Second, the two trials measured different outcomes. The 1996 trial measured symptom score and peak urinary flow rate, while the MTOPS trial measured clinical progression of BPH, described as the first occurrence of an increase over baseline of at least four points in the symptom score: acute urinary retention, kidney problems, recurrent urinary tract infection, and urinary incontinence.

A possible association between finasteride use and male breast cancer was revealed in the MTOPS trial when four cases of breast cancer were reported in men taking finasteride. This rate is nearly 200 times greater than what is seen in men in the general population.[6]

Finasteride has also been tested in a very large clinical trial called the Prostate Cancer Prevention Trial (PCPT) with mixed results.

There was a 25% relative reduction (6% absolute reduction) in cancers in healthy men taking finasteride. This means that for every 17 men treated with finasteride for 7 years, one cancer would be prevented. There was, however, a 1.7-fold increase in the risk of an aggressive tumor in those men who developed cancer.[7]

We were opposed to the PCPT at its inception because of the theoretical harm that could come from giving healthy men finasteride. Now that the potential for harm is no longer theoretical, our advice is that finasteride should not be used for prostate cancer prevention.

If your BPH symptoms are minimal, no treatment is necessary, no matter what the size of your prostate gland. If you have BPH symptoms and do not have a very enlarged gland, then an alpha-blocker such as terazosin would be the best choice. If your prostate is very enlarged, treatment with an alpha-blocker would again be the best choice. Finasteride should be used only if an alpha-blocker failed to relieve your symptoms.

Surgical procedures are also an option for men with severe symptomatic BPH, in addition to the alpha-blockers and the 5-alpha reductase inhibitors.[8]

DRUG PROFILES

Alpha-blockers

Do Not Use Until Seven Years After Release

Alfuzosin (al *foo* zoe sin)
(Do Not Use Until 2010)
UROXATRAL (Sanofi-Synthelabo)

GENERIC: not available

Limited Use

Doxazosin (*dox* a zoe sin)
CARDURA (Pfizer)

GENERIC: available

Tamsulosin (tam *soo* loh sin)
FLOMAX (Boehringer Ingelheim)

GENERIC: not available

Terazosin (ter *ay* zoe sin)
HYTRIN (Abbott)

GENERIC: available

FAMILY: Alpha-blockers

PREGNANCY WARNING

These drugs cross the placenta, exposing the fetus to the drug and causing fetal harm in animal studies, including increased fetal resorptions, decreased fetal weight, and reduced fetal survival. After birth, the drugs caused slower body weight gain, delayed appearance of features and reflexes, and pup death. Because of the potential for serious adverse effects to the fetus, these drugs should not be used by pregnant women. Alfuzosin and tamsulosin are not approved for use in women.

BREAST-FEEDING WARNING

For women who take the alpha-blockers doxazosin or terazosin to lower blood pressure:

Doxazosin accumulates in rat breast milk to a concentration 20 times greater than the level in maternal plasma. Because of the potential for serious adverse effects to the fetus, these drugs should not be used by pregnant women.

The alpha-blocker family includes five drugs: alfuzosin (UROXATRAL), doxazosin (CARDURA), prazosin (MINIPRESS), tamsulosin (FLOMAX), and terazosin (HYTRIN). Three of these drugs—doxazosin, prazosin, and tera-

We have listed these alpha-blockers as **Do Not Use** drugs for the treatment of high blood pressure. See p. 102 in Chapter 4, Drugs for Heart Conditions, for more information.

BLOOD-PRESSURE-LOWERING EFFECTS

The alpha-blocking drugs can cause a sudden drop in blood pressure, especially in the upright position, that can lead to dizziness and fainting. These adverse effects are most common with the first dose but can also occur when there is a dosage increase, or if treatment is interrupted for more than a few days. To decrease the likelihood of excessive blood pressure lowering, it is essential that treatment be started with a low dose.

---

zosin—are approved by the FDA to treat high blood pressure. Alfuzosin and tamsulosin are FDA-approved to treat benign prostatic hyperplasia (BPH), or enlarged prostate gland. Terazosin and doxazosin are approved for both high blood pressure and enlarged prostate.

Alpha-blockers relieve the symptoms of BPH by relaxing smooth muscle in the prostate. Overall, alpha-blockers appear to be similarly effective in relieving the symptoms of BPH.[8]

If your BPH symptoms are minimal, no treatment is necessary, no matter what the size of your prostate gland. If you have BPH symptoms and do not have a very enlarged gland, then an alpha-blocker such as terazosin would be the best choice. If your prostate is very enlarged, treatment with an alpha-blocker would again be the best choice.

Alfuzosin is the newest alpha-blocker on the market in the United States but has been used in Europe since 1987.[9] This drug differs from the other drugs in this family in that it must not be used in people with moderate to severe liver problems. In addition, alfuzosin must not be used together with ketoconazole (NIZORAL), itraconazole (SPORANOX), or ritonavir (NORVIR) because blood levels of alfuzosin will be increased.[10]

Alfuzosin also causes an adverse effect of the heart known as QTc interval prolongation.[10]

THE HEALTH RESEARCH GROUP'S SEVEN-YEAR RULE

You should wait at least seven years from the date of release to take any new drug unless it is one of those rare "breakthrough" drugs that offer you a documented therapeutic advantage over older proven drugs. New drugs are tested in a relatively small number of people before being released, and serious adverse effects or life-threatening drug interactions may not be detected until the new drug has been taken by hundreds of thousands of people. A number of new drugs have been withdrawn within their first seven years after release. Also, warnings about serious new adverse reactions have been added to the labeling of a number of drugs, or new drug interactions have been detected, usually within the first seven years after a drug's release.

The QTc interval is the length of time it takes the large chambers of the heart (ventricles) to electrically discharge and recharge. A prolongation of the QTc interval may lead to a type of heart rhythm disturbance, or cardiac arrhythmia, known as torsades de pointes and sudden death. *Torsades de pointes* is a French phrase that means "twisted point," describing the appearance of this rhythm disturbance on the EKG tracing.

Men with a known history of QTc prolongation or who are using drugs known to prolong the QTc interval should not take alfuzosin. The only extensive list of drugs that prolong QTc intervals is maintained by the University of Arizona Health Sciences Center: www.torsades.org.

Before You Use This Drug

Do not use if you have or have had:

- prostate cancer
- allergies to the drug or any component of the capsule or tablet
- liver problems

Tell your doctor if you have or have had:

- angina (chest pain)
- high blood pressure (symptomatic)
- previous low blood pressure from other drugs
- heart problems
- history of prolonged QTc intervals
- kidney problems

Tell your doctor about any other drugs you take, including aspirin, herbs, vitamins, and other nonprescription products.

When You Use This Drug

- Avoid alcohol.
- Try to have a companion stay with you for a few hours when you take your first dose. Move any object that would be dangerous if you fell onto it, during day or night. This includes unanchored rugs. Change positions gradually. If you are lying down, hang your legs over the side of the bed for a few minutes, then get up slowly. When getting up from a chair, stay by the chair until you are sure that you are not dizzy, especially after the first dose. If you become dizzy, sit or lie down.
- Do not drive or operate hazardous equipment until you know whether or not you become drowsy or dizzy when using an alpha-blocker, especially for the first 24 hours after the first dose, whenever a dose is increased, or when use is resumed after interruption of therapy.
- Take your blood pressure periodically.
- Tell any doctor, dentist, emergency help, pharmacist, or surgeon you see that you use an alpha-blocker.
- Rule out the presence of prostate cancer before starting the drug.
- It may take two to six weeks before you experience improvement in symptoms.

How to Use This Drug

• If you miss a dose, take it as soon as you remember, but skip it if it is almost time for the next dose. **Do not take double doses.**

• Do not share your medication with others.

• Take the drug at the same time(s) each day. If you are prescribed more than one dose per day, space the doses at equal intervals.

• Swallow alfuzosin tablet(s) whole, with food, and with the same meal each day. Do not chew or crush.

• Swallow doxazosin tablets in the morning or evening.

• Swallow tamsulosin capsule(s) whole about 30 minutes after the same meal each day, usually breakfast. Do not chew, crush, or open capsules.

• Swallow terazosin capsule(s) at bedtime.

• Store capsules or tablets at room temperature with lid on tightly. Do not expose to heat, moisture, or strong light. Keep out of reach of children.

Interactions with Other Drugs

The following drugs, biologics (e.g., vaccines, therapeutic antibodies), or foods are listed in *Evaluations of Drug Interactions* 2003 as causing "highly clinically significant" or "clinically significant" interactions when used together with any of the drugs in this section. In some sections with multiple drugs, the interaction may have been reported for one but not all drugs in this section, but we include the interaction because the drugs in this section are similar to one another. We have also included potentially serious interactions listed in the drug's FDA-approved professional package insert or in published medical journal articles. There may be other drugs, especially those in the families of drugs listed below, that also will react with this drug to cause severe adverse effects. Make sure to tell your doctor and pharmacist the drugs you are taking and tell them if you are taking any of these interacting drugs:

amlodipine, bepridil, CALAN, CARDENE, CARDIZEM, cimetidine, DIBENZYLINE, diltiazem, DYNACIRC, felodipine, ISOPTIN, isradipine, moxisylyte, nicardipine, nifedipine, nimodipine, NIMOTOP, nisoldipine, NORVASC, phenoxybenzamine, phentolamine, PLENDIL, PROCARDIA, REGITINE, SULAR, TAGAMET, VASCOR, verapamil.

For alfuzosin: itraconazole, ketoconazole, NIZORAL, NORVIR, ritonavir, SPORANOX.

Adverse Effects

Call your doctor immediately if you experience:

• blood pressure decrease
• difficulty breathing
• chest pain
• dizziness, lightheadedness, or fainting
• headache
• difficulty sleeping
• painful or prolonged erection
• fast, irregular, or pounding heartbeat
• numbness or tingling of hands and feet
• skin itching, rash, or spots
• swelling of ankles or feet
• swelling of tongue, lips, neck, or face
• uncontrollable urination
• unusual weakness or tiredness
• drowsiness
• back pain
• diarrhea
• nausea
• stuffy or runny nose
• abnormal ejaculation

Call your doctor if these symptoms continue:

• wheezing
• constipation
• diarrhea

- belching
- tenderness around eyes
- trouble swallowing
- voice changes
- heartburn
- tightness in chest
- drowsiness, fatigue, sleepiness
- dry cough or cough producing mucus
- dry mouth
- ringing in ears
- sore gums or throat
- headache
- joint pain
- hoarseness
- nasal congestion
- nausea or vomiting
- indigestion
- nervousness, restlessness, or irritability
- pain in joints, arms, back, or legs
- sexual dysfunction, such as diminished ejaculation (especially tamsulosin) or impotence
- blurred vision
- undesired weight gain (especially with doxazosin and terazosin)
- abdominal pain
- fever

Signs of overdose:

- profound drowsiness
- severe headache
- decreased heart rate
- depressed reflexes
- low blood pressure
- seizures

If you suspect an overdose, call this number to contact your poison control center: (800) 222-1222.

Periodic Tests

Ask your doctor which of these tests should be done periodically while you are taking this drug:

- blood pressure
- digital rectal exam
- peak urinary flow rate
- PSA (prostate-specific antigen)
- questionnaires on symptom relief

5-Alpha Reductase Inhibitors

Limited Use

Finasteride (fin *as* tur ide)
PROSCAR (Merck)

GENERIC: not available
FAMILY: 5-Alpha Reductase Inhibitors

PREGNANCY WARNING

RISK TO MALE FETUS

Women should not handle crushed or broken Proscar tablets when they are pregnant or may potentially be pregnant because of the possibility of absorption of finasteride and the subsequent potential risk to a male fetus. Proscar tablets are coated and will prevent contact with the active ingredient finasteride during normal handling, provided that the tablets have not been broken or crushed.

Finasteride is used to control symptoms of enlarged prostate called benign prostatic hyperplasia (BPH). Enlargement of the prostate gland impedes urination, causing a weak stream, double voiding, inability to empty the bladder completely, and urinary tract infections. BPH affects 50% of men over age 60 and 90% of men in their seventies and eighties.[2]

Finasteride blocks an enzyme called 5-alpha reductase that is necessary to convert the male sex hormone testosterone to another hormone

Do not use finasteride to prevent prostate cancer. The use of this drug for cancer prevention has resulted in more aggressive cancer in men who do develop prostate cancer (see the introduction to this chapter, p. 489).

A possible association between finasteride use and male breast cancer was revealed in a large clinical trial when four cases of breast cancer were reported in men taking finasteride. This rate is nearly 200 times greater than what is seen in men in the general population (see the introduction to this chapter, p. 489).

that causes the prostate to grow. As a result, the size of the prostate gland is decreased.

The other family of drugs approved by the FDA to treat BPH is the alpha-blockers. These drugs are preferred to finasteride and are discussed on p. 490 of this chapter.

A large clinical trial compared the effect of finasteride with terazosin in more than 1,000 men with BPH. This study lasted one year. Overall, this study concluded that terazosin was effective therapy, finasteride was not, and the combination of terazosin and finasteride was not more effective than terazosin alone. However, the researchers did find that finasteride was effective in a group of men with very large glands, while terazosin was effective in men with a very large or smaller prostate gland.[3]

Another study found that long-term use of finasteride reduces the probability of surgery for an enlarged prostate gland.[11] But, the editorial accompanying this study took a different view: "Treatment with finasteride to prevent these complications may be unwarranted for most men with symptoms of this disorder [BPH]." The editorial relates a hypothetical conversation between a man asking about finasteride and reducing the risk of prostate surgery and a very good doctor who explains the results of the study.

Patient: Doctor, my wife just read about this new drug for the prostate. She said it was like an insurance policy. You pay a little premium each day to avoid needing surgery later.

Physician: That is a good way to think about it. After four years, 13 of 100 men had

complete urine blockage or needed surgery for their prostate. A drug called finasteride reduced the chances of these problems; instead of occurring in 13 of 100 men, they occurred in 7 of 100. In other words, about 6 out of 100 men benefited after four years of taking the drug.

Patient: So 100 men paid the premium for four years and 6 of them got the benefit?

Physician: You seem to have the basic point. Those men who kept taking the drug also said that their urinary symptoms were a little better—an improvement of 2 points on a 35-point scale. But a few men taking the drug had impotence, breast tenderness, and loss of energy.[12]

If your BPH symptoms are minimal, no treatment is necessary, no matter what the size of your prostate gland. If you have BPH symptoms and do not have a very enlarged gland, then an alpha-blocker such as terazosin would be the best choice. If your prostate is more enlarged, treatment with an alpha-blocker would again be the best choice. Finasteride should be used only if an alpha-blocker fails to relieve your symptoms.

Surgical procedures are also an option for men with severe symptomatic BPH in addition to the alpha-blockers and the 5-alpha reductase inhibitors.[8]

Before You Use This Drug

Tell your doctor if you have or have had:

- allergy to finasteride or any of its components
- liver problems
- difficulties urinating

Tell your doctor about any other drugs you take, including aspirin, herbs, vitamins, and other nonprescription products.

Before you start this drug, have your doctor do a digital rectal exam and baseline PSA test, and check that you do not have conditions with similar symptoms, such as infection, prostate cancer, stricture disease, or hypotonic bladder.

When You Use This Drug

- Do not let any women who are pregnant or could become pregnant crush your tablets or touch your medication.
- Use a condom to protect any women you have intercourse with from pregnancy, since finasteride in semen can harm the fetus.
- Do not drink alcohol or coffee in the evening.
- Rule out the presence of prostate cancer before starting this drug.
- Read information about your prescription each time you refill it in case new information has become available.

How to Use This Drug

- If you miss a dose, take it as soon as you remember, but skip it if it is almost time for the next dose. **Do not take double doses.**
- Do not share your medication with others.
- Take the drug at the same time(s) each day.
- Take with or without food.
- Swallow tablets whole or crushed.
- Store at room temperature with lid on tightly. Do not store in the bathroom. Do not expose to heat, moisture, or strong light. Keep out of reach of children.

- Check with your doctor before discontinuing finasteride.

Interactions with Other Drugs

Evaluations of Drug Interactions 2003 lists no drugs, biologics (e.g., vaccines, therapeutic antibodies), or foods as causing "highly clinically significant" or "clinically significant" interactions when used together with the drugs in this section. We also found no interactions in the drugs' FDA-approved professional package inserts. However, as the number of new drugs approved for marketing increases and as more experience is gained with these drugs over time, new interactions may be discovered.

Adverse Effects

Call your doctor immediately if you experience:

- pelvic or testicular pain
- skin rash
- swelling of lips
- breast enlargement or tenderness

Call your doctor if these symptoms continue:

- abdominal pain
- back pain
- decreased amount of ejaculation
- dizziness
- gas
- headache
- impotence
- diarrhea
- testicular pain

Periodic Tests

Ask your doctor which of these tests should be done periodically while you are taking this drug:

- digital rectal examination

REFERENCES

1. Medina JJ, Parra RO, Moore RG. Benign prostatic hyperplasia (the aging prostate). *Medical Clinics of North America* 1999; 83:1213–29.

2. National Institute of Diabetes and Digestive and Kidney Diseases. Prostate Enlargement: Benign Prostatic Hyperplasia, February 1, 2004. Available at: http://kidney.niddk.nih.gov/kudiseases/pubs/prostateenlargement/index.htm#common. Accessed March 1, 2004.

3. Lepor H, Williford WO, Barry MJ, et al. The efficacy of terazosin, finasteride, or both in benign prostatic hyperplasia. Veterans Affairs Cooperative Studies Benign Prostatic Hyperplasia Study Group. *New England Journal of Medicine* 1996; 335:533–9.

4. McConnell JD, Roehrborn CG, Bautista OM, et al. The long-term effect of doxazosin, finasteride, and combination therapy on the clinical progression of benign prostatic hyperplasia. *New England Journal of Medicine* 2003; 349:2387–98.

5. Vaughan ED Jr. Medical management of benign prostatic hyperplasia—are two drugs better than one? *New England Journal of Medicine* 2003; 349:2449–51.

6. Lee SC, Ellis RJ. Male breast cancer during finasteride therapy. *Journal of the National Cancer Institute* 2004; 96:338–9.

7. Thompson IM, Goodman PJ, Tangen CM, et al. The influence of finasteride on the development of prostate cancer. *New England Journal of Medicine* 2003; 349:215–24.

8. Barry MJ, Roehrborn CG. Benign prostatic hyperplasia. *British Medical Journal* 2001; 323:1042–6.

9. Alfuzosin (uroxatral)—another alpha1-blocker for benign prostatic hyperplasia. *Medical Letter on Drugs and Therapeutics* 2004; 46:1–2.

10. *Physicians' Desk Reference.* 58th ed. Montvale, N.J.: Thomson PDR, 2004:3036–8.

11. McConnell JD, Bruskewitz R, Walsh P, et al. The effect of finasteride on the risk of acute urinary retention and the need for surgical treatment among men with benign prostatic hyperplasia. Finasteride Long-Term Efficacy and Safety Study Group. *New England Journal of Medicine* 1998; 338:557–63.

12. Wasson JH. Finasteride to prevent morbidity from benign prostatic hyperplasia. *New England Journal of Medicine* 1998; 338:612–3.

16

EYE DRUGS

GENERAL INSTRUCTIONS FOR APPLICATION OF EYE DROPS AND OINTMENT

The normal eye can hold about 10 microliters (10 millionths of a quart) of liquid. A single drop formed by an eye dropper, however, ranges from 25 to 50 microliters. What happens to the excess 15 to 40 microliters when you apply eye drops? Two things occur:

1. Medicine overflows the eyelids and runs down your face, especially if you are upright when applying the drops. This is not a very efficient use of medicine but is relatively harmless.

2. Medicine drains from the eyes into a small opening located at the inside corner of the eye. This small opening is the entrance to a duct (the nasolacrimal duct) through which tears and moisture normally leave the eye and drain into the nose (which is why your nose usually runs when you cry). In the nose, the medicine is absorbed into the blood supply and carried throughout the body, where it can affect the brain, heart, digestive system, lungs and airways, and other areas of the body, causing adverse effects.

What can be done to maximize drug absorption in the eye and minimize drug absorption through the nasal blood vessels?

1. Do not apply more than one drop of medicine within a five-minute period, regardless of whether the second drop is the same or a different drug. The eye cannot hold more than one drop at a time, so an extra drop both flushes out the first drop and is diluted by it. It also increases the amount that is absorbed through the nasal blood vessels. Therefore, always wait at least five minutes between drops to give adequate time for the drug to be absorbed by the eye.

2. Lie down when applying drops. This helps to prevent "tears" from rolling down your face and through the nasolacrimal duct. As much as 10 times more drug is lost when you are in an upright position than when you are reclining.

3. Using your thumb and middle finger (one in the corner of each eye), apply gentle pressure to the inside corner of the eye for five minutes after applying each drop, to block the medicine from draining through the nasolacrimal duct.

Compressing the duct for five minutes allows enough time for the drug to be absorbed through the eye and decreases adverse effects.

To avoid contaminating the eye drops, do not touch the applicator tip to any surface, including the eye. Store the bottle tightly closed. To ensure sterility, periodically discard used bottles of medicine. Drops can be considered safe for four weeks and ointments for three months after they have been opened.

To apply drops, first wash your hands. To increase drug absorption, it is best to lie down while applying this medicine. With the middle finger of the hand on the same side as the eye (right eye, right hand, for example), apply pressure to the inside corner of your eye to block the drainage duct. After you have begun to apply pressure with your middle finger, tilt your head back. With the index finger of the same hand, pull the lower eyelid away from the eye to form a pouch. Place a drop of medicine into the pouch, remove the index finger, and close your eyes gently, without blinking. Keep your eyes closed and continue to apply pressure for five minutes. Do not close your eyes tightly and do not blink.

To apply ointment, first wash your hands. Lie down or tilt your head back. Squeeze about a quarter to a half inch of ointment inside your lower lid without actually touching the tube to your lid. Close your eye gently and roll your eyeball in all directions while the eye is closed to evenly distribute the medicine. Wait at least 10 minutes before applying other medicines to your eyes. If you need to apply ointment and drops, it is best to put the drops in prior to the ointment, as the ointment will all but prevent absorption of the drops because of its "Vaseline"-like character.

GLAUCOMA

Glaucoma is a slowly progressing disorder in which the pressure inside the eye gradually increases. If left untreated, this elevated pressure may lead to nerve damage, decreased vision,

and blindness. In general, the higher the pressure inside the eye, the greater the chance of damaging the optic nerve (the nerve to the eye that allows us to see) and losing vision. Most people with glaucoma have no symptoms until extensive, irreversible damage to the optic nerve has occurred, so it is important to have regular eye exams as you grow older. It is also important to take your medicine regularly if you have glaucoma.

To understand what causes glaucoma, it helps to start by discussing how the eye normally works. The eye (shown on p. 500 as it would appear when cut in half) can be divided into three parts. The vitreous chamber is the large, round area behind the lens. The posterior chamber is the smaller area located behind the iris and in front and to the sides of the lens. The anterior chamber is located in front of the iris. Both the anterior and the posterior chambers are filled with a clear liquid called the aqueous humor. Normally, aqueous humor flows from the posterior chamber through the opening in the iris to the anterior chamber. It leaves the eye through a small opening, called the canal of Schlemm, at the outermost edges of the iris. In glaucoma, less aqueous humor drains from the eye, raising the pressure inside the eye. The disorder is similar to blowing up a balloon: if there is no opening for the air to flow out, the pressure in the balloon steadily increases as the balloon fills with air.

Elevated pressure inside the eye can be treated in two ways:

- increasing the amount of aqueous humor that leaves the eye through the canal of Schlemm; or
- decreasing the amount of aqueous humor that is produced.

Drugs such as dipivefrin (PROPINE), pilocarpine (ADSORBOCARPINE, ISOPTO CARPINE), and physostigmine (ESERINE) increase aqueous humor outflow from the anterior chamber, whereas acetazolamide (DIAMOX), dorzo-

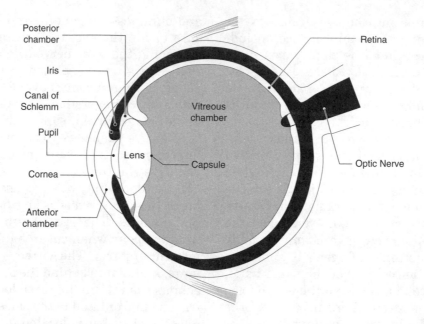

lamide (TRUSOPT), and beta-blockers such as timolol (TIMOPTIC) decrease aqueous humor production. In either case, the total amount of aqueous humor is reduced and the pressure decreased. Timolol is often used for mild glaucoma, except for older adults who have congestive heart failure, abnormal heart rhythms, asthma, or emphysema. In these patients, pilocarpine or carbonic anhydase inhibitors like dorzolamide or acetazolamide can be an alternative choice. A prostaglandin-containing drug (latanoprost [XALATAN]) is now the most widely used eye-drop product for treating glaucoma. A combination of drugs may be necessary for more severe forms. Surgery is reserved for those people who continue to have optic nerve destruction and visual loss, in spite of multiple drug therapies.

DRUG PROFILES

Glaucoma

Acetazolamide (a set a *zole* a mide)
DIAMOX (Duramed)

Methazolamide (meth a *zole* a mide)

GENERIC: available
FAMILY: Glaucoma Drugs (see p. 499)

PREGNANCY WARNING

These drugs caused fetal harm in animal studies, including limb defects in developing fetuses. Because of the potential for serious adverse effects to the fetus, these drugs should not be used by pregnant women.

BREAST-FEEDING WARNING

No information is available from either human or animal studies. However, it is likely that these drugs are excreted in human milk, and because of the potential for adverse effects in nursing infants, you should not take these drugs while nursing.

Acetazolamide and methazolamide are oral drugs used to treat glaucoma (see p. 499). These drugs belong to the carbonic anhydrase inhibitor family of medications that lower the pressure in the eye and thus improve vision in patients with glaucoma. Acetazolamide is also used to treat altitude sickness and to supplement other drugs used for seizure disorders such as epilepsy. In the past, acetazolamide was used as a diuretic (water pill) to treat high blood pressure, but it is outdated for this use because more effective drugs are now available.[1,2] Methazolamide is used long-term for open-angle glaucoma. It may be used temporarily before surgery for angle-closure (narrow-angle) glaucoma. Studies of methazolamide to control essential tremor are not yet conclusive.[3]

These drugs are cousins of sulfa drugs (see p. 702) and thiazide diuretics (see p. 60), having the potential for the same adverse effects but no action against bacteria. This family of drugs may cause kidney stones and gouty arthritis and may depress your bone marrow. Older people with decreased kidney function need to be cautious when taking these drugs. These drugs may also reduce the amount of potassium in your body. To compensate for this loss, eat foods high in potassium (see p. 160). Many individuals cannot tolerate the adverse effects of this family of drugs for a prolonged period of time.[2]

Acetazolamide has caused a few cases of hives, fever, blood cell disorders, and kidney problems.[4] Stop taking the drug and call your doctor if you experience any of these reactions.

Methazolamide can upset the gastrointestinal tract and severely deplete your levels of calcium, potassium, and other minerals. Unfortunately, stopping methazolamide does not always reverse the damage to bone marrow.[5] Those with liver disease are at an increased risk of serious liver problems when using methazolamide.[6]

Before You Use This Drug

Do not use if you have or have had:

- allergies to acetazolamide, sulfas, or thiazide diuretics
- acidosis, hyperchloremic type
- adrenal gland failure
- kidney or liver problems
- very low potassium or sodium levels
- diabetes

Tell your doctor if you have or have had:

- pregnancy or are breast-feeding
- allergies to carbonic anhydrase inhibitors
- adrenal gland problem (Addison's disease)
- diabetes
- gout
- hyperchloremic acidosis
- low blood level of sodium
- low blood level of potassium
- kidney or liver problems, including kidney stones
- liver problems, including cirrhosis
- emphysema or other chronic lung disease

Tell your doctor about any other drugs you take, including aspirin, herbs, vitamins, and other nonprescription products.

When You Use This Drug

- Do not use more often or in a higher dose than prescribed. **Do not stop taking this drug suddenly.** Your doctor must lower your dose gradually. Until you know how you react to this drug, do not drive or perform other activities requiring alertness. This drug may cause drowsiness, dizziness, lightheadedness, and/or tiredness.
- To help prevent kidney stones, drink at least six to eight glasses (eight ounces each) of fluids each day.
- **Caution diabetics:** This drug may elevate blood and urine sugar levels.

How to Use This Drug

• Follow directions for applying drops on p. 498.

• If you miss a dose, take it as soon as you remember, but skip it if it is almost time for the next dose. **Do not take double doses.**

• Do not share your medication with others.

• Take the drug at the same time(s) each day.

• Take with food or milk.

• Store at room temperature with lid on tightly. Do not store in the bathroom. Do not expose to heat, moisture, or strong light. Keep out of reach of children.

• Take with food to decrease stomach upset.

• Do not store in the bathroom. Do not expose to heat, moisture, or strong light. Do not allow to freeze.

Interactions with Other Drugs

The following drugs, biologics (e.g., vaccines, therapeutic antibodies), or foods are listed in *Evaluations of Drug Interactions* 2003 as causing "highly clinically significant" or "clinically significant" interactions when used together with any of the drugs in this section. In some sections with multiple drugs, the interaction may have been reported for one but not all drugs in this section, but we include the interaction because the drugs in this section are similar to one another. We have also included potentially serious interactions listed in the drug's FDA-approved professional package insert or in published medical journal articles. There may be other drugs, especially those in the families of drugs listed below, that also will react with this drug to cause severe adverse effects. Make sure to tell your doctor and pharmacist the drugs you are taking and tell them if you are taking any of these interacting drugs:

aspirin, AZOPT, brinzolamide, cyclosporine, dorzolamide, ECOTRIN, ESKALITH, GEN-UINE BAYER ASPIRIN, HIPREX, lithium, LITHOBID, LITHONATE, methenamine, NEORAL, quinidine, SANDIMMUNE, TOPAMAX, topiramate, TRUSOPT, UREX.

Adverse Effects

Call your doctor immediately if you experience:

• bloody or dark (acetazolamide) urine, difficult, painful, or burning urination; or sudden decrease in amount of urine

• bloody or black, tarry stools

• clumsiness, unsteadiness

• convulsions

• pale stools (acetazolamide)

• yellow eyes or skin (acetazolamide)

• dry mouth or increased thirst

• irregular heartbeat or weak pulse

• mood or mental changes

• muscle cramps, pain, or weakness

• nausea or vomiting

• nearsightedness

• unusual tiredness or weakness

• fever and sore throat

• unusual bruising or bleeding

• hives, itching, sores, or skin rash

• mental confusion or depression

• trouble breathing or shortness of breath

• ringing or buzzing in ears

• tremors in hands or feet

• vision changes

• confusion

• lower back pain

• severe muscle weakness or trembling

• shortness of breath

Call your doctor if these symptoms continue:

• constipation

• diarrhea

- dizziness or lightheadedness (methazolamide)
- drowsiness
- general feeling of discomfort or illness
- headache
- increased frequency of urination or amount of urine
- increased sensitivity of eyes to sunlight
- appetite loss
- loss of taste and smell
- metallic taste in mouth
- nausea or vomiting
- numbness, tingling, or burning in hands, fingers, feet, toes, mouth, tongue, lips, or anus
- weight loss
- impotence[7]

Periodic Tests

Ask your doctor which of these tests should be done periodically while you are taking this drug:

- complete blood count
- blood electrolyte (sodium, potassium) tests
- platelet count
- tests of kidney function and kidney stone formation

Betaxolol (bait *ax* o lole) (Eye Drops)
BETOPTIC (Alcon)
BETOPTIC S (Alcon)

Levobunolol (lev o *bewn* o lole)
BETAGAN (Allergan)

Timolol (*tim* oh lole) (Eye Drops)
TIMOPTIC (Merck)

GENERIC: available except for Betaxolol
FAMILY: Glaucoma Drugs (see p. 499)
Beta-blockers (see p. 87)

PREGNANCY WARNING

Data from animal studies indicated toxicity to developing fetuses. Use during pregnancy only for clear medical reasons. Tell your doctor if you are pregnant or thinking of becoming pregnant before you take these drugs.

BREAST-FEEDING WARNING

Timolol, taken as eye drops, was excreted into breast milk. Because it is likely that the other beta-blockers are also excreted into breast milk and because of the potential for serious adverse effects in nursing infants, you should not take these drugs while nursing.

Betaxolol, levobunolol, and timolol belong to the beta-blocker family of drugs. When used as oral tablets, both betaxolol and timolol can be used to treat heart disease. As eye drops these medications are used for the treatment of glaucoma. This profile discusses the antiglaucoma use of these drugs.

The beta-blocker family of antiglaucoma eye drops are well tolerated by most people, especially those who have cataracts or who have problems using another antiglaucoma drug called pilocarpine (see p. 514). Although these medications are prepared as eye drops, some can be absorbed from the eyes into the bloodstream and the rest of the body, and if this happens you may experience some of the general adverse effects listed under Adverse Effects. (See p. 498 for directions on how to apply eye drops.)

When used for a long time, the initial im-

If these eye drops are absorbed into the body, older people have an increased risk of hypothermia. Early signs are shivering, cold hands and feet, and memory lapse. Stay indoors, especially when it is cold and windy. Keep warm with extra clothes and blankets. If you must go outdoors, dress to protect yourself from the wind and cold. Avoid getting wet. Take along something to eat suitable to your diet, such as trail mix.

provement may diminish. Long-term use can exacerbate serious heart problems, even in people who did not previously have heart disease. Levobunolol and timolol can decrease lung function by 30%, an adverse effect not seen as much in betaxolol.[8] Very rarely, serious harm and even fatalities have occurred, mostly to those with asthma or heart problems.[9] But according to *The Medical Letter,* betaxolol may be less likely than timolol or levobunolol to have adverse effects on patients with asthma.[10] Older people are especially sensitive to the harmful effects of betaxolol. Timolol taken by mouth has been shown to cause an increased number of adrenal, lung, uterine, and breast cancers in rats. This has not been shown for the eye drops. As the effect of these drugs may diminish over time, it is sometimes necessary to supplement their use with other antiglaucoma medications such as pilocarpine, dipivefrin, or acetazolamide. Use with epinephrine is controversial.

Before You Use This Drug

Do not use if you have or have had:

- bronchial asthma
- congestive heart failure, slow heartbeat, or heart block
- previous allergic reaction to beta-blockers used for eyes
- severe chronic lung disease

Tell your doctor if you have or have had:

- allergies to drugs
- bronchitis
- diabetes
- heart problems
- low blood sugar (hypoglycemia)
- lung disorder
- myasthenia gravis
- pregnancy or are breast-feeding
- stroke
- mental depression

- emphysema or chronic bronchitis
- history of smoking
- thyroid problems
- impotence

Tell your doctor about any other drugs you take, including aspirin, herbs, vitamins, and other nonprescription products.

When You Use This Drug

- Restrict your use of caffeine, since it may add to the effect of these drugs on the heart.[11]
- **Caution diabetics:** Be aware that these drugs may mask trembling and pulse rate used to signal low blood sugar. They also may cause changes in blood glucose.
- Remove any soft contact lenses prior to administering this drug for products containing benzalkonium as a preservative.[12]
- If you plan to have any surgery, including dental, tell your doctor that you take this drug.
- Check with your doctor immediately if having eye surgery or if you get an eye injury or infection.
- Wear sunglasses and avoid too much exposure to bright light.
- Be cautious driving until the effect of the drug is complete (about two weeks)[9] and no blurred vision occurs.
- Do not take other drugs without talking to your doctor first—especially nonprescription drugs for appetite control, asthma, colds, coughs, hay fever, or sinus problems.

How to Use This Drug

- Follow directions for applying drops on p. 498.
- If you use the suspension form, shake it well first.
- Wash your hands before using this drug.
- After opening, avoid touching the tip against your eye or anything else.
- Do not share your medication with others.

- Take the drug at the same time(s) each day.
- Store at room temperature with lid on tightly. Do not store in the bathroom. Do not expose to heat, moisture, or strong light. Keep out of reach of children.
- *If you miss a dose, use the following guidelines:* If you are using betaxolol only once a day, apply the missed dose as soon as you remember, but skip it if you don't remember until the next day. If you are using any of these drugs more than once a day, apply the missed dose as soon as you remember, but skip it if it is almost time for the next dose. **Do not take double doses.**

Interactions with Other Drugs

The following drugs, biologics (e.g., vaccines, therapeutic antibodies), or foods are listed in *Evaluations of Drug Interactions* 2003 as causing "highly clinically significant" or "clinically significant" interactions when used together with any of the drugs in this section. In some sections with multiple drugs, the interaction may have been reported for one but not all drugs in this section, but we include the interaction because the drugs in this section are similar to one another. We have also included potentially serious interactions listed in the drug's FDA-approved professional package insert or in published medical journal articles. There may be other drugs, especially those in the families of drugs listed below, that also will react with this drug to cause severe adverse effects. Make sure to tell your doctor and pharmacist the drugs you are taking and tell them if you are taking any of these interacting drugs:

arbutamine, DELTASONE, prednisone.

Adverse Effects

These drugs can be absorbed into the body through the eye. All adverse effects for oral beta-blockers are possible with the eye-drop preparation.

Call your doctor immediately if you experience the following local problems:

- eyes with different-sized pupils (betaxolol)
- irritation or inflammation of eyelid (timolol)
- irritation or inflammation of eye and eyelid (levobunolol)
- irritation or inflammation of eye (betaxolol and timolol)
- droopy upper eyelid (timolol)
- eyeball discoloration (betaxolol)
- decreased corneal sensitivity
- seeing double (timolol)
- eye pain (betaxolol)
- tongue redness or irritation (betaxolol)
- blurred or decreased vision

There are, in addition, many other symptoms of systemic absorption listed under beta-blockers in Chapter 4, Drugs for Heart Conditions (see p. 87); some of these are listed below:

- coughing, wheezing, difficulty breathing
- chest pain
- hallucinations[13]
- cold hands or feet
- depression, confusion
- dizziness, fainting
- headache
- slow or irregular heartbeat
- irritation, severe swelling, or inflammation of eye or eyelids
- blurred vision or other vision changes
- difficulty swallowing or painful tongue
- unusual tiredness or weakness
- insomnia
- nausea, vomiting, or diarrhea
- droopy upper eyelid
- unsteadiness or clumsiness
- decreased sexual ability
- hair loss
- eye pain

- raw or red areas of skin
- different-size pupils or discoloration of eyeball
- skin rash, hives, or itching
- numbness or tingling of limbs
- bloody, stuffy, or runny nose
- swelling of feet, ankles, or lower legs

Call your doctor immediately if you experience the following total-body problems:

- burning or prickling feeling on body (timolol)
- chest pain (timolol)
- clumsiness or unsteadiness (levobunolol)
- confusion or mental depression (betaxolol, timolol)
- coughing, wheezing, or troubled breathing
- decreased sexual ability (timolol)
- diarrhea (timolol)
- dizziness or feeling faint
- drowsiness (timolol)
- hair loss (betaxolol, timolol)
- hallucinations (timolol)
- headache
- heart disorder (betaxolol, timolol)
- high blood pressure (timolol)
- nausea or vomiting (timolol)
- nosebleed (timolol)
- raw or red areas of the skin (betaxolol)
- ringing in ears (levobunolol)
- runny nose (timolol)
- skin rash, hives, or itching (betaxolol, timolol)
- stuffy nose (timolol)
- swelling of feet, ankles, or lower legs (betaxolol, timolol)
- systemic lupus erythematosus (timolol)
- trouble sleeping (betaxolol)
- unusual tiredness or weakness

Call your doctor if these symptoms continue:

- transient blurred vision (levobunolol and timolol gel-forming solution)

- transient stinging of eye or other eye irritation upon administration of drug (betaxolol, levobunolol)
- eyelash crusting (betaxolol)
- dryness of eye (betaxolol, timolol)
- feeling of having something in the eye (betaxolol)
- increased sensitivity of eye to light (betaxolol)
- redness, itching, stinging, burning, or watering of eye or other eye irritation

Periodic Tests

Ask your doctor which of these tests should be done periodically while you are taking this drug:

- eye pressure exams

Limited Use

Brimonidine (bri *moe* ni deen)
ALPHAGAN (Allergan)

GENERIC: not available

FAMILY: Glaucoma Drugs (see p. 499)

PREGNANCY WARNING

Brimonidine crosses the placenta, exposing the fetus to the drug. Use during pregnancy only for clear medical reasons. Tell your doctor if you are pregnant or thinking of becoming pregnant before you take this drug.

BREAST-FEEDING WARNING

Brimonidine was excreted in animal milk. Since it is likely that this drug, like many others, is excreted in human milk, you should consult with your doctor if you are planning to nurse.

Brimonidine is a drug that helps lower the pressure inside the eye to treat glaucoma. It works by decreasing the production of fluid in the eye and by increasing the flow of fluids out of the eye.

Clinical studies have shown that when used

twice daily, brimonidine is not as effective at lowering eye pressure as timolol (TIMOPTIC) (see p. 503), a beta-blocker eye drop,[14,15] or latanoprost (XALATAN) (see p. 512).[16]

When used three times daily, brimonidine was found to be as effective as dorzolamide (TRUSOPT) (see p. 510).[17]

However, dorzolamide is considered therapeutically inferior to timolol.[18] Studies on patients who need to use a second drug in addition to timolol to control their eye pressure have found that brimonidine provides more benefit than dorzolamide[19] and latanoprost when used as a combination agent.[20]

Unlike timolol, brimonidine does not worsen lung disorders such as asthma nor does it cause a decrease in heart rate like timolol. Brimonidine does cause a lowering of blood pressure during recovery from exercise and at four hours after use.[15,21]

A major drawback to brimonidine use is its tendency to cause allergic reactions, such as inflammation of the lining of the eye and eyelids, in almost 12% of users.[15]

In a clinical trial of this drug, 7% of patients had to discontinue use of brimonidine due to allergic complications.[14]

Brimonidine also commonly causes stinging, dry mouth, blurring, headache, and drowsiness.[14]

No studies have been conducted on children with brimonidine. However, one infant given the drug after approval reacted to treatment with brimonidine with severe lethargy and stupor, requiring discontinuation of the drug.[22]

Due to its therapeutic inferiority to other available antiglaucoma drugs, and its adverse effect profile, brimonidine should only be used when other treatment options have been exhausted or when a secondary drug is needed in addition to current therapy.

Before You Use This Drug

Do not use this drug if you have or have had:

- allergy to this drug or other ingredients in its formulation

Tell your doctor if you have or have had:

- allergy to drugs
- pregnancy or are breast-feeding
- decreased blood circulation to the brain
- heart disease
- kidney disease
- liver disease
- inflammation of the blood vessels
- low blood pressure
- mental depression
- Raynaud's disease

Tell your doctor about any other drugs you take, including aspirin, herbs, vitamins, and other nonprescription products.

When You Use This Drug

- Until you know how you react to this drug, do not drive or perform other activities requiring alertness. This drug may cause drowsiness.
- This drug may cause your eyes to be more sensitive to bright lights. You may need to wear sunglasses and avoid intense lights.
- Call your doctor immediately if you become faint or have a fainting episode.
- Have regular visits with your doctor to check your eye pressure.

How to Use This Drug

- Follow directions for applying drops on p. 498.
- Prevent the container from becoming contaminated. Avoid letting the tip of the container touch your eye, hands, or any other object.
- Recap the container immediately to prevent contamination and to prevent crystals from forming on the tip of the container.[23]

• Contact lenses should be removed prior to administration of this drug. Preservative in the drug product may be absorbed by the contacts; wait at least 15 minutes after putting in eye drops before inserting contacts.

• Wait at least 10 minutes between application of two different eye-drop drugs. If you miss a dose, take it as soon as you remember, but skip it if it is almost time for the next dose. **Do not take double doses.**

• Do not share your medication with others.

• Take the drug at the same time(s) each day.

• Store at room temperature with lid on tightly. Do not store in the bathroom. Do not expose to heat, moisture, or strong light. Keep out of reach of children.

Interactions with Other Drugs

The following drugs, biologics (e.g., vaccines, therapeutic antibodies), or foods are listed in *Evaluations of Drug Interactions* 2003 as causing "highly clinically significant" or "clinically significant" interactions when used together with any of the drugs in this section. In some sections with multiple drugs, the interaction may have been reported for one but not all drugs in this section, but we include the interaction because the drugs in this section are similar to one another. We have also included potentially serious interactions listed in the drug's FDA-approved professional package insert or in published medical journal articles. There may be other drugs, especially those in the families of drugs listed below, that also will react with this drug to cause severe adverse effects. Make sure to tell your doctor and pharmacist the drugs you are taking and tell them if you are taking any of these interacting drugs:

ELDEPRYL, furazolidone, isocarboxazid, MARPLAN, MATULANE, moclobemide, NARDIL, pargyline, PARNATE, phenelzine, procarbazine, selegiline, tranylcypromine.

Adverse Effects

In addition to the allergic reactions mentioned above, brimonidine can be absorbed into the blood through the eye. Therefore, use of this drug may have systemic adverse effects.

Call your doctor immediately if you experience:

- blood pressure increase
- bloody eye
- blurred vision or other change in vision
- corneal erosion
- dizziness
- eye pain or ache
- fainting
- feeling of something in eye
- headache
- itching
- mental depression
- muscle pain
- nausea or vomiting
- oozing in eye
- redness of eye or inner lining of eyelid
- runny or stuffy nose
- sneezing
- redness, swelling, and/or itching of eyelid
- tearing

Call your doctor if these symptoms continue:

- anxiety
- burning, stinging, or tearing of eye
- crusting on eyelid or corner of eye
- discoloration of white part of eye
- drowsiness or tiredness
- dryness of eye
- increased sensitivity of eye to light
- muscle weakness
- paleness of eye or inner lining of eyelid
- pounding heartbeat
- change in sense of taste
- trouble sleeping

Periodic Tests

Ask your doctor if this test should be done periodically while you are taking this drug:

- eye pressure exams

Dipivefrin (dye *pi* ve frin)
PROPINE (Allergan)

GENERIC: available

FAMILY: Glaucoma Drugs (see p. 499)

PREGNANCY WARNING

The available data from animal studies does not indicate harm in the use of dipivefrin during pregnancy. Use during pregnancy only for clear medical reasons. Tell your doctor if you are pregnant or thinking of becoming pregnant before you take this drug.

BREAST-FEEDING WARNING

No information is available from either human or animal studies. Since it is likely that this drug, like many others, is excreted in human milk, you should consult with your doctor if you are planning to nurse.

Dipivefrin is used to treat the most common form of glaucoma (see p. 499). In glaucoma, the pressure of the fluid inside the eye increases, and dipivefrin controls the pressure by reducing the amount of fluid that is produced and improving its circulation. It has not proven to be as effective in lowering intraocular pressure as pilocarpine (see p. 514), beta-blockers such as timolol (see p. 503), or carbonic anhydrase inhibitors such as dorzolamide (see p. 510). When used for a long time, the initial improvement may diminish.

Before You Use This Drug

Do not use if you have or have had:

- angle-closure glaucoma

Tell your doctor if you have or have had:

- allergies to drugs
- pregnancy or are breast-feeding
- the lens in your eye removed

Tell your doctor about any other drugs you take, including aspirin, herbs, vitamins, and other nonprescription products.

How to Use This Drug

- See directions for applying drops on p. 498.
- Wash hands immediately after applying eye drops.
- If you miss a dose, take it as soon as you remember, but skip it if it is almost time for the next dose. **Do not take double doses.**
- Do not share your medication with others.
- Take the drug at the same time(s) each day.
- Store at room temperature with lid on tightly. Do not store in the bathroom. Do not expose to heat, moisture, or strong light. Keep out of reach of children.

Interactions with Other Drugs

Evaluations of Drug Interactions 2003 lists no drugs, biologics (e.g., vaccines, therapeutic antibodies), or foods as causing "highly clinically significant" or "clinically significant" interactions when used together with the drugs in this section. We also found no interactions in the drugs' FDA-approved professional package inserts. However, as the number of new drugs approved for marketing increases and as more experience is gained with these drugs over time, new interactions may be discovered.

Adverse Effects

Call your doctor immediately if you experience:

- severe itching, pain, redness, or swelling of eye or eyelid
- skin rash or hives
- fast or irregular heartbeat
- blood pressure increase
- severe and continuing watering of eyes

Call your doctor if these symptoms continue:

- blurred vision
- burning or stinging of the eye
- headache
- increased sensitivity of eyes to light
- large pupils

Periodic Tests

Ask your doctor which of these tests should be done periodically while you are taking this drug:

- eye pressure tests
- complete eye exam, including test for visual acuity

Limited Use

Dorzolamide (dor *zole* a mide)
TRUSOPT (Merck)

Dorzolamide with Timolol
(dor *zole* a mide with *tim* oh lole)
COSOPT (Merck)

GENERIC: not available
FAMILY: Glaucoma Drugs (see p. 499)

PREGNANCY WARNING

These drugs caused fetal harm in animal studies, including malformation of the spine and delayed bone formation. Use during pregnancy only for clear medical reasons. Tell your doctor if you are pregnant or thinking of becoming pregnant before you take this drug.

BREAST-FEEDING WARNING

These drugs are excreted in human milk and caused delays in development of pups in animal studies. Because of the potential for serious adverse effects in nursing infants, you should not take these drugs while nursing.

Dorzolamide is used to treat glaucoma, especially open-angle glaucoma, and to lower pressure in the eye. This medication is also used in certain eye surgeries. Excess pressure in the eye can damage the optic nerve and cause loss of vision. Dorzolamide blocks the enzyme carbonic anhydrase, as does the oral drug acetazolamide (see p. 500). Carbonic anhydrase is present in the eyes, kidney, lungs, and stomach. Dorzolamide belongs to the family of sulfa drugs.

The usual dose is one drop in the affected eye or eyes, three times daily. Some people may be able to use dorzolamide twice daily.[24] Drugs for glaucoma usually work more quickly in people with light-colored eyes than in people with dark eyes.[24] Bitter taste is a common adverse effect to dorzolamide. If the container becomes contaminated, your eye can be damaged, or you may even suffer loss of vision. Dorzolamide does not lower pressure in the eye as much as acetazolamide or timolol.[18,25] Adverse effects are generally less likely than with oral acetazolamide. However, dorzolamide, like other eye drops, is absorbed throughout your body. Any adverse effect of sulfas or carbonic anhydrase inhibitors could occur with dorzolamide. These include rare but sometimes fatal severe allergic reactions, blood disorders, and bone marrow depression.

People who are allergic to sulfa drugs should not use dorzolamide. Dorzolamide has not been studied in people with liver problems. It is not recommended for people with narrow-angle glaucoma, kidney disease, or people who wear soft contacts. Dorzolamide is also not recommended for children, or women who are pregnant or nursing. Information about dorzolamide, particularly effects after use for more than one year, remains limited. If you stop taking dorzolamide, some of the drug may remain in your body for a few months.[24]

Timolol has two forms for different uses: Blocadren tablets for the heart (see p. 87) and Timoptic eye drops for the eyes, specifically for treating glaucoma (see p. 503).

The dorzolamide and timolol combination is a product used to lower pressure in the eye when treatment with a single antiglaucoma drug has failed to accomplish this objective.[26,27] This combination drug is as effective as applying each drug separately; however, it costs more than buying them individually. Additionally, this combination choice is far from ideal. Studies comparing brimonidine (ALPHAGAN) (see p. 506) and dorzolamide for use as combination drugs with timolol found that brimonidine is a significantly more effective second agent than dorzolamide for further lowering eye pressure in timolol users.[19,28]

The following is true for dorzolamide alone. Analogous information for timolol can be found on p. 503.

Before You Use This Drug

Do not use if you have or have had:

- allergy to dorzolamide

Tell your doctor if you have or have had:

- pregnancy or are breast-feeding[24]
- liver disorder
- kidney disorder

Tell your doctor about any other drugs you take, including aspirin, herbs, vitamins, and other nonprescription products.

The following is true for dorzolamide alone. Analogous information for timolol can be found on p. 503.

When You Use This Drug

- *If using more than one eye drug:* Wait 10 minutes between the use of two different eye preparations to prevent "washing out" of the first one.
- Be careful, since blurred vision can occur temporarily. Check with your doctor if blurred vision continues.
- Check with your doctor if you have itching, redness, or swelling of eye or eyelid.

- Eyes can be sensitive to sunlight or bright light; wear sunglasses and avoid exposure to bright light.

The following is true for dorzolamide alone. Analogous information for timolol can be found on p. 503.

How to Use This Drug

- Follow directions for applying drops on p. 498.
- Prevent the container from becoming contaminated. Avoid letting the tip of the container touch your eye, hands, or any other object.
- If you miss a dose, take it as soon as you remember, but skip it if it is almost time for the next dose. **Do not take double doses.**
- Do not share your medication with others.
- Take the drug at the same time(s) each day.
- Store at room temperature with lid on tightly. Do not store in the bathroom. Do not expose to heat, moisture, or strong light. Keep out of reach of children.

The following is true for dorzolamide alone. Analogous information for timolol can be found on p. 503.

Interactions with Other Drugs

The following drugs, biologics (e.g., vaccines, therapeutic antibodies), or foods are listed in *Evaluations of Drug Interactions* 2003 as causing "highly clinically significant" or "clinically significant" interactions when used together with any of the drugs in this section. In some sections with multiple drugs, the interaction may have been reported for one but not all drugs in this section, but we include the interaction because the drugs in this section are similar to one another. We have also included potentially serious interactions listed in the drug's FDA-approved professional package insert or in published medical journal articles. There may be other drugs, especially those in the families of drugs listed below, that also will react with this drug to cause severe adverse effects. Make sure to tell your doctor and pharmacist the drugs you are taking and tell them if you are taking any of these interacting drugs:

> acetazolamide, DIAMOX, dichlorphenamide, methazolamide, quinidine, TOPAMAX, topiramate.

> For dorzolamide with timolol, the preceding apply, plus arbutamide, DELTASONE, prednisone.

> Other possible drug interactions are: cholinesterase inhibitors, such as ambenonium (MYTELASE), edrophonium (TENSILON), neostigmine (PROSTIGMIN), or pyridostigmine (MESTINON). The effect of these drugs (often used in myasthenia gravis) may be lowered by dorzolamide.[24] When taken with diuretics there can be a greater loss of potassium.[24] Use with phenytoin (DILANTIN) may aggravate osteoporosis.[24] Salicylic acid (SALSALATE) taken with dorzolamide can lead to acidosis.[24] Also, the preservative in dorzolamide drops (benzalkonium chloride) can interact with soft contact lenses.

The following is true for dorzolamide alone. Analogous information for timolol can be found on p. 503.

Adverse Effects

Call your doctor immediately if you experience:

- blood in urine
- eye pain, tearing, and blurred vision
- itching, redness, swelling, or other signs of eye or eyelid irritation
- nausea or vomiting
- pain in side, back, or abdomen
- skin rash

Call your doctor if these symptoms continue:

- bitter or metallic taste
- blurred vision
- burning, stinging, or discomfort when medicine is applied
- dryness of eyes
- feeling of something in eye
- headache
- nausea
- sensitivity of eyes to light
- tearing of eye
- unusual tiredness or weakness

Latanoprost (la *ta* noe prost)
XALATAN (Pharmacia & Upjohn)

GENERIC: not available

FAMILY: Glaucoma Drugs (see p. 499)

PREGNANCY WARNING

Latanoprost caused fetal death in animal studies. Because of the potential for serious adverse effects to the fetus, this drug should not be used by pregnant women.

BREAST-FEEDING WARNING

No information is available from either human or animal studies. Since it is likely that this drug, like many others, is excreted in human milk, you should consult with your doctor if you are planning to nurse.

Latanoprost is a drug that helps lower the pressure inside the eye to treat glaucoma. It works by decreasing the production of fluid in the eye and by increasing the flow of fluids out of the eye.

Clinical studies suggest that latanoprost is more effective at lowering eye pressure than timolol (TIMOPTIC) (see p. 503), a beta-blocker eye drop,[29] and as effective as the combination of dorzolamide plus timolol (COSOPT) (see p. 510).[30]

Additionally, latanoprost does not share timolol's ability to aggravate lung disorders such as asthma. However, latanoprost does have several unique adverse effects, whose clinical significance are not clearly understood.

Latanoprost has been shown to darken the iris, eyelashes, and skin around the eyes and to cause lengthening and thickening of the eyelashes.[29,31,32]

Iris color changes occur in 11 to 23% of patients, and seem to happen more frequently in patients with brown-green or yellow-brown eyes.[33]

The clinical significance and long-term consequence of this color change are unknown. Latanoprost is also associated with changes to the surface of the eye.[34,35]

A case report of latanoprost-associated angina (chest pain) has been reported in the medical literature,[36] and a similar event was reported in a latanoprost clinical trial.[34]

Before You Use This Drug

Do not use this drug if you have or have had:

- allergy to latanoprost
- allergy to benzalkonium chloride, a preservative used in eye drops and contact lens solutions

Tell your doctor if you have or have had:

- eye lens removed or replaced with a prosthetic lens
- liver disease
- inflammation of the eye
- kidney disease
- macular edema
- migraine
- pregnancy or are breast-feeding

Tell your doctor about any other drugs you take, including aspirin, herbs, vitamins, and other nonprescription products.

When You Use This Drug

- Take note of any changes in eye, eyelash, or eyelid skin color. This change may be perma-

nent. Also, these changes affect only the eye under treatment, so special care is needed if you are using this drug in only one eye.
- This drug may cause your eyes to be more sensitive to bright light. You may need to wear sunglasses and avoid intense lights.
- This drug will precipitate into its solid form if it comes into contact with thimerosal, which is contained in many eye-drop and contact lens solutions. Five minutes should pass between application of this drug and any of these products.
- Have regular visits with your doctor to check eye pressure.

How to Use This Drug

- Follow directions for applying drops on p. 498.
- Prevent the container from becoming contaminated. Avoid letting the tip of the container touch your eye, hands, or any other object.
- Contact lenses should be removed prior to administration of this drug. This drug may be absorbed by soft contact lenses. Wait at least 15 minutes after using this drug before putting in contact lenses.
- Store in refrigerator until opened. Then store at room temperature for up to six weeks before discarding. Do not expose to heat or direct light.
- If you miss a dose, take it as soon as you remember, but skip it if it is almost time for the next dose. **Do not take double doses.**
- Do not share your medication with others.
- Take the drug at the same time(s) each day.
- Keep out of reach of children.

Interactions with Other Drugs

The following drugs, biologics (e.g., vaccines, therapeutic antibodies), or foods are listed in *Evaluations of Drug Interactions* 2003 as causing "highly clinically significant" or "clinically significant" interactions when used together with any of the drugs in this section. In some sections with multiple drugs, the interaction may have been reported for one but not all drugs in this section, but we include the interaction because the drugs in this section are similar to one another. We have also included potentially serious interactions listed in the drug's FDA-approved professional package insert or in published medical journal articles. There may be other drugs, especially those in the families of drugs listed below, that also will react with this drug to cause severe adverse effects. Make sure to tell your doctor and pharmacist the drugs you are taking and tell them if you are taking any of these interacting drugs:

thimerosal-containing eye medications or contact lens solutions.

Adverse Effects

In addition to causing darkening of the iris, eyelashes, and skin around the eyes and lengthening and thickening of the eyelashes, latanoprost can be absorbed into the blood through the eye, although much less than other eye drops. Therefore, use of this drug may have some adverse effects beyond the eye.

Call your doctor immediately if you experience:

- blurred vision, eye irritation, or tearing
- darkening of eyelid skin color
- discharge from eye
- double vision
- eye pain
- eyelid crusting, redness, swelling, discomfort, or pain
- fever
- increase in brown color in colored part of eye
- longer, thicker, and darker eyelashes
- muscle, joint, or back pain
- noisy breathing
- redness of eye or inside eyelid

- sensitivity of eye to light
- shortness of breath
- skin rash
- sore throat
- swelling of eye
- tightness in chest
- wheezing

Call your doctor if these symptoms continue:

- dryness of eye
- stinging of eye
- increased sensitivity to light
- itching of eye
- redness of eye or inside of eyelid
- sensation of something in the eye
- tearing

Periodic Tests

Ask your doctor if this test should be done periodically while you are taking this drug:

- eye exams

Pilocarpine (pye loe *kar* peen)
ADSORBOCARPINE, ISOPTO CARPINE
(Alcon)

GENERIC: available
FAMILY: Glaucoma Drugs (see p. 499)

PREGNANCY WARNING

Pilocarpine caused fetal harm in animal studies, including a decrease in body weight, an increase in stillbirths and skeletal changes, and decreased survival. Because of the potential for serious adverse effects to the fetus, this drug should not be used by pregnant women.

BREAST-FEEDING WARNING

No information is available from either human or animal studies. However, since it is likely that this drug, like many others, is excreted in human milk and because of the potential for serious adverse effects in nursing infants, you should not take this drug while nursing.

Pilocarpine is a drug used for treating most forms of glaucoma (see p. 499). Glaucoma is a condition in which the pressure of the fluid inside the eye increases, and pilocarpine lowers the increased pressure.

Pilocarpine makes the pupils of your eyes smaller and affects how quickly they react to light by enlarging or narrowing. Smaller pupils and their slower reaction allow less light to enter the eyes. This can hinder you from performing tasks such as driving at night. Be careful when performing such tasks. When used for a long time, the initial improvement may diminish.

Right after you use pilocarpine, your vision may be blurred, but it will clear. You might notice this more when viewing things at a distance.

Before You Use This Drug

Tell your doctor if you have or have had:

- allergy to pilocarpine
- bronchial asthma
- eye infection or inflammation
- predisposition to or previous retinal detachment
- pregnancy or are breast-feeding

Tell your doctor about any other drugs you take, including aspirin, herbs, vitamins, and other nonprescription products.

When You Use This Drug

- Wash hands immediately after application to remove any drug that may be on them.
- Have regular visits with your doctor to check your eye pressure.
- Be cautious if you have blurred vision or change in near or far vision, especially at night.

How to Use This Drug

- Follow directions for applying drops on p. 498. If you use an eye system form, follow directions that accompany it. Do not use if system is damaged or if too much medication is being released.
- Store gel and eye system forms in refrigerator. Do not store in the bathroom. Do not expose to heat, moisture, or strong light. Do not allow this drug to freeze. Keep out of reach of children.
- If you miss a dose, take it as soon as you remember, but skip it if it is almost time for the next dose. **Do not take double doses.**
- Do not share your medication with others.
- Take the drug at the same time(s) each day.

Interactions with Other Drugs

Evaluations of Drug Interactions 2003 lists no drugs, biologics (e.g., vaccines, therapeutic antibodies), or foods as causing "highly clinically significant" or "clinically significant" interactions when used together with the drugs in this section. We also found no interactions in the drugs' FDA-approved professional package inserts. However, as the number of new drugs approved for marketing increases and as more experience is gained with these drugs over time, new interactions may be discovered.

Adverse Effects

Call your doctor immediately if you experience:

- increased sweating
- muscle tremors
- nausea, vomiting, or diarrhea
- troubled breathing or wheezing
- watering of mouth
- eye pain

Call your doctor if these symptoms continue:

- blurred vision or change in near or far vision
- brow ache or headache

- irritation of eyes
- decrease in night vision

Periodic Tests

Ask your doctor which of these tests should be done periodically while you are taking this drug:

- eye pressure tests

Infection

Erythromycin Acetate (er *ith* roe my sin *a* si tate)
ILOTYCIN (Dista)

GENERIC: available

FAMILY: Macrolides

PREGNANCY WARNING

There was no evidence of toxicity in animal studies. Use during pregnancy only for clear medical reasons. Tell your doctor if you are pregnant or thinking of becoming pregnant before you take this drug.

BREAST-FEEDING WARNING

Erythromycin is excreted in human milk. Because of the potential for serious adverse effects in nursing infants, you should consult with your doctor if you are planning to nurse.

Erythromycin, an aminoglycoside antibiotic, is formulated as an ointment for the treatment of eye infections such as conjunctivitis, blepharitis, and keratitis. The Centers for Disease Control and Prevention (CDC) recommends the use of the eye ointment as one of three primary drug treatments for the prevention of gonococcal ophthalmia (gonorrhea infection of the eye) in newborns. Although erythromycin is also approved for the prevention of chlamydial infections in newborns, the CDC states: "The efficacy of these preparations in preventing chlamydial ophthalmia is less clear, and they do not eliminate nasopharyngeal colonization by *C. trachomatis.*"[37] There are reports of an association between the oral form of erythromycin and pyloric stenosis in infants. However, the association was not found with the eye form of erythromycin.[37,38]

Before You Use This Drug

- Tell your doctor if you are allergic to erythromycin, other macrolides, or any component to this medicine.

Tell your doctor about any other drugs you take, including aspirin, herbs, vitamins, and other nonprescription products.

When You Use This Drug

- Your vision may become blurry after application of the eye ointment.
- Do not wear your contact lenses while using the drug.
- Call your doctor if your eye infection does not improve within a few days or if it gets worse.
- Use all the erythromycin your doctor prescribed, even if you feel better before you finish. If you stop too soon, your symptoms could come back.

How to Use This Drug

- Follow the instructions on p. 498 for applying eye ointment correctly so that you won't absorb the drug into your body and possibly suffer serious adverse effects.
- If you miss a dose, take it as soon as you remember, but skip it if it is almost time for the next dose. **Do not take double doses.**
- Do not share your medication with others.
- Take the drug at the same time(s) each day.
- Store at room temperature with lid on tightly. Do not store in the bathroom. Do not expose to heat, moisture, or strong light. Keep out of reach of children.
- Do not let the ointment freeze.

Interactions with Other Drugs

Although there are potential drug interactions reported with the other forms of the drug, there have been no "highly clinically significant" or "clinically significant" drug interactions reported with the ocular form of erythromycin in *Evaluations of Drug Interactions* 2003. We also found no interactions in the drugs' FDA-approved professional package inserts. However, as the number of new drugs approved for marketing increases and as more experience is gained with these drugs over time, new interactions may be discovered.

Adverse Effects

Call your doctor immediately if you experience:

- eye irritation not present before therapy

Call your doctor if this symptom continues:

- eye irritation

Limited Use

Gentamicin (*jen* ta mye sin)
GARAMYCIN (Schering)

Tobramycin (*toe* bra mye sin)
TOBREX (Alcon)

GENERIC: available
FAMILY: Antibiotics (see p. 673)
Aminoglycosides

PREGNANCY WARNING

Gentamicin has been shown to depress both body and kidney weights and to harm kidney structure. Information is lacking for tobramycin. Use during pregnancy only for clear medical reasons. Tell your doctor if you are pregnant or thinking of becoming pregnant before you take these drugs.

BREAST-FEEDING WARNING

No information is available from either human or animal studies. Since it is likely that these drugs, like many others, are excreted in human milk, you should consult with your doctor if you are planning to nurse.

Gentamicin and tobramycin are used in ointment, cream, or liquid form to treat eye, ear, and skin infections. Drugs in this family (aminoglycosides) are also given intravenously in the hospital to treat serious infections, but the information on this page does not apply to this use.

Gentamicin is sometimes used on the skin to treat severe burns that are infected. This is not a recommended use. If you use gentamicin this way, you may develop bacteria that are resistant to the drug, and the injected form of gentamicin might then be ineffective if you ever received it.[4]

Before You Use This Drug

Tell your doctor if you have or have had:

- allergy to gentamicin or tobramycin
- an unusual reaction to any aminoglycoside (neomycin, for example)
- pregnancy or are breast-feeding

Tell your doctor about any other drugs you take, including aspirin, herbs, vitamins, and other nonprescription products.

When You Use This Drug

- Call your doctor if your infection does not improve within a few days or if it gets worse.
- Avoid wearing contact lenses during treatment.
- Use all the gentamicin or tobramycin your doctor prescribed, even if you feel better before you finish. If you stop too soon, your symptoms could come back.

How to Use This Drug

• Follow the instructions on p. 498 for applying eye drops and ointment correctly so that you won't absorb the drug into your body and possibly suffer serious adverse effects.

• If you miss a dose, take it as soon as you remember, but skip it if it is almost time for the next dose. **Do not take double doses.**

• Do not share your medication with others.

• Take the drug at the same time(s) each day.

• Store at room temperature with lid on tightly. Do not store in the bathroom. Do not expose to heat, moisture, or strong light. Keep out of reach of children.

Interactions with Other Drugs

The following drugs, biologics (e.g., vaccines, therapeutic antibodies), or foods are listed in *Evaluations of Drug Interactions* 2003 as causing "highly clinically significant" or "clinically significant" interactions when used together with any of the drugs in this section. In some sections with multiple drugs, the interaction may have been reported for one but not all drugs in this section, but we include the interaction because the drugs in this section are similar to one another. We have also included potentially serious interactions listed in the drug's FDA-approved professional package insert or in published medical journal articles. There may be other drugs, especially those in the families of drugs listed below, that also will react with this drug to cause severe adverse effects. Make sure to tell your doctor and pharmacist the drugs you are taking and tell them if you are taking any of these interacting drugs:

carbenicillin, cephalothin, cidofovir, GEOCILLIN, INDOCIN, indomethacin, tubocurarine, VISTIDE.

Adverse Effects

Call your doctor immediately if you experience:

• black, tarry stools
• blood in urine or stools
• eye pain, sensitivity to light, or tearing
• itching, redness, swelling, or other irritation that has appeared since you started using the drug
• seeing, hearing, or feeling things that are not there
• unusual bleeding or bruising

Call your doctor if these symptoms continue:

• burning or stinging of eyes

Signs of overdose:

• increased eye watering
• itching, redness, or swelling of the eyes or eyelids
• painful irritation of the clear front part of eye

If you suspect an overdose, call this number to contact your poison control center: (800) 222-1222.

Limited Use

Sulfacetamide (sul fa *see* ta mide)

GENERIC: available

FAMILY: Antibiotics (see p. 673)
Sulfa Drugs

PREGNANCY WARNING

Sulfacetamide caused fetal harm in children born of mothers taking the drug by mouth. Because of the potential for serious adverse effects to the fetus, this drug should not be used by pregnant women.

BREAST-FEEDING WARNING

Sulfacetamide caused harm in nursing infants when mothers took this drug by mouth. Because of the potential for adverse effects in nursing infants, you should not take this drug while nursing.

Sulfacetamide is used to treat some eye infections and is available as a liquid or an ointment. It can cause blurred vision, stinging, or burning after use. It also makes your eyes sensitive to bright light. Wearing sunglasses may help with this problem. For serious eye infections, sulfacetamide may not be as effective as other antibiotics.

Before You Use This Drug

Tell your doctor if you have or have had:

- allergies to drugs
- pregnancy or are breast-feeding
- an unusual reaction to other sulfa drugs, furosemide, thiazide diuretics (water pills), sulfonylurea (diabetes drugs), or carbonic anhydrase inhibitors

Tell your doctor about any other drugs you take, including aspirin, herbs, vitamins, and other nonprescription products.

When You Use This Drug

- Call your doctor if your symptoms do not improve in a few days.
- You may get blurred vision or stinging or burning after application.
- Use all the sulfacetamide your doctor prescribed, even if you feel better before you finish. If you stop too soon, your symptoms could come back.

How to Use This Drug

- Follow directions for applying drops on p. 498.
- Do not let the tip of the applicator touch your eye, your fingers, or anything else. It could become contaminated.
- If the drug gets dark brown, throw it away.
- If you miss a dose, take it as soon as you remember, but skip it if it is almost time for the next dose. **Do not take double doses.**

- Do not share your medication with others.
- Take the drug at the same time(s) each day.
- Store at room temperature with lid on tightly. Do not store in the bathroom. Do not expose to heat, moisture, or strong light. Keep out of reach of children.

Interactions with Other Drugs

Evaluations of Drug Interactions 2003 lists no drugs, biologics (e.g., vaccines, therapeutic antibodies), or foods as causing "highly clinically significant" or "clinically significant" interactions when used together with the drugs in this section. We also found no interactions in the drugs' FDA-approved professional package inserts. However, as the number of new drugs approved for marketing increases and as more experience is gained with these drugs over time, new interactions may be discovered.

Adverse Effects

Call your doctor immediately if you experience:

- itching, redness, or swelling not present before using this drug
- other adverse effects like those that occur with the sulfonamides (sulfa drugs). See sulfisoxazole, p. 703, for examples.

 Do Not Use

ALTERNATIVE TREATMENT:
An antibiotic alone, if necessary.

Sulfacetamide and Prednisolone
(sul fa *see* ta mide and pred *niss* oh lone)
BLEPHAMIDE (Allergan)
VASOCIDIN (Novartis)

FAMILY: Antibiotics (see p. 673)
         Corticosteroids (see p. 664)

These are eye drops that contain two drugs, sulfacetamide (see p. 519) and prednisolone (see p. 664). The drops are used to treat some eye and eyelid infections caused by bacteria or allergies. There is no persuasive proof that they are beneficial for this purpose.

This combination is like several others that contain a drug from the corticosteroid family (in this case prednisolone) and one from the antibiotic family (in this case sulfacetamide). In general, combinations like this are not recommended for treating eye infections externally.[39] Corticosteroids like prednisolone may actually be dangerous because they can hide the signs of an infection or make it spread. For serious eye infections, sulfacetamide may not be as effective as other antibiotics.

Ofloxacin (oh *floks* a sin)
OCUFLOX (Allergan)

Moxifloxacin (mox ee *floks* a sin)
VIGAMOX (Alcon)

GENERIC: not available
FAMILY: Antibiotics (see p. 673)
       Fluoroquinolones

PREGNANCY WARNING

Ofloxacin and moxifloxacin caused fetal harm in animal studies, including decreased fetal body weight and increased death when given by mouth. Because of the potential for serious adverse effects to the fetus, these drugs should not be used by pregnant women unless there is no safer substitute.

BREAST-FEEDING WARNING

These drugs are excreted in human milk. Because of the potential for serious adverse effects in nursing infants, you should not take these drugs while nursing.

> Prolonged use of any antimicrobial may result in the overgrowth of nonsusceptible organisms, including fungi.

WARNING—INCREASED RISK OF TENDINITIS AND TENDON RUPTURE WITH ALL FLUOROQUINOLONE ANTIBIOTICS

Public Citizen's Health Research Group petitioned the FDA successfully to add a warning for doctors to the labeling, or package, for all fluoroquinolone antibiotics, about the risk of tendinitis, including the possibility of complete tendon rupture.

This adverse reaction most frequently involves the Achilles tendon, the tendon that runs from the back of the heel to the calf. Rupture of the Achilles tendon may require surgical repair. Tendons in the rotator cuff (the shoulder), the hand, the biceps, and the thumb have also been involved. This reaction appears to be more common in those taking steroid drugs, in older patients, and in kidney transplant recipients but cases have occurred in people without any of these risk factors. The onset of symptoms is sudden and has occurred as soon as 24 hours after starting treatment with a fluoroquinolone. Most people have recovered completely after one to two months.

If you experience unexpected tendon pain while taking a fluoroqinolone antibiotic, stop the drug immediately, call your doctor, and rest.

Ofloxacin, a fluoroquinolone, is formulated as an eye drop and ointment for the treatment of eye infections, including conjunctivitis and corneal ulcers. Moxifloxacin, also a fluoroquinolone, is formulated only as an eye drop and is used for the treatment of bacterial conjunctivitis.

Before You Use This Drug

Do not use if you have or have had:

- allergy to ofloxacin, other fluoroquinolones, or any component to this medicine

Tell your doctor if you have or have had:

- pregnancy or are breast-feeding

Tell your doctor about any other drugs you take, including aspirin, herbs, vitamins, and other nonprescription products.

When You Use This Drug

• Stop using the drug at the first sign of a rash or an allergic reaction.
• Your eyes may sting or burn just after using. Call your doctor if this problem does not go away in a few days.
• Your vision may become blurry after application of the eye ointment.
• Your eyes may become sensitive to bright light. Wear sunglasses and avoid prolonged exposure to bright light.
• Do not wear your contact lenses while using the drug.
• Call your doctor if your eye infection does not improve within seven days or if it gets worse.
• Use all the ofloxacin your doctor prescribed, even if you feel better before you finish. If you stop too soon, your symptoms could come back.

How to Use This Drug

• Follow the instructions on p. 498 for applying eye drops correctly so that you won't absorb the drug into your body and possibly suffer serious adverse effects.
• If you miss a dose, take it as soon as you remember, but skip it if it is almost time for the next dose. **Do not take double doses.**
• Do not share your medication with others.
• Take the drug at the same time(s) each day.
• Store at room temperature with lid on tightly. Do not store in the bathroom. Do not expose to heat, moisture, or strong light. Keep out of reach of children.
• Do not let the ointment or liquid form freeze.

Interactions with Other Drugs

Although there are potential drug interactions reported with the other forms of the drug, there have been no "highly clinically significant" or "clinically significant" drug interactions reported with the ocular form of ofloxacin in *Evaluations of Drug Interactions* 2003. We also found no interactions in the drugs' FDA-approved professional package inserts. However, as the number of new drugs approved for marketing increases and as more experience is gained with these drugs over time, new interactions may be discovered.

Adverse Effects

Call your doctor immediately if you experience:

• difficulty breathing
• chest pain
• difficulty swallowing
• dizziness
• itching, rash, or hives
• swelling or puffiness of eye, lips, or face
• tightness in chest or wheezing

Call your doctor if these symptoms continue:

• blurred vision
• burning of eye
• dryness of eye
• eye pain
• feeling of something in the eye
• increased sensitivity of eye to light
• redness, irritation, or itching of eye, eyelid, or inner lining of eyelid
• tearing of eye

Inflammation

Fluorometholone (flure oh *meth* oh lone)
FML (Allergan)

GENERIC: available
FAMILY: Corticosteroids (see p. 664)

PREGNANCY WARNING

Fluorometholone caused fetal harm in animal studies, including cleft palate, deformed rib cage, deformed limbs, and deformed brain and spinal cord. Because of the potential for serious adverse effects to the fetus, this drug should not be used by pregnant women.

BREAST-FEEDING WARNING

Corticosteroids are excreted in human milk. Because of the potential for serious adverse effects in nursing infants, you should not take fluorometholone while nursing.

Fluorometholone is a steroid used to treat eye conditions that produce inflammation (swelling and redness), itching, or sensitivity. As with all drugs, you should always use the smallest dose of fluorometholone that works. You should also use it for as short a time as possible. Check with your doctor if you do not notice improvement after five to seven days of taking the drug, or if your eye condition worsens.

Corticosteroids (steroids) such as fluorometholone can cause many adverse effects, especially if you use them for a long time so that your entire body absorbs them. Steroids suppress your immune system, lowering your body's defense against disease. Because of this, if you use fluorometholone for a long time, you will be more likely to develop bacterial, fungal, parasitic, and viral infections.

Before You Use This Drug

Do not use if you have or have had:

- ocular fungal disease
- ocular tuberculosis
- ocular herpes
- ocular acute viral disease

Tell your doctor if you have or have had:

- allergies to drugs
- pregnancy or are breast-feeding
- diabetes
- glaucoma
- cataracts
- cornea or other eye disorders or infections

Tell your doctor about any other drugs you take, including aspirin, herbs, vitamins, and other nonprescription products.

When You Use This Drug

- Check with your doctor if there is no improvement after five to seven days of therapy or if condition worsens.
- *For contact lens wearers:* Check with eye doctor prior to using this drug; contact lenses should not be worn during, and possibly for a time following, applications of this drug because of an increased risk of infection.

How to Use This Drug

- Follow directions for applying drops on p. 498.
- Shake the suspension form of this drug vigorously before applying.
- Do not touch applicator tip to any surface.
- If you miss a dose, take it as soon as you remember, but skip it if it is almost time for the next dose. **Do not take double doses.**
- Do not share your medication with others.
- Take the drug at the same time(s) each day.
- Store at room temperature with lid on tightly. Do not store in the bathroom. Do not expose to heat, moisture, or strong light. Keep out of reach of children.

Interactions with Other Drugs

Evaluations of Drug Interactions 2003 lists no drugs, biologics (e.g., vaccines, therapeutic antibodies), or foods as causing "highly clinically significant" or "clinically significant" interactions when used together with the drugs in this section. We also found no interactions in the drugs' FDA-approved professional package inserts. However, as the number of new drugs approved for marketing increases and as more experience is gained with these drugs over time, new interactions may be discovered.

Adverse Effects

Call your doctor immediately if you experience:

- decreased or blurred vision
- watering eyes
- glaucoma
- high eye pressure
- optic nerve damage
- cataracts
- eye pain
- nausea
- vomiting
- eye infection

Call your doctor if these symptoms continue:

- burning, stinging, redness, or watering of the eyes
- temporary mild blurred vision (ointment)

Periodic Tests

Ask your doctor which of these tests should be done periodically while you are taking this drug:

- eye exams

Do Not Use—
except in conjunction with
cataract / intraocular lens surgery.

ALTERNATIVE TREATMENT:
An antibiotic alone, if necessary.

Neomycin and Dexamethasone
(nee oh *mye* sin and dex a *meth* a sone)

Neomycin, Polymixin B, and Dexamethasone (nee oh *mye* sin, pah lee *mix* in bee, and dex a *meth* a sone)
MAXITROL (Falcon)

FAMILY: Antibiotics (see p. 673)
Corticosteroids (see p. 664)

These are eye drops that contain two types of drugs, antibiotics (neomycin and polymixin B) and a corticosteroid (dexamethasone). The drops are used to treat some allergies or eye and eyelid infections caused by bacteria. There is no persuasive proof that they are beneficial for this purpose. However, ophthalmologists find this combination useful to prevent infections and reduce postoperative inflammation in the first few days after intraocular lens surgery.

Dexamethasone belongs to a family of drugs called corticosteroids that are used to reduce inflammation, a natural defense against infection and injury. Drugs in this family are not recommended for treating infections because they can hide the signs of an infection or make it spread.

The antibiotics in these combinations, neomycin and polymixin B, are used to fight infection. If your eye problem is being caused by a bacterial infection, an antibiotic may be needed. Otherwise, antibiotics are unnecessary and should not be used.[39]

Neomycin commonly causes skin rashes in 8% of the people who use it.[40] Using neomycin can also make it hard for you to use other drugs in its family (aminoglycoside antibiotics such as gentamicin and tobramycin, see p. 517) that may be needed later to treat serious infections.

Allergy

Olopatadine (oh loe pa *ta* deen)
PATANOL (Alcon)

GENERIC: not available
FAMILY: Antihistamines

PREGNANCY WARNING

Olopatadine caused an increase in fetal deaths in animal studies. Use during pregnancy only for clear medical reasons. Tell your doctor if you are pregnant or thinking of becoming pregnant before you take this drug.

BREAST-FEEDING WARNING

Olopatadine was excreted in human milk. Because of the potential for adverse effects in the nursing infant, you should consult with your doctor if you are planning to nurse.

Olopatadine is an eye drop used to treat allergies that affect the eye. Olopatadine works in two ways. First, it blocks the action of the allergy-causing chemical histamine, and is therefore classified as an antihistamine. Also, it prevents mast cells (the body's allergy-mediating cells) from releasing histamine.[41]

Alcon Laboratories of Fort Worth, Texas, manufacturer of Patanol, claims that its product olopatadine is superior to cromolyn (GASTROCOM), pemirolast (ALAMAST), and nedocromil (ALOCRIL) in inhibiting release of histamine from mast cells.[42]

The company alleges that clinically, olopatadine provides more effective relief from itching than nedocromil[43] and ketotifen (ZADITOR).[44] These claims have not been independently verified by the FDA and Alcon therefore cannot legally use the results of these studies in their advertising for olopatadine.

Olopatadine's manufacturer states that 7% of users describe headache when using this drug.[41]

Before You Use This Drug

Do not use if you have or have had:

- allergy to olopatadine

Tell your doctor if you have or have had:

- pregnancy or are breast-feeding
- allergy to benzalkonium

When You Use This Drug

- Check with your doctor if symptoms do not improve or if condition worsens.

Tell your doctor about any other drugs you take, including aspirin, herbs, vitamins, and other nonprescription products.

How to Use This Drug

- Follow directions for applying drops on p. 498.
- Prevent the container from becoming contaminated. Avoid letting the tip of the container touch your eye, hands, or any other object.
- Contact lenses should be removed prior to administration of this drug. This drug may be absorbed by soft contact lenses. Wait at least 15 minutes after using olopatadine before putting in contact lenses.
- If you miss a dose, take it as soon as you remember, but skip it if it is almost time for the next dose. **Do not take double doses.**
- Do not share your medication with others.
- Take the drug at the same time(s) each day.
- Store at room temperature with lid on tightly. Do not store in the bathroom. Do not expose to heat, moisture, or strong light. Keep out of reach of children.

Interactions with Other Drugs

Evaluations of Drug Interactions 2003 lists no drugs, biologics (e.g., vaccines, therapeutic antibodies), or foods as causing "highly clinically significant" or "clinically significant" interactions when used together with the drugs in this section. We also found no interactions in the drugs' FDA-approved professional package inserts. However, as the number of new drugs approved for marketing increases and as more experience is gained with these drugs over time, new interactions may be discovered.

Adverse Effects

Call your doctor if these symptoms continue:

- unusual tiredness or weakness
- headache
- burning, dryness, itching, or stinging of the eye
- change in sense of taste
- cold symptoms
- feeling of something in the eye
- redness of eye or inside of eyelid
- eye irritation or pain
- eyelid swelling
- sore throat
- stuffy or runny nose

Artificial Tears

Artificial Tears
TEARISOL (Iolab)
TEARS NATURALE (Alcon)
HYPOTEARS (CIBA Vision)

GENERIC: available
FAMILY: Artificial Tears

PREGNANCY AND BREAST-FEEDING WARNINGS
There is no information in the labels for these drugs. Consult with your doctor or pharmacist if you already are or are planning to become pregnant or to breast-feed.

Artificial tears are used to treat people who do not produce tears normally. You can also use them on a temporary basis to moisten dry eyes. Do not use artificial tears for more than three days unless your doctor has prescribed them.

Most artificial tears preparations contain either polyvinyl alcohol or a methylcellulose solution for lubrication. Methylcellulose solutions stay in your eye longer, but they tend to form crusts on the eyelids. If you use artificial tears containing polyvinyl alcohol, do not also use an eye solution containing boric acid. The combination may form gummy deposits.[45]

To avoid eye infection, irritation, and other problems, take care to prevent contamination when applying eye drops. Do not allow the applicator tip to touch anything, including your eye. After applying drops, replace the cap tightly on the bottle.

Before You Use This Drug

Tell your doctor if you have or have had:

- allergy to hydroxypropyl methylcellulose (artificial tears)

Tell your doctor about any other drugs you take, including aspirin, herbs, vitamins, and other nonprescription products.

When You Use This Drug

- If you wear hard contact lenses, take care not to float lens from eye when applying this drug.
- Check with doctor if present symptoms continue for more than three days or become worse.

How to Use This Drug

- Follow directions for applying eye drops on p. 498.
- Prevent contamination by not touching applicator tip to any surface.
- If you miss a dose, take it as soon as you remember, but skip it if it is almost time for the next dose. **Do not take double doses.**
- Do not share your medication with others.
- Take the drug at the same time(s) each day.
- Store at room temperature with lid on tightly. Do not store in the bathroom. Do not expose to heat, moisture, or strong light. Keep out of reach of children.

Interactions with Other Drugs

Evaluations of Drug Interactions 2003 lists no drugs, biologics (e.g., vaccines, therapeutic antibodies), or foods as causing "highly clinically significant" or "clinically significant" interactions when used together with the drugs in this section. We also found no interactions in the drugs' FDA-approved professional package inserts. However, as the number of new drugs approved for marketing increases and as more experience is gained with these drugs over time, new interactions may be discovered.

Adverse Effects

Call your doctor immediately if you experience:

- eye irritation that was not present before you started using artificial tears

Call your doctor if these symptoms continue:

- blurred vision
- matted or sticky eyelids

REFERENCES

1. *US PDI, Drug Information for the Health Care Provider.* 6th ed. Rockville, Md.: The United States Pharmacopeial Convention, Inc., 1986:448.

2. AMA Department of Drugs. *AMA Drug Evaluations.* 5th ed. Chicago: American Medical Association, 1983:763–4.

3. Koller WC. A new drug for treatment of essential tremor? Time will tell. *Mayo Clinic Proceedings* 1991; 66:1085–7.

4. AMA Department of Drugs. *AMA Drug Evaluations.* 5th ed. Chicago: American Medical Association, 1986:1686.

5. Moroi-Fetters SE, Metz EN, Chambers RB, et al. Aplastic anemia with platelet autoantibodies in a patient after taking methazolamide. *American Journal of Ophthalmology* 1990; 110:570–1.

6. *US PDI, Drug Information for the Health Care Provider.* 23rd ed. Rockville, Md.: The United States Pharmacopeial Convention, Inc., 2004:714–7.

7. Dukes MNG, Beeley L., eds. *Side Effects of Drugs Annual 15.* Amsterdam: Elsevier, 1991:513.

8. Dukes MNG, Beeley L., eds. *Side Effects of Drugs Annual 15.* Amsterdam: Elsevier, 1991:510.

9. *American Hospital Formulary Service Drug Information.* Bethesda, Md.: American Society of Hospital Pharmacists. 1992: 1694–7.

10. Two new beta-blockers for glaucoma. *Medical Letter on Drugs and Therapeutics* 1986; 28:45–6.

11. *US PDI, Drug Information for the Health Care Provider.* 12th ed. Rockville, Md.: The United States Pharmacopeial Convention, Inc., 1992:1757–61.

12. *US PDI, Drug Information for the Health Care Provider.* 12th ed. Rockville, Md.: The United States Pharmacopeial Convention, Inc., 1992:656–9.

13. Allen RC, Hertzmark E, Walker AM, et al. A double-masked comparison of betaxolol vs timolol in the treatment of open-angle glaucoma. *American Journal of Ophthalmology* 1986; 101:535–41.

14. Schuman JS, Horwitz B, Choplin NT, et al. A 1-year study of brimonidine twice daily in glaucoma and ocular hypertension: A controlled, randomized, multicenter clinical trial. Chronic Brimonidine Study Group. *Archives of Ophthalmology* 1997; 115:847–52.

15. Katz LJ. Brimonidine tartrate 0.2% twice daily vs timolol 0.5% twice daily: 1-year results in glaucoma patients. Brimonidine Study Group. *American Journal of Ophthalmology* 1999; 127:20–6.

16. Stewart WC, Day DG, Stewart JA, et al. The efficacy and safety of latanoprost 0.005% once daily versus brimonidine 0.2% twice daily in open-angle glaucoma or ocular hypertension. *American Journal of Ophthalmology* 2001; 131:631–5.

17. Stewart WC, Sharpe ED, Harbin TS Jr., et al. Brimonidine 0.2% versus dorzolamide 2% each given three times daily to reduce intraocular pressure. *American Journal of Ophthalmology* 2000; 129:723–7.

18. Heijl A, Strahlman E, Sverrisson T, et al. A comparison of dorzolamide and timolol in patients with pseudoexfoliation and glaucoma or ocular hypertension. *Ophthalmology* 1997; 104:137–42.

19. Simmons ST. Efficacy of brimonidine 0.2% and dorzolamide 2% as adjunctive therapy to beta-blockers in adult patients with glaucoma or ocular hypertension. *Clinical Therapeutics* 2001; 23:604–19.

20. Maus TL, Nau C, Brubaker RF. Comparison of the early effects of brimonidine and apraclonidine as topical ocular hypotensive agents. *Archives of Ophthalmology* 1999; 117:586–91.

21. Nordlund JR, Pasquale LR, Robin AL, et al. The cardiovascular, pulmonary, and ocular hypotensive effects of 0.2% brimonidine. *Archives of Ophthalmology* 1995; 113:77–83.

22. Korsch E, Grote A, Seybold M, et al. Systemic adverse effects of topical treatment with brimonidine in an infant with secondary glaucoma. *European Journal of Pediatrics* 1999; 158:685.

23. Zambarakji HJ, Spencer AF, Vernon SA. An unusual side effect of Dorzolamide. *Eye* 1997; 11(pt 3):418–9.

24. Pfeiffer N. Dorzolamide: Development and clinical application of a topical carbonic anhydrase inhibitor. *Survey of Ophthalmology* 1997; 42:137–51.

25. Maus TL, Larsson LI, McLaren JW, et al. Comparison of dorzolamide and acetazolamide as suppressors of aqueous humor flow in humans. *Archives of Ophthalmology* 1997; 115:45–9.

26. Hutzelmann J, Owens S, Shedden A, et al. Comparison of the safety and efficacy of the fixed combination of dorzolamide/timolol and the concomitant administration of dorzolamide and timolol: A clinical equivalence study. International Clinical Equivalence Study Group. *British Journal of Ophthalmology* 1998; 82:1249–53.

27. *2002 Mosby's Drug Consult.* St. Louis, Mo.: Mosby, 2002.

28. Centofanti M, Manni G, Gregori D, et al. Comparative acute effects of brimonidine 0.2% versus dorzolamide 2% combined with beta-blockers in glaucoma. *Graefe's Archive for Clinical and Experimental Ophthalmology* 2000; 238:302–5.

29. Zhang WY, Po AL, Dua HS, et al. Meta-analysis of randomised controlled trials comparing latanoprost with timolol in the treatment of patients with open angle glaucoma or ocular hypertension. *British Journal of Ophthalmology* 2001; 85:983–90.

30. Polo V, Larrosa JM, Gomez ML, et al. Latanoprost versus combined therapy with timolol plus dorzolamide: IOP-lowering effect in open-angle glaucoma. *Acta Ophthalmologica Scandinavica* 2001; 79:6–9.

31. Wand M. Latanoprost and hyperpigmentation of eyelashes. *Archives of Ophthalmology* 1997; 115:1206–8.

32. Wand M, Ritch R, Isbey EK Jr., et al. Latanoprost and periocular skin color changes. *Archives of Ophthalmology* 2001; 119:614–5.

33. Yanoff M, Duker JS. Therapy—Current Medical Management of Glaucoma. In *Ophthalmology.* London: Mosby, 2004:xxi, 1548–9.

34. Watson P, Stjernschantz J. A six-month, randomized, double-masked study comparing latanoprost with timolol in open-angle glaucoma and ocular hypertension. The Latanoprost Study Group. *Ophthalmology* 1996; 103:126–37.

35. Camras CB. Comparison of latanoprost and timolol in patients with ocular hypertension and glaucoma: A six-month masked, multicenter trial in the United States. The United States Latanoprost Study Group. *Ophthalmology* 1996; 103:138–47.

36. Mitra M, Chang B, James T. Drug points. Exacerbation of angina associated with latanoprost. *British Medical Journal* 2001; 323:783.

37. Centers for Disease Control and Prevention. Sexually transmitted diseases treatment guidelines. *Morbidity and Mortality Weekly Report* 2002; 51:RR-6. Available at: http://www.cdc.gov/STD/treatment/4-2002TG.htm#OphthalmiaNeonatorumProphylaxis. Accessed April 28, 2004.

38. Mahon BE, Rosenman MB, Kleiman MB. Maternal and infant use of erythromycin and other macrolide antibiotics as risk factors for infantile hypertrophic pyloric stenosis. *Journal of Pediatrics* 2001; 139:380–4.

39. AMA Department of Drugs. *AMA Drug Evaluations.* 1st ed. Chicago: American Medical Association, 1971:526.

40. Patrick J, Panzer JD, Derbes VJ. Neomycin sensitivity in the normal (nonatopic) individual. *Archives of Dermatology* 1970; 102:532–5.

41. *Physicians' Desk Reference.* 56th ed. Montvale, N.J.: Medical Economics Company, Inc., 2002:540–2.

42. Yanni JM, Miller ST, Gamache DA, et al. Comparative effects of topical ocular anti-allergy drugs on human conjunctival mast cells. *Annals of Allergy, Asthma, and Immunology* 1997; 79:541–5.

43. Butrus S, Greiner JV, Discepola M, et al. Comparison of the clinical efficacy and comfort of olopatadine hydrochloride 0.1% ophthalmic solution and nedocromil sodium 2% ophthalmic solution in the human conjunctival allergen challenge model. *Clinical Therapeutics* 2000; 22:1462–72.

44. Berdy GJ, Spangler DL, Bensch G, et al. A comparison of the relative efficacy and clinical performance of olopatadine hydrochloride 0.1% ophthalmic solution and ketotifen fumarate 0.025% ophthalmic solution in the conjunctival antigen challenge model. *Clinical Therapeutics* 2000; 22:826–33.

45. *Handbook of Nonprescription Drugs.* 7th ed. Washington, D.C.: American Pharmaceutical Association, 1982:425.

17

DRUGS FOR GASTROINTESTINAL DISORDERS

The purpose of the gastrointestinal (GI) tract is to extract fluid and essential nutrients from the food we eat and to eliminate wastes. All the way along the tract, food is propelled by involuntary rhythmic muscular contractions called peristalsis. From the mouth, ingested food proceeds down a straight tube called the esophagus into the stomach. It is here that the process of digestion begins, with stomach acid being secreted to break down food. Enzymes that also facilitate the breakdown of chemicals in food, permitting absorption into the bloodstream, are secreted here and in subsequent sections of the GI tract. From the stomach, food passes into the small intestine, a relatively thin, long (12 feet) tube with three distinct portions: duodenum, jejunum, and ileum. Enzymes from the pancreas and the gallbladder enter at the duodenum and have specific roles in the digestion of food. Generally, several hours later, the remaining food passes from the ileum into the large intestine or colon. The appendix is a pouch of uncertain function close to the junction between the large and small intestines. Water and some remaining nutrients are extracted in the large intestine, before the remains are excreted through the rectum as stool.

Most of the time, the GI tract functions without problems, but there are a number of ways in which the system can go awry. In this chapter, we discuss drugs for two of the most common of these (ulcers and irritable bowel syndrome) as well as drugs for certain GI symptoms (e.g., constipation, diarrhea, gas).

ULCERS AND GASTROESOPHAGEAL REFLUX DISEASE (GERD)

As mentioned, the stomach secretes acids to aid digestion. There is a sphincter at the junction between the esophagus and the stomach that is supposed to prevent these acidic stomach contents from backing up into the esophagus, which is not designed to tolerate such strong acids. When such regurgitation occurs, resulting in irritation of the esophagus, it can cause the chest pain or discomfort that is sometimes called heartburn, as well as nausea and an unpleasant taste in the mouth. The problem is typically worse after meals, when the stomach is full, and when lying down, because gravity no longer keeps the stomach contents in place.

There are nondrug treatments, with no safety concerns, and less expensive drugs that may be effective for GERD; these should be tried before you use any drugs for heartburn. First, try to avoid foods that trigger your condition (e.g., fatty foods, onions, caffeine, peppermint, and chocolate), and avoid alcohol, smoking, and tight clothing.[1]

Second, avoid food, and particularly alcohol, within two or three hours of bedtime. Third, elevate the head of the bed about six inches or sleep with extra pillows.

An ulcer is a different condition, though related to GERD in the sense that both are related to excess stomach acid. An ulcer is a pit in the lining of the GI tract (most commonly the stomach and the duodenum); the superficial cells in the lining are absent, exposing underlying tissues in the tract. Ulcers can cause significant pain, can bleed, and, in infrequent cases, can actually erode all the way through the wall of the GI tract (a perforated ulcer).

For both GERD and ulcers, it is important to avoid drug-induced causes. Aspirin, ibuprofen, and other nonsteroidal anti-inflammatory drugs (NSAIDs) (see p. 281) are known to cause ulcers. Ask your doctor if acetaminophen could be substituted for these drugs. Check with your doctor about the osteoporosis medications alendronate and risedronate (FOSAMAX and ACTONEL) (see p. 584), which irritate the esophagus.

If these measures are not effective, try simple over-the-counter (OTC) antacids such as a generic aluminum hydroxide and magnesium hydroxide product (MAALOX, MAALOX TC, see p. 533). If this does not relieve your symptoms, one of the family of stomach acid–blocking drugs known as histamine2-blockers can be tried (see p. 538). Histamine2-blockers are available in both over-the-counter and prescription strengths. If you still have not experienced adequate relief, your doctor may prescribe one of a newer family of drugs called proton pump inhibitors (PPIs). PPIs inhibit secretion of stomach acid, whereas histamine2-blockers partially prevent production of the acid. Histamine2-blockers relieve GERD pain more quickly than PPIs.[2] It is likely that most people being prescribed PPIs for GERD have not first had an adequate trial of the nondrug and other drug treatments discussed above.

A relatively new development in the treatment of ulcers is the focus on a bacterium, *Helicobacter pylori,* which has been implicated in ulcer disease.[3] *Helicobacter pylori* can be diagnosed by tests of the blood, breath, and stool, as well as through samples taken during endoscopy.[3] Doctors sometimes prescribe various combinations of antibiotics, histamine2-blockers, and PPIs to eradicate this infection. Such treatments have high success rates and low recurrence rates, but the treatment is arduous.

If at any time during any of the above treatments symptoms worsen or bleeding occurs, call your doctor.

IRRITABLE BOWEL SYNDROME (IBS)

IBS is a rather ill-defined syndrome said to affect 15% of people in Western countries.[4] For unclear reasons, it appears to affect women more often than men. The essential elements of IBS are chronic abdominal pain associated with either constipation (constipation-predominant IBS) or diarrhea (diarrhea-predominant IBS); some patients alternate between constipation and diarrhea.

IBS itself is not a life-threatening condition, although it can be debilitating. The diagnosis of IBS should be based on a set of internationally recognized symptoms known as the Rome II Criteria[4] (see box, p. 556) and requires the exclusion of treatable causes of the patient's symptoms, such as ulcerative colitis. This is especially important if the following signs of ulcerative colitis are present: onset after age 50, rectal bleeding, fever, weight loss, or anemia. There are no abnormal laboratory tests or changes in the cells of the GI tract on biopsy that can objectively establish the diagnosis of IBS. In fact, the diagnosis of IBS can only be made if all tests for other diseases that might explain the patient's symptoms are negative. For young, otherwise healthy patients, extensive testing may not be necessary.

The FDA has approved drugs for both diarrhea-predominant and constipation-predominant IBS. The former, alosetron (LOTRONEX) (see p. 555), had to be removed from the market after it caused serious constipation and a condition of decreased blood flow to the intestine called ischemic colitis. The latter, tegaserod (ZELNORM) (see p. 557), has also been associated with ischemic colitis and severe, disabling diarrhea, and it is barely effective.

Instead, we recommend that you manage IBS through a combination of dietary and drug treatments targeted at your particular symptoms. There is also a report of a successful multidisciplinary approach, including psychological counseling, to this disease.[5]

CONSTIPATION

Constipation is a significant change or persistent abnormality in bowel habits, usually with fewer than three stools per week, lumpy or hard stools, excessive straining, or incomplete emptying of the rectum. Causes include diet, body structure, complications of childbirth, a longer time for passage of intestinal contents, and certain medications (see p. 38). The latter include antacids (see p. 533), anticholinergics (see p. 617), antihistamines (see p. 360), antidepressants (see p. 184), antipsychotics (see p. 258), benzodiazepines[6] (see p. 223), diuretics (see p. 60), incontinence drugs, iron, and narcotics (see p. 282).[7] Constipation is more common in women, children, and older people. A rare condition called Hirschsprung's disease also causes constipation, is more likely to affect males, and has onset in childhood.[8] Risk factors for constipation include anal fissures, cystic fibrosis, depression, diabetes, physical abuse, eating disorders, malabsorption disorders, multiple sclerosis, Parkinson's disease, and pregnancy.[6–9]

When do you really need to take a laxative? You should not take a laxative to "clean out your system" or to make your body act more "normally." It is untrue that everyone must have a bowel movement daily. Perfectly healthy people may have from three bowel movements per week to three bowel movements per day.

If the frequency of your bowel movements has decreased, if you are having bowel movements less than three times a week, or if you are having difficulty passing stools, you are constipated, but this does not necessarily mean that you need a laxative. It is better to treat simple, occasional constipation without drugs, by eating a high-fiber diet that includes whole-grain breads and cereals, raw vegetables, raw and dried fruits, and beans, and by drinking plenty of nonalcoholic liquids (six to eight glasses per day). This type of diet will both prevent and treat constipation, and it is less costly than taking drugs. Regular exercise—at least 30 minutes per day of swimming, cycling, jogging, or brisk walking—will also help your body maintain regularity.

If you are constipated while traveling or at some other time when it is hard for you to eat properly, it may be appropriate to take a laxative for a short time. The only types of laxatives you should use for self-medication are bulk-forming laxatives such as psyllium or methylcellulose (see p. 566), or a hyperosmotic laxative such as lactulose (see p. 568). Bulk-forming laxatives usually take effect in 12 hours to three days, compared with docusate (see p. 571), which takes effect one or two days after the first dose but may require three to five days of treatment. Even bulk-forming laxatives should only be used occasionally, if possible.

DIARRHEA

Diarrhea is a change in the frequency and consistency of bowel movements and is characterized by the abnormally frequent passage of loose or watery stools. Diarrhea can be associated with underlying disease, anxiety, or infection, usually due to a virus in the intestinal tract. Diarrhea can also be a reaction to a medication, food, or alcohol. Drugs that cause diarrhea include antibiotics (see p. 673), antacids containing magnesium such as Maalox (see p. 533) and Mylanta (see p. 537), dietary supplements containing magnesium,[10] certain drugs for high blood pressure, all laxatives except the bulk-forming variety (e.g., psyllium and methylcellulose, see p. 566), and quinidine, a drug for irregular heartbeat (see p. 140). See p. 39 for a longer list of drugs that can cause diarrhea.

Acute or sudden simple diarrhea lasts only a few days and typically improves with or without medication. Even most infectious diarrhea does not require an antibiotic.

According to a telephone survey by the fed-eral Centers for Disease Control and Prevention (CDC), residents of the United States on average experience 0.72 episodes of acute diarrhea each year. The highest rates were among children under the age of five years (1.1 episodes per year), and the lowest among those 65 years and older (0.32 episodes per year),[11] although death rates per case of diarrhea are likely to be disproportionately high in older adults. Focusing on food-borne illnesses alone (not necessarily diarrhea), the CDC has also developed an estimate of 76 million illnesses, 325,000 hospitalizations, and 5,000 deaths in the United States each year.[12]

Despite the heavy promotion and frequent use of ineffective and/or dangerous prescription or over-the-counter drugs, the world standard for hydrating patients with diarrhea is oral rehydration therapy, an essentially free therapy that is at everyone's fingertips. Many of the deaths in children and older adults described above might have been prevented if the patients had been given oral rehydration solution (ORS) (see box on this page).

How to Treat Acute Simple Diarrhea

• Do not eat or drink milk and dairy products, fresh fruits and vegetables, coffee, spicy foods, or other food you do not tolerate well.

• Do not consume drinks with a high sugar content, such as grape juice, apple juice, and soft drinks, including cola, ginger ale, and sports drinks.[13]

• Do not eat highly sweetened foods such as candy, ice cream, or Jell-O because they have too much sugar, which can make the diarrhea worse.[13]

• Drink plenty of ORS (see formula in box). Once you have noticed watery diarrhea in the toilet bowl, you are probably already a liter (slightly more than a quart) dehydrated. This means you should try to catch up with the fluids you have already lost by drinking three to four eight-ounce glasses of ORS over the next several hours. Once you have caught up—this will

---

**HOW TO MAKE ORAL
REHYDRATION SOLUTION (ORS)**

To one liter (slightly more than a quart) of clean water add:

• one-half of a level teaspoon of salt

• eight level teaspoons of sugar

(Caution: Before adding the sugar, taste the drink and be sure it is less salty than tears.)

If it is available, you can add a mashed ripe banana, which also provides potassium.

be apparent because you will be well enough hydrated to pass urine—you should drink at least four additional eight-ounce glasses of ORS every 12 hours until the diarrhea stops. Patients on a fluid- or salt-restricted diet should consult their physicians concerning the use of ORS.

• Do not eat salty foods such as salty soup, potato chips, or peanuts.

• Do not take medication not prescribed or directed by your doctor or other health professional.

• Take your temperature once a day.

When to Seek Help from a Health Professional
• severe diarrhea in an older adult, particularly one who is very weak
• fever above 101°F (38.3°C)
• blood in the stools or black, tarry stools
• diarrhea for more than three days
• a drug taken under the direction of a doctor may be the cause of the diarrhea
• diarrhea accompanied by severe, incapacitating abdominal pain
• diarrhea with severe dehydration, characterized by dizziness while standing, confusion, or unresponsiveness

---

GAS

One of the miracles of modern Madison Avenue marketing is that the public is still spending money for simethicone, alone or in combination with other drugs, for gas or infant colic.

Despite the millions spent on advertising to convince us otherwise, the feeling of bloating and pain after eating is not caused by gas. There is no relation between these symptoms and the amount of gas in the intestinal tract. The use of antigas products to relieve this discomfort is inappropriate, as there is no medical need to expel gas from the body.

There are two major sources of gas in the gastrointestinal tract. The first is swallowed air that is either released in belching or continues through the intestines and must be passed as flatus. Gas is also produced in the large intestine by normal bacteria and must eventually leave the body as flatus through the rectum. Both of these processes are perfectly normal.

In 1975, *The Medical Letter on Drugs and Therapeutics,* one of the world's most respected sources of objective drug information, wrote: *"There is no convincing evidence that simethicone, alone or in combination, is effective for the treatment of flatulence [gas] associated with functional disorders of the gastrointestinal tract."* [14] Two decades later, a randomized trial of 83 infants between two and eight weeks of age with colic found no significant difference between simethicone and placebo (a look-alike dummy drug). [15] *The Medical Letter* reviewed simethicone again in 1996 and said: *"There is no convincing evidence that simethicone, alone or in combination, is effective for treatment of eructation [belching], flatulence or any other signs or symptoms of excess gastrointestinal gas."* [16] The best approach to gas is to avoid those foods you have identified as problems for you.

DRUG PROFILES

Ulcers and Gastroesophageal Reflux Disease (GERD)

Antacids

Aluminum Hydroxide (a *loo* mi num hye *drox* ide)
AMPHOJEL (Wyeth-Ayerst)

Aluminum Hydroxide and Magnesium Hydroxide (a *loo* mi num hye *drox* ide and mag *nee* zee um hye *drox* ide)
MAALOX, MAALOX TC (Novartis)

NIGHTTIME HEARTBURN TREATMENTS: TRY THESE FIRST

There are nondrug treatments, with no safety concerns, and less expensive drugs that may be effective for you; these should be tried before you use any drugs for heartburn. First, try to avoid foods that trigger your condition (e.g., fatty foods, onions, caffeine, peppermint, and chocolate), and avoid alcohol, smoking, and tight clothing.[1]

Second, avoid food, and particularly alcohol, within two or three hours of bedtime. Third, elevate the head of the bed about six inches or sleep with extra pillows.

For both heartburn and ulcers, it is important to avoid drug-induced causes. Aspirin, ibuprofen, and other nonsteroidal anti-inflammatory drugs (NSAIDs) (see p. 281) are known to cause ulcers. Ask your doctor if acetaminophen could be substituted for these drugs. Check with your doctor about the osteoporosis medications alendronate and risedronate (FOSAMAX and ACTONEL) (see p. 584), which irritate the esophagus.

If these measures are not effective, try simple over-the-counter (OTC) antacids such as a generic aluminum hydroxide and magnesium hydroxide product (MAALOX, MAALOX TC, see p. 533). If symptoms worsen or bleeding occurs, call your doctor. If this does not relieve your symptoms, one of the family of stomach acid–blocking drugs known as histamine2-blockers can be tried (see p. 538). This family includes cimetidine (TAGAMET), famotidine (PEPCID), nizatidine (AXID), and ranitidine (ZANTAC). Histamine2-blockers are available in both OTC and prescription strengths.

If the OTC histamine2-blockers do not give adequate relief of your symptoms after 14 days, it is time to consult your physician.

Aluminum Hydroxide and Magnesium Carbonate (a loo mi num hye drox ide and mag nee zee um car bon ate)
GAVISCON (GlaxoSmithKline)
GAVISCON-2 (GlaxoSmithKline)

Magaldrate (mag al drate)
RIOPAN (Whitehall-Robins)

Limited Use

Magnesium Hydroxide (mag nee zee um hye drox ide)
PHILLIPS' MILK OF MAGNESIA
(Bayer Healthcare)

GENERIC: available
FAMILY: Antacids

PREGNANCY AND BREAST-FEEDING
There is no information in the drug labels. Consult with your doctor or pharmacist.

Aluminum hydroxide and magnesium hydroxide neutralize stomach acid and are used to treat ulcers, stomach upset caused by stomach acid, and reflux esophagitis (heartburn) or gastroesophageal reflux disease (GERD). In reflux esophagitis, acidic stomach contents flow backwards up into the esophagus (the tube leading from the mouth to the stomach), causing a burning sensation under the breastbone. Magaldrate, a chemical combination of aluminum hydroxide and magnesium hydroxide, is used in the same way. Liquid antacids are considered to be more effective than solid or powdered forms.[17]

Aluminum can cause constipation, and magnesium can cause diarrhea. By combining aluminum with magnesium, these drugs reduce the problems that either substance alone can cause. However, the combination may still cause either constipation or diarrhea.

The combination of aluminum hydroxide and magnesium carbonate is only used to temporarily relieve heartburn caused by reflux esophagitis. You should not take Gaviscon or Gaviscon-2, two brand-name products that contain this combination of drugs, for ulcers or serious stomach upset due to stomach acid. They do not contain enough antacid to neutralize significant amounts of stomach acid. Instead, you should take a generic combination of aluminum hydroxide and magnesium hydroxide.

Because it loosens stools, magnesium hydroxide can also be used as a laxative. It should only be used occasionally for this purpose (see constipation, p. 531, for alternatives).

Aluminum hydroxide is also used to prevent a certain type of kidney stone. If you become constipated while using aluminum hydroxide, ask your doctor about switching to a product that contains both aluminum hydroxide and magnesium hydroxide.

If you take large doses of one of these drugs or use it for a long time, see your doctor for regular checkups. If you are treating yourself with these drugs, do not take them for more than two weeks unless you check with your doctor.

Ulcers often come back after a few months. For frequent, severe recurrences, maintenance therapy using histamine2-blockers is used. If your ulcer disease is resistant to treatment with histamine2-blockers, talk to your doctor about the antibiotic combination treatments that are used to eradicate the bacterium *Helicobacter pylori* (see p. 530). This bacterium is present in a large number of people with ulcers. The presence of this bacterium can be diagnosed with a blood, breath, or stool test in people with a history of ulcer disease.

Anyone with severe kidney disease should not use magnesium antacids, as the magnesium can build up in the blood.[18] Dialysis patients should avoid aluminum-containing antacids, as aluminum can be deposited in and weaken bone.[19]

Before You Use This Drug

Do not use if you have or have had:

- intestinal obstruction
- severely reduced kidney function

Tell your doctor if you have or have had:

- abdominal pain that is severe
- allergies to drugs
- Alzheimer's disease
- appendicitis
- bleeding from rectum or gastrointestinal tract
- bone fractures (antacids containing aluminum or magaldrate)
- colon inflammation (colitis)
- colostomy
- constipation that is severe or prolonged
- diarrhea that is prolonged
- diverticulitis
- hemorrhoids
- ileostomy
- intestinal blockage
- kidney problems
- liver problems
- pregnancy or are breast-feeding

Tell your doctor about any other drugs you take, including aspirin, herbs, vitamins, and other nonprescription products.

When You Use This Drug

- **Call your doctor immediately if you have black, tarry stools or if you vomit material that looks like coffee grounds. These are signs of a bleeding ulcer.**
- Call your doctor if you have trouble swallowing or persistent abdominal pain.
- If you are on a low-salt (low-sodium) or low-phosphate diet, ask your doctor or pharmacist to help you choose an antacid. Many brands contain these substances.
- Have regular visits with your doctor if you are taking large doses or using regularly for a long time.

- Aluminum-containing drugs may interfere with radiopharmaceutical tests; be sure to tell your doctor you are taking them.
- Keep an interval of one or two hours between taking these and other oral drugs.
- Do not take for more than two weeks unless your doctor tells you to.

How to Use This Drug

- If you miss a dose, take it as soon as you remember, but skip it if it is almost time for the next dose. **Do not take double doses.**
- Do not share your medication with others.
- Take the drug at the same time(s) each day.
- Take tablets with **a full glass (eight ounces)** of water. If you use tablets, chew them thoroughly.
- *For ulcer treatment:* Take one to three hours after meals and at bedtime for maximum effectiveness.
- Drink plenty of fluids if taking aluminum-containing antacids.
- Store at room temperature with lid on tightly. Do not store in the bathroom. Do not expose to heat, moisture, or strong light. Do not let liquid form freeze. Keep out of reach of children.

Interactions with Other Drugs

The following drugs, biologics (e.g., vaccines, therapeutic antibodies), or foods are listed in *Evaluations of Drug Interactions* 2003 as causing "highly clinically significant" or "clinically significant" interactions when used together with any of the drugs in this section. In some sections with multiple drugs, the interaction may have been reported for one but not all drugs in this section, but we include the interaction because the drugs in this section are similar to one another. We have also included potentially serious interactions listed in the drug's FDA-approved professional package insert or in published medical journal articles. There may be other drugs, especially those in the families of drugs listed below, that also will react with this drug to cause severe adverse effects. Make sure to tell your doctor and pharmacist the drugs you are taking and tell them if you are taking any of these interacting drugs:

ACTONEL, AGENERASE, ALLEGRA, amprenavir, aspirin, AVELOX, cefdinir, CELEBREX, celecoxib, CIPRO, ciprofloxacin, delavirdine, digoxin, ECOTRIN, fexofenadine, GENUINE BAYER ASPIRIN, KAYEXALATE, ketoconazole, LANOXICAPS, LANOXIN, LEVAQUIN, levofloxacin, MAXAQUIN, moxifloxacin, NIZORAL, OCUFLOX, OMNICEF, RESCRIPTOR, risedronate, SKELID, sodium polystyrene sulfonate, SUMYCIN, tetracycline, tiludronate, vitamin D_3.

Adverse Effects

Call your doctor immediately if you experience:

- appetite loss
- bone pain
- constipation that is severe
- continuing feeling of discomfort
- dizziness or lightheadedness
- fecal impaction
- headache
- irregular heartbeat
- mood or mental changes
- muscle weakness
- nausea or vomiting
- swelling of wrists, ankles, feet, or lower legs
- tiredness or weakness that is unusual
- urination that is frequent
- weight loss that is unusual

Call your doctor if these symptoms continue:

- chalky taste
- constipation
- diarrhea or laxative effect
- nausea or vomiting
- stomach cramps
- stools that are speckled or whitish

Periodic Tests

Ask your doctor which of these tests should be done periodically while you are taking this drug:

- blood aluminum, calcium, phosphate, and potassium levels
- kidney function tests

 Do Not Use

ALTERNATIVE TREATMENT:
See the box accompanying this drug profile.

Magnesium Hydroxide, Aluminum Hydroxide, and Simethicone

(mag *nee* zee um hye *drox* ide, a *loo* mi num hye *drox* ide, and sye *meth* a cone)
MYLANTA, MYLANTA-II (Johnson & Johnson/Merck)

FAMILY: Antacids

This combination of magnesium hydroxide, aluminum hydroxide, and simethicone is used both as an antacid and as an antiflatulent (antigas) drug. As an antacid, it is used to treat ulcers, serious stomach upset caused by stomach acid, and heartburn. As an antiflatulent, it is used to relieve "excess gas."

We do not recommend this widely used drug because it contains an ineffective and unnecessary ingredient, simethicone. There is no convincing evidence that simethicone, alone or in combination with other drugs, is effective in treating so-called excess gas.[16] If you need an antacid, use a combination of aluminum hydroxide and magnesium hydroxide (see p. 533). Do not waste your money on products that contain simethicone.

If you think that you suffer from "excess gas," it may be that you actually have a bloated feeling from overeating or discomfort from eating the wrong food. In this case, no antigas drug will help you because the problem has nothing to do with gas. If you do have excess gas in your

---

NIGHTTIME HEARTBURN TREATMENTS: TRY THESE FIRST

There are nondrug treatments, with no safety concerns, and less expensive drugs that may be effective for you; these should be tried before you use any drugs for heartburn. First, try to avoid foods that trigger your condition (e.g., fatty foods, onions, caffeine, peppermint, and chocolate), and avoid alcohol, smoking, and tight clothing.[1]

Second, avoid food, and particularly alcohol, within two or three hours of bedtime. Third, elevate the head of the bed about six inches or sleep with extra pillows.

For both heartburn and ulcers, it is important to avoid drug-induced causes. Aspirin, ibuprofen, and other non-steroidal anti-inflammatory drugs (NSAIDs) (see p. 281) are known to cause ulcers. Ask your doctor if acetaminophen could be substituted for these drugs. Check with your doctor about the osteoporosis medications alendronate and risedronate (FOSAMAX and ACTONEL) (see p. 584), which irritate the esophagus.

If these measures are not effective, try simple over-the-counter (OTC) antacids such as a generic aluminum hydroxide and magnesium hydroxide product (MAALOX, MAALOX TC, see p. 533). If symptoms worsen or bleeding occurs, call your doctor. If this does not relieve your symptoms, one of the family of stomach acid–blocking drugs known as histamine2-blockers can be tried (see p. 538). This family includes cimetidine (TAGAMET), famotidine (PEPCID), nizatidine (AXID), and ranitidine (ZANTAC). Histamine2-blockers are available in both OTC and prescription strengths.

If the OTC histamine2-blockers do not give adequate relief of your symptoms after 14 days, it is time to consult your physician.

stomach, the best way to treat it is to reduce the amount of air that you swallow. You can do this by cutting down on smoking, carbonated drinks, eating rapidly, and gum-chewing, which make you swallow air. A dry mouth (which may be due to anxiety or a drug you are taking) and badly fitting dentures also make you swallow more air.

Most gas is created when bacteria in the large intestine come into contact with carbohydrates, especially those found in cabbage, broccoli, and beans.[16] This bacterial action is normal, as is the passing of gas (flatus). Different people pass different amounts of gas, and passing gas is no cause for medical concern. Simethicone is not recommended for the treatment of infant colic.[20]

Histamine2-Blockers

Cimetidine (sye *met* i deen)
TAGAMET (GlaxoSmithKline)

Famotidine (fam *oat* i deen)
PEPCID (Merck)

Nizatidine (nye *zat* i deen),
AXID (Lilly)

Ranitidine (ra *nit* i deen)
ZANTAC (GlaxoSmithKline)

GENERIC: available
FAMILY: Histamine2-Blockers

PREGNANCY WARNING

There were sporadic abortions in an animal study with famotidine. There was no evidence of toxicity in animal studies with ranitidine; no data were available for cimetidine and nizatidine. Use during pregnancy only for clear medical reasons. Tell your doctor if you are pregnant or thinking of becoming pregnant before you take this drug.

BREAST-FEEDING WARNING

These drugs are excreted in human milk. Because of the potential for adverse effects in nursing infants, you should not take these drugs while nursing.

NIGHTTIME HEARTBURN TREATMENTS: TRY THESE FIRST

There are nondrug treatments, with no safety concerns, and less expensive drugs that may be effective for you; these should be tried before you use any drugs for heartburn. First, try to avoid foods that trigger your condition (e.g., fatty foods, onions, caffeine, peppermint, and chocolate), and avoid alcohol, smoking, and tight clothing.[1]

Second, avoid food, and particularly alcohol, within two or three hours of bedtime. Third, elevate the head of the bed about six inches or sleep with extra pillows.

For both heartburn and ulcers, it is important to avoid drug-induced causes. Aspirin, ibuprofen, and other nonsteroidal anti-inflammatory drugs (NSAIDs) (see p. 281) are known to cause ulcers. Ask your doctor if acetaminophen could be substituted for these drugs. Check with your doctor about the osteoporosis medications alendronate and risedronate (FOSAMAX and ACTONEL) (see p. 584), which irritate the esophagus.

If these measures are not effective, try simple over-the-counter (OTC) antacids such as a generic aluminum hydroxide and magnesium hydroxide product (MAALOX, MAALOX TC, see p. 533). If symptoms worsen or bleeding occurs, call your doctor. If this does not relieve your symptoms, one of the family of stomach acid–blocking drugs known as histamine2-blockers can be tried (see p. 538). This family includes cimetidine (TAGAMET), famotidine (PEPCID), nizatidine (AXID), and ranitidine (ZANTAC). Histamine2-blockers are available in both OTC and prescription strengths.

If the OTC histamine2-blockers do not give adequate relief of your symptoms after 14 days, it is time to consult your physician.

Cimetidine, famotidine, nizatidine, and ranitidine block the release of stomach acid and are used to treat ulcers and conditions caused by excess stomach acid. They do so by blocking the action of histamine at the histamine2-receptors in certain stomach cells that produce stomach acid. (These drugs are distinct from those that block histamine1—the drugs used for allergy (see p. 360). You should not take these drugs for minor digestive complaints such as occasional upset stomach, nausea, or heartburn, as there is no evidence that they are effective for treating those problems.

There is no valid scientific evidence that one of these histamine2-blockers is better than another. All of the histamine2-blockers are now available in nonprescription strengths.

Ulcers often come back after a few months. For frequent, severe recurrences, maintenance therapy using histamine2-blockers is used. If your ulcer disease is resistant to treatment with histamine2-blockers, talk to your doctor about the antibiotic combination treatments that are used to eradicate the bacterium *Helicobacter pylori* (see p. 530). This bacterium is present in a large number of people with ulcers. The presence of this bacterium can be diagnosed with a blood, breath, or stool test in people with a history of ulcer disease.

A possible adverse effect with these drugs is confusion.[21] Elderly people are more likely to have reduced kidney or liver function, and are thus at greater risk for this complication. **If you have reduced kidney function, your doctor should start you on a low or less frequent dose.**

If you are over 60, you should generally be taking less than the usual adult dose of these drugs, especially if you have reduced kidney or liver function. Elderly people eliminate these drugs more slowly than younger people.[22] This means that the drug stays in the body for a longer time, which puts you at a higher risk of adverse effects, particularly dizziness and confusion.[23]

Rarely, people taking cimetidine have developed bone marrow depression, a serious adverse effect in which the bone marrow is unable to produce blood cells normally. Cimetidine has been shown to cause benign tumors in the testicles of rats,[22] and it can reduce the sperm count in men (and therefore their ability to father children) if it is taken regularly for at least nine weeks.[24] Famotidine, nizatidine, and ranitidine are less likely than cimetidine to cause enlarged breasts, decreased sexual ability, and low sex drive.[25]

Cigarette smoking can delay the healing of ulcers.[26] Liquid antacids of magnesium and aluminum (see p. 534) in low doses are as effective at healing ulcers as histamine2-blockers and are less costly. However, long-term use of antacids has risks. Antacids with aluminum can cause constipation and those with magnesium can cause severe diarrhea. Those antacids should not be taken by anyone with severe kidney disease. If ulcer symptoms worsen or bleeding occurs, you should seek medical help.

Before You Use This Drug

Tell your doctor if you have or have had:

- allergies to any drugs in this class
- immune system problems
- kidney or liver problems
- phenylketonuria (chewable tablet and oral disintegrating tablet of Pepcid; effervescent, granule, and tablet forms of Zantac)
- pregnancy or are breast-feeding

Tell your doctor about any other drugs you take, including aspirin, herbs, vitamins, and other nonprescription products.

When You Use This Drug

• **Call your doctor immediately if you have black, tarry stools or if you vomit material that looks like coffee grounds. These are signs of a bleeding ulcer.**

- Call your doctor if you have trouble swallowing or persistent abdominal pain.
- Check with your doctor if your symptoms do not improve or get worse.
- If you take an antacid, take it at least 30 minutes apart from cimetidine. One source suggests taking stomach acid blockers two hours before antacids.[27]
- Do not drink alcohol or smoke.
- Avoid any food or drink that aggravates your ulcer.
- Check with your doctor before taking any aspirin, ibuprofen, or other NSAIDs. These drugs can cause or aggravate ulcers.
- Avoid exposure to organophosphate pesticides, such as Diazinon.[28]

How to Use This Drug

- If you miss a dose, take it as soon as you remember, but skip it if it is almost time for the next dose. **Do not take double doses.**
- Do not share your medication with others.
- Take the drug at the same time(s) each day.
- Take this drug for the prescribed length of time. If you stop too soon, your symptoms could come back.
- *Nonprescription strengths:* Do not take maximum daily dose for more than two weeks unless your doctor tells you to do so.
- *Prescription strengths:* If 1 dose per day, take at bedtime. If 2 doses per day, take in the morning and at bedtime. If several doses per day, take with meals and at bedtime.
- *Famotidine chewable tablets:* Chew well before swallowing.
- *Famotidine oral disintegrating tablets:* Open pack just before use and place tablet on tongue to dissolve and swallow.
- *Ranitidine effervescent granules or tablets:* Dissolve in six to eight ounces of water and drink.
- Cimetidine tablets have an odor. This is normal and no cause for concern.
- Do not store in the bathroom. Do not expose to heat, moisture, or strong light. Do not let the liquid form freeze. Keep out of reach of children.

Interactions with Other Drugs

The following drugs, biologics (e.g., vaccines, therapeutic antibodies), or foods are listed in *Evaluations of Drug Interactions* 2003 as causing "highly clinically significant" or "clinically significant" interactions when used together with any of the drugs in this section. In some sections with multiple drugs, the interaction may have been reported for one but not all drugs in this section, but we include the interaction because the drugs in this section are similar to one another. We have also included potentially serious interactions listed in the drug's FDA-approved professional package insert or in published medical journal articles. There may be other drugs, especially those in the families of drugs listed below, that also will react with this drug to cause severe adverse effects. Make sure to tell your doctor and pharmacist the drugs you are taking and tell them if you are taking any of these interacting drugs:

ADALAT, ADALAT CC, AGENERASE, alprazolam, altretamine, amitryptiline, amprenavir, ANECTINE, ANZEMET, AVENTYL, AVINZA, BICNU, carbamazepine, carmustine, chlordiazepoxide, clozapine, CLOZARIL, COGNEX, COUMADIN, delavirdine, desipramine, DIASTAT, diazepam, DILANTIN, dofetilide, dolasetron, DURAQUIN, ELAVIL, ELIXOPHYLLIN, FAZACLO, FLAGYL, flecainide, FLOMAX, GLIADEL, glipizide, GLUCOPHAGE, GLUCOTROL, GLYCET, HALCION, HEXALEN, imipramine, INDERAL, INDERAL LA, KADIAN, ketoconazole, labetalol, lercanidipine, LIBRIUM, lidocaine, MALARONE, METAGLIP, metformin, metronidazole, midazolam, miglitol, MIRAPEX, mizolastine, morphine, MS CONTIN, nifedipine, NIZORAL, NORMODYNE,

NORPRAMIN, nortryptiline, ORAMORPH, PAMELOR, PERTOFRANE, phenytoin, pramipexole, procainamide, PROCANBID, PROCARDIA, PROCARDIA XL, proguanil, PRONESTYL, propranolol, QUINAGLUTE DURA-TABS, QUINIDEX, quinidine, RE-SCRIPTOR, ROXANOL, sertraline, sildenafil, SLO-BID, succinylcholine, tacrine, TAMBOCOR, tamsulosin, TEGRETOL, THEO-24, theophylline, TIKOSYN, TOFRANIL, TRANDATE, triazolam, VALIUM, VERSED, VIAGRA, warfarin, XANAX, XYLOCAINE, ZOLOFT, ZOMIG, zolmitriptan.

Adverse Effects

Call your doctor immediately if you experience (for all histamine2-blockers):

- allergic reaction or hives
- bleeding or bruising that is unusual
- blisters on palms and soles of feet
- confusion or anxiety
- dizziness or fainting
- eyes that are red or irritated
- fever, chills, or sore throat
- general feeling of discomfort
- hallucinations
- heartbeat fast, pounding, or irregular
- joint pain
- mood or mental changes
- muscle cramps
- peeling skin
- skin that is red or itching
- tiredness or weakness that is unusual
- trouble breathing
- ulcers or white spots on lips, in mouth, or on genitals
- urination increased or decreased[29]
- yellow skin or eyes

For cimetidine:

- abdominal pain
- fever or sore throat
- joint pain
- muscle ache
- tiredness or weakness that is unusual
- vomiting

For famotidine:

- fever or sore throat
- heartbeat fast, pounding, or irregular
- joint pain
- muscle ache
- tiredness or weakness that is unusual
- wheezing or troubled breathing

For nizatidine:

- chest and back pain
- increased cough
- itching or hives
- joint pain
- skin rash
- tiredness or weakness that is unusual
- upper respiratory infections more frequent
- vision changes
- wheezing or troubled breathing

For ranitidine:

- abdominal pain
- chest and back pain
- faintness or weakness that is sudden
- fever
- heartbeat irregular or fast
- joint pain
- muscle ache
- throat sore
- tiredness or weakness that is unusual
- vision changes
- vomiting
- wheezing or troubled breathing

Call your doctor if these symptoms continue (for all histamine2-blockers):

- breasts enlarged or sore in males or females
- diarrhea
- dizziness

- drowsiness
- headache
- impotence
- muscle cramps or pain
- sexual desire decreased
- skin rash

For cimetidine:

- fever
- hair loss
- joint pain
- muscle tenderness
- skin rash or hives
- urination difficult
- urination increased or decreased

For famotidine:

- abdominal pain
- appetite loss
- constipation
- ears ringing
- hair loss
- mouth dry
- nausea
- skin dry
- sleeping difficulty
- vomiting

For nizatidine:

- abdominal pain
- constipation
- mouth dry
- nausea or vomiting
- nose running
- sleeping difficulty
- sweating increased

For ranitidine:

- abdominal pain
- constipation
- hair loss
- nausea or vomiting
- sleeping difficulty

Periodic Tests

Ask your doctor which of these tests should be done periodically while you are taking this drug:

- Vitamin B_{12} measurements

━━━━━━━━━

Proton Pump Inhibitors

Limited Use

=========

Lansoprazole (lan *sop* ra zole)
PREVACID (TAP)

Omeprazole (o *mep* ra zole)
PRILOSEC (AstraZeneca)

Do Not Use Until Seven Years After Release

=========

Pantoprazole (pan *toe* pra zole)
(Do Not Use Until 2007)
PROTONIX (Wyeth-Ayerst)

Rabeprazole (ra *be* pray zole)
(Do Not Use Until 2006)
ACIPHEX (Janssen)

GENERIC: not available except for omeprazole
FAMILY: Proton Pump Inhibitors

PREGNANCY WARNING

Omeprazole caused harm to developing fetuses in animal studies, including deaths of embryos and disruptions of pregnancies. Use these drugs during pregnancy only for clear medical reasons. Tell your doctor if you are pregnant or thinking of becoming pregnant before you take these drugs.

BREAST-FEEDING WARNING

These drugs are excreted in the milk of rats and reach levels higher than in the mother's blood. Because of the ability of these drugs to cause DNA damage and tumors in rats and mice, you should not take these drugs while nursing.

Lansoprazole, omeprazole, pantoprazole, and rabeprazole are close chemical relatives in the

THE HEALTH RESEARCH GROUP'S SEVEN-YEAR RULE

You should wait at least seven years from the date of release to take any new drug unless it is one of those rare "breakthrough" drugs that offers you a documented therapeutic advantage over older proven drugs. New drugs are tested in a relatively small number of people before being released, and serious adverse effects or life-threatening drug interactions may not be detected until the new drug has been taken by hundreds of thousands of people. A number of new drugs have been withdrawn within their first seven years after release. Also, warnings about serious new adverse reactions have been added to the labeling of a number of drugs, or new drug interactions have been detected, often within the first seven years after a drug's release.

family of ulcer drugs known as proton pump inhibitors (PPIs). These drugs are approved for short-term treatment of gastroesophageal reflux disease (GERD), and all but pantoprazole are also approved for duodenal and stomach ulcers resistant to treatment with antacids and histamine2-blockers. All the PPIs except pantoprazole are also approved for use in combination with antibiotics to treat ulcer disease caused by the bacterium *Helicobacter pylori* (see p. 530). Omeprazole is also available over-the-counter for the treatment of frequent heartburn. Most studies do not show significant differences between the different PPIs for the healing of GERD, duodenal ulcer, or *Helicobacter pylori* eradication.[30]

All four drugs are also indicated for the treatment for Zollinger-Ellison syndrome, a rare hormonal disorder characterized by excessive stomach acid production due to a stomach tumor. The PPIs do not alter the course of this syndrome.

PPIs inhibit secretion of stomach acid, whereas histamine2-blockers such as cimetidine (TAGAMET) partially prevent production of the acid (see p. 538). Histamine2-blockers relieve heartburn pain more quickly than PPIs.[2]

For ulcers, treatment takes up to six weeks; for Zollinger-Ellison syndrome, treatment is indefinite. To maintain effectiveness in treating Zollinger-Ellison syndrome, the dose may need to be increased annually.[31] After long-term treatment, vitamin B_{12} stores may be depleted in strict vegetarians and the elderly and hence might be monitored.[32,33] Long-term use may also be associated with increased acid secretion after stopping use of the PPI in patients who do not have *Helicobacter pylori* infection.[34]

Relapse of acid reflux is common. Long-term acid suppression may lead to intestinal infections.[32] It is uncertain whether long-term suppression of stomach acid may also cause stomach cancer.[35,36]

Before You Use This Drug

Tell your doctor if you have or have had:

- allergies to drugs in this class
- heart problems [37]
- *Helicobacter pylori* infection
- liver problems
- pernicious anemia [37,38]
- pregnancy or are breast-feeding

Tell your doctor about any other drugs you take, including aspirin, herbs, vitamins, and other nonprescription products.

When You Use This Drug

• **Call your doctor immediately if you have black, tarry stools or if you vomit material that looks like coffee grounds. These are signs of a bleeding ulcer.**

NIGHTTIME HEARTBURN TREATMENTS: TRY THESE FIRST

There are nondrug treatments, with no safety concerns, and less expensive drugs that may be effective for you; these should be tried before you use any drugs for heartburn. First, try to avoid foods that trigger your condition (e.g., fatty foods, onions, caffeine, peppermint, and chocolate), and avoid alcohol, smoking, and tight clothing.[1]

Second, avoid food, and particularly alcohol, within two or three hours of bedtime. Third, elevate the head of the bed about six inches or sleep with extra pillows.

For both heartburn and ulcers, it is important to avoid drug-induced causes. Aspirin, ibuprofen, and other non-steroidal anti-inflammatory drugs (NSAIDs) (see p. 281) are known to cause ulcers. Ask your doctor if acetaminophen could be substituted for these drugs. Check with your doctor about the osteoporosis medications alendronate and risedronate (FOSAMAX and ACTONEL) (see p. 584), which irritate the esophagus.

If these measures are not effective, try simple over-the-counter (OTC) antacids such as a generic aluminum hydroxide and magnesium hydroxide product (MAALOX, MAALOX TC, see p. 533). If symptoms worsen or bleeding occurs, call your doctor. If this does not relieve your symptoms, one of the family of stomach acid–blocking drugs known as histamine2-blockers can be tried (see p. 538). This family includes cimetidine (TAGAMET), famotidine (PEPCID), nizatidine (AXID), and ranitidine (ZANTAC). Histamine2-blockers are available in both OTC and prescription strengths.

If the OTC histamine2-blockers do not give adequate relief of your symptoms after 14 days, it is time to consult your physician.

• Call your doctor if you have trouble swallowing or persistent abdominal pain.

• Check with your doctor if your symptoms do not improve or get worse.

• Do not drink alcohol or smoke.

• Avoid any food or drink that aggravates your ulcer.

• Check with your doctor before taking any aspirin, ibuprofen, or other NSAIDs. These drugs can cause or aggravate ulcers.

How to Use This Drug

• If you miss a dose, take it as soon as you remember, but skip it if it is almost time for the next dose. **Do not take double doses.**

• Do not share your medication with others.

• Take the drug at the same time(s) each day.

• Swallow capsule whole. Do not crush, chew, or open the capsule.

• Take the tablet in the morning, with or without food (pantoprazole).

• Take the capsule form immediately before a meal, preferably breakfast (omeprazole, lansoprazole).

• If you cannot swallow the capsule whole, capsules may be opened and the contents mixed with apple juice (and swallowed immediately) or mixed with applesauce, jelly, or ketchup, then swallowed without chewing or crushing.

• Take antacids for pain relief for several days until pain relief begins or until your doctor tells you.

• Take the full course of therapy.

• Store at room temperature with lid on tightly. Do not store in the bathroom. Do not expose to heat, moisture, or strong light. Keep out of reach of children.

Interactions with Other Drugs

The following drugs, biologics (e.g., vaccines, therapeutic antibodies), or foods are listed in *Evaluations of Drug Interactions* 2003 as caus-

In long-term (two-year) studies in rats, all the drugs in this class caused an increase in carcinoid tumors of the stomach. Although such tumors have not yet been demonstrated in humans, using these drugs for long-term therapy is not advisable, except for the treatment of Zollinger-Ellison syndrome.

ing "highly clinically significant" or "clinically significant" interactions when used together with any of the drugs in this section. In some sections with multiple drugs, the interaction may have been reported for one but not all drugs in this section, but we include the interaction because the drugs in this section are similar to one another. We have also included potentially serious interactions listed in the drug's FDA-approved professional package insert or in published medical journal articles. There may be other drugs, especially those in the families of drugs listed below, that also will react with this drug to cause severe adverse effects. Make sure to tell your doctor and pharmacist the drugs you are taking and tell them if you are taking any of these interacting drugs:

ADALAT, ADALAT CC, BIAXIN, bismuth subsalicylate, carbamazepine, caffeine, CARAFATE, cilostazol, clarithromycin, COUMADIN, cyclosporine, DIASTAT, diazepam, DILANTIN, ELIXOPHYLLIN, ketoconazole, methotrexate, moclobemide, nifedipine, NEORAL, NIZORAL, NORVIR, PEPTO-BISMOL, phenytoin, PLETAL PREVPAC, PROCARDIA, PROCARDIA XL, ritonavir, SANDIMMUNE, SLO-BID, sucralfate, TEGRETOL, THEO-24, theophylline, TREXALL, VALIUM, warfarin.

Adverse Effects

Call your doctor immediately if you experience:

- abdominal or stomach pain
- anxiety
- appetite increased or decreased
- bleeding or bruising that is unusual
- bloody urine
- breathing interruptions
- chest pain
- chest tightness or wheezing
- chills, fever, or sore throat
- constipation
- convulsions or seizures (rabeprazole)
- cough
- depression
- diarrhea
- eye or eyelid puffiness or swelling
- hive-like swellings on eyelids, face, lips, mouth, and/or tongue
- muscle or joint pain
- nausea or vomiting
- rectal bleeding
- shortness of breath
- skin color changes in the face
- skin peeling or redness
- skin rash or itching
- thirst that is unusual
- tiredness or weakness that is unusual
- ulcers or sores on mouth that are persistent
- urination painful
- urine frequency or volume increased
- yellow eyes or skin

Call your doctor if these symptoms continue:

- abdominal pain
- anxiety
- chills
- confusion
- constipation
- cough
- diarrhea
- dizziness
- drowsiness or tiredness that is unusual
- ears buzzing or ringing
- gas
- headache

- heartburn
- hoarseness
- joint or back pain
- moving difficulty
- muscle rigidity
- nausea or vomiting
- numbness, tingling, pain, or weakness in hands or feet
- skin itchy
- sleeping difficulty
- throat sore
- vision blurred
- weakness

Signs of overdose:

- abdominal pain
- confusion
- drowsiness
- flushing
- headache
- heartbeat fast or irregular
- ill feeling
- mouth dry
- nausea or vomiting
- vision blurred

If you suspect an overdose, call this number to contact your poison control center: (800) 222-1222.

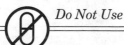 *Do Not Use*

ALTERNATIVE TREATMENT:
See the box accompanying this drug profile.

Esomeprazole (e so *mep* ra zole)
NEXIUM (AstraZeneca)

FAMILY: Proton Pump Inhibitors

Esomeprazole was approved in February 2001 as the fifth member of the proton pump inhibitor (PPI) family of drugs (see p. 542). These drugs are approved for short-term treatment of gastroesophageal reflux disease (GERD) and most are also approved for duodenal and stomach ulcers resistant to treatment with histamine2-blockers (see p. 538) and antacids. Most of the PPIs are also used in combination with antibiotics to treat ulcer disease caused by the bacterium *Helicobacter pylori* (see p. 530). Most studies do not show a significant difference between the different PPIs for the treatment of GERD, duodenal ulcer, or *Heliocobacter pylori.*[30] PPIs inhibit the secretion of stomach acid, whereas histamine2-blockers partially prevent production of acid.

In fact, patients who have been taking omeprazole (PRILOSEC) since it was approved in 1989 have been getting esomeprazole with each dose. Like many drugs, omeprazole is a mixture of two forms that are chemically identical but are "mirror images" of each other. These mirror images are called optical isomers, and esomeprazole is one of the two that make up omeprazole. Esomeprazole and omeprazole are both produced by the same company, AstraZeneca Pharmaceuticals.

In its application for marketing to the FDA, AstraZeneca claimed that esomeprazole had important advantages over omeprazole. An FDA Medical Officer was charged with reviewing the veracity of this claim. FDA reviews can be very different from the image that drug companies try to portray about their new drugs because the agency has access to research data that may never be published if it is not in the economic interests of the company. The Medical Officer stated:

The sponsor's [AstraZeneca's] conclusion that H 199/18 [esomeprazole] has been shown to provide a significant clinical advance over omeprazole in the first-line treatment of patients with acid-related disorders **is not supported by data** [emphasis in original].

. . . Specifically, there are [sic] no scientific basis for the sponsor's statement that com-

---

NIGHTTIME HEARTBURN TREATMENTS: TRY THESE FIRST

There are nondrug treatments, with no safety concerns, and less expensive drugs that may be effective for you; these should be tried before you use any drugs for heartburn. First, try to avoid foods that trigger your condition (e.g., fatty foods, onions, caffeine, peppermint, and chocolate), and avoid alcohol, smoking, and tight clothing.[1]

Second, avoid food, and particularly alcohol, within two or three hours of bedtime. Third, elevate the head of the bed about six inches or sleep with extra pillows.

For both heartburn and ulcers, it is important to avoid drug-induced causes. Aspirin, ibuprofen, and other non-steroidal anti-inflammatory drugs (NSAIDs) (see p. 281) are known to cause ulcers. Ask your doctor if acetaminophen could be substituted for these drugs. Check with your doctor about the osteoporosis medications alendronate and risedronate (FOSAMAX and ACTONEL) (see p. 584), which irritate the esophagus.

If these measures are not effective, try simple over-the-counter (OTC) antacids such as a generic aluminum hydroxide and magnesium hydroxide product (MAALOX, MAALOX TC, see p. 533). If symptoms worsen or bleeding occurs, call your doctor. If this does not relieve your symptoms, one of the family of stomach acid–blocking drugs known as histamine2-blockers can be tried (see p. 538). This family includes cimetidine (TAGAMET), famotidine (PEPCID), nizatidine (AXID), and ranitidine (ZANTAC). Histamine2-blockers are available in both OTC and prescription strengths.

If the OTC histamine2-blockers do not give adequate relief of your symptoms after 14 days, it is time to consult your physician.

---

pared to omeprazole, H 199/18 offers a faster and improved resolution of heartburn symptoms and higher rates of healing in the treatment of erosive esophagitis. The two compounds are comparable in their efficacy for this indication.[39]

The Medical Officer's final recommendation on esomeprazole was equally clear:

In addition, it is recommended not to allow the sponsor [AstraZeneca] to claim that esomeprazole magnesium has any significant clinical advantage over omeprazole in the first-line treatment of these acid-related disorders because no data in support of such a claim have been submitted.[39]

Why would an industry that claims it is so innovative engage in such tactics? Omeprazole was about to lose its patent protection. The most expedient strategy for AstraZeneca to protect its lucrative share of the PPI market was thus for the company to develop esomeprazole, a drug that would have patent protection even though it is clearly not an innovation that required much scientific ingenuity, and then get physicians to switch their omeprazole patients to esomeprazole. The result: AstraZeneca revenues stay up, the price of drugs increases, and patients derive no clinical benefit whatsoever.

We have listed esomeprazole as a **Do Not Use** drug rather than a Do Not Use Until Seven Years After Release drug not because of safety and effectiveness concerns but because there is no significant difference between this drug and omeprazole. Switching from omeprazole, which is available generically, to esomeprazole will cause the health care system economic harm. Patients with poor or nonexistent drug coverage will foot the bill that ensues from doctors being conned into prescribing esomeprazole. However, we acknowledge that particular health insurance plans may reimburse for esomeprazole and not some other PPIs that have longer track records.

Prostaglandins

Limited Use

Misoprostol (mice o *prost* all)
CYTOTEC (Searle)

GENERIC: available

FAMILY: Prostaglandins

PREGNANCY WARNING

There are literature reports of skull defects, cranial nerve palsies, facial malformations, and limb defects in women who took misoprostol during the first trimester of pregnancy. Because of the possibility of inducing an abortion, misoprostol should not be used by women who are pregnant. Patients must be advised of these properties and warned not to give the drug to others.

BREAST-FEEDING WARNING

No information is available from either human or animal studies. However, it is likely that this drug, like many others, is excreted in human milk, and because of the potential for adverse effects in nursing infants, including serious diarrhea, you should not take this drug while nursing.

Misoprostol is used to prevent stomach ulcers caused by aspirin, ibuprofen, and other non-steroidal anti-inflammatory drugs (NSAIDs) commonly used to treat arthritis (see p. 281). NSAIDs can cause serious harm, even fatalities, from bleeding in the stomach or intestines. Misoprostol is a synthetic prostaglandin drug that may protect the lining of the stomach and modestly decreases the secretion of stomach acid.

People at high risk for ulcers from NSAIDs include the elderly, people with other debilitating diseases, and those who have had an ulcer previously. **Misoprostol should only be used by those with severe arthritis who had an ulcer previously.**

Because too many people receive NSAIDs for too long, approach taking misoprostol to treat the adverse effects of NSAIDs with great caution. Many patients have conditions that can be treated with more conservative measures, or with generic acetaminophen (which does not induce stomach ulcers). Of patients chronically taking NSAIDs, 2 to 4% will develop a serious complication of an ulcer.[40] However, there is no evidence that misoprostol prevents the serious, life-threatening gastrointestinal complications associated with NSAIDs. It has only been shown to reduce the number of stomach ulcers visible through an endoscope. It has not been shown to have an effect on duodenal (part of the small instestine, not the stomach) ulcers or abdominal pain.

Before deciding to take misoprostol along with an NSAID, ask your doctor why misoprostol was prescribed and how long you could expect to take it. Ask if a different arthritis drug with a lower rate of adverse effects can be used. If you develop a duodenal (not a stomach) ulcer, one of the histamine2-blockers should be tried first.[41]

Diarrhea is a common adverse effect of misoprostol, ranging from minor to severe enough to be life-threatening.[42,43] In clinical trials the incidence of loose stools ranged from 14 to 40%. In older people, loss of fluids and minerals from diarrhea can cause heart, kidney, and mental problems.

Before You Use This Drug

Do not use if you have or have had:

- pregnancy or are breast-feeding

Tell your doctor if you have or have had:

- allergies to prostaglandins or similar drugs
- cerebral vascular disease, stroke, or transient ischemic attack
- coronary artery disease
- epilepsy heart problems
- inflammatory bowel disease

Tell your doctor about any other drugs you take, including aspirin, herbs, vitamins, and other nonprescription products.

When You Use This Drug

• **Call your doctor immediately if you have black, tarry stools or if you vomit material that looks like coffee grounds. These are signs of a bleeding ulcer.**

• Call your doctor if you have trouble swallowing or persistent abdominal pain.

• Check with your doctor if your symptoms do not improve or get worse.

• Do not drink alcohol or smoke.

• Avoid any food or drink that aggravates your ulcer.

• Stop medication immediately and check with your doctor if you suspect that you are pregnant.

• Consult your doctor if diarrhea lasts more than a week.

• Use antacids and laxatives that do not contain magnesium.

• Drink liquids to replace fluids lost by diarrhea.

How to Use This Drug

• If you miss a dose, take it as soon as you remember, but skip it if it is almost time for the next dose. **Do not take double doses.**

• Do not share your medication with others.

• Take the drug at the same time(s) each day.

• Take with or after meals or at bedtime. Take with food or milk.

• Swallow tablets whole or break in half. Take with or after meals to lessen chance of diarrhea.

• Store at room temperature with lid on tightly. Do not store in the bathroom. Do not expose to heat, moisture, or strong light. Keep out of reach of children.

Interactions with Other Drugs

Evaluations of Drug Interactions 2003 lists no drugs, biologics (e.g., vaccines, therapeutic antibodies), or foods as causing "highly clini-

cally significant" or "clinically significant" interactions when used together with the drugs in this section. We also found no interactions in the drugs' FDA-approved professional package inserts. However, as the number of new drugs approved for marketing increases and as more experience is gained with these drugs over time, new interactions may be discovered.

Adverse Effects

Call your doctor if these symptoms continue:

• abdominal or stomach cramps, or pain in lower abdomen or stomach
• confusion [44]
• constipation
• diarrhea
• gas
• headache
• heartburn, indigestion, or acid stomach
• nausea and/or vomiting
• urinary incontinence [45]
• vaginal bleeding

Signs of overdose:

• abdominal pain
• blood pressure decrease
• breathing difficulty
• diarrhea
• drowsiness
• fever
• heartbeat fast or pounding
• heartbeat slow
• seizures
• tremor

If you suspect an overdose, call this number to contact your poison control center: (800) 222-1222.

Antibiotic-containing Treatments

Amoxicillin (a mox i *sill* in)
(see p. 682)
AMOXIL (GlaxoSmithKline)

GENERIC: available

Bismuth Subsalicylate (*bis* muth sub sa *lis* a late)
PEPTO BISMOL (Procter & Gamble)

GENERIC: available

Bismuth Subsalicylate, Metronidazole, Tetracycline (*bis* muth sub sa *lis* a late, me troe *ni* da zole, tet ra *sye* kleen)
HELIDAC (Procter & Gamble)

GENERIC: available for each ingredient

Clarithromycin (kla rith ro *mye* sin)
(see p. 695)
BIAXIN (Abbott)

GENERIC: not available

Lansoprazole (lan *soe* pra zole)
(see p. 542)
PREVACID (TAP)

GENERIC: not available

Metronidazole (me troe *ni* da zole)
(see p. 725)
FLAGYL (Searle)

GENERIC: available

Omeprazole (oh *mep* ra zole)
(see p. 542)
PRILOSEC (Astra Merck)

GENERIC: available

Ranitidine (ra *ni* ti deen)
(see p. 538)
ZANTAC (Glaxo Wellcome)

GENERIC: available

Ranitidine Bismuth Citrate
(ra *ni* ti deen *bis* muth *si* trate)
TRITEC (Glaxo Wellcome)

GENERIC: not available

Tetracycline (te tra *sye* kleen)
(see p. 700)
ACHROMYCIN (Lederle)

GENERIC: available
FAMILY: Antibiotic-Containing Treatments

PREGNANCY WARNINGS FOR BISMUTH SUBSALICYLATE–CONTAINING DRUGS (PEPTO BISMOL AND HELIDAC):
Salicylates readily cross the placenta and cause birth defects in animal studies and in humans.
Pregnancy warnings for the other drugs in this group may be located with their individual profiles.

BREAST-FEEDING WARNING FOR BISMUTH SUBSALICYLATE–CONTAINING DRUGS (PEPTO BISMOL AND HELIDAC):
Salicylates are excreted in human milk. Because of the potential for serious adverse effects in nursing infants, you should not take these drugs while nursing.
Breast-feeding warnings for the other drugs in this group may be located with their individual profiles.

PREGNANCY WARNING FOR RANITIDINE BISMUTH CITRATE
No valid data are available from animal studies, as it was not tested properly. However, there is a case of injury to a human infant of a mother who took this drug for 7 days prior to and 20 days post-conception (extra number of fingers and toes). Use during pregnancy only for clear medical reasons. Tell your doctor if you are pregnant or thinking of becoming pregnant before you take this drug.

The bacterium *Helicobacter pylori* (*H. pylori*) has been implicated in causing ulcer disease. Its presence can be detected by tests of the blood, breath, and stool, as well as through samples taken during endoscopy.[3] When the bacterium, present in a large proportion of people with ulcers, is eradicated, ulcers can heal and the likelihood of recurrence is reduced. Generally, *H. pylori* is more easily eradicated in duodenal ulcers than in stomach ulcers. If you have *H. pylori* but do not have an ulcer, there is evidence that *H. pylori* may protect against the

---

FDA-APPROVED TREATMENTS FOR *HELICOBACTER PYLORI* INFECTION

Bismuth subsalicylate/metronidazole/tetracycline/ histamine2-blocker (see p. 538)

Esomeprazole/amoxicillin/clarithromycin

Lansoprazole/amoxicillin/clarithromycin

Lansoprazole/amoxicillin (if you have allergy, intolerance, or insensitivity to clarithromycin)

Omeprazole/clarithromycin

Omeprazole/amoxicillin/clarithromycin

Ranitidine bismuth citrate/clarithromycin[3]

---

symptoms of gastroesophageal reflux disease (GERD), and you should not take medicine to eradicate the bacterium.[19]

The drugs listed in this section are either antibiotics or drugs used in combination with antibiotics to treat *H. pylori* infection. Except for bismuth, each drug is discussed in detail elsewhere in this book. Antibiotic-containing combinations that have been approved by the FDA for the treatment of *H. pylori* infection are listed in the accompanying box.

If only one antibiotic is used, resistance is apt to develop and relapse to occur, particularly with metronidazole. Low doses of antibiotics can also lead to resistance. Combining a single antibiotic (amoxicillin or clarithromycin) with a proton pump inhibitor (see p. 542) still only results in less than 70% of *H. pylori* being eradicated. The FDA has thus approved a number of regimens that use two antibiotics with a proton pump inhibitor, which allows for shorter periods of therapy (10–14 days). Cure rates of about 80–85% can be expected and recurrence rates are very low.[46] There is no evidence that any one PPI is more effective than another in these combinations.[3]

Another alternative is bismuth, either as bismuth subsalicylate or in ranitidine bismuth citrate. Ranitidine bismuth citrate has been used with clarithromycin and either tetracycline or amoxicillin. Bismuth subsalicylate can be combined with metronidazole and tetracycline for two weeks and a histamine2-blocker for four weeks; this is likely to be the least expensive option. None of the regimens described in this section are approved by the FDA for indigestion or GERD.

The choice of combinations will depend on your allergies, medical condition, other medications you take, antibiotic resistance, and your likelihood of taking several drugs several times a day for up to four weeks. Some drugs must be taken with food, others on an empty stomach. The more drugs you take the more adverse reactions are possible. Prolonged use of antibiotics can cause infections by other organisms. To simplify things, some companies have packaged drugs together in the form of new combination drugs. In this case, you are paying more for convenience, because equivalent drugs are usually available generically. Some are even available without a prescription.

The following information applies to bismuth only. Analogous information on the other drugs used in these combinations can be found with the separate listings for the individual drugs.

Before You Use This Drug (see individual drugs for more detailed information)

Tell your doctor if you have or have had (for bismuth subsalicylate only):

- allergies to drugs
- bleeding or bleeding disorder
- dehydration
- diabetes (drug can affect glucose urine test results)
- dysentery
- gout
- kidney disorder
- pregnancy or are breast-feeding
- ulcers

Tell your doctor about any other drugs you take, including aspirin, herbs, vitamins, and other nonprescription products.

When You Use This Drug
(for bismuth subsalicylate only)

• You may experience darkening of tongue or grayish-black stools. These effects do not require medical attention.

How to Use This Drug
(for bismuth subsalicylate only)

• If you miss a dose, take it as soon as you remember, but skip it if it is almost time for the next dose. **Do not take double doses.**
• Do not share your medication with others.
• Take the drug at the same time(s) each day.
• Store at room temperature with lid on tightly. Do not store in the bathroom. Do not expose to heat, moisture, or strong light. Keep out of reach of children.
• Take with **a full glass (eight ounces)** of water.
• Do not chew regular tablets.
• Chewable tablets can be chewed or allowed to disintegrate in mouth before swallowing.

Interactions with Other Drugs
(for bismuth subsalicylate only)

Evaluations of Drug Interactions 2003 lists no drugs, biologics (e.g., vaccines, therapeutic antibodies), or foods as causing "highly clinically significant" or "clinically significant" interactions when used together with the drug in this section. We also found no interactions in the drug's FDA-approved professional package inserts. However, as the number of new drugs approved for marketing increases and as more experience is gained with these drugs over time, new interactions may be discovered.

Adverse Effects
(for bismuth subsalicylate only)

Call your doctor immediately if you experience:

• anxiety
• breathing that is fast or deep
• confusion
• constipation that is severe
• depression
• diarrhea that is severe or continues
• dizziness or lightheadedness
• drowsiness that is severe
• ears ringing or buzzing
• flapping movements of hands
• headache that is severe or continues
• hearing loss
• movements that are uncontrolled
• muscle spasms, especially of face, neck, and back
• muscle weakness
• nausea or vomiting that is severe or continues
• speaking difficulty or slurred speech
• stomach pain that is severe or continues
• sweating increased
• thirst increased
• trembling
• vision problems

Signs of overdose
(for bismuth subsalicylate only):

• anxiety
• breathing that is fast or deep
• confusion
• depression
• diarrhea that is severe
• dizziness or lightheadedness
• drowsiness that is severe
• ears ringing
• headache that is severe
• hearing loss
• movements that are uncontrolled
• muscle spasms

- muscle weakness
- nausea or vomiting that is severe
- speaking difficulty or slurred speech
- stomach pain
- sweating increased
- thirst increased
- trembling
- vision problems

If you suspect an overdose, call this number to contact your poison control center: (800) 222-1222.

Coating Agents

Limited Use

Sucralfate (soo *kral* fate)
CARAFATE (Hoechst Marion Roussel)

GENERIC: available
FAMILY: Coating Agents

PREGNANCY WARNING

No valid data are available for sucralfate, as it was not tested properly in animal studies. Use during pregnancy only for clear medical reasons. Tell your doctor if you are pregnant or thinking of becoming pregnant before you take this drug.

BREAST-FEEDING WARNING

No information is available from either human or animal studies. Since it is likely that this drug, like many others, is excreted in human milk, you should consult with your doctor if you are planning to nurse.

Sucralfate is used to treat and prevent ulcers in the duodenum, a part of the small intestine. After you take the drug, it forms a gummy substance that sticks to the ulcer. This protects the ulcer from stomach acid, allowing it to heal. You should not take sucralfate for minor digestive problems. Do not take sucralfate for more than 12 weeks unless your doctor tells you to. Sucralfate can cause constipation.

Before You Use This Drug

Tell your doctor if you have or have had:

- allergies to drugs
- intestinal obstruction
- kidney failure
- swallowing difficulty

Tell your doctor about any other drugs you take, including aspirin, herbs, vitamins, and other nonprescription products.

When You Use This Drug

- **Call your doctor immediately if you have black, tarry stools or if you vomit material that looks like coffee grounds. These are signs of a bleeding ulcer.**
- Call your doctor if you have trouble swallowing or persistent abdominal pain.
- Check with your doctor if your symptoms do not improve or get worse.
- Do not drink alcohol or smoke.
- Avoid any food or drink that aggravates your ulcer.
- Check with your doctor before taking any aspirin, ibuprofen, or other NSAIDs. These drugs can cause or aggravate ulcers.
- If you take antacids for ulcer pain, do not do so closer than a half hour before or after the time you take sucralfate.

How to Use This Drug

- If you miss a dose, take it as soon as you remember, but skip it if it is almost time for the next dose. **Do not take double doses.**
- Do not share your medication with others.
- Take the drug at the same time(s) each day.
- Take the full course of drug prescribed by your doctor.
- Have regular checkups with your doctor to monitor progress.
- Take on an empty stomach, at least one hour before meals, and at bedtime.

NIGHTTIME HEARTBURN TREATMENTS: TRY THESE FIRST

There are nondrug treatments, with no safety concerns, and less expensive drugs that may be effective for you; these should be tried before you use any drugs for heartburn. First, try to avoid foods that trigger your condition (e.g., fatty foods, onions, caffeine, peppermint, and chocolate), and avoid alcohol, smoking, and tight clothing.[1]

Second, avoid food, and particularly alcohol, within two or three hours of bedtime. Third, elevate the head of the bed about six inches or sleep with extra pillows.

For both heartburn and ulcers, it is important to avoid drug-induced causes. Aspirin, ibuprofen, and other non-steroidal anti-inflammatory drugs (NSAIDs) (see p. 281) are known to cause ulcers. Ask your doctor if acetaminophen could be substituted for these drugs. Check with your doctor about the osteoporosis medications alendronate and risedronate (FOSAMAX and ACTONEL) (see p. 584), which irritate the esophagus.

If these measures are not effective, try simple over-the-counter (OTC) antacids such as a generic aluminum hydroxide and magnesium hydroxide product (MAALOX, MAALOX TC, see p. 533). If symptoms worsen or bleeding occurs, call your doctor. If this does not relieve your symptoms, one of the family of stomach acid–blocking drugs known as histamine2-blockers can be tried (see p. 538). This family includes cimetidine (TAGAMET), famotidine (PEPCID), nizatidine (AXID), and ranitidine (ZANTAC). Histamine2-blockers are available in both OTC and prescription strengths.

If the OTC histamine2-blockers do not give adequate relief of your symptoms after 14 days, it is time to consult your physician.

• Do not chew tablets.

• Store at room temperature with lid on tightly. Do not store in the bathroom. Do not expose to heat, moisture, or strong light. Keep out of reach of children.

Interactions with Other Drugs

The following drugs, biologics (e.g., vaccines, therapeutic antibodies), or foods are listed in *Evaluations of Drug Interactions* 2003 as causing "highly clinically significant" or "clinically significant" interactions when used together with any of the drugs in this section. In some sections with multiple drugs, the interaction may have been reported for one but not all drugs in this section, but we include the interaction because the drugs in this section are similar to one another. We have also included potentially serious interactions listed in the drug's FDA-approved professional package insert or in published medical journal articles. There may be other drugs, especially those in the families of drugs listed below, that also will react with this drug to cause severe adverse effects. Make sure to tell your doctor and pharmacist the drugs you are taking and tell them if you are taking any of these interacting drugs:

AVELOX, DILANTIN, moxifloxacin, norfloxacin, NOROXIN, phenytoin, SKELID, tiludronate, trovafloxacin, TROVAN.

Adverse Effects

Call your doctor if these symptoms continue:

• backache
• constipation
• diarrhea
• dizziness or lightheadedness
• drowsiness
• indigestion
• mouth dry
• nausea

- skin rash, hives, or itching
- stomach cramps or pain

Periodic Tests

Ask your doctor which of these tests should be done periodically while you are taking this drug:

- blood levels of aluminum if you have kidney failure, especially if you are taking aluminum-containing antacids (see p. 533)

Irritable Bowel Syndrome (IBS)

 Do Not Use

ALTERNATIVE TREATMENT:
See the box accompanying this drug profile about alternative treatments for IBS.

Alosetron (a *loe* se tron)
LOTRONEX (GlaxoSmithKline)

FAMILY: Irritable Bowel Syndrome (IBS) Drugs

Alosetron was approved by the FDA for the management of irritable bowel syndrome (IBS) in women with diarrhea as their predominant symptom. The drug is not approved for men.

IBS itself is not a life-threatening condition, although it can be debilitating. If the major symptom is diarrhea, the condition is known as diarrhea-predominant IBS; if it is characterized by constipation, it is called constipation-predominant IBS. The diagnosis of IBS should be based on a set of internationally recognized symptoms known as the Rome II Criteria[4] (see box on p. 556) and requires exclusion of treatable causes of the patient's symptoms, such as ulcerative colitis. This is especially important if the following signs of ulcerative colitis are present: onset after age 50, rectal bleeding, fever, weight loss, or anemia. There are no abnormal laboratory tests or changes in the cells of the gastrointestinal (GI) tract on biopsy that can objectively establish the diagnosis of IBS. In fact, the diagnosis of IBS can only be made if all tests for other diseases that might explain the patient's symptoms are negative and the patient continues to have recurrent abdominal discomfort or pain associated with diarrhea, constipation, or both.

FDA BLACK BOX WARNING

Serious gastrointestinal adverse events, some fatal, have been reported with the use of LOTRONEX. These events, including ischemic colitis and serious complications of constipation, have resulted in hospitalization, blood transfusion, surgery, and death.

• Only physicians who have enrolled in GlaxoSmithKline's Prescribing Program for LOTRONEX, based on their attestation of qualifications and acceptance of responsibilities, should prescribe LOTRONEX.

• LOTRONEX is indicated only for women with severe diarrhea-predominant IBS who have failed to respond to conventional therapy. Less than 5 percent of IBS is considered severe. Before receiving the initial prescription for LOTRONEX, the patient must read the Patient-Physician Agreement.

• LOTRONEX should be discontinued immediately in patients who develop constipation or symptoms of ischemic colitis. Physicians should instruct patients to immediately report constipation or symptoms of ischemic colitis. LOTRONEX should not be resumed in patients who develop ischemic colitis. Physicians should instruct patients who report constipation to immediately contact them if the constipation does not resolve after discontinuation of LOTRONEX. Patients with resolved constipation should resume LOTRONEX only on the advice of their treating physician.

ROME II CRITERIA FOR DIAGNOSIS OF IRRITABLE BOWEL SYNDROME [4]

In the preceding 12 months, at least 12 weeks, not necessarily consecutive, of abdominal discomfort or pain that has two out of these three features:

1. Relieved with defecation.
2. Onset associated with a change in frequency of stool.
3. Onset associated with a change in form (appearance) of stool.

Symptoms that cumulatively support the diagnosis of irritable bowel syndrome:

abnormal stool frequency (for research purposes "abnormal" may be defined as greater than three bowel movements per day and less than three per week);
abnormal stool form (lumpy/hard or loose/watery);
abnormal stool passage (straining, urgency, or feeling of incomplete evacuation);
passage of mucus;
bloating or feeling of abdominal distension.

ALTERNATIVE TREATMENTS FOR IRRITABLE BOWEL SYNDROME

General measures include reducing intake of caffeine, alcohol, and fried foods. Because intolerance to lactose (milk sugar) can mimic some symptoms of irritable bowel syndrome (IBS), a test to determine if you are lactose intolerant should be done. Sorbitol, the sugar in sugarless gum or candy, should be avoided. Minimization of stress and the use of relaxation techniques have helped many people. For constipation-predominant IBS, increased dietary fiber and/or the use of psyllium or methylcellulose (see p. 566) and increased fluid intake may be helpful. For diarrhea-predominant IBS, the cautious use of loperamide (IMODIUM) (see p. 572) can be helpful.

Alosetron was withdrawn after only nine months on the market, but has since returned to the market in restricted fashion, following patient demands for the drug. The reason for withdrawal was a life-threatening adverse reaction known as ischemic colitis, a decrease in blood flow to the GI tract that can lead to bleeding, inflammation, and perforation of the intestines, sometimes leading to surgery. The condition can result in infection of the abdominal cavity that can be fatal.

Alosetron was inexplicably granted a priority or "fast track" review by the FDA. The justification for granting such a review was that the agency considered alosetron "a significant therapeutic advance" over existing therapies. In fact, alosetron was only required to be compared to a placebo, not to the alternative treatments mentioned in the accompanying box.

In truth, the drug is not much better than a placebo. In clinical trials, only 12–15% of patients actually benefited from the drug. Patients on alosetron improved their abdominal pain/discomfort scores by 0.12–0.14 points on a 4-point scale,[48,49] a trivial benefit. Most patients who improve while taking the drug are exhibiting the "placebo effect."

Four cases of ischemic colitis were identified in patients participating in clinical trials even before alosetron was approved. This was "gold standard" evidence that the drug caused a life-threatening adverse drug reaction. But the FDA chose to overlook it. In August 2000, Public Citizen petitioned to ban the drug; there had already been 26 cases of ischemic colitis.[49] We argued that the drug should be available only in a research setting. By April 2002, the FDA had 84 reports of ischemic colitis and 113 of severe constipation.[50]

The drug was removed from the market in late 2000, but reinstated under restricted conditions in June 2002 after patient groups, some funded by the pharmaceutical industry, demanded the drug's return. Patients are supposed to be female (there is no evidence alosetron is effective in men), have severe, chronic (over six months) diarrhea-predominant IBS, and have failed to respond to other therapies. Physicians are required to "self-attest" that they are qualified to diagnose and treat IBS. Both physicians and patients are required to sign consent forms, which will probably protect the manufacturer in product-liability lawsuits.

Public Citizen has argued that even such a highly restricted distribution system is likely to prove inadequate because there are no known factors to predict which women are at the greatest risk of developing ischemic colitis.[51] Therefore, there is no way to adequately warn them which symptoms may lead to this serious adverse reaction or to adequately monitor them as would be more feasible in the research setting.

With the drug back on the market, cases of ischemic colitis and severe constipation have resumed. After little over a year back on the market, with dramatically decreased sales, alosetron had already been associated with eight cases of ischemic colitis and eight serious complications of constipation.[52]

Do Not Use

ALTERNATIVE TREATMENT:
See the box accompanying this drug profile about alternative treatments for IBS.

Tegaserod (te *gas* a rod)
ZELNORM (Novartis)

FAMILY: Irritable Bowel Syndrome (IBS) Drugs

Tegaserod has been approved by the FDA for the treatment of women with IBS in whom constipation is the predominant symptom. The drug is not approved for men. The drug stimulates the 5-HT4 receptor, one of a family of serotonin receptors. Public Citizen opposed the approval of the drug based on its marginal efficacy and concerns about the induction of cysts in the ovaries.[53]

ALTERNATIVE TREATMENTS FOR IRRITABLE BOWEL SYNDROME

General measures include reducing intake of caffeine, alcohol, and fried foods. Because intolerance to lactose (milk sugar) can mimic some symptoms of irritable bowel syndrome (IBS), a test to determine if you are lactose intolerant should be done. Sorbitol, the sugar in sugarless gum or candy, should be avoided. Minimization of stress and the use of relaxation techniques have helped many people. For constipation-predominant IBS, increased dietary fiber and/or the use of psyllium or methylcellulose (see p. 566) and increased fluid intake may be helpful. For diarrhea-predominant IBS, the cautious use of loperamide (IMODIUM) (see p. 572) can be helpful.

ROME II CRITERIA FOR DIAGNOSIS OF IRRITABLE BOWEL SYNDROME [4]

In the preceding 12 months, at least 12 weeks, not necessarily consecutive, of abdominal discomfort or pain that has two out of these three features:

1. Relieved with defecation.

2. Onset associated with a change in frequency of stool.

3. Onset associated with a change in form (appearance) of stool.

Symptoms that cumulatively support the diagnosis of irritable bowel syndrome:

abnormal stool frequency (for research purposes "abnormal" may be defined as greater than three bowel movements per day and less than three per week);

abnormal stool form (lumpy/hard or loose/watery);

abnormal stool passage (straining, urgency, or feeling of incomplete evacuation);

passage of mucus;

bloating or feeling of abdominal distension.

IBS itself is not a life-threatening condition, although it can be debilitating. If the major symptom is diarrhea, the condition is known as diarrhea-predominant IBS; if it is characterized by constipation, it is called constipation-predominant IBS. The diagnosis of IBS should be based on a set of internationally recognized symptoms known as the Rome II Criteria [4] (see box) and requires exclusion of treatable causes of the patient's symptoms, such as ulcerative colitis. This is especially important if the following signs of ulcerative colitis are present: onset after age 50, rectal bleeding, fever, weight loss, or anemia. There are no abnormal laboratory tests or changes in the cells of the GI tract on biopsy that can objectively establish the diagnosis of IBS. In fact, the diagnosis of IBS can only

be made if all tests for other diseases that might explain the patient's symptoms are negative and the patient continues to have recurrent abdominal discomfort or pain associated with diarrhea, constipation, or both.

There were eight cases of ovarian cysts in women taking tegaserod during the clinical trials, compared to one in the placebo groups. Although the company ultimately convinced the FDA that these were not related to the drug, we remain concerned because tegaserod induced ovarian cysts in rats and because there are 5-HT4 receptors in human ovaries.[54] In addition, there was an increase in abdominal surgeries in patients taking tegaserod during clinical trials compared to placebo-treated patients. The increase was attributed primarily to an increase in gallbladder removals.

After marketing, new safety concerns with tegaserod arose. In April 2004, the FDA announced that the drug would be relabeled because of 21 cases of serious diarrhea and 23 cases of ischemic colitis or closely related diseases.[55]

In addition to the ovarian cysts, the diarrhea, the ischemic colitis, and the non-life-threatening nature of IBS, tegaserod also has questionable efficacy: none of the three pivotal clinical trials demonstrated effectiveness, as judged by the original, predetermined primary clinical outcome measures.[53] When it was seen, after the fact, that there was no significant improvement for either of the two original outcome measures in the first completed trial, Novartis cunningly altered the endpoints for the other two ongoing (but still blinded) trials, eliminating one measure and redefining the other in a manner that created a lower threshold for declaring improvement. However, even this manipulation produced only one pivotal trial with a statistically significant result, and that result was only half of what Novartis had expected.

In sum, tegaserod is a potentially dangerous drug of minimal efficacy used in the treatment of non-life-threatening conditions. We recommend that you not use it and try the measures outlined in the box (see p. 557) instead.

In July 2004, an FDA advisory committee recommended the approval of tegaserod for the treatment of chronic constipation in women under 65 years of age. The FDA usually follows the recommendations of its advisory committees; we recommend that you don't use this drug for any purpose.

─────

Nausea

Limited Use

Prochlorperazine (proe klor *pair* a zeen)
COMPAZINE (GlaxoSmithKline)

Promethazine (proe *meth* a zeen)
PHENERGAN (Wyeth-Ayerst)

GENERIC: available
FAMILY: Nausea Drugs

PREGNANCY WARNING

Phenothiazines cross the placenta, and there have been reports of prolonged jaundice and nervous system effects in infants of mothers who took these drugs during pregnancy. Tell your doctor if you are pregnant or thinking of becoming pregnant before you take one of these drugs.

BREAST-FEEDING WARNING

Phenothiazines are excreted in human milk. Because of the potential for serious adverse effects in nursing infants, you should not take these drugs while nursing.

Prochlorperazine and promethazine are phenothiazines used to control nausea and vomiting. Promethazine is also listed in this book as a **Do Not Use** combination drug for allergy, cough, and cold symptoms (see p. 378). Prochlorperazine is approved for treating schizophrenia, although a leading textbook says it has "questionable utility"[57] for this purpose. It has

not been proved effective in treating patients with mental retardation.

For severe nausea and vomiting, you should only be taking prochlorperazine and promethazine if you have already tried making changes in your diet (see box p. 557) and this has not worked.

Prochlorperazine and promethazine can cause serious adverse effects: drug-induced parkinsonism (see p. 30) and tardive dyskinesia (involuntary movements of parts of the body, which may last indefinitely). More information appears under Adverse Effects below. Taking large doses of these drugs or tak-

---

ANTICHOLINERGIC EFFECTS

WARNING: SPECIAL MENTAL AND PHYSICAL ADVERSE EFFECTS

Older adults are especially sensitive to the harmful anticholinergic (see Glossary, p. 889) effects of this drug. Drugs in this family should not be used unless absolutely necessary.

Mental Effects: confusion, delirium, short-term memory problems, disorientation, and impaired attention.

Physical Effects: dry mouth, constipation, difficulty urinating (especially for a man with an enlarged prostate), blurred vision, decreased sweating with increased body temperature, sexual dysfunction, and worsening of glaucoma.

Use extra care not to become overheated during exercise or hot weather while you are taking one of these medications, because overheating may result in heatstroke. Also, hot baths or saunas may make you feel dizzy or faint when you are taking this medication.

These drugs may also make you more sensitive to cold temperatures. Dress warmly during cold weather. Be careful during prolonged exposure to cold, such as in winter sports or when swimming in cold water.

Drugs used to treat cancer often cause severe nausea and vomiting, either immediately after the drug is taken or several hours later. You can treat this kind of nausea and vomiting by changing your diet or by taking an antinausea drug. You should always try dietary changes first.[56]

• Eat small, frequent meals so your stomach is never empty.

• When you get up from sleeping or resting, eat some dry crackers or toast before you start being active.

• Drink carbonated drinks or other clear liquids such as soups and gelatin.

• Eat tart foods such as lemons and pickles.

• Do not eat foods with strong smells.

ing them for a long time could increase your chance of experiencing these and other adverse effects. If you have used either of these drugs regularly for some time, ask your doctor if your drug can be changed. **If you are over 60, you should generally be taking less than the usual adult dose.**

These drugs are contraindicated in patients less than two years of age, or who weigh less than 20 pounds. Muscle spasms due to these drugs are more common in children with dehydration or acute illness.

Before You Use This Drug

Do not use if you have or have had (if taking prochlorperazine):

• blood pressure that is severely high or low
• coma
• genetic defect in drug metabolism (2D6 enzyme)
• heart or blood vessel disease
• heart rhythm problems
• long QT syndrome that you were born with
• reactions to other antipsychotics (see p. 258)

Tell your doctor if you have or have had:

• alcohol dependence
• allergic reaction to drugs
• angina
• blood disease
• bone marrow depression
• brain damage
• breast cancer
• epilepsy or seizures
• glaucoma
• heart disease
• jaundice
• kidney disease
• liver disease
• lung disease or breathing problems
• Parkinson's disease
• prostate enlarged or difficulty urinating
• Reye's syndrome
• stroke or transient ischemic attack
• ulcer of stomach or duodenum

Tell your doctor about any other drugs you take, including aspirin, herbs, vitamins, and other nonprescription products.

When You Use This Drug

• **Do not stop taking this drug suddenly. Your doctor must give you a schedule to lower your dose gradually, to prevent withdrawal symptoms** such as nausea, vomiting, stomach upset, trembling, dizziness, and symptoms of Parkinson's disease.

• Do not use over-the-counter drugs for colds or allergies.

• Do not take over-the-counter antacids or antidiarrheals within two hours of taking promethazine.

• It may take two or three weeks before you can tell that this drug is working.

• Until you know how you react to this drug, do not drive or perform other activities requiring alertness. Prochlorperazine can cause blurred vision, drowsiness, and fainting.

• To avoid heatstroke, use caution when exercising, when the weather is hot, and when taking hot baths.

• Wear protective clothing and use sunblock when outdoors and avoid use of sunlamps, tanning beds, or tanning booths. Check with your doctor if you get a severe reaction.

• Wear sunglasses to protect your eyes from ultraviolet light.

• If you have dry mouth, use sugarless gum or candy, ice, or saliva substititute and check with your doctor or dentist if this condition lasts more than two weeks.

• Do not drink alcohol or use other drugs that can cause drowsiness.

• You may feel dizzy when rising from a lying or sitting position. When getting out of bed, hang your legs over the side of the bed for a few minutes, then get up slowly. When getting up from a chair, stay by the chair until you are sure that you are not dizzy. (See p. 13.)

• If you plan to have any surgery, including dental, tell your doctor that you take this drug.

How to Use This Drug

• If you miss a dose, take it as soon as you remember, but skip it if it is almost time for the next dose. **Do not take double doses.**

• Do not share your medication with others.

• Take the drug at the same time(s) each day.

• Take with food or **a full glass (eight ounces)** of milk or water to prevent stomach upset.

• Swallow extended-release capsules whole.

• Store at room temperature with lid on tightly. Do not store in the bathroom. Do not expose to heat, moisture, or strong light. Do not let the liquid form freeze. Keep out of reach of children.

Interactions with Other Drugs

The following drugs, biologics (e.g., vaccines, therapeutic antibodies), or foods are listed in *Evaluations of Drug Interactions* 2003 as causing "highly clinically significant" or "clinically significant" interactions when used together with any of the drugs in this section. In some sections with multiple drugs, the interaction may have been reported for one but not all drugs in this section, but we include the interaction because the drugs in this section are similar to one another. We have also included potentially serious interactions listed in the drug's FDA-approved professional package insert or in published medical journal articles. There may be other drugs, especially those in the families of drugs listed below, that also will react with this drug to cause severe adverse effects. Make sure to tell your doctor and pharmacist the drugs you are taking and tell them if you are taking any of these interacting drugs:

barbiturates (e.g., phenobarbital), cabergoline, DOSTINEX, epinephrine, EPIPEN, ESIMIL, GLUCOPHAGE, guanethidine, HALFAN, halofantrine, INDERAL, INDERAL LA, ISMELIN, monoamine oxidase (MAO) inhibitors (e.g., phenelzine), metformin, NEOSPORIN, NORPRAMIN, ORAP, PARLODEL, pergolide, PERMAX, pimozide, polymyxin B, propranolol, tramadol, ULTRAM, zotepine.

Adverse Effects

Call your doctor immediately if you experience:

• **signs of tardive dyskinesia:** lip smacking, chewing movements, puffing of cheeks, rapid, darting tongue movements, uncontrolled movements of arms or legs

• **signs of parkinsonism:** difficulty speaking or swallowing, loss of balance, mask-like face, muscle spasms, stiffness of arms or legs, trembling and shaking, unusual twisting movements of body, shuffling walk

• **signs of neuroleptic malignant syndrome:** troubled or fast breathing, high or low blood pressure, increased sweating, loss of bladder control, muscle stiffness, seizures, unusual tiredness or weakness, fast heartbeat, irregular pulse, pale skin

- abdominal or stomach pain
- arms, legs, or muscles weak
- bleeding or bruising that is unusual
- breathing difficulty
- changed or blurred vision; difficulty seeing at night
- confusion
- difficulty urinating
- erections that are prolonged, painful, or inappropriate
- eyes or skin yellow
- eyes unable to move
- fainting
- fatigue
- fever
- mouth, gums, or throat sore
- muscles and joints aching
- nausea, vomiting, diarrhea
- nightmares
- restlessness or need to keep moving
- skin hot or dry
- skin rash, itching, or sunburn
- skin tanned or blue/gray discoloration
- sweating decreased

Call your doctor if these symptoms continue:

- breast swelling or pain
- constipation
- dizziness, lightheadedness
- drowsiness
- ears ringing or buzzing
- menstrual period changes
- milk, unusual secretion
- mouth dry
- mouth watering
- nasal congestion
- sexual ability decreased
- skin rash
- skin sensitivity to sun
- sweating decreased
- tongue rough or "fuzzy"
- weight gain that is unusual

Signs of overdose:

- agitation
- breathing difficulty
- confusion
- convulsions
- drowsiness, stupor, or coma
- fever
- heart rhythm disturbance
- mouth dry
- muscle weakness
- pupils dilated
- reflexes increased or decreased
- vision blurred
- vomiting

If you suspect an overdose, call this number to contact your poison control center: (800) 222-1222.

Call your doctor if these symptoms continue after you stop taking this drug:

- dizziness
- eyes unable to move
- muscle spasms of face, neck, body, arms, or legs
- nausea and vomiting
- stomach pain
- tardive dyskinesia (see glossary, p. 897)
- ticlike or twitching movements
- sticking out of tongue
- trembling of fingers and hands
- trouble breathing, speaking, or swallowing
- twisting movements of body

Periodic Tests

Ask your doctor which of these tests should be done periodically while you are taking this drug:

- complete blood count if you develop a sore throat
- glaucoma tests
- blood potassium levels
- monitoring of heart function (ECG or EKG)

- liver function tests
- urine tests for bile and bilirubin
- observation for early signs of tardive dyskinesia
- evaluation of continued need for drug
- blood pressure
- eye examinations

Limited Use

Metoclopramide (met oh *kloe* pra mide)
REGLAN (Baxter)

GENERIC: available

FAMILY: Nausea Drugs

PREGNANCY WARNING

No valid data are available from animal studies. Use during pregnancy only for clear medical reasons. Tell your doctor if you are pregnant or thinking of becoming pregnant before you take this drug.

BREAST-FEEDING WARNING

Metoclopramide is excreted in human milk. Because metoclopromide causes mammary tumors in animal studies, you should consult with your doctor if you are planning to nurse.

Metoclopramide increases the tone of the muscle at the junction of the stomach and the esophagus (the tube connecting the mouth to the stomach) and increases contractions of the stomach. For people who have a condition in which the stomach takes too long to empty (diabetic gastroparesis), it relieves symptoms such as nausea, vomiting, loss of appetite, heartburn, and a feeling of fullness after meals. It also controls reflux esophagitis, a condition in which the stomach contents flow backwards into the esophagus, causing heartburn. It prevents nausea and vomiting caused by chemotherapy for cancer. This drug should not be used to treat motion sickness or vertigo (dizziness).

If you are experiencing nausea and vomiting from cancer chemotherapy, you should try changing your diet to relieve these effects before taking a drug such as metoclopramide (see box below). There is very little experience with long-term metoclopramide use in clinical studies.[58]

Metoclopramide can cause serious adverse effects: severe drowsiness, drug-induced parkinsonism (see p. 30), and tardive dyskinesia (involuntary movements of parts of the body, which may last indefinitely). The latter two conditions can occur when the drug is used over a long period of time, especially in people with impaired kidney function. More information appears under Adverse Effects.

If you are over 60, you should generally be taking less than the usual adult dose, because older adults often do not tolerate metoclopramide well.

Before You Use This Drug

Do not use if you have or have had:

- epilepsy or seizures
- stomach or intestinal bleeding, obstruction, or perforation
- pheochromocytoma

Drugs used to treat cancer often cause severe nausea and vomiting, either immediately after the drug is taken or several hours later. You can treat this kind of nausea and vomiting by changing your diet or by taking an antinausea drug. You should always try dietary changes first.[56]

- Eat small, frequent meals so your stomach is never empty.
- When you get up from sleeping or resting, eat some dry crackers or toast before you start being active.
- Drink carbonated drinks or other clear liquids such as soups and gelatin.
- Eat tart foods such as lemons and pickles.
- Do not eat foods with strong smells.

Tell your doctor if you have or have had:

- allergies to metoclopramide, procaine, or procainamide
- asthma
- high blood pressure
- kidney problems
- mental depression
- Parkinson's disease
- pregnancy or are breast-feeding

Tell your doctor about any other drugs you take, including aspirin, herbs, vitamins, and other nonprescription products.

When You Use This Drug

- Do not drink alcohol or use other drugs that can cause drowsiness.
- Until you know how you react to this drug, do not drive or perform other activities requiring alertness.

How to Use This Drug

- If you miss a dose, take it as soon as you remember, but skip it if it is almost time for the next dose. **Do not take double doses.**
- Do not share your medication with others.
- Take the drug at the same time(s) each day.
- Take 30 minutes before meals and at bedtime for maximum effectiveness.
- *Oral solution:* Mix with liquid or semisolid food such as water, juice, soda, applesauce, or pudding.
- Store at room temperature with lid on tightly. Do not store in the bathroom. Do not expose to heat, moisture, or strong light. Do not let the liquid form freeze. Keep out of reach of children.

Interactions with Other Drugs

The following drugs, biologics (e.g., vaccines, therapeutic antibodies), or foods are listed in *Evaluations of Drug Interactions* 2003 as causing "highly clinically significant" or "clinically significant" interactions when used together with any of the drugs in this section. In some sections with multiple drugs, the interaction may have been reported for one but not all drugs in this section, but we include the interaction because the drugs in this section are similar to one another. We have also included potentially serious interactions listed in the drug's FDA-approved professional package insert or in published medical journal articles. There may be other drugs, especially those in the families of drugs listed below, that also will react with this drug to cause severe adverse effects. Make sure to tell your doctor and pharmacist the drugs you are taking and tell them if you are taking any of these interacting drugs:

acetaminophen, cabergoline, cyclosporine, digoxin, DOSTINEX, EFFEXOR, fosfomycin, LANOXICAPS, LANOXIN, levodopa, monoamine oxidase (MAO) inhibitors (e.g., phenelzine), MONUROL, NEORAL, pergolide, PERMAX, REQUIP, ropinirole, SANDIMMUNE, SINEMET, STALEVO, SUMYCIN, tetracycline, TYLENOL, venlafaxine.

Adverse Effects

Call your doctor immediately if you experience:

- **signs of tardive dyskinesia:** lip smacking, chewing movements, puffing of cheeks, rapid, darting tongue movements, uncontrolled movements of arms or legs
- **signs of parkinsonism:** difficulty speaking or swallowing, loss of balance, mask-like face, muscle spasms, stiffness of arms or legs, trembling and shaking, unusual twisting movements of body, shuffling walk
- arms or legs stiff
- blood pressure increased
- chills
- dizziness or fainting
- eyes unable to move

- fever
- headache that is severe or continued
- heartbeat that is fast or irregular
- legs aching, uncomfortable, or sensation of crawling
- muscle spasms of face, neck, and back
- nervousness, restlessness, or irritability
- paniclike sensation
- speaking or swallowing difficulty
- throat sore
- tiredness or weakness
- trembling and shaking of hands and fingers
- twisting movements of body
- twitching movements

Call your doctor if these symptoms continue:

- breast milk flow increased
- breast tenderness and swelling
- constipation or diarrhea
- depression
- dizziness
- drowsiness
- headache
- irritability
- menstruation changes
- mouth dry
- nausea
- restlessness
- skin rash
- sleeping difficulty
- tiredness or weakness that is unusual

Signs of overdose:

- confusion
- drowsiness that is severe
- hands shaking, trembling
- muscle spasms
- seizures
- ticlike, jerky movements of head and face

If you suspect an overdose, call this number to contact your poison control center: (800) 222-1222.

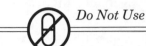

Do Not Use

ALTERNATIVE TREATMENT:
See box on dietary modifications, p. 563.

Trimethobenzamide (trye meth oh *ben* za mide)
TIGAN (King)

FAMILY: Nausea Drugs

Trimethobenzamide is approved by the FDA to relieve nausea and vomiting associated with surgery and gastroenteritis. **There is no convincing proof that it is effective.**[59] It has little or no value for preventing or treating vertigo (a form of dizziness) or motion sickness.[60]

Trimethobenzamide can hide some of the signs of an aspirin or salicylate overdose.[61] Rarely, trimethobenzamide causes convulsions, and this is more common among older users of the drug.[60] Some of the drug's hazards are magnified in children, in whom it should not be used for uncomplicated vomiting.[61]

ANTICHOLINERGIC EFFECTS

WARNING: SPECIAL MENTAL AND PHYSICAL ADVERSE EFFECTS

Older adults are especially sensitive to the harmful anticholinergic (see Glossary, p. 889) effects of this drug. Drugs in this family should not be used unless absolutely necessary.

Mental Effects: confusion, delirium, short-term memory problems, disorientation, and impaired attention.

Physical Effects: dry mouth, constipation, difficulty urinating (especially for a man with an enlarged prostate), blurred vision, decreased sweating with increased body temperature, sexual dysfunction, and worsening of glaucoma.

━━━━━━━━

Constipation

Psyllium (*sill* i yum)
METAMUCIL (Procter & Gamble)
PERDIEM (Novartis Consumer)

Methylcellulose (meth ill *sell* you loas)
CITRUCEL (GlaxoSmithKline Consumer)

GENERIC: available
FAMILY: Bulk-Forming Laxatives

PREGNANCY AND BREAST-FEEDING WARNING
There is no information in the drug labels. Consult with your doctor or pharmacist.

Psyllium and methylcellulose are laxatives that work by absorbing water and softening the stools in your intestine. The increased stool bulk stimulates the intestines to contract. Fiber that you get from food works exactly the same way. **Because a diet high in fiber, combined with plenty of nonalcoholic liquids, has the same effect as psyllium and methylcellulose, it is not usually necessary to use these drugs.** Eating high-fiber foods is preferable to taking psyllium or methylcellulose because these foods give you essential nutrients in addition to fiber. Psyllium and methylcellulose appear to be approximately equally effective.[62] Patients taking psyllium or methylcellulose appear to be less likely to pass gas than when taking another effective laxative, lactulose (see p. 568).[63]

When do you really need to take a laxative? You should not take a laxative to "clean out your system" or to make your body act more "normally." It is untrue that everyone must have a bowel movement daily. Perfectly healthy people may have from three bowel movements per week to three bowel movements per day.

If the frequency of your bowel movements has decreased, if you are having bowel movements less than three times a week, or if you are having difficulty in passing stools, you are constipated, but this does not mean that you need a laxative. It is better to treat simple, occasional constipation without drugs, by eating a high-fiber diet that includes whole-grain breads and cereals, raw vegetables, raw and dried fruits, and beans, and by drinking plenty of nonalcoholic liquids (six to eight glasses per day). This type of diet will both prevent and treat constipation, and it is less costly than taking drugs. Regular exercise—at least 30 minutes per day of swimming, cycling, jogging, or brisk walking—will also help your body maintain regularity.

If you are constipated while traveling or at some other time when it is hard for you to eat properly, it may be appropriate to take a laxative for a short time. The only types of laxatives you should use for self-medication are bulk-forming laxatives such as psyllium or methylcellulose or a hyperosmotic laxative such as lactulose. Bulk-forming laxatives usually take effect in 12 hours to three days, compared with docusate (see p. 571), which takes effect one or two days after the first dose but may require three to five days of treatment. Even bulk-forming laxatives should only be used occasionally, if possible.

If you are on a special diet such as a low-salt or low-sugar diet, ask your doctor or pharmacist to help you choose a laxative without ingredients you are trying to avoid. Some laxatives contain sugar (up to half of the product), salt (up to 250 milligrams per dose), or the artificial sweetener NutraSweet.

When added to the diet, psyllium is a safe, effective method of lowering cholesterol. If cholesterol remains high despite diet, add 10 grams of psyllium a day. Numerous studies have shown that five grams of psyllium twice a day can significantly lower total cholesterol and LDL cholesterol.[64] Psyllium, a naturally occurring vegetable fiber, is clearly safer than any of the cholesterol-lowering drugs.

Psyllium has been implicated in severe allergic reactions, typically by inhalation or by ingestion after exposure in the health care setting.[65]

Before You Use This Drug

Tell your doctor if you have or have had:

- severe abdominal pain
- allergies to drugs
- phenylketonuria (if you take the sugarless form)
- appendicitis
- colostomy
- diabetes
- heart disease
- high blood pressure
- hypertension
- ileostomy
- impacted bowel movement
- congestive heart failure
- intestinal obstruction
- kidney problems
- occupational exposure to psyllium
- rectal bleeding
- difficulty swallowing

Tell your doctor about any other drugs you take, including aspirin, herbs, vitamins, and other nonprescription products.

When You Use This Drug

- Check with your doctor to make certain your fluid intake is adequate and appropriate (e.g., four to six 8-ounce glasses of fluid daily). If you do not get enough fluids, the laxative will not work properly and may dry and harden, clogging the intestine.[66] This is especially true during hot weather or strenuous exercise. Exercise regularly, such as walking.
- Avoid alcohol and medications that may cause constipation.
- Do not use other laxatives while on psyllium or methylcellulose.
- Do not use unnecessarily (for a cold, tonic, or clean system).

- Wait at least two days without a bowel movement before considering use.
- Check with your doctor if a sudden change lasts more than two weeks.
- Avoid a laxative habit. Overuse or extended use may cause dependence.
- Do not take within two hours of taking other medicines.
- Check with your doctor if you develop a skin rash.
- **Caution diabetics:** Psyllium contains 3.5 grams of dextrose.
- Do not use for more than one week. If you have used psyllium or methylcellulose for a week, stop taking it to see if a high-fiber diet and liquids alone will work. If your constipation continues for longer than a week, call your doctor.

How to Use This Drug

- If you miss a dose, take it as soon as you remember, but skip it if it is almost time for the next dose. **Do not take double doses.**
- Do not share your medication with others.
- Take the drug at the same time(s) each day.
- Follow manufacturer's package directions.
- Drink six to eight full glasses of water each day when using any laxative.
- Take each dose with **a full glass (eight ounces)** of water or juice. Mix well.
- If you take any other drugs, take them at least two hours before or after the time you take psyllium.
- Do not expose to heat, moisture, or strong light. Keep out of reach of children.

Interactions with Other Drugs

Evaluations of Drug Interactions 2003 lists no drugs, biologics (e.g., vaccines, therapeutic antibodies), or foods as causing "highly clinically significant" or "clinically significant" interactions when used together with the drugs in this section. We also found no interactions in the drugs' FDA-approved professional package inserts. However, as the number of new drugs approved for marketing increases and as more experience is gained with these drugs over time, new interactions may be discovered.

Adverse Effects

Call your doctor immediately if you experience:

- breathing difficulty
- intestinal obstruction (cramping, bloating, nausea)
- skin rash or itching
- swallowing difficulty

Call your doctor if you continue to experience:

- stomach and/or intestinal cramping

Limited Use

Lactulose (*lak* tu lose)
CEPHULAC (Hoechst Marion Roussel)
CHRONOLAC (Hoechst Marion Roussel)

GENERIC: available

FAMILY: Hyperosmotic Laxatives

PREGNANCY WARNING

No valid data are available for lactulose, as it was not tested properly in animal studies. Use during pregnancy only for clear medical reasons. Tell your doctor if you are pregnant or thinking of becoming pregnant before you take this drug.

BREAST-FEEDING WARNING

No information is available from either human or animal studies. Since it is likely that this drug, like many others, is excreted in human milk, you should consult with your doctor if you are planning to nurse.

Lactulose is a synthetic combination of the sugars galactose and fructose. It is not well ab-

sorbed from the intestines, and the body responds by secreting water into the intestines. Drugs that reduce constipation this way are called hyperosmotic laxatives. The sugars are also fermented by bacteria in the colon, producing hydrogen gas. (Patients taking the laxatives psyllium or methylcellulose [see p. 566] appear to be less likely to pass gas than those taking lactulose.[63]) Both actions expand the colon, which responds by contracting and expelling its contents. Much of the water in the colonic contents is reabsorbed in the colon; the decreased transit time means there is less time for water reabsorption and stools are therefore softer.[7,67]

In advanced liver disease, ammonia builds up in the body and can enter the brain, causing confusion and even coma, a condition called hepatic encephalopathy. Lactulose slightly acidifies the colon and converts ammonia into ammonium, which is then passed out in the stool.[66] Lactulose is thus an accepted treatment for hepatic encephalopathy.[68]

Hyperosmotic laxatives, such as lactulose, usually take a few days to work. Doses may need adjusting for individual response.[69] Some people dislike the sweet taste.[68,70] Lactulose is usually taken orally, but it may be administered via enema or nasogastric tube in encephalopathic patients.[68] Laxatives should only be taken for a limited time. If lactulose is used for more than six months or by elderly or debilitated people, electrolytes should be monitored.[71]

When do you really need to take a laxative? You should not take a laxative to "clean out your system" or to make your body act more "normally." It is untrue that everyone must have a bowel movement daily. Perfectly healthy people may have from three bowel movements per week to three bowel movements per day.

If the frequency of your bowel movements has decreased, if you are having bowel movements less than three times a week, or if you are having difficulty in passing stools, you are constipated, but this does not mean that you need a laxative. It is better to treat simple, occasional constipation without drugs, by eating a high-fiber diet that includes whole-grain breads and cereals, raw vegetables, raw and dried fruits, and beans, and by drinking plenty of nonalcoholic liquids (six to eight glasses per day). This type of diet will both prevent and treat constipation, and it is less costly than taking drugs. Regular exercise—at least 30 minutes per day of swimming, cycling, jogging, or brisk walking—will also help your body maintain regularity.

If you are constipated while traveling or at some other time when it is hard for you to eat properly, it may be appropriate to take a laxative for a short time. The only types of laxatives you should use for self-medication are bulk-forming laxatives such as psyllium or methylcellulose (see p. 566) or a hyperosmotic laxative such as lactulose. Bulk-forming laxatives usually take effect in 12 hours to three days, compared with docusate (see p. 571), which takes effect one or two days after the first dose but may require three to five days of treatment. Even bulk-forming laxatives should only be used occasionally, if possible.

If you are on a special diet such as a low-salt or low-sugar diet, ask your doctor or pharmacist to help you choose a laxative without ingredients you are trying to avoid. Some laxatives contain sugar (up to half of the product), salt (up to 250 milligrams per dose), or the artificial sweetener NutraSweet.

People with diabetes should use lactulose cautiously. Rarely, lactulose causes gas within the bowel wall, a condition called pneumatosis intestinalis that sometimes requires surgery.[72] Infants administered lactulose are especially prone to low blood sodium and dehydration.[66] People who undergo electrocautery procedures during proctoscopy or colonoscopy risk hazard if an electrical spark triggers an explosion with hydrogen gas. Bowel cleansing for these procedures should use a nonfermentable solution.[71]

If diarrhea occurs in the course of treatment for constipation, lactulose should be stopped. Prolonged diarrhea can cause excess sodium in the blood as well as loss of potassium.[68,73]

Before You Use This Drug

Tell your doctor if you have or have had:

- abdominal pain
- allergies to drugs, including to lactose
- anorexia
- appendicitis
- blood in stools
- colon cancer, including family history
- diabetes
- diarrhea
- galactose-low diet[66]
- heart problems
- hypertension (high blood pressure)
- impaction of stool (intestinal obstruction)
- inflammatory bowel disease, including family history
- intestinal obstruction
- kidney problems
- nausea or vomiting
- pregnancy or are breast-feeding
- weight loss

Tell your doctor about any other drugs you take, including aspirin, herbs, vitamins, and other nonprescription products.

When You Use This Drug

- Check with your doctor to make certain your fluid intake is adequate and appropriate (e.g., four to six 8-ounce glasses of fluid daily). If you do not get enough fluids, the laxative will not work properly and may dry and harden, clogging the intestine.[66] This is especially true during hot weather or strenuous exercise.
- Get regular exercise, such as walking.
- Avoid alcohol and medications that may cause constipation.

• Limit use of candies, gums, and foods containing mannitol or sorbitol, as these may add to effects of lactulose.

• Do not use other laxatives while on lactulose.[66]

• Do not use unnecessarily (for a cold, tonic, or clean system).

• Wait at least two days without a bowel movement before considering use.

• Check with your doctor if a sudden change lasts more than two weeks.

• Avoid a laxative habit. Overuse or extended use may cause dependence.

• Do not use for more than one week. If you have used lactulose for a week, stop taking it to see if a high-fiber diet and liquids alone will work. If your constipation continues for longer than a week, call your doctor.

How to Use This Drug

• If you use a powder form, open the packet and dissolve contents in water, according to instructions. For liquid forms, measure your dose.

• Take with **a full glass (eight ounces)** of water. To improve flavor, mix with fruit juice, citrus-carbonated beverage, or milk. Taking with food or at bedtime may delay results.

• If you miss a dose, take it as soon as you remember, but skip it if it is almost time for the next dose. **Do not take double doses.**

• Do not share your medication with others.

• Take the drug at the same time(s) each day.

• Do not use for prolonged periods of time.

• Store at room temperature with lid on tightly. Do not store in the bathroom. Do not expose to heat, moisture, or strong light. Do not let the liquid form freeze. Keep out of reach of children.

Interactions with Other Drugs

Evaluations of Drug Interactions 2003 lists no drugs, biologics (e.g., vaccines, therapeutic antibodies), or foods as causing "highly clinically significant" or "clinically significant" interactions when used together with the drugs in this section. We also found no interactions in the drugs' FDA-approved professional package inserts. However, as the number of new drugs approved for marketing increases and as more experience is gained with these drugs over time, new interactions may be discovered.

Adverse Effects

Call your doctor immediately if you experience:

• abdominal pain
• confusion
• diarrhea that is unusual
• dizziness or lightheadedness
• heartbeat irregular
• muscle cramps
• tiredness or weakness that is unusual

Call your doctor if you continue to experience:

• appetite decreased
• bloating
• bowel habits changed suddenly and continue for two weeks
• cramping
• diarrhea
• gas
• nausea
• stomach and/or intestinal cramping
• thirst

Signs of overdose:

• abdominal cramps
• dehydration
• diarrhea

If you suspect an overdose, call this number to contact your poison control center: (800) 222-1222.

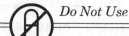 *Do Not Use*

ALTERNATIVE TREATMENT:
*See Psyllium and Methylcellulose, p. 566,
and Lactulose, p. 568.*

Docusate (*dok* yoo sate)
COLACE (Purdue)
SURFAK (Pharmacia & Upjohn)

Bisacodyl (bis a *koe* dill)
DULCOLAX (Boehringer Ingelheim)

Docusate and Casanthranol
(*dok* yoo sate and ka *san* thra nole)
DIALOSE PLUS (Johnson & Johnson
Consumer)
PERI-COLACE (Purdue)

FAMILY: Stool-Softener Laxatives
          Stimulant Laxatives

Docusate is a laxative that works by softening your stools. Docusate and other laxatives in its family can cause long-lasting damage to your intestine and can interfere with your body's use of nutrients. Docusate can also be dangerous if you are taking other drugs at the same time because it can make your body absorb the other drugs at an increased rate. There are other laxatives that are safer than docusate; we do not recommend that you use it.

Casanthranol and bisacodyl are stimulant laxatives. If you take this type of laxative for a long time, it gradually reduces your intestine's ability to work efficiently. This causes increased constipation and a disease of the large intestine called cathartic colon, in which the intestine becomes enlarged and will not move without chemical stimulation.

You should not take stool softeners or stimulant laxatives, alone or in combination, to treat simple constipation.

Many people take laxatives more often than they need to. This is dangerous for several rea-

sons. First, some laxatives can have adverse effects. Second, laxatives can be habit-forming. If you take them too often or for too long, your body will become less able to pass stools without them. This leads to a cycle of abuse in which you become dependent on laxatives and have to take them continuously. If you think you have become dependent on laxatives, talk to your doctor.

When do you really need to take a laxative? You should not take a laxative to "clean out your system" or to make your body act more "normally." It is untrue that everyone must have a bowel movement daily. Perfectly healthy people may have from three bowel movements per week to three bowel movements per day.

If the frequency of your bowel movements has decreased, if you are having bowel movements less than three times a week, or if you are having difficulty in passing stools, you are constipated, but this does not mean that you need a laxative. It is better to treat simple, occasional constipation without drugs, by eating a high-fiber diet that includes whole-grain breads and cereals, raw vegetables, raw and dried fruits, and beans, and by drinking plenty of nonalcoholic liquids (six to eight glasses per day). This type of diet will both prevent and treat constipation, and it is less costly than taking drugs. Regular exercise—at least 30 minutes per day of swimming, cycling, jogging, or brisk walking—will also help your body maintain regularity.

If you are constipated while traveling or at some other time when it is hard for you to eat properly, it may be appropriate to take a laxative for a short time. The only types of laxatives you should use for self-medication are bulk-forming laxatives such as psyllium or methylcellulose (see p. 566) or a hyperosmotic laxative such as lactulose (see p. 568). Bulk-forming laxatives usually take effect in 12 hours to three days, compared with docusate, which takes effect one or two days after the first dose but may require three to five days of treatment. Even bulk-forming laxatives should only be used occasionally, if possible.

If you are on a special diet such as a low-salt or low-sugar diet, ask your doctor or pharmacist to help you choose a laxative without ingredients you are trying to avoid. Some laxatives contain sugar (up to half of the product), salt (up to 250 milligrams per dose), or the artificial sweetener NutraSweet.

Diarrhea

Limited Use

Loperamide (loe *per* a mide)
IMODIUM (McNeil Consumer)

GENERIC: available
FAMILY: Diarrhea Drugs

PREGNANCY WARNING
No data are available for loperamide. Use during pregnancy only for clear medical reasons. Tell your doctor if you are pregnant or thinking of becoming pregnant before you take this drug.

BREAST-FEEDING WARNING
No information is available from either human or animal studies. Since it is likely that this drug, like many others, is excreted in human milk, you should consult with your doctor if you are planning to nurse.

Loperamide is used to treat severe diarrhea. It should never replace rehydration, which is the primary treatment for diarrhea. The World Health Organization has warned against the drug's use in children.[74] The U.S. Centers for Disease Control and Prevention has concluded: "Little evidence exists to support the use of non-specific drug therapy [for acute diarrhea] in children, and much information exists to the contrary."[75]

When older adults get diarrhea, they have a greater risk than younger adults of complications from the loss of fluid, sodium and potassium chloride, and other electrolytes. If you

---

ANTICHOLINERGIC EFFECTS

WARNING: SPECIAL MENTAL AND PHYSICAL ADVERSE EFFECTS

Older adults are especially sensitive to the harmful anticholinergic (see Glossary, p. 889) effects of this drug. Drugs in this family should not be used unless absolutely necessary.

Mental Effects: confusion, delirium, short-term memory problems, disorientation, and impaired attention.

Physical Effects: dry mouth, constipation, difficulty urinating (especially for a man with an enlarged prostate), blurred vision, decreased sweating with increased body temperature, sexual dysfunction, and worsening of glaucoma.

---

occasionally have short-term diarrhea, it is best to treat it without drugs using oral rehydration solution (see p. 532). If nondrug treatments do not control your diarrhea, ask your doctor if loperamide is appropriate for you.

If you use loperamide, do not take more than four 2-milligram capsules of loperamide per day (total of 8 milligrams).[76] The first dose should be two 2-milligram capsules, followed by one capsule after each episode of diarrhea until the maximum dose is reached. An overdose can depress your breathing severely and can cause coma, permanent brain damage, and sometimes death.

If you still have diarrhea after using loperamide for two days, or if you develop a fever, stop taking the drug and call your doctor.[76]

Before You Use This Drug

Do not use if you have or have had:

- allergic reaction to loperamide
- colitis that is severe
- diarrhea caused by antibiotics
- dysentery (bloody stools and fever)

Tell your doctor if you have or have had:

- condition in which constipation must be avoided
- dehydration
- infectious diarrhea
- liver problems

Tell your doctor about any other drugs you take, including aspirin, herbs, vitamins, and other nonprescription products.

When You Use This Drug

- Call your doctor immediately if diarrhea continues past two days or if you get a fever. To prevent severe constipation, stop taking this drug once your diarrhea stops.
- Call your doctor if you develop difficulty urinating.[77]
- Until you know how you react to this drug, do not drive or perform other activities requiring alertness. Loperamide may cause drowsiness.
- Have regular checkups if you use loperamide for a long time.

How to Use This Drug

- If you miss a dose, take it as soon as you remember, but skip it if it is almost time for the next dose. **Do not take double doses.**
- Do not share your medication with others.
- Take the drug at the same time(s) each day.
- Be sure you drink enough liquids.
- Store at room temperature with lid on tightly. Do not store in the bathroom. Do not expose to heat or direct light. Do not let the liquid form freeze. Keep out of reach of children.

Interactions with Other Drugs

Evaluations of Drug Interactions 2003 lists no drugs, biologics (e.g., vaccines, therapeutic antibodies), or foods as causing "highly clini-cally significant" or "clinically significant" interactions when used together with the drug in this section. We also found no interactions in the drug's FDA-approved professional package inserts. However, as the number of new drugs approved for marketing increases and as more experience is gained with these drugs over time, new interactions may be discovered.

Some other drugs that you may be taking (either over-the-counter or prescription drugs) can interact with this one, causing adverse effects. Ask your doctor what these drugs are and let him or her know if you are taking any of them.

Adverse Effects

Call your doctor immediately if you experience:

- appetite loss
- bloated feeling
- constipation
- nausea or vomiting
- skin rash
- stomach pain that is severe

Call your doctor if these symptoms continue:

- dizziness
- drowsiness
- dry mouth

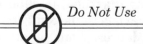

Do Not Use

ALTERNATIVE TREATMENT:
See Diarrhea, p. 532.

Diphenoxylate and Atropine
(dye fen *ox* i late and a *troe* peen)
LOMOTIL (Searle)

FAMILY: Diarrhea Drugs

This combination of diphenoxylate and atropine (see opposite page) is used to treat severe diarrhea. It should never replace rehydration, which is the primary treatment for diarrhea. **Because of serious adverse effects, we recommend that older adults not use this product.** The World Health Organization has warned against the drug's use in children.[74]

If you occasionally have short-term diarrhea, it is best to treat it without drugs using oral rehydration solution (see p. 532). If nondrug treatments do not control your diarrhea, see your doctor. The U.S. Centers for Disease Control and Prevention has concluded: "Little evidence exists to support the use of nonspecific drug therapy [for acute diarrhea] in children, and much information exists to the contrary."[75]

Diphenoxylate can depress your breathing, causing severe shortness of breath. An overdose can cause severe respiratory depression and coma, possibly leading to permanent brain damage or death.

Other Gastrointestinal Drugs

 Do Not Use

ALTERNATIVE TREATMENT:
*See Diarrhea, p. 532.
For spastic colon, see Psyllium and Methylcellulose, p. 566.*

Atropine (a *troe* peen)

Atropine, Hyoscyamine, Scopolamine, and Phenobarbital (a *troe* peen, hye oh *sye* a meen, scoe *pol* a meen, and fee noe *bar* bi tal)
DONNATAL (PBM)

Dicyclomine (dye *sye* kloe meen)
BENTYL (Axcan Scandipharm)

Hyoscyamine (hye oh *sye* a meen)
LEVSIN (Schwarz)
LEVBID (Schwarz)

FAMILY: Anticholinergics

Atropine, hyoscyamine, dicyclomine, and scopolamine are antispasmodic drugs that are used to relieve abdominal discomfort from cramping (spasms) and to control diarrhea. The use of these drugs as treatment for peptic ulcer disease has been replaced by more effective agents.[78] **All four have such severe adverse effects that older adults should not use them.** Even if you are taking only the usual adult dose, you may suffer from excitement, restlessness, drowsiness, or confusion.[79]

These drugs should never replace rehydration, which is the primary treatment for diarrhea. If you occasionally have short-term diarrhea, it is best to treat it without drugs using oral rehydration solution (see p. 532). If nondrug treatments do not control your diarrhea, see your doctor. The U.S. Centers for Disease Control and Prevention has concluded: "Little evidence exists to support the use of nonspecific

---

ANTICHOLINERGIC EFFECTS

WARNING: SPECIAL MENTAL AND PHYSICAL ADVERSE EFFECTS

Older adults are especially sensitive to the harmful anticholinergic (see Glossary, p. 889) effects of this drug. Drugs in this family should not be used unless absolutely necessary.

Mental Effects: confusion, delirium, short-term memory problems, disorientation, and impaired attention.

Physical Effects: dry mouth, constipation, difficulty urinating (especially for a man with an enlarged prostate), blurred vision, decreased sweating with increased body temperature, sexual dysfunction, and worsening of glaucoma.

One hazard of taking this drug continuously for longer than several weeks is drug-induced dependence to phenobarbital. **Do not stop taking the drug suddenly.** With the help of your doctor, work out a schedule for slowly lowering the amount of the drug you take by about 5 to 10% each day. Keep a written record of the dosage reduction schedule with you. These steps will make it much easier to become drug-free without developing distressing symptoms of drug withdrawal.

---

drug therapy [for acute diarrhea] in children, and much information exists to the contrary."[75]

The effective adult dose of dicyclomine is 160 milligrams per day, but older adults have unacceptably high rates of adverse reactions at this dose. However, there are no safety data from clinical trials longer than two weeks with doses over 80 milligrams.[80]

Donnatal is a particularly unacceptable drug, as it combines three antispasmodic drugs with a barbiturate, phenobarbital, a drug the World Health Organization has said older adults

---

The FDA has concluded that Donnatal lacks evidence of effectiveness.

---

should not take.[81] The only reason to take phenobarbital is for epilepsy, and in France this is the only use endorsed by the government.[82] You can easily become addicted to phenobarbital. If you stop taking it suddenly, you may suffer withdrawal symptoms such as anxiety, restlessness, muscle twitching, trembling hands, weakness, dizziness, vision problems, nausea, vomiting, trouble sleeping, faintness, and lightheadedness. Later, you may suffer more serious symptoms such as seizures and hallucinations. These may last for more than two weeks after you stop taking phenobarbital. The FDA has not classified Donnatal as "effective" for any indication;[83] such drugs are supposed to be removed from the market, but the FDA has failed to do so. **It is an irrational mixture of drugs that is dangerous for older adults to use.**[84]

 Do Not Use

ALTERNATIVE TREATMENT:
See Psyllium and Methylcellulose, p. 566.

Chlordiazepoxide and Clidinium
(klor dye az e *pox* ide and kli *di* nee um)
LIBRAX (Roche)

FAMILY: Anticholinergics
Benzodiazepines (see p. 223)

This combination of chlordiazepoxide (see p. 223) and clidinium is used to treat stomach and duodenal ulcers and colitis. It is said to relieve abdominal discomfort from cramping (spasms), reduce the amount of stomach acid, and relax the digestive system. However, **it is an irrational and ineffective mixture of drugs that older adults should not use.** In

ANTICHOLINERGIC EFFECTS

WARNING: SPECIAL MENTAL AND PHYSICAL ADVERSE EFFECTS

Older adults are especially sensitive to the harmful anticholinergic (see Glossary, p. 889) effects of clidinium. Drugs in this family should not be used unless absolutely necessary.

Mental Effects: confusion, delirium, short-term memory problems, disorientation, and impaired attention.

Physical Effects: dry mouth, constipation, difficulty urinating (especially for a man with an enlarged prostate), blurred vision, decreased sweating with increased body temperature, sexual dysfunction, and worsening of glaucoma.

One hazard of taking chlordiazepoxide continuously for longer than several weeks is drug dependence. **Do not stop taking your drug suddenly.** With the help of your doctor, work out a schedule for slowly lowering the amount of the drug you take by about 5 to 10% each day. Keep a written record of the dosage reduction schedule with you. These steps will make it much easier to become drug-free without developing distressing symptoms of drug withdrawal.

---

particular, the FDA has determined that this drug does not have evidence of effectiveness;[85] such drugs are supposed to be removed from the market, but the FDA has failed to do so.

One ingredient in this combination is clidinium, an antispasmodic drug. **Clidinium alone has such severe adverse effects that older adults should not use it** (see box above). Even if you are taking only the usual adult dose, you may suffer excitement, restlessness, drowsiness, or confusion.[79] Clidinium can also reduce the amount of saliva. Because saliva fights bacteria in the mouth, a decrease in the

---

The FDA has concluded that this drug lacks evidence of effectiveness.

---

amount of saliva leads to erosion of the gums and teeth, and later to dental or denture problems such as tooth decay.

The second ingredient in this combination, chlordiazepoxide, is a benzodiazepine tranquilizer. Because of this ingredient, this product is addictive. Withdrawal reactions include sweating, vomiting, tremor, abdominal pain, and seizures.

Chlordiazepoxide (sold by itself as LIBRIUM) belongs to a family of drugs called benzodiazepines (see p. 223) that can cause confusion, lack of muscle coordination leading to falls and hip fractures, and drowsiness in older adults. We believe that people 60 years of age and older should not use chlordiazepoxide. Other drugs in the benzodiazepine family are sometimes appropriate to treat anxiety or sleeping problems on a short-term basis, but, because they are addictive, they should be used only as a last resort. They should not be used to treat digestive problems.

If you are taking this combination of chlordiazepoxide and clidinium, ask your doctor to prescribe another drug. If you have used the drug continuously for several weeks or longer, ask for a dosing schedule that lowers your dose gradually.

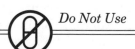 *Do Not Use*

ALTERNATIVE TREATMENT:
Reduce the causes of "excess gas" (see below).
See Gas, p. 533.

Simethicone (si *meth* i kone)
MYLICON (Johnson & Johnson/Merck)
PHAZYME (GlaxoSmithKline)

FAMILY: Antiflatulents (antigas)

Simethicone is marketed as a drug to reduce the amount of "excess gas" and the discomfort that it causes. **There is no convincing evidence that this drug, alone or combined with others, is effective for this purpose.**[16] Do not waste your money on products containing simethicone that claim to relieve "excess gas."

If you think that you suffer from "excess gas," it may be that you actually have a bloated feeling from overeating or discomfort from eating the wrong food. In this case, no antigas drug will help you because the problem has nothing to do with gas. If you do have excess gas in your stomach, the best way to treat it is to reduce the amount of air that you swallow. You can do this by cutting down on smoking, carbonated drinks, and gum chewing, which make you swallow air. A dry mouth (which may be due to anxiety or a drug you are taking) and badly fitting dentures also make you swallow more air.

Most gas in the large intestine is created when bacteria there come into contact with carbohydrates, especially those found in cabbage, broccoli, and beans.[16] This bacterial action is normal, as is the passing of gas (flatus). Different people pass different amounts of gas, and passing gas is no cause for medical concern. Simethicone is not recommended for the treatment of infant colic[86] because it is no more effective than a placebo.[15]

Sulfasalazine (sul fa *sal* a zeen)
AZULFIDINE (Pharmacia & Upjohn)

GENERIC: available
FAMILY: Anti-inflammatory Drugs

PREGNANCY WARNING

Sulfasalazine causes DNA damage in studies in rats and mice. Fetal exposure is possible, since the drug crosses the placenta. There is a potential for brain damage associated with jaundice. There is a case of severe depression of the granulocyte-producing bone marrow in an infant whose mother was taking both sulfasalazine and prednisone throughout pregnancy. Use during pregnancy only for clear medical reasons. Tell your doctor if you are pregnant or thinking of becoming pregnant before you take this drug.

BREAST-FEEDING WARNING

Sulfasalazine is excreted into breast milk and may cause hemolytic anemia in glucose-6-phosphate dehydrogenase–deficient infants as well as high bilirubin levels. Because of the potential for serious adverse effects in nursing infants, you should not take this drug while nursing.

Sulfasalazine is used to treat inflammatory bowel diseases. The two major diseases of this type are ulcerative colitis, which typically affects the colon, and Crohn's disease, which can occur anywhere in the intestine. Crohn's disease typically presents in young adulthood with weight loss, abdominal pain, anemia, and malnutrition. Ulcerative colitis typically occurs later in life. Both are associated with increased risk for colon cancer, although the risk is greater for ulcerative colitis. Sulfasalazine is also approved for the treatment of rheumatoid arthritis.

Because of the chronic nature of these conditions, sulfasalazine is usually taken for a long time. If your disease improves enough, you may be able to lower your dose to a maintenance level or even stop using the drug for periods of time. **If you have impaired kidney function, you may need to take less than the usual adult dose.** The drug should not be used in children under the age of two years.[87]

Before You Use This Drug
Do not use if you have or have had:

- gastrointestinal tract obstruction
- previous allergic reaction to sulfasalazine, sulfonamides, salicylates, furosemide, thiazide diuretics, sulfonylureas, or carbonic anhydrase inhibitors
- urinary obstruction

Tell your doctor if you have or have had:

- allergies that are severe
- asthma

- blood problems
- glucose-6-phosphate dehydrogenase deficiency
- kidney or liver problems
- porphyria
- stomach or intestinal blockage

Tell your doctor about any other drugs you take, including aspirin, herbs, vitamins, and other nonprescription products.

When You Use This Drug

- Check with your doctor to make certain your fluid intake is adequate and appropriate.
- Call your doctor if your symptoms (including diarrhea) do not improve in a month or two, or if they get worse. Schedule regular visits to your doctor to check your progress.
- Your skin or urine may turn orange-yellow in color. This is no cause for alarm.
- Take all the sulfasalazine your doctor prescribed, even if you begin to feel better. If you stop too soon, your symptoms could come back.
- Throw away outdated drugs.
- **Caution diabetics:** see p. 405.
- This drug makes you more sensitive to the sun. Stay out of the sun as much as possible, and call your doctor if you get a rash, hives, or any other skin reaction.
- You may need more folic acid than usual while taking sulfasalazine. Ask your doctor about how to get more folic acid in your diet.
- If you plan to have any surgery, including dental, tell your doctor that you take this drug.
- Have regular checkups to check on blood counts if you are on long-term therapy.
- Until you know how you react to this drug, do not drive or perform other activities requiring alertness.

How to Use This Drug

- If you miss a dose, take it as soon as you remember, but skip it if it is almost time for the next dose. **Do not take double doses.**

- Do not share your medication with others.
- Take the drug at the same time(s) each day.
- Take with **a full glass (eight ounces)** of water. Sulfasalazine can be taken right after meals or with food to lessen stomach upset.
- Swallow tablets whole.
- Take the full course of therapy.
- Store at room temperature with lid on tightly. Do not store in the bathroom. Do not expose to heat, moisture, or strong light. Do not let the liquid form freeze. Keep out of reach of children.

Interactions with Other Drugs

The following drugs, biologics (e.g., vaccines, therapeutic antibodies), or foods are listed in *Evaluations of Drug Interactions* 2003 as causing "highly clinically significant" or "clinically significant" interactions when used together with any of the drugs in this section. In some sections with multiple drugs, the interaction may have been reported for one but not all drugs in this section, but we include the interaction because the drugs in this section are similar to one another. We have also included potentially serious interactions listed in the drug's FDA-approved professional package insert or in published medical journal articles. There may be other drugs, especially those in the families of drugs listed below, that also will react with this drug to cause severe adverse effects. Make sure to tell your doctor and pharmacist the drugs you are taking and tell them if you are taking any of these interacting drugs:

digoxin, HIPREX, LANOXICAPS, LANOXIN, methenamine, potassium aminobenzoate, UREX.

Adverse Effects

Call your doctor immediately if you experience:

- appetite loss
- back, leg, or stomach pain

- bleeding or bruising that is unusual
- chest pain
- chills
- cough or difficulty breathing
- diarrhea, bloody
- eyes or skin yellow
- feeling of discomfort or illness
- fever
- fingernails, lips, or skin bluish
- headache
- itching or skin rash
- muscle or joint aches
- nausea or vomiting
- redness, blistering, peeling, or loosening of skin
- skin pale
- sore throat
- sun sensitivity
- swallowing difficulty
- tiredness or weakness that is unusual

Call your doctor if these symptoms continue:

- abdominal or stomach pain or upset
- appetite loss

- diarrhea
- nausea or vomiting

Periodic Tests

Ask your doctor which of these tests should be done periodically while you are taking this drug:

- complete blood count every two to three weeks for the first two to three months, then every three to six months.
- liver function test every two weeks for the first three months, then monthly for the second three months and then once every three months.
- proctoscopy and sigmoidoscopy
- urine tests

REFERENCES

1. Flynn CA. The evaluation and treatment of adults with gastro-esophageal reflux disease. *Journal of Family Practice* 2001; 50:57–63.

2. Over-the-counter omeprazole (prilosec OTC). *Medical Letter on Drugs and Therapeutics* 2003; 45:61–2.

3. Suerbaum S, Michetti P. *Helicobacter pylori* infection. *New England Journal of Medicine* 2002; 347:1175–86.

4. Thompson WG, Longstreth GF, Drossman DA, et al. Functional bowel disorders and functional abdominal pain. *Gut* 1999; 45(suppl 2):II43–7.

5. Gerson CD, Gerson MJ. A collaborative health care model for the treatment of irritable bowel syndrome. *Clinical Gastroenterology and Hepatology* 2003; 1:446–52.

6. Bohmer CJ, Taminiau JA, Klinkenberg-Knol EC, et al. The prevalence of constipation in institutionalized people with intellectual disability. *Journal of Intellectual Disability Research* 2001; 45:212–8.

7. Lembo A, Camilleri M. Chronic constipation. *New England Journal of Medicine* 2003; 349:1360–8.

8. Rubin GP. Childhood constipation. *American Family Physician* 2003; 67:1041–2.

9. Tytgat GN, Heading RC, Muller-Lissner S, et al. Contemporary understanding and management of reflux and constipation in the general population and pregnancy: A consensus meeting. *Alimentary Pharmacology and Therapeutics* 2003; 18:291–301.

10. Fine KD, Santa Ana CA, Fordtran JS. Diagnosis of magnesium-induced diarrhea. *New England Journal of Medicine* 1991; 324:1012–7.

11. Imhoff B, Morse D, Shiferaw B, et al. Burden of self-reported acute diarrheal illness in FoodNet surveillance areas, 1998–1999. *Clinical Infectious Diseases* 2004; 38(suppl 3):S219–26.

12. Mead PS, Slutsker L, Dietz V, et al. Food-related illness and death in the United States. *Emerging Infectious Diseases* 1999; 5:607–25.

13. *Training Manual for Treatment and Prevention of Childhood Diarrhea with Oral Rehydration Therapy, Proper Nutrition and Hygiene.* Columbia, Md.: International Child Health Foundation, 1992.

14. Simethicone for discomfort caused by gastrointestinal gas. *Medical Letter on Drugs and Therapeutics* 1975; 17:80.

15. Metcalf TJ, Irons TG, Sher LD, et al. Simethicone in the treatment of infant colic: A randomized, placebo-controlled, multicenter trial. *Pediatrics* 1994; 94:29–34.

16. Simethicone for gastrointestinal gas. *Medical Letter on Drugs and Therapeutics* 1996; 38:57–8.

17. *USP DI, Drug Information for the Health Care Professional.* Greenwood Village, Colo.: MICROMEDEX, 2003:194.

18. *USP DI, Drug Information for the Health Care Professional.* Greenwood Village, Colo.: MICROMEDEX, 2003:198.

19. *Physicians' Desk Reference for Nonprescription Drugs and Dietary Supplements.* 25th ed. Montvale, N.J.: Thompson PDR, 2004:700–1.

20. *USP DI, Drug Information for the Health Care Professional.* Greenwood Village, Colo.: MICROMEDEX, 2003:2461.

21. Karlstadt RG, Palmer RH. Unrecognized drug interactions with famotidine and nizatidine. *Archives of Internal Medicine* 1991; 151:810.

22. Vestal RE, ed. *Drug Treatment in the Elderly.* Sydney, Australia: ADIS Health Science Press, 1984:250.

23. *USP DI, Drug Information for the Health Care Professional.* Greenwood Village, Colo.: MICROMEDEX, 2003:1483.

24. Van Thiel DH, Gavaler JS, Smith WI Jr., et al. Hypothalamic-pituitary-gonadal dysfunction in men using cimetidine. *New England Journal of Medicine* 1979; 300:1012–5.

25. *USP DI, Drug Information for the Health Care Professional.* Greenwood Village, Colo.: MICROMEDEX, 2003:1485.

26. *USP DI, Drug Information for the Health Care Professional.* Greenwood Village, Colo.: MICROMEDEX, 2003:1486.

27. Lipsy RJ, Fennerty B, Fagan TC. Clinical review of histamine2 receptor antagonists. *Archives of Internal Medicine* 1990; 150:745–51.

28. According to University of Texas (Dallas) expert on drug toxicity Dr. Thomas L. Kurt, MD, MPH, cimetidine can interfere with the body's clearance of organophosphate pesticides because it inhibits the liver enzyme that breaks them down. As a result, there can be increased levels of pesticides in the body.

29. Fisher AA, Le Couteur DG. Nephrotoxicity and hepatotoxicity of histamine H2 receptor antagonists. *Drug Safety* 2001; 24:39–57.

30. Stedman CA, Barclay ML. Comparison of the pharmacokinetics, acid suppression and efficacy of proton pump inhibitors [review article]. *Alimentary Pharmacology and Therapeutics* 2000; 14:963–78.

31. *Cecil Textbook of Medicine.* 21st ed. Philadelphia: W. B. Saunders Company, 2000:684–5.

32. Laine L, Ahnen D, McClain C, et al. Potential gastrointestinal effects of long-term acid suppression with proton pump inhibitors [review article]. *Alimentary Pharmacology and Therapeutics* 2000; 14:651–68.

33. Reilly JP. Safety profile of the proton-pump inhibitors. *American Journal of Health-System Pharmacy* 1999; 56:S11–7.

34. Gillen D, Wirz AA, Ardill JE, et al. Rebound hypersecretion after omeprazole and its relation to on-treatment acid suppression and *Helicobacter pylori* status. *Gastroenterology* 1999; 116:239–47.

35. Gillen D, McColl KE. Problems associated with the clinical use of proton pump inhibitors. *Pharmacology and Toxicology* 2001; 89:281–6.

36. Kuipers EJ, Meuwissen SG. The efficacy and safety of long-term omeprazole treatment for gastroesophageal reflux disease. *Gastroenterology* 2000; 118:795–8.

37. Langman MJ. Omeprazole. *British Medical Journal* 1991; 303:481–2.

38. Lind T, Cederberg C, Olausson M, et al. Omeprazole in elderly duodenal ulcer patients: Relationship between reduction in gastric acid secretion and fasting plasma gastrin. *European Journal of Clinical Pharmacology* 1991; 40:557–60.

39. FDA Medical Officer Review of Esomeprazole, September 21, 2000:171–4.

40. *Physicians' Desk Reference.* 58th ed. Montvale, N.J.: Thomson PDR, 2004:2903.

41. Rubin W. Medical treatment of peptic ulcer disease. *Medical Clinics of North America* 1991; 75:981–98.

42. Gabriel SE. Is misoprostol prophylaxis indicated for NSAID induced adverse gastrointestinal events? An epidemiologic opinion. *Journal of Rheumatology* 1991; 18:958–61.

43. Kornbluth A, Gupta R, Gerson CD. Life-threatening diarrhea after short-term misoprostol use in a patient with Crohn ileocolitis. *Annals of Internal Medicine* 1990; 113:474–5.

44. Morton MR, Robbins ME. Delirium in an elderly woman possibly associated with administration of misoprostol. *DICP, The Annals of Pharmacotherapy* 1991; 25:133–4.

45. Fossaluzza V, Di Benedetto P, Zampa A, et al. Misoprostol-

induced urinary incontinence. *Journal of Internal Medicine* 1991; 230:463–4.

46. Laheij RJ, Rossum LG, Jansen JB, et al. Evaluation of treatment regimens to cure *Helicobacter pylori* infection—a meta-analysis. *Alimentary Pharmacology and Therapeutics* 1999; 13:857–64.

47. *Physicians' Desk Reference*. 58th ed. Montvale, N.J.: Thomson PDR, 2004:1564.

48. Barbehenn E, Lurie P, Wolfe SM. Alosetron for irritable bowel syndrome. *The Lancet* 2000; 356:2009–10.

49. Barbehenn E, Lurie P, Sasich L, Wolfe SM. Petition to the Food and Drug Administration to remove Lotronex from the market (Health Research Group Publication #1533), August 31, 2000. Available at: http://www.citizen.org/publications/release.cfm?ID=6734.

50. Moynihan R. Alosetron: A case study in regulatory capture, or a victory for patients' rights? *British Medical Journal* 2002; 325:592–5.

51. Barbehenn E, Lurie P, Wolfe SM. Letter to the FDA concerning a memo from their Office of Post-marketing Drug Risk Assessment (OPDRA) on the dangers of Lotronex (Health Research Group Publication #1566), April 18, 2001. Available at: http://www.citizen.org/publications/release.cfm?ID=6767&secID=1667&catID=126.

52. Wolfe SM. Testimony before FDA's Drug Safety Advisory Committee Hearing Concerning Alosetron (Health Research Group Publication #1697), May 5, 2004. Available at: http://www.citizen.org/publications/release.cfm?ID=7314.

53. Barbehenn E, Lurie P, Wolfe SM. Letter to the Food and Drug Administration urging that it not approve tegaserod (Health Research Group Publication #1561), March 22, 2001. Available at: http://www.citizen.org/publications/release.cfm?ID=6764.

54. Bach T, Syversveen T, Kvingedal AM, et al. 5HT4(a) and 5-HT4(b) receptors have nearly identical pharmacology and are both expressed in human atrium and ventricle. *Naunyn-Schmiedeberg's Archives of Pharmacology* 2001; 363:146–60.

55. Food and Drug Administration. Questions and Answers on Zelnorm (tegaserod maleate), April 28, 2004. Available at: http://www.fda.gov/cder/drug/infopage/zelnorm/zelnorm_QA.htm.

56. Fong NL. Chemotherapy and Nutritional Management. In *Nutritional Management of the Cancer Patient*. New York: Raven Press, 1979.

57. Hardman JG, Limbird LE, Gilman AG, eds. *The Pharmacological Basis of Therapeutics*. New York: McGraw-Hill, 2001:500.

58. Lata PF, Pigarelli DL. Chronic metoclopramide therapy for diabetic gastroparesis. *Annals of Pharmacotherapy* 2003; 37:122–6.

59. Drugs for relief of nausea and vomiting. *Medical Letter on Drugs and Therapeutics* 1974; 16:46–8.

60. AMA Department of Drugs. *AMA Drug Evaluations*. Chicago: American Medical Association, 1974:594.

61. *USP DI, Drug Information for the Health Care Professional*. Greenwood Village, Colo.: MICROMEDEX, 2003:2658.

62. Hamilton JW, Wagner J, Burdick BB, et al. Clinical evaluation of methylcellulose as a bulk laxative. *Digestive Diseases and Sciences* 1988; 33:993–8.

63. Zumarraga L, Levitt MD, Suarez F. Absence of gaseous symptoms during ingestion of commercial fibre preparations. *Alimentary Pharmacology and Therapeutics* 1997; 11:1067–72.

64. Levin EG, Miller VT, Muesing RA, et al. Comparison of psyllium hydrophilic mucilloid and cellulose as adjuncts to a prudent diet in the treatment of mild to moderate hypercholesterolemia. *Archives of Internal Medicine* 1990; 150:1822–7.

65. Khalili B, Bardana EJ Jr., Yunginger JW. Psyllium-associated anaphylaxis and death: A case report and review of the literature. *Annals of Allergy Asthma & Immunology* 2003; 91:579–84.

66. *Drug Facts and Comparisons*. St. Louis, Mo.: Wolters Kluwer Health, Inc., 2000:1166.

67. *USP DI, Drug Information for the Health Care Professional*. Greenwood Village, Colo.: MICROMEDEX, 2003:1662.

68. Blei AT, Cordoba J. Hepatic Encephalopathy. *American Journal of Gastroenterology* 2001; 96:1968–76.

69. Clausen MR, Jorgensen J, Mortensen PB. Comparison of diarrhea induced by ingestion of fructooligosaccharide Idolax and disaccharide lactulose: Role of osmolarity versus fermentation of malabsorbed carbohydrate. *Digestive Diseases and Sciences* 1998; 43:2696–707.

70. Cheetham MJ, Cohen CR, Kamm MA, et al. A randomized, controlled trial of diathermy hemorrhoidectomy vs. stapled hemorrhoidectomy in an intended day-care setting with longer-term follow-up. *Diseases of the Colon and Rectum* 2003; 46:491–7.

71. *Physicians' Desk Reference*. 58th ed. Montvale, N.J.: Thomson PDR, 2004:962.

72. Goodman RA, Riley TR III. Lactulose-induced pneumatosis intestinalis and pneumoperitoneum. *Digestive Diseases and Sciences* 2001; 46:2549–53.

73. Xing JH, Soffer EE. Adverse effects of laxatives. *Diseases of the Colon and Rectum* 2001; 44:1201–9.

74. *The Rational Use of Drugs in the Management of Acute Diarrhea in Children*. Geneva: World Health Organization, 1990.

75. Duggan C, Santosham M, Glass RI. The management of acute diarrhea in children: Oral rehydration, maintenance, and nutritional therapy. Centers for Disease Control and Prevention. *MMWR Recommendations and Reports* 1992; 41:1–20.

76. *USP DI, Drug Information for the Health Care Professional*. Greenwood Village, Colo.: MICROMEDEX, 2003:1760.

77. Urinary retention with loperamide. *Prescrire International* 2002; 11:50.

78. *USP DI, Drug Information for the Health Care Professional*. Greenwood Village, Colo.: MICROMEDEX, 2003:225.

79. *USP DI, Drug Information for the Health Care Professional*. Greenwood Village, Colo.: MICROMEDEX, 2003:228.

80. *Physicians' Desk Reference*. 52nd ed. Montvale, N.J.: Medical Economics Company, 1998:1199.

81. *Drugs for the Elderly*. 2nd ed. Copenhagen: World Health Organization, 1997:29.

82. Phenobarbital for mild sedation: Market withdrawal. *Prescrire International* 2001; 10:120.

83. *Physicians' Desk Reference*. 52nd ed. Montvale, N.J.: Medical Economics Company, 1998:2414.

84. AMA Department of Drugs. *AMA Drug Evaluations*. Chicago: American Medical Association, 1974:594.

85. *Physicians' Desk Reference*. 52nd ed. Montvale, N.J.: Medical Economics Company, 1998:2521.

86. *USP DI, Drug Information for the Health Care Professional*. Greenwood Village, Colo.: MICROMEDEX, 2003:2461.

87. *USP DI, Drug Information for the Health Care Professional*. Greenwood Village, Colo.: MICROMEDEX, 2003:2484.

18

DRUGS FOR OSTEOPOROSIS

Estrogens are no longer approved by the FDA for the treatment of osteoporosis. The FDA now requires a statement in the professional product labeling for estrogens that estrogen therapy for the prevention of osteoporosis should only be considered for women at significant risk of osteoporosis and that nonestrogen medications should be carefully considered.

Osteoporosis is a reduction in bone mass and weakening of bone architecture that increases the susceptibility of bone to fracture. Bone is a living tissue that is constantly being broken down and resynthesized at 1 to 2 million microscopic sites in the adult skeleton. Osteoporosis occurs when the rate of breakdown is faster than the rate of resynthesis.[1]

Osteoporosis occurs in both sexes but is more frequent in women after menopause. One measure of susceptibility to fracture is bone mineral density (BMD), which is measured by X-ray absorption. The results are given (for women) in terms of the decrease in density from that of the average 35-year-old. The decrease in BMD and its relation to fracture applies to the whole population of women and does not tell whether an individual will have a fracture, only that they are in a population of higher risk.

It is important to realize that BMD is only one of many risk factors for fracture: others include "smoking, early menopause, lack of physical exercise, especially weight-bearing exercise, family history, personal history of fracture, a tendency to fall, and alcohol abuse" as well as glucocorticoid use.[2] On the other hand, physical activity increases bone mass, density, and strength and can improve balance and coordination even in old, frail people.[3]

The site of fracture is important in terms of consequences: hip fractures cause more severe and long-term problems than those of arms, back (vertebral), or wrist, yet the drugs available have greater effectiveness at these latter sites. The patient needs to take into account the drug's risks, as described in the drug profiles below, along with a possible benefit. This is especially true for vertebral fractures that are often used to measure the efficacy of a drug yet are frequently unaccompanied by any symptoms.

The history of the treatment or prevention of osteoporosis is strewn with drugs such as estrogens—discussed below—and others in this chapter with marginal effectiveness or with risks clearly outweighing the benefits.

THE GREAT FAILED HORMONE REPLACEMENT EXPERIMENT

For the last several decades, much attention in the osteoporosis field has been lavished on the acclaimed ability of hormone replacement therapy (HRT) to prevent osteoporosis. In 1991, Public Citizen's Health Research Group wrote, "Female replacement hormones may someday be remembered as the most recklessly prescribed and dangerous drugs of this century."[4] In 2002, the results of the Women's Health Initiative (WHI), a large, long-term, clinical trial sponsored by the National Institutes of Health, finally confirmed that the risks of hormone replacement therapy (HRT) outweighed its benefits.[5]

The WHI trial enrolled 27,000 healthy postmenopausal women between 1993 and 1998 with the goal of seeing whether HRT would help prevent heart disease and hip fractures. The trial was divided into two parts: 11,000 women with a previous hysterectomy were randomized to get either estrogen alone or a placebo; 16,600 women were randomized to get estrogen plus medroxyprogesterone (or a commercially available combination of the two with the brand name Prempro) or a placebo. The trial was originally scheduled to conclude in 2005, but both parts were stopped early because of the increase in serious adverse events.

In the estrogen plus medroxyprogesterone arm, the main reason for stopping the trial early was an increased risk of invasive breast cancer in women receiving HRT, as opposed to those on placebo. This risk, combined with an increase in adverse cardiovascular events, such as increased coronary heart disease, stroke, and pulmonary embolism that began in the first year of HRT treatment, outweighed the benefit of an increase in BMD and a decrease in hip fractures. A later analysis of the WHI study found that there was no benefit with HRT even in the subgroup of women considered to be at high risk of fracture.[6]

In the estrogen-alone part of the trial (in women who had had a hysterectomy and thus were not at risk for uterine cancer, which can be caused by estrogen), the main reason for stopping was the lack of an effect on heart disease (either increase or decrease), the major question being evaluated. The increased risk of stroke outweighed the benefit of a decrease in hip fracture risk.[7] Thus, neither estrogen alone nor estrogen combined with progesterone is now recommended for prevention of osteoporosis.

A SAFER APPROACH: EXERCISE, CALCIUM, AND VITAMIN D SUPPLEMENTATION

The mainstays for decreasing the risk of postmenopausal osteoporosis are weight-bearing exercise and adequate calcium and vitamin D intake. Regular exercise, particularly weight bearing, is most protective and can be as simple as daily walking and climbing stairs. On average, postmenopausal women require 1,500 milligrams per day of elemental calcium. Vitamin D supplementation of 400 to 800 international units (IU) per day may also be required to ensure adequate daily intake in postmenopausal women. Calcium and vitamin D are discussed in greater detail in Chapter 27, Vitamins and Minerals.

Some of the best sources of calcium are dietary. The following table lists the elemental calcium content, in milligrams, of some common foods.[8]

CALCIUM CONTENT OF SOME FOODS

Food	Serving Size	Calcium Content (milligrams)
Milk, skim	1 cup	302
Yogurt (low-fat, fruit-flavored)	8 ounces	300
Gruyere cheese	1 ounce	287
Swiss cheese	1 ounce	272
Figs, dried	10 figs	269
Tofu, raw, firm	½ cup	258
Calcium-fortified cereals	¾ cup	250
Cheddar cheese	1 ounce	204
Calcium-fortified orange juice	6 ounces	200
Mozzarella cheese, part-skim	1 ounce	183
Collards, cooked from frozen, chopped	½ cup	179
American cheese, processed	1 ounce	174
Black strap molasses	1 tablespoon	172
Creamed cottage cheese	1 cup	126
Sardines, canned in oil	2 sardines	92
Parmesan cheese, grated	1 tablespoon	69
Mustard greens	½ cup	52
Kale, boiled	½ cup	47
Broccoli, boiled	½ cup	36

DRUG PROFILES

Bisphosphonates

Limited Use

Alendronate (a *len* dro nate)
FOSAMAX (Merck)

Do Not Use Until Seven Years After Release

Risedronate (ris *ed* roe nate)
(Do Not Use Until 2007)
ACTONEL (Procter & Gamble)

GENERIC: not available
FAMILY: Bisphosphonates

PREGNANCY WARNING

The bisphosphonates caused fetal harm in animal studies, including interference with bone formation. Because of the potential for serious adverse effects to the fetus, these drugs should not be used by pregnant women.

BREAST-FEEDING WARNING

No data are available about the excretion of bisphosphonates in milk. However, since bisphosphonates interfere with bone formation and remain in bones for an extremely long time (years), you should not nurse while taking these drugs.

Bisphosphonates for Osteoporosis and Paget's Disease

Bisphosphonates are approved to treat osteoporosis in both men and postmenopausal women, in osteoporosis caused by corticosteroids (but they should not be used for this purpose; see boxes), and Paget's disease. For

THE HEALTH RESEARCH GROUP'S SEVEN-YEAR RULE

You should wait at least seven years from the date of marketing to take any new drug unless it is one of those rare "breakthrough" drugs that offers you a documented therapeutic advantage over older proven drugs. New drugs are tested in a relatively small number of people before being approved, and serious adverse effects or life-threatening drug interactions may not be detected until the new drug has been taken by hundreds of thousands of people. A number of new drugs have been withdrawn within the first seven years after approval. Also, serious new adverse reaction warnings have been added to the labeling of a number of drugs, or new drug interactions have been detected, often within a drug's first seven years on the market.

DO NOT USE

ALENDRONATE AND RISEDRONATE FOR THE TREATMENT OF GLUCOCORTICOID (STEROID)-INDUCED OSTEOPOROSIS

Each year, millions of people are prescribed steroids such as prednisone, prednisolone, or other similar anti-inflammatory steroids for treatment of autoimmune diseases such as lupus, rheumatoid arthritis, asthma, ulcerative colitis, muscle disorders, skin conditions, or other diseases. When the use of these drugs exceeds a very short period of time, osteoporosis can result, because these steroids inhibit the formation of new bone. The way, or mechanism, by which this happens is very different from the mechanism whereby postmenopausal osteoporosis occurs.[9]

Despite this important difference, Merck, seeking to significantly increase its market for this drug, conducted studies to see if alendronate, previously approved for postmenopausal osteoporosis, could also be approved for preventing steroid-induced osteoporosis. The fact that the FDA, unfortunately, approved this new use almost five years ago represents a triumph of Merck pressure, with complicity by top FDA officials, over medical evidence and against the recommendation for nonapproval by the FDA physician primarily responsible for reviewing the studies concerning this new indication.[10]

Alendronate improved bone mineral density (BMD) in the spine, although not as much as it does in postmenopausal osteoporosis, and reduced the occurrence of vertebral fractures. Although there was a reduction in vertebral fractures, there was a barely measurable improvement in total height (stature) of only 1.5 millimeters (less than one-sixteenth of an inch.[10] Most disturbingly, it actually *increased* the total incidence of nonvertebral fractures, such as those of the foot, pelvis, ankle, and hip.[9] The FDA medical officer who opposed this approval correctly described these latter, nonvertebral fractures as more serious, more painful, and more incapacitating than vertebral fractures.[9] Other problems identified in the review included the fact that alendronate causes esophageal ulcers and irritation and, compared to a placebo, increases the risk of abdominal pain. The FDA medical officer concluded, in recommending against approval, that the drug represents "very small returns for the inconvenience and the costs and risks of taking this drug."[11]

women at risk of developing osteoporosis, alendronate and risedronate are also approved to prevent osteoporosis.

Alendronate and risedronate belong to a class of drugs called bisphosphonates, which act on bone. They inhibit activity of the bone cells that resorb bone, and because resorption and synthesis are linked, they decrease bone turnover (synthesis and breakdown). Osteoporosis can develop in the elderly as well as in people who take corticosteroids such as prednisone (DELTASONE) or prednisolone (METICORTEN) for extended periods of time for conditions such as asthma, skin disorders, or arthritis.

Clinical Data (Alendronate)

Alendronate has been shown to reduce the risk of hip fracture by 1% in women who had previously experienced at least one vertebral fracture (2% of women on placebo had hip fractures versus 1% of women on alendronate, a 50% relative reduction). We are still waiting for the results of a study evaluating the effects of alendronate on hip fracture in postmenopausal women who have never experienced a vertebral fracture. Most women who took the placebo (over 85%) in the three-year clinical trials did not have a fracture of any

---

WHAT YOU CAN DO TO PREVENT OSTEOPOROSIS

DIET AND EXERCISE

Many women are not at risk of developing hip or other types of fractures. Women who are thin or small-boned, particularly if they are Asian or white, and women who drink more than two alcoholic drinks per day are at higher risk of osteoporosis. Black women, heavy women, and women who get lots of exercise are at a lower risk. There are steps women can take to prevent osteoporosis; for instance, a lot of calcium in the diet from early adulthood and weight-bearing exercise such as jogging, walking, tennis, and bicycling. You should be receiving from 800 to 1,200 milligrams of calcium per day in your diet, depending on your age. Women who are postmenopausal require an average of 1,500 milligrams per day of calcium (see calcium table, p. 584). These two steps (diet and exercise) are enough to prevent osteoporosis in many adults.

THINGS YOU CAN DO TO PREVENT FALLS

Falls, of course, will increase your chances of a fracture. Ask your doctor to review your continued need for and dose of any drug that causes you to be dizzy or drowsy. Check p. 33 for drugs that can cause falls. Check your home for situations that can lead to falls such as areas that are not well lit or loose rugs on hardwood floors.

(2) those who had been on 5 milligrams per day for 10 years, and (3) those who had been on 10 milligrams per day for 10 years. The main study endpoint was bone mineral density (BMD) at the lumbar spine, not fractures.[12]

Although there were increases in BMD with increasing dose, this increase was not related to fracture rate: the 5 milligram group had eight times the increase in BMD of the spine of the discontinued group but twice the number of new vertebral fractures. Women who had discontinued the drug for five years had about the same number of fractures as those taking 10 milligrams for five years. (New "fractures" were defined by examining radiographs and measuring loss of height of the vertebrae.) As noted in the drug profile for raloxifene, BMD and fracture reduction are not clearly related (see p. 589); that appears here as well. Yet, women are often treated based on BMD alone.

Questions raised in an accompanying commentary to the 10-year trial include worries about what happens to bone structure with continuing increases in BMD, since there is evidence from animal studies that with time, bones become more brittle and susceptible to fracture. Unfortunately, at what point that occurs in people is unknown. Thus, it is unknown how long women should stay on alendronate as well as how long benefits might last after the drug is stopped.[13]

Clinical Data (Risedronate)

Risedronate, like alendronate, is associated with a modestly favorable effect on the risk for vertebral fracture, a type of spinal fracture that may or may not be symptomatic. The absolute reduction in the risk of a new vertebral fracture in women taking risedronate is 5% compared to women taking an inactive placebo. The most benefit was seen in women with two or more vertebral fractures before they started taking risedronate.[14]

type. Fewer studies have been done on men taking alendronate.

A recent update on alendronate use for up to 10 years has left many questions unanswered. Three groups of postmenopausal women were studied: (1) those who had been on alendronate for 5 years and been discontinued for 5 years,

A published study sponsored by Procter & Gamble, the maker of risedronate, suggests that risedronate may reduce the risk of hip fracture, the most serious consequence of osteoporosis, in elderly women with low bone mineral density by about 1% (the same result as alendronate).[15] However, this study has been criticized on a number of grounds, including the fact that follow-up information was not available for 3,324 of the 9,331 women in the study.[16] This could have biased the results in favor of risedronate by leaving out women who had fractures.

Risedronate is retained in bones for many years, but long-term effects are still not known. Concern exists because some bisphosphonates increase the occurrence of spontaneous fractures in animals.[17]

Common Problems When Taking Bisphosphonates

Since bisphosphonates can irritate the esophagus (the tube that connects the mouth and stomach), causing ulcers and bleeding, they must be taken with water on an empty stomach. Stay upright for at least half an hour to ensure that the tablet does not get stuck in your esophagus before reaching the stomach. You should not eat or drink anything but water during this half hour to get the maximum absorption of the drug.

Common adverse effects include stomach pain, nausea, indigestion, constipation, and diarrhea.[18] Rare adverse effects include changes in vision.[19] Bisphosphonates are retained in bones for many years, even after patients stop taking them.[20,21] Uncertainty exists as to when therapy should begin and how long it should continue, as well as the impact on nonspinal fractures for those with low risk.[22]

Bisphosphonates are not to be used by people with mild osteoporosis, with severe kidney problems, or in women before menopause. It should not be given to people with dementia or who are otherwise unable to follow the instructions on how to take the medication. Bisphosphonates should not be used in pregnant or breast-feeding women. Safety and effectiveness is not known in children under the age of 18 years.

For use in Paget's disease, alendronate is given daily for six months. If a relapse occurs, alendronate is sometimes resumed; risedronate is given for two months and repeated if necessary.

Before You Use This Drug

Do not use if you have or have had:

- frequent heartburn
- reflux disease
- hiatal hernia
- throat problems
- difficulty swallowing
- ulcers
- kidney problems
- sensitivity to alendronate or risedronate
- pregnancy or are breast-feeding
- low calcium levels or vitamin D deficiency
- inability to sit or stand for 30 minutes

Tell your doctor if you have or have had:

- allergies
- Crohn's disease

Tell your doctor about any other drugs you take, including aspirin, herbs, vitamins, and other nonprescription products.

When You Use This Drug

- Get regular, preferably weight-bearing exercise, such as bicycling, jogging, tennis, or walking.
- Eat a diet adequate in calcium. You may need to take a calcium supplement. If you do not live in a sunny climate, you may need to take vi-

tamin D, particularly during the winter or if you do not go outdoors.

• Prevent falls by using handrails on stairs, adequate lighting, and avoiding throw rugs and electric cords in your path. Use proper lifting techniques.

• Avoid alcohol and sedatives, which increase the risk of falls and fractures.

• Stop smoking, which increases the risk of osteoporosis.

• If a relative or friend takes alendronate at an institution, check that the timing and method for taking alendronate (as described below) is correct and followed closely.

How to Use This Drug

• On arising or soon after, sit or stand, then swallow tablet with a full six- to eight-ounce glass of plain water. Do not chew or suck on tablets. Take on an empty stomach. Wait at least 30 minutes before taking any food, beverage (including mineral water, coffee, tea, or orange juice), or medication. Do not take any other medications or dietary supplements during this time.

• Stay upright, standing or sitting, for at least 30 minutes after a dose of alendronate.

• If you miss a daily dose, skip it. If you miss a weekly dose, take it the morning after you remember. **Do not take double doses.**

• Do not take at bedtime or before getting up for the day.

• Wait at least one-half hour after taking alendronate before taking any calcium supplement. A good practice is to take calcium with the evening meal.

• Do not share your medication with others.

• Take the drug at the same time(s) each day.

• Store tablets at room temperature with lid on tightly. Do not store in the bathroom. Do not expose to heat, moisture, or strong light. Keep out of reach of children.

Interactions with Other Drugs

The following drugs, biologics (e.g., vaccines, therapeutic antibodies), or foods are listed in *Evaluations of Drug Interactions* 2003 as causing "highly clinically significant" or "clinically significant" interactions when used together with any of the drugs in this section. In some sections with multiple drugs, the interaction may have been reported for one but not all drugs in this section, but we include the interaction because the drugs in this section are similar to one another. We have also included potentially serious interactions listed in the drug's FDA-approved professional package insert or in published medical journal articles. There may be other drugs, especially those in the families of drugs listed below, that also will react with this drug to cause severe adverse effects. Make sure to tell your doctor and pharmacist the drugs you are taking and tell them if you are taking any of these interacting drugs:

antacids, calcium supplements, iron supplements, NAPROSYN, naproxen, sodium bicarbonate, TUMS, zinc carbonate, zinc sulfate.

Be especially careful of taking aspirin- and salicylate-containing products. Beware that aspirin is one of the ingredients in many combination drug products and may increase adverse reactions. Read your drug labels and/or ask your pharmacist. Examples include: aspirin, ECOTRIN, EMPIRIN.

Adverse Effects

Call your doctor immediately if you experience:

• abdominal pain
• abnormal bleeding
• heartburn
• nausea or vomiting
• muscle pain

- skin rash
- swallowing difficulty
- throat irritated or painful

Call your doctor if these symptoms continue:

- abdomen feels full or bloated
- constipation
- diarrhea
- gas
- headache
- nausea
- tastes altered
- vision changes

Signs of overdose:

- upset stomach
- heartburn
- esophagitis
- gastritis
- ulcer

If you suspect an overdose, call this number to contact your poison control center: (800) 222-1222.

Periodic Tests

Ask your doctor which of these tests should be done periodically while you are taking this drug:

- bone mineral density
- alkaline phosphatase level in serum
- calcium and creatinine serum levels
- urinary hydroxyproline
- urinary collagen (N-telopeptide, type 1)

Selective Estrogen Receptor Modulators (SERMs)

Do Not Use Until Seven Years After Release

Raloxifene (ra *lox* i feen)
(Do Not Use Until 2006)
EVISTA (Lilly)

GENERIC: not available

FAMILY: Selective Estrogen Receptor Modulators (SERMs)

PREGNANCY WARNING

Raloxifene caused delayed or abnormal development and/or death in the young of animals exposed to it during pregnancy. If you are pregnant or thinking of becoming pregnant, you should not take raloxifene because of the potential danger to the fetus.

BREAST-FEEDING WARNING

It is likely that this drug, like many others, is excreted in human milk, and because of the potential for adverse effects in nursing infants, you should not take this drug while nursing.

Raloxifene is approved for the prevention and treatment of osteoporosis in women past menopause. It belongs to the family of drugs known as selective estrogen receptor modulators (SERMs), which act like estrogen in bone and some other tissues but antagonize estrogen in reproductive tissues.[26] Whether this is important in terms of long-term adverse effects is unknown.

In a three-year treatment study in postmenopausal women, raloxifene increased bone mineral density of the lumbar spine and hip (the only two sites measured). However, of these two sites, raloxifene decreased the risk of frac-

THE HEALTH RESEARCH GROUP'S SEVEN-YEAR RULE

You should wait at least seven years from the date of marketing to take any new drug unless it is one of those rare "breakthrough" drugs that offer you a documented therapeutic advantage over older proven drugs. New drugs are tested in a relatively small number of people before being approved, and serious adverse effects or life-threatening drug interactions may not be detected until the new drug has been taken by hundreds of thousands of people. A number of new drugs have been withdrawn within the first seven years after approval. Also, serious new adverse reaction warnings have been added to the labeling of a number of drugs, or new drug interactions have been detected, often within a drug's first seven years on the market.

WARNING: BLOOD CLOTS[23-25]

The benefits of raloxifene are offset by the serious adverse effect of increased risk of venous thromboembolic events, or blood clots that form in the veins and may break off and travel to the lungs. The 2.5-fold increase in the risk for blood clots in women treated with raloxifene was similar to that reported for women on hormone replacement therapy. Women with a history of blood clots in their veins should not use raloxifene.

tures only in the spine. Indeed, the authors state that, as in previous studies, "the effect of fracture reduction is not clearly related to the increase in bone mineral density."[27] Of 12 kinds of nonspinal fractures tracked in this study, only ankle fractures were statistically reduced (1.1% versus 0.7%, a difference of only 0.4%). There was no reduction in the incidence of fractures of the hip, the site of most importance.[23,25,28]

Raloxifene had the most effect on the risk of spinal fracture. For the group of patients without a history of spinal fractures, the incidence of new spinal fractures, as detected by X-ray, was reduced by 2.4% (spinal fractures occurred in 4.3% of placebo patients and 1.9% of raloxifene-treated patients) for a relative risk reduction of 55%, the number most often seen in descriptions of this study. In the group of patients who had had a previous spinal fracture, there was a 6% reduction in spinal fractures as detected by X-ray: 20% in the placebo group and 14% in the raloxifene-treated group.[29]

The group of patients most in need of treatment were those who had had a painful spinal fracture (not just one found on X-ray). Here the difference between treated and untreated was only 1.3% (3.1% of placebo patients and 1.8% of raloxifene-treated had new painful spinal fractures over three years).[29]

Commonly reported adverse effects of raloxifene included hot flashes and leg cramps. Hot flashes are especially common in women near menopause, and raloxifene increases their incidence. Other adverse effects included flu symptoms, peripheral edema, fluid in the endometrial cavity, and high blood sugar. Raloxifene should not be taken by women until after menopause. Safety and effectiveness have not been studied in men or children. Long-term effects of raloxifene, such as safety for more than two years or effects on the pituitary gland, are unknown.

When raloxifene is compared to other drugs used for osteoporosis, the bisphosphonates are more effective both in increasing bone mineral density and reducing the risk of fractures.

Before You Use This Drug

Do not use if you have or have had:

- deep vein thrombosis
- pulmonary embolism
- retinal vein thrombosis

WHAT YOU CAN DO TO PREVENT OSTEOPOROSIS

DIET AND EXERCISE

Many women are not at risk of developing hip or other types of fractures. Women who are thin or small-boned, particularly if they are Asian or white, and women who drink more than two alcoholic drinks per day are at higher risk of osteoporosis. Black women, heavy women, and women who get lots of exercise are at a lower risk. There are steps women can take to prevent osteoporosis; for instance, a lot of calcium in the diet from early adulthood and weight-bearing exercise such as jogging, walking, tennis, and bicycling. You should be receiving from 800 to 1,200 milligrams of calcium per day in your diet, depending on your age. Women who are postmenopausal require an average of 1,500 milligrams per day of calcium (see calcium table, p. 584). These two steps (diet and exercise) are enough to prevent osteoporosis in many adults.

THINGS YOU CAN DO TO PREVENT FALLS

Falls, of course, will increase your chances of a fracture. Ask your doctor to review your continued need for and dose of any drug that causes you to be dizzy or drowsy. Check p. 33 for drugs that can cause falls. Check your home for situations that can lead to falls such as areas that are not well lit or loose rugs on hardwood floors.

Tell your doctor if you have or have had:

- allergies
- cancer
- congestive heart failure
- diabetes[25]
- liver problems, such as cirrhosis
- pregnancy or are breast-feeding

Tell your doctor about any other drugs you take, including aspirin, herbs, vitamins, and other nonprescription products.

When You Use This Drug

- Get regular, preferably weight-bearing exercise, such as bicycling, jogging, tennis, or walking.
- Eat a diet adequate in calcium. You may need to take a calcium supplement. If you do not live in a sunny climate, you may need to take vitamin D, particularly during the winter or if you do not go outdoors.
- Avoid alcohol and sedatives, which increase the risk of falls and fractures.

- Stop smoking, which increases the risk of osteoporosis.
- Prevent falls by using handrails on stairs, adequate lighting, and avoiding throw rugs and electric cords in your path. Use proper lifting techniques.
- Ask your doctor whether to continue raloxifene if you will be inactive for long periods, such as on an extensive plane trip.
- See your doctor regularly.
- Stop your medication immediately and check with your doctor if you suspect you might be pregnant.
- Tell your doctor if you have vaginal bleeding, breast pain, or swelling of hands or feet.
- Tell any doctor, dentist, emergency help, pharmacist, or surgeon you see that you take raloxifene. If you have planned surgery, including dental, your doctor will usually discontinue raloxifene 72 hours prior to the surgery. Raloxifene should not be resumed until after you are able to be up and walking around.

How to Use This Drug

- If you miss a dose, take it as soon as you remember, but skip it if it is almost time for the next dose. **Do not take double doses.**
- Do not share your medication with others.
- Take the drug at the same time(s) each day.
- Take with or without food.
- Store tablets at room temperature with lid on tightly. Do not store in the bathroom. Do not expose to heat, moisture, or strong light. Keep out of reach of children.

Interactions with Other Drugs

The following drugs, biologics (e.g., vaccines, therapeutic antibodies), or foods are listed in *Evaluations of Drug Interactions* 2003 as causing "highly clinically significant" or "clinically significant" interactions when used together with any of the drugs in this section. In some sections with multiple drugs, the interaction may have been reported for one but not all drugs in this section, but we include the interaction because the drugs in this section are similar to one another. We have also included potentially serious interactions listed in the drug's FDA-approved professional package insert or in published medical journal articles. There may be other drugs, especially those in the families of drugs listed below, that also will react with this drug to cause severe adverse effects. Make sure to tell your doctor and pharmacist the drugs you are taking and tell them if you are taking any of these interacting drugs:

chlorotrianisene, cholestyramine, conjugated estrogens, DELESTROGEN, DES, diethylstilbestrol, esterified estrogens, ESTINYL, ESTRACE, ESTRADERM, estradiol, estradiol transdermal, estriol, estrogens, estrone, estropipate, ethinyl estradiol, MENEST, mestranol, NORETHINDRONE, NORINYL, OGEN, ORTHO-EST, ORTHO-NOVUM, polyestradiol, PREMARIN, LOCHOLEST, QUESTRAN, quinestrol

If you take these drugs your doctor may or may not change your doses: COUMADIN, diazepam, diazoxide, lidocaine, VALIUM, warfarin, XYLOCAINE.

Adverse Effects

Call your doctor immediately if you experience:

- severely painful abdomen
- appetite loss
- breast pain
- difficulty breathing
- chest pain
- coughing up blood
- severe diarrhea
- endometrial disorder
- flulike symptoms, such as body aches or pains, cough, fever, hoarseness or voice loss, runny nose, sinus congestion, dry or sore throat
- headache or migraine headache
- incoordination
- infection
- leg cramps
- numbness in arms, chest, or legs
- pneumonia
- skin rash
- difficulty swallowing
- swelling of ankles, feet, or hands
- difficult, painful, or burning urination, or bloody or cloudy urine
- vaginal bleeding or itching
- vision changes
- weakness

Call your doctor if you continue to experience:

- mental depression
- gas
- hot flashes
- indigestion
- trouble sleeping
- pain in muscles or joints

- nausea or vomiting
- profuse sweating
- swollen joints
- white vaginal discharge
- unexplained weight gain

Periodic Tests

Ask your doctor which of these tests should be done periodically while you are taking this drug:

- physical exam with special attention to breasts and uterus
- triglycerides blood test
- bone mineral density

Hormones

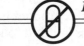 *Do Not Use*

ALTERNATIVE TREATMENT:
See Alendronate, p. 684.

Calcitonin (kal si *toe* nin)
(Calcitonin-Salmon)
MIACALCIN Injection (Novartis)
MIACALCIN Nasal Spray (Novartis)

FAMILY: Hormones

Calcitonin is a hormone produced by thyroid glands of mammals and fish. Synthetic forms have been made of the hormones from humans, pigs, salmon, and eels. Calcitonin is used to treat moderate to severe Paget's disease, high levels of calcium in the blood (such as occur with cancer), and osteoporosis in women five years or more after menopause.

The regulatory history of calcitonin in the treatment of postmenopausal osteoporosis provides a rare insight into drug regulation at the FDA.[30] Keep the following facts in mind as you read the calcitonin history:

1. FDA guidelines issued in 1994 emphasized documenting the efficacy of a drug in reducing fractures before it is approved for the treatment of osteoporosis. Since 1995, the FDA has approved three drugs under these guidelines, alendronate (see p. 584), raloxifene (see p. 589), and risedronate (see p. 584), for the treatment of osteoporosis. Note that conjugated estrogens are no longer approved for the treatment of postmenopausal osteoporosis.

2. Approximately 2.8 million prescriptions for calcitonin nasal spray were dispensed in 2003 at a retail cost of over $200 million, without evidence that the drug reduces the risk of fracture.

In the late 1970s, a new drug application (NDA) was submitted to the FDA, seeking approval of injectable calcitonin for treatment of post-menopausal osteoporosis. The FDA's review of the clinical data submitted by the company was not favorable, and the drug was not approved. Although there was a suggestion that daily subcutaneous (under the skin) or intramuscular injections of 100 international units (IU) of calcitonin increased total body calcium as compared with no treatment, the fact that the drug had no effect on bone mineral content in the radius (the small forearm bone) was of concern to FDA scientists.

The FDA's Endocrinologic and Metabolic Drugs Advisory Committee, made up of outside advisors, met in the autumn of 1981 to review calcitonin's NDA. The drug's failure to increase bone mineral content of the radius (forearm) was judged to be expected, since calcitonin's effect was most pronounced in the type of bone found in the vertebrae of the spine, and the radius was known to be composed mostly of a different type of bone. The advisory committee dismissed any potential clinical relevance of calcitonin's failure to increase mineral content of the radius.

The committee next shifted its attention to the effect of calcitonin on total body calcium.

Concern was expressed about the decreased rate of accrual of total body calcium during the second year of treatment with calcitonin. Several members of the committee were also uneasy about the absence of fracture data and questioned the legitimacy of total body calcium as a "surrogate endpoint" (a fill-in) for actual evidence that the drug reduced fracture risk.

As a vote on approval of calcitonin drew near, a spokesman for the company asked the FDA if the advisory committee could suggest that approval be contingent on the company agreeing to do a phase IV (postapproval) study examining the effects of calcitonin on fractures. A senior FDA member reminded the advisory committee that recommendations for a new drug's approval should be based on the available evidence. Phase IV [postapproval] studies were not intended to be used to "clarify substantial points of safety and effectiveness."

Half the committee members present voted yes and half no when asked if evidence supported approval of calcitonin for the treatment of osteoporosis. Through the efforts of the chairman it was learned that a member of the committee who left the meeting early was in favor of calcitonin's approval.

The FDA approved calcitonin in 1984 for treatment of postmenopausal osteoporosis subject to a phase IV study. Within a year, a phase IV fracture study was under way. After four years, only 151 of the proposed 300 women had been enrolled, and 77 of those had dropped out of the study. An early analysis of the study found an imbalance between the calcitonin and control groups in the average number of vertebral fractures at the beginning of the study. A vertebral fracture may not be noticed clinically and may only be identified in a spinal X-ray. The results from this study were deemed unreliable, and calcitonin's efficacy in reducing fracture remained unknown. After the failed fracture study, the company decided against attempting a second one. The use of injectable calcitonin for osteoporosis has since declined.

By the early 1990s, the development of calcitonin nasal spray was under way by Novartis. The company sponsored a large clinical trial known as the Prevent Reoccurrence of Osteoporotic Fractures, or PROOF trial. This five-year trial compared the effects of 100 IU, 200 IU, and 400 IU of calcitonin nasal spray to a placebo on incidence of vertebral fractures.

In 1994, another FDA advisory committee met to discuss the results from studies of calcitonin nasal spray, but not the yet-to-be-completed PROOF trial. The results from five clinical trials lasting one to two years and including about 550 patients were presented to the committee. The advisory committee found that the potential benefits of calcitonin nasal spray outweighed the potential risks and recommended its approval.

The FDA subsequently approved the drug for the treatment of postmenopausal osteoporosis in women who were more than five years postmenopausal. The drug's professional product labeling or package insert plainly stated that "the evidence of efficacy [was] based on increases in spinal bone mineral density," not fracture data.

Reports from small studies began to be published of calcitonin's efficacy in reducing the risk of fractures. One study reported an increased risk of fracture in patients receiving calcitonin. Then, after 20 years of anticipation for conclusive proof that calcitonin reduces the risk of fracture, the results of the PROOF trial were finally published in late 2000.[31]

The results of the PROOF trial were disappointing. Although the 200 IU dose of calcitonin nasal spray was found to statistically significantly decrease risk of new vertebral fractures, no fracture efficacy was shown for the 100 IU or 400 IU dosages. However, the 400 IU dose was the only dose associated with a significant increase in spinal bone mineral density. A National Institutes of Health osteoporosis consensus panel summarized the results of the PROOF trial in the following manner: "The absence of dose response, a 60 percent dropout rate, and the lack of strong supporting data from BMD [bone mineral density] and markers decrease confidence in the fracture risk data."

The calcitonin history concluded diplomatically: *"after 30 years of clinical experience, calcitonin's effect on fracture risk is uncertain. As the 40th anniversary of calcitonin's discovery approaches, perhaps it is time for all interested parties to reassess this drug's role in treatment of patients with osteoporosis."* [14]

Our conclusion would be more to the point: after 30 years of clinical experience, there is no clear evidence that calcitonin reduces the risk of fracture. In the absence of such evidence, calcitonin should no longer be prescribed for the treatment of patients with osteoporosis.

Parathyroid Hormone

 Do Not Use

ALTERNATIVE TREATMENT:
See Alendronate, p. 684.

Teriparatide (terr ih *par* a tyd)
FORTEO Injection (Lilly)

FAMILY: Parathyroid Hormones

Teriparatide was approved by the FDA in November 2002 for the treatment of osteoporosis in postmenopausal women who are at high risk for fracture and to increase bone mass in men with osteoporosis, who are also at high risk for fracture.

This drug is a shortened version of the human parathyroid hormone, the hormone that is the primary regulator of calcium and phosphate metabolism in bone and kidney. It is produced by recombinant DNA technology and has 34 amino acids that are identical in sequence to human parathyroid hormone. The drug is administered by subcutaneous (under the skin)

FDA BLACK BOX WARNING

In male and female rats, teriparatide caused an increase in the incidence of osteosarcoma (a malignant bone tumor) that was dependent on dose and treatment duration. The effect was observed at systemic exposures to teriparatide ranging from 3 to 60 times the exposure in humans given a 20-mcg dose. Because of the uncertain relevance of the rat osteosarcoma finding to humans, teriparatide should be prescribed only to patients for whom the potential benefits are considered to outweigh the potential risk. Teriparatide should not be prescribed for patients who are at increased baseline risk for osteosarcoma (including those with Paget's disease of bone or unexplained elevations of alkaline phosphatase, open epiphyses [open bone plates], or prior radiation therapy involving the skeleton).

injection daily and is approved for a maximum of two years of use.

In women, the treatment outcome that was used to approve teriparatide was the occurrence of new, X-ray-diagnosed fractures of the vertebrae (the bones that make up the spine), referred to as vertebral fractures. Vertebral fractures are not broken bones in the common use of the phrase; rather, they are defined as changes in the height of previously undeformed vertebrae seen on X-ray. Many such fractures are not symptomatic.

Women who were defined as being at high risk for fracture were those with at least one vertebral fracture before being treated with teriparatide.

Notice that teriparatide is not approved to treat osteoporosis in men, but rather to increase bone mass in those with osteoporosis who are at high risk for fracture. The definition of men at high risk for fracture is the same as for women, at least one vertebral fracture. The drug does increase bone mass in men, but there are no data available at this time showing that teriparatide reduces the risk of fracture in men. In our opinion, the FDA should not have approved this drug for use in men without evidence that it reduces their fracture risk.

Teriparatide was approved with a number of severe conditions and restrictions on its distribution and promotion because it caused osteosarcoma, a type of bone cancer, in laboratory animals. The professional product labeling or package insert for the drug contains a black-box warning about osteosarcoma. A black-box warning is the strongest type of warning that the FDA can require on a drug's labeling. It is extremely unusual to see a new drug marketed with a black-box warning.

Pharmacists must also distribute FDA-approved information written specifically for patients (known as a Medication Guide) with each new and refill prescription for teriparatide. The FDA can require a Medication Guide for those drugs that present a significant public health problem or when patients need additional information to use a drug safely and effectively. At this time, Medication Guides are required for only a small handful of drugs.

The drug's manufacturer also committed to the establishment of a postapproval safety surveillance program to evaluate whether there is an association between treatment with teriparatide and the occurrence of osteosarcoma in patients, since it was shown to cause this bone cancer in animals. Data collection for the program was to begin within 90 days after the first marketed use of teriparatide. Progress reports are to be submitted to the FDA at six months, one year, and annually thereafter. The program is to last for 10 years. We have serious concerns about this program, as described in the FDA's approval letter for teriparatide. It remains to be seen whether or not, as the program is planned, it will actually be able to detect a link between the drug and osteosarcoma (if one exists) in a timely manner.

In addition, the manufacturer agreed to re-stricted initial marketing of teriparatide by a limited sales force with no direct-to-consumer (DTC) advertising, and restrictions on the distribution of free samples of the drug. Further, the company agreed to conduct a physician education program to emphasize that teriparatide is approved only to treat patients at high risk for osteoporotic fractures.

Because of our concerns about the safety of this drug in relation to its effectiveness, Public Citizen's Health Research Group testified before the FDA's Endocrinologic Drugs Advisory Committee on July 27, 2001, to urge that the drug not be approved.[32]

We testified that the ability of teriparatide to cause cancer—in this case osteosarcoma—in rats was some of the most striking animal carcinogenicity data we had ever seen. Tumors developed in the animals at even the lowest dose level of teriparatide administered, which was only three times the drug levels in humans.

In effectiveness studies, when teriparatide given with calcium and vitamin D was compared with placebo given with calcium and vitamin D, the risk of one or more new vertebral fractures was reduced from 14% in women given the placebo to 5% in those given teriparatide. Thus, the absolute difference in the risk of a new vertebral fracture with teriparatide compared to placebo was 9.3%. The risk of a new vertebral fracture with teriparatide relative to the risk with placebo was 65%. This result was statistically significant.

Using the absolute difference in risk of a new vertebral fracture, the number of patients that need to be treated with teriparatide for a period of 19 months—the length of the effectiveness studies—to prevent one new vertebral fracture can be calculated and is 11 patients.

There is no direct comparison between teriparatide and the very popular and heavily promoted osteoporosis drug alendronate (see p. 584); however, a study published in the medical journal *The Lancet* in 1996 provides some basis for a comparison.[33] In women similar to those in the teriparatide studies, the number that needed to be treated with alendronate to prevent one new vertebral fracture after 36 months was 14. This information is only given for context; the most valid type of information would be a direct head-to-head comparison of teriparatide to alendronate, which has not been done at this time.

One direct comparison of teriparatide to alendronate is available: cost. A 30-day supply of teriparatide is $515.79 at drugstore.com, while 30 alendronate 10 milligram tablets, enough for 30 days, are $65.16. This is a difference of over $5,400 for one year of treatment.

The following table is taken from the FDA-approved professional product labeling for teriparatide and summarizes the sites of fractures, other than vertebral fractures, in women given teriparatide versus a placebo. There were 541 women in the teriparatide group and 544 in the placebo group. The number of fractures at a particular site is given, and the percentage of the group represented by that number is reported in parentheses.

There are a number of groups of patients that should not use teriparatide, primarily those with an increased baseline risk of osteosarcoma, including:

- Paget's disease of the bone
- unexplained high levels of alkaline phosphatase in the blood, which may mean the presence of Paget's disease (if you are not sure, ask your doctor)
- children or growing young adults
- patients who have had radiation therapy involving the bones

In addition, patients who have ever been diagnosed with bone cancer or other cancers that have spread (metastasized) to the bones, have a bone disease other than osteoporosis, have too much calcium in the blood (hypercalcemia), or are pregnant or nursing should not use teriparatide.

Other common adverse reactions seen with teriparatide in clinical trials include nausea, dizziness, leg cramps, and headache. Redness and swelling have also occurred at the injection site. Low blood pressure (orthostatic hypotension) that can lead to fainting has been seen with the first few doses of teriparatide. Elevations of calcium levels in both the blood and urine have also been reported.

FRACTURE SITE	TERIPARATIDE	PLACEBO
Wrist	2 (0.4%)	7 (1.3%)
Ribs	3 (0.6%)	5 (0.9%)
Hip	1 (0.2%)	4 (0.7%)
Ankle/Foot	1 (0.2%)	4 (0.7%)
Humerus (arm bone)	2 (0.4%)	2 (0.4%)
Pelvis	0	3 (0.6%)
Other	6 (1.1%)	8 (1.5%)
Total	15 (2.7%)	33 (6.0%)

REFERENCES

1. Rodan GA, Martin TJ. Therapeutic approaches to bone diseases. *Science* 2000; 289:1508–14.

2. Fracture prevention in elderly women: Treatment of osteoporosis is one approach, together with physical exercise and fall prevention. *Prescrire International* 1998; 7:155–9.

3. Kannus P. Preventing osteoporosis, falls, and fractures among elderly people. Promotion of lifelong physical activity is essential. *British Medical Journal* 1999; 318:205–6.

4. Wolfe SM, Jones RD. *Women's Health Alert.* New York: Addison-Wesley, 1991:193–222.

5. Writing Group for the Women's Health Initiative Investigators. Risks and benefits of estrogen plus progestin in healthy postmenopausal women. *Journal of the American Medical Association* 2002; 288:321–33.

6. Cauley JA, Robbins J, Chen Z, et al. Effects of estrogen plus progestin on risk of fracture and bone mineral density. *Journal of the American Medical Association* 2003; 290:1729–38.

7. FDA Plans to Evaluate Results of Women's Health Initiative Study for Estrogen-Alone Therapy, March 2, 2004. Available at: http://www.fda.gov/bbs/topics/ANSWERS/2004/ANS01281.html.

8. Calcium supplements. *The Medical Letter on Drugs and Therapeutics* 2000; 42:29–31.

9. Troendle G. Food and Drug Administration Medical Officer Review of Alendronate (Fosamax) for the Treatment of Glucocorticoid Induced Osteoporosis, March 12, 1998. Available at: http://www.fda.gov/cder/approval/index.htm. Accessed February 18, 2004.

10. Troendle G. Food and Drug Administration Medical Officer's Review of Response to Approvable Letter for Alendronate (Fosamax) for the Treatment of Glucocorticoid Induced Osteoporosis, June 14, 1999:1–22. Available at: http://www.fda.gov/cder/approval/index.htm. Accessed February 18, 2004.

11. Troendle G. Food and Drug Administration Medical Officer's Comments on Alendronate (Fosamax) Professional Product Labeling, June 16, 1999. Available at: http://www.fda.gov/cder/approval/index .htm. Accessed February 18, 2004.

12. Bone HG, Hosking D, Devogelaer JP, et al. Ten years' experience with alendronate for osteoporosis in postmenopausal women. *New England Journal of Medicine* 2004; 350:1189–99.

13. Strewler GJ. Decimal point—osteoporosis therapy at the 10-year mark. *New England Journal of Medicine* 2004; 350:1172–4.

14. Colman E. Food and Drug Administration Medical Officer Review of Risedronate (Actonel), August 10, 1999:66.

15. McClung MR, Geusens P, Miller PD, et al. Effect of risedronate on the risk of hip fracture in elderly women. Hip Intervention Program Study Group. *New England Journal of Medicine* 2001; 344:333–40.

16. Goodman RL. The effect of risedronate on the risk of hip fracture in elderly women. *New England Journal of Medicine* 2001; 344:1720–1.

17. Papapoulos SE. Bisphosphonates: Pharmacology and use in the treatment of osteoporosis. In *Osteoporosis.* 1st ed. Marcus R, Feldman D, Kelsey J, eds. San Diego: Academic Press, 1996:1209–30.

18. Kherani RB, Papaioannou A, Adachi JD. Long-term tolerability of the bisphosphonates in postmenopausal osteoporosis: A comparative review. *Drug Safety* 2002; 25:781–90.

19. Ocular adverse effects of alendronic acid. *Prescrire International* 2002; 10:82.

20. Greenspan SL, Emkey RD, Bone HG, et al. Significant differential effects of alendronate, estrogen, or combination therapy on the rate of bone loss after discontinuation of treatment of postmenopausal osteoporosis. A randomized, double-blind, placebo-controlled trial. *Annals of Internal Medicine* 2002; 137:875–83.

21. Tuck SP, Francis RM. Osteoporosis. *Postgraduate Medical Journal* 2002; 78:526–32.

22. Cranney A, Guyatt G, Griffith L, et al. Meta-analyses of therapies for postmenopausal osteoporosis. IX: Summary of meta-analyses of therapies for postmenopausal osteoporosis. *Endocrine Review* 2002; 23:570–8.

23. Cranney A, Tugwell P, Zytaruk N, et al. Meta-analyses of therapies for postmenopausal osteoporosis. IV: Meta-analysis of raloxifene for the prevention and treatment of postmenopausal osteoporosis. *Endocrine Review* 2002; 23:524–8.

24. Gluck O, Maricic M. Raloxifene: Recent information on skeletal and non-skeletal effects. *Current Opinion in Rheumatology* 2002; 14:429–32.

25. Raloxifene and prevention of vertebral fracture. *Prescrire International* 2000; 9:190–1.

26. Vignali M, Infantino M, Matrone R, et al. Endometriosis: Novel etiopathogenetic concepts and clinical perspectives. *Fertility and Sterility* 2002; 78:665–78.

27. Ettinger B, Black DM, Mitlak BH, et al. Reduction of vertebral fracture risk in postmenopausal women with osteoporosis treated with raloxifene: Results from a 3-year randomized clinical trial. Multiple Outcomes of Raloxifene Evaluation (MORE) Investigators. *Journal of the American Medical Association* 1999; 282:637–45.

28. Riggs BL, Hartmann LC. Selective estrogen-receptor modulators—mechanisms of action and application to clinical practice. *New England Journal of Medicine* 2003; 348:618–29.

29. *Physicians' Desk Reference.* 58th ed. Montvale, N.J.: Thomson PDR, 2004:1804–8.

30. Colman E, Hedin R, Swann J, et al. A brief history of calcitonin. *The Lancet* 2002; 359:885–6.

31. Chesnut CH III, Silverman S, Andriano K, et al. A randomized trial of nasal spray salmon calcitonin in postmenopausal women with established osteoporosis: The prevent recurrence of osteoporotic fractures study. PROOF Study Group. *American Journal of Medicine* 2000; 109:267–76.

32. Public Citizen's Health Research Group. Statement to the Food and Drug Administration's Endocrinologic and Metabolic Drugs Advisory Committee Not to Approve Teriparatide (Forteo), July 27, 2001. Available at: http://www.citizen.org/publications/release.cfm?ID=6787. Accessed December 5, 2003.

33. Black DM, Cummings SR, Karpf DB, et al. Randomised trial of effect of alendronate on risk of fracture in women with existing vertebral fractures. Fracture Intervention Trial Research Group. *The Lancet* 1996; 348:1535–41.

19

DRUGS FOR ALZHEIMER'S DISEASE

OVERVIEW

The strategy to sell Alzheimer's disease (AD) drugs is based on hope, fear, and guilt: hope that one of these drugs might "work," fear that if one of these drugs is not started quickly, all will be lost; and guilt if family members have not made the decision to "fight" the disease with expensive, sometimes dangerous, drugs.

The strategy is working. According to a front-page article in the April 7, 2004, *New York Times* that questions the actual benefits of these drugs, "A million Americans take them, at an overall cost of $1.2 billion a year." A professor at Johns Hopkins University School of Medicine who is an expert in Alzheimer's disease was quoted in the article. He placed the value of the current crop of Alzheimer's drugs in perspective when he said, "You can name 11 fruits in a

> At this time, there are no safe and effective treatments that substantially alter the progression of Alzheimer's disease.

minute instead of 10. Is that worth 120 bucks a month?"[1]

Recent reviews by the U.S. Preventive Services Task Force and the American Academy of Neurology are appropriately skeptical of the use of these drugs. The Alzheimer's Disease Assessment Scale—Cognitive Subscale (ADAS-Cog) is the main test used to measure cognitive improvement in patients with Alzheimer's disease and it consists of a 70-point measure of cognitive functioning. For the four cholinesterase inhibitor drugs discussed in this chapter, the average improvement between patients being given one of the drugs and those patients randomized to get a placebo was 1.36 to 3.4 points out of a total of 70 points.[2] This statistically significant but clinically questionable result is in accord with the above-mentioned improvement in remembering fruits. The task force also thought that the effect of the drugs on physical function, assessed by activities of daily living, is inconclusive.

The American Academy of Neurology concluded that these drugs (cholinesterase inhibitors) "should be considered in patients with mild to moderate AD although studies suggest a small average degree of benefit." They further pointed out, referring to all drugs, not just the cholinesterase inhibitors, that "there is no standard approach to determining the effect size of antidementia agents."[3] Some careful clinicians who use these drugs will give them a two-month trial and will discontinue the drugs if no improvement is seen.

Alzheimer's disease is a progressive deterioration of the brain that significantly impairs cognition and the ability to perform daily activities. It is the most common cause of dementia among the elderly, accounting for 50 to 60% of all dementia cases.[4,5] Currently, 4.5 million people in the United States suffer with the disease, and by year 2050, an estimated 11.3 million to 16 million Americans will have AD.[6]

In general, there are two forms of Alzheimer's disease: familial and sporadic.[5] Familial Alzheimer's disease, known also as early-onset, is a rare form of this disorder occurring before the age of 60. The sporadic form, known also as late-onset Alzheimer's disease, is the most common form of the disorder and occurs after 60 years of age.

It is not understood what causes Alzheimer's disease. However, there are several factors that play a role in its development, including advanced age, family history, and genetics.[4,7] The greatest risk factor for Alzheimer's disease is age. Over 10% of individuals 65 years and older have Alzheimer's disease and nearly half of those over 85 years of age are affected with the disease as well.[6] Family history is another factor that increases the risk up to two to three times.[5]

Research has identified a genetic link for Alzheimer's disease. Three genes were identified to be associated with the development of early-onset Alzheimer's: presenilin 1, presenilin 2, and amyloid precursor protein.[7] Another gene coding for apolipoprotein E-4 (ApoE-4), which is involved in cholesterol transport, may also be a factor in the development of late-onset Alzheimer's.[7,8] An estimated 35 to 60% of patients with late-onset Alzheimer's possess at least one copy of the ApoE-4 gene.[5]

With the gradual loss of brain cells, common symptoms associated with Alzheimer's disease include memory loss, difficulty performing familiar tasks, language problems, disorientation to time and place, problems with abstract thinking, misplacing things, changes in mood or behavior, changes in personality, and loss of initiative.[5]

A definitive diagnosis of Alzheimer's disease is determined only by examination of brain tissue upon autopsy.[4] Therefore, a possible or probable diagnosis of Alzheimer's disease may be determined through a complete medical history, physical assessment, neurologic and mental evaluation, laboratory tests, and radiologic findings.[7] No one test that can diagnose Alzheimer's disease exists at this time.[6] The disease progression for Alzheimer's varies from 3 to 20 years after the onset with an average life span of 8 to 10 years after the diagnosis.[9]

There are no medical treatments to cure or stop the progression of Alzheimer's disease. Current drug therapy includes four drugs known as acetylcholinesterase inhibitors. These are donepezil (ARICEPT), rivastigmine (EXELON), galantamine (REMINYL), and tacrine (COGNEX). These drugs increase the level of acetylcholine, a brain transmitter, with the assumption that this might improve Alzheimer's-associated dementia.

The newest drug for treating Alzheimer's, memantine (NAMENDA), was approved by the FDA in 2003 for the treatment of moderate to severe dementia of the Alzheimer's type. It works in a different way from the acetylcholinesterase inhibitors by blocking a receptor called the N-methyl-D-aspartate (NMDA) receptor. Memantine is not a new drug; it has been used in Europe since the 1980s. Although approved for moderate to severe dementia, without comparative studies it is unclear whether memantine is even as effective, let alone more effective, than acetylcholinesterase inhibitors for moderately severe dementia.[10] Furthermore, the data for memantine's efficacy on severe AD is weak.[10]

Although these drugs show statistically significant improvements on certain memory and thinking tests, it is unclear how a few extra points on a mental exam relates to an Alzheimer's disease patient's daily functioning in the real world. These drugs do not change the underlying course of the disease, but rather they have a modest effect on cognition and global impression scales for a minority of Alzheimer's disease patients.

DRUG PROFILES

Cholinesterase Inhibitors

Do Not Use

ALTERNATIVE TREATMENT:
At this time, there are no safe and effective treatments that substantially alter the progression of Alzheimer's disease.

Donepezil (doe *ne* pe zil)
ARICEPT (Pfizer)

Tacrine (*ta* crin)
COGNEX (Parke-Davis)

FAMILY: Cholinesterase Inhibitors

Tacrine was the first drug approved by the FDA exclusively for Alzheimer's disease, and donepezil the second. The action of both drugs is to inhibit the enzyme that breaks down acetylcholine, a brain transmitter, a deficiency of which has been thought to play a role in Alzheimer's disease.

Tacrine

The major clinical trial evaluating tacrine found a statistically significant reduction in the decline of cognitive function in patients taking the drug compared to those taking a placebo (inactive sugar pill).[11] The editorial accompanying this clinical trial stated that the differences between the placebo and tacrine groups, although statistically significant, were "clinically trivial."[12] The editors of the internationally respected *Medical Letter on Drugs and Therapeutics,* an independent source of drug information, said: *"Tacrine appears to improve or slow the decline in various test scores in a minority of patients with mild to moderate Alzheimer's disease, but there is no evidence from controlled trials that its use leads to substantial functional improvement. The drug can cause hepatic [liver] injury and may inhibit the metabolism of other drugs."*[13]

Prescrire International, a respected independent source of drug information, found in their review of the drug that "it is impossible to confirm that tacrine has any real clinical efficacy." Also covered in this review were the results of a French study involving 5,000 patients in which nearly half the patients who received tacrine had elevations in liver enzymes, an early sign of potential liver toxicity.[14]

Tacrine is still produced, although sales have slumped to the point where the drug's original maker, Parke-Davis, has suspended promoting the drug to doctors and discontinued patient support programs. Tacrine is now distributed by a new company, though it is still manufactured by Parke-Davis.

Donepezil

Donepezil, like tacrine, has shown a modest positive effect compared with a placebo, and the differences between the donepezil and placebo groups were statistically significant. The most common adverse effects of donepezil have been nausea, diarrhea, and vomiting. Insomnia, fatigue, muscle cramps, and loss of appetite have also been reported by donepezil users. So far, the effect of serious liver injury that is present with tacrine has not been seen with donepezil.

The *Medical Letter* editors in their 1997 review of donepezil said: "There is no evidence that use of either donepezil or tacrine leads to substantial functional improvement or prevents the progression of the disease."[15]

Prescrire International's 1998 review of donepezil found that "the effects of donepezil are moderate and visible only on psychometric scales [surveys]; the possible clinical benefit is unknown. In the long term, donepezil only delays cognitive deterioration by a few months."[16]

A statistical summary of clinical trials, known as a meta-analysis, of donepezil conducted by the prestigious Cochrane Collaboration in 2003 found that in selected patients with mild or moderate Alzheimer's disease treated for periods of 12, 24, or 52 weeks: "Donepezil produced modest improvements in cognitive function and study clinicians rated global clinical state more positively in treated patients. No improvements were present on patient self-assessed quality of life and data on many important outcomes are not available. The practical importance of these changes to patients and carers [care givers] is unclear."[17]

A study published in the July 2003 issue of the *Journal of the American Geriatrics Society* funded by Pfizer, the producer of donepezil, concluded that the use of donepezil delayed the placement of Alzheimer's disease patients in nursing homes by about two years.[18] This study became the basis of advertising placed in leading medical journals such as the *Journal of the American Medical Association* and the *Journal of the American Geriatrics Society*.

If the conclusion of the July 2003 *Journal of the American Geriatrics Society* study were based on a randomized, placebo-controlled trial, the scientific gold standard for medical research, wherein 50% of the patients got donepezil and the other 50% were randomly assigned to be given a placebo, it would be a major public health breakthrough and a cause for celebration. Unfortunately, it is not based on such a study and is not any cause for celebration.

Buried in the middle of this study cited in the medical journal ads is the statement that since it is an observational study (observing two different groups of people), "the current investigation . . . could not prove conclusively that taking effective doses of donepezil delayed nursing home placement."[18] The study further stated that the only way to prove this finding of delayed nursing home placement would be to do a randomized double-blind placebo-controlled prospective trial that would assure that the two groups were completely comparable. Similarly buried in the copy of the ads is the statement that in all "studies of this type, results [delayed nursing home placement] may be attributed to various factors."[18]

Two letters to the editor of the *Journal of the American Geriatrics Society* by experts in Alzheimer's disease were extremely critical of the quality of the study and its conclusions. In one, the author concluded that this study "is plainly insufficient to justify a claim for treatment [with donepezil] to prevent nursing home treatment."[19] The other letter concluded by stating: "Would it be churlish to wonder out loud how this paper is different from an advertisement?"[20]

Donepezil has been deceptively oversold to physicians and patients, perpetuating the exploitation of patients with Alzheimer's disease and their families.

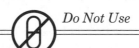 *Do Not Use*

ALTERNATIVE TREATMENT:
At this time, there are no safe and effective treatments that substantially alter the progression of Alzheimer's disease.

Galantamine (ga *lan* ta meen)
REMINYL (Janssen)

Rivastigmine (riv a *stig* meen)
EXELON (Novartis)

FAMILY: Cholinesterase Inhibitors

Rivastigmine and galantamine are the third and fourth drugs, respectively, to be approved by the FDA for the treatment of mild to moderate Alzheimer's disease dementia. The two older drugs are tacrine (COGNEX) and donepezil (ARICEPT).

These drugs work by inhibiting the enzyme acetylcholinesterase and are generally referred to as cholinesterase inhibitors. They increase levels of acetylcholine with the assumption that this might improve Alzheimer's-associated dementia.

Rivastigmine

The FDA medical officer reviewing the data submitted by Novartis to support the approval of rivastigmine commented: "Although there [are] no direct ("head-to-head") comparisons [that] have been carried out, there is no clear indication Exelon has any advantages over donepezil."[21]

The medical officer goes on to say in his review of rivastigmine: "The key elements of the risk-benefit equation in the case of Exelon are as follows:

• The very modest efficacy of the drug [is] most apparent at higher doses which are also the doses at which the common and troublesome adverse events occur,
• The lack of any readily apparent advantage, and the presence of several readily apparent disadvantages, when Exelon is compared to donepezil,
• The very high incidence of nausea [47%], vomiting [31%] and anorexia [loss of appetite], and their potentially serious consequences, especially in this population. The consequences of vomiting are potentially serious regardless of whether episodes are short-lived and nonrecurrent, or frequent."

He concludes his review: "I recommend that this application not be approved on the grounds that the risks of using the drug outweigh the possible benefits."[21]

The editors of *The Medical Letter on Drugs and Therapeutics*, a highly respected independent source of drug information written for physicians and pharmacists, concluded their review of rivastigmine by saying: "As with tacrine and donepezil, there is no convincing evidence that rivastigmine markedly improves quality of life in patients with Alzheimer's disease, or substantially alters progression of the disease."[22]

A similar conclusion was recently reached by *The Drug and Therapeutics Bulletin,* the British equivalent of *The Medical Letter:* "We remain unconvinced of the value of currently available cholinesterase inhibitors in clinical practice."[23]

In January 2001 the following warning was added in boldface to the professional product labeling or package insert for rivastigmine because of severe gastrointestinal (GI) adverse reactions:[24]

WARNING

GASTROINTESTINAL
ADVERSE REACTIONS

Exelon (rivastigmine tartrate) use is associated with significant gastrointestinal adverse reactions, including nausea and vomiting, anorexia, and weight loss. For this reason, patients should always be started at a dose of 1.5 mg BID [twice daily] and titrated to their maintenance dose. If treatment is interrupted for longer than several days, treatment should be reinitiated with the lowest daily dose to reduce the possibility of severe vomiting and its potentially serious sequelae (e.g., there has been one post marketing report of severe vomiting with esophageal [tube that runs from the mouth to stomach] rupture following inappropriate reinitiation of treatment with a 4.5-mg dose after 8 weeks of treatment interruption).

Galantamine

The same FDA medical officer who reviewed rivastigmine also reviewed galantamine and recommended its approval. However, he stated: "It should again be noted that the beneficial effects of Reminyl are small, and similar to those of other cholinesterase inhibitors; only a small minority of patients actually improve in relation to baseline; and the efficacy of galantamine (REMINYL) beyond six months of treatment is uncertain, as randomized controlled studies longer than six months in duration have not been carried out. There is also no evidence that galantamine has a disease-modifying effect, and at least some evidence that it may not."[25]

The *Medical Letter* editors' opinion of galantamine was similar to their opinion of the other cholinesterase inhibitors used to treat Alzheimer's disease: "Galantamine produces modest improvements in measures of cognition and functioning in patients with mild to moderate Alzheimer's disease. Gastrointestinal symptoms have been the most common adverse effects. Whether galantamine offers any advantage over donepezil or rivastigmine remains to be established by comparative trials."[22]

NMDA Receptor Inhibitor

Do Not Use

ALTERNATIVE TREATMENT:
At this time, there are no safe and effective treatments that substantially alter the progression of Alzheimer's disease.

Memantine (me *man* teen)
NAMENDA (Forest)

FAMILY: N-methyl-D-aspartate (NMDA) Receptor Inhibitors

Memantine is the first drug approved by the FDA for the treatment of moderate to severe Alzheimer's disease dementia. Other drugs approved for the treatment of Alzheimer's are specifically approved only for mild to moderately severe dementia.

One theory is that Alzheimer's disease may be caused, in part, by overactivation of N-methyl-D-aspartate (NMDA) receptors by the brain transmitter glutamate, which may add to the destruction of nerve cells. Memantine is postulated to work by blocking the NMDA receptors from binding to glutamate, thereby preventing cell death.[26]

Memantine is not a new drug. It has been marketed in Europe since the 1980s. Since 1982, it has been sold for the treatment of parkinsonism, cerebral and peripheral spasticity, and organic brain syndrome in Germany under the brand name Akatinol. In 2002, the European Union approved memantine for the treatment of Alzheimer's disease. The original drug application for United States approval was submitted in July 2002 and then resubmitted in December with an additional study.[27] The FDA ultimately approved memantine in October 2003.[28]

The chemical structure of memantine is nearly identical to that of amantadine (SYMMETREL) (see p. 762), differing by only two carbon atoms. Amatadine is also an NMDA inhibitor[29] and is approved by the FDA for the prevention and treatment of influenza A, Parkinson's disease, and drug-induced movement disorder.[30]

In a French medical journal review of memantine, the editors of *Prescrire International,* a highly respected source of independent drug information, state: "Data on the effects of memantine in severe Alzheimer's disease are sparse and weak."[10]

In the UK, the editors of *The Drug and Therapeutics Bulletin,* also a highly respected source of independent drug information, concluded their review of the drug by saying: "On published evidence, memantine produces, at best, only a small reduction in the rate of deterioration in global, functional, and cognitive scales in such patients. Whether this translates into important changes in quality of life or how long the effects last is unclear."[31]

The FDA guidelines for approval of drugs to treat Alzheimer's disease require that studies demonstrate a statistically significant effect on two primary outcome measures: (1) cognitive function; and (2) global patient functioning or activities of daily function. The FDA medical officer reviewing the data submitted by Forest Laboratories states: "There was a small effect size [difference] between memantine treated and placebo treated groups on cognitive improvement."[26]

He continued to comment on the measures of global functioning: "Only a small minority of patients treated with memantine showed even a minimal or moderate improvement, with no patients showing a marked improvement, and the most common response being no change."[26]

Furthermore, an analysis by the FDA statistician of a subgroup of patients showed memantine failed to demonstrate a significant effect on patient global function for severe dementia of the Alzheimer's type.[26]

Although memantine shows a modest effect on improvement compared with placebo for moderately severe Alzheimer's disease, the effectiveness of memantine has not been compared with any of the acetylcholinesterase inhibitors.

The effect of memantine on the progression of the disease is summed up in the drug's professional product labeling or package insert, which states: "At this time, there is no evidence that memantine prevents or slows neurodegeneration in patients with Alzheimer's disease."[29]

One highly touted study purports to show that the use of memantine causes significant decrease in caregiver time with Alzheimer's disease. Although this study allegedly randomized patients to get either memantine or a placebo, there were statistically significant differences between the patients who eventually got the placebo and those who eventually were given memantine *before* the study began. Thus, any conclusions about the positive effects of the drug are, at the least, highly suspect.[32]

Common adverse effects reported with memantine include dizziness, headache, constipation, pain, and difficult breathing, which are believed to be related to the dose of the drug. Three reports of inflammation of the pancreas and four cases of renal failure were reported from ongoing trials. Of the renal failure reports, the treatment assignments remain blinded for three cases. From post-marketing surveillance, two cases of a severe skin reaction called epidermal necrolysis, one case of bone marrow failure to make blood cells, and one case of liver failure were reported.[27]

Since memantine is already marketed in Germany, the company has received 73 adverse event reports for 48 patients, including seizures, high blood pressure, circulatory failure, jerky movements, bullous rash, pruritis, nervousness, tremors, aggressive reactions, and nausea.[10]

Ergot Derivatives

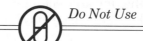 *Do Not Use*

ALTERNATIVE TREATMENT:
At this time, there are no safe and effective treatments that substantially alter the progression of Alzheimer's disease.

Ergoloid Mesylates (er goe loid *mess* i lates)
HYDERGINE, HYDERGINE LC (Novartis)

FAMILY: Ergot Derivatives

Ergoloid mesylates was first marketed in the United States in November 1953. Over the years this drug has been misleadingly promoted and advertised as effective treatment for "those who would be considered to suffer from some ill-defined process related to aging" and as "the only product for Alzheimer's dementia."[33] The reality is very different.

The term "dementia" describes a collection of symptoms including confusion, disorientation, apathy, and memory loss. More than 60 disorders can cause dementia.[34] Alzheimer's dementia, which is not reversible, accounts for about 50 to 60% of the cases of dementia.[35] A smaller percentage of dementias are reversible.

A 1990 study, published in *The New England Journal of Medicine,*[36] shows ergoloid mesylates to be totally ineffective for mild to moderate Alzheimer's, and to actually accelerate patients' mental deterioration. This study was more carefully designed than previous research showing ergoloid mesylates to be effective. Potential participants underwent a rigorous evaluation at the start of the study to screen out those patients whose dementia was due to a medical or psychiatric problem other than Alzheimer's. More patients were studied (39 took ergoloid mesylates, and 41 took placebo), and the trial was continued for longer (24 weeks) than most previous studies.

Subjects taking Hydergine LC, at the recommended dose of one milligram three times daily, did worse than the control group on one measure of appropriate behavior and one measure of IQ. The authors said that the drug may either be directly toxic to the brain or somehow accelerate the progression of Alzheimer's.

A 1991 review on geriatric medicine published in *The Journal of the American Medical Association* found that "one widely used treatment [for Alzheimer's] (ergoloid mesylates) has been convincingly demonstrated to be of no value. This trial [referring to the study discussed above], along with the absence of a convincing pathophysiologic basis for its use, indicates that this treatment should be abandoned."[8]

Ergoloid mesylates remain on a well-recognized list of drugs that are inappropriate for use in older adults.[37]

A person showing signs of dementia should be completely tested to see whether he or she is suffering from one of the dementias that can be cured. These tests include complete physical, neurological, and psychiatric examinations as well as a chest X-ray, CT scan, and blood tests. In addition, many cases of dementia are caused or worsened by prescription drugs such as tranquilizers and sleeping pills (see p. 166). If you are taking one of these drugs, ask your doctor about stopping or changing your prescription.

If, after testing, a physician determines that a person has Alzheimer's dementia, a health care team—including a doctor, a nurse, and a social worker experienced in working with dementia—can offer practical suggestions to increase the person's safety and comfort at home, and can discuss alternative care options. Efforts to improve the mental and physical state of older or senile adults are most beneficial if they address social, physical, nutritional, psychological, occupational, and recreational needs.[38]

REFERENCES

1. Grady D. Nominal Benefits Seen in Drugs for Alzheimer's Disease. *New York Times,* April 7, 2003:A1.

2. Boustani M, Peterson B, Hanson L, et al. Screening for dementia in primary care: A summary of the evidence for the U.S. Preventive Services Task Force. *Annals of Internal Medicine* 2003; 138:927–37.

3. Doody RS, Stevens JC, Beck C, et al. Practice parameter: Management of dementia (an evidence-based review). Report of the Quality Standards Subcommittee of the American Academy of Neurology. *Neurology* 2001; 56:1154–66.

4. Goetz CG. *Textbook of Clinical Neurology.* 2nd ed. Philadelphia: Elsevier Science, 2003:682–92.

5. Alzheimer's Organization, 2004. Available at: www.alz.org. Accessed April 13, 2004.

6. Hebert LE, Scherr PA, Bienias JL, et al. Alzheimer disease in the US population: Prevalence estimates using the 2000 census. *Archives of Neurology* 2003; 60:1119–22.

7. Goldman L, Bennett JC. *Cecil Textbook of Medicine.* 21st ed. Philadelphia: WB Saunders Company, 2000:2042–4.

8. Larson EB. Geriatric medicine. *Journal of the American Medical Association* 1991; 265:3125–6.

9. Alzheimer's Disease Education Referral Center, 2004. Available at: www.alz.org. Accessed April 13, 2004.

10. Memantine: New preparation. Poor evaluation and uncertain benefit in Alzheimer's disease. *Prescrire International* 2003; 12:203–5.

11. Davis KL, Thal LJ, Gamzu ER, et al. A double-blind, placebo-controlled multicenter study of tacrine for Alzheimer's disease. The Tacrine Collaborative Study Group. *New England Journal of Medicine* 1992; 327:1253–9.

12. Growdon JH. Treatment for Alzheimer's disease? *New England Journal of Medicine* 1992; 327:1306–8.

13. Tacrine for Alzheimer's disease. *Medical Letter on Drugs and Therapeutics* 1993; 35:87–8.

14. Tacrine: A second look. An outdated drug to be discarded. *Prescrire International* 1999; 8:16–8.

15. Donepezil (Aricept) for Alzheimer's disease. *Medical Letter on Drugs and Therapeutics* 1997; 39:53–4.

16. Donepezil: New preparation. Moderate efficacy in Alzheimer's disease. *Prescrire International* 1998; 7:146–7.

17. Birks JS, Melzer D, Beppu H. Donepezil for mild and moderate Alzheimer's disease. *Cochrane Database of Systematic Reviews* 2003; CD001190.

18. Geldmacher DS, Provenzano G, McRae T, et al. Donepezil is associated with delayed nursing home placement in patients with Alzheimer's disease. *Journal of the American Geriatrics Society* 2003; 51:937–44.

19. Finucane TE. Another advertisement for donepezil. *Journal of the American Geriatrics Society* 2004; 52:843.

20. Karlawish JH. Donepezil delay to nursing home placement study is flawed. *Journal of the American Geriatrics Society* 2004; 52:845.

21. Mani RB. Food and Drug Administration Medical Officer Review of Rivastigmine (Exelon), April 7, 2000.

22. Rivastigmine (Exelon) for Alzheimer's disease. *Medical Letter on Drugs and Therapeutics* 2000; 42:93–4.

23. Rivastigmine for Alzheimer's disease. *Drug and Therapeutics Bulletin* 2000; 38:15–6.

24. Bess AL. Dear Health Care Provider Letter—Rivastigmine (Exelon), January 26, 2001.

25. Mani RB. Food and Drug Administration—Medical Officer Review of Galantamine (Reminyl), November 29, 2000.

26. Mani RB. Food and Drug Administration—Final Briefing Document for Advisory Committee Meeting—Efficacy Review of Memantine (Namenda), August 19, 2003. Available at: http://www.fda.gov/ohrms/dockets/ac/03/briefing/3979B1_05_FDA-Efficacy%20Review.pdf.

27. Boehm G. Food and Drug Administration New Drug Application Safety Review—Memantine (Namenda), August 20, 2003. Available at: http://www.fda.gov/ohrms/dockets/ac/03/briefing/3979B1_04_FDA-Safety%20Review.pdf.

28. The Pink Sheet. *Forest Namenda Clears FDA: Alzheimer Drug Shipments or Begin in December,* October 20, 2003:3.

29. Namenda (memantine) Professional Product Labeling, October 1, 2003. Available at: http://www.namenda.com/pdf/namenda_pi.pdf. Accessed April 26, 2004.

30. *Physicians' Desk Reference.* 58th ed. Montvale, N.J.: Thomson PDR, 2004:1247–9.

31. Memantine for dementia? *Drug and Therapeutics Bulletin* 2003; 41:73–6.

32. Wimo A, Winblad B, Stoffler A, et al. Resource utilisation and cost analysis of memantine in patients with moderate to severe Alzheimer's disease. *Pharmacoeconomics* 2003; 21:327–40.

33. Boehm G. Advertisment for Hydergine. *Journal of the American Medical Association* 1985; 254:2233.

34. Haase GR. Disease presenting as dementia. In *Dementia.* 2nd ed. Wells CE, ed. Philadelpha: FA Davis, 1977:27–67.

35. Smith JS, Kiloh LG. The investigation of dementia: Results in 200 consecutive admissions. *The Lancet* 1981; 1:824–7.

36. Thompson TL, Filley CM, Mitchell WD, et al. Lack of efficacy of hydergine in patients with Alzheimer's disease. *New England Journal of Medicine* 1990; 323:445–8.

37. Fick DM, Cooper JW, Wade WE, et al. Updating the Beers criteria for potentially inappropriate medication use in older adults: Results of a US consensus panel of experts. *Archives of Internal Medicine* 2003; 163:2716–24.

38. Hydergine for cerebral arteriosclerosis. *Medical Letter on Drugs and Therapeutics* 1974; 16:21–2.

20

DRUGS FOR ERECTILE DYSFUNCTION

OVERVIEW

The three drugs covered in this chapter for the treatment of erectile dysfunction (ED) are vardenafil (LEVITRA), tadalafil (CIALIS), and sildenafil (VIAGRA). All work in a similar way and are members of the family of drugs known as phosphodiesterase inhibitors.

A recent review article[1] on the diagnosis and treatment of ED offers good advice about distinguishing it from other types of sexual dysfunction. "The most important component of diagnosing erectile dysfunction is obtaining a complete medical and sexual history. It is important to distinguish the condition from other sexual dysfunctions, such as premature ejaculation and loss of libido."

This review continues, saying: "The circumstances surrounding erectile dysfunction may be helpful in determining whether a situational or nonorganic factor is involved. Sudden onset, maintenance of nocturnal erections, presence of psychological problems and concurrent major life events or relationship issues may be associated with nonorganic erectile dysfunction. Concurrent medical illnesses and any medications the patient may be taking should be reviewed. Erectile dysfunction is often a component of generalized medical illness and may represent the initial presentation of cardiovascular disease or diabetes. The history may also reveal certain reversible or modifiable risk factors, such as tobacco use or inadequate diabetes control."

A number of drugs can cause sexual dysfunction in both women and men. These drugs are listed on p. 34 in Chapter 3 of this book.

Determining the potential benefits of vardenafil, tadalafil, or sildenafil is much more complex than for drugs that are used to treat cancer, heart disease, or high blood pressure, for example, where one of the potential benefits may be increased survival or avoidance of a heart attack or stroke. It is unlikely that untreated ED contributes to decreased survival, even though it may contribute to emotional distress and strained relationships. Weighing the potential benefits of these drugs involves the interactions in a private relationship based on human emotions and a couple's perception of their quality of life.

There will be many men without erectile dysfunction who will want to try these drugs, seeking to increase their sexual performance. This can only be regarded as risky behavior.

DRUG PROFILES

Phosphodiesterase Inhibitors

Limited Use

Sildenafil (sil *den* a fil)
VIAGRA (Pfizer)

Do Not Use Until Seven Years After Release

Tadalafil (ta *dal* a fil)
(Do Not Use Until 2011)
CIALIS (Lilly)

Vardenafil (var *den* a fil)
(Do Not Use Until 2011)
LEVITRA (Bayer)

GENERIC: not available

FAMILY: Phosphodiesterase Inhibitors

PREGNANCY WARNING

In animal studies, tadalafil crossed the placenta and exposed the fetus to the drug. Fewer pups survived from mothers treated with either tadalafil or vardenafil and there were delays in physical development of pups. Because of the potential for serious adverse effects to the fetus, these drugs should not be used by pregnant women.

BREAST-FEEDING WARNING

Tadalafil and vardenafil are excreted in animal milk at concentrations 2- to 10-fold higher than mother's plasma. Sildenafil levels were not measured in animal milk. It is likely that these drugs, like many others, are also excreted in human milk and, because of the potential for serious adverse effects in nursing infants, you should not take these drugs while nursing.

Vardenafil and tadalafil join sildenafil as the second and third oral drugs approved by the FDA to treat erectile dysfunction. All three drugs work the same way by inhibiting an enzyme known as phosphodiesterase type 5. Inhibition of this enzyme causes relaxation of

THE HEALTH RESEARCH GROUP'S SEVEN-YEAR RULE

You should wait at least seven years from the date of release to take any new drug unless it is one of those rare "breakthrough" drugs that offer you a documented therapeutic advantage over older proven drugs. New drugs are tested in a relatively small number of people before being released, and serious adverse effects or life-threatening drug interactions may not be detected until the new drug has been taken by hundreds of thousands of people. A number of new drugs have been withdrawn within their first seven years after release. Also, warnings about serious new adverse reactions have been added to the labeling of a number of drugs, or new drug interactions have been detected, usually within the first seven years after a drug's release.

smooth muscles and increased blood flow to the penis.

Many commonly used drugs can interfere with sexual function in both men and women, causing loss of libido, or can interfere with erection or ejaculation in men, or can delay or prevent orgasm in women. Drug-related adverse effects on sexual function may be difficult to distinguish from the effects of depression or disease, but most are reversible when drug use is stopped and sometimes when dosage is decreased. See p. 34 in Chapter 3 for a list of drugs that can interfere with sexual function.

In general, vardenafil, tadalafil, and sildenafil also should not be used in combination with the alpha-blocker family of drugs, which are used to treat high blood pressure and enlarged prostate (benign prostatic hyperplasia). These drugs include alfuzosin (UROXATRAL), doxazosin (CARDURA), prazosin (MINIPRESS), tamsulosin (FLOMAX), and terazosin (HYTRIN). Using alpha-blockers with these three erectile dysfunction drugs can cause a

---

DRUGS THAT SHOULD NOT BE USED WITH
VARDENAFIL, TADALAFIL, OR SILDENAFIL

NITROGLYCERIN-CONTAINING DRUGS

Deponit; Minitran; Nitrek; Nitro-Bid; Nitrocine; Nitro-Derm; Nitro Disc; Nitro-Dur; Nitrogard; Nitroglycerin; Nitroglycerin T/R; Nitroglyn; Nitrol Ointment; Nitrolan; Nitrolingual Spray; Nitrong; Nitropar; Nitropress; Nitro-prex; Nitro SA; Nitrospan; Nitrostat; Nitro Transdermal; Nitro-Trans System; Nitro-Time; Transderm-Nitro; Tridil.

ISOSORBIDE MONONITRATE–CONTAINING DRUGS

Dilatrate-SR; Imdur; ISMO; Isosorbide Mononitrate; Iso-bid; Isordil; Isordil Tembids; Isosorbide Dinitrate; Isosorbide Dinitrate LA; Isosorbide Nitrate; Monoket; Sorbitrate; Sorbitrate SA.

ALPHA-BLOCKERS

alfuzosin (UROXATRAL), doxazosin (CARDURA), prazosin (MINIPRESS), tamsulosin (FLOMAX), terazosin (HYTRIN).

ILLICIT SUBSTANCES CONTAINING NITRATES

Amyl nitrate or nitrite that goes by various names, including "poppers" and butyl nitrate.

---

dangerously low blood pressure that could lead ultimately to a stroke or heart attack.

The professional product labeling or package insert for tadalafil says not to take the drug with alpha-blockers other than tamsulosin.[2] The professional labeling for sildenafil says that the drug should not be taken in a dose greater than 25 milligrams at the same time (within four hours) of a dose of any alpha-blocker.[3] We advise consumers to be more cautious than this and avoid these erectile dysfunction drugs if they are taking an alpha-blocker.

There are a number of medical conditions in which vardenafil, tadalafil, and sildenafil should be used with caution, or not at all, because of the potential for an adverse outcome. These are:

- heart problems such as angina, heart failure, irregular heartbeats, or a heart attack;

ask your doctor if it is safe for you to have sexual activity
- low blood pressure or high blood pressure that is not controlled
- stroke
- liver problems
- kidney problems or dialysis
- retinitis pigmentosa, a rare genetic (runs in families) eye disease
- stomach ulcers
- bleeding problem, deformed penis shape, or Peyronie's disease
- erection that has lasted more than four hours
- blood cell problems such as sickle cell anemia, multiple myeloma, or leukemia

Vardenafil is unique among these three drugs in that there are precautions in the drug's professional product labeling about a condition known as QTc interval prolongation.[4] This is an abnormality in the heart's electrical conduction that can lead to fatal heart rhythm disturbances.

The QT interval is the length of time it takes the ventricles (large chambers of the heart) to discharge and recharge electrically. The QTc interval is measured on an electrocardiogram (EKG or ECG) in milliseconds (msec); the subscript "c" indicates that the QT interval has been corrected for the patient's heart rate. Prolongation of the QT interval can lead to heart rhythm disturbances (cardiac arrhythmias) such as torsades de pointes. *Torsades de pointes* is a French phrase meaning "twisted point," describing the appearance of this type of rhythm disturbance on the EKG tracing.

Men with congenital QT prolongation and those taking drugs for heart rhythm disturbances such as amiodarone (CORDARONE), procainamide (PROCANBID), quinidine (DURAQUIN, QUINAGLUTE DURA-TABS, QUINIDEX), and sotalol (BETAPACE) should not take vardenafil.

There are legitimate reasons for using the erectile dysfunction drugs when other causes of erectile dysfunction have been ruled out. However, when these drugs are used for recreational purposes by men who do not need them, the risks of the drugs always outweigh the benefits.

Before You Use This Drug

Do not use if you have or have had:

- unstable angina
- allergy to a phosphodiesterase inhibitor or any components of the tablets
- angina during sexual intercourse
- heart failure within the last three months
- severe heart failure
- retinal disorders
- uncontrolled high blood pressure
- low blood pressure
- stroke within the last six months

- heart attack within the past 90 days
- severe heart rhythm problems
- severe renal disorder
- severe liver disorder

Tell your doctor if you have or have had:

- penis abnormalities or disorder
- retinal disorder (retinitis pigmentosa)
- peptic ulcer
- heart or blood vessel disease
- bleeding disorder
- blood disorder
- liver disease
- stroke
- kidney disorder
- leukemia
- sickle cell anemia
- multiple myeloma

Tell your doctor about any other drugs you take, including aspirin, herbs, vitamins, and other nonprescription products.

When You Use This Drug

- Do not drink substantial amounts of alcohol.
- Be aware that these drugs do not protect against sexually transmitted diseases.
- Get immediate medical help if chest pain occurs after taking the drug.
- Get immediate medical help if an erection lasts longer than four hours.
- Know which other medicines cannot be taken along with these drugs, such as nitrates and alpha-blockers.
- Do not take any other drugs for impotence when you are taking one of these.

How to Use This Drug

- Read the patient package information before you start taking this drug.
- Drug begins to work within 30 minutes after taking it and its effect continues for up to 4

hours (sildenafil and vardenafil); tardenafil's effectiveness lasts up to 36 hours.

- Drug should be taken about one hour before sexual activity.
- Do not share your medication with others.
- These drugs can be taken with or without food.
- Store at room temperature with lid on tightly. Do not store in the bathroom. Do not expose to heat, moisture, or strong light. Keep out of reach of children.

Interactions with Other Drugs

The following drugs, biologics (e.g., vaccines, therapeutic antibodies), or foods are listed in *Evaluations of Drug Interactions* 2003 as causing "highly clinically significant" or "clinically significant" interactions when used together with any of the drugs in this section. In some sections with multiple drugs, the interaction may have been reported for one but not all drugs in this section, but we include the interaction because the drugs in this section are similar to one another. We have also included potentially serious interactions listed in the drug's FDA-approved professional package insert or in published medical journal articles. There may be other drugs, especially those in the families of drugs listed below, that also will react with this drug to cause severe adverse effects. Make sure to tell your doctor and pharmacist the drugs you are taking and tell them if you are taking any of these interacting drugs:

AGENERASE, amlodipine, amprenavir, amyl nitrate, cimetidine, CRIXIVAN, DE-PONIT, EES, erythrityl tetranitrate, ERYTHROCIN, erythromycin, FORTO-VASE, ILOSONE, IMDUR, indinivir, INVIRASE, ISMO, ISORDIL, isosorbide, itraconazole, ketoconazole, MINITRAN, nelfinavir, NIPRIDE, nitric oxide, NITRO-BID, NITRO-DUR, NITRODISC, nitroglycerin, NITROPRESS, nitroprusside, NITROSTAT, NIZORAL, NORVASC, NORVIR, pentaerythritol tetranitrate, PRIFTIN, RIFADIN, rifampin, rifapentine, RIMACTANE, ritonavir, saquinavir, SORBITRATE, SPORANOX, TAGAMET, TRANSDERM-NITRO, VIRACEPT.

See the box accompanying this drug profile for other drugs that should not be taken in combination with vardenafil, tadalafil, or sildenafil.

Adverse Effects

Call your doctor immediately if you experience:

- arm, back, or jaw pain
- bladder pain (sildenafil)
- any change in vision, including blurred vision, temporary vision loss, or color changes
- any change in eyes, including eye pain, bleeding, or swelling
- back and muscle pain
- change in heart rhythm
- breast enlargement (sildenafil)
- chest pain, heaviness, tightness, or discomfort
- chills
- cloudy or bloody urine (sildenafil)
- confusion
- deafness (sildenafil)
- dizziness
- drowsiness (sildenafil)
- faintness or lightheadedness
- fast or irregular heartbeat
- fever
- headache
- hoarseness (vardenafil)
- increased or decreased frequency of or painful urination (more likely with sildenafil)
- rash, hives, or itching of skin
- muscle weakness, aching, or cramping

- nausea or vomiting
- nervousness
- numbness of hands
- painful or swollen joints
- prolonged, painful, or inappropriate erection of the penis
- ringing or buzzing in the ears
- runny nose
- seizures (sildenafil)
- shortness of breath
- skin dryness, redness, scaling, or peeling
- sleep disturbances
- speech slurred
- swallowing difficulty
- sweating
- swelling of hands, feet, or lower legs
- swelling of eyelids, eyes, face, lips, or tongue
- thirst increased
- throat dry or sore
- unusual tiredness or weakness
- wheezing

Call your doctor if these symptoms continue:

- diarrhea
- indigestion, belching, or heartburn
- flushing
- headache
- nasal congestion
- abnormal dreams (sildenafil)
- abnormal sexual response
- acid or sour stomach
- anxiety (sildenafil)
- reduced appetite (vardenafil)
- asthma (sildenafil)
- back pain (tadalafil, vardenafil)
- belching
- bloody nose
- burning feeling in chest or stomach
- chills (vardenafil)
- clumsiness, unsteadiness, lack of coordination (sildenafil)
- cough
- difficulty moving

- difficulty seeing at night (vardenafil)
- dizziness
- dry mouth
- dry throat (tadalafil)
- ear pain (sildenafil)
- increased erection (tadalafil)
- increased sensitivity of eyes to sunlight (vardenafil)
- swelling of eyes or face (tadalafil, vardenafil)
- redness, pain, dryness, itching, burning, tearing, or swelling of eye, eyelid, or inner lining of eyelid (tadalafil, vardenafil)
- fatigue or sleepiness
- feelings of burning, crawling, itching, numbness, prickling, or tingling
- fever
- generalized pain or discomfort
- swollen, sore, or bleeding gums (sildenafil)
- hearing loss (vardenafil)
- heartburn (tadalafil, vardenafil)
- hoarseness (sildenafil, tadalafil)
- indigestion
- insomnia
- lack or loss of strength (tadalafil, vardenafil)
- limb pain (tadalafil)
- sores, ulcers, or white spots on lips, inside of mouth, or tongue
- mental depression (sildenafil)
- increased skin sensitivity to sunlight, resulting in sunburn (vardenafil)
- muscle or joint pain
- muscle tone changes
- nausea or vomiting
- swollen and tender neck glands (tadalafil)
- neck pain
- rectal bleeding (sildenafil)
- ringing in ears (sildenafil, vardenafil)
- shortness of breath or wheezing
- skin rash or itching
- stomach discomfort, upset, or pain following meals
- difficulty swallowing
- sweating

- swollen joints
- increased thirst (sildenafil)
- throat pain or burning
- reduced touch and pain sensations
- blurred, dimmed, or changed vision (including color vision)

- voice changes
- sinus problems (vardenafil)
- urinary frequency changes (sildenafil)

REFERENCES

1. Fazio L, Brock G. Erectile dysfunction: Management update. *Canadian Medical Association Journal* 2004; 170:1429–37.

2. Cialis (Tadalafil) Professional Product Labeling, November 1, 2003. Available at: http://www.fda.gov/cder/foi/label/2003/021368lbl.pdf. Accessed May 4, 2004.

3. *Physicians' Desk Reference.* 58th ed. Montvale, N.J.: Thomson PDR, 2004:2662–5.

4. Levitra (Vardenafil) Professional Product Labeling, August 1, 2003. Available at: http://www.univgraph.com/bayer/inserts/levitra.pdf. Accessed May 4, 2004.

21

DRUGS FOR URINARY DISORDERS

URINARY SYSTEM

The urinary system serves the function of ridding the body of certain toxic or unnecessary waste products. It begins in the kidney, where blood containing these toxins passes through a sieve-like structure, resulting in the retention in the filtered blood of all the needed elements. The remaining, unneeded chemicals pass from the kidneys as a liquid (urine) down two tubes (one for each kidney) called the ureters and into the bladder. There the urine waits until the bladder, which is actually a muscle, contracts and the urine is passed from the body through a single tube called the urethra during urination.

Most of the time this system works well, but problems may occur, especially in the elderly. One problem is that the muscles in the bladder may contract sporadically, leading to a loss of urine (incontinence). Typically the patient experiences these contractions as a sudden urge to urinate, and may not make it to the bathroom in time; this is called urge incontinence. Drug treatment for this condition seeks to prevent stimulation of the bladder muscles.

Alternatively, the bladder may be unable to contract adequately and urine thus accumulates in the bladder (urinary retention). Sometimes the bladder is so full it overflows, a condition called overflow incontinence. Drug treatment for this condition seeks to increase bladder contractions to aid urination.

Another form of incontinence is stress incontinence. This form of incontinence, not infrequent after childbirth, is a result of damage to the muscles in the pelvis. In this condition, a cough or a sneeze results in the leakage of urine. Muscle-strengthening exercises and, rarely, surgery are among the approaches to this condition.

It is important to distinguish between urge incontinence, overflow incontinence, stress incontinence, and a fourth form of incontinence called functional incontinence (incontinence due to ambulatory difficulties or inadequate access to a toilet), as each has different treatments.

Another common affliction of the urinary tract system is an infection called a urinary tract infection (UTI). If a UTI ascends the urinary tract it can enter the kidneys and cause lasting damage. The antibiotics that treat UTIs are discussed in Chapter 24; in this chapter we discuss a drug that is claimed to act as a painkiller for the urinary tract, especially during infections.

DRUG PROFILES

Anticholinergics

Limited Use

Oxybutynin (ox i *byoo* ti nin)
DITROPAN (Alza)
DITROPAN XL (Alza)
OXYTROL TRANSDERMAL SYSTEM (Watson)

GENERIC: available for non-extended-release oral forms

Tolterodine (*tole* tear oh deen)
DETROL (Pharmacia & Upjohn)
DETROL LA (Pharmacia & Upjohn)

GENERIC: not available
FAMILY: Anticholinergics

PREGNANCY WARNING

Tolterodine caused fetal harm in animal studies, including an increased incidence of cleft palate, abdominal hemorrhage, and various skeletal abnormalities. There do not appear to be adequate animal studies on oxybutynin. Because of the potential for serious adverse effects to the fetus, these drugs should not be used by pregnant women.

BREAST-FEEDING WARNING

Tolterodine is excreted in animal milk, and it is likely that this also occurs in humans. Information was lacking on oxybutynin. Because of the potential for serious adverse effects in nursing infants, you should not take these drugs while nursing.

Both oxybutynin and tolterodine are approved by the FDA to treat urge urinary incontinence (loss of bladder control due to sporadic contractions of the bladder muscle) and frequent urination. The drugs decrease the spasms in the bladder that produce these symptoms and increase the bladder's ability to hold urine. Although oxybutynin is used by some doctors to treat disorders of the stomach and intestines, it has not been proved effective for this purpose.

ANTICHOLINERGIC EFFECTS

WARNING: SPECIAL MENTAL AND PHYSICAL ADVERSE EFFECTS

Older adults are especially sensitive to the harmful anticholinergic (see Glossary, p. 889) effects of drugs such as oxybutynin and tolterodine. Drugs in this family should not be used unless absolutely necessary.

Mental Effects: confusion, delirium, short-term memory problems, disorientation, and impaired attention.

Physical Effects: dry mouth, constipation, difficulty urinating (especially for a man with an enlarged prostate), blurred vision, decreased sweating with increased body temperature, sexual dysfunction, and worsening of glaucoma.

These drugs are in the family known as anticholinergic agents. Such drugs block the effects of acetylcholine, a substance produced by the body that is responsible for certain nervous system (parasympathetic) activities. Drugs with anticholinergic effects (including antidepressants, antihistamines, antipsychotics, drugs for intestinal problems, antiparkinsonians) all inhibit the secretion of acid in the stomach; slow the passage of food through the digestive system; inhibit the production of saliva, sweat, and lung secretions; and increase heart rate and blood pressure. Adverse effects of these drugs thus include dry mouth, constipation, difficulty urinating, and decreased sweating. Other adverse effects are described in the accompanying box. Because both the effectiveness and the adverse effect profile of the drugs are related to their anticholinergic activity, more effective drugs or doses are likely to be more toxic. The drugs are contraindicated in patients with inability to urinate (urinary retention), gastric retention, or narrow-angle glaucoma.

Oxybutynin was first approved in 1975. For

years it dominated the incontinence market. It is now available as a less expensive generic. In 1998, tolterodine was approved by the FDA for the same indications. Reflecting the new competition in the market, Pharmacia & Upjohn, tolterodine's manufacturer, was twice cited by the FDA for overstating the benefits of the drug.[1]

In clinical trials, both drugs performed better than a placebo, although the extent of the drugs' effectiveness is disappointing. For example, in one trial comparing short-acting versions of the drugs, after subtracting the effects of the placebo, tolterodine reduced the number of episodes of incontinence per day by 0.5, compared to a reduction of 0.8 for oxybutynin.[1] A type of statistical summary of clinical trials known as a meta-analysis found tolterodine and oxybutynin to be clinically similar. Oxybutynin was statistically significantly more effective, but tolterodine was better tolerated.[2] Similarly, the editors of The Medical Letter on Drugs and Therapeutics concluded their review of tolterodine by saying, "Tolterodine appears to be tolerated better than older drugs for treatment of overactive bladder, but it may be less effective."[3]

Since the arrival of tolterodine, we have seen the marketing of extended-release versions of both oxybutynin (DITROPAN XL) and tolterodine (DETROL LA), as well as a skin patch (OXYTROL) that delivers oxybutynin and is applied every three to four days. All seek to improve patient compliance with the drugs by reducing the number of doses per day and to keep drug levels in the blood more stable. This might reduce anticholinergic adverse effects by avoiding the ups and downs associated with intermittent drug dosing. Indeed, clinical trials show that dry mouth, in particular, is less common with the extended-release formulations. However, as The Medical Letter points out, "Both the tolerability and the effectiveness of these drugs are related to their [anticholinergic] activity. The less dry mouth, the less effec-

tive they are likely to be. None of them are as effective as advertisements to the public have suggested."[4]

When the oxybutynin patch was introduced, The Medical Letter had a similar reaction: "Oxybutynin delivered transdermally may cause less dry mouth than when it is taken orally, but it may be less effective for incontinence, and itching at the application site can be a problem."[5] Here is why the authors reached that conclusion. In the first of two clinical trials described in the drug's product labeling, patch oxybutynin was compared to placebo in patients experiencing about 5.1 episodes of incontinence per day. At the end of 12 weeks, there was an average reduction in incontinence episodes of 3.0 per day in patients using the patch, compared to 2.7 in patients on placebo.[6] In the second study in the labeling, patients who had previously responded to an anticholinergic drug and had approximately 4.9 incontinence episodes per day were studied for 12 weeks. The average daily reduction in incontinence episodes was 2.9 in the patch-treated group, compared to 2.1 in the placebo group.[7] These are not major differences.

There are also effective nondrug treatments available to manage urge urinary incontinence. In our view, a proper trial of these should precede drug treatment whenever possible. The first randomized trial of behavioral treatment compared to a drug (oxybutynin) was conducted in older women and actually showed the behavioral intervention to be more effective. Behavioral treatment (four treatments including biofeedback on contraction of pelvic muscles) reduced the number of incontinence episodes by 81% compared with 69% for oxybutynin and 39% for placebo. The authors concluded, "Behavioral treatment is a safe and effective conservative intervention that should be made more readily available to patients as a first-line treatment for urge and mixed incontinence."[8] A follow-up study in which patients were given the option of adding the other treatment (biofeedback for the oxybutynin group and oxybutynin for the biofeedback group) suggested that the combination is more effective than either treatment alone.[9] The least invasive or dangerous treatment should be tried first, and for many forms of urinary incontinence this is behavioral treatment rather than drugs.

Importantly, there are a number of drugs that can cause loss of bladder control. A list of these drugs can be found on p. 41.

Before You Use This Drug

Do not use if you have or have had:

- allergy to tolterodine or oxybutynin
- glaucoma, narrow-angle, that is not controlled
- pregnancy or are breast-feeding
- stomach empties slowly
- urinary retention

Tell your doctor if you have or have had:

- abdominal obstruction or disease
- allergies to drugs
- bladder obstruction
- bleeding that is severe (oxybutynin)
- diarrhea
- dry mouth that is severe and continuing
- glaucoma, narrow-angle, controlled
- heart disease
- heartbeat that is rapid
- hiatal hernia with heartburn (oxybutynin)
- high blood pressure (oxybutynin)
- kidney problems
- liver problems
- myasthenia gravis (oxybutynin)
- prostate that is enlarged
- reflux from the stomach
- thyroid gland that is overactive (hyperthyroidism) (oxybutynin)
- toxemia of pregnancy/preeclampsia (oxybutynin)
- ulcerative colitis that is severe (oxybutynin)

Tell your doctor about any other drugs you take, including aspirin, herbs, vitamins, and other nonprescription products.

When You Use This Drug

- Until you know how you react to this drug, do not drive or perform other activities requiring alertness.
- Do not drink alcoholic beverages.
- Wear sunglasses if bothered by sunlight.
- Do not exercise in hot weather.
- Be aware that you are especially susceptible to glaucoma if you are over 40 years old.

How to Use This Drug

- If you miss a dose, take it as soon as you remember, but skip it if it is almost time for the next dose. **Do not take double doses.**
- Do not share your medication with others.
- Take the drug at the same time(s) each day.
- Take with **a full glass (eight ounces) of water** or take with food or milk if stomach irritation occurs (oxybutynin).
- Take with **a full glass (eight ounces) of water** (tolterodine).
- Do not break, chew, or crush extended-release forms.
- If you have dry mouth, use sugarless candy or gum, ice, or saliva substitute; check with your doctor or dentist if dry mouth continues for more than two weeks.
- Store at room temperature with lid on tightly. Do not store in the bathroom. Do not expose to heat, moisture, or strong light. Keep out of reach of children.

Interactions with Other Drugs

The following drugs, biologics (e.g., vaccines, therapeutic antibodies), or foods are listed in *Evaluations of Drug Interactions* 2003 as causing "highly clinically significant" or "clinically significant" interactions when used together with any of the drugs in this section. In some sections with multiple drugs, the interaction may have been reported for one but not all drugs in this section, but we include the interaction because the drugs in this section are similar to one another. We have also included potentially serious interactions listed in the drug's FDA-approved professional package insert or in published medical journal articles. There may be other drugs, especially those in the families of drugs listed below, that also will react with this drug to cause severe adverse effects. Make sure to tell your doctor and pharmacist the drugs you are taking and tell them if you are taking any of these interacting drugs:

BIAXIN, clarithromycin, COUMADIN, DIFLUCAN, ERYCETTE, erythromycin, fluconazole, fluoxetine, itraconazole, ketoconazole, miconazole, MONISTAT, NIZORAL, PCE, PROZAC, SPORANOX, warfarin.

Adverse Effects

Call your doctor immediately if you experience:

- eye pain
- rash or hives
- urination problems: difficult, painful, or burning urination; increased frequency of urination; bloody or cloudy urine
- vision that is abnormal, including difficulty in adjusting to distances

Call your doctor if these symptoms continue:

- breast milk flow decreased (oxybutynin)
- chest pain (tolterodine)
- constipation
- diarrhea
- dizziness (tolterodine)
- drowsiness

- eyes dry
- eyes sensitive to light
- headache
- mouth, nose, and throat dry
- nausea
- sexual ability decreased
- sleeping difficulty
- swallowing difficulty
- sweating decreased
- tiredness or weakness that is unusual
- urination difficult
- vomiting

Signs of overdose for oxybutynin:

- breathing difficulty or shortness of breath
- clumsiness or unsteadiness
- confusion
- dizziness
- drowsiness that is severe
- face flushed or red
- fever
- hallucinations
- heartbeat that is rapid
- nervousness, restlessness, excitement, or irritability that is unusual

If you suspect an overdose, call this number to contact your poison control center: (800) 222-1222.

Periodic Tests

Ask your doctor which of these tests should be done periodically while you are taking this drug:

- cystometry (a test for pressure in the urinary bladder)

Cholinergics

Limited Use

Bethanechol (be *than* e kole)
URECHOLINE (Odyssey)

GENERIC: available
FAMILY: Cholinergics

PREGNANCY WARNING

No data are available for bethanechol from either animal or human studies. Use during pregnancy only for clear medical reasons. Tell your doctor if you are pregnant or thinking of becoming pregnant before you take this drug.

BREAST-FEEDING WARNING

No information is available from either human or animal studies. Since it is likely that this drug, like many others, is excreted in human milk, you should consult with your doctor if you are planning to nurse.

Under certain circumstances (e.g., after spinal cord injury, surgery, or childbirth), urine accumulates in the bladder, which cannot be emptied. This is a potentially serious condition, because in addition to the obvious discomfort, the bladder can even rupture in rare cases. Bethanechol helps stimulate the emptying of the bladder by causing the bladder to contract. The contraction of the bladder is stimulated by a neurotransmitter called acetylcholine, and bethanechol performs the same function as acetylcholine; for this reason it is known as a cholinergic drug. However, its use has generally been replaced by more effective agents.[10]

Although some doctors use the drug to prevent the backward flow of stomach contents into the esophagus (reflux esophagitis), evidence to support this use is very limited[11] and the FDA has not approved the drug for this purpose. This condition, also known as Gastroesophageal reflux disease (GERD), and its treatment are discussed on p. 529.

The drug should not be used if the bladder or gastrointestinal wall may be weak, as the increased contractions may lead to rupture. Such conditions include mechanical obstruction, surgery, and inflammation.

Importantly, there are a number of drugs that can cause urinary retention. A list of these drugs can be found on p. 41.

Before You Use This Drug

Tell your doctor if you have or have had:

- allergy to bethanechol
- asthma
- bladder disorder or obstruction
- blood pressure that is high or low
- constipation
- coronary artery disease
- epilepsy
- heart problems
- hyperthyroidism (overactive thyroid gland)
- intestinal disorder or obstruction
- Parkinson's disease
- peritonitis
- pregnancy or are breast-feeding
- recent surgery to the abdomen
- recent surgery to the urinary bladder
- sweating that is excessive
- ulcer of the stomach or duodenum

Tell your doctor about any other drugs you take, including aspirin, herbs, vitamins, and other nonprescription products.

When You Use This Drug

- You may feel dizzy when rising from a lying or sitting position. When getting out of bed, hang your legs over the side of the bed for a few minutes, then get up slowly. When getting up from a chair, stay by the chair until you are sure that you are not dizzy. (See p. 13.)

How to Use This Drug

• If you miss a dose, take it as soon as you remember, but skip it if it is two or more hours after the time you would have taken it. **Do not take double doses.**

• Do not share your medication with others.

• Take the drug at the same time(s) each day.

• Do not eat or drink for about an hour before or after taking this medication.

Interactions with Other Drugs

Evaluations of Drug Interactions 2003 lists no drugs, biologics (e.g., vaccines, therapeutic antibodies), or foods as causing "highly clinically significant" or "clinically significant" interactions when used together with the drugs in this section. We also found no interactions in the drugs' FDA-approved professional package inserts. However, as the number of new drugs approved for marketing increases and as more experience is gained with these drugs over time, new interactions may be discovered.

Adverse Effects

Call your doctor immediately if you experience:

• shortness of breath, wheezing, or chest tightness

Call your doctor if these symptoms continue:

• belching
• diarrhea
• dizziness or lightheadedness
• faint feeling
• headache
• mouth watering
• nausea or vomiting
• nervousness
• seizures

• skin red, flushed, or feeling warm
• sleeping difficulty
• stomach discomfort or pain
• sweating increased
• urinate, frequent urge to
• vision changes

Urinary Tract Analgesics

Do Not Use

ALTERNATIVE TREATMENT:
Drink plenty of fluids and treat the cause of the pain, such as the urinary tract infection.

Phenazopyridine (fen az oh *peer* i deen)
PYRIDIUM (Warner-Chilcott)

FAMILY: Urinary Tract Analgesics (Painkillers)

Phenazopyridine is approved by the FDA to treat pain, burning, and other symptoms when the lower part of the urinary tract (bladder and urethra) is irritated due to an infection or surgery. Much of its apparent effectiveness appears to derive from the fact that it turns the urine reddish-orange, making patients more likely to conclude that the drug is having an effect. Because older people's kidneys eliminate drugs less effectively than younger people's, this drug can stay in an older person's system much longer than it should and can build up until it reaches dangerously high levels in the bloodstream. This can lead to harmful adverse effects such as anemia and liver damage. In addition, according to the World Health Organization's International Agency for Research on Cancer, phenazopyridine can cause cancer.[12]

Despite the drug's questionable effectiveness (the FDA recommends not using it for more than two days)[13] and its propensity to cause cancer, the drug is available over the counter (OTC). Misuse of the OTC versions (e.g., Azo-

Standard, Prodium, Uristat) is rife: 51% of patients used the drug inappropriately and 38% used it as a substitute for medical care.[14]

Phenazopyridine is also sometimes combined with antibiotics in prescription drugs, although the National Academy of Sciences has concluded that the evidence for the effectiveness of these combinations is lacking.[15]

Instead of prescribing this drug to relieve pain and irritation, a physician should find and treat the cause of the pain and irritation and use conventional painkillers if necessary.

REFERENCES

1. Tolterodine (DETROL)—another drug for urinary incontinence. *Worst Pills, Best Pills News* 1999; 5:44–6.

2. Harvey MA, Baker K, Wells GA. Tolterodine versus oxybutynin in the treatment of urge urinary incontinence: A meta-analysis. *American Journal of Obstetrics and Gynecology* 2001; 185:56–61.

3. Tolterodine for overactive bladder. *Medical Letter on Drugs and Therapeutics* 1998; 40:101–2.

4. Detrol LA and Ditropan XL for overactive bladder. *Medical Letter on Drugs and Therapeutics* 2001; 43:28.

5. Oxybutynin transdermal (Oxytrol) for overactive bladder. *Medical Letter on Drugs and Therapeutics* 2003; 45:38–9.

6. Dmochowski RR, Davila GW, Zinner NR, et al. Efficacy and safety of transdermal oxybutynin in patients with urge and mixed urinary incontinence. *Journal of Urology* 2002; 168:580–6.

7. Dmochowski RR, Sand PK, Zinner NR, et al. Comparative efficacy and safety of transdermal oxybutynin and oral tolterodine versus placebo in previously treated patients with urge and mixed urinary incontinence. *Urology* 2003; 62:237–42.

8. Burgio KL, Locher JL, Goode PS, et al. Behavioral vs drug treatment for urge urinary incontinence in older women: A randomized controlled trial. *Journal of the American Medical Association* 1998; 280:1995–2000.

9. Burgio KL, Locher JL, Goode PS. Combined behavioral and drug therapy for urge incontinence in older women. *Journal of the American Geriatric Society* 2000; 48:370–4.

10. *USP DI, Drug Information for the Health Care Professional.* Greenwood Village, Colo.: MICROMEDEX, 2003:569.

11. Drugs for esophageal reflux. *Medical Letter on Drugs and Therapeutics* 1980; 22:26–8.

12. *International Agency for Research on Cancer Monographs on the Evaluation of the Carcinogenic Risk to Humans: Some Pharmaceutical Drugs.* Lyon, France: International Agency for Research on Cancer, 1980:163.

13. *Physicians' Desk Reference.* 54th ed. Montvale, N.J.: Medical Economics Company, 2000:3164.

14. Shi CW, Asch SM, Fielder E, et al. Usage patterns of over-the-counter phenazopyridine (pyridium). *Journal of General Internal Medicine* 2003; 18:281–7.

15. *Physicians' Desk Reference.* 58th ed. Montvale, N.J.: Thomson PDR, 2004:2654.

22

DRUGS FOR NEUROLOGICAL DISORDERS

DRUG PROFILES

Parkinson's Disease

 Do Not Use

ALTERNATIVE TREATMENT:
*See other drugs for Parkinson's disease
in this section.*

Benztropine (*benz* troe peen)

Trihexyphenidyl (try hex ee *fen* i dill)

FAMILY: Drugs for Parkinson's Disease

Trihexyphenidyl and benztropine are approved by the FDA for the symptoms of Parkinson's disease and to manage the drug-induced movement disorders that may result from some of the drugs used to treat serious mental illness.

Drugs like trihexyphenidyl and benztropine, also known as anticholinergics, were the first drugs available for the symptomatic treatment of Parkinson's disease.[1]

These drugs should not be used to treat Parkinson's disease because they can cause several serious anticholinergic adverse effects (see Glossary, p. 889)—more frequently in older adults. These effects include memory impairment, confusion, hallucinations, and retention of urine.

A major statistical summary of clinical trials, known as a meta-analysis, concluded: *"As monotherapy or as an adjunct to other antiparkinsonian drugs, anticholinergics are more effective than placebo in improving motor function in Parkinson's disease. Neuropsychiatric and cognitive adverse events occur more frequently on anticholinergics than on placebo and are a more common reason for withdrawal than lack of efficacy."*[1]

An Australian review of treating Parkinson's disease in older patients concluded: *"Anticholinergic drugs such as benztropine and benzhexol [British generic name for trihexyphenidyl] are best avoided because of the high risk of major side effects."*[2]

If you have symptoms of parkinsonism (tremor, rigid muscles, and disturbances in posture, walking, balance, speech, swallowing, and muscle strength), there is a good chance that they are caused by a drug you are taking. As many as half of older adults with symptoms of parkinsonism may have developed them as adverse effects of a drug. A list of drugs that can

> Trihexyphenidyl and benztropine are appropriate drugs to manage the drug-induced movement disorders that may be seen with the use of drugs for treating serious mental illness (see p. 625).

ANTICHOLINERGIC EFFECTS

WARNING: SPECIAL MENTAL AND PHYSICAL ADVERSE EFFECTS

Older adults are especially sensitive to the harmful anticholinergic (see Glossary, p. 889) effects of this drug. Drugs in this family should not be used unless absolutely necessary.

Mental Effects: confusion, delirium, short-term memory problems, disorientation, and impaired attention.

Physical Effects: dry mouth, constipation, difficulty urinating (especially for a man with an enlarged prostate), blurred vision, decreased sweating with increased body temperature, sexual dysfunction, and worsening of glaucoma.

DO NOT USE BROMOCRIPTINE FOR POSTPARTUM BREAST ENGORGEMENT

This drug has caused heart attacks, strokes, and seizures in young, healthy women who were prescribed bromocriptine to suppress lactation after giving birth (postpartum lactation suppression) when safer, more effective nondrug measures were available.

The Health Research Group ultimately had to file suit against the FDA to remove postpartum lactation suppression as an approved use for bromocriptine in 1995.

cause symptoms of parkinsonism appears on p. 30. If you take any of the drugs on this list, discuss the possibility of drug-induced parkinsonism with your doctor and ask to have your prescription changed or stopped.

Limited Use

Bromocriptine (broe moe *krip* teen)
PARLODEL (Novartis)

GENERIC: available
FAMILY: Drugs for Parkinson's Disease

PREGNANCY WARNING

Ergot alkaloids can cause fetal harm when administered to a pregnant woman. If you are pregnant or suspect that you may be pregnant, you should not take this drug.

BREAST-FEEDING WARNING

Ergot alkaloids are excreted in human milk. Because of the potential for serious adverse effects in nursing infants, you should not take this drug while nursing.

Bromocriptine is derived from "ergot," and has several uses. Here we discuss its use for Parkin-

son's disease, for which it is the second-choice drug, after a combination of levodopa and carbidopa (see p. 631). If you have Parkinson's disease, your doctor should first try levodopa with carbidopa and should prescribe bromocriptine only if the combination drug does not decrease your symptoms or if it causes too many adverse effects. Bromocriptine often works best when given with levodopa. If you are over 60, you should generally be taking less than the usual adult dose.

In older adults, bromocriptine often causes dizziness, nausea, constipation, and tingling in fingers or toes when exposed to the cold. It can also cause more serious adverse effects called choreiform movements—unusual and uncontrolled movements in the body, face, tongue, arms, hands, and upper body. About 25% of bromocriptine users in all age groups experience this adverse effect. If you have any of these symptoms, especially if they are severe or persistent, call your doctor and ask if your dose of bromocriptine should be reduced. Do not take less bromocriptine than your doctor prescribed unless he or she instructs you to do so.

If you have symptoms of parkinsonism (tremor, rigid muscles, and disturbances in posture, walking, balance, speech, swallowing, and

HEAT STRESS ALERT

This drug can affect your body's ability to adjust to heat, putting you at risk of "heat stress." If you live alone, ask a friend to check on you several times during the day. Early signs of heat stress are dizziness, lightheadedness, faintness, and slightly high temperature. Call your doctor if you have any of these signs. Drink more fluids (water, fruit and vegetable juices) than usual—even if you're not thirsty—unless your doctor has told you otherwise. Do not drink alcohol.

muscle strength), there is a good chance that they are caused by a drug you are taking. As many as half of older adults with symptoms of parkinsonism may have developed them as adverse effects of a drug. A list of drugs that can cause symptoms of parkinsonism appears on p. 30. If you take any of the drugs on this list, discuss the possibility of drug-induced parkinsonism with your doctor and ask to have your prescription changed or stopped.

Before You Use This Drug

Do not use if you have or have had:

- pregnancy or are breast-feeding

Tell your doctor if you have or have had:

- allergies to bromocriptine or other ergot alkaloids
- liver problems
- mental illness
- high blood pressure

Tell your doctor about any other drugs you take, including aspirin, herbs, vitamins, and other nonprescription products.

When You Use This Drug

- Do not use more or less often or in a higher or lower dose than prescribed. Higher doses in-

crease the risk of adverse effects, while lower doses may worsen symptoms of parkinsonism.
- Until you know how you react to this drug, do not drive or perform other activities requiring alertness. Bromocriptine can cause drowsiness and lightheadedness.
- You may feel dizzy when rising from a lying or sitting position. When getting out of bed, hang your legs over the side of the bed for a few minutes, then get up slowly. When getting up from a chair, stay by the chair until you are sure that you are not dizzy. (See p. 13.)
- Do not drink alcohol while using this drug.
- If you get dry mouth, use sugarless gum or candy, ice, or saliva substitute. Check with your doctor or dentist if dry mouth continues for more than two weeks.
- Have regular checkups with your doctor to monitor progress.

How to Use This Drug

- Take with food or milk.
- Store at room temperature with lid on tightly. Do not store in the bathroom. Do not expose to heat, moisture, or strong light. Keep out of reach of children.
- If you miss a dose, take it as soon as you remember, but skip it if it is more than four hours since the last dose. Do not take double doses.
- Do not share your medication with others.
- Take the drug at the same time(s) each day.

Interactions with Other Drugs

The following drugs, biologics (e.g., vaccines, therapeutic antibodies), or foods are listed in *Evaluations of Drug Interactions* 2003 as causing "highly clinically significant" or "clinically significant" interactions when used together with any of the drugs in this section. In some sections with multiple drugs, the interaction may have been reported for one but not all drugs in this section, but we include the inter-

action because the drugs in this section are
similar to one another. We have also included
potentially serious interactions listed in the
drug's FDA-approved professional package insert or in published medical journal articles.
There may be other drugs, especially those in
the families of drugs listed below, that also will
react with this drug to cause severe adverse
effects. Make sure to tell your doctor and
pharmacist the drugs you are taking and tell
them if you are taking any of these interacting
drugs:

CRIXIVAN, delavirdine, efavirenz, FORTO-
VASE, HALDOL, haloperidol, indinavir, IN-
VIRASE, MAXALT, MELLARIL, MERIDIA,
metoclopramide, ORAP, pimozide, REGLAN,
REQUIP, RESCRIPTOR, rizatriptan, ropinirole, saquinavir, sibutramine, SUSTIVA,
thioridazine.

Adverse Effects

Call your doctor immediately if you experi-
ence:

- confusion
- uncontrolled body movements, particularly
  of the face, tongue, arms, hands, head, and
  upper body
- hallucinations
- severe chest pain
- fainting
- fast heartbeat
- increased sweating
- continuing or severe nausea and vomiting
- nervousness
- unexplained shortness of breath
- weakness
- atypical headache
- blurred vision or temporary blindness
- black, tarry stools
- bloody vomit
- severe or continuing abdominal or stomach
  pain
- increased frequency of urination

- loss of appetite
- lower back pain

Call your doctor if these symptoms con-
tinue:

- dizziness or lightheadedness
- nausea
- constipation
- diarrhea
- drowsiness or tiredness
- dry mouth
- nighttime leg cramps
- appetite loss
- mental depression
- tingling or pain in fingers or toes when exposed to cold
- stomach pain
- stuffy nose
- vomiting

Periodic Tests

Ask your doctor which of these tests should
be done periodically while you are taking
this drug:

- blood pressure

Limited Use

Entacapone (in *tack* a pohn)
COMTAN (Novartis)

Entacapone with levodopa and carbidopa
STALEVO (Novartis)

GENERIC: not available

If you are taking the combination of entacapone with levodopa and carbidopa, refer to information about levodopa
with carbidopa on p.631.

FAMILY: Drugs for Parkinson's Disease
         Catechol-O-Methyltransferase (COMT) Inhibitors

These drugs caused fetal harm in animal studies, including abortions, resorptions and decreased fetal weights, as well as malformed eyes, viscera, and skeleton. Because of the potential for serious adverse effects to the fetus, these drugs should not be used by pregnant women.

These drugs are excreted in animal milk. It is likely that these drugs, like many others, are also excreted in human milk. Because of the potential for serious adverse effects in nursing infants, you should not take these drugs while nursing.

Entacapone was approved by the FDA in October 1999 to be used along with the combination levodopa and carbidopa (SINEMET) (see p. 631) to treat Parkinson's disease in patients who experience the signs and symptoms of end-of-dose "wearing off." Entacapone's effectiveness has not been systematically evaluated in patients with Parkinson's disease who do not experience end-of-dose "wearing off."[3]

Entacapone is not used alone. Rather, it is used to improve the response to the medication levodopa (see p. 631), which is used to treat parkinsonism. Various strengths of levodopa are combined with the drug carbidopa in a formulation called Sinemet. Various strengths of levodopa and carbidopa are also combined with entacapone in a formulation called Stalevo.

When people with parkinsonism take levodopa, it replenishes dopamine and controls involuntary movements. However, after a few years levodopa is less effective, leading to imbalance and gait-freeze.[4-6] Changes in the dose of levodopa or the interval between doses alone may improve control. If the effect of wearing off before the next dose persists, then several other measures are considered to improve control of Parkinson's. Wearing off is sometimes signaled by curled toes or inverted foot. Other measures to prevent wearing off of levodopa include other drugs, physical therapy, and surgery.

Entacapone inhibits the enzyme COMT (catechol-O-methyltransferase), which breaks down levodopa, allowing levodopa to stay in the body, especially the brain, longer, preventing wearing off of levodopa.[4,7,8] This improves more balanced mobility and the ability to perform daily living activities.[9-11] Since entacapone increases levodopa levels, more adverse effects of levodopa are seen. These include involuntary movements, nausea, and occurrence of hallucination.

Tolcapone (see p. 637), another COMT inhibitor, available in the United States, is listed as a **Do Not Use** drug because of its liver toxicity.

Although entacapone can help improve muscle control, it can damage muscles and cause involuntary movement of muscles that seem contorted, or repetitive movements of face, tongue, or arms and legs. Some people develop hallucinations. A sudden drop in blood pressure may occur when changing position.[3]

The Medical Letter, a highly respected source of independent drug information for physicians and pharmacists, found entacapone to be "modestly effective in prolonging the effectiveness of levodopa in Parkinson's disease patients with 'wearing-off' motor fluctuations."[12]

The Medical Letter reviewed Stalevo in their May 2004 issue and expressed concern about the ease of use of this fixed-dose combination of three drugs: "Because of the fixed dose of entacapone, only one Stalevo tablet can be taken at each dosing interval. Stalevo tablets (which are not scored) should not be cut in half; doing so would reduce the dose of entacapone by half, which may be ineffective. Patients requiring more than 150 mg of levodopa per dose would have to take an additional carbidopa/levodopa pill. Those who are on different doses of levodopa through the day may require different Stalevo prescriptions for each one. This might cause more confusion because Stalevo pills, although shaped differently, are all the same color. Finally, patients who take controlled-release levodopa preparations (which are only 70% as bioavailable as immediate-release) plus entacapone cannot easily be switched to Stalevo.[13]

The following sections refer only to enta-capone; see p. 631 for levodopa and car-bidopa.

Before You Use This Drug

Do not use if you have or have had:

- allergy to entacapone

Tell your doctor if you have or have had:

- low blood pressure
- fainting spells
- involuntary movements
- liver problems
- pregnancy or are breast-feeding

Tell your doctor about any other drugs you take, including aspirin, herbs, vitamins, and other nonprescription products.

When You Use This Drug

- Have regular visits to your doctor to monitor progress.
- Do not drive or operate equipment requiring alertness until you know whether or not you develop dizziness, drowsiness, hallucinations, involuntary muscle movements, or change in blood pressure.
- Change positions gradually when going from lying down to sitting, or sitting to standing.
- Tell any doctor, dentist, emergency help, pharmacist, or surgeon you see that you use entacapone.
- Always take this drug with levodopa/carbidopa; never take it by itself.
- Check with your doctor before discontinuing this drug; gradual dosage reduction may be needed.
- Drug may cause urine to turn brownish-orange. There is no need to contact your doctor if this happens.

How to Use This Drug

- Take at the same times of day that you take levodopa/carbidopa. Take with or without food, but be consistent.
- If you miss a dose, take it as soon as you remember, but skip it if it is almost time for the next dose. **Do not take double doses.**
- Do not share your medication with others.
- Take the drug at the same time(s) each day.
- Store at room temperature with lid on tightly. Do not store in the bathroom. Do not expose to heat, moisture, or strong light. Keep out of reach of children.

Interactions with Other Drugs

The following drugs, biologics (e.g., vaccines, therapeutic antibodies), or foods are listed in *Evaluations of Drug Interactions* 2003 as causing "highly clinically significant" or "clinically significant" interactions when used together with any of the drugs in this section. In some sections with multiple drugs, the interaction may have been reported for one but not all drugs in this section, but we include the interaction because the drugs in this section are similar to one another. We have also included potentially serious interactions listed in the drug's FDA-approved professional package insert or in published medical journal articles. There may be other drugs, especially those in the families of drugs listed below, that also will react with this drug to cause severe adverse effects. Make sure to tell your doctor and pharmacist the drugs you are taking and tell them if you are taking any of these interacting drugs:

ALDOMET, amitriptyline, amoxapine, ANAFRANIL, apomorphine, AVENTYL, clomipramine, desipramine, dobutamine, DOBUTREX, dopamine, doxepin, EFFEXOR, ELAVIL, ELDEPRYL, furazolidone, hypericum, imipramine, iron supplements, isocarboxazid, isoproterenol, ISUPREL, LEVOPHED, LUDIOMIL, maprotiline,

MARPLAN, MATULANE, methyldopa, moclobemide, NARDIL, norepinephrine, NORPRAMIN, nortriptyline, pargyline, PARNATE, phenelzine, procarbazine, protriptyline, selegiline, SINEQUAN, SURMONTIL, TOFRANIL, tranylcypromine, trimipramine, venlafaxine, VIVACTIL.

Adverse Effects

Call your doctor immediately if you experience:

- twitching
- twisting
- uncontrolled repetitive movements of tongue, lips, face, arms, or legs
- hallucinations
- hyperactivity
- increase in body movements
- absence of or decrease in body movements
- fever
- chills
- cough or hoarseness
- lower back or side pain
- painful or difficult urination
- confusion
- shortness of breath
- muscle cramps
- pain
- stiffness
- weakness
- unusual tiredness

Call your doctor if these symptoms continue:

- abdominal pain
- small red spots on skin
- bruising
- sleepiness or unusual drowsiness
- increased sweating
- acid or sour stomach
- anxiety
- back pain
- belching
- burning feeling in chest or stomach

- constipation
- diarrhea
- difficult or labored breathing
- dizziness
- dry mouth
- fatigue
- heartburn
- indigestion
- irritability
- loss of strength or energy
- muscle pain or weakness
- nausea
- nervousness
- passing gas
- restlessness
- shortness of breath
- stomach discomfort, upset, or pain
- tenderness in stomach area
- tightness in chest
- tremor
- unusual weak feeling
- vomiting
- wheezing
- unusual or unpleasant taste in mouth

Levodopa and Carbidopa (*lee* voe doe pa and *kar* bi doe pa)
SINEMET (Bristol-Myers Squibb)
SINEMET CR (Bristol-Myers Squibb)

GENERIC: available

FAMILY: Drugs for Parkinson's Disease

PREGNANCY WARNING

Levodopa and carbidopa caused fetal harm in animal studies, including malformations and death. Because of the potential for serious adverse effects to the fetus, this drug should not be used by pregnant women.

BREAST-FEEDING WARNING

No information is available from either human or animal studies. Since it is likely that this drug, like many others, is excreted in human milk, and because of the potential for adverse effects in nursing infants, you should not take this drug while nursing.

The combination of levodopa and carbidopa is used to treat Parkinson's disease, a condition that produces tremor (shaking), rigid muscles, and disturbances in posture, walking, balance, speech, swallowing, and muscle strength. This is the better choice for treating Parkinson's disease than levodopa alone, because carbidopa prevents the breakdown of levodopa in the body.

The editors of *The Medical Letter,* a respected independent source of drug information, say that "the combination of these two drugs is the most effective treatment available for symptomatic relief of Parkinson's disease." [14]

Levodopa is effective for the majority of patients during the first two to five years of therapy. As the course of the disease progresses, the duration of benefit of a dose becomes shorter. This is known as the "wearing off" effect. Some patients develop sudden, unpredictable fluctuations between being able to move and not being able to move. This is referred to as the "on-off" effect.[14]

If you take levodopa alone, you should avoid foods and vitamins that contain vitamin B_6 (pyridoxine), since this vitamin can destroy the drug's effectiveness. To keep your intake of vitamin B_6 down, you should avoid multiple vitamins, avocados, beans, peas, sweet potatoes, dry skim milk, oatmeal, pork, bacon, beef liver, tuna, and cereals fortified with vitamin B_6. If you take carbidopa and levodopa, you do not need to worry about this.

If you have symptoms of parkinsonism (tremor, rigid muscles, and disturbances in posture, walking, balance, speech, swallowing, and muscle strength), there is a good chance that they are caused by a drug you are taking. As many as half of older adults with symptoms of parkinsonism may have developed them as adverse effects of a drug. A list of drugs that can cause symptoms of parkinsonism appears on p. 30. If you take any of the drugs on this list, discuss the possibility of drug-induced parkinsonism with your doctor and ask to have your prescription changed or stopped.

Before You Use This Drug

Tell your doctor if you have or have had:

- allergies to carbidopa and/or levodopa
- pregnancy or are breast-feeding
- bronchial emphysema, asthma, or other chronic lung disease
- heart or blood vessel disease
- diabetes
- hormone problems
- skin cancer
- glaucoma
- stomach ulcer
- seizure disorder or epilepsy
- kidney disease
- liver problems
- mental depression or psychosis

Tell your doctor about any other drugs you take, including aspirin, herbs, vitamins, and other nonprescription products.

When You Use This Drug

- Maximum effectiveness of drug may not occur for several weeks or months after starting therapy.
- Until you know how you react to this drug, do not drive or perform other activities requiring alertness. This drug can cause faintness and lightheadedness.
- You may feel dizzy when rising from a lying or sitting position. When getting out of bed, hang your legs over the side of the bed for a few minutes, then get up slowly. When getting up from a chair, stay by the chair until you are sure that you are not dizzy. (See p. 13.)
- **Caution diabetics:** This drug may interfere with urine tests for sugar and ketones.
- If you plan to have any surgery, including dental, tell your doctor that you take this drug.
- You may experience difficulty in retaining full dentures.
- Drug may darken urine, saliva, or sweat.

How to Use This Drug

• Take with meals or snacks for the first few months until tolerance for the stomach side effects occurs. Then, take with water only. Do not eat or drink for about an hour before taking this medication. An empty stomach is necessary for this drug to be absorbed maximally.

• If you miss a dose, take it as soon as you remember, but skip it if it is within two hours of the next dose. **Do not take double doses.**

• Do not share your medication with others.

• Take the drug at the same time(s) each day.

• Store at room temperature with lid on tightly. Do not store in the bathroom. Do not expose to heat, moisture, or strong light. Keep out of reach of children.

Interactions with Other Drugs

The following drugs, biologics (e.g., vaccines, therapeutic antibodies), or foods are listed in *Evaluations of Drug Interactions* 2003 as causing "highly clinically significant" or "clinically significant" interactions when used together with any of the drugs in this section. In some sections with multiple drugs, the interaction may have been reported for one but not all drugs in this section, but we include the interaction because the drugs in this section are similar to one another. We have also included potentially serious interactions listed in the drug's FDA-approved professional package insert or in published medical journal articles. There may be other drugs, especially those in the families of drugs listed below, that also will react with this drug to cause severe adverse effects. Make sure to tell your doctor and pharmacist the drugs you are taking and tell them if you are taking any of these interacting drugs:

amitriptyline, chlorpromazine, DILANTIN, ELAVIL, HALDOL, haloperidol, INH, iron supplements, isoniazid, metoclopramide, NARDIL, phenelzine, phenytoin, pyridoxine (vitamin B⁶), REGLAN, RISPERDAL, risperidone, selegiline, THORAZINE.

Adverse Effects

Call your doctor immediately if you experience:

• agitation
• anxiety
• clumsiness or unsteadiness
• clenching or grinding of teeth
• unusual and uncontrolled body movements, including of the face, tongue, arms, hands, head, and upper body
• confusion
• abnormal thinking
• dizziness
• difficulty swallowing
• false sense of well-being
• unusual tiredness or weakness
• feeling faint
• hallucinations
• increased hand tremor
• general feeling of discomfort or illness
• nausea or vomiting
• numbness, burning, tingling, or prickling sensations
• excessive mouth watering
• increased eyelid blinking or spasm
• blurred vision
• fast, irregular, or pounding heartbeat
• double vision
• hot flashes
• dilated pupils
• mood or mental changes
• dizziness or lightheadedness when getting up from a lying or sitting position
• skin rash
• difficulty opening mouth
• unusual weight gain or loss
• appetite loss
• loss of urinary bladder control
• difficulty urinating
• chills

- fever
- sore throat
- stomach pain
- facial swelling
- swelling of feet or lower legs
- bloody or black, tarry stools
- vomiting blood or vomit that looks like coffee grounds
- back or leg pain
- pale skin
- high blood pressure
- inability to move eyeballs
- prolonged, painful, or inappropriate penile erection
- convulsions

Call your doctor if these symptoms continue:

- abdominal pain
- appetite loss
- dry mouth
- passing gas
- nightmares
- constipation
- diarrhea
- skin flushing
- headache
- hiccups
- increased sweating
- trouble sleeping
- muscle twitching
- unusual tiredness or weakness

Signs of overdose:

- increased eyelid blinking or spasms

If you suspect an overdose, call this number to contact your poison control center: (800) 222-1222.

Periodic Tests

Ask your doctor which of these tests should be done periodically while you are taking this drug:

- complete blood count
- liver function tests
- kidney function tests
- eye pressure tests
- cardiovascular monitoring

Limited Use

Selegiline (sell *edge* ell lean) (also known as Deprenyl) **ELDEPRYL** (Somerset)

GENERIC: not available

FAMILY: Drugs for Parkinson's Disease

PREGNANCY WARNING

Selegiline caused fetal harm in animal studies, including a decrease in body weight and pup survival after birth. Because of the potential for serious adverse effects to the fetus, this drug should not be used by pregnant women.

BREAST-FEEDING WARNING

No information is available from either human or animal studies. It is likely that this drug, like many others, is also excreted in human milk, and because of the potential for serious adverse effects in nursing infants, you should not take this drug while nursing.

Selegiline is approved by the FDA as an adjunct in the management of Parkinson's disease in patients being treated with levodopa and carbidopa (SINEMET) (see p. 631) who exhibit deterioration in the quality of their response to this treatment. There is no evidence from controlled studies that selegiline has any beneficial effect in the absence of concurrent levodopa therapy.[15]

Selegiline belongs to a group of drugs called monoamine oxidase (MAO) inhibitors. Serious adverse effects and the severe dietary restrictions required when taking type A MAO inhibitors curtailed use of these drugs for depression. Selegiline is a type B MAO inhibitor purported to have fewer adverse effects. However, the same adverse effects can occur, espe-

---

BEWARE OF COMPOUNDING PHARMACISTS

Selegiline, or deprenyl, is being promoted by compounding pharmacists to improve memory, slow the loss of sexual capacity, and increase life span.

Drugs compounded by pharmacists are not FDA-approved. They have not been shown to be safe or effective for use and are produced in facilities that do not have to meet Good Manufacturing Practice guidelines.

---

cially at high doses.[16] In order to reduce adverse effects, it is a good practice to start with a low dose of selegiline, then increase the dose gradually.[17,18]

Originally, selegiline was thought to be most useful in the early stages of Parkinson's disease to slow the advance of the disease and to delay the need to institute levodopa. This practice has not proved to be effective.[19] Now selegiline is used only as adjunctive treatment in some patients. Selegiline is not recommended for those in the advanced stages of Parkinson's disease or with dementia.[17,20] Mental adverse effects are of special concern in the elderly.[21]

If you have symptoms of parkinsonism (tremor, rigid muscles, and disturbances in posture, walking, balance, speech, swallowing, and muscle strength), there is a good chance that they are caused by a drug you are taking. As many as half of older adults with symptoms of parkinsonism may have developed them as adverse effects of a drug. A list of drugs that can cause symptoms of parkinsonism appears on p. 30. If you take any of the drugs on this list, discuss the possibility of drug-induced parkinsonism with your doctor and ask to have your prescription changed or stopped.

Before You Use This Drug

Tell your doctor if you have or have had:

- pregnancy or are breast-feeding
- allergy to selegiline
- stomach ulcers
- excessive tremor
- profound dementia
- severe mental problems
- uncontrolled movements of tongue, lips, face, trunk, or extremities

Tell your doctor about any other drugs you take, including aspirin, herbs, vitamins, and other nonprescription products.

When You Use This Drug

- If taking 20 milligrams or more of selegiline a day, avoid tyramine-containing foods, such as aged cheese, fava or broad bean pods, yeast/protein extracts, smoked or pickled meats—including fish and poultry, bologna, pepperoni, salami, summer sausage—other fermented meat, sauerkraut, overripe fruit, beer, reduced-alcohol and alcohol-free beer and wine, red and white wines, sherry, liqueurs.
- Avoid alcoholic beverages.
- Avoid large quantities of caffeine-containing drinks.
- Avoid nonprescription cough and cold drugs.
- Avoid the painkiller meperidine (DEMEROL).
- Be cautious when getting up suddenly.
- Check with your doctor or hospital emergency room if you have a hypertensive crisis: severe chest pain, enlarged pupils, fast or slow heartbeat, severe headache, increased sweating (possible with fever or cold), clammy skin, nausea or vomiting, stiff or sore neck.
- If mouth is dry, use sugarless candy or gum, ice, or saliva substitute. If dry mouth continues for more than two weeks, check with doctor or dentist.

• If you discontinue this drug, the preceding dietary restrictions must be continued for at least two weeks.

How to Use This Drug

• If you miss a dose, take it as soon as you remember, but skip it if it is almost time for the next dose. **Do not take double doses.**
• Do not share your medication with others.
• Take the drug at the same time(s) each day.
• Store at room temperature with lid on tightly. Do not store in the bathroom. Do not expose to heat, moisture, or strong light. Keep out of reach of children.

Interactions with Other Drugs

The following drugs, biologics (e.g., vaccines, therapeutic antibodies), or foods are listed in *Evaluations of Drug Interactions* 2003 as causing "highly clinically significant" or "clinically significant" interactions when used together with any of the drugs in this section. In some sections with multiple drugs, the interaction may have been reported for one but not all drugs in this section, but we include the interaction because the drugs in this section are similar to one another. We have also included potentially serious interactions listed in the drug's FDA-approved professional package insert or in published medical journal articles. There may be other drugs, especially those in the families of drugs listed below, that also will react with this drug to cause severe adverse effects. Make sure to tell your doctor and pharmacist the drugs you are taking and tell them if you are taking any of these interacting drugs:

ALPHAGAN P, brimonidine, bupropion, CELEXA, citalopram, COMTAN, DELSYM, DEMEROL, dextromethorphan, entacapone, fluoxetine, imipramine, IMITREX, meperidine, MERIDIA, mirtazapine, nefazodone, PROZAC, reboxetine, REMERON, SERZONE, sibutramine, sumatriptan, TOFRANIL, tramadol, ULTRAM, WELLBUTRIN, ZYBAN.

Adverse Effects

Call your doctor immediately if you experience:

• increase in unusual body movements
• mood or other mental changes
• new, increased, or severe chest pain
• irregular heartbeat
• wheezing, breathing difficulty, or tightness in chest
• swelling of feet or lower legs
• difficulty speaking
• loss of balance control
• uncontrolled movements, especially of face, neck, arms, legs, and back
• restlessness or desire to keep moving
• twisting body movements
• bloody or black, tarry stools
• severe stomach pain
• vomiting blood or vomit that looks like coffee grounds
• hallucinations
• severe headache
• severe high blood pressure
• dizziness or lightheadedness
• difficult or frequent urination
• lip smacking or puckering
• puffing of cheeks
• rapid or wormlike movements of tongue
• uncontrolled chewing movements
• enlarged pupils
• fast or slow heartbeat
• increased sensitivity of eyes to light
• increased sweating, possibly with fever or cold, clammy skin
• severe nausea or vomiting
• stiff or sore neck

Call your doctor if these symptoms continue:

- abdominal or stomach pain
- dizziness or faintness
- dry mouth
- trouble sleeping
- nausea or vomiting
- anxiety, nervousness, or restlessness
- increased inability to move
- sudden closing of eyelids
- blurred or double vision
- body aches or back or leg pain
- slowed movements
- chills
- constipation or diarrhea
- increased sweating
- drowsiness
- headache
- heartburn
- high or low blood pressure
- impaired memory
- slow or difficult urination
- frequent urge to urinate
- irritability
- appetite loss
- weight loss
- muscle cramps or numbness of fingers or toes
- fast or pounding heartbeat
- burning lips or mouth
- burning in throat
- increased sensitivity of skin and eyes to sunlight
- skin rash
- ringing or buzzing in ears
- changes in sense of taste
- unusual feeling of well-being
- unusual tiredness or weakness
- teeth grinding, clenching, or gnashing
- sudden jerky body movements

Signs of overdose:

- agitation or irritability
- chest pain
- convulsions
- cool, clammy skin
- increased sweating

- severe dizziness or faintness
- fast or irregular pulse
- high or low blood pressure
- high fever
- severe spasm where head and heels are bent backward and the body arches forward
- troubled breathing
- lockjaw

If you suspect an overdose, call this number to contact your poison control center: (800) 222-1222.

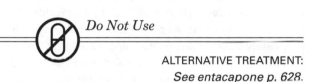

Do Not Use

ALTERNATIVE TREATMENT:
See entacapone p. 628.

Tolcapone (*tole* ka pone)
TASMAR (Roche)

FAMILY: Drugs for Parkinson's Disease
Catechol-O-Methyltransferase (COMT) Inhibitors

Tolcapone was approved by the FDA in January 1998 for the treatment of Parkinson's disease in conjunction with other drugs such as levodopa and carbidopa (SINEMET). After less than one year on the market, in November 1998, the FDA required new warnings in the drug's professional product labeling or package insert about cases of liver failure, some resulting in death, associated with the use of tolcapone.[22]

On November 17, 1998, one day after the FDA's announcement, the European Medicines Evaluation Agency announced that the sale of tolcapone would be suspended in European markets.[23] Tolcapone was first marketed in Europe in June 1997, six months before the FDA cleared it for United States use. The liver toxicity warning was strengthened in Europe on October 16, 1998, one month before the same change was made in this country.

FDA BLACK BOX WARNING

Because of the risk of potentially fatal, acute fulminant liver failure, TASMAR (tolcapone) should ordinarily be used in patients with Parkinson's disease on l-dopa/carbidopa who are experiencing symptom fluctuations and are not responding satisfactorily to or are not appropriate candidates for other adjunctive therapies.

Because of the risk of liver injury and because TASMAR, when it is effective, provides an observable symptomatic benefit, the patient who fails to show substantial clinical benefit within 3 weeks of initiation of treatment, should be withdrawn from TASMAR.

TASMAR therapy should not be initiated if the patient exhibits clinical evidence of liver disease or two SGPT/ALT or SGOT/AST values greater than the upper limit of normal. Patients with severe dyskinesia or dystonia should be treated with caution.

Patients who develop evidence of hepatocellular injury [liver toxicity] while on TASMAR and are withdrawn from the drug for any reason may be at increased risk for liver injury if TASMAR is reintroduced. Accordingly, such patients should not ordinarily be considered for retreatment.

Cases of severe hepatocellular injury, including fulminant liver failure resulting in death, have been reported in postmarketing use. As of October 1998, 3 cases of fatal fulminant hepatic failure have been reported from approximately 60,000 patients providing about 40,000 patient years of worldwide use. This incidence may be 10- to 100-fold higher than the background incidence in the general population. Underreporting of cases may lead to significant underestimation of the increased risk associated with the use of TASMAR.

A prescriber who elects to use TASMAR in face of the increased risk of liver injury is strongly advised to monitor patients for evidence of emergent liver injury. Patients should be advised of the need for self-monitoring for both the classical signs of liver disease (eg, clay colored stools, jaundice) and the nonspecific ones (eg, fatigue, loss of appetite, lethargy).

Although a program of frequent laboratory monitoring for evidence of hepatocellular injury is deemed essential, it is not clear that baseline and periodic monitoring of liver enzymes will prevent the occurrence of fulminant liver failure. However, it is generally believed that early detection of drug-induced hepatic injury along with immediate withdrawal of the suspect drug enhances the likelihood for recovery. It is also widely held, without a robust body of evidence, that patients with preexisting hepatic disease are more vulnerable to hepatotoxins. Accordingly, the following liver monitoring program is recommended.

Before starting treatment with TASMAR, the physician should conduct appropriate tests to exclude the presence of liver disease. In patients determined to be appropriate candidates for treatment with TASMAR, serum glutamic-pyruvic transaminase (SGPT/ALT) and serum glutamic-oxaloacetic transaminase (SGOT/AST) levels should be determined at baseline and then every 2 weeks for the first year of therapy, every 4 weeks for the next 6 months, and then every 8 weeks thereafter. If the dose is increased to 200 mg tid [3 times a day] liver enzyme monitoring should take place before increasing the dose and then be reinitiated at the frequency above.

TASMAR should be discontinued if SGPT/ALT or SGOT/AST exceeds the upper limit of normal or if clinical signs and symptoms suggest the onset of hepatic failure (persistent nausea, fatigue, lethargy, anorexia, jaundice, dark urine, pruritus, and right upper quadrant tenderness).

Tolcapone's labeling now cautions that the drug should be reserved for use in patients who do not respond to or who are not appropriate candidates for other available treatments. A boxed warning also advises that in light of the severe liver toxicity, if a patient fails to show a substantial clinical benefit within the first three weeks of use, treatment should be withdrawn. The complete text of tolcapone's boxed warning precedes this profile.

The actual number of people killed or injured by tolcapone is unknown because the FDA's postmarketing safety surveillance system relies largely on health professionals' voluntary reports of adverse drug reactions. There is no law or regulatory requirement for the reporting of adverse reactions. Consequently, the FDA estimates that only about 10% of actual incidents get reported.

Using the FDA's adverse drug reaction database, we estimate that through the third quarter of 2001 there had been 21 cases of severe liver toxicity reported with tolcapone. Eight of these cases resulted in death.

The new labeling also includes an informed consent document that doctors are advised to use when prescribing tolcapone. Patients are asked to initial the following five statements:[24]

1. The patient understands that tolcapone is used to treat certain types of patients with Parkinson's disease and the doctor has told the patient that he/she is this type of patient.

2. The patient understands there is a serious risk of severe liver failure, which may be potentially fatal, in using tolcapone.

3. The patient understands that there are no laboratory tests that will predict an increased risk of fatal liver failure.

4. The patient understands that he/she should have recommended blood tests before treatment with tolcapone is begun or continued, on a schedule of every two weeks for the first year, then every four weeks for the next six months, and then every eight weeks thereafter while taking tolcapone. The patient understands that although the blood tests may help detect liver failure if it develops, it may do so only after significant, irreversible, and potentially fatal damage has already occurred.

5. The patient understands the need to report any unusual symptoms to the doctor and be especially aware of persistent nausea, fatigue,

lethargy, decreased appetite, jaundice (yellowing of the skin or whites of the eyes), dark urine, itchiness, or right-side abdominal pain (the location of the liver), all typical symptoms of liver toxicity.

Very troubling is the fact that tolcapone's original professional product labeling raised a red flag about the risk of liver toxicity, indicating that this possibility was well known before the drug was approved.[25] In clinical trials conducted before approval, approximately 1% of patients taking 100 milligrams three times a day and 3% taking twice that dose had liver-enzyme elevations three times the upper limit of normal. Such blood-level elevations are an early indicator of potential liver toxicity.

In reading the labeling for tolcapone, it appears that there is no way that this drug can be used safely. Liver toxicity testing is now required every two weeks for the first year that the drug is used. We have never seen another drug that requires such intensive testing to detect the development of an adverse drug reaction. Even this exhaustive level of testing may not detect liver damage soon enough to prevent significant, irreversible, and potentially fatal liver damage.

Epilepsy

Carbamazepine (kar ba *maz* e peen)
TEGRETOL (Novartis)

GENERIC: available

FAMILY: Drugs for Epilepsy
Drugs for Trigeminal Neuralgia

PREGNANCY WARNING

Carbamazepine crosses the placenta in pregnant women and causes malformations, including spina bifida and heart defects. Taking more than one drug for epilepsy increases the risk. Tell your doctor if you are pregnant or thinking of becoming pregnant before you take this drug.

BREAST-FEEDING WARNING

Carbamazepine is excreted in human milk. Because of the potential for serious adverse effects in nursing infants, you should not take this drug while nursing.

Carbamazepine is used to treat some forms of epilepsy (partial and generalized tonic-clonic [grand mal] seizures) and to treat a form of excruciating facial pain called trigeminal neuralgia or tic douloureux. This drug is not a simple painkiller and should not be used to treat general aches or pains. *The Medical Letter on Drugs and Therapeutics* has long listed carbamazepine as the mainstay of treatment for trigeminal neuralgia.[26]

If you are over 60, you will generally need to take less than the usual adult dose. Ask your doctor about starting with a daily dose of 50 milligrams to prevent harmful adverse effects, especially mental confusion and slowed pulse.

Call your doctor if either of these adverse effects occurs. If you are taking carbamazepine for neuralgia, your doctor should try reducing your dose every few months to see if a smaller dose will relieve your symptoms.

Carbamazepine can cause serious, and sometimes fatal, blood cell abnormalities in some people. These disorders can usually be treated if detected early. If you are taking carbamazepine and have any of the following symptoms, call your doctor immediately: fever and sore throat, ulcers in the mouth, easy bruising, or skin rashes.[27] Before you start using carbamazepine, you should have a complete blood count to be certain that you don't have any potential blood abnormalities that could be worsened by the drug.

Carbamazepine causes malignant liver tumors in female rats and benign tumors of the testicles in male rats.[28]

FDA BLACK BOX WARNING

APLASTIC ANEMIA AND AGRANULOCYTOSIS [bone marrow toxicity] HAVE BEEN REPORTED IN ASSOCIATION WITH THE USE OF TEGRETOL. DATA FROM A POPULATION-BASED CASE CONTROL STUDY DEMONSTRATE THAT THE RISK OF DEVELOPING THESE REACTIONS IS 5–8 TIMES GREATER THAN IN THE GENERAL POPULATION. HOWEVER, THE OVERALL RISK OF THESE REACTIONS IN THE UNTREATED GENERAL POPULATION IS LOW, APPROXIMATELY SIX PATIENTS PER ONE MILLION POPULATION PER YEAR FOR AGRANULOCYTOSIS AND TWO PATIENTS PER ONE MILLION POPULATION PER YEAR FOR APLASTIC ANEMIA.

ALTHOUGH REPORTS OF TRANSIENT OR PERSISTENT DECREASED PLATELET OR WHITE BLOOD CELL COUNTS ARE NOT UNCOMMON IN ASSOCIATION WITH THE USE OF TEGRETOL, DATA ARE NOT AVAILABLE TO ESTIMATE ACCURATELY THEIR INCIDENCE OR OUTCOME. HOWEVER, THE VAST MAJORITY OF THE CASES OF LEUKOPENIA HAVE NOT PROGRESSED TO THE MORE SERIOUS CONDITIONS OF APLASTIC ANEMIA OR AGRANULOCYTOSIS.

BECAUSE OF THE VERY LOW INCIDENCE OF AGRANULOCYTOSIS AND APLASTIC ANEMIA, THE VAST MAJORITY OF MINOR HEMATOLOGIC CHANGES OBSERVED IN MONITORING OF PATIENTS ON TEGRETOL ARE UNLIKELY TO SIGNAL THE OCCURRENCE OF EITHER ABNORMALITY. NONETHELESS, COMPLETE PRETREATMENT HEMATOLOGICAL TESTING SHOULD BE OBTAINED AS A BASELINE. IF A PATIENT IN THE COURSE OF TREATMENT EXHIBITS LOW OR DECREASED WHITE BLOOD CELL OR PLATELET COUNTS, THE PATIENT SHOULD BE MONITORED CLOSELY. DISCONTINUATION OF THE DRUG SHOULD BE CONSIDERED IF ANY EVIDENCE OF SIGNIFICANT BONE MARROW DEPRESSION DEVELOPS.

Before You Use This Drug

Do not use if you have or have had:

- certain types of seizures (atypical or generalized absence seizures, atonic seizures, or myoclonic seizures)
- heart block
- blood disorders
- bone marrow depression

Tell your doctor if you have or have had:

- allergies or reaction to carbamazepine or to tricyclic antidepressants
- pregnancy or are breast-feeding
- previous use of this drug
- heart problems
- diabetes
- glaucoma
- alcohol dependence
- liver problems
- low amount of salt in the blood
- retention of urine
- kidney problems
- anemia
- behavioral problems

Tell your doctor about any other drugs you take, including aspirin, herbs, vitamins, and other nonprescription products.

When You Use This Drug

- Until you know how you react to this drug, do not drive or perform other activities requiring alertness. Carbamazepine can cause dizziness, drowsiness, and lack of muscle coordination.
- Schedule regular visits with your doctor to check your progress.
- Wear a medical identification bracelet or carry a card stating that you take carbamazepine.
- If you plan to have any surgery, including dental, tell your doctor that you take this drug.

- Use proper oral hygiene.
- Avoid alcoholic drinks.
- **Caution diabetics:** Carbamazepine may increase urine sugar concentration.
- Wear sunscreen when outdoors.
- If using oral contraceptives, use another method of birth control instead.
- This drug may interfere with pregnancy tests.

How to Use This Drug

- Take with food.
- Store at room temperature with lid on tightly. Do not store in the bathroom. Do not expose to heat, moisture, or strong light. Keep out of reach of children.
- If you miss a dose, take it as soon as you remember, but skip it if it is almost time for the next dose. **Do not take double doses.**
- Do not share your medication with others.
- Take the drug at the same time(s) each day.
- Do not suddenly stop taking without checking with your doctor to find out if you need to taper off this drug.

Interactions with Other Drugs

The following drugs, biologics (e.g., vaccines, therapeutic antibodies), or foods are listed in *Evaluations of Drug Interactions* 2003 as causing "highly clinically significant" or "clinically significant" interactions when used together with any of the drugs in this section. In some sections with multiple drugs, the interaction may have been reported for one but not all drugs in this section, but we include the interaction because the drugs in this section are similar to one another. We have also included potentially serious interactions listed in the drug's FDA-approved professional package insert or in published medical journal articles. There may be other drugs, especially those in the families of drugs listed below, that also will react with this drug to cause severe adverse effects. Make sure to tell your doctor and pharmacist the drugs you are taking and tell them if you are taking any of these interacting drugs:

alcohol, CALAN SR, charcoal, cimetidine, clozapine, CLOZARIL, COVERA-HS, CRIXI-VAN, cyclosporine, danazol, DANOCRINE, DARVON, DARVON-N, DECADRON, delavirdine, DEPAKENE/DEPAKOTE, dexamethasone, dicumarol, divalproex/valproic acid, doxycycline, EES, ELIXOPHYLLIN, ERYTHROCIN, erythromycin, ESKALITH, felbamate, FELBATOL, FLAGYL, GABITRIL, HALDOL, haloperidol, HEXADROL, ILOSONE, indinavir, INH, isoniazid, ISOPTIN SR, lithium, ketorolac, LITHOBID, LITHONATE, metronidazole, NEORAL, olanzapine, oral contraceptives, oxcarbazepine, propoxyphene, RESCRIPTOR, SANDIMMUNE, sertindole, SLO-BID, TAGAMET, THEO-24, theophylline, tiagabine, ticlodipine, TOPAMAX, topiramate, TORADOL, TRILEPTAL, verapamil, VERELAN, VIBRAMYCIN, VINCASAR, vincristine, ZYPREXA.

The use of carbamazepine in combination with the monoamine oxidase (MAO) inhibitor antidepressants is not recommended. The MAO inhibitors include drugs such as isocarboxazid (MARPLAN), phenelzine (NARDIL), and tranylcypromine (PARNATE).

Adverse Effects

Call your doctor immediately if you experience:

- behavioral changes
- black, tarry stools
- blood in urine or stools
- blurred or double vision
- bone or joint pain
- chest pain
- chills
- confusion, agitation, or hostility
- continuous back-and-forth eye movements
- continuous headache
- cough or hoarseness
- cramps in abdomen or muscles
- swelling of face, hands, feet, or lower legs
- fainting
- fast, slow, pounding, or irregular heartbeat
- fever
- low or high blood pressure
- lower back or side pain
- mental depression with restlessness and nervousness
- painful or difficult urination
- pinpoint red spots on skin
- rapid weight gain
- rigidity
- increase in seizure frequency
- severe diarrhea
- severe nausea and vomiting
- shortness of breath, troubled breathing, wheezing, or tightness in chest
- skin rash, hives, or itching
- sore throat
- sores, ulcers, or white spots on lips or in mouth
- difficulty speaking or slurred speech
- swollen or painful glands
- unusual bleeding, bruising, or nosebleeds
- unusual drowsiness or tiredness
- unusual weakness
- ringing, buzzing, or other unexplained sounds in the ears
- trembling
- uncontrolled body movements
- hallucinations
- darkened urine
- pale stools
- yellow eyes or skin
- frequent urination
- sudden decrease in amount of urine

- numbness, tingling, pain, or weakness in hands and feet
- pain or bluish color of leg or foot

Call your doctor if these symptoms continue:

- clumsiness or unsteadiness
- confusion
- mild dizziness or lightheadedness
- mild drowsiness
- mild nausea or vomiting
- aching joints, muscles, or leg cramps
- hair loss
- appetite loss
- constipation
- increased sweating
- diarrhea
- dry mouth
- irritation or soreness of tongue or mouth
- headache
- increased sensitivity of skin to sunlight
- sexual problems in males
- stomach pain or discomfort
- unusual tiredness or weakness

Signs of overdose:

- sudden decrease in amount of urine
- fast or irregular heartbeat
- convulsions
- severe dizziness
- severe drowsiness
- poor control of body movements
- overactive reflexes, followed by underactive reflexes
- low or high blood pressure
- motor restlessness
- muscle twitching
- large pupils
- severe nausea or vomiting
- clumsiness or unsteadiness
- abnormal body movements
- body spasms where head and heels are bent backward and body is bowed forward
- irregular, slow, or shallow breathing
- fainting
- tremor

If you suspect an overdose, call this number to contact your poison control center: (800) 222-1222.

Periodic Tests

Ask your doctor which of these tests should be done periodically while you are taking this drug:

- blood levels of carbamazepine
- complete blood count, including platelet counts
- kidney function tests
- liver function tests
- eye tests
- complete urinalysis
- calcium concentrations in blood
- iron blood levels
- heart exam
- electrolyte levels

Clonazepam (clawn *az* ah pam)
KLONOPIN (Roche)

GENERIC: available

FAMILY: Drugs for Epilepsy
Drugs for Panic Disorder
Benzodiazepines (see p. 166)

PREGNANCY WARNING

Clonazepam caused fetal malformations in animal studies, including cleft palate, open eyelid, fused backbone, and limb defects. Taking more than one drug for epilepsy increases the risk. Tell your doctor if you are pregnant or thinking of becoming pregnant before you take this drug.

BREAST-FEEDING WARNING

Clonazepam is excreted in human milk. Because of the potential for adverse effects in nursing infants, you should not take this drug while nursing.

Clonazepam is approved by the FDA for the control of several types of seizures in which my-

One hazard of taking this drug continuously for longer than several weeks is drug-induced dependence. **Do not stop taking your drug suddenly.** With the help of your doctor, work out a schedule for slowly lowering the amount of the drug you take by about 5 to 10% each day. Keep a written record of the dosage reduction schedule with you. These steps will make it much easier to become drug free without developing distressing symptoms of drug withdrawal.

oclonus is a major element. Myoclonus refers to brusque, lightninglike movements of a muscle or part of a muscle, sometimes sufficiently strong enough to move an entire limb. Usually, other anticonvulsants are needed as well, to control the nonmyoclonic elements of the seizure. Clonazepam is also approved for panic disorder.[29]

Clonazepam is one of the benzodiazepine drugs (see p. 223), the best known of which are Valium, Xanax, Librium, and Halcion. Elderly people are usually more sensitive to the central nervous system effects of these drugs.

Before You Use This Drug

Tell your doctor if you have or have had:

- allergies to drugs
- pregnancy or are breast-feeding
- alcoholism
- coma
- shock
- a history of drug abuse or dependence
- epilepsy or seizures
- glaucoma
- liver problems
- severe mental depression
- myasthenia gravis
- brain disorder
- severe lung disease
- mental disorder
- kidney problem
- sleep disorder
- hyperactivity
- low albumin level
- porphyria

Tell your doctor about any other drugs you take, including aspirin, herbs, vitamins, and other nonprescription products.

When You Use This Drug

- Do not drink alcohol or use other drugs that can cause drowsiness.
- Do not increase the dose of this drug if it seems less effective after a few weeks; check with your doctor.
- Check with your doctor before discontinuing this drug, as gradual dosage reduction may be necessary.
- Have regular visits to your doctor during both initial and prolonged therapy.
- Check with your doctor if physical or psychological dependence is suspected.
- Get medical help at once if you suspect an overdose.
- Until you know how you react to this drug, do not drive or perform other activities requiring alertness.
- You may feel dizzy when rising from a lying or sitting position. If you are lying down, hang your legs over the side of the bed for a few minutes, then get up slowly. When getting up from a chair, stay by the chair until you are sure that you are not dizzy. (See p. 13.)
- Carry medical identification stating your condition and that you are taking clonazepam.
- If you plan to have any surgery, including dental, tell your doctor that you take this drug.

How to Use This Drug

- If you miss a dose, take it as soon as you remember, but skip it if it is almost time for the next dose. **Do not take double doses.**

- Do not share your medication with others.
- Take the drug at the same time(s) each day.
- Store at room temperature with lid on tightly. Do not store in the bathroom. Do not expose to heat, moisture, or strong light. Keep out of reach of children.

Interactions with Other Drugs

The following drugs, biologics (e.g., vaccines, therapeutic antibodies), or foods are listed in *Evaluations of Drug Interactions* 2003 as causing "highly clinically significant" or "clinically significant" interactions when used together with any of the drugs in this section. In some sections with multiple drugs, the interaction may have been reported for one but not all drugs in this section, but we include the interaction because the drugs in this section are similar to one another. We have also included potentially serious interactions listed in the drug's FDA-approved professional package insert or in published medical journal articles. There may be other drugs, especially those in the families of drugs listed below, that also will react with this drug to cause severe adverse effects. Make sure to tell your doctor and pharmacist the drugs you are taking and tell them if you are taking any of these interacting drugs:

BENADRYL, carbamazepine, cimetidine, digoxin, DILANTIN, diphenhydramine, itraconazole, KETALAR, ketamine, ketoconazole, LANOXICAPS, LANOXIN, LUMINAL, NIZORAL, NORVIR, phenobarbital, phenytoin, ritonavir, SOLFOTON, SOMINEX FORMULA, SPORANOX, TAGAMET, TEGRETOL.

Additionally, the *United States Pharmacopeia Drug Information* 2003 lists central nervous system depressant (CNS) drugs including alcohol, antidepressants, antihistamines, antipsychotics, some blood pressure medications (reserpine, methyldopa, beta-blockers), motion sickness medications, muscle relaxants, narcotics, sedatives, sleeping pills and tranquilizers, as well as MS CONTIN, morphine, and ROXANOL as having interactions of major significance.

Adverse Effects

Call your doctor immediately if you experience:

- lack of memory of events taking place after taking drug
- anxiety
- confusion
- mental depression
- fast, pounding, or irregular heartbeat
- abnormal thinking
- false beliefs
- loss of sense of reality
- disorientation
- skin rash or itching
- behavior changes
- chills, fever, and sore throat
- unusual tiredness or weakness
- ulcers or sores in mouth or throat
- unusual bleeding or bruising
- uncontrolled body movements, including of the eyes
- yellow eyes or skin
- low blood pressure
- muscle weakness
- agitation, unusual excitement, irritability, or nervousness
- aggressive behavior, hostility, or rage
- hallucinations
- trouble sleeping
- seizures

Call your doctor if these symptoms continue:

- clumsiness or unsteadiness
- dizziness or lightheadedness
- drowsiness

- slurred speech
- abdominal or stomach cramps or pain
- blurred vision or other vision problems
- changes in sexual desire or ability
- constipation
- diarrhea
- dry mouth or increased thirst
- false sense of well-being
- headache
- increased bronchial secretions or mouth watering
- muscle spasm
- nausea or vomiting
- urination problems
- trembling or shaking
- unusual tiredness or weakness

Call your doctor if these symptoms continue after you stop taking this drug:

- trouble sleeping
- irritability
- nervousness
- abdominal or stomach cramps
- muscle cramps
- confusion
- loss of sense of reality
- increased sweating
- mental depression
- nausea or vomiting
- increased sense of hearing
- increased sensitivity to touch and pain
- tingling, burning, or prickly sensations
- sensitivity of eyes to light
- fast or pounding heartbeat
- trembling or shaking
- hallucinations
- paranoia
- convulsions

Signs of overdose:

- continuing confusion
- decreased reflexes
- severe drowsiness or coma
- seizures
- shakiness

- slow heartbeat
- continuing slurred speech
- staggering
- difficulty breathing
- severe weakness

If you suspect an overdose, call this number to contact your poison control center: (800) 222-1222.

Periodic Tests

Ask your doctor which of these tests should be done periodically while you are taking this drug:

- reassessment of the need for clonazepam

Divalproex (dye *val* pro ex)
DEPAKOTE (Abbott)
DEPAKOTE CP (Abbott)
DEPAKOTE CR (Abbott)

GENERIC: not available

Valproic Acid (val *pro* ic acid)
DEPAKENE (Abbott)

GENERIC: available
FAMILY: Drugs for Epilepsy
Drugs to Prevent Migraine Headache
Drugs for Mania

PREGNANCY WARNING

Valproic acid caused serious harm to human infants born to mothers taking this drug during pregnancy. Such infants have been born with damage to the heart, blood vessels, skull, and spinal cord. Infants have died after birth from liver failure following use of valproic acid by their mothers during pregnancy. Because of the potential for serious adverse effects to the fetus, this drug should not be used by pregnant women.

BREAST-FEEDING WARNING

Valproic acid is excreted in human milk. Because of the potential for serious adverse effects in nursing infants, you should not take valproic acid while nursing.

FDA BLACK BOX WARNING

HEPATOTOXICITY (LIVER TOXICITY)

HEPATIC FAILURE RESULTING IN FATALITIES HAS OCCURRED IN PATIENTS RECEIVING VALPROIC ACID AND ITS DERIVATIVES. EXPERIENCE HAS INDICATED THAT CHILDREN UNDER THE AGE OF TWO YEARS ARE AT A CONSIDERABLY INCREASED RISK OF DEVELOPING FATAL HEPATOTOXICITY, ESPECIALLY THOSE ON MULTIPLE ANTICONVULSANTS, THOSE WITH CONGENITAL METABOLIC DISORDERS, THOSE WITH SEVERE SEIZURE DISORDERS ACCOMPANIED BY MENTAL RETARDATION, AND THOSE WITH ORGANIC BRAIN DISEASE. WHEN DEPAKOTE IS USED IN THIS PATIENT GROUP, IT SHOULD BE USED WITH EXTREME CAUTION AND AS A SOLE AGENT. THE BENEFITS OF THERAPY SHOULD BE WEIGHED AGAINST THE RISKS. ABOVE THIS AGE GROUP, EXPERIENCE IN EPILEPSY HAS INDICATED THAT THE INCIDENCE OF FATAL HEPATOTOXICITY DECREASES CONSIDERABLY IN PROGRESSIVELY OLDER PATIENT GROUPS.

THESE INCIDENTS USUALLY HAVE OCCURRED DURING THE FIRST SIX MONTHS OF TREATMENT. SERIOUS OR FATAL HEPATOTOXICITY MAY BE PRECEDED BY NON-SPECIFIC SYMPTOMS SUCH AS MALAISE, WEAKNESS, LETHARGY, FACIAL EDEMA, ANOREXIA, AND VOMITING. IN PATIENTS WITH EPILEPSY, A LOSS OF SEIZURE CONTROL MAY ALSO OCCUR. PATIENTS SHOULD BE MONITORED CLOSELY FOR APPEARANCE OF THESE SYMPTOMS. LIVER FUNCTION TESTS SHOULD BE PERFORMED PRIOR TO THERAPY AND AT FREQUENT INTERVALS THEREAFTER, ESPECIALLY DURING THE FIRST SIX MONTHS.

TERATOGENICITY

VALPROATE CAN PRODUCE TERATOGENIC EFFECTS SUCH AS NEURAL TUBE DEFECTS (E.G., SPINA BIFIDA). ACCORDINGLY, THE USE OF DEPAKOTE TABLETS IN WOMEN OF CHILDBEARING POTENTIAL REQUIRES THAT THE BENEFITS OF ITS USE BE WEIGHED AGAINST THE RISK OF INJURY TO THE FETUS. THIS IS ESPECIALLY IMPORTANT WHEN THE TREATMENT OF A SPONTANEOUSLY REVERSIBLE CONDITION NOT ORDINARILY ASSOCIATED WITH PERMANENT INJURY OR RISK OF DEATH (E.G., MIGRAINE) IS CONTEMPLATED.

AN INFORMATION SHEET DESCRIBING THE TERATOGENIC POTENTIAL OF VALPROATE IS AVAILABLE FOR PATIENTS.

PANCREATITIS (INFLAMMATION OF THE PANCREAS)

CASES OF LIFE-THREATENING PANCREATITIS HAVE BEEN REPORTED IN BOTH CHILDREN AND ADULTS RECEIVING VALPROATE. SOME OF THE CASES HAVE BEEN DESCRIBED AS HEMORRHAGIC WITH A RAPID PROGRESSION FROM INITIAL SYMPTOMS TO DEATH. CASES HAVE BEEN REPORTED SHORTLY AFTER INITIAL USE AS WELL AS AFTER SEVERAL YEARS OF USE. PATIENTS AND GUARDIANS SHOULD BE WARNED THAT ABDOMINAL PAIN, NAUSEA, VOMITING, AND/OR ANOREXIA CAN BE SYMPTOMS OF PANCREATITIS THAT REQUIRE PROMPT MEDICAL EVALUATION. IF PANCREATITIS IS DIAGNOSED, VALPROATE SHOULD ORDINARILY BE DISCONTINUED. ALTERNATIVE TREATMENT FOR THE UNDERLYING MEDICAL CONDITION SHOULD BE INITIATED AS CLINICALLY INDICATED.

Divalproex is essentially two molecules of valproic acid hooked together. Divalproex is approved by the FDA to treat certain types of epilepsy, to prevent migraine headaches, and to manage manic episodes associated with bipolar disorder.[30] Valproic acid, however, is approved only for epilepsy.[31]

The professional product labeling or package inserts for divalproex and valproic acid are required by the FDA to have a black-box warning about liver toxicity, birth defects, and inflammation of the pancreas. A black-box warning is the strongest type of warning that the FDA can require. It appears at the beginning of this drug profile.

Before You Use This Drug

Do not use if you have or have had:

- liver disease

Tell your doctor if you have or have had:

- allergies to valproic acid, divalproex, or valproate
- pregnancy or are breast-feeding
- kidney problems
- liver problems
- blood disease
- brain disease
- low albumin in blood
- diabetes

Tell your doctor about any other drugs you take, including aspirin, herbs, vitamins, and other nonprescription products.

When You Use This Drug

- Have regular visits with your doctor to check your progress.
- Check with your doctor before you discontinue this drug.
- Do not drink alcohol or use other drugs that can cause drowsiness.

- Until you know how you react to this drug, do not drive or perform other activities that require alertness.
- If you plan to have any surgery, including dental, tell your doctor that you take this drug.
- This drug may interfere with thyroid tests.
- Carry medical identification card or bracelet stating that you are taking this drug.
- **Caution diabetics:** When testing for urine ketones, there is the possibility of false-positive test results.

How to Use This Drug

- Store at room temperature with lid on tightly. Do not store in the bathroom. Do not expose to heat, moisture, or strong light. Keep out of reach of children.
- If you miss a dose and are taking one dose a day, take it as soon as you remember, but skip it if it is almost time for the next dose. **Do not take double doses.** If you miss a dose and are taking two or more doses a day, take if remembered within six hours; then take remaining doses at evenly spaced intervals.
- Do not share your medication with others.
- Take the drug at the same time(s) each day.
- Take with food or milk.
- *For valproic acid capsules:* Do not break, chew, or crush capsules.
- *For divalproex delayed-release capsules:* Do not chew or crush this drug. Capsules may be opened and the contents mixed with applesauce, jelly, or ketchup, then swallowed immediately without chewing.
- *For divalproex delayed-release tablets:* Do not break, chew, or crush long-acting forms of this drug.

Interactions with Other Drugs

The following drugs, biologics (e.g., vaccines, therapeutic antibodies), or foods are listed in

Evaluations of Drug Interactions 2003 as causing "highly clinically significant" or "clinically significant" interactions when used together with any of the drugs in this section. In some sections with multiple drugs, the interaction may have been reported for one but not all drugs in this section, but we include the interaction because the drugs in this section are similar to one another. We have also included potentially serious interactions listed in the drug's FDA-approved professional package insert or in published medical journal articles. There may be other drugs, especially those in the families of drugs listed below, that also will react with this drug to cause severe adverse effects. Make sure to tell your doctor and pharmacist the drugs you are taking and tell them if you are taking any of these interacting drugs:

amitriptyline, aspirin, carbamazepine, COUMADIN, diazepam, DILANTIN, ECOTRIN, EES, ELAVIL, ERYTHROCIN, erythromycin, ethosuximide, felbamate, FELBATOL, GABITRIL, GENUINE BAYER ASPIRIN, LAMICTAL, lamotrigene, LUMINAL, MYSOLINE, nortriptyline, ORINASE, oxcarbazepine, PAMELOR, phenobarbital, phenytoin, primidone, RETROVIR, RIFADIN, rifampin, RIMACTANE, SOLFOTON, TEGRETOL, tiagabine, tolbutamide, TRILEPTAL, VALIUM, warfarin, ZARONTIN, zidovudine (AZT).

Adverse Effects

Call your doctor immediately if you experience:

- behavior, mood, or mental changes
- increased seizure frequency
- appetite loss
- continuing nausea or vomiting
- facial swelling
- tiredness or weakness
- yellow eyes or skin
- double vision
- continuous, uncontrolled back-and-forth or rolling eye movements
- appearance of spots before eyes
- severe abdominal or stomach cramps
- unusual bleeding or bruising

Call your doctor if these symptoms continue:

- mild abdominal or stomach cramps
- appetite loss
- change in menstrual periods
- diarrhea
- hair loss
- indigestion
- nausea and vomiting
- trembling of hands and arms
- unusual weight loss or gain
- clumsiness or unsteadiness
- constipation
- dizziness
- drowsiness
- headache
- skin rash
- unusual excitement, restlessness, or irritability

Periodic Tests

Ask your doctor which of these tests should be done periodically while you are taking this drug:

- blood levels of ammonia
- bleeding time determinations
- complete blood count
- kidney function determination
- liver function tests, especially during the first six months of taking this drug
- blood levels of valproate

Limited Use

Gabapentin (ga ba *pen* tin)
NEURONTIN (Pfizer)

GENERIC: not available

FAMILY: Drugs for Epilepsy
Drugs to Prevent Pain after Shingles
(Postherpetic Neuralgia)

PREGNANCY WARNING

Gabapentin caused fetal harm in animal studies, including delayed formation of the bones of the skull, back, arms, and legs and malformation of the kidney. Because of the potential for serious adverse effects to the fetus, this drug should not be used by pregnant women.

BREAST-FEEDING WARNING

Gabapentin is excreted in human milk. Because of the potential for serious adverse effects in nursing infants, you should not take this drug while nursing.

Gabapentin is approved by the FDA for use, in combination with older seizure medications, for a relatively rare type of seizure disorder known as partial seizure, and pain after an episode of shingles known as postherpetic neuralgia.[33] The potential number of patients needing gabapentin for these two uses is limited, yet over 15.6 million prescriptions were dispensed for this drug in 2003. Gabapentin was originally marketed by Parke-Davis, a subsidiary of Warner-Lambert, which in turn was acquired by Pfizer, in 2000.

On March 14, 2002, the *New York Times* revealed that the manufacturer of gabapentin illegally promoted the drug to prescribing physicians for at least 11 "off-label" (unapproved) medical conditions, using their own employees, often physicians, euphemistically called "medical liaisons," as the messengers.[34] Apparently, much of the "evidence" for the safety and effectiveness of gabapentin for these 11 unapproved uses was fabricated by the drug's manufacturer. The fabrications involved paying physicians for the use of their names as authors of medical journal articles on unapproved uses for

The manufacturer of Neurontin plead guilty on May 13, 2004, to criminal and civil charges and agreed to pay $430 million in penalties for the illegal promotion of the drug for uses that were not shown to be safe and effective.[32]

gabapentin—articles that had actually been written by others working under the direction of the company's marketing department.

The company's promotional strategy for gabapentin became public as the result of a lawsuit and the release of court papers.[35] The questionable uses for gabapentin are:

1. **Bipolar Disorder:** Psychiatrists were told that early results from trials evaluating gabapentin in the treatment of bipolar disorder indicated a 90% response rate when the drug was started at 900 milligrams per day and increased to 4,800 milligrams per day. No such results existed. In fact, the only type of clinical trial being conducted at the time was a pilot study. According to court documents, Parke-Davis was in possession of clinical data indicating that increasing the dose did not increase gabapentin's effect. The FDA-approved dosage for gabapentin in adults is 900 to 1,800 milligrams per day.

Any data regarding gabapentin in bipolar disorder were anecdotal and of unclear scientific value. Most of the published reports on the use of gabapentin in bipolar disorder had been written and sponsored by Parke-Davis, a fact that was hidden. Medical liaisons of the company were trained to tell psychiatrists that there were no reports of adverse reactions with gabapentin when used in psychiatric illness. In fact, such reports *had* been given to Parke-Davis by health care professionals, but the company attempted to hide this information from physicians.

2. **Pain Syndromes, Peripheral Neuropathy, and Diabetic Neuropathy:** Parke-

Davis medical liaisons were instructed to report that "leaks" from clinical trials demonstrated that gabapentin was highly effective in the treatment of a number of pain syndromes and that a 90% response rate in the management of pain was being reported. No such evidence existed. Medical liaisons were trained to claim support for these findings as a result of inside information despite the fact that no such information existed. The only basis for these claims was anecdotal evidence of minimal, if any, scientific value. Many of the published case reports, according to the court papers, had been created and sponsored by Parke-Davis in articles that frequently hid the company's involvement in the creation of the article. The company's payment for the creation of these case reports was also concealed.

3. **Treatment of Epilepsy Alone (as Monotherapy):** Medical liaisons were strongly encouraged to push neurologists to prescribe gabapentin as the only drug to treat epilepsy, in spite of the fact that studies found it safe and effective only when used in combination with other seizure drugs. Neurologists were told that substantial evidence supported the company's claim that gabapentin was effective when used alone for seizure. In fact, at the time the court papers were filed, Parke-Davis knew that clinical trials using gabapentin alone in seizure were inconclusive. One of Parke-Davis's clinical trials showed that gabapentin alone was *not* effective. The vast majority of patients in the study taking gabapentin were unable to continue with gabapentin alone. In the same study, there was no significant difference between doses of 600, 1,200, and 2,400 milligrams. Nevertheless, Parke-Davis continued to urge doctors to use higher doses than approved by the FDA.

In 1997, the FDA rejected the company's application for approval of gabapentin as monotherapy in the treatment of seizures.

4. **Reflex Sympathetic Dystrophy (RSD):** Physicians were informed that extensive evidence demonstrated the efficacy of gabapentin in the treatment of RSD, a condition of pain and tenderness following traumatic injury to a limb. Again, the only evidence was in anecdotal reports of little or no scientific value. The Parke-Davis medical liaisons were trained to imply that case reports, most of which had been created or sponsored by the company, were actually scientifically valid studies.

5. **Attention Deficit Disorder (ADD):** Pediatricians were told that gabapentin was effective for the treatment of ADD. No hard data to support this claim existed—only occasional anecdotal evidence. Parke-Davis medical liaisons were trained to report that large numbers of physicians had success in treating ADD with gabapentin when no such case reports existed.

6. **Restless Leg Syndrome (RLS):** This is another condition in which company medical liaisons were trained to refer to a growing body of evidence relating to RLS when no such scientific data existed. The only reports were anecdotal, the majority of which had been sponsored or created by Parke-Davis.

7. **Trigeminal Neuralgia:** The company represented gabapentin as a treatment for trigeminal neuralgia, a syndrome of severe bursts of facial pain, when no scientific data supported this claim—only occasional anecdotal reports. No evidence was available that gabapentin was as effective as currently available and less expensive painkillers.

8. **Post-Herpetic Neuralgia (PHN):** This is a syndrome of severe pain following a herpes virus infection that causes shingles. Physicians were told that 75 to 80% of all PHN patients were successfully treated with gabapentin. Again, no clinical trial data supported such a claim at the time.

The FDA did approve gabapentin for PHN in June 2002. Two studies of gabapentin in PHN have been published[36,37] showing a modest effect for the drug compared to placebo. We will reserve our opinion on the therapeutic value of gabapentin in PHN until the FDA makes their reviews of the drug publicly available.

9. **Essential Tremor Periodic Limb Movement:** No scientific data supported Parke-Davis's claim that gabapentin was effective for this disorder, just anecdotal reports of dubious scientific value.

10. **Migraine:** Claims that gabapentin was effective in the treatment of migraine headache were made by company medical liaisons and were alleged to be based on early results from clinical trials. Pilot studies had been suggested and undertaken, but no early results existed to support these claims. The data were purely anecdotal and most case reports were either created or sponsored by Parke-Davis.

11. **Drug and Alcohol Withdrawal Seizures:** It was suggested by the company that gabapentin be used in the treatment of drug and alcohol withdrawal seizures despite the lack of any evidence supporting the use of the drug for these conditions.

Parke-Davis's made-up uses for gabapentin turned the drug into a "blockbuster"—the Wall Street description for any drug that brings in $1 billion a year or more.

The court papers offer a remarkable insight into the ethics (or lack thereof) of a major multinational pharmaceutical company. A senior marketing executive at Parke-Davis was quoted during a meeting as saying to medical liaisons: *"Pain management, now that's money. Monotherapy, that's money. We don't want to share these patients with everybody, we want them on Neurontin only. We want their whole drug budget, not a quarter, not half, the whole thing. . . . That's where we need to be holding their hand and whispering in their ear: 'Neurontin for pain, Neurontin for bipolar, Neurontin for monotherapy, Neurontin for everything . . .' I don't want to hear that safety crap either, have you tried Neurontin, every one of you should take one just to see there is nothing [that the drug is safe], it's a great drug."*

If you or a family member are taking gabapentin for one of the 10 unapproved uses listed above, you and the prescribing doctor should evaluate your need for gabapentin.

Before You Use This Drug

Tell your doctor if you have or have had:

- allergies to gabapentin or any ingredient in the formulation
- kidney disease
- pregnancy or are breast-feeding

Tell your doctor about any other drugs you take, including aspirin, herbs, vitamins, and other nonprescription products.

When You Use This Drug

- Do not drink alcohol or use other drugs that can cause drowsiness.
- Until you know how you react to this drug, do not drive or perform other activities requiring alertness. Gabapentin can cause dizziness, blurred vision, drowsiness, and lack of muscle coordination.
- Schedule regular visits with your doctor to check your progress, especially for the first few months you take gabapentin.
- Do not stop taking this drug without consulting your doctor about gradually reducing the dosage.

How to Use This Drug

- Gabapentin should not be taken for at least two hours after any antacid is used.
- Take with or without food.
- If you miss a dose of gabapentin, take it as soon as possible. However, if it is less than two hours until your next dose, take the missed dose right away, and take the next dose one to two hours later. Then go back to your regular dosing schedule. **Do not take double doses.**

• Do not exceed a 12-hour interval between any two doses while on a three-times-a-day dosing schedule.

• Do not share your medication with others.

• Take the drug at the same time(s) each day.

• Store capsules and tablets at room temperature with lid on tightly. Do not store in the bathroom. Do not expose to heat, moisture, or strong light. Keep out of reach of children.

• *Immediately before use:* Tablets or capsules may be mixed in with food or drink. Capsules may be opened and the contents mixed with applesauce, jelly, or ketchup, then swallowed without chewing.

• Store the liquid form of the drug in the refrigerator, but keep it from freezing. Also dissolve each dose as needed; do not dissolve ahead of time.

Interactions with Other Drugs

Evaluations of Drug Interactions 2003 lists no drugs, biologics (e.g., vaccines, therapeutic antibodies), or foods as causing "highly clinically significant" or "clinically significant" interactions when used together with the drugs in this section. We also found no interactions in the drugs' FDA-approved professional package inserts. However, as the number of new drugs approved for marketing increases and as more experience is gained with these drugs over time, new interactions may be discovered.

Adverse Effects

Call your doctor immediately if you experience:

• clumsiness or unsteadiness
• continuous, uncontrolled, back-and-forth, and/or rolling eye movements
• memory loss
• depression, irritability, or other mood or mental changes
• fever

• chills
• cough or hoarseness
• lower back or side pain
• painful or difficult urination

Call your doctor if these symptoms continue:

• weakness or loss of strength
• dizziness
• fatigue
• muscle ache or pain
• swelling of hands, feet, or lower legs
• drowsiness
• trembling or shaking
• blurred or double vision
• dry mouth or throat
• slurred speech
• frequent urination
• constipation
• diarrhea
• nausea or vomiting
• indigestion
• headache
• low blood pressure
• decreased sexual desire or ability
• trouble sleeping
• runny nose
• noise in ears
• twitching
• weight gain

Signs of overdose:

• diarrhea
• double vision
• slurred speech
• sluggishness
• drowsiness

If you suspect an overdose, call this number to contact your poison control center: (800) 222-1222.

Limited Use

Phenobarbital (fee noe *bar* bi tal)

GENERIC: available

FAMILY: Drugs for Epilepsy
Barbiturates (see p. 326)

PREGNANCY WARNING

A number of reports suggest an association between the use of phenobarbital by women with epilepsy and malformations in their infants, including spina bifida and heart defects. Taking more than one drug for epilepsy increases the risk. Tell your doctor if you are pregnant or thinking of becoming pregnant before you take this drug.

BREAST-FEEDING WARNING

Phenobarbital is excreted in human milk. Because of the potential for serious adverse effects in nursing infants, you should not take this drug while nursing.

Phenobarbital is of limited benefit to older adults because it is addictive and has potentially serious adverse effects. You should not be taking it to promote sleep, relieve nervousness or anxiety, lower blood pressure, or reduce pain. Like other barbiturates, it is commonly misused as a painkiller, despite the fact that it can actually increase your sensation of, and reaction to, pain. You should only be taking phenobarbital to control convulsions (seizures). For this purpose, you can take it at doses well below those that cause you to go to sleep.

If your kidney or liver function is impaired, you need to take less than the usual adult dose of phenobarbital. Phenobarbital causes liver cancer in mice and rats.

Before You Use This Drug

Do not use if you have or have had:

- porphyria
- pregnancy or are breast-feeding

Tell your doctor if you have or have had:

- allergies to barbiturates
- severe anemia

One hazard of taking this drug continuously for longer than several weeks is drug-induced dependence. **Do not stop taking your drug suddenly.** With the help of your doctor, work out a schedule for slowly lowering the amount of the drug you take by about 5 to 10% each day. Keep a written record of the dosage reduction schedule with you. These steps will make it much easier to become drug free without developing distressing symptoms of drug withdrawal.

- asthma or other breathing difficulties
- diabetes
- liver problems
- history of drug abuse or dependence
- abnormally increased and sometimes uncontrollable activity or muscular movements
- overactive thyroid (hyperthyroidism)
- adrenal gland problems
- mental depression or suicidal tendencies
- pain (acute or chronic)
- kidney problems
- weakness or feebleness

Tell your doctor about any other drugs you take, including aspirin, herbs, vitamins, and other nonprescription products.

When You Use This Drug

- Have regular visits with your doctor to check on your progress.
- Do not suddenly stop taking this drug without checking with your doctor to find out if you need to taper off.
- Until you know how you react to this drug, do not drive or perform other activities requiring alertness. Phenobarbital may cause drowsiness, dizziness, and lightheadedness.
- Do not drink alcohol or use other drugs that can cause drowsiness.
- If physical or psychological dependence is suspected, check with your doctor.

- Get emergency help at once if you suspect an overdose.
- If taking oral contraceptives, use another or additional birth control method.

How to Use This Drug

- If you miss a dose, take it as soon as you remember, but skip it if it is almost time for the next dose. **Do not take double doses.**
- Do not share your medication with others.
- Take the drug at the same time(s) each day.
- Do not increase the dose if the drug seems ineffective without checking with your doctor first.
- If you stop taking this medication, remember that adverse effects can still last for several weeks or months.
- *Extended-release form:* Swallow capsule or tablet whole.
- Store at room temperature with lid on tightly. Do not store in the bathroom. Do not expose to heat, moisture, or strong light. Keep out of reach of children.

Interactions with Other Drugs

The following drugs, biologics (e.g., vaccines, therapeutic antibodies), or foods are listed in *Evaluations of Drug Interactions* 2003 as causing "highly clinically significant" or "clinically significant" interactions when used together with any of the drugs in this section. In some sections with multiple drugs, the interaction may have been reported for one but not all drugs in this section, but we include the interaction because the drugs in this section are similar to one another. We have also included potentially serious interactions listed in the drug's FDA-approved professional package insert or in published medical journal articles. There may be other drugs, especially those in the families of drugs listed below, that also will react with this drug to cause severe adverse effects. Make sure to tell your doctor and pharmacist the drugs you are taking and tell them if you are taking any of these interacting drugs:

AGENERASE, alcohol, amprenavir, chlorpromazine, COUMADIN, CRYSTODIGIN, cyclosporine, DECADRON, delavirdine, DEPAKENE/DEPAKOTE, dexamethasone, digitoxin, divalproex/valproic acid, doxycycline, DURAQUIN, ELIXOPHYLLIN, FLAGYL, FORTOVASE, GABITRIL, HEXADROL, INVIRASE, LOPRESSOR, methoxyflurane, metoprolol, metronidazole, nelfinavir, NEORAL, NORVIR, oral contraceptives, oxcarbazepine, PENTHRANE, QUINAGLUTE DURA-TABS, QUINIDEX, quinidine, RESCRIPTOR, ritonavir, SANDIMMUNE, saquinavir, SLO-BID, THEO-24, theophylline, THORAZINE, tiagabine, TOPROL XL, TRILEPTAL, VIBRAMYCIN, valproic acid, VIRACEPT, warfarin.

Adverse Effects

Call your doctor immediately if you experience:

- confusion
- mental depression
- unusual excitement
- sore throat and/or fever
- skin rash or hives
- swelling of eyelids, face, or lips
- wheezing or chest tightness
- red, thickened, or scaly skin
- hallucinations
- unusual tiredness or weakness
- bleeding sores on lips
- chest pain
- muscle or joint pain
- painful sores, ulcers, or white spots in mouth
- unusual bleeding or bruising
- yellow eyes or skin
- bone pain, tenderness, or aching

- appetite loss
- weight loss

Call your doctor if these symptoms continue:

- clumsiness or unsteadiness
- dizziness or lightheadedness
- drowsiness
- "hangover" feeling
- anxiety or nervousness
- constipation
- faintness
- headache
- irritability
- nausea or vomiting
- nightmares or trouble sleeping

Call your doctor if these symptoms continue after you stop taking this drug:

- anxiety or restlessness
- muscle twitching
- hand trembling
- weakness
- dizziness
- vision problems
- nausea
- vomiting
- trouble sleeping
- increased dreaming or nightmares
- faintness
- lightheadedness
- convulsions
- hallucinations

Signs of overdose:

- severe confusion
- decrease in or loss of reflexes
- severe drowsiness
- fever
- low body temperature
- shortness of breath or troubled breathing
- slow heartbeat
- slurred speech
- staggering

- unusual eye movements
- severe weakness

If you suspect an overdose, call this number to contact your poison control center: (800) 222-1222.

Periodic Tests

Ask your doctor which of these tests should be done periodically while you are taking this drug:

- complete blood count
- liver function tests
- kidney function tests
- blood levels of phenobarbital (when used as an anticonvulsant)
- folate concentrations
- bone marrow function

Phenytoin (*fen* i toyn)
DILANTIN (Parke-Davis)

GENERIC: available
FAMILY: Drugs for Epilepsy

PREGNANCY WARNING

Phenytoin has caused serious harm to human infants born to mothers taking this drug during pregnancy. Such infants have been born with cleft palate, damage to the heart, a small head, and mental deficiency. There have been reports of cancer in children whose mothers took phenytoin during pregnancy. Because of the potential for serious adverse effects to the fetus, this drug should not be used by pregnant women.

BREAST-FEEDING WARNING

Phenytoin is excreted in human milk. Because of the potential for serious adverse effects in nursing infants, you should not take this drug while nursing.

Phenytoin is approved by the FDA to treat most forms of epilepsy. If you are taking phenytoin, you should adhere strictly to the prescribed dosing schedule and inform the prescribing physician of any situation in which it is not possible to take the drug as prescribed, for example, surgery. Your physician should be notified if a skin rash develops.

Good dental hygiene is important in order to minimize the development of gingival hyperplasia (gum overgrowth) and its complications.

Before You Use This Drug

Do not use if you have or have had:

- heart disease

Tell your doctor if you have or have had:

- allergies to drugs
- pregnancy or are breast-feeding
- alcohol dependence
- blood cell abnormalities
- diabetes
- fever above 101°F for longer than 24 hours
- liver problems
- hcart or blood vesssel disease
- porphyria
- kidney problems
- thyroid problems
- systemic lupus erythematosus

Tell your doctor about any other drugs you take, including aspirin, herbs, vitamins, and other nonprescription products.

When You Use This Drug

- Schedule regular visits with your doctor to check your progress.
- Check with your doctor before taking other drugs.
- Until you know how you react to this drug, do not drive or perform other activities requiring alertness. Phenytoin can cause dizziness, blurred vision, drowsiness, and lack of muscle coordination.
- Do not drink alcohol.
- Do not take this drug within two to three hours of taking an antacid or drug for diarrhea.
- Do not change brands or dosage forms of this drug without checking with your doctor.

- Do not suddenly stop taking this drug without checking with your doctor to find out if you need to taper off the drug.
- Schedule frequent visits with your dentist to have your teeth cleaned, to prevent enlarged, tender, and bleeding gums.
- Wear a medical identification bracelet or carry a card stating that you take phenytoin.
- There is a possible interference with some laboratory tests.
- If you plan to have any surgery, including dental, tell your doctor that you take this drug.
- If using oral contraceptives, use a different or additional birth control method.

How to Use This Drug

- Do not share your medication with others.
- Take the drug at the same time(s) each day.
- If you miss a dose and you are supposed to take the drug once a day, take as soon as possible unless it is the next day, then continue on schedule. **Do not take double doses.** If you are supposed to take the drug several times a day, take the missed dose as soon as possible unless within four hours of next scheduled dose, then continue on regular schedule. **Do not take double doses.** Check with your doctor if doses are missed for two or more days in a row.
- Take with food.
- Store at room temperature with lid on tightly. Do not store in the bathroom. Do not expose to heat, moisture, or strong light. Keep out of reach of children.
- *For liquid dosage form:* Shake well and use an accurate measuring spoon, a plastic syringe, or a small graduated cup.
- *For chewable tablets:* Chew or crush tablets or swallow them whole.
- *For capsules:* Swallow capsule whole.

Interactions with Other Drugs

The following drugs, biologics (e.g., vaccines, therapeutic antibodies), or foods are listed in

Evaluations of Drug Interactions 2003 as causing "highly clinically significant" or "clinically significant" interactions when used together with any of the drugs in this section. In some sections with multiple drugs, the interaction may have been reported for one but not all drugs in this section, but we include the interaction because the drugs in this section are similar to one another. We have also included potentially serious interactions listed in the drug's FDA-approved professional package insert or in published medical journal articles. There may be other drugs, especially those in the families of drugs listed below, that also will react with this drug to cause severe adverse effects. Make sure to tell your doctor and pharmacist the drugs you are taking and tell them if you are taking any of these interacting drugs:

8-MOP, ADALAT, ADALAT CC, ADVIL, AGENERASE, alcohol, ALERMINE, allopurinol, amiodarone, amprenavir, ANTABUSE, azapropazone, BICNU, CALCIFEROL, CAMPTOSAR, CARAFATE, carmustine, charcoal, chloramphenicol, CHLOROMYCETIN, chlorpheniramine, CHLOR-TRIMETON, cimetidine, CIPRO, ciprofloxacin, clopidogrel, CORDARONE, cyclosporine, DECADRON, delavirdine, DEPAKENE/DEPAKOTE, dexamethasone, diazoxide, dicumarol, DIFLUCAN, digitalis, digoxin, disopyramide, disulfiram, divalproex/valproic acid, dopamine, doxycycline, DURAQUIN, ELIXOPHYLLIN, ergocalciferol, felbamate, FELBATOL, fluconazole, fluoxetine, folic acid, FOLICET, FOLVITE, FORTOVASE, GABITRIL, GANTANOL, GLUCOPHAGE, HEXADROL, ibuprofen, INH, INTROPIN, INVIRASE, irinotecan, isoniazid, ketorolac, LANOXICAPS, LANOXIN, metformin, methotrexate, methoxsalen, miconazole, MONISTAT-DERM, MONISTAT 7, MOTRIN, MYSO-LINE, nelfinavir, NEORAL, nifedipine, NORPACE, NORVIR, omeprazole, oral contraceptives, OXSORALEN, oxcarbazepine, PLAVIX, PRIFTIN, PRILOSEC, primidone, PROCARDIA, PROCARDIA XL, PROGLYCEM, PROLOPRIM, PROZAC, quetiapine, QUINAGLUTE DURA-TABS, QUINIDEX, quinidine, RESCRIPTOR, RIFADIN, rifampin, RIMACTANE, rifapentine, ritonavir, SANDIMMUNE, saquinavir, SEROQUEL, sertindole, SLO-BID, sucralfate, sulfamethizole, sulfamethoxazole, TAGAMET, THEO-24, theophylline, THIOSULFIL, tiagabine, ticlodipine, TICLID, TOPAMAX, topiramate, TORADOL, TRILEPTAL, trimethoprim, TRIMPEX, valproic acid, VELBAN, VIBRAMYCIN, vinblastine, VIRACEPT, vitamin D, ZYLOPRIM.

Adverse Effects

Call your doctor immediately if you experience:

- appetite and weight loss
- painful, tingling, or numb hands or feet
- bleeding, tender, or enlarged gums
- difficulty breathing
- chills
- clumsiness or unsteadiness
- chest discomfort
- confusion
- dark urine
- defects in intelligence, short-term memory, learning ability, or attention
- dizziness
- fever
- hand trembling
- headache
- joint pain
- light gray stools
- muscle pain
- nausea or vomiting

- nosebleeds or other unusual bleeding or bruising
- restlessness or agitation
- severe stomach pain
- skin rash or itching
- slurred speech or stuttering
- sore throat
- uncontrolled movements of eyes, hands, arms, legs, lips, tongue, or cheeks
- unusual excitement, nervousness, or irritability
- unusual tiredness or weakness
- yellow eyes or skin
- penile pain
- bone disorders or fractures

Call your doctor if these symptoms continue:

- constipation
- mild dizziness
- mild drowsiness
- nausea and vomiting
- enlargement of facial features
- swelling of breasts in males
- headache
- unusual and excessive hair growth on body and face
- trouble sleeping
- muscle twitching

Signs of overdose:

- clumsiness or unsteadiness
- staggering walk
- blurred or double vision
- severe confusion
- severe dizziness or drowsiness
- stuttering
- slurred speech
- blood pressure changes
- nausea and vomiting
- continuous, uncontrolled back-and-forth and/or rolling eye movements
- seizures

- tremor
- unusual tiredness or weakness

If you suspect an overdose, call this number to contact your poison control center: (800) 222-1222.

Periodic Tests

Ask your doctor which of these tests should be done periodically while you are taking this drug:

- blood levels of phenytoin
- electroencephalogram (EEG)
- complete blood and platelet count
- thyroid function tests
- dental exam, every three months
- liver function tests
- blood levels of calcium
- blood levels of albumin
- respiratory function tests
- blood pressure
- blood levels of folate
- blood levels of phosphate
- cardiac function tests
- physical exam

Spasticity

Limited Use

Tizanidine (tye *zan* i dine)
ZANAFLEX (Elan)

GENERIC: not available
FAMILY: Drugs for Spasticity

PREGNANCY WARNING
Tizanidine caused fetal death and developmental retardation in animal studies. Because of the potential for serious adverse effects to the fetus, this drug should not be used by pregnant women.

Tizanidine is approved by the FDA for the management of spasticity in conditions such as multiple sclerosis and spinal cord injury. It has been available in Japan and Europe since 1985 for use as a short-term muscle relaxant.[38]

This drug is related chemically to the blood-pressure-lowering drug clonidine (CATAPRES) (see p. 107).[39] Because tizanidine can lower blood pressure, it must be used cautiously in combination with blood-pressure-lowering drugs. Even when used alone, dizziness, lightheadedness, or fainting may be experienced when getting up suddenly from a sitting or lying position because of the blood-pressure-lowering effect of this drug.

Elevated liver function tests (LFT) greater than three times the upper limit of what is considered normal were seen in approximately 5% of patients participating in controlled clinical trials. This level of LFT elevation is an early indicator of possible liver toxicity. In postmarketing reports, three deaths from liver failure have been associated with the use of tizanidine. LFT monitoring should be done before and during the first six months of tizanidine treatment.[39]

Sedation was reported by 48% of patients taking tizanidine in clinical trials. In 10% of these cases, the sedation was described as severe.

A statistical summary of clinical trials, called a meta-anaylsis, examined the comparative effectiveness and tolerability of various antispasticity drugs in multiple sclerosis patients, including tizanidine. Because the use of these agents in multiple sclerosis is poorly documented, no recommendations could be made on which drug is the best.[40]

Before You Use This Drug

Tell your doctor if you have or have had:

- kidney disease
- allergy to tizanidine
- liver disease
- pregnancy or are breast-feeding

Tell your doctor about any other drugs you take, including aspirin, herbs, vitamins, and other nonprescription products.

When You Use This Drug

- Schedule regular visits with your doctor to check your progress.
- Until you know how you react to this drug, do not drive or perform other activities that require alertness.
- Do not drink alcohol or use other drugs that can cause drowsiness.
- Chew sugarless gum, candy, or ice, or use a saliva substitute if you develop dryness in your mouth. If dryness continues more than two weeks, check with your doctor or dentist.
- You may feel dizzy when rising from a lying or sitting position. When getting out of bed, hang your feet over the side of the bed for a few minutes, then get up slowly. When getting out of a chair, stay by the chair until you are sure that you are not dizzy. (See p. 13.)
- Do not suddenly stop taking this drug without checking with your doctor to find out if you need to taper off.

How to Use This Drug

- If you miss a dose, take it if it is within an hour of the missed dose, but skip it if you don't remember until later. **Do not take double doses.**
- Do not share your medication with others.
- Take the drug at the same time(s) each day.
- Store at room temperature with lid on

tightly. Do not store in the bathroom. Do not expose to heat, moisture, or strong light. Keep out of reach of children.

Interactions with Other Drugs

The following drugs, biologics (e.g., vaccines, therapeutic antibodies), or foods are listed in *Evaluations of Drug Interactions* 2003 as causing "highly clinically significant" or "clinically significant" interactions when used together with any of the drugs in this section. In some sections with multiple drugs, the interaction may have been reported for one but not all drugs in this section, but we include the interaction because the drugs in this section are similar to one another. We have also included potentially serious interactions listed in the drug's FDA-approved professional package insert or in published medical journal articles. There may be other drugs, especially those in the families of drugs listed below, that also will react with this drug to cause severe adverse effects. Make sure to tell your doctor and pharmacist the drugs you are taking and tell them if you are taking any of these interacting drugs:

> alcohol, any blood-pressure-lowering medications, oral contraceptives, or phenytoin (DILANTIN).

Adverse Effects

Call you doctor immediately if you experience:

- nervousness
- tingling, burning, or prickling sensations
- fever
- appetite loss
- nausea or vomiting
- yellow eyes or skin
- skin sores
- painful or burning urination

- irregular heartbeat
- unusual tiredness or weakness
- chills, fever, or sore throat
- black, tarry stools
- bloody vomit
- coldness
- dry, puffy skin
- weight gain
- mood or mental changes, including false beliefs
- hallucinations
- kidney stones
- seizures
- fainting
- cough
- blurred vision
- eye pain

Call your doctor if these symptoms continue:

- anxiety
- neck pain
- unusual tiredness or weakness
- back pain
- constipation
- depression
- dizziness or lightheadedness
- drowsiness or sleepiness
- dry mouth
- uncontrolled body movements
- heartburn
- diarrhea
- stomach pain
- vomiting
- muscle spasms or weakness
- increased sweating
- sore throat
- runny nose
- skin rash
- difficulty speaking
- hair loss
- arthritis
- warm, swollen, and tender body areas
- dry skin

- difficulty swallowing
- swelling of feet or lower legs
- migraine headache
- mood or mental changes, including agitation
- unusual feeling of well-being
- trembling or shaking
- weight loss

Signs of overdose:

- difficulty breathing

If you suspect an overdose, call this number to contact your poison control center: (800) 222-1222.

Periodic Tests

Ask your doctor which of these tests should be done periodically while you are taking this drug:

- liver function tests

REFERENCES

1. Katzenschlager R, Sampaio C, Costa J, et al. Anticholinergics for symptomatic management of Parkinson's disease. *Cochrane Database of Systematic Reviews* 2003:CD003735.

2. Chan DK. The art of treating Parkinson disease in the older patient. *Australian Family Physician* 2003; 32:927–31.

3. Comtan (Entacapone) Professional Product Labeling, March 1, 2002. Available at: http://www.pharma.us.novartis.com/product/pi/pdf/comtan.pdf.

4. Fenelon G, Gimenez-Roldan S, Montastruc JL, et al. Efficacy and tolerability of entacapone in patients with Parkinson's disease treated with levodopa plus a dopamine agonist and experiencing wearing-off motor fluctuations. A randomized, double-blind, multicentre study. *Journal of Neural Transmission* 2003; 110:239–51.

5. Ahlskog JE. Medical treatment of later-stage motor problems of Parkinson disease. *Mayo Clinic Proceedings* 1999; 74:1239–54.

6. Najib J. Entacapone: A catechol-O-methyltransferase inhibitor for the adjunctive treatment of Parkinson's disease. *Clinical Therapeutics* 2001; 23:802–32.

7. Rinne UK, Larsen JP, Siden A, et al. Entacapone enhances the response to levodopa in parkinsonian patients with motor fluctuations. Nomecomt Study Group. *Neurology* 1998; 51:1309–14.

8. Kaakkola S. Clinical pharmacology, therapeutic use and potential of COMT inhibitors in Parkinson's disease. *Drugs* 2000; 59:1233–50.

9. Kupsch A, Trottenberg T, Bremen D. Levodopa therapy with entacapone in daily clinical practice: Results of a post-marketing surveillance study. *Current Medical Research and Opinions* 2004; 20:115–20.

10. Heikkinen H, Nutt JG, LeWitt PA, et al. The effects of different repeated doses of entacapone on the pharmacokinetics of L-Dopa and on the clinical response to L-Dopa in Parkinson's disease. *Clinical Neuropharmacology* 2001; 24:150–7.

11. Brooks DJ, Sagar H. Entacapone is beneficial in both fluctuating and non-fluctuating patients with Parkinson's disease: A randomised, placebo controlled, double blind, six month study. *Journal of Neurology, Neurosurgery, and Psychiatry* 2003; 74:1071–9.

12. Entacapone for Parkinson's disease. *Medical Letter on Drugs and Therapeutics* 2000; 42:7–8.

13. Stalevo for Parkinson's Disease. *Medical Letter on Drugs and Therapeutics* 2004; 46:39–40.

14. Treatment Guidelines from the *Medical Letter:* Drugs for Parkinson's Disease, June 1, 2004:41–6.

15. Eldepryl (Selegiline) Professional Product Labeling, July 1, 1998. Available at: http://www.somersetpharm.com/products/product_labeling.html.

16. Dukes MNG, Beeley L. eds. *Side Effects of Drugs Annual* 14. Amsterdam: Elsevier, 1990:11–2.

17. Boyson SJ. Psychiatric effects of selegiline. *Archives of Neurology* 1991; 48:902.

18. Deprenyl for the treatment of early Parkinson's disease. *New England Journal of Medicine* 1990; 322:1526–8.

19. Parkinson Study Group. Impact of deprenyl and tocopherol treatment on Parkinson's disease in DATATOP patients requiring levodopa. *Annals of Neurology* 1996; 39:37–45.

20. Gilman AG, Rall TW, Nies AS, Taylor P, eds. *The Pharmacological Basis of Therapeutics.* 8th ed. New York: Pergamon Press, 1990:475.

21. Marsden CD. Parkinson's disease. *The Lancet* 1990; 335:948–52.

22. Food and Drug Administration. FDA Talk Paper: New Warnings for Parkinson's Drug Tasmar, November 16, 1998. Available at: http://www.fda.gov/bbs/topics/ANSWERS/ANS00924.html.

23. Roche Media Release. Tasmar Label Change in the U.S.: Suspension in the European Union, November 17, 1998.

24. *Physicians' Desk Reference.* 56th ed. Montvale, N.J.: Medical Economics Company, Inc., 2002:3010–5.

25. *Physicians' Desk Reference.* 56th ed. Montvale, N.J.: Medical Economics Company, Inc., 1999:3010–5.

26. Carbamazepine (tegretol)—trigeminal neuralgia and other uses. *Medical Letter on Drugs and Therapeutics* 1973; 15:95–6.

27. *Physicians' Desk Reference.* 40th ed. Oradell, N.J.: Medical Economics Company, Inc., 1986:900.

28. *US PDI, Drug Information for the Health Care Provider.* 6th ed. Rockville, Md.: The United States Pharmacopeial Convention, Inc., 1986:441.

29. *Physicians' Desk Reference.* 58th ed. Montvale, N.J.: Thomson PDR, 2004:2920–3.

30. *Physicians' Desk Reference.* 58th ed. Montvale, N.J.: Thomson PDR, 2004:430–4.

31. *Physicians' Desk Reference.* 58th ed. Montvale, N.J.: Thomson PDR, 2004:425–30.

32. United States Department of Justice District of Massachusetts. Warner-Lambert to Pay $430 Million to Resolve Criminal & Civil Health Care Liability Relating to Off-Label Promotion, press release, May 13, 2004.

33. *Physicians' Desk Reference.* 58th ed. Montvale, N.J.: Thomson PDR, 2004:2559–64.

34. Petersen M. Whistle-blower says marketers broke the rules to push a drug. *New York Times,* March 14, 2002:C1.

35. United States District Court for the District of Massachusetts. United States ex Rel. David Franklin v Pfizer, Inc., et al. Civil Action No. 96-11651-PBS. Available at: http://www.citizen.org/documents/1638attach.pdf.

36. Rice AS, Maton S. Gabapentin in postherpetic neuralgia: A randomised, double blind, placebo controlled study. *Pain* 2001; 94:215–24.

37. Rowbotham M, Harden N, Stacey B, et al. Gabapentin for the treatment of postherpetic neuralgia: A randomized controlled trial. *Journal of the American Medical Association* 1998; 280:1837–42.

38. Tizanidine for spasticity. *Medical Letter on Drugs and Therapeutics* 1997; 39:62–3.

39. *Physicians' Desk Reference.* 56th ed. Montvale, N.J.: Medical Economics Company, Inc., 2002:1305–6.

40. Shakespeare DT, Boggild M, Young C. Anti-spasticity agents for multiple sclerosis. *Cochrane Database of Systematic Reviews* 2003:CD001332.

23

ADRENAL STEROIDS

WHAT ARE ADRENAL STEROIDS?

Adrenal steroids are a class of hormones that regulate vital body functions. Hormones are chemicals produced in one organ in the body that then travel through the bloodstream to have an effect on organs elsewhere in the body. The steroids discussed in this chapter are produced by the adrenal glands, small organs weighing about one-sixth of an ounce that are located on top of the kidneys.

There are three types of adrenal steroids: mineralocorticoids, which maintain sodium and potassium balance in the body, glucocorticoids, and male sex steroids (although most male sex hormones are produced in the testicles). Mineralocorticoids and glucocorticoids are sometimes referred to jointly as corticosteroids, a term we do not use in this chapter. Male sex steroids (androgens) are also used, often illegally, as the so-called anabolic steroids used by athletes in the hope of enhancing performance. This chapter only considers glucocorticoids.

Glucocorticoids affect carbohydrate, protein, and fat metabolism, support normal heart and blood vessel function, influence mood and sleep patterns, and maintain normal muscle strength. They also inhibit the body's inflammatory response to acute or chronic disease and infection. Prescription glucocorticoids are either identical to or a synthetic version of the adrenal hormones. They are given to either replace the body's glucocorticoids when the adrenal glands are diseased or to suppress inflammation in diseases such as arthritis or asthma.

Glucocorticoids are taken in many different dosage forms. Nasal, ophthalmic (eye), topical (skin), and inhaler forms have been developed to deliver the drugs directly to the affected area, thus minimizing adverse effects. This chapter considers only oral (by mouth) and topical glucocorticoids; nasal glucocorticoids are discussed on p. 379, inhaled versions on p. 394, and eye forms on p. 521. Injectable forms of glucocorticoids as well as formulations for the ear also exist but are not discussed in this book. Some glucocorticoids have more than one formulation; we discuss the form that predominates in the marketplace.

DRUG PROFILES

Oral Adrenal Steroids

Dexamethasone (dex a *meth* a sone)
DECADRON (Merck)
HEXADROL (Organon USA)
MYMETHASONE (Morton Grove)

Hydrocortisone (hye droe *kor* ti sone)
CORTEF (Pharmacia & Upjohn)
HYDROCORTONE (Merck)

Methylprednisolone (meth il pred *niss* oh lone)
MEDROL (Pharmacia & Upjohn)

Prednisolone (pred *niss* oh lone)
PRELONE (Teva)

Prednisone (*pred* ni sone)
DELTASONE (Pharmacia & Upjohn)

GENERIC: available

FAMILY: Adrenal Steroids

PREGNANCY WARNING

Glucocorticoids cross the placenta and expose the fetus to the drug. Because of the potential for serious adverse effects to the fetus, including cleft palate, spontaneous abortions, and growth retardation, these drugs should not be used by pregnant women.

BREAST-FEEDING WARNING

Glucocorticoids are excreted in human milk. Because of the potential for serious adverse effects in nursing infants, including growth suppression and inhibition of steroid production in the infant, you should not take these drugs while nursing.

Glucocorticoids, one of the groups of adrenal steroids (see discussion on p. 664), are used to treat asthma, bronchitis, allergies, and other breathing problems; conditions that produce inflammation, such as arthritis and other joint and muscle disorders; skin conditions; and certain cancers, hormonal disorders, and infections. For several of these conditions (e.g., asthma), these drugs can be extremely effective and even lifesaving. For others (e.g., allergies, arthritis), they are best not used as initial therapy and should instead be saved for more severe cases. Unfortunately, some physicians still prescribe oral glucocorticoids too widely. For example, some pediatricians use the drugs for a variety of ear, nose, and throat conditions, despite the absence of evidence to support most such uses.[1] Similarly, glucocorticoids can be effective in the treatment of rheumatoid arthritis, but their place in therapy remains controversial; other drugs should be used first.[2]

Drugs taken by mouth (orally) are distributed throughout the body—to areas that require treatment as well as to those that do not. Because the entire body is exposed to the drug's action, there can be unnecessary adverse effects. For this reason, if the drug can be delivered directly to the site of action (e.g., eye, lung, skin), this is generally preferred. For similar reasons, the oral glucocorticoids should be used at the lowest effective dose and for the shortest duration possible.

Adverse effects from oral glucocorticoids can be minimized further by using alternate-day therapy. If you will be taking oral steroids on a long-term basis, ask your doctor about switching to alternate-day therapy. The body's own glucocorticoids are released primarily in the early morning hours between 4:00 A.M. and 8:00 A.M., with very little being released in the evenings. These variations help to set your body's clock and to establish sleep and waking cycles. Therefore, for the least disruption of your body's natural rhythms, a single daily dose or an alternate-day dose should be taken in the morning prior to 8:00 A.M.

If you take an oral glucocorticoid every day or every other day, you will need one that stays in the body long enough. Adrenal steroids are divided into short-acting (e.g., hydrocortisone), intermediate-acting (e.g., methylprednisolone, prednisolone, prednisone), and long-acting glucocorticoids (e.g., dexamethasone). For the conditions discussed in this chapter, intermediate-acting glucocorticoids will usually be the most appropriate choice,[3] and prednisone is the one used most frequently.

Glucocorticoids suppress your immune system, lowering your defenses against disease and making you more vulnerable to infections. If you use these drugs for a long time, you increase your risk of getting bacterial, viral, parasitic, and fungal infections. For this reason, avoid exposure to chicken pox and measles, in particular, if you are taking these drugs.

Glucocorticoids can also cause osteoporosis— even if used short-term or at low doses[4]—fluid retention, and high blood pressure. These adverse effects are all more common in the elderly.

Glucocorticoid users are also more prone to gastrointestinal ulcers and psychiatric disturbances ranging from confusion to depression to psychosis. They cause glaucoma and cataracts and slow wound healing. More commonly, they lead to weight gain and high blood sugar. The drugs should not be used if body-wide fungal or threadworm infection is present. Live virus vaccines (e.g., smallpox, oral polio virus) should not be administered to patients on high doses of glucocorticoids.

If you no longer need an oral glucocorticoid, your doctor should slowly reduce your dose over several weeks, unless you have only been taking the medication for less than a week. This is done to avoid a withdrawal syndrome (muscle and joint pain, fever) and, rarely, the absence of or reduction in adrenal function (due to previous suppression by the glucocorticoid), a serious medical problem.

In sum, these are useful drugs that are sometimes overprescribed but whose toxicity can be minimized if they are prescribed and taken properly.

Before You Use This Drug

Tell your doctor if you have or have had:

- albumin levels in blood that are low
- allergy to adrenal steroids
- blood pressure that is elevated
- chicken pox (existing or recent)
- cholesterol that is elevated
- cold sores
- colitis
- diabetes

- diverticulitis
- fungal infection throughout the body
- glaucoma
- heart disease
- herpes eye infection
- HIV or AIDS
- infection
- kidney disease
- liver disease
- lupus
- measles (existing or recent)
- myasthenia gravis
- osteoporosis
- pregnancy or are breast-feeding
- psychosis
- stomach ulcer, esophagitis, or gastritis
- surgery or serious injury that is recent
- threadworm infection
- thyroid problems
- tuberculosis

Tell your doctor about any other drugs you take, including aspirin, herbs, vitamins, and other nonprescription products.

When You Use This Drug

- If you plan to have any surgery, including dental, tell your doctor that you take this drug.
- Do not drink alcohol; it may increase the chance of ulcers.
- Check with doctor before discontinuing medicine.
- This drug may increase blood glucose concentrations in patients with diabetes.
- See doctor regularly to check progress during and following therapy.

For patients on long-term therapy:

- Possible need for
  - salt restriction
  - potassium supplements
  - calorie restriction
  - increased protein in diet

- eye exams
- caution when receiving skin tests

• Carry a medical identification card or bracelet indicating use of this drug.

• Tell your doctor if you get a serious infection or injury.

• Avoid exposure to persons who have chicken pox or measles, or who have just had an oral polio virus vaccine. Tell your doctor immediately if contact occurs.

• Check with your doctor before getting any vaccinations.

How to Use This Drug

- Do not share your medication with others.
- Take the drug at the same time(s) each day.
- Swallow capsules whole.
- Do not take more drug than prescribed.
- Take with food.

• Store at room temperature with lid on tightly. Do not store in the bathroom. Do not expose to heat, moisture, or strong light. Keep out of reach of children.

• Do not suddenly stop taking this drug without checking with your doctor to find out if you need to taper off. Gradual dosage reduction may be necessary. Check with your doctor if symptoms recur or worsen when the dose is decreased or therapy discontinued.

• If you miss a dose and your dosing schedule is every other day, take as soon as possible if remembered the same morning. If you remember later, then take the next morning and skip a day. If your dosing schedule is once a day, take the dose as soon as you remember, but skip it if it is almost time for the next dose. **Do not take double doses.** If your dosing schedule is several times a day, take the dose as soon as possible. Take double the dose if it's time for the next dose.

Interactions with Other Drugs

The following drugs, biologics (e.g., vaccines, therapeutic antibodies), or foods are listed in *Evaluations of Drug Interactions* 2003 as causing "highly clinically significant" or "clinically significant" interactions when used together with any of the drugs in this section. In some sections with multiple drugs, the interaction may have been reported for one but not all drugs in this section, but we include the interaction because the drugs in this section are similar to one another. We have also included potentially serious interactions listed in the drug's FDA-approved professional package insert or in published medical journal articles. There may be other drugs, especially those in the families of drugs listed below, that also will react with this drug to cause severe adverse effects. Make sure to tell your doctor and pharmacist the drugs you are taking and tell them if you are taking any of these interacting drugs:

aminogluthethimide, aspirin, BLOCADREN, carbamazepine, COUMADIN, CRIXIVAN, cyclosporine, CYTADREN, digoxin, DILANTIN, E-BASE, ECOTRIN, E-MYCIN, ephedrine, ERYC, ERY-TAB, erythromycin, FORTOVASE, GENUINE BAYER ASPIRIN, GLUCOPHAGE, hormonal contraceptives, interleukin-2, INVIRASE, ketoconazole, LANOXICAPS, LANOXIN, metformin, NIZORAL, NORVIR, PCE, phenobarbital, phenytoin, potassium-depleting diuretics (e.g., hydrochlorothiazide, see p. 60), RIFADIN, rifampin, RIMACTANE, ritonavir, SANDIMMUNE, saquinavir, TAO, TEGRETOL, THALOMID, thalidomide, timolol, TIMOPTIC, troleandomycin, warfarin.

Adverse Effects

Call your doctor immediately if you experience:

- allergic reaction
- blindness that is sudden
- breathing difficulty

- confusion
- depression
- disorientation
- excitement
- false sense of well-being
- hallucinations
- heart problems
- leg swelling
- mistaken feelings of self-importance or sense of being mistreated
- mood swings
- paranoia
- restlessness
- skin rash or hives
- thirst increased
- urination that is frequent
- vision that is decreased or blurred

Call your doctor if these symptoms continue:

- appetite increased
- dizziness, sensation of spinning, or light-headedness
- flushing of face or cheeks
- headache
- hiccups
- indigestion
- joint pain
- nausea
- nervousness or restlessness
- skin color changes
- sleeping difficulty
- sweating increased
- vomiting
- weight gain

Call your doctor immediately if you experience these symptoms during long-term use:

- acne
- apathy
- appetite loss
- blood pressure decreased
- blood pressure elevated
- bone fractures
- breathing difficulty

- bruising that is unusual
- burning, tingling, or prickly sensations in any part of the body
- cataracts
- coma
- confusion
- eye pain
- eyes red
- eyes sensitive to light
- eyes tearing
- face rounder
- fainting
- glaucoma
- growth suppression in children
- hair growth increase
- headache
- heart problems
- hip or shoulder pain
- lightheadedness
- lines on the skin of arms, face, legs, trunk or groin that are reddish or purplish
- menstrual irregularities
- muscle cramps or pain
- muscle weakness
- nausea
- osteoporosis
- pain in back, ribs, arms, or legs
- seizures
- skin that is thin and shiny
- sleeping difficulty
- stomach pain
- stools that are bloody or black, tarry
- swelling of feet or lower legs
- tendon rupture
- tiredness or weakness that is unusual
- vision blurry or gradual loss of vision
- vomiting
- weight gain that is unusual
- wounds that will not heal

Call your doctor if these symptoms continue after you stop taking this drug:

- abdominal or back pain
- appetite loss that is prolonged
- breathing difficulty

- dizziness
- fainting
- fever
- headaches that are frequent or continuing
- muscle or joint pain
- nausea
- reappearance of disease symptoms
- tiredness or weakness that is unusual
- vomiting
- weight loss that is rapid

Periodic Tests

Ask your doctor which of these tests should be done periodically while you are taking this drug:

- adrenal function tests
- blood in stool
- electrolytes
- eye exam
- glucose testing in blood or urine
- prothrombin time, for patients receiving anticoagulants

Topical Adrenal Steroids

Betamethasone (bay ta *meth* a sone)
ALPHATREX (Savage)
DIPROLENE (Schering)
DIPROSONE (Schering)

Desoximetasone (des ox i *met* a sone)
TOPICORT (Medicis)

Fluocinolone (floo oh *sin* oh lone)
SYNALAR (Medicis)

Fluocinonide (floo oh *sin* oh nide)
LIDEX, LIDEX-E (Medicis)

Hydrocortisone (hye dro *kor* ti sone)
ALA-CORT (Del Ray Labs)

HI-COR (C and M Pharma)
HYTONE (Dermik Labs)
PENECORT (Allergan Herbert)
SYNACORT (Medicis)

Triamcinolone (trye am *sin* oh lone)
ARISTOCORT (Fujisawa)
KENALOG (Apothecon)
TRIACET (Teva)
TRIDERM (Del Ray Labs)

GENERIC: available
FAMILY: Adrenal Steroids

PREGNANCY WARNING

Glucocorticoids were absorbed through the skin and caused harm to fetuses (malformations) in animal studies. Because of the potential for serious adverse effects to the fetus, these drugs should not be used by pregnant women.

BREAST-FEEDING WARNING

Glucocorticoids are excreted in human milk. Because of the potential for serious adverse effects in nursing infants, you should not take these drugs while nursing.

These drugs are applied to the skin (topical use) and are commonly used to reduce inflammation (redness and swelling) and relieve itching caused by many kinds of skin conditions (e.g., eczema, psoriasis, seborrheic dermatitis).

There are two major categories of glucocorticoid (see explanation, p. 664) preparations that are applied to the skin: those that contain fluorine and those that do not. In general, fluorinated versions (e.g., fluocinonide) are more effective than those that are not fluorinated (e.g., hydrocortisone). However, the fluorinated preparations are more likely to cause adverse effects such as skin thinning (particularly on the face, armpits, and groin), loss of pigment, and acne. In general, one should use the least potent preparation that is effective. Fluorinated glucocorticoids, in particular, should not be used for prolonged periods on the face or around the eye. Higher-strength glucocorticoids, in particular, should be spread in a very thin layer, covering only the area requiring treatment. For most conditions, applying the medication once daily will suffice.[5] If the area that you are treating becomes irritated, stop using the drug and call your doctor. More potent versions should be avoided in children whenever possible.

Adverse effects beyond the skin, due to absorption into the blood system, are related to the amount and strength of drug used and can pose a problem when large areas of skin, especially in children, are treated. In principle, any adverse effect that can be caused by an oral glucocorticoid (see p. 664) could also result from topical use. However, such effects are rare if these preparations are used correctly.

For a given formulation, ointments are likely to be more effective than creams or lotions. However, some people find ointments too greasy, especially for hairy areas. In this case, a cream, lotion, or gel may come into better contact with the skin.

Sometimes doctors use occlusive techniques (e.g., gloves, plastic film) to cover the topical glucocorticoid. While this increases effectiveness, it also leads to more absorption into the body and potentially to more adverse effects. These techniques should be used only with a physician's order.

Hydrocortisone (CORTAID) can now be purchased without a prescription in two strengths, 0.25% and 0.50%. However, the lowest concentration of this drug that is generally considered effective is 0.50%.

Some manufacturers combine topical glucocorticoids with topical antifungals (e.g., betamethasone and clotrimazole [LOTRISONE]). Such products are discussed on p. 743.

Before You Use This Drug

Tell your doctor if you have or have had:

- allergies to glucocorticoids
- infection at treatment site
- pregnancy or are breast-feeding
- skin disorder

Tell your doctor about any other drugs you take, including aspirin, herbs, vitamins, and other nonprescription products.

When You Use This Drug

- Check with your doctor if symptoms do not improve within one week or get worse.
- You may experience stinging when this drug is applied. You do not need to call your doctor if this happens.

How to Use This Drug

- If you miss a dose, take it as soon as you remember, but skip it if it is almost time for the next dose. **Do not take double doses.**
- Do not share your medication with others.
- Take the drug at the same time(s) each day.
- Store at room temperature with lid on tightly. Do not store in the bathroom. Do not expose to heat, moisture, or strong light. Keep out of reach of children.
- Keep drug away from eyes.
- Do not bandage or otherwise wrap the treated skin area without your doctor's permission.
- *For foams:* Do not smoke while using; do not use near an open flame.
- *For aerosols:*
  - Do not smoke while using; do not use near an open flame.
  - Do not breathe spray vapors.
  - Do not get spray in eyes.

Interactions with Other Drugs

In general, any interaction that might occur with an oral glucocorticoid is theoretically possible with a topical formulation. However, the frequency and severity of such interactions are likely to be reduced and can be reduced further by the measures mentioned in this section. See p. 667 for a list of interactions reported for oral glucocorticoid drugs.

Adverse Effects

Call your doctor immediately if you experience:

- acne or oily skin
- appetite loss
- backache
- blood-containing blisters
- blood pressure increase
- bruising that is unusual
- depression
- eye pain
- face rounder
- finger numbness
- hair follicles are painful, itchy, red, and have pus-containing blisters
- hair growth increased
- hair loss
- heartbeat irregular
- irritability
- lines on the skin of the arms, face, legs, trunk, or groin that are reddish or purplish
- menstrual irregularities
- muscle cramps or pain
- muscle weakness
- nausea
- sexual desire or ability decreased in men
- skin burning and itching and/or pinsized red blisters
- skin color changes
- skin infection
- skin irritation around mouth
- skin sensitivity increased
- skin thinning and bruising
- skin with raised, dark red, wartlike spots
- stomach bloating, burning, cramping, or pain
- swelling of feet or lower legs
- tiredness or weakness that is unusual
- vision blurring or loss
- vomiting
- weakness of arms and legs
- weight gain that is rapid
- weight loss

With long-term use of more potent formulations or if substantial absorption occurs:

- cataracts
- diabetes
- glaucoma
- tuberculosis

Call your doctor if these symptoms continue:

- burning, dry, irritated, itching, or red skin (mild; transient)
- skin lesions with increased redness or scaling (mild; temporary)
- skin rash (minor; transient)

Signs of overdose:

- backache
- depression
- face rounder
- irritability
- menstrual irregularities
- sexual desire or ability in men decreased
- tiredness or weakness that is unusual

If you suspect an overdose, call this number to contact your poison control center: (800) 222-1222.

Periodic Tests

Ask your doctor which of these tests should be done periodically while you are taking this drug:

- adrenal function tests

REFERENCES

1. Steroid therapy of acute ENT infections: Rarely indicated. *Prescrire International* 2001; 10:185–7.

2. Drugs for rheumatoid arthritis. *Medical Letter on Drugs and Therapeutics* 2000; 42:57–64.

3. Isselbacker, KJ, Braunwald E, Wilson JD, et al, eds. *Harrison's Principles of Internal Medicine.* 13th ed. New York: McGraw-Hill, 1994:1974.

4. Laan RF, van Riel PL, van Erning LJ, et al. Vertebral osteoporosis in rheumatoid arthritis patients: Effect of low dose prednisone therapy. *British Journal of Rheumatology* 1992; 31:91–6.

5. Topical steroids for atopic dermatitis in primary care. *Drug and Therapeutics Bulletin* 2003; 41:5–8.

24

DRUGS FOR INFECTIONS

ANTIBIOTICS

Antibiotics (drugs used to treat bacterial infections) are overwhelmingly misprescribed in the United States. Despite congressional hearings and numerous academic studies on this issue, it has become the general consensus that 40 to 60% of all antibiotics in this country are misprescribed. New studies continue to confirm the fact that a large proportion of antibiotic prescribing for both children and adults continues to be inappropriate.[1,2] To put it simply, a large proportion of antibiotics are prescribed in situations in which the infection cannot be treated by any antibiotic, or another, more effective and appropriate antibiotic should be used instead. This should be a major concern, since the misprescribing of antibiotics poses some real dangers to the population at large, as well as to the individuals taking them, especially older adults.

Widespread Misprescribing of Antibiotics

Colds and Bronchitis

Two recently published studies, based on nationwide data from office visits for children and adults, have decisively documented the expensive and dangerous massive overprescribing of antibiotics for conditions that, because of their viral origin, do not respond to these drugs. Forty-four percent of children under 18 years old were given antibiotics for treatment of a cold and 75% for treatment of bronchitis. Similarly, 51% of people 18 or older were treated with antibiotics for colds and 66% for bronchitis. Despite the lack of evidence of any benefit for most people from these treatments, more than 23 million prescriptions a year were written for colds, bronchitis, and upper respiratory infections. This accounted for approximately one-fifth of all prescriptions for antibiotics written for children or adults.[1,2]

Sore Throats

Sore throats are one of the leading causes of visits to doctors, with more than 10 million such visits a year. The only kind of sore throat that merits treatment with an antibiotic is a bacterial sore throat caused by group A beta-hemolytic streptococci, the so-called strep throat. Although only approximately 10% of adults seen by a doctor for a sore throat actually have a strep throat, 75% of patients with sore throats seen by doctors are prescribed an antibiotic.[3] Though the likelihood that a sore throat in a child is a strep throat is somewhat higher, perhaps 25%, the majority of children are also treated with antibiotics.

Bladder Infections

In a recent study of more than 13,000 women going to a doctor because of a bladder infection, more than 95% of whom had an acute bladder infection, not a recurrent one, only 37% were prescribed the preferred treatment for this condition, the combination antibiotic trimethoprim/sulfamethoxazole (sometimes prescribed by the brand name Bactrim or Septra. Almost as many (32%) were prescribed one of the heavily promoted fluoroquinolones such as ciprofloxacin (CIPRO), which are not the first-choice drug for bladder infections. Using such drugs when there is a better alternative contributes to the rapidly increasing and health-threatening problem of resistance to antibiotics, whereby when the fluoroquinolones are actually needed, people may be infected with bacteria that are resistant to them (see below). The recommended duration of treatment for an acute bladder infection is three days of the antibiotic,

and yet less than 10% of the prescriptions were for three days. The most common duration of treatment was 10 days, followed by seven and five days. Thus, in addition to using the wrong antibiotic most of the time, the duration of therapy was too long most of the time.[4]

FDA WARNING ON UNNECESSARY ANTIBIOTIC PRESCRIBING[5]

To reduce the development of drug-resistant bacteria and maintain the effectiveness of this antibacterial drug product and other antibacterial drugs, this drug product should be used only to treat or prevent infections that are proven or strongly suspected to be caused by susceptible bacteria. When culture and susceptibility information are available, they should be considered in selecting or modifying antimicrobial therapy. In the absence of such data, local epidemiology and susceptibility patterns may contribute to the empiric selection of therapy. Prescribing this antibacterial drug product in the absence of a proven or strongly suspected bacterial infection [for] a prophylactic indication is unlikely to provide benefit to the patient and increases the risk of the development of drug-resistant bacteria.

Problems from Misuse of Antibiotics

The problems resulting from misuse are adverse effects from the drugs, exposure to additional complications from ineffective treatment of an infection, and bacterial resistance to antibiotics. In addition, misprescribing is a waste of money.

Adverse Effects

Although the numbers of adverse effects and problems with antibiotics are often low compared with other drugs, there are still some serious adverse effects that can occur. For example, an allergic reaction to penicillin can cause death, although this is uncommon. Use of antibiotics taken by mouth can cause stomach irritation and diarrhea, which can progress to a more severe condition caused by intestinal bacteria that are difficult to kill.

Other antibiotics can cause problems with the liver and kidneys, which is a real concern when prescribing for older adults. The best way to avoid these adverse effects is not to use antibiotics unless they are indicated and to avoid especially dangerous ones whenever possible. This is not the current practice, however.

Chloramphenicol (see p. 733), for example, is one antibiotic that has a particular danger. In rare instances, this drug can cause irreversible bone marrow depression, which can be fatal. In 1983, 49% of all prescriptions of chloramphenicol were for conditions in which the drug was clearly not indicated, such as tonsillitis and infection prevention after surgery. This meant that half the prescriptions for chloramphenicol unnecessarily exposed people to a serious danger. Now, fortunately, it is rarely used (see p. 733).

Exposure to Additional Complications

As discussed above, antibiotics are often misused to treat the common cold, flu, or other acute respiratory illnesses that should not be treated with any antibiotic. Since both the cold and the flu are caused by viruses, there is absolutely no possible way antibiotics can help cure these diseases or speed up the natural cure. They can, however, make a person more susceptible to a dangerous bacterial superinfection, such as pneumonia, which could be resistant to the antibiotic the person is taking. Patients should not insist that their doctors prescribe antibiotics for trivial conditions such as colds.

Other microorganisms that are not killed by the antibiotics can cause an infection, such as candidiasis, a fungal infection. Oral candidiasis

is fairly common in older adults who wear dentures. A sore mouth or tongue, or soreness of the vagina, are possible symptoms.

Bacterial Resistance

This is becoming an ever-expanding problem. After antibiotics are used for a period of time, certain bacteria develop methods that enable them to become resistant to some antibiotics. The resistant bacteria are the ones that survive after antibiotic treatment, and over time they become the dominant force via a process of natural selection.

In a current campaign to educate doctors and the public about the seriousness of the problem of antibacterial resistance, the Federal Centers for Disease Control has published these worrisome statistics:

Drug-resistant pathogens are a growing threat to all people, especially in health care settings.

• Each year nearly 2 million patients in the United States get an infection in a hospital.
• Of those patients, about 90,000 die as a result of their infection.
• More than 70% of the bacteria that cause hospital-acquired infections are resistant to at least one of the drugs most commonly used to treat them.
• Persons infected with drug-resistant organisms are more likely to have longer hospital stays and require treatment with second- or third-choice drugs that may be less effective, more toxic, and/or more expensive.[6]

For example, the staphylococcus, a common bacterium causing skin infections, used to be exquisitely sensitive to penicillin when the drug was first introduced. Twenty years later, penicillin was no longer anywhere near as effective against the staphylococcus. A new drug, called methicillin, was designed to combat the "staph bug," and it was widely used. Over time, strains of methicillin-resistant "super-staph" (MRSA) have also emerged.

At a recent government-sponsored conference on antibiotic resistance, some alarming data were presented on the rapid rise in resistance to antibiotics of some common bacterial causes of life-threatening illness and death. For example, the odds that staph aureus will be resistant to a once extremely useful antibiotic, methicillin (MRSA), have increased from about 4% in 1980 to over 55% in 2000. Thus, clearly related to the wanton misprescribing of antibiotics to people who do not have bacterial infections or the wrong antibiotic to those who do have infections (see p. 673), there has been a more than 13-fold increase in resistance. For another common cause of bacterial illness and death, enterococcus, resistance of vancomycin (VRE) has increased from about 1% in 1988 to about 27% in 2000, a 27-fold increase.[7]

The consequences of increased bacterial resistance to antibiotics are very serious: infections with staph aureus resistant to methicillin (MRSA) can cause ventilator-assisted pneumonia, and blood infections associated with catheters in people in intensive care units (ICUs). In ICU patients, infections with VRE are taking the form of abdominal or blood infections. The authors of this review on the impact of antibiotic resistance summarized the possible outcomes caused by antibiotic-resistant organisms:[8]

- increased mortality
- prolonged length of hospital stay
- need for more costly therapy and management
- medical complications

These examples illustrate that newer, improved antibiotics are not the final answer to bacterial resistance. If new antibiotics are developed but then overused, bacteria will find new ways to develop resistance, rendering those drugs ineffective.

Many bacteria in the hospital setting have now become resistant to multiple antibiotics, and, as a result, infections with these bacteria have become a very dangerous occurrence. The only way to help stop the development of bacterial resistance is by discouraging the gross misuse and overuse of antibiotics. It makes sense to use these "magic bullets," especially the newer ones, only when necessary so that their power will still be effective when it is truly needed.

Thus, there are both dangers and benefits to antibiotics. When you have an infection that can be cured with the proper antibiotic, the benefit of taking the drug is much, much greater than its dangers. But since there are dangers, there are compelling reasons to avoid unnecessary use of antibiotics and to select the safest and most effective ones.

Avoiding Unnecessary Use of Antibiotics

There are several basic principles that should be followed in determining the correct antibiotic:

1. Establish that an antibiotic is necessary. This means that your infection has to be the type that can be effectively treated by an antibiotic. Antibiotics are used specifically to treat bacterial infections. Antibiotics do not treat viral infections, such as the common cold. (Although there has been some heartening progress in the development of specific antiviral agents such as amantadine and acyclovir, ribavirin, AZT, and other drugs for HIV infections, viral infections, for the most part, cannot be treated with drugs.)

2. Choose the correct antibiotic. It must be effective against the most likely organisms that can cause your infection. In our drug profiles on individual antibiotics, we state the types of infections for which each antibiotic is best suited.

3. Take a culture before using an antibiotic. A culture should be taken from the site where you have an infection, such as your throat, sputum, urine, or blood, and then grown to determine the specific organism that is causing your infection and whether it is susceptible to the preferred antibiotic. For example, if you have a urinary tract infection, the doctor should take a urine specimen and send it for culture before treating your infection. This does not mean that your infection cannot be treated right away, only that a culture is sent before you start antibiotics. In this way, if your infection persists, your doctor can determine which alternative antibiotic can be used against the bacteria. Your doctor may find out that you do not have an infection and do not require antibiotics.

4. Consider the cost of the antibiotic. This should be done when everything else is equal. If several antibiotics are equally effective, their cost should be taken into consideration when selecting a drug to use. Newer drugs on patent are much more expensive than older antibiotics that have been on the market for some time. For example, the oral cephalosporin cefuroxime (CEFTIN) is often used to treat urinary tract infections. There is no advantage to using this drug instead of a generic drug such as trimethoprim and sulfamethoxazole. Cefuroxime, however, costs 12 times as much for two weeks of treatment.[9] Clearly, in the case of a simple infection, the less expensive drug for the shorter period of time is preferred as an initial choice.

The Importance of Completing a Full Course of Therapy

It is important with any antibiotic to take the entire amount of the drug that your doctor prescribes. Often, after the first few days of taking antibiotics, you will begin to feel better. Perhaps you think that you do not have to finish your course of treatment, since you are, after all, feeling healthy. This is not the case, however. The length of the regimen that your doctor prescribes for you is designed to eliminate all of the bacteria that are causing your illness. If you do

not take all of your medication, the bacteria will not be completely eliminated and can quickly multiply, causing another infection. This infection may then be resistant to the original antibiotic.

In general, antibiotics taken by mouth are preferred if you do not require hospitalization and can take the pills without any problem. There is usually no advantage to having an injection of an antibiotic except in certain clinical situations.

Newer Versus Older Antibiotics

Remember, newer antibiotics are more expensive than the older ones. They should be used only when an advantage can be shown over older antibiotics—for example, if the new antibiotic is more active against resistant bacteria.

In summary, antibiotics can make a world of difference when the right antibiotic is chosen for the right situation. Unfortunately, in the United States and most of the rest of the world today, this is only being done a minority of the time. Questioning your doctor about why he or she is prescribing an antibiotic is a step in the right direction toward safer and better antibiotic use.

PENICILLINS AND CEPHALOSPORINS

Penicillins are a group of antibiotics used to kill bacteria or prevent infections. They are probably the least toxic of all the antibiotics. The penicillins are some of the most commonly prescribed antibiotics and are often the drugs of choice for people who are not allergic to them.

Cephalosporins are relatives of the penicillins and have a similar, if slightly expanded, range of action. They have a good safety record,[10] but certain problems can occur with their use. Diarrhea is the most common adverse effect, and it may become so bad that treatment must be stopped.

Following is a list of the penicillins and cephalosporins that are discussed in this book (generic and BRAND names). It does not identify the ones that are given mainly as injections or intravenously, most of which are used primarily in the hospital.

Penicillins (Oral)
- amoxicillin (AMOXIL)
- amoxicillin and clavulanate (AUGMEN-TIN)
- ampicillin (OMNIPEN)
- cloxacillin
- dicloxacillin (DYCILL, DYNAPEN)
- penicillin G
- penicillin (VK)

Cephalosporins (Oral)
- cefaclor (CECLOR)
- cefadroxil (DURICEF)
- cefditoren (SPECTRACEF)
- cefixime (SUPRAX)
- cefpodoxime (VANTIN)
- cefprozil (CEFZIL)
- cefuroxime axetil (CEFTIN)
- cephalexin (KEFLEX)
- cephradine (VELOSEF)
- loracarbef (LORABID)

Types of Allergic Reactions

Allergic reactions are the most common adverse effects observed with penicillins. Between 5 and 10% of the general public are allergic to them. If you are allergic to penicillins, you should carry a card or wear an ID bracelet stating that you are allergic. Make sure to tell your doctor if you think you have an allergy to penicillins so that the information will be recorded.

There are three kinds of allergic reactions to penicillins: immediate, accelerated, and delayed.

Immediate reactions, also known as anaphylaxis, usually happen within 20 minutes of receiving the drug. Symptoms range from skin rash and itching to swelling, difficulty breathing, and even death. Immediate anaphylactic reactions are very rare, occurring in less than 1% of the people who are allergic to penicillins.[11]

Accelerated reactions usually happen between 20 minutes and two days after taking penicillins. Itching, rash, and fever are some of the symptoms.

Delayed reactions usually happen at least two days to one month after taking penicillins. Symptoms can include fever, feeling sick or uncomfortable, skin rash, muscle or joint pain, or pain in the abdomen.

Similar allergies can occur in people who take cephalosporins, since the drugs are related to penicillins. If you experience any of the above symptoms, call your doctor immediately. Although penicillin and cephalosporin allergies are more common in people who have had such a reaction previously, they also can occur in people who have repeatedly taken penicillins without prior incident.

Some people who are allergic to a penicillin may also be allergic to a cephalosporin; this occurs about 5% of the time. Cephalosporins should not be used for people who have had immediate reactions to penicillins. People who have had delayed reactions, such as a rash, should discuss with their doctors whether they should take a cephalosporin.

In older adults, caution must be used with high intravenous or intramuscular doses of penicillins and cephalosporins to prevent damage to the nervous system resulting in seizures, drowsiness, and confusion.[12] The dose of most penicillins and cephalosporins must be reduced when the kidneys do not function normally in order to prevent other complications. For example, a normal dose of 20 million units of penicillin G potassium injection in someone with kidney problems could potentially lead to a severe or even fatal increase of potassium (hyperkalemia). Older adults and people with decreased kidney function are more likely to have damage to the kidney when a cephalosporin and an aminoglycoside antibiotic (gentamicin, tobramycin, and neomycin, for example) are used at the same time.

Almost any antibiotic can cause antibiotic-associated colitis (inflammation of the colon). Clindamycin, lincomycin, and ampicillin are thought to cause this disease most frequently. Other penicillins and cephalosporins are implicated less often, but this reaction is still common. Risk of this disease seems to increase with the age of the user.

Dosage Forms, Effects, and Uses

Oral forms of cefaclor, a cephalosporin, and most penicillins should be taken on an empty stomach (one hour before or two hours after meals) with a full glass (eight ounces) of water. Most other cephalosporins and amoxicillin can be taken on a full stomach. Try to take your doses at evenly spaced times during the day and night so that the amount of drug in your body will stay constant. Store liquid forms in the refrigerator, but do not allow them to freeze. Capsules may be opened to facilitate swallowing. Oral penicillins and cephalosporins may cause nausea, vomiting, or diarrhea.

Injectable forms of penicillins and cephalosporins can cause pain and swelling at the site of injection. Diabetics may not absorb these drugs well when they are given in the muscle. Tell your doctor if you are on a salt-restricted (sodium-restricted) diet, because injected penicillins and cephalosporins contain sodium. People who have congestive heart failure may have a hard time getting rid of extra sodium.[12]

People who are elderly, have poor nutrition, or are alcoholic may have a greater risk of developing bleeding problems (blood takes longer to clot, for example) that are associated with some of the cephalosporins.[13] Vitamin K supplements, as pills or injections, may prevent this complication.

Cephalosporins are often used to prevent in-fections caused by surgery. In most operations where an artificial part is used, such as open heart surgery, and in gynecologic and gastrointestinal surgery, the use of cephalosporins before surgery is generally justified.[14] For many operations, an older cephalosporin, such as cephalexin (KEFLEX), is preferred. An exception to this is pelvic and gastrointestinal surgery, for which cefoxitin (MEFOXIN) may be a better choice.[15]

Loracarbef is another expensive alternative for treatment of respiratory, urinary tract, and skin infections. For acute pharyngitis, penicillin remains the drug of choice. For skin or soft-tissue infections, there is no reason to use loracarbef rather than dicloxacillin, cephalexin, or cephradine.[16] Cefprozil may be used as an alternative to cefaclor and cefuroxime axetil for treatment of otitis media or bronchitis. The same can be said for cefprozil as for loracarbef. For acute pharyngitis and skin infections, there is no reason to use cefprozil rather than dicloxacillin, cephalexin, or cephradine.[16] However, in treating strep pharyngitis (strep throat), there is some evidence that second-generation oral cephalosporins such as cefpodoxime can be used for a shorter period of time.

Cephalosporins are widely overused in the United States. They are not the first-choice drugs to treat most infections. Usually when a cephalosporin is chosen to treat an infection, an equally effective and less expensive antibiotic is available. The newer cephalosporins are relatively expensive, but some of them have become the drugs of choice for some serious infections.[17]

FLUOROQUINOLONES

The following fluoroquinolones (generic and BRAND names) are discussed in this book:

- ciprofloxacin (CIPRO, CILOXAN)
- enoxacin (PENETREX)

- gatifloxacin (TEQUIN)
- gemifloxacin (FACTIVE)
- levofloxacin (LEVAQUIN)
- lomefloxacin (MAXAQUIN)
- moxifloxacin (AVELOX)
- norfloxacin (NOROXIN, CHIBROXIN)
- ofloxacin (FLOXIN, OCUFLOX)
- sparfloxacin (ZAGAM)
- trovafloxacin (TROVAN)

One of the biggest-selling and most overprescribed classes of drugs in the United States is the family called fluoroquinolones. One clue that a drug your doctor wants to give you is in this class is the fact that the generic names of all such drugs approved in the United States include the sequence floxacin. These drugs have been alternatives for individuals allergic to, or with infections resistant to, other antibiotics. Some fluoroquinolones are commonly misprescribed for colds, sore throats, bladder infections, or community-acquired (as opposed to hospital-acquired) pneumonia. Whereas fluoroquinolones such as levofloxacin (LEVAQUIN) may be appropriate for treating community-acquired pneumonia, the fluoroquinolone ciprofloxacin (CIPRO) should not be prescribed for this purpose.

No antibiotic should be prescribed for the common cold, and penicillin or—if allergic—erythromycin is the drug of choice for a strep throat. In the past no fluoroquinolone has been the drug of choice for treatment of bronchitis or pneumonia that could be caused by pneumococcal bacteria, the most common cause of community-acquired pneumonia. Unfortunately, due to the inappropriate overuse of older, safer, and less expensive antibiotics and depending on the resistance of the pneumococcal bacteria in the area in which you live, your physician may prescribe one of the newer fluoroquinolones if you have community-acquired pneumonia.

A recent study illustrates the rampant, out-of-control dangers of misprescribing and overprescribing fluoroquinolone antibiotics, one of the most heavily advertised and expensive groups of antibiotics. In a study of the use of these drugs in the emergency rooms of two academic medical centers, 100 consecutive patients who were prescribed a fluoroquinolone were studied to find out if the use was appropriate according to the guidelines used at those institutions. Of the 100 patients, 81 (81%) were given the antibiotic for an inappropriate use, including 43 (53% of the 81 patients) for whom another antibiotic was the first-line treatment and 27 (33%) in whom there was no evidence of an infection. Of the 19 patients for whom the prescribing of this class of antibiotics was appropriate, only one patient was prescribed the right dose for the correct length of time.[18]

With very few exceptions, fluoroquinolones are not the drug of choice for other infections. A seven-day course of treatment with one of the fluoroquinolone drugs can be 7 to 21 times more expensive than equally effective (for most infections) treatment with other drugs, for example generic ampicillin or trimethoprim/sulfamethoxazole (BACTRIM/SEPTRA). Both resistance and allergy to one drug in this family usually cross to the rest of the fluoroquinolones and sometimes even occur during therapy.[19,20] Overgrowth of normal bacteria may cause yeast infections, especially when antibiotics are used for long periods. The fluoroquinolones can cause central nervous system problems and psychosis.[21] Severe, even fatal, allergic reactions have happened after just one dose. Collapse of the circulatory system has occurred. As a group, the fluoroquinolones are expensive, resistance

In mid-1992, only a few months after it was initially approved for release in the United States, Abbott's Omniflox, generic name temafloxacin, was pulled off the market worldwide because of an unacceptably high number of cases of serious anemia, kidney failure, and life-threatening anaphylactic (allergic) shock resulting in a number of deaths.

WARNING: INCREASED RISK OF TENDINITIS AND TENDON RUPTURE WITH ALL FLUOROQUINOLONE ANTIBIOTICS

Public Citizen's Health Research Group petitioned the FDA successfully to add a warning for doctors to the labeling or package for all fluoroquinolone antibiotics about the risk of tendinitis, including the possibility of complete tendon rupture.

This adverse reaction most frequently involves the Achilles tendon, the tendon that runs from the back of the heel to the calf. Rupture of the Achilles tendon may require surgical repair. Tendons in the rotator cuff (the shoulder), the hand, the biceps, and the thumb have also been involved. This reaction appears to be more common in those taking steroid drugs, in older patients, and in kidney transplant recipients, but cases have occurred in people without any of these risk factors. The onset of symptoms is sudden and has occurred as soon as 24 hours after starting treatment with a fluoroquinolone. Most people have recovered completely after one to two months.

If you experience unexpected tendon pain while taking a fluoroquinolone antibiotic, stop the drug immediately, call your doctor, and rest.

---

is increasing, and many effective alternatives are available.[22] The use of fluoroquinolones in animal feed is a major reason for resistance developing.

TETRACYCLINES

Tetracyclines are rarely the antibiotics of choice to treat bacterial infections that are common in older adults. In general, tetracyclines are used to treat such infections as urethritis (inflammation of the urinary tract), prostate infections, pelvic inflammatory disease, acne, Rocky Mountain spotted fever, recurrent bronchitis in people with chronic lung disease, "walking" pneumonia, and other miscellaneous infections.[23]

Considerations When Prescribing for Older Adults

Since a decrease in kidney function is one of the normal changes associated with the aging process, tetracyclines must be used with this in mind. With the exception of doxycycline, these drugs should not be used for someone with impaired kidney function, as they can damage the kidneys further. Tetracyclines also can cause liver damage. This is more likely to happen when they are injected into the blood (intravenously) in people who already have liver or kidney impairment.[24]

Dosage Forms, Uses, and Effects

The oral forms—tablet, capsule, suspension—should be taken with a full glass (eight ounces) of water. The last dose of the day should be taken at least an hour before bedtime.[25] Esophageal ulcers (irritation of the esophagus, the tube leading from the throat to the stomach) have occurred in people who have taken doxycycline at bedtime with insufficient water to wash it down. Liquid forms should be shaken well before use. Do not freeze them. Try to take your doses at evenly spaced times during the day and night so that the amount of drug in your body will stay constant. If you miss a dose, take it as soon as possible. If it is almost time for the next dose and you are supposed to take your medicine

- once a day, space missed dose and next dose about 12 hours apart.
- twice a day, space missed dose and next dose about six hours apart.
- three or more times a day, space missed dose and next dose about three hours apart or double the next dose.

Go back to your regular schedule after following the instructions above.

The injected forms should only be used when the oral forms are not adequate or not tolerated, as they are very painful. The intravenous forms should be used only when the oral forms are not appropriate, as severe vein inflammation or clotting commonly occurs.[26]

Tetracyclines applied externally as ointments or creams are of little value except for treatment of some eye infections and possibly some skin conditions. Two types of eye (ophthalmic) preparations are available—ointment and drops. (See p. 498 for directions on applying eye preparations.)

Sometimes when tetracyclines are used, microbes that are not killed by these drugs cause infection. An example is candidiasis, a fungal infection. (Some of its symptoms are sore mouth and tongue and itching in the genital or rectal area.) Candidiasis in the mouth is fairly common in older adults who wear dentures.

Tell your doctor that you take a tetracycline before you have any tests done. These drugs may interfere with your urine test results. Talk to your doctor before you change your diet or any medication.

DRUG PROFILES

Bacterial Infection

Penicillins

Amoxicillin (a mox i *sill* in)
AMOXIL (GlaxoSmithKline)

Amoxicillin and Clavulanate
(a mox i *sill* in and clav *yew* lan ate)
AUGMENTIN (GlaxoSmithKline)

Ampicillin (am pi *sill* in)
OMNIPEN (Wyeth-Ayerst)

GENERIC: available for amoxicillin; not available for amoxicillin and clavulanate
FAMILY: Penicillins (see p. 677)

PREGNANCY WARNING

No valid data are available for these drugs, as they were not tested properly in animal studies. Use during pregnancy only for clear medical reasons. Tell your doctor if you are pregnant or thinking of becoming pregnant before you take this drug.

BREAST-FEEDING WARNING

These drugs are excreted in human milk. Because of the potential for adverse effects in nursing infants, you should not take these drugs while nursing.

Amoxicillin is used to treat certain infections caused by bacteria, such as ear, sinus, and bladder infections. It is also prescribed for bronchitis in people with chronic lung disease and for gonorrhea. A second drug, clavulanate, is sometimes combined with amoxicillin. It helps amoxicillin work better by preventing bacteria from resisting the drug. Amoxicillin will not help a cold or the flu.

If you have kidney disease, you may need to take less than the usual adult dose of amoxicillin. In rare instances older people may develop hepatitis if taking the combination of amoxicillin and clavulanate. This is reversible, but the hepatitis often does not occur until after the drug is stopped.[30,31]

Ampicillin is an older form of amoxicillin. Many people who take ampicillin develop a slight skin rash. This may or may not be a sign that you are allergic to the drug. If you get a skin rash, call your doctor. Some of ampicillin's adverse effects can appear as much as a month after you stop taking it.

Before You Use This Drug

Do not use if you have or have had:

- allergy to penicillins
- liver disease (for amoxicillin and clavulanate)

Antibiotic-associated diarrhea (AAD) is quite common and its incidence varies from 5% to 20% of patients depending on which antibiotic they are taking although practically all antibiotics have been associated with AAD. Fortunately, most cases are mild and self-limited, ending with the cessation of use of the offending antibiotic. The antibiotics most commonly associated with this mild form of AAD include ampicillin, amoxicillin, cephalosporins and clindamycin.[27] There have been studies in children or adults in which the use of prophylactic yogurt in people using antibiotics has significantly reduced the occurrence or severity of AAD.[28,29] However, 10 to 20% of all patients who get AAD (0.5 to 4% of patients using antibiotics) will get the more severe form of AAD known as pseudomembranous colitis (see below). If you are taking any antibiotic and develop diarrhea after starting to use the drug, call your physician to discuss whether another antibiotic should be used and to discuss the need for rehydration due to the fluid losses from the diarrhea.

Pseudomembranous colitis has been reported with nearly all antibacterial agents and may range in severity from mild to life-threatening. Therefore, it is important to consider this diagnosis in patients who present with diarrhea subsequent to the administration of antibacterial agents.

Because antibiotic therapy has been associated with severe colitis which may end fatally, it should be reserved for serious infections where less toxic antimicrobial agents are inappropriate, as described in the **INDICATIONS AND USAGE** section. It should not be used in patients with nonbacterial infections such as most upper respiratory tract infections. Treatment with antibacterial agents alters the normal flora of the colon and may permit over-growth of clostridia. Studies indicate that a toxin produced by *Clostridium difficile* is one primary cause of "antibiotic-associated colitis."

After the diagnosis of pseudomembranous colitis has been established, therapeutic measures should be initiated. Mild cases of pseudomembranous colitis usually respond to drug discontinuation alone. In moderate to severe cases, consideration should be given to management with fluids and electrolytes, protein supplementation, and treatment with an antibacterial drug clinically effective against *C. difficile* colitis.

Diarrhea, colitis, and pseudomembranous colitis have been observed to begin up to several weeks following cessation of therapy.

Tell your doctor if you have or have had:

- allergies to drugs (see p. 678 for examples)
- history of allergies, such as asthma, eczema, or hay fever
- stomach or intestinal disease
- kidney disease
- infectious mononucleosis
- bleeding disorder
- heart disease
- cystic fibrosis
- phenylketonuria (chewable tablets of amoxicillin and clavulanate)
- diabetes (certain diabetes tests are affected)
- pregnancy or are breast-feeding

Tell your doctor about any other drugs you take, including aspirin, herbs, vitamins, and other nonprescription products.

When You Use This Drug

- Check with your doctor if there is no improvement within a few days or if symptoms become worse.
- If you get severe diarrhea, check with your doctor before taking any antidiarrheals.
- If you plan to have any surgery, including dental, tell your doctor that you take this drug.
- Possibly use an alternate or additional method of contraception if you are taking estrogen-containing oral contraceptives.

- **Caution diabetics:** These drugs may interfere with glucose urine tests.

How to Use This Drug

- If you miss a dose, take it as soon as you remember, but skip it if it is almost time for the next dose. **Do not take double doses.**
- Do not share your medication with others.
- Take the drug at the same time(s) each day.
- *For ampicillin:* Take the drug with water only. Do not eat or drink for about an hour before taking this medication.
- Amoxicillin and amoxicillin with clavulanate may be taken with or without food.
- Take this drug for the prescribed length of time. If you stop too soon, your symptoms could come back.
- For tablets, store at room temperature with lid on tightly. Do not store in the bathroom. Do not expose to heat, moisture, or strong light. Keep out of reach of children.

Interactions with Other Drugs

The following drugs, biologics (e.g., vaccines, therapeutic antibodies), or foods are listed in *Evaluations of Drug Interactions* 2003 as causing "highly clinically significant" or "clinically significant" interactions when used together with any of the drugs in this section. In some sections with multiple drugs, the interaction may have been reported for one but not all drugs in this section, but we include the interaction because the drugs in this section are similar to one another. We have also included potentially serious interactions listed in the drug's FDA-approved professional package insert or in published medical journal articles. There may be other drugs, especially those in the families of drugs listed below, that also will react with this drug to cause severe adverse effects. Make sure to tell your doctor and pharmacist the drugs you are taking and tell them if you are taking any of these interacting drugs:

COUMADIN, GARAMYCIN, gentamicin, heparin, oral contraceptives, warfarin.

Adverse Effects

Call your doctor immediately if you experience:

- severe asthma (wheezing)
- extreme weakness
- nausea or vomiting
- rash
- fast or irregular breathing
- puffiness or swelling around the face
- shortness of breath
- severe decrease in blood pressure
- red, scaly skin
- joint pain
- fever
- hives or itching
- sore throat and fever
- anxiety or confusion
- depression
- seizures
- decrease in amount of urine
- pain, cramps, or bloating in abdomen or stomach
- severe, watery diarrhea (may contain blood)
- dark urine
- yellow eyes or skin
- light-colored stools
- loss of appetite
- dizziness or headache
- joint pain
- unusual bleeding or bruising
- vaginal itching or discharge (for amoxicillin and clavulanate)
- swelling of face, fingers, or lower legs (for amoxicillin and clavulanate)
- blistering, peeling, or loosening of skin (for amoxicillin and clavulanate)

Call your doctor if these symptoms continue:

- mild diarrhea
- nausea or vomiting
- headache
- white patches on mouth and/or tongue
- vaginal itching or discharge
- gas (for amoxicillin and clavulanate)
- stomach pain (for amoxicillin and clavulanate)

Periodic Tests

Ask your doctor which of these tests should be done periodically while you are taking this drug:

- blood tests
- stool exam
- liver and kidney tests

Cloxacillin (klox a *sill* in)

Dicloxacillin (dye klox a *sill* in)
DYCILL (GlaxoSmithKline)
DYNAPEN (Apothecon)

GENERIC: available
FAMILY: Penicillins (see p. 677)

PREGNANCY WARNING
Members of the penicillin family of drugs cross the placenta and expose the fetus to the drug. Use during pregnancy only for clear medical reasons. Tell your doctor if you are pregnant or thinking of becoming pregnant before you take these drugs.

BREAST-FEEDING WARNING
Members of the penicillin family of drugs are excreted in human milk. Because of the potential for adverse effects in nursing infants, you should not take these drugs while nursing.

Cloxacillin and dicloxacillin are used to treat bacterial infections that are resistant to penicillin, such as certain infections of the skin, soft tissue (such as puncture wounds or deep cuts), and joints, and to prevent infection after hip surgery. Your doctor should usually do lab tests before prescribing either of these drugs and should prescribe one of them only if tests show that the bacteria causing your infection are resistant to penicillin. If the bacteria are not resistant to penicillin, your doctor should prescribe penicillin instead. These drugs will not help a cold or the flu.

Cloxacillin and dicloxacillin should be used with caution in people who are over age 70, or people with impaired kidney function.[32]

Before You Use This Drug

Do not use this drug if you have or have had:

- allergy to penicillins (see p. 678 for examples)

Tell your doctor if you have or have had:

- allergies to drugs
- general history of other allergies
- stomach or intestinal disease
- kidney disease
- congestive heart failure
- infectious mononucleosis
- bleeding disorder
- cystic fibrosis
- diabetes (certain diabetes tests are affected)
- pregnancy or are breast-feeding

Tell your doctor about any other drugs you take, including aspirin, herbs, vitamins, and other nonprescription products.

When You Use This Drug

- Check with your doctor if there is no improvement within a few days.
- If you plan to have any surgery, including dental, tell your doctor that you take this drug.
- If you get severe diarrhea, check with your doctor before taking any antidiarrheals.

Antibiotic-associated diarrhea (AAD) is quite common and its incidence varies from 5% to 20% of patients depending on which antibiotic they are taking although practically all antibiotics have been associated with AAD. Fortunately, most cases are mild and self-limited, ending with the cessation of use of the offending antibiotic. The antibiotics most commonly associated with this mild form of AAD include ampicillin, amoxicillin, cephalosporins and clindamycin.[27] There have been studies in children or adults in which the use of prophylactic yogurt in people using antibiotics has significantly reduced the occurrence or severity of AAD.[28,29] However, 10 to 20% of all patients who get AAD (0.5 to 4% of patients using antibiotics) will get the more severe form of AAD known as pseudomembranous colitis (see below). If you are taking any antibiotic and develop diarrhea after starting to use the drug, call your physician to discuss whether another antibiotic should be used and to discuss the need for rehydration due to the fluid losses from the diarrhea.

Pseudomembranous colitis has been reported with nearly all antibacterial agents and may range in severity from mild to life-threatening. Therefore, it is important to consider this diagnosis in patients who present with diarrhea subsequent to the administration of antibacterial agents.

Because antibiotic therapy has been associated with severe colitis which may end fatally, it should be reserved for serious infections where less toxic antimicrobial agents are inappropriate, as described in the **INDICATIONS AND USAGE** section. It should not be used in patients with nonbacterial infections such as most upper respiratory tract infections. Treatment with antibacterial agents alters the normal flora of the colon and may permit over-growth of clostridia. Studies indicate that a toxin produced by *Clostridium difficile* is one primary cause of "antibiotic-associated colitis."

After the diagnosis of pseudomembranous colitis has been established, therapeutic measures should be initiated. Mild cases of pseudomembranous colitis usually respond to drug discontinuation alone. In moderate to severe cases, consideration should be given to management with fluids and electrolytes, protein supplementation, and treatment with an antibacterial drug clinically effective against *C. difficile* colitis.

Diarrhea, colitis, and pseudomembranous colitis have been observed to begin up to several weeks following cessation of therapy.

• Possibly use an alternate or additional method of contraception if you are taking estrogen-containing oral contraceptives.

• **Caution diabetics:** These drugs may interfere with glucose urine tests.

How to Use This Drug

• If you miss a dose, take it as soon as you remember, but skip it if it is almost time for the next dose. **Do not take double doses.**

• Do not share your medication with others.

• Take the drug at the same time(s) each day.

• Take with water only. Do not eat or drink for about an hour before taking this medication.

• Take the drug for the prescribed length of time. If you stop too soon, your symptoms could come back.

• *For tablets:* Store at room temperature with lid on tightly. Do not store in the bathroom. Do not expose to heat, moisture, or strong light. Keep out of reach of children.

Interactions with Other Drugs

The following drugs, biologics (e.g., vaccines, therapeutic antibodies), or foods are listed in *Evaluations of Drug Interactions* 2003 as causing "highly clinically significant" or "clinically significant" interactions when used together with any of the drugs in this section. In some sections with multiple drugs, the interaction may have been reported for one but not all

drugs in this section, but we include the interaction because the drugs in this section are similar to one another. We have also included potentially serious interactions listed in the drug's FDA-approved professional package insert or in published medical journal articles. There may be other drugs, especially those in the families of drugs listed below, that also will react with this drug to cause severe adverse effects. Make sure to tell your doctor and pharmacist the drugs you are taking and tell them if you are taking any of these interacting drugs:

ALDACTONE, aspirin—high dose, cholestyramine, COUMADIN, enalapril, estrogen-containing oral contraceptives, GARAMYCIN, gentamicin, GENUINE BAYER ASPIRIN, heparin, methotrexate, potassium supplements, QUESTRAN, spironolactone, VASOTEC, warfarin.

Adverse Effects

Call your doctor immediately if you experience:

- severe asthma (wheezing)
- extreme weakness
- nausea or vomiting
- pain, cramps, or bloating in the abdomen or stomach
- severe, watery diarrhea (may contain blood)
- fever
- increased thirst
- abnormal weakness or tiredness
- abnormal weight loss
- skin rash, hives, or itching
- sore throat
- seizure
- decreased amount of urine
- depression
- pain at site of injection
- unusual bleeding or bruising
- yellow eyes or skin
- lightheadedness or fainting

- puffiness or swelling around face
- decrease in blood pressure
- red or scaly skin
- joint pain

Call your doctor if these symptoms continue:

- mild diarrhea
- nausea or vomiting
- sore mouth or tongue
- white patches on mouth or tongue
- vaginal itching or discharge
- headache

Penicillin G (pen i *sill* in *gee*)

Penicillin V (pen i *sill* in *vee*)

GENERIC: available

FAMILY: Penicillins (see p. 677)

PREGNANCY WARNING

There was no evidence of toxicity in animal studies. Use during pregnancy only for clear medical reasons. Tell your doctor if you are pregnant or thinking of becoming pregnant before you take this drug.

BREAST-FEEDING WARNING

Penicillin G is excreted in human milk. You should consult with your doctor if you are planning to nurse.

These two forms of penicillin are taken by mouth (orally). They are used to treat some infections caused by bacteria, including strep throat, some other oral (mouth) infections, and skin infections. Your doctor may also prescribe oral penicillin for you to take at home if you are just getting out of the hospital and were getting antibiotic shots while there. Penicillin will not help if you have a cold or the flu.

If you are taking penicillin by mouth, penicillin V is the better form to take because your body absorbs it better. If you have kidney damage, you may need to take less than the usual adult dose.

Antibiotic-associated diarrhea (AAD) is quite common and its incidence varies from 5% to 20% of patients depending on which antibiotic they are taking although practically all antibiotics have been associated with AAD. Fortunately, most cases are mild and self-limited, ending with the cessation of use of the offending antibiotic. The antibiotics most commonly associated with this mild form of AAD include ampicillin, amoxicillin, cephalosporins and clindamycin.[27] There have been studies in children or adults in which the use of prophylactic yogurt in people using antibiotics has significantly reduced the occurrence or severity of AAD.[28,29] However, 10 to 20% of all patients who get AAD (0.5 to 4% of patients using antibiotics) will get the more severe form of AAD known as pseudomembranous colitis (see below). If you are taking any antibiotic and develop diarrhea after starting to use the drug, call your physician to discuss whether another antibiotic should be used and to discuss the need for rehydration due to the fluid losses from the diarrhea.

Pseudomembranous colitis has been reported with nearly all antibacterial agents and may range in severity from mild to life-threatening. Therefore, it is important to consider this diagnosis in patients who present with diarrhea subsequent to the administration of antibacterial agents.

Because antibiotic therapy has been associated with severe colitis which may end fatally, it should be reserved for serious infections where less toxic antimicrobial agents are inappropriate, as described in the **INDICATIONS AND USAGE** section. It should not be used in patients with nonbacterial infections such as most upper respiratory tract infections. Treatment with antibacterial agents alters the normal flora of the colon and may permit over-growth of clostridia. Studies indicate that a toxin produced by *Clostridium difficile* is one primary cause of "antibiotic-associated colitis."

After the diagnosis of pseudomembranous colitis has been established, therapeutic measures should be initiated. Mild cases of pseudomembranous colitis usually respond to drug discontinuation alone. In moderate to severe cases, consideration should be given to management with fluids and electrolytes, protein supplementation, and treatment with an antibacterial drug clinically effective against *C. difficile* colitis.

Diarrhea, colitis, and pseudomembranous colitis have been observed to begin up to several weeks following cessation of therapy.

Before You Use This Drug

Do not use this drug if you have or have had:

- allergy to penicillins (see p. 678 for examples)

Tell your doctor if you have or have had:

- pregnancy or are breast-feeding
- allergies to drugs
- general history of other allergies
- stomach or intestinal disease
- kidney disease
- bleeding disorder
- heart disease
- high blood pressure
- infectious mononucleosis
- cystic fibrosis

Tell your doctor about any other drugs you take, including aspirin, herbs, vitamins, and other nonprescription products.

When You Use This Drug

- Check with your doctor if there is no improvement within a few days.
- If you get severe diarrhea, check with your doctor before taking any antidiarrheals.
- If you plan to have any surgery, including dental, tell your doctor that you take this drug.

• Possibly use an alternate or additional method of contraception if taking estrogen-containing oral contraceptives.

• **Caution diabetics:** These drugs may interfere with glucose urine tests.

How to Use This Drug

• If you miss a dose, take it as soon as you remember, but skip it if it is almost time for the next dose. **Do not take double doses.**

• Do not share your medication with others.

• Take the drug at the same time(s) each day.

• Penicillin G should be taken with water only. Do not eat or drink for about an hour before taking this medication.

• Penicillin V can be taken with or without food.

• Take this drug for the prescribed length of time. If you stop too soon, your symptoms could come back.

• Store tablets at room temperature with lid on tightly. Do not store in the bathroom. Do not expose to heat, moisture, or strong light. Keep out of reach of children.

Interactions with Other Drugs

The following drugs, biologics (e.g., vaccines, therapeutic antibodies), or foods are listed in *Evaluations of Drug Interactions* 2003 as causing "highly clinically significant" or "clinically significant" interactions when used together with any of the drugs in this section. In some sections with multiple drugs, the interaction may have been reported for one but not all drugs in this section, but we include the interaction because the drugs in this section are similar to one another. We have also included potentially serious interactions listed in the drug's FDA-approved professional package insert or in published medical journal articles. There may be other drugs, especially those in the families of drugs listed below, that also will react with this drug to cause severe adverse effects. Make sure to tell your doctor and pharmacist the drugs you are taking and tell them if you are taking any of these interacting drugs:

ALDACTONE, aspirin—high dose, cholestyramine, COUMADIN, enalapril, estrogen-containing oral contraceptives, GARAMYCIN, gentamicin, GENUINE BAYER ASPIRIN, heparin, methotrexate, potassium supplements, QUESTRAN, spironolactone, VASOTEC, warfarin.

Adverse Effects

Call your doctor immediately if you experience:

• severe asthma (wheezing)
• extreme weakness
• nausea or vomiting
• pain, cramps, or bloating in the abdomen or stomach
• severe, watery diarrhea (may contain blood)
• fever
• increased thirst
• abnormal weakness or tiredness
• abnormal weight loss
• skin rash, hives, or itching
• sore throat
• seizure
• decreased amount of urine
• depression
• pain at site of injection
• unusual bleeding or bruising
• yellow eyes or skin
• lightheadedness or fainting
• puffiness or swelling around face
• decrease in blood pressure
• red or scaly skin
• joint pain

Call your doctor if these symptoms continue:

• mild diarrhea
• nausea or vomiting
• sore mouth or tongue

- white patches on mouth or tongue
- vaginal itching and discharge

Cephalosporins

Cefaclor (*sef* a klor)
CECLOR (Lilly)

Cefadroxil (sef a *drox* il)
DURICEF (Warner-Chilcott)

Cefditoren (sef da *tor* en)
SPECTRACEF (Purdue Pharma LP)

Cefpodoxime (sef pode *ox* eem)
VANTIN (Pharmacia & Upjohn)

Cephalexin (sef a *lex* in)
KEFLEX (Lilly)

Cephradine (*sef* ra deen)
VELOSEF (Apothecon)

Limited Use

Cefixime (sef *ix* eem)
SUPRAX (Lupin)

Cefprozil (sef *proe* zil)
CEFZIL (Bristol-Myers Squibb)

Cefuroxime Axetil (sef fyoor *ox* eem *ax* i til)
CEFTIN (GlaxoSmithKline)

Loracarbef (loe ra *kar* bef)
LORABID (King)

GENERIC: available
FAMILY: Cephalosporins (see p. 677)

PREGNANCY WARNING

No valid data are available for these drugs, as they were not tested properly in animal studies. Use during pregnancy only for clear medical reasons. Tell your doctor if you are pregnant or thinking of becoming pregnant before you take these drugs.

BREAST-FEEDING WARNING

These drugs are excreted in human milk. Because of the potential for serious adverse effects in nursing infants, you should consult with your doctor if you are planning to nurse.

The cephalosporin antibiotics are used in the treatment of infections caused by bacteria. They work by killing bacteria or preventing their growth. These drugs are used to treat infections in many different parts of the body. They are sometimes given with other antibiotics. Some cephalosporins given by injection are also used to prevent infections before, during, and after surgery. However, cephalosporins will not work for colds, flu, or other virus infections.[33]

These antibiotics may cause stomach or abdominal cramps and pain; abdominal tenderness; watery diarrhea that may also be bloody; and fever. These drugs may also cause skin reactions, seizures, decrease in urine output, joint pain, loss of appetite, and nausea or vomiting.[33]

Before You Use This Drug

Do not use if you have or have had:

- previous allergic reaction to penicillins or cephalosporins

Tell your doctor if you have or have had:

- allergies to drugs
- a reaction to any penicillin or cephalosporin (see p. 677 for examples)
- stomach or intestinal disease
- kidney or liver disease
- carnitine deficiency (cefditorin increases carnitine excretion)
- history of bleeding disorder
- phenylketonuria (when using cefprozil)
- pregnancy or are breast-feeding

Tell your doctor about any other drugs you take, including aspirin, herbs, vitamins, and other nonprescription products.

Antibiotic-associated diarrhea (AAD) is quite common and its incidence varies from 5% to 20% of patients depending on which antibiotic they are taking although practically all antibiotics have been associated with AAD. Fortunately, most cases are mild and self-limited, ending with the cessation of use of the offending antibiotic. The antibiotics most commonly associated with this mild form of AAD include ampicillin, amoxicillin, cephalosporins and clindamycin.[27] There have been studies in children or adults in which the use of prophylactic yogurt in people using antibiotics has significantly reduced the occurrence or severity of AAD.[28,29] However, 10 to 20% of all patients who get AAD (0.5 to 4% of patients using antibiotics) will get the more severe form of AAD known as pseudomembranous colitis (see below). If you are taking any antibiotic and develop diarrhea after starting to use the drug, call your physician to discuss whether another antibiotic should be used and to discuss the need for rehydration due to the fluid losses from the diarrhea.

Pseudomembranous colitis has been reported with nearly all antibacterial agents and may range in severity from mild to life-threatening. Therefore, it is important to consider this diagnosis in patients who present with diarrhea subsequent to the administration of antibacterial agents.

Because antibiotic therapy has been associated with severe colitis which may end fatally, it should be reserved for serious infections where less toxic antimicrobial agents are inappropriate, as described in the **INDICATIONS AND USAGE** section. It should not be used in patients with nonbacterial infections such as most upper respiratory tract infections. Treatment with antibacterial agents alters the normal flora of the colon and may permit over-growth of clostridia. Studies indicate that a toxin produced by *Clostridium difficile* is one primary cause of "antibiotic-associated colitis."

After the diagnosis of pseudomembranous colitis has been established, therapeutic measures should be initiated. Mild cases of pseudomembranous colitis usually respond to drug discontinuation alone. In moderate to severe cases, consideration should be given to management with fluids and electrolytes, protein supplementation, and treatment with an antibacterial drug clinically effective against *C. difficile* colitis.

Diarrhea, colitis, and pseudomembranous colitis have been observed to begin up to several weeks following cessation of therapy.

When You Use This Drug

• Check with your doctor if there is no improvement of symptoms within a few days.

• If you get severe diarrhea, check with your doctor before taking any antidiarrheals.

• If you plan to have any surgery, including dental, tell your doctor that you take this drug.

• Do not take antacids within one hour of taking cefaclor.

• Take this drug for the prescribed length of time. If you stop too soon, your symptoms could come back.

• **Caution diabetics:** These drugs can interfere with the glucose urine test.

How to Use This Drug

• If you miss a dose, take it as soon as you remember, but skip it if it is almost time for the next dose. **Do not take double doses.**

• Do not share your medication with others.

• Take the drug at the same time(s) each day. Take at evenly spaced times.

• Take cefaclor extended-release tablets, cefditoren, and cefuroxime axetil oral suspension with food. Take loracarbef one hour before or two hours after food. Other cephalosporin tablets may be taken with or without food. Take with food if stomach irritation occurs.

• Do not take oral suspensions after expiration date.

• *For tablets:* Store at room temperature with lid on tightly. Do not store in the bathroom. Do not expose to heat, moisture, or strong light. Keep out of reach of children.

Interactions with Other Drugs

The following drugs, biologics (e.g., vaccines, therapeutic antibodies), or foods are listed in *Evaluations of Drug Interactions* 2003 as causing "highly clinically significant" or "clinically significant" interactions when used together with any of the drugs in this section. In some sections with multiple drugs, the interaction may have been reported for one but not all drugs in this section, but we include the interaction because the drugs in this section are similar to one another. We have also included potentially serious interactions listed in the drug's FDA-approved professional package insert or in published medical journal articles. There may be other drugs, especially those in the families of drugs listed below, that also will react with this drug to cause severe adverse effects. Make sure to tell your doctor and pharmacist the drugs you are taking and tell them if you are taking any of these interacting drugs:

> alcohol, BENEMID, COUMADIN, GARAMYCIN, gentamicin, probenecid, warfarin.

Adverse Effects

Call your doctor immediately if you experience:

- severe asthma (wheezing)
- unusual tiredness or weakness
- abdominal pain
- rash
- pain, cramps, or bloating in the abdomen or stomach
- severe, watery diarrhea (may contain blood)

- fever
- difficulty breathing
- hearing loss
- abnormal tiredness
- dizziness or headache
- joint pain
- skin rash, hives, itching, blistering, peeling, or loosening
- swelling at site of injection
- unusual bleeding or bruising
- seizures
- decrease in amount of urine
- yellowing of eyes and skin
- dizziness, drowsiness, insomnia, nervousness (loracarbef)

Call your doctor if these symptoms continue:

- mild diarrhea
- abdominal cramps
- nausea or vomiting
- headache
- sore mouth or tongue
- mild stomach pain
- vaginal itching and discharge

Call your doctor if these symptoms continue after you stop taking this drug:

- severe abdominal cramps and pain
- abdominal tenderness
- watery and severe diarrhea (may be bloody)
- fever

Periodic Tests

Ask your doctor which of these tests should be done periodically while you are taking this drug:

- bleeding time
- prothrombin time
- stool exam

Macrolides

Erythromycin (eh rith roe *mye* sin)
ERYTHROCIN (Abbott)
EES (Abbott)

GENERIC: available
FAMILY: Macrolides

PREGNANCY WARNING

No data is available for erythromycin, as it was not tested properly in animal studies. Use during pregnancy only for clear medical reasons. Tell your doctor if you are pregnant or thinking of becoming pregnant before you take this drug.

BREAST-FEEDING WARNING

Erythromycin is excreted in human milk. Because of the potential for serious adverse effects in nursing infants, you should not take this drug while nursing.

Erythromycin is used in the treatment of infections caused by bacteria. They work by killing bacteria or preventing their growth. This drug is used to treat infections in many different parts of the body. Erythromycin will not work for colds, flu, or other virus infections.

Erythromycin is one of the safest antibiotics available. However, people who use a particular type of erythromycin called erythromycin estolate are about 20 times more likely to suffer liver damage (toxicity) from the drug than people who use other forms.[34] Therefore, you should not take erythromycin estolate (see p. 697).[23] If you have liver disease, you should be taking less than the usual adult dose of erythromycin.

Antibiotic-associated diarrhea (AAD) is quite common and its incidence varies from 5% to 20% of patients depending on which antibiotic they are taking although practically all antibiotics have been associated with AAD. Fortunately, most cases are mild and self-limited, ending with the cessation of use of the offending antibiotic. The antibiotics most commonly associated with this mild form of AAD include ampicillin, amoxicillin, cephalosporins and clindamycin.[27] There have been studies in children or adults in which the use of prophylactic yogurt in people using antibiotics has significantly reduced the occurrence or severity of AAD.[28,29] However, 10 to 20% of all patients who get AAD (0.5 to 4% of patients using antibiotics) will get the more severe form of AAD known as pseudomembranous colitis (see below). If you are taking any antibiotic and develop diarrhea after starting to use the drug, call your physician to discuss whether another antibiotic should be used and to discuss the need for rehydration due to the fluid losses from the diarrhea.

Pseudomembranous colitis has been reported with nearly all antibacterial agents and may range in severity from mild to life-threatening. Therefore, it is important to consider this diagnosis in patients who present with diarrhea subsequent to the administration of antibacterial agents.

Because antibiotic therapy has been associated with severe colitis which may end fatally, it should be reserved for serious infections where less toxic antimicrobial agents are inappropriate, as described in the **INDICATIONS AND USAGE** section. It should not be used in patients with nonbacterial infections such as most upper respiratory tract infections. Treatment with antibacterial agents alters the normal flora of the colon and may permit over-growth of clostridia. Studies indicate that a toxin produced by *Clostridium difficile* is one primary cause of "antibiotic-associated colitis."

After the diagnosis of pseudomembranous colitis has been established, therapeutic measures should be initiated. Mild cases of pseudomembranous colitis usually respond to drug discontinuation alone. In moderate to severe cases, consideration should be given to management with fluids and electrolytes, protein supplementation, and treatment with an antibacterial drug clinically effective against *C. difficile* colitis.

Diarrhea, colitis, and pseudomembranous colitis have been observed to begin up to several weeks following cessation of therapy.

Before You Use This Drug

Tell your doctor if you have or have had:

- allergies to erythromycin
- an unusual reaction to erythromycin
- heart or liver problems
- hearing loss
- pregnancy or are breast-feeding

Tell your doctor about any other drugs you take, including aspirin, herbs, vitamins, and other nonprescription products.

When You Use This Drug

- Check with your doctor if there is no improvement within a few days.
- If you plan to have any surgery, including dental, tell your doctor that you take this drug.

How to Use This Drug

- If you miss a dose, take it as soon as you remember, but skip it if it is almost time for the next dose. **Do not take double doses.**
- Do not share your medication with others.
- Take the drug at the same time(s) each day.
- Take this drug for the prescribed length of time. If you stop too soon, your symptoms could come back.
- Take with **a full glass (eight ounces) of water** on an empty stomach. If stomach irritation occurs, take with food.
- Store at room temperature with lid on tightly. Do not store in the bathroom. Do not expose to heat, moisture, or strong light. Keep out of reach of children.

Interactions with Other Drugs

The following drugs, biologics (e.g., vaccines, therapeutic antibodies), or foods are listed in *Evaluations of Drug Interactions* 2003 as causing "highly clinically significant" or "clinically significant" interactions when used together with any of the drugs in this section. In some sections with multiple drugs, the interaction may have been reported for one but not all drugs in this section, but we include the interaction because the drugs in this section are similar to one another. We have also included potentially serious interactions listed in the drug's FDA-approved professional package insert or in published medical journal articles. There may be other drugs, especially those in the families of drugs listed below, that also will react with this drug to cause severe adverse effects. Make sure to tell your doctor and pharmacist the drugs you are taking and tell them if you are taking any of these interacting drugs:

ACCOLATE, ALFENTA, alfentanil, atorvastatin, AVELOX, carbamazepine, cilostazol, clozapine, CLOZARIL, COUMADIN, cyclosporine, DEPAKENE/DEPAKOTE, DETROL, digoxin, disopyramide, docetaxel, ELIXOPHYLLIN, ERGOMAR, ERGOSTAT, ergotamine, FARESTON, HALCION, LANOXICAPS, LANOXIN, LIPITOR, lovastatin, MEDROL, methylprednisolone, MEVACOR, midazolam, mizolastine, moxifloxacin, NEORAL, NORPACE, NORVIR, ORAP, pimozide, PLETAL, PROGRAF, ritonavir, SANDIMMUNE, sildenafil, SLO-BID, tacrolimus, TAXOTERE, TEGRETOL, THEO-24, theophylline, tolterodine, toremifene, triazolam, TUBARINE, tubocurarine, valproic acid, VERSED, VIAGRA, VIGAMOX, warfarin, zafirlukast.

Adverse Effects

Call your doctor immediately if you experience:

- severe, watery diarrhea (may contain blood)
- severe stomach pain
- abnormal tiredness or weakness
- yellow eyes or skin
- temporary hearing loss
- fever
- nausea or vomiting
- skin rash, redness, or itching

- pain, swelling, or redness at site of injection
- irregular or slow heart rate
- recurrent fainting

Call your doctor if these symptoms continue:

- sore mouth or tongue
- white patches in mouth or tongue
- mild abdominal or stomach cramping and discomfort
- vaginal itching and discharge
- diarrhea
- nausea or vomiting

Periodic Tests

Ask your doctor which of these tests should be done periodically while you are taking this drug:

- electrocardiogram (ECG or EKG)
- liver function determinations

Limited Use

Azithromycin (a zyth row *my* sin)
ZITHROMAX (Pfizer)

Clarithromycin (cla rith roe *my* sin)
BIAXIN (Abbott)

GENERIC: not available
FAMILY: Macrolides

PREGNANCY WARNING

Clarithromycin caused fetal harm in animal studies, including heart and blood vessel defects, growth retardation, and cleft palate. Azithromycin was not tested properly. Because of the potential for serious adverse effects to the fetus, these drugs should not be used by pregnant women.

BREAST-FEEDING WARNING

Other drugs in this class are excreted in human milk. It is likely that these drugs are also excreted in human milk. Because of the potential for serious adverse effects in nursing infants, you should not take these drugs while nursing.

Azithromycin and clarithromycin are approved by the FDA to treat bacterial infections in many parts of the body.[35],[36] These drugs will not help a cold but may be effective in the treatment of bronchitis and sinusitis.[37]

Azithromycin and clarithromycin belong to the same family of antibiotics as erythromycin (see p. 693). For many infections these drugs are similar in effectiveness to amoxicillin (see p. 682) and erythromycin. However, azithromycin and clarithromycin cost much more than these alternative antibiotics. Some experts recommend that they be reserved, in most instances, to treat AIDS-related infections.

Before You Use This Drug

Do not use if you have or have had:

- hypersensitivity to clarithromycin, azithromycin, or erythromycin

Tell your doctor if you have or have had:

- kidney or liver problems
- pregnancy or are breast-feeding

Tell your doctor about any other drugs you take, including aspirin, herbs, vitamins, and other nonprescription products.

When You Use This Drug

- Check with your doctor if there is no improvement within a few days or if condition becomes worse.
- If you plan to have any surgery, including dental, tell your doctor that you take this drug.
- Do not take with pimozide.

How to Use This Drug

- If you miss a dose, take it as soon as you remember, but skip it if it is almost time for the next dose. **Do not take double doses.**

Antibiotic-associated diarrhea (AAD) is quite common and its incidence varies from 5% to 20% of patients depending on which antibiotic they are taking although practically all antibiotics have been associated with AAD. Fortunately, most cases are mild and self-limited, ending with the cessation of use of the offending antibiotic. The antibiotics most commonly associated with this mild form of AAD include ampicillin, amoxicillin, cephalosporins, and clindamycin.[27] There have been studies in children or adults in which the use of prophylactic yogurt in people using antibiotics has significantly reduced the occurrence or severity of AAD.[28,29] However, 10 to 20% of all patients who get AAD (0.5 to 4% of patients using antibiotics) will get the more severe form of AAD known as pseudomembranous colitis (see below). If you are taking any antibiotic and develop diarrhea after starting to use the drug, call your physician to discuss whether another antibiotic should be used and to discuss the need for rehydration due to the fluid losses from the diarrhea.

Pseudomembranous colitis has been reported with nearly all antibacterial agents and may range in severity from mild to life-threatening. Therefore, it is important to consider this diagnosis in patients who present with diarrhea subsequent to the administration of antibacterial agents.

Because antibiotic therapy has been associated with severe colitis which may end fatally, it should be reserved for serious infections where less toxic antimicrobial agents are inappropriate, as described in the **INDICATIONS AND USAGE** section. It should not be used in patients with nonbacterial infections such as most upper respiratory tract infections. Treatment with antibacterial agents alters the normal flora of the colon and may permit over-growth of clostridia. Studies indicate that a toxin produced by *Clostridium difficile* is one primary cause of "antibiotic-associated colitis."

After the diagnosis of pseudomembranous colitis has been established, therapeutic measures should be initiated. Mild cases of pseudomembranous colitis usually respond to drug discontinuation alone. In moderate to severe cases, consideration should be given to management with fluids and electrolytes, protein supplementation, and treatment with an antibacterial drug clinically effective against *C. difficile* colitis.

Diarrhea, colitis, and pseudomembranous colitis have been observed to begin up to several weeks following cessation of therapy.

• Do not share your medication with others.

• Take the drug at the same time(s) each day.

• Take this drug for the prescribed length of time. If you stop too soon, your symptoms could come back.

• *Azithromycin capsules:* Take with water only. Do not eat for about an hour before or two hours after taking this medication.

• *Azithromycin tablets:* Take with or without food.

• *Clarithromycin:* Take with or without food.

• Store at room temperature with lid on tightly. Do not store in the bathroom. Do not expose to heat, moisture, or strong light. Keep out of reach of children.

Interactions with Other Drugs

The following drugs, biologics (e.g., vaccines, therapeutic antibodies), or foods are listed in *Evaluations of Drug Interactions* 2003 as causing "highly clinically significant" or "clinically significant" interactions when used together with any of the drugs in this section. In some sections with multiple drugs, the interaction may have been reported for one but not all drugs in this section, but we include the interaction because the drugs in this section are similar to one another. We have also included potentially serious interactions listed in the drug's FDA-approved professional package insert or in published medical journal articles.

There may be other drugs, especially those in the families of drugs listed below, that also will react with this drug to cause severe adverse effects. Make sure to tell your doctor and pharmacist the drugs you are taking and tell them if you are taking any of these interacting drugs:

ALFENTA, alfentanil, alprazolam, bromocriptine, carbamazepine, cilostazol, COUMADIN, cyclosporine, delavirdine, DETROL, digoxin, disopyramide, efavirenz, ELIXOPHYLLIN, ERGOMAR, ERGOSTAT, ergotamine, FORTOVASE, HALCION, INVIRASE, LANOXICAPS, LANOXIN, lovastatin, MEDROL, methylprednisolone, MEVACOR, mizolastine, MYCOBUTIN, nelfinavir, NEORAL, NORPACE, NORVIR, ORAP, PARLODEL, pimozide, PLETAL, PRANDIN, PRIFTIN, quinidine, QUINIDEX, repaglinide, RESCRIPTOR, RETROVIR, rifabutin, rifapentine, ritonavir, SANDIMMUNE, saquinavir, sildenafil, simvastatin, SLO-BID, SUSTIVA, tacrolimus, TEGRETOL, THEO-24, theophylline, tolterodine, triazolam, VIAGRA, VIRACEPT, warfarin, XANAX, zidovudine, ZOCOR.

Adverse Effects

Call your doctor immediately if you experience:

- severe, watery diarrhea (may be bloody)
- skin rash or itching
- difficulty breathing
- fever
- nausea or vomiting
- abdominal tenderness
- abdominal or stomach cramps or pain
- joint pain
- swelling of face, mouth, neck, hands, or feet
- yellow eyes or skin
- unusual bleeding or bruising

Call your doctor if these symptoms continue:

- abdominal or stomach pain
- dizziness
- mild diarrhea
- headache
- nausea or vomiting
- abnormal sense of taste (clarithromycin)

 Do Not Use

ALTERNATIVE TREATMENT:
See Erythromycin, p. 693.

Erythromycin Estolate
(eh rith roe *my* sin *ess* to late)

FAMILY: Macrolides

Erythromycin is one of the safest antibiotics available. However, people who use a particular type of erythromycin called erythromycin estolate (ILOSONE) are about 20 times more likely to suffer liver damage (toxicity) from the drug than people who use other forms.[34] Therefore, you should not take erythromycin estolate (ILOSONE).[23] If you have liver disease, you should be taking less than the usual adult dose of erythromycin.

Ketolides

 Do Not Use

ALTERNATIVE TREATMENT:
See Erythromycin, p. 693 Azithromycin, p. 695, and Clarithromycin, p. 695. These are safer antibiotics approved to treat the same infections as this drug.

Telithromycin (tel ith roe *mye* sin)
KETEK (Aventis)

FAMILY: Ketolides

Telithromycin was approved by the FDA in April 2004 for the treatment of mild to moderate community-acquired pneumonia, acute bacterial exacerbation of chronic bronchitis, and acute bacterial sinusitis. The chemical structure of telithromycin, which is classed as a ketolide, is similar to the macrolide drug family, which includes erythromycin (see p. 693), clarithromycin (see p. 695.), and azithromycin (see p. 695).

Telithromycin is approved by the FDA for treatment of community-acquired pneumonia due to multidrug-resistant *Streptococcus pneumoniae* (MDRSP). MDRSP includes penicillin-resistant *S. pneumoniae* and those bacteria that are also resistant to two or more of the following antibiotics: penicillin (see p. 677), second-generation cephalosporins (see p. 690), the macrolides mentioned above, tetracyclines (see p. 681), and trimethoprim/sulfamethoxazole (see p. 703). Levofloxacin, a fluoroquinolone (see p. 710), is currently approved for treatment against *S. pneumoniae* resistant to penicillin; however, at this time there is no agent other than telithromycin approved for treatment against *S. pneumoniae* resistant to erythromycin or to any other macrolide in the United States.

Telithromycin has undergone a long drug approval process with the FDA. The makers of telithromycin, Aventis Pharmaceuticals, submitted the new drug application (NDA) in March of 2000. The drug went through two advisory committee reviews because of efficacy and safety issues before it was approved in April of 2004. Since 2001, telithromycin has been marketed in Germany, Spain, Italy, Brazil, and Mexico.[38] It is also marketed in Canada and the UK.

In the original application, Aventis requested approval to market for four indications: tonsillopharyngitis (tonsillitis), acute worsening of bronchitis, sinusitis, and community-acquired pneumonia. Tonsillopharyngitis was not approved by the FDA based on the agency's guidelines for the efficacy of first-line claims for antibiotics. The clinical success rate must be at least 85%, according to the FDA's guidelines, for a first-line claim. Telithromycin failed to show the 85% success rate for the treatment of tonsillopharyngitis. Interestingly, the rule of thumb did not apply to the other three indications, which were later approved.[39,40]

The Anti-infective Drug Advisory Committee was unable to make a unanimous decision about the efficacy and safety of telithromycin. Some members believed there was insufficient evidence to prove the efficacy of telithromycin for the treatment of acute worsening of chronic bronchitis, since one of the leading causes of the illness, the bacteria *Haemophilus influenzae,* was only 60 to 77% eradicated by the drug.[41,42] Furthermore, one member even questioned the efficacy of the other drugs compared to telithromycin in clinical studies, which led to her disapproval for all three indications: "The data at hand does not establish the efficacy of the comparators [drug being compared to telithromycin] . . . without data in front of us establishing the efficacy of the comparators, the data in front of us does not establish efficacy of this drug [telithromycin]."[43]

The committee was also split in its decision about the effectiveness of telithromycin against MDRSP. Telithromcyin cure rates were 90% for erythromycin-resistant *S. pneumoniae,* 70% for penicillin-resistant *S. pneumoniae,* and 68.8% for penicillin plus erythromycin–resistant *S. pneumoniae.*[44] The evidence of its efficacy for patients with MDRSP and severe infection was based on a small number of patients and demands further evaluation.[44] Drug-resistant *S. pneumoniae* frequently respond to drugs they are supposedly resistant to, even cases of bacteremic pneumonia.

Most of the adverse effects for telithromycin are similar to those for other macrolides, mainly headache, dizziness, nausea, and diarrhea. But telithromycin also has a risk for heart, liver, and eye toxicity. Data from a large

U.S. safety study, number 3014, was submitted to the FDA following the first approvable letter. However, the major weakness of the trial was its design, which may have led to an underestimation of reported adverse events and limited the collection and completeness of information about each adverse drug reaction.[45]

Telithromycin causes QT prolongation, and the prolongation increases with increasing doses of the drug. QT prolongation may develop into a life-threatening heart rhythm disturbance known as torsades de pointes. Two cases of torsades de pointes were reported at the Anti-infective Drug Advisory Committee meeting, and the events were suspected to be drug related.[46,47] QT prolongation is also reported with some other macrolides, fluoroquinolones, and cephalosporin antibiotics.

Another concern with telithromycin, liver toxicity, is reported with macrolides as well. At the time of the January 8, 2003, advisory committee meeting, the FDA had received 54 reports of liver adverse event reports with telithromycin from countries in which the drug had been marketed, of which 19 were categorized as serious.[48]

Blurred vision that significantly impaired patients' ability to perform daily activities was reported during clinical trials.[49] The visual disturbances mainly occurred in women and the young. Visual side effects occurred 1 to 3 hours after a dose and the effect lasted up to 20 hours.[49] From countries in which the drug was first marketed, the FDA has received reports of 167 visual adverse events, of which 42 were categorized as serious. Telithromycin appears to cause more visual disturbances compared to macrolides already on the market.

Other concerns with telithromycin include vasculitis (inflammation of blood vessels) and worsening of myasthenia gravis, which has resulted in one fatality.[50,51]

Telithromycin has been shown to be no more effective than other antibiotics: amoxicillin, cefuroxime, clarithromycin, or trovafloxacin. Furthermore, the adverse-effect profile is no better than for macrolides already on the market, it is possibly less safe, and there is a higher risk for drug interactions. The only factor that sets telithromycin apart from the rest is the FDA-approved use for treatment against macrolide-resistant *S. pneumoniae*. The clinical importance of macrolide resistance is up for debate. Although there is an increase in macrolide-resistant pneumococci in the United States, the number of clinical failures has not risen.[52]

Research has found no difference in deaths for pneumonia patients infected with drug-sensitive or -resistant bacteria after controlling for other risk factors, except patients with resistant bacteria have a more prolonged hospital stay.[53] The guidelines established by the Infectious Diseases Society of America states: "A macrolide plus a beta lactam is recommended for initial empiric treatment of outpatients in whom resistance is an issue and for hospitalized patients."[52] In addition, experts believe the type of macrolide resistance found in the United States may be overcome by increasing the dose of the drug.

Some may feel very excited at the development of a "new" antibiotic and a "new" drug class and may argue that there is a need for more drugs. We would argue that we do not need more drugs, we need better drugs, and telithromycin is a drug that should not have been approved by the FDA.

We agree with the editors of the highly respected French drug journal *Prescrire International* who stated that "telithromycin is a needless addition to the other macrolides."[51]

Tetracyclines

Limited Use

Doxycycline (dox i *sye* kleen)
VIBRAMYCIN (Pfizer)

Minocycline (my noe *sye* kleen)

Tetracycline (te tra *sye* kleen)

GENERIC: available
FAMILY: Tetracyclines (see p. 681)

PREGNANCY WARNING

These drugs caused harm to developing fetuses in animal studies, including abnormal skeletal development. Use during pregnancy only if no other drugs will suffice. Tell your doctor if you are pregnant or thinking of becoming pregnant before you take these drugs.

BREAST-FEEDING WARNING

Drugs in the tetracycline class are excreted in human milk. Because of the risk for permanent discoloration of teeth (yellow-gray-brown) in children who have nursed, you should not take these drugs while nursing.

The tetracyclines are used to treat infections and to help control acne. These drugs will not work for colds, flu, or other virus infections.[54]

Before You Use This Drug

Tell your doctor if you have or have had:

- pregnancy or are breast-feeding
- allergies to drugs
- an unusual reaction to tetracyclines or local anesthetics (e.g., lidocaine)
- liver or kidney problems
- asthma
- diabetes insipidus

Tell your doctor about any other drugs you take, including aspirin, herbs, vitamins, and other nonprescription products.

When You Use This Drug

- If you plan to have any surgery, including dental, tell your doctor that you take this drug.
- Check with your doctor if there is no improvement of symptoms within a few days (or a few weeks or months for acne patients).
- Avoid concurrent use of a tetracycline and antacid.
- Avoid concurrent use of a tetracycline and iron.
- Avoid being in the sun.
- If you experience dizziness, lightheadedness, or unsteadiness, do not drive or operate dangerous machinery.
- Use an alternate or additional method of contraception if concurrently taking estrogen-containing oral contraceptives.

How to Use This Drug

- If you miss a dose, take it as soon as you remember, but skip it if it is almost time for the next dose. **Do not take double doses.**
- Do not share your medication with others.
- Take the drug at the same time(s) each day.
- In general, take with **a full glass (eight ounces) of water** while in an upright position.
- Doxycycline and minocycline may be taken with food or milk if stomach irritation occurs.
- Avoid concurrent use of milk or dairy products with tetracycline. If stomach irritation occurs, take with food.
- *For tablets:* Store at room temperature with lid on tightly. Do not store in the bathroom. Do not expose to heat, moisture, or strong light. Keep out of reach of children.
- Take this drug for the prescribed length of time. If you stop too soon, your symptoms could come back.
- Discard outdated medication.

Interactions with Other Drugs

The following drugs, biologics (e.g., vaccines, therapeutic antibodies), or foods are listed in *Evaluations of Drug Interactions* 2003 as causing "highly clinically significant" or "clinically significant" interactions when used together with any of the drugs in this section. In some sections with multiple drugs, the interaction may have been reported for one but not all

Antibiotic-associated diarrhea (AAD) is quite common and its incidence varies from 5% to 20% of patients depending on which antibiotic they are taking although practically all antibiotics have been associated with AAD. Fortunately, most cases are mild and self-limited, ending with the cessation of use of the offending antibiotic. The antibiotics most commonly associated with this mild form of AAD include ampicillin, amoxicillin, cephalosporins and clindamycin.[27] There have been studies in children or adults in which the use of prophylactic yogurt in people using antibiotics has significantly reduced the occurrence or severity of AAD.[28,29] However, 10 to 20% of all patients who get AAD (0.5 to 4% of patients using antibiotics) will get the more severe form of AAD known as pseudomembranous colitis (see below). If you are taking any antibiotic and develop diarrhea after starting to use the drug, call your physician to discuss whether another antibiotic should be used and to discuss the need for rehydration due to the fluid losses from the diarrhea.

Pseudomembranous colitis has been reported with nearly all antibacterial agents and may range in severity from mild to life-threatening. Therefore, it is important to consider this diagnosis in patients who present with diarrhea subsequent to the administration of antibacterial agents.

Because antibiotic therapy has been associated with severe colitis which may end fatally, it should be reserved for serious infections where less toxic antimicrobial agents are inappropriate, as described in the **INDICATIONS AND USAGE** section. It should not be used in patients with nonbacterial infections such as most upper respiratory tract infections. Treatment with antibacterial agents alters the normal flora of the colon and may permit over-growth of clostridia. Studies indicate that a toxin produced by *Clostridium difficile* is one primary cause of "antibiotic-associated colitis."

After the diagnosis of pseudomembranous colitis has been established, therapeutic measures should be initiated. Mild cases of pseudomembranous colitis usually respond to drug discontinuation alone. In moderate to severe cases, consideration should be given to management with fluids and electrolytes, protein supplementation, and treatment with an antibacterial drug clinically effective against *C. difficile* colitis.

Diarrhea, colitis, and pseudomembranous colitis have been observed to begin up to several weeks following cessation of therapy.

drugs in this section, but we include the interaction because the drugs in this section are similar to one another. We have also included potentially serious interactions listed in the drug's FDA-approved professional package insert or in published medical journal articles. There may be other drugs, especially those in the families of drugs listed below, that also will react with this drug to cause severe adverse effects. Make sure to tell your doctor and pharmacist the drugs you are taking and tell them if you are taking any of these interacting drugs:

aluminum hydroxide, AMPHOJEL, calcium carbonate, carbamazepine, CALTRATE, certoparin, COUMADIN, digoxin, DILANTIN, ESKALITH, FEOSOL, FERGON, ferrous gluconate, ferrous sulfate, LANOXIN, lithium, LUMINAL, MAALOX, magnesium hydroxide, methoxyflurane, oral contraceptives, OS-CAL 500, phenobarbital, phenytoin, PHILLIPS' MILK OF MAGNESIA, PRIFTIN, rifapentine, SLOW FE, SOLFOTON, TEGRETOL, warfarin.

Adverse Effects

Call your doctor immediately if you experience:

- skin rash or increased skin sensitivity to the sun

> ### WARNING
>
> The use of tetracyclines during tooth development (last half of pregnancy, infancy, and childhood to the age of eight years) may cause permanent discoloration of the teeth.

- changes in vision
- increased frequency of urination or amount of urine
- increased thirst
- yellowing or increased pigmentation of skin
- abdominal pain
- nausea or vomiting
- widening of soft spot on head (infants)
- staining of teeth (children)
- headache
- loss of appetite

Call your doctor if these symptoms continue:

- stomach irritation or cramps
- diarrhea
- darkened or discolored tongue
- itching in the genital or rectal area
- sore mouth or tongue
- dizziness, lightheadedness, or unsteadiness

Sulfonamides

Silver Sulfadiazine (sul fa *dye* a zeen)
SILVADENE (King)

GENERIC: available
FAMILY: Sulfonamides

PREGNANCY WARNING

No data are available for silver sulfadiazine, as it was not tested properly in animal studies. Use during pregnancy only for clear medical reasons. Tell your doctor if you are pregnant or thinking of becoming pregnant before you take this drug.

BREAST-FEEDING WARNING

No information is available from either human or animal studies. However, this class of drug, the sulfonamides, is known to be excreted in human milk and to cause harm to the nursing infant. Because of the potential for serious adverse effects in nursing infants, you should not take this drug while nursing.

Silver sulfadiazine is a cream that is used on burns to prevent and treat infection. It is almost always used in the hospital. If you have decreased kidney and/or liver function, you may need to use less than the usual adult dose to prevent dangerous levels of this drug from accumulating in your body. When you use this cream on burns over large areas of your body, your doctor should be carefully watching your kidney function and the levels of the drug in your body, and your urine should be tested for sulfa crystals.

Before You Use This Drug

Tell your doctor if you have or have had:

- pregnancy or are breast-feeding
- glucose-6-phosphate dehydrogenase (G6PD) deficiency
- kidney or liver problems
- blood problems
- porphyria

Tell your doctor about any other drugs you take, including aspirin, herbs, vitamins, and other nonprescription products.

When You Use This Drug

- If you plan to have any surgery, including dental, tell your doctor that you take this drug.
- Check with your doctor if there is no improvement within a few days or weeks (for more serious burns or burns over more extensive areas).

How to Use This Drug

- If you miss a dose, apply it as soon as you remember, but skip it if it is almost time for the next dose. **Do not take double doses.**

- Do not share your medication with others.
- Take this drug for the prescribed length of time.
- Clean affected areas before applying.
- Apply the drug at the same time(s) each day, wearing a sterile glove. Apply a thin layer and keep affected areas covered with the medication at all times.
- Reapply after bathing, showering, or use of a whirlpool bath.
- After applying, cover with a dressing or leave uncovered.
- Store at room temperature with cap on tightly. Do not store in the bathroom. Do not expose to heat, moisture, or strong light. Keep out of reach of children.

Interactions with Other Drugs

Some other drugs that you may be taking (either over-the-counter or prescription drugs) can interact with this one, causing adverse effects. Ask your doctor what these drugs are and let him or her know if you are taking any of them.

cimetidine, TAGAMET.

Adverse Effects

Call your doctor immediately if you experience:

- skin burning, itching, peeling, or rash
- red skin lesions, often with purple center
- intense itching of burn wounds
- worsening of condition or no improvement
- increased sensitivity to the sun
- bloody or cloudy urine
- greatly decreased frequency of urination or amount
- painful or difficult urination
- shortness of breath
- chills, cough, fever, or sore throat
- unusual bleeding or bruising

- tiredness
- sores, ulcers, or white spots on lips or in mouth
- unusual bleeding or bruising
- blue-green to black skin

Call your doctor if these symptoms continue:

- burning feeling on treated areas
- brownish-gray skin discoloration
- skin rash or itching

Because silver sulfadiazine is absorbed into the body, you may have other adverse effects that occur with the sulfonamides (sulfa drugs). See sulfisoxazole, below, for examples.

Periodic Tests

Ask your doctor which of these tests should be done periodically while you are taking this drug:

- complete blood count
- serum sulfadiazine concentrations
- urinalysis

Sulfisoxazole (sul fi *sox* a zole)
GANTRISIN (Roche)

Trimethoprim and sulfamethoxazole
(trye *meth* oh prim and sul fa meth *ox* a zole)
BACTRIM (Women First Healthcare)
SEPTRA (Monarch)
COTRIM (Teva)

GENERIC: available
FAMILY: Sulfonamides
Sulfonamides with Synthetic Antibacterial

PREGNANCY WARNING
Sulfisoxazole caused harm to developing fetuses in animal studies, including cleft palates, malformations, brain damage, and death. Because of the potential for serious adverse effects to the fetus, these drugs should not be used by pregnant women.

Sulfisoxazole is used to treat urinary tract infections and some other infections. If you have kidney or liver damage, you should take less than the usual adult dose. Sulfisoxazole will not help a cold or the flu.

Sulfisoxazole is available in several forms. It is often taken by mouth. Another form is a vaginal cream that is used to treat vaginitis, but there is no evidence that this is an effective treatment. For eye infections, there is an eye ointment and eye solution, which are similar to sulfacetamide (see p. 518).

Trimethoprim with sulfamethoxazole is a combination of the synthetic antibacterial trimethoprim and the sulfa drug sulfamethoxazole. This combination of drugs is commonly used to treat urinary tract infections but is also approved to treat bacterial infections in other parts of the body.

Deaths have been associated with the use of sulfonamides due to severe skin reactions that include Stevens-Johnson syndrome, toxic epidermal necrolysis, fulminant hepatic necrosis (liver toxicity), and bone marrow toxicity. Products such as trimethoprim with sulfamethoxazole should be discontinued at the first appearance of skin rash or any sign of an adverse reaction.[55]

Practice measures to prevent urinary tract infections. Drink plenty of fluids, especially water. While cranberry juice is unreliable as a cure for urinary tract infections, the juice may reduce odor from incontinence.[56] Practice meticulous hygiene. After using the toilet, wipe backward, not forward, then wash your hands. Prepare and store foods properly, especially when traveling, to prevent diarrhea. Restrict caffeine, which widens the urethra. Indwelling catheters invite urinary tract infections. However, unless there are symptoms of urinary infection, it is not always necessary to take medication just because bacteria are found in a urine test.[57] Women are particularly prone to repeated urinary tract infections. If urinary tract symptoms occur often, ask your doctor about keeping a supply of medication on hand. Ideally, the antibiotic you use should be the most effective, least toxic, and least costly.[34,37]

Before You Use This Drug

Do not use if you have or have had allergy to:

- sulfonamides
- furosemide
- thiazide diuretics
- sulfonylureas
- carbonic anhydrase inhibitors (see p. 501)

Tell your doctor if you have or have had:

- pregnancy or are breast-feeding
- allergies to drugs
- glucose-6-phosphate dehydrogenase deficiency
- kidney or liver disease
- porphyria
- anemia or other blood problems

Tell your doctor about any other drugs you take, including aspirin, herbs, vitamins, and other nonprescription products.

When You Use This Drug

- If you plan to have any surgery, including dental, tell your doctor that you take this drug.
- Check with your doctor if there is no improvement within a few days.
- Have regular visits with your doctor to check your blood.
- Protect yourself from the sun.
- If you get dizzy, do not drive or operate heavy machinery.

How to Use This Drug

• If you miss a dose, take it as soon as you remember, but skip it if it is almost time for the next dose. **Do not take double doses.**
• Do not share your medication with others.
• Take the drug at the same time(s) each day.
• Maintain adequate fluid intake.
• Take this drug for the prescribed length of time. If you stop too soon, your symptoms could come back.
• Take with **a full glass (eight ounces) of water** and maintain adequate fluid levels.
• *For tablets:* Store at room temperature with lid on tightly. Do not store in the bathroom. Do not expose to heat, moisture, or strong light. Keep out of reach of children.

Interactions with Other Drugs

The following drugs, biologics (e.g., vaccines, therapeutic antibodies), or foods are listed in *Evaluations of Drug Interactions* 2003 as causing "highly clinically significant" or "clinically significant" interactions when used together with any of the drugs in this section. In some sections with multiple drugs, the interaction may have been reported for one but not all drugs in this section, but we include the interaction because the drugs in this section are similar to one another. We have also included potentially serious interactions listed in the drug's FDA-approved professional package insert or in published medical journal articles. There may be other drugs, especially those in the families of drugs listed below, that also will react with this drug to cause severe adverse effects. Make sure to tell your doctor and pharmacist the drugs you are taking and tell them if you are taking any of these interacting drugs:

aminobenzoate, COUMADIN, DILANTIN, GLUCOPHAGE, GLUCOVANCE, HIPREX, METAGLIP, metformin, methenamine, methotrexate, ORINASE, phenytoin, thiopental, tolbutamide, TREXALL DOSE PACK, UREX, warfarin.

Adverse Effects

Call your doctor immediately if you experience:

• increased sensitivity of skin to the sun (increased sunburn)
• skin rash or red, itching, blistering, or peeling skin
• aching joints and muscles
• difficulty swallowing
• fever
• pale skin
• sore throat
• abnormal bleeding or bruising
• abnormal tiredness or weakness
• yellow eyes or skin
• lower back pain
• increased thirst
• difficulty urinating
• blood in urine
• painful urination
• greatly increased or decreased frequency of urination
• severe abdominal or stomach cramps
• watery and severe diarrhea (may be bloody)
• mood or mental changes
• swelling of neck
• confusion, hallucinations
• loss of appetite

Call your doctor if these symptoms continue:

• diarrhea
• dizziness
• headache
• tiredness
• loss of appetite
• nausea or vomiting

Periodic Tests

Ask your doctor which of these tests should be done periodically while you are taking this drug:

- complete blood count
- urinalysis

Fluoroquinolones

 Do Not Use

ALTERNATIVE TREATMENT:
Numerous other, safer antibiotics are approved to treat the same infections as this drug (see p. 679).

Moxifloxacin (mox i *flox* a sin)
AVELOX (Bayer Corporation)

Sparfloxacin (spar *flox* a sin)
ZAGAM (Mylan)

Gatifloxacin (gat if *flox* a sin)
TEQUIN (Bristol-Myers Squibb)

FAMILY: Fluoroquinolones (see p. 679)

Moxifloxacin

This antibiotic was approved by the FDA on December 10, 1999, and became the ninth member of the family of antibiotics known as fluoroquinolone antibiotics. Ciprofloxacin (CIPRO), the best-known member of this family, is also made by the Bayer Corporation.

We list moxifloxacin as **Do Not Use** because of its effect on electrical conduction in the heart (known as QT prolongation), which can cause potentially fatal heart rhythm disturbances. The QTc interval is the length of time it takes the large chambers of the heart (ventricles) to electrically discharge and recharge. A prolongation of the QTc interval can lead to a type of heart rhythm disturbance, or cardiac arrhythmia, known as torsades de pointes and sudden death. The QTc interval is measured by an electrocardiogram (EKG or ECG) in milliseconds (msec). The lowercase "c" indicates that the QT interval has been corrected for the patient's heart rate. *Torsades de pointes* is a French phrase that means "twisted point," describing the appearance of this rhythm disturbance on the EKG tracing.

The FDA's Anti-infective Drugs Advisory Committee voted seven to three to recommend approval of the drug if its professional product labeling or package insert warned of heart prob-

---

WARNING: INCREASED RISK OF TENDINITIS AND TENDON RUPTURE WITH ALL FLUOROQUINOLONE ANTIBIOTICS

Public Citizen's Health Research Group petitioned the FDA to add a warning for doctors to the labeling or package for all fluoroquinolone antibiotics about the risk of tendinitis, including the possibility of complete tendon rupture.

This adverse reaction most frequently involves the Achilles tendon, the tendon that runs from the back of the heel to the calf. Rupture of the Achilles tendon may require surgical repair. Tendons in the rotator cuff (the shoulder), the hand, the biceps, and the thumb have also been involved. This reaction appears to be more common in those taking steroid drugs, in older patients, and in kidney transplant recipients, but cases have occurred in people without any of these risk factors. The onset of symptoms is sudden and has occurred as soon as 24 hours after starting treatment with a fluoroquinolone. Most people have recovered completely after one to two months.

If you experience unexpected tendon pain while taking a fluoroquinolone antibiotic, stop the drug immediately, call your doctor, and rest.

Antibiotic-associated diarrhea (AAD) is quite common and its incidence varies from 5% to 20% of patients depending on which antibiotic they are taking although practically all antibiotics have been associated with AAD. Fortunately, most cases are mild and self-limited, ending with the cessation of use of the offending antibiotic. The antibiotics most commonly associated with this mild form of AAD include ampicillin, amoxicillin, cephalosporins and clindamycin.[27] There have been studies in children or adults in which the use of prophylactic yogurt in people using antibiotics has significantly reduced the occurrence or severity of AAD.[28,29] However, 10 to 20% of all patients who get AAD (0.5 to 4% of patients using antibiotics) will get the more severe form of AAD known as pseudomembranous colitis (see below). If you are taking any antibiotic and develop diarrhea after starting to use the drug, call your physician to discuss whether another antibiotic should be used and to discuss the need for rehydration due to the fluid losses from the diarrhea.

Pseudomembranous colitis has been reported with nearly all antibacterial agents and may range in severity from mild to life-threatening. Therefore, it is important to consider this diagnosis in patients who present with diarrhea subsequent to the administration of antibacterial agents.

Because antibiotic therapy has been associated with severe colitis which may end fatally, it should be reserved for serious infections where less toxic antimicrobial agents are inappropriate, as described in the **INDICATIONS AND USAGE** section. It should not be used in patients with nonbacterial infections such as most upper respiratory tract infections. Treatment with antibacterial agents alters the normal flora of the colon and may permit over-growth of clostridia. Studies indicate that a toxin produced by *Clostridium difficile* is one primary cause of "antibiotic-associated colitis."

After the diagnosis of pseudomembranous colitis has been established, therapeutic measures should be initiated. Mild cases of pseudomembranous colitis usually respond to drug discontinuation alone. In moderate to severe cases, consideration should be given to management with fluids and electrolytes, protein supplementation, and treatment with an antibacterial drug clinically effective against *C. difficile* colitis.

Diarrhea, colitis, and pseudomembranous colitis have been observed to begin up to several weeks following cessation of therapy.

lems. One concerned committee member who voted against the drug's approval said: "I think there are enough things that really haven't been answered [about moxifloxacin]. . . . and I'm not sure I see what this drug adds to drugs we already have that's so unique that we need this drug, that we absolutely need it, and we need it now for some indication [use]."[75]

We agree with this committee member's assessment of moxifloxacin. There are numerous antibiotics available that can be used to treat the same infections as moxifloxacin and do not alter the heart's QT interval. We do not need *more* new drugs; we need *better* new drugs that

are safer and more effective than those we already have. Unfortunately, there is nothing in U.S. drug law that requires a new drug to be either safer or more effective than drugs already on the market.

The FDA did heed the advisory committee's advice and required a boldface warning notifying doctors and pharmacists of moxifloxacin's heart problems and potentially life-threatening drug interactions. Regrettably, there is still no requirement to inform the only group at risk of adverse drug reactions from moxifloxacin—the patients for whom the drug is prescribed.

The text of the FDA warning reads:

WARNINGS

THE SAFETY AND EFFECTIVENESS OF MOXIFLOXACIN IN PEDIATRIC PATIENTS, ADOLESCENTS (LESS THAN 18 YEARS OF AGE), PREGNANT WOMEN, AND LACTATING WOMEN HAVE NOT BEEN ESTABLISHED. MOXIFLOXACIN HAS BEEN SHOWN TO PROLONG THE QT INTERVAL OF THE ELECTROCARDIOGRAM [EKG or ECG] IN SOME PATIENTS. THE DRUG SHOULD BE AVOIDED IN PATIENTS WITH KNOWN PROLONGATION OF THE QT INTERVAL, PATIENTS WITH UNCORRECTED HYPOKALEMIA AND PATIENTS RECEIVING CLASS IA (E.G. QUINIDINE, PROCAINAMIDE) OR CLASS III (E.G. AMIODARONE, SOTALOL) ANTIARRHYTHMIC AGENTS, DUE TO THE LACK OF CLINICAL EXPERIENCE WITH THE DRUG IN THESE PATIENT POPULATIONS.[3]

Moxifloxacin should not be prescribed along with certain drugs used to treat heart rhythm disturbances. These are: amiodarone (CORDARONE), bretylium, disopyramide (NORPACE), moricizine (ETHMOZINE), procainamide (PROCANBID), quinidine (DURAQUIN, QUINAGLUTE DURA-TABS, QUINIDEX), and sotalol (BETAPACE).

Moxifloxacin should not be used by people with prolonged QT intervals or by those with low blood levels of potassium (hypokalemia).

In the FDA's adverse drug reaction database that covers the period from the drug's approval through the second quarter of 2001, there are 24 reports of rhythm disturbances of the large chamber of the heart (the ventricles); 23 reports of QT prolongation, and 3 reports of torsades de pointes. Some patients experienced more than one of these problems. Actual instances are probably much greater, because the FDA conservatively estimates that only 1 in 10 serious adverse drug reactions are reported to the agency.

The professional product labeling for moxifloxacin also warns that the drug has not been studied with other drugs that prolong the QT interval and should be used with caution when given together with drugs such as erythromycin (EES, ERYTHROCIN), antipsychotic drugs such as thioridazine (MELLARIL), and tricyclic antidepressants such as amitriptyline (ELAVIL) and imipramine (TOFRANIL). We do not think it is worth the risk of taking moxifloxacin together with these drugs when there are other antibiotics that can be used safely.

The labeling also states that the effect of moxifloxacin in patients with inherited prolongation of the QT interval has not been studied; however, it is expected that these individuals may be more susceptible to drug-induced QT prolongation. The only way to know if you have inherited QT prolongation is by having an electrocardiogram done by your doctor. Moxifloxacin's labeling also says that because of limited clinical experience, the drug should be used with caution in patients with conditions that increase the risk of heart rhythm disturbances, such as a clinically significant slow heart rate (bradycardia), and acute blockage or narrowing of the blood vessels in the heart known as myocardial ischemia. We think moxifloxacin should also be avoided if you have these conditions.

Moxifloxacin shares the potential for many other serious adverse effects with the other members of the fluoroquinolone family of antibiotics. Convulsions have been reported in patients receiving fluoroquinolones. They can also cause central nervous system (CNS) adverse effects including dizziness, confusion, tremors, hallucinations, depression, and sometimes suicidal thoughts or acts. These adverse reactions may occur following the first dose. The use of nonsteroidal anti-inflammatory drugs such as ibuprofen (MOTRIN), celecoxib (CELEBREX), and rofecoxib (VIOXX) with a fluoroquinolone antibiotic may increase the risk of CNS stimulation and convulsions.

Sparfloxacin

This fluoroquinolone antibiotic was cleared for marketing by the FDA in December 1996.

Sparfloxacin must not be used in individuals with a history of hypersensitivity or photosensitivity reactions. Torsades de pointes, a life-threatening heart rhythm disturbance, has been reported in patients receiving sparfloxacin together with disopyramide (NORPACE) and amiodarone (CORDARONE). Consequently, sparfloxacin should not be used in individuals receiving these drugs as well as other QTc-prolonging drugs used to treat heart rhythm disturbances reported to cause torsades de pointes, such as quinidine (QUINAGLUTE DURA-TABS), procainamide (PROCANBID), sotalol (BETAPACE), and bepridil (VASCOR). Sparfloxacin is contraindicated in patients with known QTc prolongation.[76]

It is essential for patients to avoid exposure to the sun, bright natural light, and UV rays throughout the entire duration of treatment and for five days after treatment with sparfloxacin is stopped. Sparfloxacin is contraindicated in patients whose lifestyle or employment will not permit compliance with required safety precautions concerning phototoxicity.[76]

Gatifloxacin

The approval of gatifloxacin (TEQUIN) in October 2001 brought to nine the number of fluoroquinolone antibiotics on the market, and this drug joins sparfloxacin (ZAGAM) and moxifloxacin (AVELOX) as fluoroquinolones that can cause a dangerous abnormality in the heart's electrical conduction known as QT prolongation that can lead to fatal heart rhythm disturbances such as torsades de pointes.

The European Agency for the Evaluation of Medicinal Products in a press release dated April 26, 2002, indicated that a review of gatifloxacin "was initiated because of safety and efficacy concerns." The exact nature of these concerns was not revealed but may involve the drug's association with QT prolongation.

The QT interval is the length of time it takes the ventricles (large chambers of the heart) to discharge and recharge electrically. Prolongation of the QT interval can lead to disturbances (called cardiac arrhythmias) such as torsades de pointes. The QTc interval is measured on an electrocardiogram (EKG or ECG) in milliseconds (msec). The lowercase "c" indicates that the QT interval has been corrected for the patient's heart rate. *Torsades de pointes* is a French phrase that means "twisted point"; it describes the appearance of this type of rhythm disturbance on the EKG tracing.

The professional product labeling or package insert for gatifloxacin carries the following boldface warning:

WARNINGS
THE SAFETY AND EFFECTIVENESS OF GATIFLOXACIN IN PEDIATRIC PATIENTS, ADOLESCENTS (LESS THAN 18 YEARS OF AGE), PREGNANT WOMEN, AND LACTATING WOMEN HAVE NOT BEEN ESTABLISHED. GATIFLOXACIN MAY HAVE THE POTENTIAL TO PROLONG THE QTc INTERVAL OF THE ELECTROCARDIOGRAM IN SOME PATIENTS. DUE TO THE LACK OF CLINICAL EXPERIENCE, GATIFLOXACIN SHOULD BE AVOIDED IN PATIENTS WITH KNOWN PROLONGATION OF THE QTc INTERVAL, PATIENTS WITH UNCORRECTED HYPOKALEMIA (LOW BLOOD POTASSIUM LEVELS), AND PATIENTS RECEIVING CLASS 1A 9E.G., QUINIDINE, PROCAINAMIDE) OR CLASS III 9E.G., AMIODARONE, SOTALOL) ANTIARRHYTHMIC AGENTS.

Gatifloxacin must not be used together with certain drugs given to treat heart rhythm disturbances. These are amiodarone (CORDARONE), bretylium, disopyramide (NORPACE), mori-cizine (ETHMOZINE), procainamide (PROCAN-BID), quinidine (QUINAGLUTE DURA-TABS, QUINIDEX), and sotalol (BETAPACE).

The professional product labeling for gati-floxacin also warns that it has not been studied in combination with other drugs that pro-long the QT interval and should be used with caution when given with drugs such as erythro-mycin (EES), antipsychotic drugs such as thioridazine (MELLARIL), and tricyclic antide-pressants such as amitriptyline (ELAVIL) and imipramine (TOFRANIL). We do not think it is worth the risk of taking gatifloxacin together with these drugs when there are other antibi-otics just as effective and safer.

The editors of a highly respected independent source of drug information written for doctors and pharmacists, *The Medical Letter on Drugs and Therapeutics,* concluded their review of gatifloxacin by saying it may be more *"active than levofloxacin [LEVAQUIN in a test tube] against pneumococci, but there is no evidence of any clinical advantage over the older drug. It is too early to tell whether any of the unexpected se-rious adverse effects that have limited use of some fluoroquinolones will occur with these new agents."*[77]

Limited Use

Ciprofloxacin (sip roe *flox* a sin)
CIPRO (Bayer)

Levofloxacin (lee voe *flox* a sin)
LEVAQUIN (Ortho-McNeil)

Lomefloxacin (loe me *flox* a sin)
MAXAQUIN (Pharmacia)

Ofloxacin (oe *flox* a sin)
FLOXIN (Ortho-McNeil)

GENERIC: not available
FAMILY: Fluoroquinolones (see p. 679)

PREGNANCY WARNING

Fluoroquinolones caused fetal harm in animal studies, in-cluding decreased body weights and malformed bones as well as an increased risk of death. Because of the potential for serious adverse effects to the fetus, these drugs should not be used by pregnant women.

BREAST-FEEDING WARNING

Fluoroquinolones are excreted in human milk. Because of the potential for serious adverse effects in nursing infants, you should not take these drugs while nursing.

The fluoroquinolone family of antibiotics are used to treat bacterial infections in many dif-ferent parts of the body. They work by killing bacteria or preventing their growth. The fluoro-quinolones will not work for colds, flu, or other virus infections.[78]

The *Journal of the American Medical As-sociation* reports widespread misuse of the fluo-roquinolone ciprofloxacin. Ciprofloxacin is inappropriate for common sinus and ear infec-tions and community-acquired pneumonias. For most pneumonias and streptococcal infec-tions, penicillin or a cephalosporin remain drugs of choice.[79]

A recent study illustrates the rampant, out-of-control misprescribing and overprescribing of fluoroquinolone antibiotics. In a study of the use of these drugs in the emergency rooms of two academic medical centers, 100 consecutive patients who were prescribed a fluoroquinolone were studied to find out if the use was appropri-ate according to the guidelines used at those institutions. Of the 100 patients, 81 (81%) were given the antibiotic for an inappropriate use, including 43 (53% of the 81 patients) for whom another antibiotic was the first-line treatment, and 27 (33%) in whom there was no evidence of an infection. Of the 19 patients for whom the prescribing of this class of antibiotics was appropriate, only one patient was pre-scribed the right dose for the correct length of time.[18]

Antibiotic-associated diarrhea (AAD) is quite common and its incidence varies from 5% to 20% of patients depending on which antibiotic they are taking although practically all antibiotics have been associated with AAD. Fortunately, most cases are mild and self-limited, ending with the cessation of use of the offending antibiotic. The antibiotics most commonly associated with this mild form of AAD include ampicillin, amoxicillin, cephalosporins and clindamycin.[27] There have been studies in children or adults in which the use of prophylactic yogurt in people using antibiotics has significantly reduced the occurrence or severity of AAD.[28,29] However, 10 to 20% of all patients who get AAD (0.5 to 4% of patients using antibiotics) will get the more severe form of AAD known as pseudomembranous colitis (see below). If you are taking any antibiotic and develop diarrhea after starting to use the drug, call your physician to discuss whether another antibiotic should be used and to discuss the need for rehydration due to the fluid losses from the diarrhea.

Pseudomembranous colitis has been reported with nearly all antibacterial agents and may range in severity from mild to life-threatening. Therefore, it is important to consider this diagnosis in patients who present with diarrhea subsequent to the administration of antibacterial agents.

Because antibiotic therapy has been associated with severe colitis which may end fatally, it should be reserved for serious infections where less toxic antimicrobial agents are inappropriate, as described in the **INDICATIONS AND USAGE** section. It should not be used in patients with nonbacterial infections such as most upper respiratory tract infections. Treatment with antibacterial agents alters the normal flora of the colon and may permit over-growth of clostridia. Studies indicate that a toxin produced by *Clostridium difficile* is one primary cause of "antibiotic-associated colitis."

After the diagnosis of pseudomembranous colitis has been established, therapeutic measures should be initiated. Mild cases of pseudomembranous colitis usually respond to drug discontinuation alone. In moderate to severe cases, consideration should be given to management with fluids and electrolytes, protein supplementation, and treatment with an antibacterial drug clinically effective against *C. difficile* colitis.

Diarrhea, colitis, and pseudomembranous colitis have been observed to begin up to several weeks following cessation of therapy.

Before You Use This Drug

Do not use if you have or have had:

- allergies to fluoroquinolones or quinolone-type drugs
- photosensitivity
- inflammation or rupture of tendons

Tell your doctor if you have or have had:

- epilepsy or seizures
- kidney and liver problems (ciprofloxacin)
- liver problems (ofloxacin)
- kidney problems
- myasthenia gravis[80]
- an implanted metal device[81]
- brain or spinal cord disease
- slow heart rate (levofloxacin)
- diabetes (levofloxacin)
- low potassium blood level (levofloxacin)
- pregnancy or are breast-feeding

Tell your doctor about any other drugs you take, including aspirin, herbs, vitamins, and other nonprescription products. It is especially important you tell your doctor if you take any heart drug (see p. 45).

When You Use This Drug

- Do not drive or perform other activities that require alertness because this drug may make you drowsy, dizzy, or lightheaded.
- If you plan to have any surgery, including dental, tell your doctor that you take this drug.

WARNING

Extreme caution should be used when fluoroquinolones such as ciprofloxacin are to be prescribed in conjunction with aminophylline or theophylline, particularly in elderly patients. Aminophylline or theophylline doses should be adjusted, perhaps reduced by 30 to 50% at the start of fluoroquinolone therapy. The reduction in dose must be guided by the clinical conditions of the patient, the use of other medications, and the baseline level of the aminophylline or theophylline in the blood. In addition, blood aminophylline or theophylline levels should be obtained following the initiation of a fluoroquinolone no later than two days into therapy.

- Check with your doctor if there is no improvement of symptoms within a few days.
- Protect yourself from sunburn. Do not use a sunlamp.
- Stop taking ciprofloxacin at the first sign or symptom of blistering, itching, rash, or redness of skin or sensation of skin burning or swelling. Check with your doctor.
- If you get a skin reaction to the sun, avoid further sunlight and artificial light until reaction has stopped or for five days, whichever is longer.
- Call your doctor and discontinue the drug if you get pain, inflammation, or rupture of a tendon.
- **Caution diabetics:** call your doctor and discontinue drug if you have a hypoglycemic episode.
- *For oral forms of this drug:* Do not take this drug and antacids or sucralfate (CARAFATE) at the same time. Take six hours before or two hours after ciprofloxacin. Ask your doctor or pharmacist how long you have to wait for the drug that you are taking.

How to Use This Drug

- If you miss a dose, take it as soon as you remember, but skip it if it is almost time for the next dose. **Do not take double doses.**
- Do not share your medication with others.
- Take the drug at the same time(s) each day.
- Drink plenty of fluids.
- Take with **a full glass (eight ounces) of water.**
- Take with or without food.
- Take this drug for the prescribed length of time. If you stop too soon, your symptoms could come back.
- Store at room temperature with lid on tightly. Do not store in the bathroom. Do not expose to heat, moisture, or strong light. Keep out of reach of children.

Interactions with Other Drugs

The following drugs, biologics (e.g., vaccines, therapeutic antibodies), or foods are listed in *Evaluations of Drug Interactions* 2003 as causing "highly clinically significant" or "clinically significant" interactions when used together with any of the drugs in this section. In some sections with multiple drugs, the interaction may have been reported for one but not all drugs in this section, but we include the interaction because the drugs in this section are similar to one another. We have also included potentially serious interactions listed in the drug's FDA-approved professional package insert or in published medical journal articles. There may be other drugs, especially those in the families of drugs listed below, that also will react with this drug to cause severe adverse effects. Make sure to tell your doctor and pharmacist the drugs you are taking and tell them if you are taking any of these interacting drugs:

aluminum hydroxide, AMPHOJEL, caffeine (beverages or drugs), calcium carbonate, CALTRATE, CARAFATE, COUMADIN,

WARNING: INCREASED RISK OF TENDINITIS AND TENDON RUPTURE WITH ALL FLUOROQUINOLONE ANTIBIOTICS

Public Citizen's Health Research Group petitioned the FDA successfully to add a warning for doctors to the labeling or package for all fluoroquinolone antibiotics about the risk of tendinitis, including the possibility of complete tendon rupture.

This adverse reaction most frequently involves the Achilles tendon, the tendon that runs from the back of the heel to the calf. Rupture of the Achilles tendon may require surgical repair. Tendons in the rotator cuff (the shoulder), the hand, the biceps, and the thumb have also been involved. This reaction appears to be more common in those taking steroid drugs, in older patients, and in kidney transplant recipients, but cases have occurred in people without any of these risk factors. The onset of symptoms is sudden and has occurred as soon as 24 hours after starting treatment with a fluoroquinolone. Most people have recovered completely after one to two months.

If you experience unexpected tendon pain while taking a fluoroquinolone antibiotic, stop the drug immediately, call your doctor, and rest.

cyclosporine, DIABETA, DILANTIN, ELIXOPHYLLIN, FEOSOL, ferrous sulfate and other iron preparations, glyburide, MAALOX, magnesium hydroxide, methotrexate, MEXATE, NEORAL, OS-CAL 500, phenytoin, PHILLIPS' MILK OF MAGNESIA, PRIFTIN, REQUIP, rifapentine, ropinirole, SANDIMMUNE, SLOW FE, sucralfate, THEO-24, theophylline, warfarin, zinc preparations.

Adverse Effects

Call your doctor immediately if you experience:

- watery and severe or bloody diarrhea
- agitation
- dizziness
- sensation of skin burning
- joint pain
- fast or irregular heartbeat
- fainting
- blood in urine
- dark or amber urine
- loss of appetite
- stomach pain
- yellow eyes or skin
- difficulty breathing
- confusion, hallucinations
- fever
- skin rash, itching, redness, or peeling
- seizure
- swelling of face, neck, calves, or lower legs
- tremors
- blurred vision
- pain in calves radiating to heels
- heartbeat change

For levofloxacin (in addition to above):

- sharp drop in blood pressure
- coma
- bleeding gums
- failure of heart, lungs, kidneys, and/or liver

Call your doctor if these symptoms continue:

- dizziness, lightheadedness
- drowsiness
- headache
- nervousness
- difficulty sleeping
- insomnia, restlessness
- nausea or vomiting
- mild diarrhea
- mild pain in abdomen, stomach, or joints
- vaginal pain or discharge
- increased sensitivity of skin to sunlight

Call your doctor if these symptoms continue after you stop taking this drug:

- severe abdominal or stomach cramps
- abdominal tenderness
- watery and severe diarrhea
- pain in calves radiating to heels
- sensation of skin burning
- skin rash, itching, redness, or peeling
- swelling of face, neck, calves, or lower legs

Periodic Tests

Ask your doctor which of these tests should be done periodically while you are taking this drug:

- bleeding times

Limited Use

Norfloxacin (nor *flox* a sin)
NOROXIN TABLETS (Merck)

GENERIC: available

FAMILY: Fluoroquinolones (see p. 679)

PREGNANCY WARNING

Fluoroquinolones caused fetal harm in animal studies, including decreased body weights and malformed bones as well as an increased risk of death. Because of the potential for serious adverse effects to the fetus, these drugs should not be used by pregnant women.

BREAST-FEEDING WARNING

Fluoroquinolones are excreted in human milk. Because of the potential for serious adverse effects in nursing infants, you should not take these drugs while nursing.

Norfloxacin kills bacteria and can cure infections caused by susceptible organisms. Oral norfloxacin differs from the other fluoroquinolone antibiotics in that it is used only to treat infections in the urinary tract, prostate gland, and sexually transmitted diseases.[82] Drops of norfloxacin are used to treat eye infections.

Elderly people have suffered more severe adverse effects, fatalities, and harmful interactions from norfloxacin.[83,84] Since in people over age 65 norfloxacin is excreted more slowly, a lower dose is usually used.

A seven-day course of norfloxacin costs 5 to 10 times more than drugs such as amoxicillin (see p. 682) or trimethoprim and sulfamethoxazole (see p. 703), which are equally effective for most infections. Both resistance and allergy to one drug in this family usually cross to the rest of the fluoroquinolones and sometimes even occur during therapy.[19,20] Overgrowth of normal bacteria may cause yeast infections, especially when antibiotics are used for long periods. The fluoroquinolones can cause central nervous system reactions and psychosis.[21] Severe, even fatal, allergic reactions have happened after just one dose. Collapse of the circulatory system has occurred. As a group fluoroquinolones are expensive, resistance is increasing, and effective alternatives are available.[85]

The same adverse effects of norfloxacin can result from either oral tablets or eye drops.

Practice measures to prevent urinary tract infections. Drink plenty of fluids, especially water. While cranberry juice is unreliable as a cure for urinary tract infections, the juice may reduce odor from incontinence.[56] Practice meticulous hygiene. After using the toilet, wipe backward, not forward, then wash your hands. Prepare and store foods properly, especially when traveling, to prevent diarrhea. Restrict caffeine, which widens the urethra. Indwelling catheters invite urinary tract infections. However, unless there are symptoms of urinary infection, it is not always necessary to take medication just because bacteria are found in a urine test.[57] Women are particularly prone to repeated urinary tract infections. If urinary tract symptoms occur often, ask your doctor about keeping a supply of medication on hand. Ideally, the antibiotic you use should be the most effective, least toxic, and least costly.[37,60]

Antibiotic-associated diarrhea (AAD) is quite common and its incidence varies from 5% to 20% of patients depending on which antibiotic they are taking although practically all antibiotics have been associated with AAD. Fortunately, most cases are mild and self-limited, ending with the cessation of use of the offending antibiotic. The antibiotics most commonly associated with this mild form of AAD include ampicillin, amoxicillin, cephalosporins and clindamycin.[27] There have been studies in children or adults in which the use of prophylactic yogurt in people using antibiotics has significantly reduced the occurrence or severity of AAD.[28,29] However, 10 to 20% of all patients who get AAD (0.5 to 4% of patients using antibiotics) will get the more severe form of AAD known as pseudomembranous colitis (see below). If you are taking any antibiotic and develop diarrhea after starting to use the drug, call your physician to discuss whether another antibiotic should be used and to discuss the need for rehydration due to the fluid losses from the diarrhea.

Pseudomembranous colitis has been reported with nearly all antibacterial agents and may range in severity from mild to life-threatening. Therefore, it is important to consider this diagnosis in patients who present with diarrhea subsequent to the administration of antibacterial agents.

Because antibiotic therapy has been associated with severe colitis which may end fatally, it should be reserved for serious infections where less toxic antimicrobial agents are inappropriate, as described in the **INDICATIONS AND USAGE** section. It should not be used in patients with nonbacterial infections such as most upper respiratory tract infections. Treatment with antibacterial agents alters the normal flora of the colon and may permit over-growth of clostridia. Studies indicate that a toxin produced by *Clostridium difficile* is one primary cause of "antibiotic-associated colitis."

After the diagnosis of pseudomembranous colitis has been established, therapeutic measures should be initiated. Mild cases of pseudomembranous colitis usually respond to drug discontinuation alone. In moderate to severe cases, consideration should be given to management with fluids and electrolytes, protein supplementation, and treatment with an antibacterial drug clinically effective against *C. difficile* colitis.

Diarrhea, colitis, and pseudomembranous colitis have been observed to begin up to several weeks following cessation of therapy.

Before You Use This Drug

Do not use if you have or have had:

- allergies to fluoroquinolones or quinolone-type drugs
- photosensitivity
- inflammation or rupture of tendons

Tell your doctor if you have or have had:

- allergies to drugs
- epilepsy or seizures
- liver problems
- kidney problems
- myasthenia gravis[80]
- an implanted metal device[81]
- brain or spinal cord disease
- heart disorder
- diabetes
- low potassium blood level
- pregnancy or are breast-feeding

Tell your doctor about any other drugs you take, including aspirin, herbs, vitamins, and other nonprescription products. It is especially important you tell your doctor if you take any heart drug (see p. 45).

When You Use This Drug

- Check with your doctor if there is no improvement of symptoms within a few days.
- Do not drive or perform other activities

that require alertness because this drug may make you drowsy, dizzy, or lightheaded.

• If you plan to have any surgery, including dental, tell your doctor that you take this drug.

• Protect yourself from sunburn. Do not use a sunlamp.

• If you get a skin reaction to the sun, avoid further sunlight and artificial light until reaction has stopped or for five days, whichever is longer.

• Call your doctor and discontinue the drug if you get pain, inflammation, or rupture of a tendon.

• **Caution diabetics:** Call your doctor and discontinue drug if you have a hypoglycemic episode.

• *For oral forms of this drug:* Do not take this drug and antacids or sucralfate (CARAFATE) at the same time. You have to wait two hours after taking an antacid or sucralfate before you can take norfloxacin; you also have to wait two hours after taking norfloxacin before you can take an antacid or sucralfate.

• Call your doctor and discontinue the drug if you get pain, inflammation, or rupture of a tendon.

How to Use This Drug

• If you miss a dose, take it as soon as you remember, but skip it if it is almost time for the next dose. **Do not take double doses.**

• Do not share your medication with others.

• Take the drug at the same time(s) each day.

• Take this drug for the prescribed length of time. If you stop too soon, your symptoms could come back.

• Drink plenty of fluids.

• Take with **a full glass (eight ounces) of water.**

• Take with or without food.

• Store at room temperature with lid on tightly. Do not store in the bathroom. Do not expose to heat, moisture, or strong light. Keep out of reach of children.

Interactions with Other Drugs

The following drugs, biologics (e.g., vaccines, therapeutic antibodies), or foods are listed in *Evaluations of Drug Interactions* 2003 as causing "highly clinically significant" or "clinically significant" interactions when used together with any of the drugs in this section. In some sections with multiple drugs, the interaction may have been reported for one but not all drugs in this section, but we include the interaction because the drugs in this section are similar to one another. We have also included potentially serious interactions listed in the drug's FDA-approved professional package insert or in published medical journal articles. There may be other drugs, especially those in the families of drugs listed below, that also will react with this drug to cause severe adverse effects. Make sure to tell your doctor and pharmacist the drugs you are taking and tell them if you are taking any of these interacting drugs:

aluminum hydroxide, AMPHOJEL, caffeine (beverages, drugs), CARAFATE, cyclosporine, FEOSOL, FERGON, ferrous gluconate, ferrous sulfate, MAALOX, magnesium hydroxide, NEORAL, PHILLIPS' MILK OF MAGNESIA, SANDIMMUNE, SLOW FE, sucralfate.

A report in the *Archives of Internal Medicine* adds interaction with COUMADIN (warfarin) as the one most frequently reported in older people.[83]

Caution should be taken when the following drugs are used with this one (see warning box): aminophylline, ELIXOPHYLLIN, SLO-BID, SOMOPHYLLIN, SOMOPHYLLIN-DF, THEO-24, theophylline.

Adverse Effects

*Call your doctor immediately if you experi-
ence:*

- severe or bloody diarrhea
- agitation
- difficulty breathing
- confusion, hallucinations
- fever
- skin rash, itching, redness, or peeling
- seizure
- swelling of face, neck, calves, or lower legs
- tremors
- blurred vision
- pain at site of injection
- pain in calves radiating to heels
- heartbeat change

*Call your doctor if these symptoms con-
tinue:*

- dizziness, lightheadedness
- drowsiness
- headache
- insomnia, restlessness
- nausea or vomiting
- diarrhea
- pain in abdomen, stomach, or joints
- increased sensitivity of skin to sunlight

*Call your doctor if these symptoms con-
tinue after you stop taking this drug:*

- severe abdominal or stomach cramps
- abdominal tenderness
- watery and severe diarrhea
- pain in calves radiating to heels
- sensation of skin burning
- skin rash, itching, redness, or peeling
- swelling of face, neck, calves, or lower legs

Periodic Tests

*Ask your doctor which of these tests should
be done periodically while you are taking
this drug:*

- bleeding times

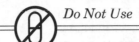

Do Not Use

ALTERNATIVE TREATMENT:
*Numerous other, safer antibiotics are approved to
treat the same infections as this drug (see p. 679).*

Trovafloxacin (troe va *flox* a sin)
TROVAN (Pfizer)

FAMILY: Fluoroquinolones (see p. 679)

Trovafloxacin was approved by the FDA in December 1997 and became the ninth member of
the fluoroquinolone family of antibiotics available in the United States. Shortly after the approval of the drug in the United States,
European drug regulatory authorities issued a
public statement on May 25, 1999, about serious, severe, and unpredictable liver injuries associated with the use of trovafloxacin.

We petitioned the FDA on June 3, 1999, to immediately remove this dangerous drug from the
market.

On June 9, 1999, the FDA issued a public
health advisory about trovafloxacin.[86] The FDA
has received reports of over 100 cases of clinically symptomatic liver toxicity in patients receiving trovafloxacin. Some of these patients
developed serious liver injury leading to liver
transplant and death or both. At the present
time, the FDA was aware of 14 cases of acute
liver failure that were strongly associated with
trovafloxacin exposure. Four of these patients
required liver transplant (one of whom subsequently died). Five additional patients died of
liver-related illness. Three patients recovered
without transplantation, and the final outcome
is still pending on two patients. These numbers
of patients with acute liver failure, although
few, represent a rate that appears to be significantly higher than would be expected to
occur idiopathically in the general population—
despite the under-reporting of cases that gener-

WARNING: INCREASED RISK OF TENDINITIS AND TENDON RUPTURE WITH ALL FLUOROQUINOLONE ANTIBIOTICS

Public Citizen's Health Research Group petitioned the FDA to add a warning for doctors to the labeling or package for all fluoroquinolone antibiotics about the risk of tendinitis, including the possibility of complete tendon rupture.

This adverse reaction most frequently involves the Achilles tendon, the tendon that runs from the back of the heel to the calf. Rupture of the Achilles tendon may require surgical repair. Tendons in the rotator cuff (the shoulder), the hand, the biceps, and the thumb have also been involved. This reaction appears to be more common in those taking steroid drugs, in older patients, and in kidney transplant recipients, but cases have occurred in people without any of these risk factors. The onset of symptoms is sudden and has occurred as soon as 24 hours after starting treatment with a fluoroquinolone. Most people have recovered completely after one to two months.

If you experience unexpected tendon pain while taking a fluoroquinolone antibiotic, stop the drug immediately, call your doctor, and rest.

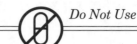

Do Not Use

ALTERNATIVE TREATMENT:
Numerous other, safer antibiotics are approved to treat the same infections as this drug (see p. 679).

Gemifloxacin (gem i *flox* a sin)
FACTIVE (Oscient Pharmaceuticals)

FAMILY: Fluroquinolones (see p. 679)

Gemifloxacin was approved by the FDA in April 2003 and became the tenth member of the fluoroquinolone family of antibiotics on the market in the United States. Marketing rights for the drug in North America belong to GeneSoft Pharmaceuticals Inc. of California, who licensed gemifloxacin from LG Life Sciences Ltd., a company based in Korea.

The primary sources of information for this drug profile are the FDA's evaluations of data and clinical trials submitted by GeneSoft in support of gemifloxacin's approval. These evaluations were posted on the FDA's Web site at www.fda.gov/ohrms/dockets/ac/03/briefing/3931b1.htm prior to the March 4, 2003, Anti-Infective Drugs Advisory Committee meeting in which gemifloxacin's safety and effectiveness were reviewed.

GeneSoft originally submitted its application to the FDA for gemifloxacin in December 1999. In the original application, the company sought approval for the treatment of adults for three types of respiratory tract infections: (1) community-acquired pneumonia; (2) acute bacterial exacerbation (worsening) of chronic bronchitis; and (3) acute bacterial sinusitis (sinus infection). In addition, GeneSoft wanted the drug approved for two types of urinary tract infections: (1) uncomplicated urinary tract infection and (2) complicated urinary tract infection.

Ultimately gemifloxacin was approved for

ally occurs with our postmarketing surveillance system.

Trovafloxacin-associated liver failure appears to be unpredictable. It has been reported with both short-term (as little as two days' exposure) and longer-term drug exposure; therefore the efficacy of liver function monitoring in acceptably managing this risk is uncertain.

The FDA restricted the distribution of trovafloxacin, mainly to hospitals, while the drug was banned from the markets in every other country in which it had been approved.

WARNING: INCREASED RISK OF TENDINITIS AND TENDON RUPTURE WITH ALL FLUOROQUINOLONE ANTIBIOTICS

Public Citizen's Health Research Group petitioned the FDA to add a warning for doctors to the labeling or package for all fluoroquinolone antibiotics about the risk of tendinitis, including the possibility of complete tendon rupture.

This adverse reaction most frequently involves the Achilles tendon, the tendon that runs from the back of the heel to the calf. Rupture of the Achilles tendon may require surgical repair. Tendons in the rotator cuff (the shoulder), the hand, the biceps, and the thumb have also been involved. This reaction appears to be more common in those taking steroid drugs, in older patients, and in kidney transplant recipients, but cases have occurred in people without any of these risk factors. The onset of symptoms is sudden and has occurred as soon as 24 hours after starting treatment with a fluoroquinolone. Most people have recovered completely after one to two months.

If you experience unexpected tendon pain while taking a fluoroquinolone antibiotic, stop the drug immediately, call your doctor, and rest.

only two infections, community-acquired pneumonia and acute bacterial exacerbation of chronic bronchitis. Treatment is limited to seven days for community-acquired pneumonia and five days for acute bacterial exacerbation of chronic bronchitis because of the increased risk of adverse drug reactions with a longer duration of treatment.[87]

During the course of the FDA's review of gemifloxacin, significant questions arose regarding the drug's safety. The questions involved the higher than expected rate of rash reported in patients receiving gemifloxacin and related questions regarding how the drug caused rash, the potential for cross-sensitization with other fluoroquinolone antibiotics, and the possibility that the frequent occurrence of rash may foreshadow a risk for more serious skin drug reactions. Also, there were unresolved questions regarding gemifloxacin's liver safety and concern over the potential for the drug to alter the heart's electrical conduction that could lead to dangerous heart rhythm disturbances.

Each of the three major safety issues with gemifloxacin—rash, potential liver toxicity, and the possibility of heart rhythm disturbance—are discussed below.

Rash

As mentioned above, during the initial review of gemifloxacin, a higher than expected rate of rash was noted in the clinical trials. The rates of rash ranged from less than 1% to higher than 25%, depending upon the population or subset of patients being analyzed. Analyses of the rash data have shown that females under 40, and a duration of treatment greater than seven days, are associated with an increased risk of rash.

GeneSoft addressed the rash issue by conducting an additional study of gemifloxacin compared to ciprofloxacin (CIPRO), an older, very popular fluoroquinolone, in healthy women who appeared to be at the greatest risk of developing a rash, those under 40 years of age and taking the drug for longer than 10 days. We have serious questions about the ethics of conducting a clinical trial in normal women to see how many rashes could be induced.

At the end of the study, rash had appeared in 31.7% of women given gemifloxacin and in 4.3% of the women receiving ciprofloxacin. This is a greater than sevenfold difference in the risk of rash between the two drugs.

It was found that 80% of women who developed a rash did so on days 8, 9, or 10 of the study. Over 25% of these women had a rash covering greater than 60% of their body, and 7.3 percent were classified as having a severe rash, whereas none of the women taking ciprofloxacin had a rash classified as severe. In addition, there were 16 cases of mucous membrane involvement among the 260 women who developed a rash from gemifloxacin (6.2%), and none in the seven women who developed a rash from ciprofloxacin.

Gemifloxacin's professional product labeling or package insert instructs physicians to warn patients to stop taking the drug and call the prescribing physician if a rash develops.[87]

Potential for Liver Toxicity

In doses greater than the FDA-approved 320 milligrams daily, gemifloxacin produced elevations in blood levels of liver enzymes. Such elevations can be an early sign of liver toxicity. In studies submitted to the FDA in women who received a single dose of 640 milligrams of gemifloxacin, double the dose finally approved of 320 milligrams, there was a greater proportion of patients who developed elevations of liver enzymes compared to women receiving ciprofloxacin.

Gemifloxacin's professional product labeling carries the following precautionary warning: "The recommended dose of gemifloxacin 320 mg daily should not be exceeded and the recommended length of therapy should not be exceeded."[87]

QT Interval Prolongation

The QT interval is the length of time it takes the large chambers of the heart (ventricles) to electrically discharge and recharge. A prolongation of the QT interval can lead to heart rhythm disturbances, or cardiac arrhythmias, such as torsades de pointes and other life-threatening arrhythmias. *Torsades de pointes* is a French phrase that means "twisted point," describing the appearance of this type of rhythm disturbance on the EKG tracing. The QTc interval is measured by an electrocardiogram (EKG or ECG) in milliseconds (msec). The lowercase "c"

indicates that the QT interval has been corrected for the patient's heart rate.

QT interval prolongation is seen with other fluoroquinolone antibiotics, and there was enough concern at the FDA that the following bolded warning was required in professional product labeling for gemifloxacin:

WARNINGS
THE SAFETY AND EFFECTIVENESS OF FACTIVE IN CHILDREN, ADOLESCENTS (LESS THAN 18 YEARS OF AGE), PREGNANT WOMEN, AND LACTATING WOMEN HAVE NOT BEEN ESTABLISHED. QT EFFECTS: GEMIFLOXACIN MAY PROLONG THE QT INTERVAL IN SOME PATIENTS. GEMIFLOXACIN SHOULD BE AVOIDED IN PATIENTS WITH A HISTORY OF PROLONGATION OF THE QTc INTERVAL, PATIENTS WITH UNCORRECTED ELECTROLYTE DISORDERS (HYPOKALEMIA [low blood levels of potassium] OR HYPOMAGNESEMIA [low blood levels of magnesium]), AND PATIENTS RECEIVING CLASS IA (E.G., QUINIDINE, PROCAINAMIDE) OR CLASS III (E.G., AMIODARONE, SOTALOL) ANTIARRHYTHMIC AGENTS.

The table below lists the generic and brand names of the drugs for heart rhythm disturbances (antiarrhymthics) referred to in the warning above.

GENERIC NAME	BRAND NAME(S)
Class IA Antiarrhythmic Drugs	
disopyramide	NORPACE
procainamide	PROCANBID
moricizine	ETHMOZINE
quinidine	DURAQUIN, QUINIDEX, QUINAGLUTE
Class III Antiarrhythmic Drugs	
bretylium	
amiodarone	CORDARONE
sotalol	BETAPACE

Gemifloxacin is a drug that should not have been approved and should not be used.

Other Drugs for Bacterial Infection

Trimethoprim (trye *meth* o prim)
PROLOPRIM (Monarch)

GENERIC: available
FAMILY: Other Drugs for Bacterial Infection

PREGNANCY WARNING

This drug crossed the placenta and caused malformations in developing fetuses in animal studies. Use during pregnancy only for clear medical reasons. Tell your doctor if you are pregnant or thinking of becoming pregnant before you take this drug.

BREAST-FEEDING WARNING

Trimethoprim is excreted in human milk at concentrations equal to or greater than the mother's serum and may interfere with folic acid metabolism in nursing infants. Because of the potential for serious adverse effects in nursing infants, you should not take this drug while nursing.

Trimethoprim is approved by the FDA for the treatment of initial episodes of uncomplicated urinary tract infections.[58] It will not help a cold or the flu.

If you have severe kidney impairment, you should use caution in taking trimethoprim.[59] If you have impaired kidney function, you may need to take less than the usual adult dose. While taking trimethoprim, you may suffer a rash or itching.

Practice measures to prevent urinary tract infections. Drink plenty of fluids, especially water. While cranberry juice is unreliable as a cure for urinary tract infections, the juice may reduce odor from incontinence.[56] Practice meticulous hygiene. After using the toilet, wipe backward, not forward, then wash your hands. Prepare and store foods properly, especially when traveling, to prevent diarrhea. Restrict caffeine, which widens the urethra. Indwelling catheters invite urinary tract infections. However, unless there are symptoms of urinary infection, it is not always necessary to take medication just because bacteria are found in a urine test.[57] Women are particularly prone to repeated urinary tract infections. If urinary tract symptoms occur often, ask your doctor about keeping a supply of medication on hand. Ideally, the antibiotic you use should be the most effective, least toxic, and least costly.[37,60]

Before You Use This Drug

Tell your doctor if you have or have had:

- pregnancy or are breast-feeding
- an unusual reaction to trimethoprim
- folic acid (folate) deficiency
- kidney or liver problems
- anemia

Tell your doctor about any other drugs you take, including aspirin, herbs, vitamins, and other nonprescription products.

When You Use This Drug

- If you plan to have any surgery, including dental, tell your doctor that you take this drug.
- Check with your doctor or dentist concerning proper technique in taking care of your teeth.
- Check with your doctor if there is no improvement within a few days.
- Have regular visits with your doctor to check on your progress.
- If you take trimethoprim for a long time, ask your doctor if you need a folic acid supplement.
- Stay out of the sun.

How to Use This Drug

- If you miss a dose, take it as soon as you remember, but skip it if it is almost time for the next dose. **Do not take double doses.**
- Do not share your medication with others.
- Take the drug at the same time(s) each day.

- Take without food unless you have stomach irritation, then take with food.
- *For tablets:* Store at room temperature with lid on tightly. Do not store in the bathroom. Do not expose to heat, moisture, or strong light. Keep out of reach of children.
- Take this drug for the prescribed length of time. If you stop too soon, your symptoms could come back.

Interactions with Other Drugs

The following drugs, biologics (e.g., vaccines, therapeutic antibodies), or foods are listed in *Evaluations of Drug Interactions* 2003 as causing "highly clinically significant" or "clinically significant" interactions when used together with any of the drugs in this section. In some sections with multiple drugs, the interaction may have been reported for one but not all drugs in this section, but we include the interaction because the drugs in this section are similar to one another. We have also included potentially serious interactions listed in the drug's FDA-approved professional package insert or in published medical journal articles. There may be other drugs, especially those in the families of drugs listed below, that also will react with this drug to cause severe adverse effects. Make sure to tell your doctor and pharmacist the drugs you are taking and tell them if you are taking any of these interacting drugs:

COUMADIN, DILANTIN, dofetilide, methotrexate, phenytoin, TREXALL DOSE PACK, TIKOSYN, warfarin.

Adverse Effects

Call your doctor immediately if you experience:

- chills, fever, or sore throat
- abnormal bleeding or bruising
- abnormal paleness, tiredness, or weakness
- bluish fingernails, lips, or skin
- trouble breathing
- headache
- nausea
- neck stiffness
- shortness of breath
- swelling of face
- changes in facial skin color
- pale skin
- skin rash or itching
- joint and muscle pain
- skin red, blistering, or peeling
- redness, swelling, or soreness of tongue
- black, tarry stools
- blood in urine
- pinpoint red spots on skin
- red skin lesions, often with a purple center

Call your doctor if these symptoms continue:

- unusual taste in mouth
- diarrhea
- loss of appetite
- nausea or vomiting
- sore mouth or tongue
- stomach cramps or pain
- headache

Signs of overdose:

- chills
- fever
- sore throat
- unusual tiredness or weakness
- unusual bleeding or bruising
- black, tarry stools
- blood in urine
- pinpoint red spots on skin
- confusion
- dizziness
- headache
- depression
- nausea or vomiting

If you suspect an overdose, call this number to contact your poison control center: (800) 222-1222.

Periodic Tests

Ask your doctor which of these tests should be done periodically while you are taking this drug:

- complete blood count

———————

Limited Use

Clindamycin (klin da *mye* sin)
CLEOCIN (Pharmacia & Upjohn)

GENERIC: available
FAMILY: Other Drugs for Bacterial Infection

PREGNANCY WARNING

No valid data is available for clindamycin, as it was not tested properly in animal studies. However, because of the potential for serious adverse effects to the fetus, this drug should not be used by pregnant women.

BREAST-FEEDING WARNING

Clindamycin is excreted in human milk. Because of the potential for serious adverse effects in nursing infants, you should not take this drug while nursing.

Clindamycin is used to treat life-threatening infections[61] that do not respond to penicillin or other antibiotics, such as bone or abdominal infections. Clindamycin will not help a cold or the flu, and it is too dangerous to use for sore throats and other upper respiratory infections.

Clindamycin can have serious adverse effects. It can cause serious inflammation of the large intestine, abdominal cramps, and severe diarrhea, sometimes with passage of blood and mucus. These adverse effects can happen up to several weeks after you stop using the drug. Because of the possibility of these serious adverse effects, your doctor should prescribe a drug less toxic than clindamycin if at all possible. If you are taking clindamycin, watch closely for the serious adverse effects listed. If any occur, call your doctor immediately, stop taking clindamycin, and do not take any other medication to treat your adverse effects. When you take antidiarrheal drugs to treat diarrhea caused by clindamycin, they can prolong or worsen the diarrhea instead of helping.

If you have combined liver and kidney disease, you should take less than the usual adult dose of clindamycin.

Before You Use This Drug

Tell your doctor if you have or have had:

- allergies to drugs
- an unusual reaction to doxorubicin or lincomycin
- kidney or liver problems
- stomach or intestinal disease
- pregnancy or are breast-feeding

Tell your doctor about any other drugs you take, including aspirin, herbs, vitamins, and other nonprescription products.

When You Use This Drug

- If you plan to have any surgery, including dental, tell your doctor that you take this drug.
- Check with your doctor if there is no improvement within a few days.
- Have regular visits with your doctor to check on your progress.
- If you get severe diarrhea, check with your doctor before taking any antidiarrheals.

How to Use This Drug

- If you miss a dose, take it as soon as you remember, but skip it if it is almost time for the next dose. **Do not take double doses.**
- Do not share your medication with others.
- Take the drug at the same time(s) each day. Space doses evenly.
- Take this drug for the prescribed length of time. If you stop too soon, your symptoms could come back.

Antibiotic-associated diarrhea (AAD) is quite common and its incidence varies from 5% to 20% of patients depending on which antibiotic they are taking although practically all antibiotics have been associated with AAD. Fortunately, most cases are mild and self-limited, ending with the cessation of use of the offending antibiotic .The antibiotics most commonly associated with this mild form of AAD include ampicillin, amoxicillin, cephalosporins and clindamycin.[27] There have been studies in children or adults in which the use of prophylactic yogurt in people using antibiotics has significantly reduced the occurrence or severity of AAD.[28,29] However, 10 to 20% of all patients who get AAD (0.5 to 4% of patients using antibiotics) will get the more severe form of AAD known as pseudomembranous colitis (see below). If you are taking any antibiotic and develop diarrhea after starting to use the drug, call your physician to discuss whether another antibiotic should be used and to discuss the need for rehydration due to the fluid losses from the diarrhea.

Pseudomembranous colitis has been reported with nearly all antibacterial agents and may range in severity from mild to life-threatening. Therefore, it is important to consider this diagnosis in patients who present with diarrhea subsequent to the administration of antibacterial agents.

Because antibiotic therapy has been associated with severe colitis which may end fatally, it should be reserved for serious infections where less toxic antimicrobial agents are inappropriate, as described in the **INDICATIONS AND USAGE** section. It should not be used in patients with nonbacterial infections such as most upper respiratory tract infections. Treatment with antibacterial agents alters the normal flora of the colon and may permit over-growth of clostridia. Studies indicate that a toxin produced by *Clostridium difficile* is one primary cause of "antibiotic-associated colitis."

After the diagnosis of pseudomembranous colitis has been established, therapeutic measures should be initiated. Mild cases of pseudomembranous colitis usually respond to drug discontinuation alone. In moderate to severe cases, consideration should be given to management with fluids and electrolytes, protein supplementation, and treatment with an antibacterial drug clinically effective against *C. difficile* colitis.

Diarrhea, colitis, and pseudomembranous colitis have been observed to begin up to several weeks following cessation of therapy with clindamycin.

- Take with **a full glass (eight ounces) of water** or with meals.
- Do not take solution after expiration date.
- *For tablets:* Store at room temperature with lid on tightly. Do not store in the bathroom. Do not expose to heat, moisture, or strong light. Keep out of reach of children

Interactions with Other Drugs

The following drugs, biologics (e.g., vaccines, therapeutic antibodies), or foods are listed in *Evaluations of Drug Interactions* 2003 as causing "highly clinically significant" or "clinically significant" interactions when used together with any of the drugs in this section. In some sections with multiple drugs, the interaction may have been reported for one but not all drugs in this section, but we include the interaction because the drugs in this section are similar to one another. We have also included potentially serious interactions listed in the drug's FDA-approved professional package insert or in published medical journal articles. There may be other drugs, especially those in the families of drugs listed below, that also will react with this drug to cause severe adverse effects. Make sure to tell your doctor and pharmacist the drugs you are taking and tell them if you are taking any of these interacting drugs:

EES, erythromycin, ether, FORTOVASE, INVIRASE, pancuronium, PAVULON, saquinavir.

Adverse Effects

Call your doctor immediately if you experience:

- severe stomach cramps or abdominal pain
- abdominal tenderness
- severe, watery diarrhea (may contain blood)
- fever and sore throat
- skin rash, redness, or itching
- unusual bleeding or bruising

Call your doctor if these symptoms continue:

- diarrhea
- abdominal pain
- nausea or vomiting
- itching in the genital or rectal area

Call your doctor if these symptoms continue after you stop taking this drug:

- severe stomach cramps or abdominal pain
- abdominal tenderness
- severe, watery diarrhea (may contain blood)

Periodic Tests

Ask your doctor which of these tests should be done periodically while you are taking this drug:

- colonoscopy and/or protosigmoidoscopy
- stool examinations

Limited Use

Metronidazole (me troe *ni* da zole)
FLAGYL (Searle)

GENERIC: available
FAMILY: Other Drugs for Bacterial Infection

PREGNANCY WARNING
Metronidazole crosses the placenta and rapidly enters the fetal blood system. Because the drug causes cancer and has the potential for causing serious adverse effects in the fetus, it should not be used by pregnant women.

BREAST-FEEDING WARNING
Metronidazole is excreted in human milk. Because of the potential for serious adverse effects in nursing infants, you should not take this drug while nursing.

FDA BLACK BOX WARNING

Metronidazole has been shown to be carcinogenic in mice and rats. Unnecessary use of the drug should be avoided. Its use should be reserved for the conditions described in the Indications and Usage section below [of the professional product labeling].[62]

Metronidazole is used to treat some serious infections caused by bacteria or protozoa, including trichomonas, amoebiasis, giardiasis, and pseudomembranous colitis caused by clostridia from taking other antibiotics. This drug will not help a cold or the flu.

Metronidazole has been shown to cause cancer in mice and rats. It can cause genetic damage in human cells.[63] Because of this connection, you should only be using metronidazole if you have a serious infection. Doctors sometimes prescribe metronidazole for a vaginal infection called trichomonas ("trich"), but you should not be using this drug for this kind of infection until you have tried other treatments such as taking a tub bath twice a day, wearing cotton underwear, and not wearing panty hose. If you have tried these treatments and you still have symptoms of a trichomonas infection, then metronidazole may be prescribed.[64]

If you are taking metronidazole for a vaginal trichomonas infection, it is best to use the form that must be taken for one day only. If you are taking metronidazole for any reason and you have kidney or severe liver impairment, you may need to take less than the usual adult dose.[65]

The information in this profile deals mostly with the forms of metronidazole taken by mouth—tablets and capsules.

Before You Use This Drug

Tell your doctor if you have or have had:

- allergies to drugs
- an unusual reaction to metronidazole
- disease of the central nervous system
- epilepsy or seizures
- severe liver disease
- blood problems
- heart problems
- pregnancy or are breast-feeding
- known or previously unrecognized candidiasis

Tell your doctor about any other drugs you take, especially an anticoagulant such as warfarin or heparin, and including aspirin, herbs, vitamins, and other nonprescription products.

When You Use This Drug

- Do not drink alcohol while taking this drug or for at least three days after stopping the drug, because it can have a serious interaction with alcohol.
- If you plan to have any surgery, including dental, tell your doctor that you take this drug.
- If dry mouth occurs, use sugarless gum or sucking candy; check with your dentist if dry mouth continues for more than two weeks.
- *For treatment of giardiasis:* Have a follow-up visit with your doctor.
- *For treatment for trichomonas:* Male sexual partner may also need treatment and should use a condom while female partner is being treated.
- Until you know how you react to this drug, do not drive or perform other activities requiring alertness.
- Metronidazole may cause your urine to get darker. This is normal and not dangerous.

- Check with your doctor if there is no improvement within a few days.

How to Use This Drug

- Take this drug for the prescribed length of time. If you stop too soon, your symptoms could come back.
- If you miss a dose, take it as soon as you remember, but skip it if it is almost time for the next dose. **Do not take double doses.**
- Do not share your medication with others.
- Take the drug at the same time(s) each day.
- *For regular tablets:* Take with food or milk.
- *For extended-release tablets:* Take with water only. Do not eat or drink for about an hour before taking this medication.
- *For tablets and capsules:* Store at room temperature with lid on tightly. Do not store in the bathroom. Do not expose to heat, moisture, or strong light. Keep out of reach of children.

Interactions with Other Drugs

The following drugs, biologics (e.g., vaccines, therapeutic antibodies), or foods are listed in *Evaluations of Drug Interactions* 2003 as causing "highly clinically significant" or "clinically significant" interactions when used together with any of the drugs in this section. In some sections with multiple drugs, the interaction may have been reported for one but not all drugs in this section, but we include the interaction because the drugs in this section are similar to one another. We have also included potentially serious interactions listed in the drug's FDA-approved professional package insert or in published medical journal articles. There may be other drugs, especially those in the families of drugs listed below, that also will react with this drug to cause severe adverse effects. Make sure to tell your doctor and pharmacist the drugs you are taking and tell them if you are taking any of these interacting drugs:

alcohol, ANTABUSE, ARALEN, carbamazepine, chloroquine, cimetidine, COUMADIN, DILANTIN, disulfiram, EFUDEX, ESKALITH, fluorouracil, lithium, LITHOBID, LITHONATE, LUMINAL, phenobarbital, phenytoin, SOLFOTON, TAGAMET, TEGRETOL, warfarin.

Adverse Effects

Call your doctor immediately if you experience:

- numbness, tingling, pain, or weakness in hands or feet
- unusual bleeding or bruising
- clumsiness or unsteadiness
- seizures
- confusion, irritability, depression, weakness, or trouble sleeping
- mood or mental changes
- frequent or painful urination
- inability to control urine flow
- skin rash, redness, hives, or itching
- sore throat or fever
- new vaginal dryness, discharge, or irritation
- pain, tenderness, redness, or swelling over skin after injection
- severe abdominal or back pain
- anorexia
- nausea or vomiting
- black, tarry stools
- blood in urine
- pinpoint red spots on skin

Call your doctor if these symptoms continue:

- nausea or vomiting
- diarrhea (even if you stopped taking the drug a month ago)
- dizziness or lightheadedness
- headache
- loss of appetite
- stomach cramps or pain

- sore mouth or tongue
- problems urinating
- dry mouth
- bad taste in mouth
- dark urine

Signs of overdose:

- nausea or vomiting
- seizures
- clumsiness or unsteadiness
- numbness, tingling, pain, or weakness in hands or feet

If you suspect an overdose, call this number to contact your poison control center: (800) 222-1222.

Periodic Tests

Ask your doctor which of these tests should be done periodically while you are taking this drug:

- stool examinations (for giardiasis)

Limited Use

Mupirocin (mu *pir* o sin)
BACTROBAN ointment (GlaxoSmithKline)

GENERIC: available
FAMILY: Other Drugs for Bacterial Infection

PREGNANCY WARNING

There was no evidence of toxicity in animal studies. Tell your doctor if you are pregnant or thinking of becoming pregnant before you take this drug.

BREAST-FEEDING WARNING

No information is available from either human or animal studies. Since it is likely that this drug, like many others, is excreted in human milk, you should consult with your doctor if you are planning to nurse.

Mupirocin is approved by the FDA to treat Staph and Strep skin infections.[66] A review concluded that penicillin or erythromycin should be used to treat nonbullous to (simple) impetigo,[67] and some doctors prefer to use oral antibiotics to treat it. If the impetigo affects only a small skin area and you prefer not to take oral therapy, consider mupirocin.

Resistance and secondary infection with mupirocin can occur with prolonged use.[57,68] Mupirocin is for external use, so do not use if you have extensive broken skin or burns, since you could absorb the drug internally and cause kidney problems.[69]

Before You Use This Drug

Tell your doctor if you have or have had:

- allergies to drugs or polyethylene glycol (PEG)

When You Use This Drug

- Call your doctor if no improvement occurs within three to five days.
- Use all the mupirocin your doctor prescribed, even if you feel better before you run out. If you stop too soon, your symptoms could come back.

How to Use This Drug

- Wash the affected area with soap and water, then dry.
- Rub a small amount gently onto the skin. To avoid rubbing ointment off the skin and to protect your clothing, you may cover the site with a gauze dressing.
- If you miss a dose, apply it as soon as you remember, but skip it if it is almost time for the next application. **Do not apply double doses.**
- Do not use in the eyes.
- Recap the tube. Store at room temperature. Keep out of reach of children.

Interactions with Other Drugs

Evaluations of Drug Interactions 2003 lists no drugs, biologics (e.g., vaccines, therapeutic antibodies), or foods as causing "highly clinically significant" or "clinically significant" interactions when used together with the drugs in this section. We also found no interactions in the drugs' FDA-approved professional package inserts. However, as the number of new drugs approved for marketing increases and as more experience is gained with these drugs over time, new interactions may be discovered.

When using topical products it is advisable not to apply other topical preparations, including cosmetics, to the same site. This prevents interactions that could irritate your skin.

Adverse Reactions

Call your doctor if these symptoms appear:

- dry skin
- nausea
- skin rash, swelling, burning, itching, or pain
- abdominal pain
- dizziness
- sores in mouth or on lips

 Do Not Use If Over 60 Years of Age

Nitrofurantoin (nye troe *fyoor* an toyn)
MACRODANTIN (Procter & Gamble)
FURADANTIN (First Horizon)
MACROBID (Procter & Gamble)

FAMILY: Other Drugs for Bacterial Infection

BREAST-FEEDING WARNING

Nitrofurantoin is excreted in human milk. Because of the potential for serious adverse effects in nursing infants, you should not take this drug while nursing.

PREGNANCY WARNING

Nitrofurantoin caused fetal harm in animal studies, including growth retardation and malformations. Nitrofurantoin also caused lung tumors in the offspring of female mice treated with this drug. Because of the potential for serious adverse effects to the fetus, this drug should not be used by pregnant women.

Nitrofurantoin is used to treat certain urinary tract infections.[70] It is a dangerous drug and should not be used in older adults. People over 60 who take this drug have such a high risk of harmful adverse effects that the World Health Organization has said older adults should not use it.[71]

Because your kidneys normally work less effectively as you grow older, they do not eliminate this drug from your body fast enough. Because of this, nitrofurantoin accumulates to dangerously high levels in your bloodstream, causing adverse effects. Two of the possible adverse effects, a nerve disease called peripheral neuropathy and scarring of the lungs, may be irreversible, and deaths from these adverse effects have been reported.[72] You can almost always take another drug that will be just as effective as nitrofurantoin and much safer. If you are taking this drug, ask your doctor to change your prescription.

The professional product labeling or package

Antibiotic-associated diarrhea (AAD) is quite common and its incidence varies from 5% to 20% of patients depending on which antibiotic they are taking although practically all antibiotics have been associated with AAD. Fortunately, most cases are mild and self-limited, ending with the cessation of use of the offending antibiotic. The antibiotics most commonly associated with this mild form of AAD include ampicillin, amoxicillin, cephalosporins and clindamycin.[27] There have been studies in children or adults in which the use of prophylactic yogurt in people using antibiotics has significantly reduced the occurrence or severity of AAD.[28,29] However, 10 to 20% of all patients who get AAD (0.5 to 4% of patients using antibiotics) will get the more severe form of AAD known as pseudomembranous colitis (see below). If you are taking any antibiotic and develop diarrhea after starting to use the drug, call your physician to discuss whether another antibiotic should be used and to discuss the need for rehydration due to the fluid losses from the diarrhea.

Pseudomembranous colitis has been reported with nearly all antibacterial agents and may range in severity from mild to life-threatening. Therefore, it is important to consider this diagnosis in patients who present with diarrhea subsequent to the administration of antibacterial agents.

Because antibiotic therapy has been associated with severe colitis which may end fatally, it should be reserved for serious infections where less toxic antimicrobial agents are inappropriate, as described in the **INDICATIONS AND USAGE** section. It should not be used in patients with nonbacterial infections such as most upper respiratory tract infections. Treatment with antibacterial agents alters the normal flora of the colon and may permit over-growth of clostridia. Studies indicate that a toxin produced by *Clostridium difficile* is one primary cause of "antibiotic-associated colitis."

After the diagnosis of pseudomembranous colitis has been established, therapeutic measures should be initiated. Mild cases of pseudomembranous colitis usually respond to drug discontinuation alone. In moderate to severe cases, consideration should be given to management with fluids and electrolytes, protein supplementation, and treatment with an antibacterial drug clinically effective against *C. difficile* colitis.

Diarrhea, colitis, and pseudomembranous colitis have been observed to begin up to several weeks following cessation of therapy.

insert for nitrofurantoin carries the following bolded warning about lung toxicity:

ACUTE, SUBACUTE, OR CHRONIC PULMONARY REACTIONS HAVE BEEN OBSERVED IN PATIENTS TREATED WITH NITROFURANTOIN. IF THESE REACTIONS OCCUR, MACRODANTIN SHOULD BE DISCONTINUED AND APPROPRIATE MEASURES TAKEN. REPORTS HAVE CITED PULMONARY REACTIONS AS A CONTRIBUTING CAUSE OF DEATH.

CHRONIC PULMONARY REACTIONS (DIFFUSE INTERSTITIAL PNEUMONITIS OR PULMONARY FIBROSIS, OR BOTH) CAN DEVELOP INSIDIOUSLY. THESE REACTIONS OCCUR RARELY AND GENERALLY IN PATIENTS RECEIVING THERAPY FOR SIX MONTHS OR LONGER. CLOSE MONITORING OF THE PULMONARY CONDITION OF PATIENTS RECEIVING LONG-TERM THERAPY IS WARRANTED AND REQUIRES THAT THE BENEFITS OF THERAPY BE WEIGHED AGAINST POTENTIAL RISKS.[70]

The New Zealand Centre for Adverse Reactions Monitoring (CARM) reviewed reports of nitrofurantoin-induced lung toxicity in May 2002 after receiving a case of fatal lung toxicity resulting from long-term nitrofurantoin treatment. The patient was a 67-year-old woman with a history of severe rheumatoid arthritis who developed a cough after 20 months of nitrofurantoin treatment taken for severe recurrent urinary tract infections. Nitrofurantoin was continued for a further six months before it was stopped when lung toxicity was diagnosed. She died three months later.

In the CARM database, 34% of the nitrofurantoin adverse reaction reports involve the respiratory system. Half of these reflect lung tissue damage, including nine reports of pulmonary fibrosis. Twenty-six reports for respiratory system adverse effects were the result of chronic nitrofurantoin treatment.

Practice measures to prevent urinary tract infections. Drink plenty of fluids, especially water. While cranberry juice is unreliable as a cure for urinary tract infections, the juice may reduce odor from incontinence.[56] Practice meticulous hygiene. After using the toilet, wipe backward, not forward, then wash your hands. Prepare and store foods properly, especially when traveling, to prevent diarrhea. Restrict caffeine, which widens the urethra. Indwelling catheters invite urinary tract infections. However, unless there are symptoms of urinary infection, it is not always necessary to take medication just because bacteria are found in a urine test.[57] Women are particularly prone to repeated urinary tract infections. If urinary tract symptoms occur often, ask your doctor about keeping a supply of medication on hand. Ideally, the antibiotic you use should be the most effective, least toxic, and least costly.[37,60]

Before You Use This Drug

Tell your doctor if you have or have had:

- anemia
- pregnancy or are breast-feeding
- disease that has severely weakened you
- diabetes
- electrolyte imbalance
- vitamin B deficiency
- G6PD deficiency
- allergy to nitrofurantoin
- peripheral neuropathy (muscle weakness and atrophy, pain, and numbness)
- lung disease
- kidney disease

Tell your doctor about any other drugs you take, including aspirin, herbs, vitamins, and other nonprescription products.

When You Use This Drug

- If you plan to have any surgery, including dental, tell your doctor that you take this drug.

• Check with your doctor if there is no improvement within a few days.

• If using this drug for long-term therapy, have regular visits with your doctor to check your progress.

• You may experience rust-yellow or brown urine and/or temporary hair loss when you use this drug. You do not need to call your doctor if you experience these symptoms.

How to Use This Drug

• Take this drug for the prescribed length of time. If you stop too soon, your symptoms could come back.

• If you miss a dose, take it as soon as you remember, but skip it if it is almost time for the next dose. **Do not take double doses.**

• Do not share your medication with others.

• Take the drug at the same time(s) each day.

• Take with food or milk.

• *For oral liquid:*
  • Shake well before each dose.
  • Use a specially marked measuring spoon or other device.
  • The liquid may be mixed with water, milk, or fruit juices.

• *For extended-release capsules:*
  • Do not break, chew, or crush long-acting forms of this drug.
  • Store at room temperature with lid on tightly. Do not store in the bathroom. Do not expose to heat, moisture, or strong light. Keep out of reach of children.

Interactions with Other Drugs

Evaluations of Drug Interactions 2003 lists no drugs, biologics (e.g., vaccines, therapeutic antibodies), or foods as causing "highly clinically significant" or "clinically significant" interactions when used together with the drugs in this section. We also found no interactions in the drugs' FDA-approved professional package inserts. However, as the number of new drugs approved for marketing increases and as more experience is gained with these drugs over time, new interactions may be discovered.

antacids containing magnesium trisilicate, BENEMID, probenecid.

Adverse Effects

Call your doctor immediately if you experience:

• shortness of breath
• swelling of face, mouth, hands, or feet
• changes in facial skin color
• sudden trouble in swallowing or breathing
• hoarseness
• joint pain
• chills
• fever shortly after onset of therapy
• skin rash
• muscle pain
• itching
• hives
• chest pain
• cough
• general feeling of discomfort or illness
• sore throat
• unusual tiredness or weakness
• unusual bleeding or bruising
• pale or black, tarry stools
• blood in urine or stools
• pinpoint red spots on skin
• dizziness
• drowsiness
• headache
• burning, numbness, tingling, or painful sensations in arms, legs, hands, or feet
• weakness in arms, hands, legs, or feet
• wheezing or chest tightness
• sores, ulcer, or white spots on lips or in mouth
• swollen or painful glands
• appetite loss
• nausea or vomiting

- visual changes, blurred vision, or loss of vision, with or without eye pain
- blue skin color
- pale skin
- yellow eyes or skin
- dark urine
- continual severe abdominal or stomach pain or cramps
- continuous unpleasant breath odor
- vomiting blood
- severe watery diarrhea (may be bloody)
- confusion
- mental depression
- mood or mental changes
- blistering, peeling, or loosening of skin and mucous membranes
- red, thickened, or scaly skin
- red skin lesions, often with a purple center

Call your doctor if these symptoms continue:

- abdominal or stomach pain or upset
- diarrhea
- gas
- appetite loss
- nausea or vomiting
- headache

Call your doctor if these symptoms continue after you stop taking this drug:

- severe abdominal or stomach cramps or pain
- fever
- severe watery diarrhea (may be bloody)

Periodic Tests

Ask your doctor which of these tests should be done periodically while you are taking this drug:

- liver function tests
- kidney function tests
- lung function tests

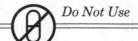

Do Not Use

ALTERNATIVE TREATMENT:
See Ampicillin, p. 682, Trimethoprim, p. 721, and Trimethoprim and Sulfamethoxazole, p. 703.

Atropine, Hyoscyamine, Methenamine, Methylene Blue, Phenyl Salicylate, and Benzoic Acid (*a* troe peen, hye oh *sye* a meen, meth *en* a meen, *meth* i leen blew, *fen* ill sa *li* si late, ben *zoe* ik *a* sid)
URISED (PolyMedica)

FAMILY: Other Drugs for Bacterial Infection
Antispasmodics
Salicylates

This combination of six drugs, atropine (see p. 574), hyoscyamine, methenamine, methylene blue, phenyl salicylate, and benzoic acid, is used to treat symptoms of urinary tract infections. This combination of drugs is irrational and too complex, and it should not be used. Part of the problem is that because the dosage of each indi-

---

ANTICHOLINERGIC EFFECTS

WARNING: SPECIAL MENTAL AND PHYSICAL ADVERSE EFFECTS

Older adults are especially sensitive to the harmful anticholinergic (see Glossary, p. 889) effects of this drug. Drugs in this family should not be used unless absolutely necessary.

Mental Effects: confusion, delirium, short-term memory problems, disorientation, and impaired attention.

Physical Effects: dry mouth, constipation, difficulty urinating (especially for a man with an enlarged prostate), blurred vision, decreased sweating with increased body temperature, sexual dysfunction, and worsening of glaucoma.

vidual drug is fixed, your doctor cannot adjust dosages to ensure that the product will be safe and effective. And one drug in this combination, atropine, causes adverse effects so severe that people over 60 should not take it at all.

Some of the ingredients in this product may cause excitement, agitation, drowsiness, or confusion in older adults, even at the usual dose. Call your doctor if you have any of these symptoms. Also, in people over 40, this drug may cause glaucoma, an eye disease that often remains hidden.

Practice measures to prevent urinary tract infections. Drink plenty of fluids, especially water. While cranberry juice is unreliable as a cure for urinary tract infections, the juice may reduce odor from incontinence.[56] Practice meticulous hygiene. After using the toilet, wipe backward, not forward, then wash your hands. Prepare and store foods properly, especially when traveling, to prevent diarrhea. Restrict caffeine, which widens the urethra. Indwelling catheters invite urinary tract infections. However, unless there are symptoms of urinary infection, it is not always necessary to take medication just because bacteria are found in a urine test.[57] Women are particularly prone to repeated urinary tract infections. If urinary

tract symptoms occur often, ask your doctor about keeping a supply of medication on hand. Ideally, the antibiotic you use should be the most effective, least toxic, and least costly.[37,60]

Do Not Use (Except in the Hospital)

ALTERNATIVE TREATMENT:
*If needed (outside the hospital),
take a less toxic antibiotic.*

Chloramphenicol (klor am *fen* i kole)
CHLOROMYCETIN (Parke-Davis)

FAMILY: Other Drugs for Bacterial Infection

Although chloramphenicol is effective in treating many conditions, it should be used only in a very limited number of situations because it is so dangerous. It can cause an irreversible depression of the bone marrow (where blood cells and platelets are produced), which usually results in death. It can also cause less serious reversible bone marrow depression.

Chloramphenicol should be used to treat serious diseases for which there is no better antibi-

---

Antibiotic-associated diarrhea (AAD) is quite common and its incidence varies from 5% to 20% of patients depending on which antibiotic they are taking although practically all antibiotics have been associated with AAD. Fortunately, most cases are mild and self-limited, ending with the cessation of use of the offending antibiotic. The antibiotics most commonly associated with this mild form of AAD include ampicillin, amoxicillin, cephalosporins and clindamycin.[27] There have been studies in children or adults in which the use of prophylactic yogurt in people using antibiotics has significantly reduced the occurrence or severity of AAD.[28,29] However, 10 to 20% of all patients who get AAD (0.5 to 4% of patients using antibiotics) will get the more severe form of AAD known as pseudomembranous colitis (see below). If you are taking any antibiotic and develop diarrhea after starting to use the drug, call your physician to discuss whether another antibiotic should be used and to discuss the need for rehydration due to the fluid losses from the diarrhea.

Pseudomembranous colitis has been reported with nearly all antibacterial agents and may range in severity from mild to life-threatening. Therefore, it is important to consider this diagnosis in patients who present with diarrhea subsequent to the administration of antibacterial agents.

(continued on page 734)

(continued from page 733)

Because antibiotic therapy has been associated with severe colitis which may end fatally, it should be reserved for serious infections where less toxic antimicrobial agents are inappropriate, as described in the **INDICATIONS AND USAGE** section. It should not be used in patients with nonbacterial infections such as most upper respiratory tract infections. Treatment with antibacterial agents alters the normal flora of the colon and may permit over-growth of clostridia. Studies indicate that a toxin produced by *Clostridium difficile* is one primary cause of "antibiotic-associated colitis."

After the diagnosis of pseudomembranous colitis has been established, therapeutic measures should be initiated. Mild cases of pseudomembranous colitis usually respond to drug discontinuation alone. In moderate to severe cases, consideration should be given to management with fluids and electrolytes, protein supplementation, and treatment with an antibacterial drug clinically effective against *C. difficile* colitis.

Diarrhea, colitis, and pseudomembranous colitis have been observed to begin up to several weeks following cessation of therapy.

otic available. Most of these diseases require hospital treatment, so there is rarely any reason to take chloramphenicol at home. The only exception is that you may need to take it at home to finish treatment that was begun in the hospital. The oral use of the drug almost always provides excellent blood levels, and intravenous or injected use of chloramphenicol only needs to be used if the intestines are not working or if the patient is comatose.

Oral chloramphenicol (taken by mouth) is usually prescribed inappropriately to treat trivial infections.[73] Chloramphenicol should not be used for minor infections, and it will not help a cold or the flu.

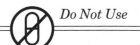

Do Not Use

ALTERNATIVE TREATMENT:
Clean the infected area well and take antibiotics by mouth or as injections, if necessary.

Neomycin, Polymyxin B, and Bacitracin
(nee oh *mye* sin, pol i *mix* in B, and bass i *tray* sin)
NEOSPORIN MAXIMUM STRENGTH OINTMENT (Monarch)

Neomycin, Polymyxin B, and Hydrocortisone (nee oh *mye* sin, pol i *mix* in B, and hye dro *court* i sone)
CORTISPORIN EAR DROPS (OTIC) (Monarch)

FAMILY: Other Drugs for Bacterial Infection
           Topical Adrenal Steroids

The combination of the three antibiotics, neomycin, polymyxin B, and bacitracin is used to treat a wide variety of skin infections. It is also used to prevent infection in burns or broken skin. It is available as an aerosol spray, powder, and ointment.

There is no satisfactory evidence that antibiotics applied directly to wounds (as opposed to injected or swallowed) help healing or prevent infection. Uninfected, well-cleaned wounds usually heal by themselves. If a wound is infected and antibiotics are needed, they should be given by mouth or by injection.

Despite the controversy over external use of antibiotics, dermatologists (skin doctors) often prescribe this combination drug to treat some superficial skin infections, such as inflammation of hair follicles (folliculitis) and impetigo.

Neomycin commonly causes skin rashes in 8% of the people who use it.[74] Using neomycin can also make it hard for you to use other drugs in its family (aminoglycoside antibiotics, such as gentamicin and tobramycin, see p. 517) that may be needed later for serious infections.

Tuberculosis

Isoniazid (eye soe *nye* a zid)
INH

GENERIC: available
FAMILY: Other Drugs for Bacterial Infection

PREGNANCY WARNING

Isoniazid crossed the placental barrier and caused harm to developing fetuses in animal studies. Because of the potential for serious adverse effects to the fetus, this drug should not be used by pregnant women.

BREAST-FEEDING WARNING

Isoniazid is excreted in human milk. Because of the potential for serious adverse effects in nursing infants, you should not take this drug while nursing.

Isoniazid is used to treat and prevent tuberculosis (TB). If you are an older adult who has had a positive TB skin test, you do not necessarily need preventive treatment for TB. You should be treated only if you are at special risk, for example, if you have cancer, if you are taking high doses of corticosteroid drugs on a long-term basis, or if you had a negative TB skin test until recently. If you have sudden, serious liver disease, you should not get preventive TB treatment.

Isoniazid can cause serious damage to your liver. Some people who have taken this drug, especially people over age 50, have developed severe and even fatal hepatitis (a liver disease).

FDA BLACK BOX WARNING

Severe and sometimes fatal hepatitis associated with isoniazid therapy may occur and may develop even after many months of treatment. The risk of developing hepatitis is age related. Approximate case rates by age are: 0 per 1,000 for persons under 20 years of age, 3 per 1,000 for persons in the 20–34 year age group, 12 per 1,000 for persons in the 35–49 year age group, 23 per 1,000 for persons in the 50–64 year age group, and 8 per 1,000 for persons over 65 years of age. The risk of hepatitis is increased with daily consumption of alcohol. Precise data to provide a fatality rate for isoniazid-related hepatitis is not available; however, in a U.S. Public Health Service Surveillance Study of 13,838 persons taking isoniazid, there were 8 deaths among 174 cases of hepatitis.

Therefore, patients given isoniazid should be carefully monitored and interviewed at monthly intervals. Serum transaminase concentration becomes elevated in about 10–20% of patients, usually during the first few months of therapy, but it can occur at any time. Usually enzyme levels return to normal despite continuance of drug, but in some cases progressive liver dysfunction occurs. Patients should be instructed to report immediately any of the prodromal symptoms of hepatitis, such as fatigue, weakness, malaise, anorexia, nausea, or vomiting. If these symptoms appear or if signs suggestive of hepatic damage are detected, isoniazid should be discontinued promptly, since continued use of the drug in these cases has been reported to cause a more severe form of liver damage.

Patients with tuberculosis should be given appropriate treatment with alternative drugs. If isoniazid must be reinstituted, it should be reinstituted only after symptoms and laboratory abnormalities have cleared. The drug should be restarted in very small and gradually increasing doses and should be withdrawn immediately if there is any indication of recurrent liver involvement. Treatment should be deferred in persons with acute hepatic diseases.[88]

> ### WARNING
>
> If you have nausea, vomiting, yellow eyes, dark urine, unexplained fatigue, or abdominal pain, stop taking this medication and call your doctor immediately. These are symptoms of possible liver toxicity.

You are more likely to get hepatitis if you drink alcohol daily, so do not drink while taking this drug. Call your doctor immediately if you have any of the symptoms of hepatitis: fatigue, weakness, malaise (vague feeling of being unwell), loss of appetite, nausea, vomiting, or yellow eyes or skin. Schedule monthly visits with your doctor while taking this drug. If you have impaired liver function or severe kidney failure, you should probably be taking less than the usual adult dose of isoniazid.

A small number of people using isoniazid develop nerve pain and tenderness in their hands and feet. Taking 15 to 50 milligrams of vitamin B_6 every day can prevent this problem. If necessary, your doctor can give you a prescription for vitamin B_6 along with the isoniazid prescription.

Before You Use This Drug

Tell your doctor if you have or have had:

- pregnancy or are breast-feeding
- an unusual reaction to isoniazid, ethionamide, pyrazinamide, niacin, or other chemically related drugs
- liver problems
- alcohol dependence
- epilepsy or seizures
- severe kidney disease
- diabetes (drug can affect test results)

Tell your doctor about any other drugs you take, including aspirin, herbs, vitamins, and other nonprescription products.

When You Use This Drug

- Do not drink alcohol.
- You may need more vitamin B_6 and niacin than usual. Ask your doctor.
- If you plan to have any surgery, including dental, tell your doctor that you take this drug.
- Check with your doctor if you have flushing after eating cheese or fish.
- Have regular visits with your eye doctor if you have problems with vision.
- Check with your doctor immediately if you have loss of appetite, nausea or vomiting, or unusual tiredness or weakness.
- Check with your doctor if there is no improvement within two to three weeks.

How to Use This Drug

- If you miss a dose, take it as soon as you remember, but skip it if it is almost time for the next dose. **Do not take double doses.**
- Do not share your medication with others.
- Take the drug at the same time(s) each day.
- Take with food if gastrointestinal irritation occurs.
- If you take aluminum-containing antacids, take them at least one hour before or after you take your isoniazid.
- Take pyridoxine to prevent or minimize nerve problems
- Take this drug for the prescribed length of time, which may be six months to two years. If you stop too soon, your symptoms could come back.
- Store at room temperature with lid on tightly. Do not store in the bathroom. Do not expose to heat, moisture, or strong light. Keep out of reach of children.

Interactions with Other Drugs

The following drugs, biologics (e.g., vaccines, therapeutic antibodies), or foods are listed in *Evaluations of Drug Interactions* 2003 as causing "highly clinically significant" or "clinically

WARNING

There have been a number of case reports of liver damage involving a possible drug interaction between isoniazid, a medication used to prevent and treat tuberculosis, and acetaminophen, an over-the-counter painkiller and the active ingredient in Tylenol. Isoniazid alone, especially as people get older, has been documented to cause liver damage. Acetaminophen, alone in large doses or probably in combination with alcohol, also increases the risk of liver damage. The combination of acetaminophen with isoniazid, according to the authors of these case reports, may also be dangerous.

If you are taking isoniazid for tuberculosis or have a positive TB skin test and are using the drug, consult your physician before using acetaminophen or any combination product containing acetaminophen. Discuss alternatives to acetaminophen with your physician.

significant" interactions when used together with any of the drugs in this section. In some sections with multiple drugs, the interaction may have been reported for one but not all drugs in this section, but we include the interaction because the drugs in this section are similar to one another. We have also included potentially serious interactions listed in the drug's FDA-approved professional package insert or in published medical journal articles. There may be other drugs, especially those in the families of drugs listed below, that also will react with this drug to cause severe adverse effects. Make sure to tell your doctor and pharmacist the drugs you are taking and tell them if you are taking any of these interacting drugs:

carbamazepine, DILANTIN, GLU-COPHAGE, GLUCOVANCE, itraconazole, METAGLIP, metformin, phenytoin, RIFADIN, rifampin, RIMACTANE, SPORANOX, TEGRETOL.

The following acetaminophen-containing drugs should not be taken with isoniazid (see warning box): acetaminophen, ESGIC, FIORICET, PERCOCET, TYLENOL, TYLENOL NO. 3, TYLOX, VICODIN.

Adverse Effects

Call your doctor immediately if you experience:

- numbness, tingling, pain, or weakness in hands or feet
- clumsiness or unsteadiness
- dark urine
- yellow eyes or skin
- loss of appetite
- light-colored stools
- headache
- pain in stomach or abdomen
- unexplained fatigue
- nausea or vomiting
- abnormal tiredness or weakness
- blurred or changed vision
- seizures
- fever or sore throat
- joint pain
- depression, mood, or other mental changes
- skin rash
- **Caution diabetics:** Isoniazide may increase blood sugar.
- unusual bleeding or bruising

Call your doctor if these symptoms continue:

- nausea or vomiting
- diarrhea
- stomach pain

Signs of overdose:

- severe nausea or vomiting
- dizziness
- slurred speech
- unusual tiredness or weakness
- seizures

- confusion
- coma

If you suspect an overdose, call this number to contact your poison control center: (800) 222-1222.

Periodic Tests

Ask your doctor which of these tests should be done periodically while you are taking this drug:

- liver function tests, before treatment and regularly thereafter (during nine months of treatment, you should have them at the end of months one, three, six, and nine)
- ophthalmologic exams

Rifampin (rif *am* pin)
RIMACTANE (Sandoz)
RIFADIN (Aventis)

GENERIC: not available

FAMILY: Drugs for Tuberculosis

PREGNANCY WARNING

Rifampin caused harm to developing fetuses in animal studies including cleft palate, spina bifida, brittle bones, and death. When taken during the last few weeks of pregnancy, rifampin can cause hemorrhaging in both the mother and infant. Because of the potential for serious adverse effects, this drug should not be used by pregnant women.

BREAST-FEEDING WARNING

No information is available from either human or animal studies. Since it is likely that this drug, like many others, is excreted in human milk, and because rifampin caused tumors in animals, you should not take this drug while nursing.

Rifampin is used together with other drugs to treat tuberculosis (TB). Rifampin and isoniazid are the most effective drugs to fight TB.[89]

If you test positive for TB in a skin test but do not have a confirmed case of the disease, and your doctor decides you need preventive treat-

ment, your treatment will probably be isoniazid (see p. 735) alone. If you are carrying a type of bacteria called meningitis but you have no symptoms, you may be prescribed a short course of rifampin alone.

Some people have developed severe and even fatal liver disease while taking rifampin. You increase your risk of liver disease if you drink alcohol daily, so do not drink while taking this drug. Call your doctor immediately if you have any symptoms of liver disease: fatigue, weakness, malaise (vague feeling of being unwell), loss of appetite, nausea, vomiting, or yellow eyes or skin. If you have impaired liver function, you will probably need to take less than the usual adult dose of rifampin.

Before You Use This Drug

Tell your doctor if you have or have had:

- pregnancy or are breast-feeding
- unusual reaction to rifampin
- alcohol dependence
- liver problems

Tell your doctor about any other drugs you take, including aspirin, herbs, vitamins, and other nonprescription products.

When You Use This Drug

- Do not drink alcohol.
- If you plan to have any surgery, including dental, tell your doctor that you take this drug.
- Check with your doctor if there is no improvement within two to three weeks.
- Check with your doctor immediately if you have loss of appetite, nausea or vomiting, or unusual tiredness or weakness.
- Check with your doctor or dentist about proper oral hygiene.
- Rifampin causes urine, feces, saliva, spit, sweat, and tears to turn reddish-orange to reddish-brown. It may permanently discolor soft

contact lenses. You do not need to call your doctor about this effect.

• Use an alternative method of contraception if taking estrogen-containing oral contraceptives.

How to Use This Drug

• If you miss a dose, take it as soon as you remember, but skip it if it is almost time for the next dose. **Do not take double doses.**
• Do not share your medication with others.
• Take the drug at the same time(s) each day.
• Take this drug for the prescribed length of time, which may be months or years. If you stop too soon, your symptoms could come back.
• Take with **a full glass (eight ounces) of water.** Take with or without food.
• Store at room temperature with lid on tightly. Do not store in the bathroom. Do not expose to heat, moisture, or strong light. Keep out of reach of children.

Interactions with Other Drugs

The following drugs, biologics (e.g., vaccines, therapeutic antibodies), or foods are listed in *Evaluations of Drug Interactions* 2003 as causing "highly clinically significant" or "clinically significant" interactions when used together with any of the drugs in this section. In some sections with multiple drugs, the interaction may have been reported for one but not all drugs in this section, but we include the interaction because the drugs in this section are similar to one another. We have also included potentially serious interactions listed in the drug's FDA-approved professional package insert or in published medical journal articles. There may be other drugs, especially those in the families of drugs listed below, that also will react with this drug to cause severe adverse effects. Make sure to tell your doctor and pharmacist the drugs you are taking and tell them if you are taking any of these interacting drugs:

AGENERASE, AMBIEN, amiodarone, amprenavir, ANZEMET, CALAN SR, CATAPRES, chloramphenicol, CHLOROMYCETIN, clonidine, clozapine, CLOZARIL, CORDARONE, COUMADIN, COVERA-HS, COZAAR, CRIXIVAN, CRYSTODIGIN, cyclosporine, delavirdine, digitoxin, digoxin, DILANTIN, dolasetron, DOLOPHINE, DURAQUIN, ELIXOPHYLLIN, FLUOTHANE, FORTOVASE, HALDOL, haloperidol, halothane, indinavir, INH, INVIRASE, isoniazid, ISOPTIN SR, ketoconazole, LANOXICAPS, LANOXIN, LOPRESSOR, losartan, methadone, METHADOSE, metoprolol, METRETON, nelfinavir, NEORAL, nevirapine, NIZORAL, NORVIR, oral contraceptives, phenytoin, PRANDIN, PRED FORTE, prednisolone, PROGRAF, pyrazinamide, QUINAGLUTE DURA-TABS, QUINIDEX, quinidine, RAPAMUNE, repaglinide, RESCRIPTOR, ritonavir, RETROVIR, RIFATER, RIFAMATE, rofecoxib, SANDIMMUNE, saquinavir, sildenafil, sirolimus, SLO-BID, tacrolimus, THEO-24, theophylline, TOPROL XL, verapamil, VERELAN, VIAGRA, VIOXX, VIRACEPT, VIRAMUNE, warfarin, zidovudine (AZT), zolpidem.

Adverse Effects

Call your doctor immediately if you experience:

• fever
• chills
• trouble breathing
• dizziness
• headache
• muscle or joint aches
• shivering
• skin rash
• itching
• confusion or inability to concentrate
• loss of appetite

- nausea or vomiting
- abnormal tiredness or weakness
- bloody or cloudy urine
- noticeable decrease in frequency of urination or amount of urine
- sore throat
- abnormal bruising or bleeding
- yellow eyes or skin

Call your doctor if these symptoms continue:

- diarrhea
- stomach cramps
- sore mouth or tongue
- blurred or changed vision

Signs of overdose:

- reddish color of skin, mouth, or eyes
- swelling around the eyes or face
- itching over whole body
- mental changes

If you suspect an overdose, call this number to contact your poison control center: (800) 222-1222.

Periodic Tests

Ask your doctor which of these tests should be done periodically while you are taking this drug:

- liver function tests

━━━━━━━━

Fungal Infection

Clotrimazole (kloe *trim* a zole)
MYCELEX (Bayer)
LOTRIMIN (Schering Plough)
GYNE-LOTRIMIN (Schering Plough)

Miconazole (my *kon* a zole)
MONISTAT-DERM (Johnson & Johnson)
MONISTAT 7 (Advanced Care Products)

MONISTAT 3 (Advanced Care Products)
MONISTAT 1 (Personal Products)

Nystatin (nye *sta* tin)
MYCOSTATIN (Bristol-Myers Squibb)

GENERIC: available
FAMILY: Drugs for Fungal Infections

PREGNANCY WARNING

There was no evidence of toxicity in animal studies using dermal application. Use during pregnancy only for clear medical reasons. Tell your doctor if you are pregnant or thinking of becoming pregnant before you take this drug.

BREAST-FEEDING WARNING

No information is available from either human or animal studies. Since it is likely that this drug, like many others, is excreted in human milk, you should consult with your doctor if you are planning to nurse.

These drugs are used to treat yeast or fungal infections in various parts of the body. For skin infections, you may be given a cream, lotion, or liquid to apply externally; for vaginal infections, vaginal cream or tablets placed in the vagina; and for mouth and throat infections, lozenges placed in the mouth.

Mild vaginal infections are often self-limiting.[90] For some women, a bland cream (without drugs) relieves symptoms until infection spontaneously goes away.[91] Preventive measures include less sugar in the diet, and avoiding tight-fitting pants and panty hose. Cotton is preferable to synthetics.[92] Dry the vaginal area thoroughly after bathing or swimming.

Before You Use This Drug

Tell your doctor if you have or have had:

- pregnancy or are breast-feeding
- allergies to drugs
- unusual reaction to clotrimazole, miconazole, or nystatin

Tell your doctor about any other drugs you take, including aspirin, herbs, vitamins, and other nonprescription products.

When You Use This Drug

• If you plan to have any surgery, including dental, tell your doctor that you take this drug.

• Call your doctor if your symptoms do not improve in three days.

• For vaginal use, protect clothing by wearing a sanitary napkin, cotton panties, and only freshly washed underclothes.

• Avoid use of latex products (condoms, diaphragms), which can be damaged by the oils in the drug during treatment and for three days afterward.

• Check with your doctor before douching between doses.

• Apply enough to cover the affected skin and the surrounding area and rub in gently.

• Do not use an airtight bandage unless your doctor recommends it.

• Avoid getting this drug in your eyes.

How to Use This Drug

• If you miss a dose, take it as soon as you remember, but skip the dose if it is almost time for the next dose. **Do not take double doses.**

• Do not share your medication with others.

• Take the drug at the same time(s) each day.

• Take this drug for the prescribed length of time, even if menstruation occurs (for vaginal use). If you stop too soon, your symptoms could come back.

• Store at room temperature with cap on tightly. Do not store in the bathroom. Do not expose to heat, moisture or strong light. Keep out of reach of children.

Interactions with Other Drugs

Some other drugs that you may be taking (either over-the-counter or prescription drugs) can interact with this one, causing adverse effects. Ask your doctor what these drugs are and let him or her know if you are taking any of them.

When using topical products it is advisable not to apply other topical preparations, including cosmetics, to the same site. This prevents interactions that could irritate your skin.

Adverse Effects

Call your doctor immediately if you experience:

• vaginal burning, itching, discharge, or other irritation not present before therapy
• skin rash or hives

Call your doctor if these symptoms continue:

• abdominal or stomach cramps
• burning or irritation of penis of sexual partner
• headache

Fluconazole (flew *kon* a zole)
DIFLUCAN (Pfizer)

GENERIC: not available
FAMILY: Drugs for Fungal Infections

PREGNANCY WARNING

Fluconazole has caused harm to developing fetuses in animal studies, including bone abnormalities of the skull. There have been reports of multiple congenital abnormalities in children born to mothers taking fluconazole. Because of the potential for serious adverse effects to the fetus, this drug should not be used by pregnant women.

BREAST-FEEDING WARNING

Fluconazole is excreted in human milk. Because of the potential for adverse effects in nursing infants, you should not take this drug while nursing.

Fluconazole is used to treat severe fungal infections, such as meningitis and infections of the mouth or esophagus such as candidia.[94,95] Often these infections occur when another condition, such as cancer, organ transplant, or HIV infection, reduces your immunity to infections. The drug should not be used to treat trivial fungal skin infections.

WARNINGS

---

(1) Hepatic [liver] injury: DIFLUCAN has been associated with rare cases of serious hepatic toxicity, including fatalities primarily in patients with serious underlying medical conditions. In cases of DIFLUCAN-associated hepatotoxicity [liver toxicity], no obvious relationship to total daily dose, duration of therapy, sex or age of the patient has been observed. DIFLUCAN hepatotoxicity has usually, but not always, been reversible on discontinuation of therapy. Patients who develop abnormal liver function tests during DIFLUCAN therapy should be monitored for the development of more severe hepatic injury. DIFLUCAN should be discontinued if clinical signs and symptoms consistent with liver disease develop that may be attributable to DIFLUCAN.

(2) Anaphylaxis [severe allergic reaction]: In rare cases, anaphylaxis has been reported.

(3) Dermatologic [skin] : Patients have rarely developed exfoliative skin disorders during treatment with DIFLUCAN. In patients with serious underlying diseases (predominantly AIDS and malignancy), these have rarely resulted in a fatal outcome. Patients who develop rashes during treatment with DIFLUCAN should be monitored closely and the drug discontinued if lesions progress.[93]

Fluconazole is also approved by the FDA to treat vaginal yeast infections (vaginal candidiasis) in a single dose of 150 milligrams.[93]

Before You Use This Drug

Do not use if you have or have had:

- allergy to azole antifungals
- congestive heart failure

Tell your doctor if you have or have had:

- pregnancy or are breast-feeding
- lack of stomach acid

- kidney or liver problems
- alcohol abuse

Tell your doctor about any other drugs you take, including aspirin, herbs, vitamins, and other nonprescription products.

When You Use This Drug

- If you plan to have any surgery, including dental, tell your doctor that you take this drug.
- Check with your doctor if there is no improvement within a few days.

How to Use This Drug

- If you miss a dose, take it as soon as you remember, but skip it if it is almost time for the next dose. **Do not take double doses.**
- Do not share your medication with others.
- Take the drug at the same time(s) each day.
- Take this drug for the prescribed length of time. If you stop too soon, your symptoms could come back.
- Take with or without food.
- Store at room temperature with lid on tightly. Do not store in the bathroom. Do not expose to heat, moisture, or strong light. Keep out of reach of children.

Interactions with Other Drugs

The following drugs, biologics (e.g., vaccines, therapeutic antibodies), or foods are listed in *Evaluations of Drug Interactions* 2003 as causing "highly clinically significant" or "clinically significant" interactions when used together with any of the drugs in this section. In some sections with multiple drugs, the interaction may have been reported for one but not all drugs in this section, but we include the interaction because the drugs in this section are similar to one another. We have also included potentially serious interactions listed in the drug's FDA-approved professional package insert or in published medical journal articles. There may be other drugs, especially those in the families of drugs listed below, that also will react with this drug to cause severe adverse effects. Make sure to tell your doctor and pharmacist the drugs you are taking and tell them if you are taking any of these interacting drugs:

amitriptyline, CELEBREX, celecoxib, cilostazol, COUMADIN, cyclosporine, DECADRON, DETROL, dexamethasone, DILANTIN, DURAQUIN, ELAVIL, glipizide, GLUCOTROL, HEXADROL, lovastatin, MEVACOR, mizolastine, NEORAL, phenytoin, PLETAL, PRIFTIN, PROGRAF, QUINAGLUTE DURA-TABS, QUINIDEX, quinidine, RETROVIR, RIFADIN, rifampin, rifapentine, RIMACTANE, SANDIMMUNE, simvastatin, tacrolimus, tolterodine, warfarin, zidovudine, ZOCOR.

Adverse Effects

Call your doctor immediately if you experience:

- unusual bleeding or bruising
- stomach pain
- fever and chills
- sore throat
- skin rash
- yellowing of eyes or skin
- reddened, blistering, itching, or peeling skin or mucous membranes
- dark or amber-colored urine
- loss of appetite
- pale stools
- unusual tiredness or weakness

Call your doctor if these symptoms continue:

- abdominal pain
- dizziness
- drowsiness

- fatigue
- headache
- nausea or vomiting
- diarrhea
- constipation
- loss of appetite
- decreased sexual ability
- menstrual irregularities
- increased sensitivity of eyes to light
- enlarged breasts in men

Periodic Tests

Ask your doctor which of these tests should be done periodically while you are taking this drug:

- blood creatinine levels
- blood urea nitrogen (BUN)
- liver function tests
- potassium levels

 Do Not Use

ALTERNATIVE TREATMENT: *See Clotrimazole, p. 740, and Betamethasone, p. 669.*

Betamethasone and Clotrimazole
(bay ta *meth* a sone and kloe *trim* a zole)
LOTRISONE CREAM (Schering)

FAMILY: Drugs for Fungal Infections
Topical Adrenal Steroids

FDA BLACK BOX WARNING

FOR TOPICAL USE ONLY, NOT FOR OPHTHALMIC, ORAL, OR FOR INTRAVAGINAL USE, NOT RECOMMENDED FOR PATIENTS UNDER THE AGE OF 17 YEARS AND NOT RECOMMENDED FOR DIAPER DERMATITIS.[96]

The FDA's Dermatologic and Ophthalmic Drugs Advisory Committee met on June 29, 2000, to discuss, among other issues, the safety labeling for Lotrisone, which contains the potent steroid betamethasone and clotrimazole, an antifungal agent. The committee recommended that a prominent warning should be added to the tube and box of the product to inform parents that Lotrisone should not be used in children under 12 or for the treatment of diaper rash.

This combination drug is approved by the FDA for the topical treatment of athlete's foot, ringworm of the scalp and body, and jock itch due to several different types of fungi. Its approved use is for periods of two to four weeks, depending on the type of infection. Lotrisone's professional product labeling states: "Effective treatment without the risks associated with topical corticosteroid [betamethasone] use may be obtained using a topical antifungal agent [such as clotrimazole] that does not contain a corticosteroid, especially for noninflammatory tinea infections."[96]

The drug was first cleared for sale in July 1984 and in 2000 5.4 million prescriptions were dispensed for Lotrisone, ranking it as the 76th most frequently prescribed drug in the United States. The advent of the new warning recommended by the advisory committee has caused the drug to dip to 140th place with 2.8 million prescriptions in 2001. Lotrisone has since fallen off the list of the most frequently prescribed drugs in the United States.

The basis for the advisory committee's recommendation was that the safety and efficacy of Lotrisone had not been proven for children under 12 or for diaper rash. Several of the advisory committee members noted that many doctors are not aware that betamethasone is a potent steroid that can cause serious and permanent adverse effects in children because it is readily absorbed through the skin.

In preparation for the June 2000 meeting, the FDA's Office of Postmarketing Drug Risk Assessment was asked to provide an analysis of all adverse drug reactions reported to the agency since the drug was first marketed. The agency had received 344 reports of adverse events due to Lotrisone by the time of the committee meeting, many of which reported more than one event, leading to a total of 761 reactions. It must always be kept in mind that the FDA believes that only about 1 in 10 adverse reactions is reported. The three most common adverse reactions reported were that Lotrisone was not effective (19%), skin reactions (10%), and aggravation of the original condition for which the drug was prescribed (8.5%).[97]

The original professional product labeling or package insert for Lotrisone stated that the drug had not been shown to be safe and effective in children less than 12 years old.[98] The drug was relabeled in 1991 to say: "The use of LOTRISONE Cream in diaper dermatitis [diaper rash] is not recommended."[99] Despite these facts, using data from a market research firm, the FDA estimated that between 1992 and 1997 approximately 20% of all Lotrisone prescriptions were for children under 12 years of age and 7.2% of these were for children 1 year old or younger. When a drug is prescribed for a use that is not approved, or in an age group in which the drug has not been tested, this is termed an "off-label" use. This type of use can present significant safety problems, since there is, by definition, a lack of evidence that the benefits outweigh the risks.

In children one year old or younger, Lotrisone was most commonly prescribed for the treatment of a yeastlike fungus (candidiasis) of the skin and nails that accounted for 37.7% of its use. Diaper rash accounted for 29.3% of its use, and fungal infections of the body, head, or groin, 8.6% of prescriptions in this age group. All of these uses are off-label.

A serious adverse reaction, growth retardation, was seen in a 1-year-old child treated for diaper rash for 27 weeks. There were 12 adverse reaction reports in children 2 to 6 years old and 19 in the 7 to 12 age group.

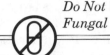

Do Not Use (Except for Serious Fungal Infection)

ALTERNATIVE TREATMENT:
Nail fungus is a cosmetic, not a medical, problem; no treatment recommended.

Itraconazole (i tra'*koe* na zole)
SPORANOX (Janssen)

Terbinafine (ter *bin* a feen)
LAMISIL (Novartis)

FAMILY: Drugs for Fungal Infections

The FDA issued a public health advisory on May 9, 2001, about itraconazole and terbinafine when used to treat nail fungus (onychomycosis). Itraconazole had been associated with the development of congestive heart failure and liver toxicity. Liver toxicity had also been seen with terbinafine.[100]

Itraconazole was first approved to treat serious fungal infections in people with compromised immune systems, such as AIDS patients, and terbinafine was previously available only for topical use. Both drugs are now being heavily promoted directly to consumers for the treatment of toenail fungus, with or without involvement of the fingernails. Fungal infections of the nails are generally resistant to topical treatment.

Itraconazole

The FDA reviewed 94 cases through April 2001 in which itraconazole-treated patients developed congestive heart failure. In 58 of the 94 cases, the FDA believes that itraconazole contributed to or may have been the cause of the congestive heart failure. Death was reported in 13 cases. The FDA also examined 24 cases of liver failure possibly associated with the use of itraconazole, including 11 deaths.[100]

FDA staff, writing in the medical journal *The*

FDA BLACK BOX WARNING

CONGESTIVE HEART FAILURE

SPORANOX (itraconazole) Capsules should not be administered for the treatment of onychomycosis [nail fungus] in patients with evidence of ventricular dysfunction such as congestive heart failure (CHF) or a history of CHF. If signs or symptoms of congestive heart failure occur during administration of SPORANOX Capsules, discontinue administration. When itraconazole was administered intravenously to dogs and healthy human volunteers, negative inotropic [strength of the heart's contraction] effects were seen.

Drug Interactions: Coadministration of pimozide, quinidine, dofetilide, or levacetylmethadol (levomethadyl) with SPORANOX® (itraconazole) Capsules, Injection or Oral Solution is contraindicated. SPORANOX, a potent cytochrome P450 3A4 isoenzyme system (CYP3A4) inhibitor, may increase plasma concentrations of drugs metabolized by this pathway. Serious cardiovascular events, including QT prolongation, torsades de pointes, ventricular tachycardia, cardiac arrest, and/or sudden death have occurred in patients using pimozide, levacetylmethadol (levomethadyl), or quinidine concomitantly with SPORANOX and/or other CYP3A4 inhibitors.

Lancet, more completely described the 58 potential cases of congestive heart failure associated with itraconazole. The median age was 57 years, the youngest was 15 years old, 65% were female, and 50% were receiving itraconazole for fungal nail infection. Information on the onset of symptoms of congestive heart failure was available for 42 patients. Of these patients, the median onset of symptoms was 10 days after starting the drug and ranged from 1 to 210 days.[101]

Terbinafine

Through April 2001, the FDA had reviewed 16 possible terbinafine-associated cases of liver failure, including 11 deaths and two patients who underwent liver transplants.[100]

The professional product labeling or package insert now carries the following warning about liver failure: "Rare cases of liver failure, some leading to death or liver transplant, have occurred with use of LAMISIL (terbinafine hydrochloride tablets) Tablets for the treatment of onychomycosis in individuals with and without pre-existing liver disease."[102]

Other serious adverse effects have been reported with terbinafine. These include liver and bone marrow toxicity, and changes in the lens and retina of the eye.[103] The relapse of toenail fungus with terbinafine is reported to be about 15%.[104]

The editors of *The Medical Letter on Drugs and Therapeutics,* the internationally respected, independent source of drug information written for doctors and pharmacists, said: "The advisability of taking either of these expensive drugs [itraconazole or terbinafine] for months to treat an infection that is mainly cosmetic and may relapse is unclear."[103] Our warning to consumers is stronger: using these drugs for a cosmetic condition is risky.

fection called candidiasis. However, one of its ingredients, triamcinolone, may actually be dangerous to an infection because drugs in its family can hide the signs of an infection or make it spread. Therefore, this drug product is an irrational combination for treating an infection. Instead, your doctor should prescribe nystatin alone.

If you have a fungal skin infection that is inflamed, itching, or scaly, it may be appropriate to use hydrocortisone (see p. 669) in addition to an antifungal ointment such as nystatin for a few days. Each drug should be applied separately in a ratio determined by your doctor.

This drug, sold under the brand name Mycolog II, also has an older form called Mycolog cream. Mycolog cream is a combination of neomycin and gramicidin, and it should not be used either. Neomycin commonly causes skin rashes in 8% of the people who use it.[74] Using neomycin can also make it hard for you to use other drugs in its family (aminoglycoside antibiotics, such as gentamicin and tobramycin, see p. 617) that may be needed later for serious infections.[74]

Ⓧ *Do Not Use*

ALTERNATIVE TREATMENT:
See Clotrimazole, p. 740, and Miconazole, p. 740.

Terconazole (tir *kone* a zole)
TERAZOL 3 VAGINAL CREAM OR SUPPOSITORIES (Ortho-McNeil)
TERAZOL 7 VAGINAL CREAM (Ortho-McNeil)

FAMILY: Drugs for Fungal Infections

Terconazole is used to treat vaginal fungal infections. It is equally as effective as some other antifungal creams (for example clotrimazole and miconazole), but it is absorbed into the body much more than these drugs and can cause flu-like symptoms of headache, chills, fever, and a drop in blood pressure.[105,106]

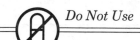

Ⓧ *Do Not Use*

ALTERNATIVE TREATMENT:
Separate antifungal and corticosteroid ointments or creams.

Nystatin and Triamcinolone
(nye *sta* tin and trye am *sin* oh lone)
MYCOLOG II (Apothecon)

FAMILY: Drugs for Fungal Infections
           Topical Adrenal Steroids

This combination of nystatin (see p. 740) and triamcinolone (see pp. 379 and 669) is commonly prescribed by dermatologists (skin doctors) to treat fungal skin infections, such as the yeast in-

Following vaginal administration of terconazole, absorption ranged from 5 to 8% in three hysterectomized subjects and from 12% to 16% in two non-hysterectomized patients with tubal ligations.[107]

If you are using this drug, or if your doctor recommends it, ask your doctor to change your prescription.

Mild vaginal infections are often self-limiting.[90] For some women a bland cream (without drugs) relieves symptoms until infection spontaneously goes away.[91] Preventive measures include less sugar in the diet and avoiding tight-fitting pants and panty hose. Cotton is preferable to synthetics.[92] Dry the vaginal area thoroughly after bathing or swimming.

Parasitic Infection

Mebendazole (meb en dah zoll)
VERMOX (McNeil)

GENERIC: not available

FAMILY: Drugs for Parasitic Infections

PREGNANCY WARNING

Mebendazole caused malformations and death in developing fetuses in animal studies. Because of the potential for serious adverse effects to the fetus, this drug should not be used by pregnant women.

BREAST-FEEDING WARNING

No information is available from either human or animal studies. However, it is likely that this drug, like many others, is excreted in human milk. If you need to take mebendazole for several weeks, as opposed to a few days, you should consult with your doctor if you are planning to nurse.

Mebendazole is approved by the FDA for treatment of pinworm, whipworm, roundworm, and hookworm.[108] The independent source of drug information for health professionals, *The Medical Letter on Drugs and Therapeutics,* lists mebendazole as the drug of choice for pinworm, whipworm, roundworm, and hookworm.[109]

It is very important that these conditions be treated, since if worms escape from the intestines, they can be quite disturbing under the skin, and dangerous in the heart, mouth, liver, or joints.[110,111] Masses of roundworms have blocked the intestines or bile duct during therapy.[112] In high doses mebendazole has suppressed the bone marrow. Mebendazole is not approved in the United States for tapeworm or hydatid diseases. Effectiveness of mebendazole depends on whether the infestation is minor or severe, how long it takes worms to pass through your digestive tract, whether or not you have diarrhea, and the susceptibility of the worms. It may take a few days for the body to expel dead forms in the stool.

Length of therapy varies from three days to several months, according to the type and number of parasites. At times treatment needs to be repeated at least once. In severe infections, use of mebendazole may prevent the need for a blood transfusion or surgery. Compared to some other pinworm medicine, mebendazole has an advantage of not staining clothing or bedding.

You may be more susceptible to parasites if you take immunosuppressant drugs or corticosteroids.[111] Several measures can prevent infestation. Wear shoes. Do not go barefoot where human or animal feces may be on the ground, including beaches, children's sandboxes, and fertilized gardens. Wash fruits and vegetables thoroughly. Eat meat that is completely cooked. Wash your hands before preparing food, eating, and after going to the toilet. Use sanitary conditions to dispose of human feces. Be cautious when traveling to areas with dense shade, high humidity, and sandy soil, coupled with poor sanitation.

Before You Use This Drug

Tell your doctor if you have or have had:

- pregnancy or are breast-feeding:
- allergies to drugs
- Crohn's disease

- inflammatory bowel disease
- liver disease
- ulcerative colitis

Tell your doctor of activities, places, or work that may have exposed you to parasites, especially if you have:

- lived or traveled in tropical or subtropical areas, especially the southeastern United States, the Caribbean, Central and South America, the Philippines, Africa, Thailand, Vietnam, Burma, Turkey, and Eastern Europe
- worked in agriculture, mining, plumbing, tunneling, or with foreign missions, immigrants, refugees, or foreign visitors
- been duck hunting

Tell your doctor about any other drugs you take, including aspirin, herbs, vitamins, and other nonprescription products.

When You Use This Drug

- If you plan to have any surgery, including dental, tell your doctor that you take this drug.
- Check with your doctor if there is no improvement within a few days.
- Have regular visits with your doctor to check on progress.
- Check with your doctor as to whether you need iron supplements (for hookworms or whipworms).
- After treatment, wash all bedding and nightclothes thoroughly to prevent reinfection.

How to Use This Drug

- If you miss a dose, take it as soon as you remember, but skip it if it is almost time for the next dose. **Do not take double doses.**
- Do not share your medication with others.
- Take the drug at the same time(s) each day.
- Take with or without food. Check with your doctor to see whether you should take with a high-fat meal.

- This medication can be broken, chewed, or crushed.
- Capsules may be opened and the contents mixed with applesauce, jelly, or ketchup, then swallowed.
- If on high-dose therapy, take with a fatty meal.
- Take this drug for the prescribed length of time. If you stop too soon, your symptoms could come back.
- Treat all household members at the same time (pinworms).
- Store at room temperature with lid on tightly. Do not store in the bathroom. Do not expose to heat, moisture, or strong light. Keep out of reach of children.

Interactions with Other Drugs

Evaluations of Drug Interactions 2003 lists no drugs, biologics (e.g., vaccines, therapeutic antibodies), or foods as causing "highly clinically significant" or "clinically significant" interactions when used together with the drugs in this section. We also found no interactions in the drugs' FDA-approved professional package inserts. However, as the number of new drugs approved for marketing increases and as more experience is gained with these drugs over time, new interactions may be discovered.

Adverse Effects

Call your doctor immediately if you experience:

- fever
- skin rash or itching
- sore throat
- unusual tiredness or weakness

Call your doctor if these symptoms continue:

- abdominal pain or upset
- diarrhea
- dizziness

- hair loss
- headache
- nausea or vomiting

Periodic Tests

Ask your doctor which of these tests should be done periodically while you are taking this drug:

- complete blood count (if on high-dose therapy)
- perianal exam (for pinworms)
- stool exam

 Do Not Use

ALTERNATIVE TREATMENT:
Nonprescription Permethrin (NIX).

Lindane (*lynn* dane) (gamma benzene hexachloride)

FAMILY: Drugs for Parasitic Infection

Lindane shampoo is available to treat head lice, while lindane cream and lotion are available to treat scabies. Outbreaks of head lice are commonplace in day care centers, schools, and nursing homes. Scabies is epidemic in nursing homes, homeless shelters, and among people with AIDS.

Treatment of lice or scabies with lindane is neither safe nor effective. Lindane is a pesticide of the organochlorine type, in the same group as DDT. Although the Environmental Protection Agency drastically cut the amount of lindane used in industry and agriculture, this toxin is still available. Workers exposed to lindane for a long time may eventually develop damage to their bone marrow, kidneys, liver, or reproductive organs.[113] Lindane is classified as a carcinogen. Even individuals who use lindane briefly

---

FDA BLACK BOX WARNINGS

Lindane Lotion [shampoo] should only be used in patients who cannot tolerate or have failed first-line treatment with safer medications for the treatment of scabies [lice]. (See INDICATIONS AND USAGE.)

NEUROLOGIC TOXICITY

Seizures and deaths have been reported following Lindane Lotion [shampoo] use with repeat or prolonged application, but also in rare cases following a single application used according to directions. Lindane Lotion [shampoo] should be used with caution for infants, children, the elderly, and individuals with other skin conditions (e.g, atopic dermatitis, psoriasis) and in those who weigh < 110 lbs (50 kg) as they may be at risk of serious neurotoxicity.

CONTRAINDICATIONS

Lindane Lotion [shampoo] is contraindicated in premature infants and individuals with known uncontrolled seizure disorders.

PROPER USE

Instruct patients on the proper use of Lindane Lotion [shampoo], the amount to apply, how long to leave it on, and avoiding re-treatment. Inform patients that itching occurs after the successful killing of scabies [lice] and is not necessarily an indication for re-treatment with Lindane Lotion [shampoo].

---

for lice or scabies, as well as people whose work exposes them to lindane, can experience rashes, dizziness, or convulsions. Vomiting, muscle cramps, nervousness, unsteadiness, and fast heartbeat have also been reported.

Lindane is readily absorbed through the skin, particularly skin that is broken or has residues of oils on it. Crusts formed in Norwegian scabies increase absorption of lindane even more.[114] The Centers for Disease Control and Prevention recommends that bathing prior to applying lindane lotion be avoided, since toxicity is increased.[115] Lindane is contraindicated for premature infants. Children and the elderly are particularly prone to convulsions from lindane.[115] A further tragedy associated with lindane is misuse in infants and children. Lindane has been left on the skin 12 hours or longer without being washed off.[116] Such misuse has been fatal to some children.

A review of clinical tests of head lice products found that in the few well-designed studies, lindane proved so ineffective that continued use could not be justified.[117] While no pediculicide is 100% effective, failure was at least eight times more likely with lindane than with permethrin (NIX). Lack of effectiveness encourages repeat applications. Prolonged use of lindane has lowered production of red blood cells. Concern also exists because some mites are now resistant to lindane; lice are suspected of developing resistance to lindane, as well as to alternative medications.

In 1995 Public Citizen filed a petition with the FDA to ban lindane.[116] The FDA later strengthened the safety labeling requirements for lindane.

In March 2003, the FDA issued a public health advisory about lindane.[118] The agency announced that a black-box warning would be required on the professional product labeling of the drug. A black-box warning is the strongest type of warning that the FDA can require on a drug's professional labeling. Also, pharmacists would be required to distribute a medication guide, written specifically for patients, with each lindane prescription. At this time, only drugs that pose serious public health concerns are required to be dispensed with a medication guide.

Viral Infection

Acyclovir (ay *sye* kloe veer)
ZOVIRAX (GlaxoSmithKline)

Valacyclovir (val ay *sye* kloe veer)
VALTREX (GlaxoSmithKline)

GENERIC: not available
FAMILY: Drugs for Viral Infections

PREGNANCY WARNING

No valid data are available for these drugs, as they were not tested adequately in animal studies. Use during pregnancy only for clear medical reasons. Tell your doctor if you are pregnant or thinking of becoming pregnant before you take these drugs.

BREAST-FEEDING WARNING

Acyclovir is excreted at very high levels in human milk; no data exists for valacyclovir, but it is probably similar to acyclovir. Because of the potential for serious adverse effects in nursing infants, you should not take these drugs while nursing.

After oral administration, valacyclovir is rapidly broken down to acyclovir in the intestine and liver.[119] Oral acyclovir is approved by the FDA for shingles (herpes zoster), genital herpes, and chicken pox.[120] The ointment form of acyclovir is approved for the initial management of genital herpes and in limited non-life-threatening herpes infection of the mucous membranes in patients with problems with their immune systems.[121] Acyclovir cream is approved by the FDA for cold sores. The duration of cold sores was reduced on average by only one-half day.[122]

Oral valacyclovir is FDA-approved for shingles, genital herpes, and the treatment of cold sores.[119] The editors of *The Medical Letter,* a respected independent source of drug information for health professionals, found that valacyclovir only "modestly" shortened the duration of a cold sore by about one day.[123]

Before You Use This Drug

Tell your doctor if you have or have had:

- pregnancy or are breast-feeding
- allergies to acyclovir or valacyclovir
- nerve disease
- dehydration
- bone marrow transplant
- kidney transplant
- HIV
- kidney or liver disease

Tell your doctor about any other drugs you take, including aspirin, herbs, vitamins, and other nonprescription products.

When You Use This Drug

- If you plan to have any surgery, including dental, tell your doctor that you take this drug.
- Check with your doctor if there is no improvement within a few days.
- Keep affected areas clean and dry; wear loose clothing.
- Use of a condom may help to prevent transmission of herpes.

How to Use This Drug

- If you miss a dose, take it as soon as you remember, but skip it if it is almost time for the next dose. **Do not take double doses.**
- Do not share your medication with others.
- Take the drug at the same time(s) each day.
- Take with **a full glass (eight ounces) of water.**
- Take with or without food.
- Take this drug for the prescribed length of time. If you stop too soon, your symptoms could come back.
- For treatment of shingles, herpes simplex, or genital herpes, start drug as soon as possible after symptoms appear.
- For treatment of chicken pox, start within 24 hours of onset of rash.

- Store at room temperature with lid on tightly. Do not store in the bathroom. Do not expose to heat, moisture, or strong light. Keep out of reach of children.

Interactions with Other Drugs

Evaluations of Drug Interactions 2003 lists no drugs, biologics (e.g., vaccines, therapeutic antibodies), or foods as causing "highly clinically significant" or "clinically significant" interactions when used together with the drugs in this section. We also found no interactions in the drugs' FDA-approved professional package inserts. However, as the number of new drugs approved for marketing increases and as more experience is gained with these drugs over time, new interactions may be discovered.

Adverse Effects

Call your doctor immediately if you experience:

- rash or hives
- blood in urine
- confusion or hallucinations
- trembling
- abdominal pain
- lower back pain
- difficulty breathing
- decreased frequency or amount of urination
- nausea or vomiting
- loss of appetite
- chills, fever, or sore throat
- black, tarry stools
- pinpoint red spots on skin
- unusual bleeding or bruising
- chest pain
- diarrhea
- unusual thirst
- seizures
- unusual tiredness or weakness
- faintness or lightheadedness

- swelling of hands, feet, or lower legs
- changes in vision
- painful menstruation

Call your doctor if these symptoms continue:

- diarrhea
- dizziness
- headache
- joint pain
- nausea or vomiting
- acne
- trouble sleeping
- general feeling of discomfort or illness
- muscle pain
- burning, tingling, or prickling sensations
- mood or mental changes

Signs of overdose:

- coma
- nervousness or restlessness
- lower back or side pain
- decreased amount of urine
- decreased frequency of urination
- hallucinations
- seizures
- tremors

If you suspect an overdose, call this number to contact your poison control center: (800) 222-1222.

Periodic Tests

Ask your doctor which of these tests should be done periodically while you are taking this drug:

- kidney function tests (during long-term, continuous treatment)
- blood urea nitrogen and creatinine serum tests

Amantadine (a *man* ta deen)
SYMMETREL (Endo)

GENERIC: available

FAMILY: Drugs for Viral Infections
Drugs for Parkinson's Disease

PREGNANCY WARNING

This drug caused harm to developing fetuses in animal studies, including malformations and death. Because of the potential for serious adverse effects to the fetus, this drug should not be used by pregnant women.

BREAST-FEEDING WARNING

Amantadine is excreted in human milk. Because of the potential for serious adverse effects in nursing infants, you should not take this drug while nursing.

Amantadine is approved by the FDA to prevent and treat influenza A, Parkinson's disease, and drug-induced movement disorders.[124] If you are over 60, you will probably need to take less than the usual adult dose. For use against flu, a lower dose of no more than 100 milligrams is recommended for older people, even less if your kidney function is impaired or you are underweight.[125,126]

For flu (influenza) prevention, it is best to get a flu shot early in the season. However, if you cannot get a flu shot because it is unavailable, or you have a medical condition that prevents it, you can use amantadine. During outbreaks of the flu, amantadine may be prescribed in addition to earlier flu shots. For amantadine to be effective against the flu, you must take it within 48 hours of your first flu symptoms.[127]

Your doctor may also prescribe amantadine if you have Parkinson's disease, usually as a supplement to another drug. A combination of two drugs called levodopa and carbidopa (see p. 631) is the best treatment for Parkinson's disease. Amantadine is often effective only for a limited time (less than six months), and it often produces adverse effects such as confusion, lightheadedness, hallucinations, and anxiety, which reduce its usefulness.[128] When you are taking amantadine, especially if you are a woman, the skin of your legs may become mottled (this is known as livedo reticularis). This will go away when you stop taking the drug.

If you have symptoms of parkinsonism, you should know that they might be caused by a drug that you are taking for another problem. As many as half of older adults with these symptoms may have developed them as an adverse effect of one of their drugs. A list of drugs that can cause symptoms of parkinsonism appears on p. 30. If you are taking any of the drugs on this list, discuss the possibility of drug-induced parkinsonism with your doctor and ask to have your prescription changed or stopped.

Before You Use This Drug

Tell your doctor if you have or have had:

- allergy to amantadine
- blood vessel disease of the brain
- congestive heart failure
- eczema (recurring)
- heart disease
- swelling of feet and ankles
- kidney disease
- mental illness or substance abuse
- seizures, epilepsy
- stomach ulcers
- pregnancy or are breast-feeding

Tell your doctor about any other drugs you take, including aspirin, herbs, vitamins, and other nonprescription products.

When You Use This Drug

- Check with your doctor if there is no improvement within a few days.
- Until you know how you react to this drug, do not drive or perform other activities requiring alertness. Amantadine can cause fainting, confusion, or impaired vision.
- Check with your doctor immediately if thoughts of suicide occur.

- You may feel dizzy when rising from a lying or sitting position. If you are lying down, hang your legs over the side of the bed for a few minutes, then get up slowly. When getting up from a chair, stay by the chair until you are sure that you are not dizzy. (See p. 13.)
- Do not drink alcohol.
- If you get dry mouth, use sugarless candy or gum, ice, or saliva substitute. Check with your doctor or dentist if this lasts more than two weeks.

How to Use This Drug

- If you miss a dose, take it as soon as you remember, but skip it if it is almost time for the next dose. **Do not take double doses.**
- Space doses evenly.
- Do not share your medication with others.
- Take the drug at the same time(s) each day.
- Take this drug for the prescribed length of time. If you stop too soon, your symptoms could come back.
- Store at room temperature with lid on tightly. Do not store in the bathroom. Do not expose to heat, moisture, or strong light. Keep out of reach of children.

Interactions with Other Drugs

Evaluations of Drug Interactions 2003 lists no drugs, biologics (e.g., vaccines, therapeutic antibodies), or foods as causing "highly clinically significant" or "clinically significant" interactions when used together with the drugs in this section. We also found no interactions in the drugs' FDA-approved professional package inserts. However, as the number of new drugs approved for marketing increases and as more experience is gained with these drugs over time, new interactions may be discovered.

Adverse Effects

Call your doctor immediately if you experience:

- confusion or hallucinations
- depression
- thoughts of or attempts at suicide
- severe mood or mental changes
- difficulty urinating
- fainting
- slurred speech
- memory loss
- increased blood pressure
- uncontrolled rolling of eyes
- fever, chills, or sore throat
- swelling of feet or lower legs
- shortness of breath
- rapid weight gain
- skin rash
- vision changes
- lack of coordination
- irritation and swelling of the eye

Call your doctor if these symptoms continue:

- difficulty concentrating
- dizziness or lightheadedness
- diarrhea
- irritability
- loss of appetite
- nausea or vomiting
- agitation, anxiety, or nervousness
- red, blotchy spots on skin
- nightmares
- trouble sleeping
- constipation
- dry mouth, nose, and throat
- headache
- unusual tiredness or weakness
- decreased sexual ability

Signs of overdose:

- shortness of breath
- heart rate changes
- aggressive behavior
- agitation
- anxiety
- stumbling
- coma

- confusion
- delirium
- disorientation
- fear
- hallucinations
- trouble sleeping
- lethargy
- hypertension
- fever
- seizures

If you suspect an overdose, call this number to contact your poison control center: (800) 222-1222.

Periodic Tests

Ask your doctor which of these tests should be done periodically while you are taking this drug:

- monitoring for an increase in seizures (if you have or have had epilepsy or seizures)

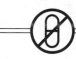 *Do Not Use*

ALTERNATIVE TREATMENT:
See Amantadine (SYMMETREL), p. 752.

Oseltamivir (oh sel *tam* i veer)
TAMIFLU (Roche)

Zanamivir (zan *am* e veer)
RELENZA (GlaxoSmithKline)

FAMILY: Drugs for Viral Infections

Oseltamivir

Oseltamivir was approved by the FDA in October 1999 and followed zanamivir (RELENZA) (see below) as the second drug cleared to treat uncomplicated flu infections in people who have had symptoms of the flu for no longer than two days.

A yearly flu vaccination remains the safest and least expensive way to fight the flu for those who are candidates for the vaccine.

If you have a high fever (greater than 101°F or 38.3°C) accompanied by shaking chills and are coughing up thick phlegm, or if coughing or breathing deeply causes sharp chest pain, you may have pneumonia and should consult your doctor for diagnosis and appropriate treatment.

The director of the FDA's Division of Antiviral Drug Products describes the effect of oseltamivir as "modest" in terms of reducing the duration of the flu, about 1.3 days, and notes that "the clinical relevance of the modest treatment benefit is a highly subjective question."[129] In our opinion, because of its limited effect on the duration of the flu, the cost of oseltamivir outweighs the "benefit" in the treatment of an illness that is self-limited in the vast majority of people.

In clinical studies, there was no difference in the incidence of complications of the flu between patients taking oseltamivir and those taking a placebo. The effectiveness and safety of oseltamivir in the treatment of patients with chronic heart or respiratory disease is unknown.[130]

In November 2000, oseltamivir received further FDA approval to prevent flu. The drug must be started within two days of close contact with a flu-infected individual. Oseltamivir is approved to be taken for up to 42 days to prevent the flu, but protection only lasts as long as the drug is being taken. The safety and effectiveness of repeated courses of prevention has not been studied.[130]

The editors of *Prescrire International,* a highly regarded French source of independent drug information for health professionals, found: "Oseltamivir is only moderately effective at preventing influenza, and there is no evidence that it differs from amantadine [see p. 752] in this respect. In patients with suspected influenza during an epidemic, the effects of oseltamivir are also moderate, and similar to those of zanamivir and amantadine. No impact on the frequency of complications has been shown in adults or children at risk."[131]

Zanamivir

Zanamivir was reviewed by the FDA's Antiviral Drug Advisory Committee on February 24, 1999. This committee of 17 outside experts was asked by the FDA: "Does the information presented by the applicant [Glaxo Wellcome] support the safety and effectiveness of zanamivir for treatment of influenza?" The committee voted 13 to 4 that it did not.[132] One committee member remarked during the meeting: "There isn't sufficient efficacy to warrant me recommending this drug [zanamivir] for my family or myself."[132]

Despite this vote, the FDA approved zanamivir in July 1999. At the time the drug was approved for marketing, only one clinical trial comparing the drug to a placebo had been published showing a statistical benefit for zanamivir compared to no treatment at all. This study was conducted in the southern hemisphere, primarily Australia, and according to the company's interpretation showed that zanamivir shortened the time to alleviation of flu symptoms by a median of 1.5 days compared to a placebo.[133] When we obtained the FDA's reviews of zanamivir through the Freedom of Information Act, we found that, in fact, two additional studies had been submitted to the FDA by Glaxo Wellcome, not just one.

The largest of the trials submitted by Glaxo Wellcome, and one of the two not yet published, is of most interest. Conducted in North America, this trial showed that the median difference in improvement between zanamivir and placebo was one day, a difference that is not statistically significant. The third and smallest trial, conducted in the European Union, found the largest treatment effect between zanamivir and placebo: 2.5 days, a difference that is statistically significant.

But the European Union study had problems. It was originally designed to enroll about 500 volunteer subjects but could only manage 356. Most study centers enrolled small numbers of subjects and the estimates of treatment effect varied markedly among centers. Surprisingly, it was found that in subjects who did not have confirmed flu, there was a shorter median time to alleviation of symptoms with zanamivir than with the placebo, and it was unclear whether this was due to chance, to false-negative flu diagnoses, or to some other reason.

The FDA statistical reviewer for the drug concluded his evaluation by saying, "Zanamivir has not been shown to be effective in this country [the United States] for the treatment of influenza, and in my opinion therefore should not be approved." [134]

In January 2000, the FDA issued a public health advisory that included a warning about prescribing zanamivir to patients with underlying asthma or chronic obstructive pulmonary disease (COPD). [135] The agency had received several reports of deterioration of respiratory function following the use of zanamivir in patients with underlying asthma or COPD.

The professional product labeling for zanamivir now carries the following warning:

BRONCHOSPASM AND DECLINE IN LUNG FUNCTION HAVE BEEN REPORTED IN SOME PATIENTS RECEIVING RELENZA. MANY BUT NOT ALL OF THESE PATIENTS HAD UNDERLYING AIRWAYS DISEASE SUCH AS ASTHMA OR CHRONIC OBSTRUCTIVE PULMONARY DISEASE. BECAUSE OF THE RISK OF SERIOUS ADVERSE EVENTS AND BECAUSE EFFICACY HAS NOT BEEN DEMONSTRATED IN THIS POPULATION, RELENZA IS NOT GENERALLY RECOMMENDED FOR TREATMENT OF PATIENTS WITH UNDERLYING AIRWAYS DISEASE. SOME PATIENTS WITH SERIOUS ADVERSE EVENTS DURING TREATMENT WITH RELENZA HAVE HAD FATAL OUTCOMES, ALTHOUGH CAUSALITY WAS DIFFICULT TO ASSESS.

RELENZA SHOULD BE DISCONTINUED IN ANY PATIENT WHO DEVELOPS BRONCHOSPASM OR DECLINE IN RESPIRATORY FUNCTION; IMMEDIATE TREATMENT AND HOSPITALIZATION MAY BE REQUIRED.

No matter how small the risk of an adverse reaction with a minimally effective or ineffective drug, those risks always outweigh the lack of a significant benefit. This is the case with zanamivir.

In their review of zanamivir, the editors of the independent French drug bulletin *Prescrire International* found that: [136]

1. Zanamivir shortens the duration of symptoms of suspected influenza by only about a day.

2. Zanamivir has not been shown to reduce antibiotic prescribing, or the incidence of complications necessitating hospitalization.

3. Zanamivir has no proven efficacy in preventing the spread of influenza by a treated patient.

4. Zanamivir inhalation can induce bronchospasm.

REFERENCES

1. Nyquist AC, Gonzales R, Steiner JF, et al. Antibiotic prescribing for children with colds, upper respiratory tract infections, and bronchitis. *Journal of the American Medical Association* 1998; 279:875–7.

2. Gonzales R, Steiner JF, Sande MA. Antibiotic prescribing for adults with colds, upper respiratory tract infections, and bronchitis by ambulatory care physicians. *Journal of the American Medical Association* 1997; 278:901–4.

3. *Physicians' Desk Reference.* 56th ed. Montvale, N.J.: Medical Economics Company, 2002:879–83.

4. McEwen LN, Farjo R, Foxman B. Antibiotic prescribing for cystitis: How well does it match published guidelines? *Annals of Epidemiology* 2003; 13:479–83.

5. Food and Drug Administration. Labeling Requirements for Systemic Antibacterial Drug Products. 21 CFR Part 201, February 6, 2003. Available at: http://www.fda.gov/OHRMS/Dockets/98fr/oon-1463-nfr00001.pdf.

6. Centers for Disease Control. Campaign to Prevent Antimicrobial Resistance in Healthcare Settings, 2004. Available at: http://www.cdc.gov/drugresistance/healthcare/problem.htm.

7. Scheld WM. FDA/IDSA/ISAP Working Group on Antimicrobial Resistance and Drug Development, April 15, 2004. Available at: http://www.fda.gov/cder/drug/antimicrobial/FDAIDSAISAPPresentations/Mike%20Scheld_files/frame.htm.

8. Niederman MS. Impact of antibiotic resistance on clinical outcomes and the cost of care. *Critical Care Medicine* 2001; 29:N114–20.

9. Cefprozil. *Medical Letter on Drugs and Therapeutics* 1992; 34:63–4.

10. Gleckman RA, Esposito AL. Antibiotics in the elderly: Skating on therapeutic thin ice. *Geriatrics* 1980; 35:26–7.

11. Philp JR. Untoward effects of antimicrobial drugs. Prevention and control. *Postgraduate Medicine* 1971; 50:193–200.

12. Moellering RC Jr. Factors influencing the clinical use of antimicrobial agents in elderly patients. *Geriatrics* 1978; 33:83–91.

13. Beam TR Jr. The third generation of cephalosporins. Part II. *Rational Drug Therapeutics* 1982; 16:1–5.

14. DiPiro JT, Bowden TA Jr., Hooks VH III. Prophylactic parenteral cephalosporins in surgery. Are the newer agents better? *Journal of the American Medical Association* 1984; 252:3277–9.

15. Antimicrobial prophylaxis for surgery. *Medical Letter on Drugs and Therapeutics* 1985; 27:105–8.

16. Loracarbef. *Medical Letter on Drugs and Therapeutics* 1992; 34:87–8.

17. The choice of antimicrobial drugs. *Medical Letter on Drugs and Therapeutics* 1986; 28:33–5.

18. Lautenbach E, Larosa LA, Kasbekar N, et al. Fluoroquinolone utilization in the emergency departments of academic medical centers: Prevalence of, and risk factors for, inappropriate use. *Archives of Internal Medicine* 2003; 163:601–5.

19. *American Hospital Formulary Service Drug Information.* Bethesda, Md.: American Society of Hospital Pharmacists, 1992: 2352–62.

20. Todd PA, Faulds D. Ofloxacin. A reappraisal of its antimicrobial activity, pharmacology and therapeutic use. *Drugs* 1991; 42:825–76.

21. Ofloxacin. *Medical Letter on Drugs and Therapeutics* 1991; 33:71–3.

22. The choice of antibacterial drugs. *Medical Letter on Drugs and Therapeutics* 1998; 40:33–42.

23. Orland MJ, Saltman R, eds. *Manual of Medical Therapeutics.* 25th ed. Boston: Little, Brown, and Company, 1985:205.

24. AMA Department of Drugs. *AMA Drug Evaluations.* 5th ed. Chicago: American Medical Association, 1983:1674.

25. Kastrup EK, ed. *Facts and Comparisons.* St. Louis: JB Lippincott and Co., 1987:341.

26. *American Hospital Formulary Service Drug Information.* Bethesda, Md.: American Society of Hospital Pharmacists, 1996:355–65.

27. Bergogne-Berezin E. Treatment and prevention of antibiotic associated diarrhea. *International Journal of Antimicrobial Agents* 2000; 16:521–6.

28. Vanderhoof JA, Whitney DB, Antonson DL, et al. Lactobacillus GG in the prevention of antibiotic-associated diarrhea in children. *Journal of Pediatrics* 1999; 135:564–8.

29. Siitonen S, Vapaatalo H, Salminen S, et al. Effect of Lactobacillus GG yoghurt in prevention of antibiotic associated diarrhoea. *Annals of Medicine* 1990; 22:57–9.

30. Larrey D, Vial T, Micaleff A, et al. Hepatitis associated with amoxycillin-clavulanic acid combination report of 15 cases. *Gut* 1992; 33:368–71.

31. Reddy KR, Brillant P, Schiff ER. Amoxicillin-clavulanate potassium-associated cholestasis. *Gastroenterology* 1989; 96:1135–41.

32. Hedstrom SA, Hybbinette CH. Nephrotoxicity in isoxazolylpenicillin prophylaxis in hip surgery. *Acta Orthopaedica Scandinavica* 1988; 59:144–7.

33. US PDI Volume II: *Advice for the Patient.* 23rd ed. Greenwood Village, Colo.: MICROMEDEX, 2004:384–90.

34. *46 Federal Register 14355,* February 27, 1981.

35. *Physicians' Desk Reference.* 58th ed. Montvale, N.J.: Thomson PDR, 2004:408–17.

36. *Physicians' Desk Reference.* 58th ed. Montvale, N.J.: Thomson PDR, 2004:2675–82.

37. Schubert ML, Sanyal AJ, Wong ES. Antibiotic prophylaxis for prevention of spontaneous bacterial peritonitis? *Gastroenterology* 1991; 101:550–2.

38. Food and Drug Administration. Briefing Package—Anti-infective Drugs Advisory Committee, January 8, 2003:49. Available at: http://www.fda.gov/ohrms/dockets/ac/03/briefing/3919B1_02_B-FDA%20Master%20Copy.pdf.

39. Food and Drug Administration. Anti-infective Drugs Advisory Committee, January 8, 2003:26. Available at: http://www.fda.gov/ohrms/dockets/ac/03/transcripts/3919T1.pdf.

40. Food and Drug Administration. Anti-infective Drugs Advisory Committee, January 8, 2003:15. Available at: http://www.fda.gov/ohrms/dockets/ac/03/transcripts/3919T1.pdf.

41. Food and Drug Administration. Anti-infective Drugs Advisory Committee, January 8, 2003:269–72. Available at: http://www.fda.gov/ohrms/dockets/ac/03/transcripts/3919T1.pdf.

42. Food and Drug Administration Briefing Package—Anti-infective Drugs Advisory Committee, January 8, 2003:29–30. Available at: http://www.fda.gov/ohrms/dockets/ac/03/briefing/3919B1_02_B-FDA%20Master%20copy.pdf.

43. Food and Drug Administration. Anti-infective Drugs Advisory Committee, January 8, 2003:263, 271. http://www.fda.gov/ohrms/dockets/ac/03/transcripts/3919T1.pdf.

44. Food and Drug Administration Briefing Package—Anti-infective Drug Advisory Committee, January 8, 2003:25, 26. Avail-

able at: http://www.fda.gov/ohrms/dockets/ac/03/briefing/3919B1_02_ B-FDA%20Master%20copy.pdf.

45. Food and Drug Administration Briefing Package—Anti-infective Drugs Advisory Committee, January 8, 2003:42. Available at: http://www.fda.gov/ohrms/dockets/ac/03/briefing/3919B1_02_B-FDA %20Master%20copy.pdf.

46. Food and Drug Administration Briefing Package—Anti-infective Drugs Advisory Committee, January 8, 2003:84. Available at: http://www.fda.gov/ohrms/dockets/ac/03/briefing/3919B1_02_ B-FDA%20Master%20copy.pdf.

47. Food and Drug Administration. Anti-infective Drugs Advisory Committee, January 8, 2003:193–4. Available at: http://www.fda.gov/ ohrms/dockets/ac/03/transcripts/3919T1.pdf.

48. Food and Drug Administration Briefing Package—Anti-infective Drugs Advisory Committee, January 8, 2003:52. Available at: http://www.fda.gov/ohrms/dockets/ac/03/briefing/3919B1_02_ B-FDA%20Master%20copy.pdf.

49. Food and Drug Administration Briefing Package—Anti-infective Drugs Advisory Committee, January 8, 2003:86. Available at: http://www.fda.gov/ohrms/dockets/ac/03/briefing/3919B1_02_ B-FDA%20Master%20copy.pdf.

50. Telithromycin and myasthenia. *Prescrire International* 2004; 13:21.

51. Telithromycin: New preparation. A needless addition to the other macrolides. *Prescrire International* 2003; 12:8–11.

52. Mandell LA, Bartlett JG, Dowell SF, et al. Update of practice guidelines for the management of community-acquired pneumonia in immunocompetent adults. *Clinical Infectious Diseases* 2003; 37:1405–33.

53. Niederman MS, Mandell LA, Anzueto A, et al. Guidelines for the management of adults with community-acquired pneumonia. Diagnosis, assessment of severity, antimicrobial therapy, and prevention. *American Journal of Respiratory and Critical Care Medicine* 2001; 163:1730–54.

54. US PDI Volume II: *Advice for the Patient.* 23rd ed. Greenwood Village, Colo.: MICROMEDEX, 2004:1477–81.

55. *Physicians' Desk Reference.* 58th ed. Montvale, N.J.: Thomson PDR, 2004:2178–89.

56. Marderosian AD, Liberti L. *Natural Product Medicine.* Philadelphia, Pa.: George F. Stickley Co., 1988:282.

57. AMA Department of Drugs. *AMA Drug Evaluations.* Chicago: American Medical Association, 1992.

58. Proloprim (Trimethoprim) Professional Product Labeling, April 1, 2002. Available at: http://www.fda.gov/cder/foi/label/2002/ 17943s16lbl.pdf. Accessed June 14, 2004.

59. *Physicians' Desk Reference.* 40th ed. Oradell, N.J.: Medical Economics, 1986:759.

60. Sarma PS, Durairaj P. Randomized treatment of patients with typhoid and paratyphoid fevers using norfloxacin or chloramphenicol. *Transactions of the Royal Society of Tropical Medicine and Hygiene* 1991; 85:670–1.

61. *Physicians' Desk Reference.* 58th ed. Montvale, N.J.: Thomson PDR, 2004:2731–2.

62. Flagyl (Metronidazole) Professional Product Labeling, August 1, 2003. Available at: http://www.fda.gov/cder/foi/label/2004/12623slr059_ flagyl_lbl.pdf. Accessed June 15, 2004.

63. Bendesky A, Menendez D, Ostrosky-Wegman P. Is metronidazole carcinogenic? *Mutation Research* 2002; 511:133–44.

64. Is flagyl dangerous? *Medical Letter on Drugs and Therapeutics* 1975; 17:53–4.

65. AMA Department of Drugs. *AMA Drug Evaluations.* 5th ed. Chicago: American Medical Association, 1983:1717.

66. *Physicians' Desk Reference.* 58th ed. Montvale, N.J.: Thomson PDR, 2004:1459–61.

67. Feder HM Jr., Abrahamian LM, Grant-Kels JM. Is penicillin still the drug of choice for non-bullous impetigo? *The Lancet* 1991; 338:803–5.

68. Slocombe B, Perry C. The antimicrobial activity of mupirocin—an update on resistance. *Journal of Hospital Infection* 1991; 19(suppl B):19–25.

69. *USP DI, Drug Information for the Health Care Professional.* 12th ed. Rockville, Md.: The United States Pharmacopeial Convention, 1992:1963–4.

70. *Physicians' Desk Reference.* 58th ed. Montvale, N.J.: Thomson PDR, 2004:2837–9.

71. *Drug Treatment in the Elderly.* 2nd ed. Copenhagen, Denmark: World Health Organizaion, 1997.

72. *Physicians' Desk Reference.* 40th ed. Oradell, N.J.: Medical Economics, 1986:1278.

73. Ray WA, Federspiel CF, Schaffner W. Prescribing of chloramphenicol in ambulatory practice. An epidemiologic study among Tennessee Medicaid recipients. *Annals of Internal Medicine* 1976; 84:266–70.

74. Patrick J, Panzer JD, Derbes VJ. Neomycin sensitivity in the normal (nonatopic) individual. *Archives of Dermatology* 1970; 102:532–5.

75. Danner RM. Statement before the FDA Anti-Infective Drug Advisory Committee, October 21, 1999:249–50.

76. Zagam (Sparfloxacin) Professional Product Labeling, April 4, 2003. Available at: http://www.fda.gov/cder/foi/label/2003/020677s 006lbl.pdf. Accessed June 11, 2004.

77. Gatifloxacin and moxifloxacin: Two new fluoroquinolones. *Medical Letter on Drugs and Therapeutics* 2000; 42:15–7.

78. US PDI Volume II: *Advice for the Patient.* 23rd ed. Greenwood Village, Colo.: MICROMEDEX, 2004:764–8.

79. Frieden TR, Mangi RJ. Inappropriate use of oral ciprofloxacin. *Journal of the American Medical Association* 1990; 264:1438–40.

80. Mumford CJ, Ginsberg L. Ciprofloxacin and myasthenia gravis. *British Medical Journal* 1990; 301:818.

81. *American Hospital Formulary Service Drug Information.* Bethesda, Md.: American Society of Hospital Pharmacists, 1992:417–26.

82. Noroxin (Norfloxacin) Professional Product Labeling, April 1, 2001. Available at: http://www.merck.com/product/usa/pi_circulars/n/ noroxin/noroxin_pi.pdf.

83. Jolson HM, Tanner LA, Green L, et al. Adverse reaction reporting of interaction between warfarin and fluoroquinolones. *Archives of Internal Medicine* 1991; 151:1003–4.

84. Dukes MNG, Beely L, eds. *Side Effects of Drugs Annual* 15. Amsterdam: Elsevier, 1991;312–3.

85. Two new fluoroquinolones. *Medical Letter on Drugs and Therapeutics* 1992; 34:58–60.

86. Food and Drug Administration. Public Health Advisory—Trovan (Trovafloxacin/Alatrofloxacin Mesylate), June 9, 1999. Available at: http://www.fda.gov/cder/news/trovan/trovan-advisory.htm.

87. Factive (gemifloxacin) Professional Product Labeling, February 1, 2004. Available at: http://www.factive.com/global/pdfs/Feb_6_ Marketing_PI.pdf. Accessed May 1, 2004.

88. *Physicians' Desk Reference.* 58th ed. Montvale, N.J.: Thomson PDR, 2004:764–5.

89. *Physicians' Desk Reference.* 58th ed. Montvale, N.J.: Thomson PDR, 2004:761–4.

90. Thomason JL. Clinical evaluation of terconazole. United States experience. *Journal of Reproductive Medicine* 1989; 34:597–601.

91. Doering PL, Santiago TM. Drugs for treatment of vulvovaginal candidiasis: Comparative efficacy of agents and regimens. *DICP, The Annals of Pharmacotherapy* 1990; 24:1078–83.

92. *US PDI, Drug Information for the Health Care Professional.* 12th ed. Rockville, Md.: The United States Pharmacopeial Convention, 1992;1558–62.

93. Diflucan (Fluconazole) Professional Product Labeling, June 1, 2003. Available at: http://www.diflucan.com/. Accessed June 9, 2004.

94. Brown AE. Overview of fungal infections in cancer patients. *Seminars in Oncology* 1990; 17:2–5.

95. Evans TG, Mayer J, Cohen S, et al. Fluconazole failure in the treatment of invasive mycoses. *Journal of Infectious Diseases* 1991; 164:1232–5.

96. Lotrisone (Betamethasone and Clotrimazole) Professional Product Labeling, March 10, 2003. Available at: http://www.fda.gov/cder/foi/labcl/2003/18827slr025_lotrisone_lbl.pdf. Accessed June 9, 2004.

97. LaGrenade L, Vega A. Executive Summary: Lotrisone and adverse events. Office of Postmarketing Drug Risk Assessment, Food and Drug Administration, March 9, 1999.

98. *Physicians' Desk Reference.* 39th ed. Oradell, N.J.: Medical Economics Company, 1985:1859–60.

99. *Physicians' Desk Reference.* 45th ed. Oradell, N.J.: Medical Economics Company, 1991:2003–4.

100. Food and Drug Administration. Public Health Advisory: The Safety of Sporanox Capsules and Lamisil Tablets for the Treatment of Onychomycosis, May 9, 2001. Available at: http://www.fda.gov/cder/drug/advisory/sporanox-lamisil/advisory.htm.

101. Ahmad SR, Singer SJ, Leissa BG. Congestive heart failure associated with itraconazole. *The Lancet* 2001; 357:1766–7.

102. Lamisil (Terbinafine) Professional Product Labeling, March 1, 2004. Available at: http://www.pharma.us.novartis.com/product/pi/pdf/Lamisil_tablets.pdf. Accessed June 8, 2004.

103. Terbinafine for onychomycosis. *Medical Letter on Drugs and Therapeutics* 1996; 38:72–4.

104. *Physicians' Desk Reference.* 52nd ed. Montvale, N.J.: Medical Economics Co., 1998:1861.

105. Hirsch HA. Clinical evaluation of terconazole. European experience. *Journal of Reproductive Medicine* 1989; 34:593–6.

106. Moebius UM. Influenza-like syndrome after terconazole. *The Lancet* 1988; 2:966–7.

107. Terazole (Terconazole) Professional Product Labeling, March 1, 2001. Available at: http://www.fda.gov/cder/foi/label/2003/019641s016lbl.pdf. Accessed June 8, 2004.

108. *Physicians' Desk Reference.* 58th ed. Montvale, N.J.: Thomson PDR, 2004:1898.

109. Drugs for parasitic infections. *Medical Letter on Drugs and Therapeutics* 1998; 40:1–12.

110. Chippaux JP. Mebendazole treatment of dracunculiasis. *Transactions of the Royal Society of Tropical Medicine and Hygiene* 1991; 85:280.

111. Walden J. Parasitic diseases. Other roundworms. Trichuris, hookworm, and Strongyloides. *Primary Care* 1991; 18:53–74.

112. Gilman AG, Rall TW, Nies AS, Taylor P, eds. *The Pharmacological Basis of Therapeutics.* 8th ed. New York: Pergamon Press, 1990.971.

113. Grasela TH Jr., Dreis MW. An evaluation of the quinolone-theophylline interaction using the Food and Drug Administration spontaneous reporting system. *Archives of Internal Medicine* 1992; 152:617–21.

114. *Physicians' Desk Reference.* 50th ed. Montvale, N.J.: Medical Economics Company, 1996:582–4.

115. Tenenbein M. Seizures after lindane therapy. *Journal of the American Geriatrics Society* 1991; 39:394–5.

116. Public Citizen Petition to FDA to Immediately Ban Lindane, June 15, 1995.

117. Vander Stichele RH, Dezeure EM, Bogaert MG. Systematic review of clinical efficacy of topical treatments for head lice. *British Medical Journal* 1995; 311:604–8.

118. Food and Drug Administration Public Health Advisory: Safety of Topical Lindane Products for the Treatment of Scabies and Lice, March 28, 2003. Available at: http://www.fda.gov/cder/drug/infopage/lindane/lindanePHA.htm.

119. *Physicians' Desk Reference.* 58th ed. Montvale, N.J.: Thomson PDR, 2004:1653–5.

120. *Physicians' Desk Reference.* 58th ed. Montvale, N.J.: Thomson PDR, 2004:1683–5.

121. *Physicians' Desk Reference.* 58th ed. Montvale, N.J.: Thomson PDR, 2004:990–1685.

122. *Physicians' Desk Reference.* 58th ed. Montvale, N.J.: Thomson PDR, 2004:990.

123. Valacyclovir (valtrex) for herpes labialis. *Medical Letter on Drugs and Therapeutics* 2002; 44:95–6.

124. *Physicians' Desk Reference.* 58th ed. Montvale, N.J.: Thomson PDR, 2004:1247–9.

125. Degelau J, Somani S, Cooper SL, et al. Occurrence of adverse effects and high amantadine concentrations with influenza prophylaxis in the nursing home. *Journal of the American Geriatrics Society* 1990; 38:428–32.

126. Stange KC, Little DW, Blatnik B. Adverse reactions to amantadine prophylaxis of influenza in a retirement home. *Journal of the American Geriatrics Society* 1991; 39:700–5.

127. AMA Department of Drugs. *AMA Drug Evaluations.* 5th ed. Chicago: American Medical Association, 1983:1457.

128. Vestal RE, ed. *Drug Treatment in the Elderly.* Sydney, Australia: ADIS Health Science Press, 1984:311.

129. Jolson HM. Food and Drug Administration, Division Director Memorandum on Tamiflu (Oseltamivir), October 25, 1999.

130. *Physicians' Desk Reference.* 56th ed. Montvale, N.J.: Medical Economics Company, 2002:3008–10.

131. Oseltamivir: New preparation. An antiviral agent with little impact on influenza. *Prescrire International* 2003; 12:85–8.

132. Food and Drug Administration, Center for Drug Evaluation and Research. Summary Minutes, Antiviral Drugs Advisory Committee. February 24, 1999. Available at: http://www.fda.gov/ohrms/dockets/ac/99/meeting/3496ml.pdf.

133. The MIST (Management of Influenza in the Southern Hemisphere Trialists) Study Group. Randomised trial of efficacy and safety of inhaled zanamivir in treatment of influenza A and B virus infections. *The Lancet* 1998; 352:1877–81.

134. Elashoff M. FDA Statistical Review of Relenza, February 24, 1999.

135. Food and Drug Administration. Public Health Advisory: Safe and Appropriate Use of Influenza Drugs, January 12, 2000. Available at: http://www.fda.gov/cder/drug/advisory/influenza.htm.

136. Zanamivir: A second look. Still no tangible impact on influenza. *Prescrire International* 2001;10: 175–7.

25

HORMONES

HORMONE REPLACEMENT THERAPY

We hope that by now most women have heard that the first part of a large, long-term, government-sponsored clinical trial evaluating hormone replacement therapy (HRT), the Women's Health Initiative (WHI), was halted prematurely. The bottom line from this trial is that long-term, HRT's risks outweigh its benefits.

In 1991, the Health Research Group published the Women's Health Alert. The largest chapter in the book was on hormone replacement therapy (HRT). By then, the evidence was clear that these drugs caused breast cancer, and very serious doubts had been raised about their ability to protect against heart disease. The first sentence in this chapter began: *Female replacement hormones may someday be remembered as the most recklessly prescribed and dangerous drugs of this century.*

The part, or arm, of the trial that was first stopped involved 16,608 women who were taking conjugated estrogens (PREMARIN) with medroxyprogesterone (PROVERA) or a combination of the two as a single pill, with the brand name PREMPRO.

The main reason for stopping was an increased risk of invasive breast cancer in women receiving HRT after 5.2 years of treatment. This increase in breast cancer, combined with an increase in cardiovascular events that began in the first year of HRT treatment and persisted, clearly outweighed the benefits, among which were a reduced incidence of colon cancer and hip fractures.

A breakdown of the risks and benefits of HRT is given in the table below. The type of risk is shown in the left-hand column. The middle column gives the size of the risks of HRT, all serious and potentially life-threatening. The numbers represent the increased number of women out of 10,000 using HRT for one year who will experience one of the listed

Health Event	Risks: Increase per 10,000 Women Using HRT for One Year	Benefits: Decrease per 10,000 Women Using HRT for One Year
Heart Attacks	7	—
Strokes	8	—
Breast Cancer	8	—
Blood Clots in Lungs	8	—
Colorectal Cancer	—	6
Hip Fractures	—	5

health events compared to those women taking an inactive placebo. The right-hand column shows the benefits of HRT. The numbers represent women who will not experience the listed health events compared to those taking a placebo.

The risk of harm to an individual woman is not that large, but the risks are extremely serious. There are 31 serious adverse effects per 10,000 women using HRT per year. On the other hand, there are 11 fewer cases of colorectal cancer and hip fracture per 10,000 women taking HRT per year. Clearly, there are almost three times as many negative outcomes as positive ones.

At the time of the WHI, approximately 38% of postmenopausal women in the United States were using HRT, and from a public health perspective, the harm is quite substantial. For every 1 million women using HRT for one year, there is an increase of 3,100 potentially life-threatening adverse events, namely heart attacks, strokes, blood clots, and breast cancer. A conservative estimate of the total number of women who have been using HRT is 5 million. This translates to an increase of 15,500 of these serious adverse events per year because of the use of HRT.

After the initial results from the WHI, new data from the same study found that HRT significantly increased the risk of dementia, and the FDA subsequently requested manufacturers to update labeling for hormone therapy products (estrogen and combination estrogen and progestin products) for use by postmenopausal women with data from the Women's Health Initiative Memory Study (WHIMS). WHIMS reported an increased risk of dementia in women 65 and older and also showed that estrogen with progestin (PREMPRO) failed to prevent mild cognitive impairment (memory loss). (WHIMS is a substudy of the WHI conducted by the National Institutes of Health.)

Most recently, the part of the WHI that involved giving estrogen alone was also halted and then published. These were women who had had a hysterectomy and therefore did not need the protection from estrogen-induced uterine cancer provided by adding a progesterone-like drug to the estrogen.

For the outcomes significantly affected by estrogen alone, there was an absolute excess risk of 12 additional strokes per 10,000 person-years and an absolute risk reduction of 6 fewer hip fractures per 10,000 person-years. The conclusion was that estrogen alone should not be recommended for chronic disease prevention in postmenopausal women.

The adverse economic impact of HRT on the health care system because of all of the diseases caused by HRT is enormous. This cost must be added to the amount spent each year on HRT. In 2001, the combined sales for conjugated estrogens and conjugated estrogens in combination with medroxyprogesterone exceeded $2 billion.

The FDA-approved uses for hormone replacement therapy include relief of menopausal symptoms and prevention of osteoporosis but do not include treatment of osteoporosis. Long-term use has been in vogue to prevent a range of chronic conditions, especially heart disease. The use of HRT to prevent chronic diseases are referred to as "off-label" uses because data have not been presented to the FDA to show that the drug is safe and effective for these conditions.

How Did the Estrogen Vogue Begin and Why Did It Continue?

The *New York Times* explored this question in a July 10, 2002, article. Robert Wilson, MD (who died in 1989), wrote a best seller in 1966 with the title *Feminine Forever*. He traveled around the country promoting the book, telling doctors and women that estrogen could keep women young, healthy, and attractive. The logic was simple, and when uncritically accepted, it was taken to mean that women need only top up with a little estrogen to be young again.

In the *Times* article, Dr. Wilson's son was quoted as saying that Wyeth-Ayerst, the manufacturer of Premarin and Prempro, had paid all the doctor's expenses of writing *Feminine Forever* and furthermore paid him to lecture to women's groups. Contacted for confirmation, Wyeth-Ayerst said it could not confirm the story because it was so long ago.

In 1990, Wyeth-Ayerst requested FDA approval for Premarin to be used as protection against heart disease. The company's request was not based on randomized controlled trials such as the Women's Health Initiative's, but rather on observational research, a study design that is excellent for raising research questions that, in turn, must be validated by randomized controlled trials. The FDA's advisory committee recommended approval, but the FDA refused the advice, saying that better data were needed.

Reliance on the positive results of observational studies elevated HRT to the status of a standard of practice for preventing heart disease, and HRT remained one of the most frequently prescribed drugs in the United States year after year.

The overdue demise of long-term HRT has sparked new activity on the part of the medical marketplace jackals, alternative medicine practitioners, compounding pharmacists, and the dietary supplement industry, all ready to offer women "proven" natural substitutes for HRT.

Shortly after the results of the Women's Health Initiative study were made public, one particularly disreputable and unethical compounding pharmacist posted a press release on her Web site with the following caption:

Natural Hormones—Safe and Effective Alternative to Prempro

Remarkably, a number of women have apparently embraced such "pitches" with no or significantly less evidence of safety and effectiveness than there was for HRT. Medically, if a drug sounds too good to be true, it usually is.

You should not be using hormone replacement therapy for any reason other than its very short-term use to control the symptoms of menopause, for as short a time as possible. Otherwise, the benefits are outweighed by the increased risks of heart attacks, strokes, breast cancer, and blood clots in the lungs.

DRUG PROFILES

Estrogens

Limited Use

Conjugated Estrogens (*con* ju gate ed *es* troe jenz)
PREMARIN (Wyeth)

Estradiol Transdermal (es *tra* di ole trans *der* mal)
CLIMARA (Berlex)

Synthetic Conjugated Estrogens
(sin *the* tik *con* ju gate ed *es* troe jenz)
CENESTIN (Duramed)

GENERIC: not available
FAMILY: Estrogens

BREAST-FEEDING WARNING
Estrogens decrease the quantity and quality of breast milk. Estrogens are also excreted in breast milk and capable of causing harm to nursing infants. Because of the potential for serious adverse effects in nursing infants, you should not take these drugs while nursing.

PREGNANCY WARNING

Because of the potential for serious adverse effects to the fetus, estrogens should not be used by pregnant women.

FDA BLACK BOX WARNING

ESTROGENS INCREASE THE RISK OF ENDOMETRIAL CANCER

Close clinical surveillance of all women taking estrogens is important. Adequate diagnostic measures, including endometrial sampling when indicated, should be undertaken to rule out malignancy in all cases of undiagnosed persistent or recurring abnormal vaginal bleeding. There is no evidence that the use of "natural" estrogens results in a different endometrial risk profile than synthetic estrogens of equivalent estrogen dose.

ESTROGENS INCREASE THE RISK OF BREAST CANCER, CARDIOVASCULAR DISEASE, AND DEMENTIA

Estrogens with or without progestins should not be used for the prevention of cardiovascular disease, since the best evidence is that they increase the risk of cardiovascular disease.

The Women's Health Initiative (WHI) study reported increased risks of myocardial infarction, stroke, invasive breast cancer, pulmonary emboli, and deep vein thrombosis in postmenopausal women (50 to 79 years of age) during five years of treatment with conjugated estrogens (0.625 milligrams) combined with medroxyprogesterone acetate (2.5 milligrams) relative to placebo.

The Women's Health Initiative Memory Study (WHIMS), a substudy of WHI, reported increased risk of developing probable dementia in postmenopausal women 65 years of age or older during four years of treatment with conjugated estrogens plus medroxyprogesterone acetate relative to placebo. It is unknown whether this finding applies to younger postmenopausal women or to women taking estrogen-alone therapy.

Other doses of conjugated estrogens and medroxyprogesterone acetate, and other combinations and dosage forms of estrogens and progestins, were not studied in the WHI clinical trials and, in the absence of comparable data, these risks should be assumed to be similar. Because of these risks, estrogens with or without progestins should be prescribed at the lowest effective doses and for the shortest duration consistent with treatment goals and risks for the individual woman.

These three estrogen products are FDA-approved to manage the symptoms of menopause. Premarin and Climara are also approved to prevent osteoporosis. However, estrogens are no longer approved by the FDA for the treatment of osteoporosis. If Premarin and Climara are prescribed solely for the prevention of postmenopausal osteoporosis, treatment should only be considered for women at significant risk of osteoporosis and for whom nonestrogen medications are not considered to be appropriate.[1,2] See Chapter 18, Drugs for Osteoporosis, p. 582.

The mainstays for decreasing the risk of postmenopausal osteoporosis are weight-bearing exercise, adequate calcium and vitamin D intake, and, when needed, treatment with drugs. Postmenopausal women require an average of 1,500 milligrams per day of elemental calcium. Therefore, when not contraindicated, calcium supplementation may be helpful for women with suboptimal dietary intake. Vitamin D supplementation of 400–800 international units (IU) per day may also be required to ensure adequate daily intake in postmenopausal women.[1,2]

The Canadian Task Force on Preventive Health Care recommends "against the use of combined estrogen-progestin therapy and estrogen-only therapy for the primary prevention of chronic diseases in menopausal women." For the management of the symptoms of meno-

---

BEWARE OF COMPOUNDING PHARMACISTS SELLING BIOIDENTICAL HORMONE REPLACEMENT THERAPIES, CLAIMING THAT THEY ARE SAFE

Pharmacy compound products are not approved by the FDA and their quality is questionable, as they are not produced in facilities meeting good manufacturing practice (GMP) guidelines.

---

pause, this task force recommends: "If the risks are acceptable to the woman and her physician, therapy of as short a duration as possible, and at as low a dose as possible, may be indicated."[3] We agree.

The North American Menopause Society (NAMS) has issued its position on the management of hot flashes in postmenopausal women. Lifestyle-related strategies such as keeping the core body temperature cool, participating in regular exercise, and using paced respiration have shown some effectiveness for mild hot flashes without adverse effects.[4]

The NAMS found that among nonprescription remedies, clinical trial results are insufficient to either support or refute the efficacy of soy foods and isoflavone supplements (from either soy or red clover), black cohosh (see p. 830), or vitamin E. Single clinical trials have found no benefit for dong quai, evening primrose oil, ginseng, a Chinese herbal mixture, acupuncture, or magnet therapy for hot flashes.[4]

There is little evidence to support the effectiveness of topical progesterone cream for hot flashes (see oral progesterone, p. 766). A number of prescription drugs have been tried for hot flashes, but none are approved by the FDA for this use.

The NAMS recommends for moderate to severe hot flashes treatment with oral estrogen, either alone or combined with a progestin or in the form of estrogen-progestin oral contraceptives.[4] These treatments are effective.

Before You Use This Drug

Do not use if you have or have had:

- blood-clotting disorder (does not apply to cream preparations)
- abnormal and undiagnosed vaginal bleeding
- cancer
- allergy to parabens or other components (cream preparations)

Tell your doctor if you have or have had:

- pregnancy or are breast-feeding
- allergies to drugs
- endometriosis
- gallstones or gallbladder disease (oral; patch)
- liver disease
- jaundice (oral; patch)
- high cholesterol or triglycerides (oral; patch)
- pancreatitis (oral; patch)
- high levels of calcium in the blood (oral; patch)
- uterine fibroids
- blood-clotting problems
- vaginal problems (cream)

Tell your doctor about any other drugs you take, including aspirin, herbs, vitamins, and other nonprescription products.

When You Use This Drug

- Perform regular breast self-examinations.
- See your doctor on a regular basis.
- Stop drug immediately if you think you are pregnant.
- Do not use latex condoms for up to 72 hours after using this drug because oils in the cream can weaken the condom (cream).
- Use cream after sexual intercourse, not before (cream).
- Full therapeutic effect can take three to four months to appear (cream).
- Have regular dental examinations (oral; patch).

- Menstrual bleeding may begin again, but if you are on continuous therapy, it will stop by 10 months (oral; patch)
- Bleeding during a menstrual cycle may occur during the first three months of therapy (oral; patch)

How to Use This Drug

- If you miss a dose, take it as soon as you remember, but skip it if it is almost time for the next dose. **Do not take double doses.**
- Do not share your medication with others.
- Take the drug at the same time(s) each day.
- Store at room temperature with lid or cap on tightly. Do not store in the bathroom. Do not expose to heat, moisture, or strong light. Keep out of reach of children.

For oral:

- Take with food or milk.

For patch:

- Wash hands immediately before and after administration.
- Apply patch to clean, dry, nonoily, hairless, intact skin.
- Follow manufacturer's instructions as to where on skin to apply patch.
- Do not apply to breasts.
- Press patch firmly in place.
- Reapply patch if it comes loose, or discard and apply a new one.
- To prevent skin irritation, rotate patch application sites.

Interactions with Other Drugs

The following drugs, biologics (e.g., vaccines, therapeutic antibodies), or foods are listed in *Evaluations of Drug Interactions* 2003 as causing "highly clinically significant" or "clinically significant" interactions when used together with any of the drugs in this section. In some sections with multiple drugs, the interaction may have been reported for one but not all drugs in this section, but we include the interaction because the drugs in this section are similar to one another. We have also included potentially serious interactions listed in the drug's FDA-approved professional package insert or in published medical journal articles. There may be other drugs, especially those in the families of drugs listed below, that also will react with this drug to cause severe adverse effects. Make sure to tell your doctor and pharmacist the drugs you are taking and tell them if you are taking any of these interacting drugs:

BIAXIN, carbamazepine, clarithromycin, EES, erythromycin, EVISTA, grapefruit juice, *Hypericum perforatum,* itraconazole, ketoconazole, LUMINAL, NIZORAL, NORVIR, phenobarbital, raloxifene, RIFADIN, rifampin, RIMACTANE, ritonavir, SPORANOX, St. John's wort, TEGRETOL.

Adverse Effects

Call your doctor immediately if you experience:

- breast pain or enlargement
- rapid weight gain (patch; oral)
- swelling of feet and lower legs (patch; oral)
- stopping of menstrual bleeding (patch; oral)
- breakthrough menstrual bleeding (patch; oral)
- prolonged or heavy menstrual bleeding (patch; oral)
- breast lumps (patch; oral)
- breast discharge (patch; oral)
- stomach, side, or abdominal pain (patch; oral)
- yellow eyes or skin (patch; oral)

Call your doctor if these symptoms continue:

- abdominal cramping or bloating (patch; oral)
- loss of appetite (patch; oral)
- nausea (patch; oral)
- skin irritation and redness (patch)

- mild diarrhea (patch; oral)
- mild dizziness (patch; oral)
- mild headache (patch; oral)
- intolerance to wearing contact lenses (patch; oral)
- increased sexual response (patch; oral)
- migraine headaches (patch; oral)
- vomiting (patch; oral)

Periodic Tests

Ask your doctor which of these tests should be done periodically while you are taking this drug:

- breast examination
- mammogram
- Pap test
- physical examination
- endometrial biopsy
- blood pressure (patch; oral)
- liver function test (patch; oral)
- lipid levels (patch; oral)

Progestins

Limited Use

Progesterone (proe *jes* ter one)
PROMETRIUM (Solvay)

GENERIC: not available
FAMILY: Progestins

BREAST-FEEDING WARNING
Progestins are excreted in human milk. Because of the potential for adverse effects in nursing infants, you should not take these drugs while nursing.

This drug is approved by the FDA to prevent endometrial hyperplasia (changes in the cells of the lining of the uterus that may be precancerous) in women who are taking conjugated estrogens and to treat women who have amenorrhea (lack of menstruation for three months).[5]

> ## PREGNANCY WARNING
>
> The progestins have caused genital abnormalities in both male and female infants born to mothers taking these drugs during pregnancy. Because of the potential for serious adverse effects to the fetus, these drugs should not be used by pregnant women.

Progesterone belongs to a family of drugs called progestins. Progestins include synthetic modifications of naturally occurring progesterone, which are available in several forms administered by different routes and approved to treat different conditions. Prometrium, an oral capsule, is identical to human progesterone but is synthesized starting from plant sources.[5]

Progesterone should not be used in a number of situations. These include during pregnancy; in women who have blood clots or a history of having blood clots, severe liver problems, cancer of the breast or genital organs, undiagnosed vaginal bleeding, or missed abortion; or as a diagnostic test for pregnancy.

Progesterone can mask onset of menopause. It may precipitate attacks of porphyria, a rare enzyme deficiency, which is particularly prevalent among Scandinavian women. Symptoms are pain in the abdomen, arms, back, and legs and muscle weakness.

A common adverse effect is drowsiness, which may decline over time. It may cause edema (swelling of ankles and feet), which may be aggravated by epilepsy, migraine, asthma, or heart or kidney dysfunction.

There is no evidence that progesterone is effective for premenstrual syndrome (PMS).[6]

Before You Use This Drug

Do not use if you have or have had:

- abnormal and undiagnosed vaginal bleeding
- undiagnosed urinary tract bleeding

> Prometrium capsules contain peanut oil and should never be used by patients allergic to peanuts.

- breast cancer, known or suspected
- inflammation of the veins
- blood clots
- pregnancy or are breast-feeding
- allergy to progestins
- allergy to peanuts
- liver disease

Tell your doctor if you have or have had:

- asthma
- stroke
- osteoporosis
- epilepsy
- high blood pressure
- migraine headaches
- kidney disease
- liver disease
- high cholesterol levels
- mental depression or convulsions
- diabetes
- pulmonary embolism
- disease of the heart or blood vessels

Tell your doctor about any other drugs you take, including aspirin, herbs, vitamins, and other nonprescription products.

When You Use This Drug

- Have regular checkups with your doctor.
- Caution when driving or doing things requiring alertness, because progesterone may cause dizziness or drowsiness for one to four hours after dose.
- Check with your doctor immediately if breakthrough bleeding continues for longer than three months or if your period is delayed by 45 days.
- Check with your doctor immediately if you

suspect you may be pregnant or a menstrual period is missed.
- Check with your dentist if tenderness, swelling, or bleeding of gums occurs.
- Tell your doctor you are taking this drug if you are scheduled for laboratory tests, as some may be affected by taking progestins.

How to Use This Drug

- Read the patient instructions.
- If you miss a dose, take it as soon as you remember, but skip it if it is almost time for the next dose. **Do not take double doses.**
- Do not share your medication with others.
- Take the drug at the same time(s) each day.
- Store at room temperature with lid on tightly. Do not store in the bathroom. Do not expose to heat, moisture, or strong light. Keep out of reach of children.

Interactions with Other Drugs

Evaluations of Drug Interactions 2003 lists no drugs, biologics (e.g., vaccines, therapeutic antibodies), or foods as causing "highly clinically significant" or "clinically significant" interactions when used together with the drugs in this section. We also found no interactions in the drugs' FDA-approved professional package inserts. However, as the number of new drugs approved for marketing increases and as more

> **BEWARE OF COMPOUNDING PHARMACISTS**
>
> Progesterone capsules are promoted by compounding pharmacists for various uses.
>
> Drugs compounded by pharmacists are not FDA-approved. They have not been shown to be safe or effective for use and are produced in facilities that do not have to meet good manufacturing practice guidelines.

experience is gained with these drugs over time, new interactions may be discovered.

Adverse Effects

Call your doctor immediately if you experience:

- stopping of menstrual periods
- medium to heavy bleeding between regular monthly periods
- spotting (light bleeding between regular monthly periods)
- increased amount of menstrual bleeding at regular monthly periods
- unexpected or increased flow of breast milk
- mental depression
- dry mouth
- frequent urination
- loss of appetite
- unusual thirst
- skin rash
- headache or migraine
- loss of or change in speech, coordination, or vision
- pain or numbness in chest, arm, or leg
- unexplained shortness of breath, sudden and severe

Call your doctor if these symptoms continue:

- dizziness
- drowsiness
- bloating or swelling of ankles or feet
- acne
- breast pain or tenderness
- hot flashes
- trouble sleeping
- loss of sexual desire
- loss or gain of body, facial, or scalp hair
- brown spots on exposed skin
- nervousness
- unusual tiredness or weakness
- unusual or rapid weight gain
- nausea

Periodic Tests

Ask your doctor which of these tests should be done periodically while you are taking this drug:

- breast exams
- Pap test
- physical exams

Anti-Estrogens

Limited Use

Tamoxifen (ta *mox* i fen)
NOLVADEX (AstraZeneca)

GENERIC: available

FAMILY: Anti-Estrogens

PREGNANCY WARNING

Tamoxifen caused fetal harm in animal studies, including abortions, premature delivery, and death. Because of the potential for serious adverse effects to the fetus, this drug should not be used by pregnant women.

BREAST-FEEDING WARNING

No information is available from either human or animal studies. However, it is likely that this drug is excreted in human milk, and because of the potential for serious adverse effects in nursing infants, you should not take this drug while nursing.

Tamoxifen was approved by the FDA in 1977 and is now approved to be used in several different situations involving breast cancer.[8] In October 1998, the drug received approval for the reduction in breast cancer incidence in women at high risk of developing the disease. High risk was defined as a five-year predicted risk of breast cancer of at least 1.67%.

Confusion soon erupted over whether the FDA approved tamoxifen for all women 60 years of age and older, without other risk factors for breast cancer. The news media was initially reporting that regardless of other factors, all

FDA BLACK BOX WARNING

WARNING—For Women with Ductal Carcinoma in Situ (DCIS) and Women at High Risk for Breast Cancer: Serious and life-threatening events associated with NOLVADEX in the risk reduction setting (women at high risk for cancer and women with DCIS) include uterine malignancies, stroke, and pulmonary embolism. Incidence rates for these events were estimated from the NSABP P-1 trial [a major clinical trial involving tamoxifen[7]].

Uterine malignancies [cancers] consist of both endometrial adenocarcinoma (incidence rate per 1,000 women-years of 2.20 for NOLVADEX vs. 0.71 for placebo) and uterine sarcoma (incidence rate per 1,000 women-years of 0.17 for NOLVADEX vs. 0.0 for placebo). For stroke, the incidence rate per 1,000 women-years was 1.43 for NOLVADEX vs. 1.00 for placebo. For pulmonary embolism, the incidence rate per 1,000 women-years was 0.75 for NOLVADEX vs. 0.25 for placebo.

Some of the strokes, pulmonary emboli, and uterine malignancies were fatal.

Health care providers should discuss the potential benefits versus the potential risks of these serious events with women at high risk of breast cancer and women with DCIS considering NOLVADEX to reduce their risk of developing breast cancer.

The benefits of NOLVADEX outweigh its risks in women already diagnosed with breast cancer.[8]

women 60 and older were at a five-year predicted risk of 1.67% (in the high-risk category) for developing breast cancer and thus were eligible to receive tamoxifen. This is not the case: **Not all women over 60 are at a high risk of developing breast cancer and not all women over 60 should be receiving tamoxifen to reduce the risk of breast cancer.**

In June 2002, the FDA required a black-box warning, the strongest type of warning that the agency can require, on the professional product label for the drug. The warning concerns increased risk of sometimes fatal uterine cancers, stroke, and blood clots in the lungs (pulmonary embolism) in women at high risk of breast cancer who use the drug to reduce the incidence of breast cancer and in women with a form of breast cancer called ductal carcinoma in situ (DCIS). DCIS is characterized by abnormal cells that involve only the lining of a duct. Such cells have not yet spread outside the duct to other breast tissues. It is a noninvasive cancer that can become invasive in some cases.

Endometrial cancer, involving the lining of the uterus, is the most common form of cancer in this organ, accounting for approximately 95% of all uterine cancers. Uterine sarcoma is a rare cancer of the body of the uterus, accounting for 2 to 5% of all uterine cancers. Because it is usually diagnosed at a more advanced stage than other uterine tumors, women diagnosed usually have a poorer outcome and shorter survival than others.

The June 2002 labeling change was aimed at women who are considering tamoxifen as a way to reduce the incidence of breast cancer or those with DCIS for whom a survival benefit of the drug has not been demonstrated. At this time, the known benefits of tamoxifen outweigh its risks in women already diagnosed with other kinds of breast cancer.

Evidence of the risk of uterine sarcoma with tamoxifen use, leading to the FDA's black-box warning decision, came in a letter to the *New England Journal of Medicine* from FDA staff in June 2002.[9] The FDA found that between 1978, when tamoxifen was first approved in the United States, and April 2001, there were 43 cases of uterine sarcoma reported to the agency or published in the medical literature. In addition, this cancer was reported to have developed in 116 women in other countries who had used tamoxifen for breast cancer.

The large clinical trial (over 13,000 women) that was used to gain approval for tamoxifen in reducing breast cancer incidence in high-risk women compared tamoxifen to a placebo over a period of five years.[7]

The incidence of breast cancer was reduced by 2.9 cases per year out of 1,000 women using tamoxifen. However, there was an excess of 1.4 cases of endometrial cancer per year out of 1,000 women taking tamoxifen. For blood clot in the lungs, blood clot in the veins, and stroke, the number of excess cases of these serious adverse drug reactions with tamoxifen compared to placebo was 0.5, 0.5, and 0.4 cases per year out of 1,000 women taking tamoxifen, respectively. Overall, there was an excess of 2.8 cases of a potentially life-threatening adverse drug reaction per year out of 1,000 women on tamoxifen. Said another way, for each reduction of one case in the incidence of breast cancer, there was about one case of a potentially life-threatening drug reaction with the use of tamoxifen.

In this study, the benefit of tamoxifen equaled its serious risks—it was a wash. However, there was also an increased risk of cataracts and cataract surgery in women using tamoxifen.

Before You Use This Drug

Do not use if you have or have had:

- blood-clotting problems
- pregnancy or are breast-feeding

Tell your doctor if you have or have had:

- allergy to tamoxifen
- blood disorder
- cataracts or other vision problems
- high cholesterol

Tell your doctor about any other drugs you take, including aspirin, herbs, vitamins, and other nonprescription products. Ask for exams of your eyes[10] and for a test to detect endometrial cancer before you start to take tamoxifen.[11]

When You Use This Drug

- See your doctor regularly for close monitoring while taking this drug.
- Continue taking this drug even if you get an upset stomach. However, check with your doctor if vomiting occurs shortly after drug is taken.
- Take analgesics if needed for pain, which often occurs when tamoxifen is started but then subsides.
- *For women:* Tamoxifen may increase fertility. Do not become pregnant. Use barrier or nonhormonal contraceptives. Tell your doctor immediately if you suspect you are pregnant.

How to Use This Drug

- If you miss a dose, take it as soon as you remember, but skip it if it is almost time for the next dose. **Do not take double doses.**
- Do not share your medication with others.
- Take the drug at the same time(s) each day.
- Store at room temperature with lid on tightly. Do not store in the bathroom. Do not expose to heat, moisture, or strong light. Keep out of reach of children.

Interactions with Other Drugs

The following drugs, biologics (e.g., vaccines, therapeutic antibodies), or foods are listed in *Evaluations of Drug Interactions* 2003 as causing "highly clinically significant" or "clinically significant" interactions when used together with any of the drugs in this section. In some sections with multiple drugs, the interaction may have been reported for one but not all drugs in this section, but we include the interaction because the drugs in this section are similar to one another. We have also included potentially serious interactions listed in the drug's FDA-approved professional package insert or in published medical journal articles. There may be other drugs, especially those in the families of drugs listed below, that also will react with this drug to cause severe adverse effects. Make sure to tell your doctor and pharmacist the drugs you are taking and tell them if you are taking any of these interacting drugs:

aminoglutethimide, AVELOX, clopidogrel, COUMADIN, CYTADREN,[12] ESTRADERM, estrogen, moxifloxacin, NORVIR, PLAVIX, PREMARIN, ritonavir, warfarin.

Adverse Effects

Call your doctor immediately if you experience:

For both women and men:

- confusion
- blistering, peeling, or loosening of skin and mucous membranes
- blurred vision
- yellowing of skin or eyes
- shortness of breath
- swelling or pain in legs
- weakness or sleepiness

For women:

- pain or pressure in pelvis
- change in vaginal discharge
- bleeding

Call your doctor if these symptoms continue:

For both men and women:

- headache
- mild nausea or vomiting
- skin rash or dryness
- transient bone pain

For women:

- hot flashes
- weight gain
- changes in menstrual periods
- itching in genital area
- vaginal discharge

For men:

- impotence or decreased interest in sex

Periodic Tests

Ask your doctor which of these tests should be done periodically while you are taking this drug:

For both women and men:

- blood levels of calcium
- blood levels of cholesterol and triglycerides
- complete blood count
- liver function tests
- eye exams

For women:

- gynecologic examinations

For women taking the drug to reduce the risk of breast cancer:

- breast examinations
- mammograms

Hormone Combinations

Limited Use

Conjugated estrogens with medroxyprogesterone (*con* joo gay ted *ess* troe jenz with me *drox* ee proe *jes* te rone)
PREMPRO (Wyeth)
PREMPHASE (Wyeth)

GENERIC: not available

Ethinyl Estradiol with Norethindrone
(*eth* in il es tra *dye* ole with nor *eth* in drone)
FEMHRT (Warner-Chilcott)

GENERIC: available
FAMILY: Estrogen-Progestin Combinations

BREAST-FEEDING WARNING
Estrogens are excreted in breast milk and have caused adverse effects in nursing infants. These drugs may also decrease the amount and quality of breast milk. Because of the potential for adverse effects in nursing infants, you should not take these drugs while nursing.

PREGNANCY WARNING

Because of the potential for serious adverse effects to the fetus, these drugs should not be used by women with known or suspected pregnancy.

These three combination estrogen with progestin products are approved by the FDA to manage the symptoms of menopause. These drugs are also approved to prevent osteoporosis. However, estrogens are no longer approved for the treatment of osteoporosis. If they are prescribed solely for the prevention of postmenopausal osteoporosis, treatment should only be considered for women at significant risk of osteoporosis and for whom nonestrogen medications are not considered to be appropriate.[29, 30]

The mainstays for decreasing the risk of postmenopausal osteoporosis are weight-bearing exercise, adequate calcium and vitamin D intake, and, when needed, treatment with drugs. Postmenopausal women require an average of 1,500 milligrams per day of elemental calcium. Therefore, when not contraindicated, calcium supplementation may be helpful for women with suboptimal dietary intake. Vitamin D supplementation of 400–800 international units per day may also be required to ensure adequate daily intake in postmenopausal women. [29, 30]

The progestins medroxyprogesterone and norethindrone are added to the estrogen component of these products to reduce the risk of uterine cancer in women who have an intact uterus.

The Canadian Task Force on Preventive Health Care recommends "against the use of combined estrogen-progestin therapy and estrogen-only therapy for the primary prevention of chronic diseases in menopausal women." For the management of the symptoms of menopause, this task force recommends, "If the risks are acceptable to the woman and her physician, therapy of as short a duration as possible, and at as low a dose as possible, may be indicated."[3] We agree.

The North American Menopause Society (NAMS) has issued its position on the management of hot flashes in postmenopausal women. For mild hot flashes, lifestyle-related strategies such as keeping the core body temperature cool, participating in regular exercise, and using paced respiration have shown some effectiveness without adverse effects.[4]

The NAMS found that, among nonprescription remedies, clinical trial results are insufficient to either support or refute the efficacy of soy foods and isoflavone supplements (soy or red clover), black cohosh, or vitamin E for hot flashes. Single clinical trials have found no benefit for dong quai, evening primrose oil, ginseng, acupuncture, or magnet therapy.[4]

Before You Use This Drug

Do not use if you have or have had:

- pregnancy or are breast-feeding
- allergy to estrogens or progestins
- abnormal or undiagnosed vaginal bleeding
- severe liver disease, including liver tumors
- high level of calcium in your blood
- breast cancer
- known or suspected cancer that is estrogen dependent
- vein inflammation
- blood-clotting disorder

Tell your doctor if you have or have had:

- asthma
- heart problems
- epilepsy
- high blood pressure
- migraine headaches
- severe kidney disease
- diabetes
- endometriosis
- gallbladder or gallstone problems
- liver disease
- jaundice
- porphyria
- high cholesterol

ESTROGENS INCREASE THE RISK OF BREAST CANCER, CARDIOVASCULAR DISEASE, AND DEMENTIA

Estrogens with or without progestins should not be used for the prevention of cardiovascular disease, since the best evidence is that they increase the risk of cardivascular disease.

The Women's Health Initiative (WHI) study reported increased risks of myocardial infarction, stroke, invasive breast cancer, pulmonary emboli, and deep vein thrombosis in postmenopausal women (50 to 79 years of age) during five years of treatment with conjugated estrogens (0.625 milligrams) combined with medroxyprogesterone acetate (2.5 milligrams) relative to placebo.

The Women's Health Initiative Memory Study (WHIMS), a substudy of WHI, reported increased risk of developing probable dementia in postmenopausal women 65 years of age or older during four years of treatment with conjugated estrogens plus medroxyprogesterone acetate relative to placebo. It is unknown whether this finding applies to younger postmenopausal women or to women taking estrogen-alone therapy.

Other doses of conjugated estrogens and medroxyprogesterone acetate, and other combinations and dosage forms of estrogens and progestins, were not studied in the WHI clinical trials, and in the absence of comparable data, these risks should be assumed to be similar. Because of these risks, estrogens with or without progestins should be prescribed at the lowest effective doses and for the shortest duration consistent with treatment goals and risks for the individual woman.

- pancreas disease
- fibroids in uterus
- blood-clotting disorder
- inflammation of veins
- stroke or circulatory brain disorder
- clot in lungs
- clot in eyes

When You Use This Drug

- See your doctor at least once a year.
- Do breast self-exams.
- Tell your doctor if you find any unusual breast lumps or discharge.
- Menstrual bleeding may begin again, but with continuous therapy it will stop by 10 months.
- Vaginal bleeding between menstrual periods will occur for the first three months after starting this drug; do not stop taking the drug. However, you should check with your doctor immediately if vaginal bleeding is unusual or continuous, if you miss a period, or you think you are pregnant.
- If you are scheduled for any lab tests, tell your doctor that you are taking this drug.

How to Use This Drug

- Read the patient directions.
- If you miss a dose, take it as soon as you remember, but skip it if it is almost time for the next dose. **Do not take double doses.**
- Do not share your medication with others.
- Take the drug at the same time(s) each day.
- If taking combination therapy, take each drug at the right time.
- *For conjugated estrogens with medroxyprogesterone:* Take with food if nausea occurs, especially for the first few weeks after starting this drug.
- Store at room temperature with lid on tightly. Do not store in the bathroom. Do not expose to heat, moisture, or strong light. Keep out of reach of children.

Interactions with Other Drugs

The following drugs, biologics (e.g., vaccines, therapeutic antibodies), or foods are listed in *Evaluations of Drug Interactions* 2003 as causing "highly clinically significant" or "clinically

significant" interactions when used together with any of the drugs in this section. In some sections with multiple drugs, the interaction may have been reported for one but not all drugs in this section, but we include the interaction because the drugs in this section are similar to one another. We have also included potentially serious interactions listed in the drug's FDA-approved professional package insert or in published medical journal articles. There may be other drugs, especially those in the families of drugs listed below, that also will react with this drug to cause severe adverse effects. Make sure to tell your doctor and pharmacist the drugs you are taking and tell them if you are taking any of these interacting drugs:

EVISTA, nelfinavir, NORVIR, raloxifene, ritonavir, VIRACEPT.

Adverse Effects

Call your doctor immediately if you experience:

- sudden loss of coordination (ethinyl estradiol with norethindrone acetate)
- chest, leg, or groin pain (ethinyl estradiol with norethindrone acetate)
- no menstrual period (conjugated estrogens with medroxyprogesterone)
- breast pain or tenderness (ethinyl estradiol with norethindrone acetate)

BEWARE OF COMPOUNDING PHARMACISTS SELLING BIOIDENTICAL HORMONE REPLACEMENT THERAPIES, CLAIMING THAT THEY ARE SAFE

Pharmacy compound products are not approved by the FDA and their quality is questionable, as they are not produced in facilities meeting good manufacturing practice (GMP) guidelines.

- high blood pressure (ethinyl estradiol with norethindrone acetate)
- dizziness or lightheadedness (ethinyl estradiol with norethindrone acetate)
- headache, severe and sudden (ethinyl estradiol with norethindrone acetate)
- swelling of feet and lower legs (ethinyl estradiol with norethindrone acetate)
- rapid weight gain (ethinyl estradiol with norethindrone acetate)
- cough, fever, sneezing, or sore throat (ethinyl estradiol with norethindrone acetate)
- change in menstrual period, including menstruating at the wrong time, change in amount of flow, breakthrough bleeding, or spotting (conjugated estrogens with medroxyprogesterone)
- vaginal bleeding (ethinyl estradiol with norethindrone acetate)
- pelvic pain or pressure (ethinyl estradiol with norethindrone acetate)
- vaginal itching or irritation
- thick, white vaginal discharge (conjugated estrogens with medroxyprogesterone)
- change in vaginal discharge (ethinyl estradiol with norethindrone acetate)
- nausea or vomiting (ethinyl estradiol with norethindrone acetate)
- breast lumps
- breast discharge
- skin rash (conjugated estrogens with medroxyprogesterone)
- yellow eyes or skin
- stomach, side, or abdomen pain or tenderness
- sudden shortness of breath (ethinyl estradiol with norethindrone acetate)
- sudden slurred speech (ethinyl estradiol with norethindrone acetate)
- sudden vision changes (ethinyl estradiol with norethindrone acetate)
- weakness or numbness in arm or leg (ethinyl estradiol with norethindrone acetate)

Call your doctor if these symptoms continue:

- abdominal pain or cramping (conjugated estrogens with medroxyprogesterone)
- joint or back pain
- flulike symptoms (ethinyl estradiol with norethindrone acetate)
- breast enlargement, pain, or tenderness (conjugated estrogens with medroxyprogesterone)
- diarrhea (conjugated estrogens with medroxyprogesterone)
- dizziness
- stomach discomfort following meals (conjugated estrogens with medroxyprogesterone)
- painful menstrual periods (conjugated estrogens with medroxyprogesterone)
- passing of gas
- increase in amount of clear, vaginal discharge (conjugated estrogens with medroxyprogesterone)
- vaginal discharge (ethinyl estradiol with norethindrone acetate)
- mental depression
- nausea
- itching
- unusual tiredness
- headaches
- tense or aching muscles
- increase in sexual desire (conjugated estrogens with medroxyprogesterone)
- bloating or swelling of face, ankles, or feet (conjugated estrogens with medroxyprogesterone)
- unusual weight gain or loss (conjugated estrogens with medroxyprogesterone)
- mood changes or nervousness (conjugated estrogens with medroxyprogesterone)
- trouble sleeping
- vomiting (conjugated estrogens with medroxyprogesterone)

Signs of overdose (ethinyl estradiol with norethindrone acetate):

- nausea or vomiting
- having a menstrual period

If you suspect an overdose, call this number to contact your poison control center: (800) 222-1222.

Periodic Tests

Ask your doctor which of these tests should be done periodically while you are taking this drug:

- blood pressure measurements
- physical exam
- breast exam or mammogram
- evaluation of endometrium (mucous membrane lining the uterus)
- liver function tests
- cholesterol levels
- Pap test

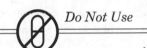

Do Not Use

ALTERNATIVE TREATMENT:
See conjugated estrogens, p. 762.

Esterified Estrogens with Methyltestosterone
(ess *terr* i fyed *ess* tro jenz with *meth* yl tes *toss* ter one)
ESTRATEST, ESTRATEST H.S. (Solvay)

FAMILY: Estrogen-Androgen Combinations

On April 10, 2003, the FDA announced that it was beginning legal procedures to remove the marketing authorizations for combination drug products containing estrogen and androgen, female and male hormones, respectively. Estrogen and androgen combination products had been approved for the treatment of moderate to severe "hot flashes" (vasomotor symptoms) associated with menopause in women whose symptoms were not improved by estrogen alone.

The only estrogen-androgen combination product remaining on the U.S. market is esterified estrogens with methyltestosterone (ESTRATEST, ESTRATEST H.S.).

FDA BLACK BOX WARNINGS

1. Estrogens have been reported to increase the risk of endometrial carcinoma.

Three independent case control studies have reported an increased risk of endometrial cancer in postmenopausal women exposed to exogenous estrogens for prolonged periods.[13–15] This risk was independent of the other known risk factors for endometrial cancer. These studies are further supported by the finding that incidence rates of endometrial cancer have increased sharply since 1969 in eight different areas of the United States with population-based cancer reporting systems, an increase which may be related to the rapidly expanding use of estrogens during the last decade.[16]

The three case control studies reported that the risk of endometrial cancer in estrogen users was about 4.5 to 13.9 times greater than in nonusers. The risk appears to depend on both duration of treatment[13] and on estrogen dose.[15] In view of these findings, when estrogens are used for the treatment of menopausal symptoms, the lowest dose that will control symptoms should be utilized and medication should be discontinued as soon as possible. When prolonged treatment is medically indicated, the patient should be reassessed on at least a semiannual basis to determine the need for continued therapy. Although the evidence must be considered preliminary, one study suggests that cyclic administration of low doses of estrogen may carry less risk than continuous administration;[15] it therefore appears prudent to utilize such a regimen.

Close clinical surveillance of all women taking estrogens is important. In all cases of undiagnosed persistent or recurring abnormal vaginal bleeding, adequate diagnostic measures should be undertaken to rule out malignancy. There is no evidence at present that "natural" estrogens are more or less hazardous than "synthetic" estrogens at equiestrogenic doses.

2. Estrogens should not be used during pregnancy.

The use of female sex hormones, both estrogens and progestogens, during early pregnancy may seriously damage the offspring. It has been shown that females exposed in utero to diethylstilbestrol, a non-steroidal estrogen, have an increased risk of developing in later life a form of vaginal or cervical cancer that is ordinarily extremely rare.[17,18] This risk has been estimated as not greater than 4 per 1000 exposures.[19] Furthermore, a high percentage of such exposed women (from 30 to 90 percent) have been found to have vaginal adenosis,[20–24] epithelial changes of the vagina and cervix. Although these changes are histologically benign, it is not known whether they are precursors of malignancy. Although similar data are not available with the use of other estrogens, it cannot be presumed they would not induce similar changes.

Several reports suggest an association between intrauterine exposure to female sex hormones and congenital anomalies, including congenital heart defects and limb reduction defects.[25–28] One case control study[28] estimated a 4.7-fold increased risk of limb reduction defects in infants exposed in utero to sex hormones (oral contraceptives, hormone withdrawal tests for pregnancy, or attempted treatment for threatened abortion). Some of these exposures were very short and involved only a few days of treatment. The data suggest that the risk of limb reduction defects in exposed fetuses is somewhat less than 1 per 1000.

In the past, female sex hormones have been used during pregnancy in an attempt to treat threatened or habitual abortion. There is considerable evidence that estrogens are ineffective for these indications, and there is no evidence from well controlled studies that progestogens are effective for these uses.

If ESTRATEST or ESTRATEST H.S. is used during pregnancy, or if the patient becomes pregnant while taking this drug, she should be apprised of the potential risks to the fetus, and the advisability of pregnancy continuation.

(continued on p. 777)

(continued from p. 776)

3. Cardiovascular and other risks.

ESTRATEST® and ESTRATEST® H.S. Tablets do not contain a progestin. ESTRATEST® and ESTRATEST® H.S. Tablets are an Estrogen/Androgen product.

Estrogens with or without progestins should not be used for the prevention of cardiovascular disease.

The Women's Health Initiative (WHI) study reported increased risks of myocardial infarction, stroke, invasive breast cancer, pulmonary emboli, and deep vein thrombosis in postmenopausal women during 5 years of treatment with conjugated equine estrogens (CE 0.625 mg) combined with medroxyprogesterone acetate (MPA 2.5 mg) relative to placebo. Other doses of conjugated estrogens with medroxyprogesterone and other combinations of estrogens and progestins were not studied in the WHI and, in the absence of comparable data, these risks should be assumed to be similar. Because of these risks, estrogens with or without progestins should be prescribed at the lowest effective doses and for the shortest duration consistent with treatment goals and risks for the individual woman.

Estrogen-only drugs are approved for the treatment of moderate to severe hot flashes associated with menopause. The FDA is taking this action because it no longer believes that there is substantial evidence that androgens contribute to the effectiveness of these combination products in treating hot flashes in menopausal women who do not find relief from these symptoms when using estrogens alone.

The legal standard for approving a drug in the United States is substantial evidence that the drug is safe and effective for its intended use. The standard used for approving combination products is that the combination must be shown to be more effective than the individual ingredients. The weight of the evidence now shows that estrogen-androgen combination drugs are not superior to estrogen in reducing the vasomotor symptoms of menopause.

If the androgen in estrogen-androgen combination products does not result in a benefit for women, then all that is left from the androgen are its risks, and these risks are not insignificant. The FDA's thinking at this time is that androgen can reverse the favorable impact of estrogen on cholesterol and triglycerides (fats in the blood). Androgen is also associated with abnormal hairiness, acne, deepening of the voice, and hair loss in women.

We agree with the FDA's decision to remove the marketing authorizations for combination drug products containing estrogen and androgen; however, the issue over the effectiveness of these combinations goes back for decades, and this action by the FDA is long overdue.

The FDA has had a long-standing policy to allow the continued marketing of drug products while matters such as these are being resolved, provided there is no documented serious public health or safety issue associated with such products. In our opinion this policy is irresponsible. It is pro-business, not pro–public health and safety. There is no justification for leaving products on the market when there are questions of effectiveness, as with the estrogen-androgen combinations.

You should consult your physician if you are now using an estrogen-androgen combination product to control the vasomotor symptoms of menopause.

Do not succumb to promotions of compounding pharmacists, and the physicians that work with them, who claim the estrogen and androgen products they prepare in their back rooms are effective and without adverse effects.

REFERENCES

1. Cenestin (Synthetic Conjugated Estrogens, A) Professional Product Labeling, February 1, 2004. Available at: http://www.cenestin.com/pi.html. Accessed May 19, 2004.

2. Premarin (Conjugated Estrogens) Professional Product Labeling, March 28, 2004. Available at: http://www.wyeth.com/content/ShowLabeling.asp?id=131. Accessed May 19, 2004.

3. Wathen CN, Feig DS, Feightner JW, et al. Hormone replacement therapy for the primary prevention of chronic diseases: Recommendation statement from the Canadian Task Force on Preventive Health Care. *Canadian Medical Association Journal* 2004; 170:1535–7.

4. Treatment of menopause-associated vasomotor symptoms: Position statement of The North American Menopause Society. *Menopause* 2004; 11:11–33.

5. *Physicians' Desk Reference.* 58th ed. Montvale, N.J.: Thomson PDR, 2004: 3170–3.

6. *USP-DI, Drug Information for the Health Care Professional.* 23rd ed. Rockville, Md.: Thomson PDR, 2004.

7. Fisher B, Costantino JP, Wickerham DL, et al. Tamoxifen for prevention of breast cancer: Report of the National Surgical Adjuvant Breast and Bowel Project P-1 Study. *Journal of the National Cancer Institute* 1998; 90:1371–88.

8. Nolvadex (Tamoxifen) Professional Product Labeling, June 1, 2003. Available at: http://www.nolvadex.com/consumer/home.asp. Accessed May 23, 2004.

9. Wysowski DK, Honig SF, Beitz J. Uterine sarcoma associated with tamoxifen use. *New England Journal of Medicine* 2002; 346:1832–3.

10. Nayfield SG, Gorin MB. Tamoxifen-associated eye disease. A review. *Journal of Clinical Oncology* 1996; 14:1018–26.

11. Jordan VC. An overview of considerations for the testing of tamoxifen as a preventive for breast cancer. *Annals of the New York Academy of Sciences* 1995; 768:141–7.

12. Hansten PD, Horn JR. *Hansten and Horn's Drug Interactions, Analysis and Management.* Vancouver, Wash.: Applied Therapeutics, 1997:26.

13. Ziel HK, Finkle WD. Increased risk of endometrial carcinoma among users of conjugated estrogens. *New England Journal of Medicine* 1975; 293:1167–70.

14. Smith DC, Prentice R, Thompson DJ, et al. Association of exogenous estrogen and endometrial carcinoma. *New England Journal of Medicine* 1975; 293:1164–7.

15. Mack TM, Pike MC, Henderson BE, et al. Estrogens and endometrial cancer in a retirement community. *New England Journal of Medicine* 1976; 294:1262–7.

16. Weiss NS, Szekely DR, Austin DF. Increasing incidence of endometrial cancer in the United States. *New England Journal of Medicine* 1976; 294:1259–62.

17. Herbst AL, Ulfelder H, Poskanzer DC. Adenocarcinoma of the vagina. Association of maternal stilbestrol therapy with tumor appearance in young women. *New England Journal of Medicine* 1971; 284:878–81.

18. Greenwald P, Barlow JJ, Nasca PC, et al. Vaginal cancer after maternal treatment with synthetic estrogens. *New England Journal of Medicine* 1971; 285:390–2.

19. Lanier AP, Noller KL, Decker DG, et al. Cancer and stilbestrol. A follow-up of 1,719 persons exposed to estrogens in utero and born 1943–1959. *Mayo Clinic Proceedings* 1973; 48:793–9.

20. Stafl A, Mattingly RF, Foley DV, et al. Clinical diagnosis of vaginal adenosis. *Obstetrics and Gynecology* 1974; 43:118–28.

21. Herbst AL, Poskanzer DC, Robboy SJ, et al. Prenatal exposure to stilbestrol. A prospective comparison of exposed female offspring with unexposed controls. *New England Journal of Medicine* 1975; 292:334–9.

22. Herbst AL, Robboy SJ, Macdonald GJ, et al. The effects of local progesterone on stilbestrol-associated vaginal adenosis. *American Journal of Obstetrics and Gynecology* 1974; 118:607–15.

23. Herbst AL, Kurman RJ, Scully RE. Vaginal and cervical abnormalities after exposure to stilbestrol in utero. *Obstetrics and Gynecology* 1972; 40:287–98.

24. Sherman AI, Goldrath M, Berlin A, et al. Cervical-vaginal adenosis after in utero exposure to synthetic estrogens. *Obstetrics and Gynecology* 1974; 44:531–45.

25. Gal I, Kirman B, Stern J. Hormonal pregnancy tests and congenital malformation. *Nature* 1967; 216:83.

26. Levy EP, Cohen A, Fraser FC. Hormone treatment during pregnancy and congenital heart defects. *The Lancet* 1973; 1:611.

27. Nora JJ, Nora AH. Birth defects and oral contraceptives. *The Lancet* 1973; 1:941–2.

28. Janerich DT, Piper JM, Glebatis DM. Oral contraceptives and congenital limb-reduction defects. *New England Journal of Medicine* 1974; 291:697–700.

29. Conjugated Estrogens with Medroxyprogesterone (Prempro, Premphase) Professional Product Labeling, 2004. Available at: http://www.wyeth.com/content/ShowLabeling.asp?id=133. Accessed May 27, 2004.

30. Ethinyl Estradiol with Norethindrone (FEMHRT) Professional Product Labeling, January 5, 2004. Available at: http://www.fda.gov/cder/foi/label/2004/21065slr009_femhrt_lbl.pdf. Accessed May 27, 2004.

26

DRUGS FOR SMOKING CESSATION

YOU CAN QUIT SMOKING

There is no question that smoking involves a physical addiction to nicotine as well as psychological "addiction" to the patterns of smoking in certain circumstances or situations. Unless attention is paid to both of these kinds of addiction, the chance of success in stopping smoking will not be as good as it could be.

An informative government pamphlet entitled "You Can Quit Smoking" is available online at http://surgeongeneral.gov/tobacco/quits.pdf or by calling toll-free (800) 358-9295. In addition to the information in the drug profiles on specific smoking cessation products, we are reprinting significant portions of the pamphlet below.

Nicotine: A Powerful Addiction

If you have tried to quit smoking, you know how hard it can be. It is hard because nicotine is a very addictive drug. For some people, it can be as addictive as heroin or cocaine. Quitting is hard. Usually people make 2 or 3 tries, or more, before finally being able to quit. Each time you try to quit, you can learn about what helps and what hurts.

QUITTING TAKES HARD WORK AND A LOT OF EFFORT, BUT—YOU CAN QUIT SMOKING.

Good Reasons for Quitting

Quitting smoking is one of the most important things you will ever do:

- You will live longer and live better.
- Quitting will lower your chance of having a heart attack, stroke, or cancer.
- If you are pregnant, quitting smoking will improve your chances of having a healthy baby.
- The people you live with, especially your children, will be healthier.
- You will have extra money to spend on things other than cigarettes.

Five Keys for Quitting

Studies have shown that these five steps will help you quit and quit for good. You have the best chances of quitting if you use them together:

1. Get ready.
2. Get support.
3. Learn new skills and behaviors.
4. Get medication and use it correctly.
5. Be prepared for relapse or difficult situations.

1. Get Ready

Set a quit date.
Change your environment.
—Get rid of ALL cigarettes and ashtrays in your home, car, and place of work.
—Don't let people smoke in your home.
Review your past attempts to quit. Think about what worked and what did not.
Once you quit, don't smoke—NOT EVEN A PUFF!

2. Get Support and Encouragement

Studies have shown that you have a better chance of being successful if you have help. You can get support in many ways: Tell your family, friends, and coworkers that you are going to quit and want their support. Ask them not to smoke around you or leave cigarettes out. Talk to your health care provider (for example, doctor, dentist, nurse, pharmacist, psychologist, or smoking counselor).

Get individual, group, or telephone counseling. The more counseling you have, the better your chances are of quitting. Programs are given at local hospitals and health centers. Call your local health department for information about programs in your area.

3. Learn New Skills and Behaviors

Try to distract yourself from urges to smoke. Talk to someone, go for a walk, or get busy with a task. When you first try to quit, change your routine. Use a different route to work. Drink tea instead of coffee. Eat breakfast in a different place. Do something to reduce your stress. Take a hot bath, exercise, or read a book. Plan something enjoyable to do every day. Drink a lot of water and other fluids.

4. Get Medication and Use It Correctly

Medications can help you stop smoking and lessen the urge to smoke. The U.S. Food and Drug Administration (FDA) has approved five medications to help you quit smoking:
—Bupropion SR—available by prescription
—Nicotine gum—available over-the-counter
—Nicotine inhaler—available by prescription
—Nicotine nasal spray—available by prescription
—Nicotine patch—available by prescription and over-the-counter

Ask your health care provider for advice and carefully read the information on the package. All of these medications will more or less double your chances of quitting and quitting for good. Everyone who is trying to quit may benefit from using a medication. If you are pregnant or trying to become pregnant, nursing, under age 18, smoking fewer than 10 cigarettes per day, or have a medical condition, talk to your doctor or other health care provider before taking medications.

5. Be Prepared for Relapse or Difficult Situations

Most relapses occur within the first three months after quitting. Don't be discouraged if you start smoking again. Remember, most people try several times before they finally quit. Here are some difficult situations to watch for.

Alcohol. Avoid drinking alcohol. Drinking lowers your chances of success.

Other smokers. Being around smoking can make you want to smoke.

Weight gain. Many smokers will gain weight when they quit, usually less than 10 pounds. Eat a healthy diet and stay active. Don't let weight gain distract you from your main goal—quitting smoking. Some quit-smoking medications may help delay weight gain.

Bad mood or depression. There are a lot of ways to improve your mood other than smoking. If you are having problems with any of these situations, talk to your doctor or other health care provider.

Special Situations or Conditions

Studies suggest that everyone can quit smoking. Your situation or condition can give you a special reason to quit.

Pregnant women / new mothers: By quitting, you protect your baby's health and your own.

Hospitalized patients: By quitting, you reduce health problems and help healing.

Heart attack patients: By quitting, you reduce your risk of a second heart attack.

Lung, head, and neck cancer patients: By quitting, you reduce your chance of a second cancer.

Parents of children and adolescents: By quitting, you protect your children and adolescents from illnesses caused by second-hand smoke.

Questions to Think About

Think about the following questions before you try to stop smoking. You may want to talk about your answers with your health care provider.

1. Why do you want to quit?

2. When you tried to quit in the past, what helped and what didn't?

3. What will be the most difficult situations for you after you quit? How will you plan to handle them?

4. Who can help you through the tough times? Your family? Friends? Health care provider?

5. What pleasures do you get from smoking? What ways can you still get pleasure if you quit?

Here are some questions to ask your health care provider.

1. How can you help me to be successful at quitting?

2. What medication do you think would be best for me and how should I take it?

3. What should I do if I need more help?

4. What is smoking withdrawal like? How can I get information on withdrawal?

DRUG PROFILES

Nicotine Products

Limited Use

Nicotine (*nick* o teen)
HABITROL (Novartis)
NICODERM (Aventis)
NICORETTE (GlaxoSmithKline)
NICOTROL (Pharmacia & Upjohn)
PROSTEP (Aveva)

GENERIC: available
FAMILY: Nicotine Products

PREGNANCY WARNING

Because smoking is extremely dangerous to the developing fetus, the safest thing you can do is not smoke while pregnant (or afterward). Educational and behavioral methods to quit smoking are the best choice. If you cannot stop smoking on your own, use this medicine, if advised to do so by your doctor.

BREAST-FEEDING WARNING

No information is available from either human or animal studies. However, since nicotine is excreted into breast milk and could harm your infant, you should consult with your doctor if you are planning to nurse.

Nicotine, whether in a patch, gum, inhaler, or nasal spray, is used to assist in quitting smoking. This is the same nicotine found in tobacco, pesticides, and some foods. In these products, nicotine serves as a temporary aid to giving up smoking by reducing physical withdrawal symptoms. However, unless the nicotine product is accompanied by a smoking cessation program, the drug works no better than a placebo,[1] because it is treating only the physical, not the psychological addiction.

Withdrawal signs from smoking include fatigue, headache, slowed heart rate, hunger, difficulty concentrating, irritability, and dreams about smoking. These symptoms start about

---

WARNING

Nicotine has only been shown to be effective when used as an aid to a comprehensive smoking cessation program. Since the above products contain nicotine, do not continue to smoke while using them.

---

two hours after the last cigarette, increase for 24 hours, then decrease over several days or weeks.[2] Signs of withdrawal do not require medical attention. Even people who have severe withdrawal are able to quit successfully.[3,4]

Aids are simple to use and can lull you into unrealistic expectations. To be effective, the use of nicotine products must be accompanied by changes in behavior. Set a quit date, learn ways to cope with urges to smoke (particularly in the morning, with company, and in response to advertising), and plan ways to cope with relapses.[5] Learn how to deal with anger, anxiety, depression, stress, and tension without smoking. People who smoke are more apt to have a history of being depressed.[6] In addition, those who are anxious or depressed tend to have severe withdrawal.[3,7] Without learning these coping skills, the patch does not work any better than a nonmedicated Band-Aid. While these aids eliminate smoke, they still contain nicotine. If you continue to smoke while using nicotine replacements, you risk serious heart disease.[1] Success rates of stopping smoking by using nicotine replacements are low, especially after six months or a year.[8-13] However, smokers who try slow withdrawal are apt to smoke less if they do resume smoking.[2,13]

Nicotine gum continues to satisfy and reinforce oral habits and may lessen weight gain.[14] The gum is harder and thicker than regular chewing gums and can loosen dental work. Not everyone masters the chewing technique. Patches are easier to use. The 16-hour patch mimics patterns of smoking, but the 24-hour patches may get you through the strong urge to smoke in the morning. Both types can irritate your skin. Overall, the various patches do not differ in the rate of people who quit smoking.[15-17]

You must also gradually stop using nicotine-containing products to prevent addiction to these nicotine products. Quitting smoking reduces your chances of bronchitis, cancers (especially of the lung, mouth, throat, and voice box), emphysema, heart disease, duodenal ulcers, and dulled sense of smell and taste. People who smoke and take psychotropic drugs often require higher doses of the nicotine and are more apt to have serious adverse effects from the psychotropic drugs, such as akathisia (involuntary restlessness, such as rocking from foot to foot).[18,19] Typically, the amount of weight gain after stopping smoking is a minimal health risk compared to the risks of smoking.[14]

Although most people quit smoking without the aid of organized programs, we recommend such a program, especially if you are using these products. Nicotine replacement is not appropriate for light smokers. A number of nonprescription aids to smoking cessation are also available, including plain chewing gum. According to one study, these work just as well as nicotine replacements for light smokers, in the absence of a comprehensive smoking cessation program.[20] These also are only temporary aids and must be augmented by changes in behavior to be successful.

Before You Use This Drug

Do not use if you have or have had:

- allergy or hypersensitivity to nicotine
- allergy or hypersensitivity to menthol (nicotine inhaler)
- severe or worsening angina
- life-threatening heart rhythm problems
- recent heart attack
- recent stroke
- pregnancy (nicotine inhaler)

- chronic nasal disorders (nicotine nasal spray)
  - allergy
  - nasal polyps
  - stuffy nose
  - sinus problems

Tell your doctor if you have or have had:

- pregnancy or are breast-feeding
- allergies to drugs
- angina
- heart problems
- Buerger's disease
- Prinzmetal's angina
- Raynaud's disease
- asthma
- chronic obstructive pulmonary disease (nicotine inhaler)
- diabetes
- hyperthyroidism
- pheochromocytoma
- liver problems
- high blood pressure
- peptic ulcer
- common cold (nicotine nasal spray)
- stuffy nose (nicotine nasal spray)
- dental problems (nicotine gum)
- temporomandibular (TMJ) disorder (nicotine gum)
- esophagitis (nicotine gum)
- throat or mouth inflammation (nicotine gum)
- skin disease (nicotine patch)

Tell your doctor about any other drugs you take, including aspirin, herbs, vitamins, and other nonprescription products.

When You Use This Drug

For all forms of nicotine replacement therapy:

- Do not smoke.
- Do not use during pregnancy.
- Participate in a smoking cessation program.

- Read patient directions carefully before using.

For nicotine inhaler:

- Gradually reduce use of the nicotine inhaler by keeping a record and showing that daily usage is being reduced.
- Do not use for more than six months.

For nicotine nasal spray:

- Continue use of spray for at least one week to adapt to the irritant effects of the spray.
- Taper off use of spray by using only half a dose at a time.
- Skip doses by not medicating every hour.
- Gradually reduce use of the nicotine spray by keeping a record and showing that daily usage is being reduced.
- Set a date for stopping use of spray.
- Do not use for more than three months.
- Avoid contact with skin, mouth, eyes, and ears.

For nicotine gum:

- Do not chew more than 24 pieces a day.
- Do not use for more than six months.
- Reduce number of pieces of nicotine gum chewed each day over a two- to three-month period.
- Do not use if you experience excessive sticking of gum to dental work.
- Carry nicotine gum at all times during therapy.
- Use hard sugarless candy between doses of nicotine gum to help alleviate urge to smoke.

For nicotine patch:

- Do not use for more than 12 weeks. Consult with your doctor if you need the patch for a longer time.
- If you get abnormal dreams, remove the patch at bedtime and put a new one on when you awake the next day.
- Call your doctor if you have an allergic reaction; do not apply a new patch. If you do have

an allergic reaction to the patch, you could also have a similar reaction to cigarettes or other products containing nicotine.

How to Use This Drug

- **Do not take double doses.**
- Do not share your medication with others.

For nicotine nasal spray:

- Avoid contact of spray with skin, mouth, eyes, and ears.
- Store at room temperature with lid on tightly. Do not store in the bathroom. Do not expose to heat, moisture, or strong light. Keep out of reach of children.

For nicotine gum:

- Use gum only when there is an urge to smoke.
- Chew gum slowly and intermittently for 30 minutes.
- Chew gum several times, then "park" it between cheek and gums; chew again after tingling sensation subsides.
- Do not chew too fast.
- Do not chew more than one piece of gum at a time.
- Do not chew more than one piece within an hour.
- Do not drink acidic beverages (citrus juices, coffee, soft drinks, or tea) within 15 minutes before or while chewing gum.

For nicotine patch:

- Keep patch in sealed pouch until ready to apply to skin.
- Do not trim or cut patch.
- Apply to clean, dry, healthy skin on upper arm or torso that is free of oil, hair, scars, cuts, burns, or irritation.
- Press patch firmly in place with palm of hand for about 10 seconds, making sure there is good contact around the edges.
- Keep patch on during showering, bathing, or swimming.
- Replace patch if it falls off.
- Wash hands with plain water after handling patches; do not use soap.
- Alternate application sites.
- Do not keep patch on for more than 24 hours.
- After patch removal, fold used patch in half with adhesive sides together and replace in protective pouch.
- Remove patch during strenuous exercise to prevent increased nicotine absorption.

Interactions with Other Drugs

Evaluations of Drug Interactions 2003 lists no drugs, biologics (e.g., vaccines, therapeutic antibodies), or foods as causing "highly clinically significant" or "clinically significant" interactions when used together with the drugs in this section. We also found no interactions in the drugs' FDA-approved professional package inserts. However, as the number of new drugs approved for marketing increases and as more experience is gained with these drugs over time, new interactions may be discovered.

Adverse Effects

Call your doctor immediately if you experience:

- injury or irritation to mouth, teeth, or dental work (nicotine gum)
- feelings of physical dependence
- joint pain
- muscle pain
- swelling of gums, mouth, or tongue
- tingling in arms, legs, hands, or feet
- confusion
- nasal blister or ulcer (nasal spray)
- numbness of nose or mouth (nasal spray)
- difficulty swallowing
- throat dryness or pain

- burning, tingling, or prickly sensations in nose, mouth, or head
- amnesia
- bronchitis
- bronchospasm
- difficulty speaking
- swelling of feet or lower legs
- blood-containing blisters on skin
- fever
- chills
- headache or migraine headache
- nausea or vomiting
- runny nose
- shortness of breath
- chest tightness
- difficulty breathing
- wheezing
- skin rash or redness
- itching
- hives
- tearing of eyes
- fast heartbeat
- irregular heartbeat
- high blood pressure

Call your doctor if these symptoms continue:

- difficulty sleeping
- abnormal dreams
- vomiting
- dizziness or lightheadedness
- increased appetite
- cough
- indigestion
- headache
- earache
- mouth and throat irritation
- stuffy nose
- runny nose
- nosebleed
- sneezing
- sinus problems
- back pain
- change in sense of taste
- diarrhea

- constipation
- watery eyes
- burning or irritation in eyes
- abdominal pain
- acne
- change in sense of smell
- menstrual problems
- facial flushing
- gum problems
- hoarseness
- itching
- vision changes
- dry mouth
- increased sputum production
- fever
- flatulence
- flulike symptoms
- hiccups
- nausea
- general pain
- pain in jaw and back
- sensation of burning, numbness, tightness, tingling, warmth, or heat
- tooth disorder
- drowsiness
- loss of appetite
- muscle or joint pain
- sweating
- irritability or nervousness

For nicotine nasal spray:

- Contact physician if nasal irritant effects of spray do not go away after one week.

For nicotine gum:

- belching
- increased mouth watering
- jaw muscle ache

For nicotine patch:

- redness, itching, or burning at application site

Call your doctor if these symptoms continue after you stop taking this drug:

- anxiety
- dizziness
- feelings of drug dependence
- mental depression
- muscle pain
- difficulty sleeping
- unusual tiredness or weakness

Signs of overdose:

- abdominal pain
- slow, fast, or irregular heartbeat
- cold sweat
- confusion
- difficulty breathing
- respiratory failure
- heart failure
- diarrhea
- disturbed hearing or vision
- dizziness
- extreme exhaustion
- headache
- low blood pressure
- nausea or vomiting
- pale skin
- excessive salivation
- seizures
- tremors
- weakness
- fainting

If you suspect an overdose, call this number to contact your poison control center: (800) 222-1222.

Other Drugs for Smoking Cessation

Limited Use

Bupropion (byu *pro* pee on)
ZYBAN (Glaxo Wellcome)

GENERIC: not available
FAMILY: Other Drugs for Smoking Cessation

PREGNANCY WARNING

Because smoking is extremely dangerous to the developing fetus, the safest thing you can do is not smoke while pregnant (or afterward). Educational and behavioral methods to quit smoking are the first choice. If you cannot stop smoking on your own, use this medicine, if advised to do so by your doctor. However, bupropion crosses the placenta, exposing the fetus to the drug. Tell your doctor if you are pregnant or thinking of becoming pregnant before you take this drug.

BREAST-FEEDING WARNING

Bupropion and its metabolites are excreted at high levels in human milk and have caused serious adverse reactions, including seizures, in the infant. Because of the potential for adverse effects in nursing infants, you should not take this drug while nursing.

Because the use of bupropion is associated with an increased risk of seizures, doses over 300 milligrams per day for smoking cessation should not be used. The risk of seizures is also related to patient factors, clinical situation, and other drugs that are being taken together with bupropion, which must be considered in selection of patients for treatment with this drug. Bupropion should be discontinued and not restarted in patients who experience a seizure while on treatment.

The seizure rate associated with doses of sustained-release bupropion up to 300 milligrams per day is approximately 0.1% (1/1,000). This incidence was prospectively determined during an eight-week treatment exposure in approximately 3,100 depressed patients. Data for the immediate-release formulation of bupropion revealed a seizure incidence of approximately 0.4% (4/1,000) in depressed patients treated at doses in a range of 300 to 450 milligrams per day. In addition, the estimated seizure incidence increases almost 10-fold between 450 and 600 milligrams per day.

Predisposing factors that may increase the risk of seizure with bupropion use include history of head trauma or prior seizure, central nervous system (CNS) tumor, the presence of severe hepatic (liver) cirrhosis, and concomitant medications that lower seizure threshold.

Situations associated with an increased seizure risk include, among others, excessive use of alcohol or sedatives (including benzodiazepines); addiction to opiates, cocaine, or stimulants; use of over-the-counter stimulants and anorectics; and diabetes treated with oral hypoglycemics or insulin.

Many drugs, for example, antipsychotics, antidepressants, theophylline, and systemic steroids, are known to lower seizure threshold. Bupropion should be used with extreme caution in patients with severe hepatic cirrhosis. In these patients a reduced frequency of dosing is required, as peak bupropion levels are substantially increased, and accumulation is likely to occur in such patients to a greater extent than usual. The dose should not exceed 150 milligrams every other day in these patients.[21]

Before You Use This Drug

Do not use if you have or have had:

- eating disorders, such as anorexia or bulimia
- seizures

Tell your doctor if you have or have had:

- pregnancy or are breast-feeding
- allergies to drugs
- bipolar disorder (manic depression)
- brain tumor
- head injury
- neurologic disease
- seizures
- drug abuse
- heart disease
- liver disease
- kidney disease
- high blood pressure
- psychosis

Tell your doctor about any other drugs you take, including aspirin, herbs, vitamins, and other nonprescription products; buprorion comes under different brand names, including Wellbutrin and Zyban.

When You Use This Drug

- Participate in a smoking cessation program.
- Until you know how you react to this drug, do not drive or perform other activities requiring alertness.
- Do not drink alcohol.
- Do not take bupropion under different brand names at the same time that you are taking it for smoking cessation.

How to Use This Drug

• If you miss a dose, take it as soon as you remember, but skip it if it is almost time for the next dose. **Do not take double doses.**

• Do not share your medication with others.

• Take the drug at the same time(s) each day.

• Take with or without food.

• Do not break, chew, or crush long-acting forms of this drug.

• Store at room temperature with lid on tightly. Do not store in the bathroom. Do not expose to heat, moisture, or strong light. Keep out of reach of children.

• Take doses of prompt-release tablets at least four hours apart.

• Take doses of extended-release tablets at least eight hours apart.

• Take this drug for seven or more days prior to the date on which smoking will be stopped.

Interactions with Other Drugs

The following drugs, biologics (e.g., vaccines, therapeutic antibodies), or foods are listed in *Evaluations of Drug Interactions* 2003 as causing "highly clinically significant" or "clinically significant" interactions when used together with any of the drugs in this section. In some sections with multiple drugs, the interaction may have been reported for one but not all drugs in this section, but we include the interaction because the drugs in this section are similar to one another. We have also included potentially serious interactions listed in the drug's FDA-approved professional package insert or in published medical journal articles. There may be other drugs, especially those in the families of drugs listed below, that also will react with this drug to cause severe adverse effects. Make sure to tell your doctor and pharmacist the drugs you are taking and tell them if you are taking any of these interacting drugs:

At least two weeks should elapse after you stop taking a monoamine oxidase (MAO) inhibitor and before you start taking bupropion. The same is true if you stop taking bupropion and then start one of these MAO inhibitors: deprenyl, ELDEPRYL, EUTONYL, furazolidone, FUROXONE, isocarboxazid, MARPLAN, MATULANE, NARDIL, PARNATE, phenelzine, procarbazine, selegiline, tranylcypromine.

AVENTYL, carbamazepine, cyclophosphamide, CYTOXIN, desipramine, DILANTIN, flecainide, fluoxetine, HALDOL, haloperidol, imipramine, LOPRESSOR, MELLARIL, metoprolol, NORFLEX, NORPRAMINE, nortriptyline, orphenadrine, paroxetine, PAXIL, phenobarbital, phenytoin, propafenone, PROZAC, RISPERDAL, risperidone, RYTHMOL, sertraline, TAMBOCOR, TEGRETOL, thioridazine, TOFRANIL, ZOLOFT.

Taking bupropion with other drugs that also affect the central nervous system adds to adverse effects, including risk of seizures: alcohol, amitriptyline, chlorpromazine, clozapine, CLOZARIL, DESYREL, ELAVIL, fluoxetine, HALDOL, haloperidol, lithium, LITHOBID, LITHONATE, loxapine, LOXITANE, LUDIOMIL, maprotiline, meclobemide, MOBAN, molindone, NAVANE, NORVIR, pargyline, PROZAC, ritonavir, thiothixene, THORAZINE, trazodone.

Adverse Effects

Call your doctor immediately if you experience:

• agitation
• anxiety
• severe headache
• skin rash, hives, or itching
• ringing in ears
• fainting
• confusion
• delusions

- hallucinations
- paranoia
- trouble concentrating
- seizures

Call your doctor if these symptoms continue:

- abdominal pain
- decrease in appetite
- constipation
- dizziness
- dry mouth
- increased sweating
- insomnia
- muscle pain
- nausea or vomiting
- sore throat
- tremor
- unusual weight loss
- blurred vision
- drowsiness
- fast or irregular heartbeat

- change in sense of taste
- unusual feeling of well-being
- frequent urination

Signs of overdose:

- hallucinations
- loss of consciousness
- nausea or vomiting
- seizures
- fast heartbeat

If you suspect an overdose, call this number to contact your poison control center: (800) 222-1222.

Periodic Tests

Ask your doctor which of these tests should be done periodically while you are taking this drug:

- supervision for suicidal tendencies
- blood pressure

REFERENCES

1. Wolfe S. Testimony at Food and Drug Administration Advisory Committee Hearing on Nicotine Patches, July 14, 1992.

2. Gunther V, Gritsch S, Meise U. Smoking cessation—gradual or sudden stopping? *Drug and Alcohol Dependence* 1992; 29:231–6.

3. West R. The focus and conduct of clinical trials. *British Journal of Addiction* 1991; 86:663–6.

4. West R. The 'nicotine replacement paradox' in smoking cessation: How does nicotine gum really work? *British Journal of Addiction* 1992; 87:165–7.

5. Morgan GD, Villagra VG. The nicotine transdermal patch: A cautionary note. *Annals of Internal Medicine* 1992; 116:424.

6. Benowitz NL. Cigarette smoking and nicotine addiction. *Medical Clinics of North America* 1992; 76:415–37.

7. Breslau N, Kilbey MM, Andreski P. Nicotine withdrawal symptoms and psychiatric disorders: Findings from an epidemiologic study of young adults. *American Journal of Psychiatry* 1992; 149:464–9.

8. Nicotine patches. *Medical Letter on Drugs and Therapeutics* 1992; 34:37–8.

9. *American Hospital Formulary Service Drug Information.* Bethesda, Md.: American Society of Hospital Pharmacists, 1992.

10. Russell MA, Jarvis MJ. Skin patches to prevent lung cancer. *European Journal of Cancer* 1991; 27:223–4.

11. Sawe U. From smoking behaviour to nicotine addiction: The history of research. *Journal of the Royal Society of Medicine* 1992; 85:184.

12. Tonnesen P, Norregaard J, Simonsen K, et al. A double-blind trial of a 16-hour transdermal nicotine patch in smoking cessation. *New England Journal of Medicine* 1991; 325:311–5.

13. Transdermal Nicotine Study Group. Transdermal nicotine for smoking cessation. Six-month results from two multicenter controlled clinical trials. *Journal of the American Medical Association* 1991; 266:3133–8.

14. Perkins KA. Metabolic effects of cigarette smoking. *Journal of Applied Physiology* 1992; 72:401–9.

15. Glover ED. Transdermal nicotine patch for smoking cessation. *New England Journal of Medicine* 1992; 326:344.

16. Rich JD. Transdermal nicotine patch for smoking cessation. *New England Journal of Medicine* 1992; 326:344–5.

17. Varma JR. Transdermal nicotine patch for smoking cessation. *New England Journal of Medicine* 1992; 326:344.

18. Kirch DG. Where there's smoke . . . nicotine and psychiatric disorders. *Biological Psychiatry* 1991; 30:107–8.

19. Menza MA, Grossman N, Van Horn M, et al. Smoking and movement disorders in psychiatric patients. *Biological Psychiatry* 1991; 30:109–15.

20. Jensen EJ, Schmidt E, Pedersen B, et al. Effect on smoking cessation of silver acetate, nicotine and ordinary chewing gum. Influence of smoking history. *Psychopharmacology* 1991; 104:470–4.

21. *Physicians' Desk Reference.* 58th ed. Montvale, N.J.: Thomson PDR, 2004:1687–92.

27

VITAMINS AND MINERALS

For the first time since the book *Worst Pills, Best Pills* was initially published in 1988, we have added an entirely new chapter called Dietary Supplements (see p. 824). That chapter contains information on the 13 biggest-selling dietary supplements, such as ginseng, St. John's wort, gingko biloba, and 10 others, all derived from botanical (herbal) preparations except for chondroitin sulfate/glucosamine and Coenzyme Q_{10}, which are of animal origin.

This chapter, however, is limited to those supplements that are vitamins or minerals and covers the same products, with important updates, discussed in the earlier editions of this book.

Based on data from 2002, the most recent year for which such data are available, there were $7.7 billion in sales of vitamin and mineral supplements,[1,2] projected to increase to $8.4 billion by 2005. The biggest-selling products were multiple vitamins, calcium, B vitamins, vitamin E, and vitamin C, these products alone accounting for 76% of total vitamin and mineral sales in 2002.

The chapter greatly benefits from a recent government-sponsored exhaustive review in the UK, *Safe Upper Levels for Vitamins and Minerals,* concerning safety issues related to these vitamins and minerals, both in dietary intake and in the form of supplements.[3] The report tackles the most frequently heard complaint about rigorously examining the safety of vitamins and minerals: "It has been argued that since vitamins and minerals are essential for human health, it is not appropriate to assess them in the same way in which other chemicals added to food are assessed. However, since there is much evidence that excessive intakes of some vitamins and minerals can cause harm, it is not appropriate to exclude essential nutrients from the safety assessment that is applied to other chemical substances [such as food additives] which are added to foods."

In a number of the profiles on specific vitamins and minerals, information from this report is quoted directly.

One promotional strategy of supplement suppliers is to make people worry about whether they are getting enough nutrients. But do most people really need to take vitamins and minerals to supplement their diets? Or are they a waste of money? Are there better alternatives to taking supplements to ensure adequate nutrition? This section will attempt to answer these questions and help you sort through the fact and fiction surrounding nutritional supplements.

CAUSES OF VITAMIN AND MINERAL DEFICIENCIES

It is a fact that some people do have vitamin and mineral deficiencies, usually older adults. They fall into three categories:

1. People who do not eat enough food—fewer than 1,500 calories a day.

2. People who eat enough food but have an unbalanced, low-quality diet, often deficient in fruits and vegetables.

3. People who have medical problems or take drugs that contribute to vitamin and mineral deficiencies.

Too Few Calories

The most common cause of inadequate nutrition is eating too few calories. A diet that provides less than 1,500 calories a day does not ensure an adequate intake of all necessary nutrients. This can occur at all ages but is a particular problem in older adults. There are special reasons why this can happen.

Physical changes occur with aging. A decrease in the sensitivity of smell and taste results in food not tasting as good, and a subsequent loss of appetite. Dental problems may make eating more difficult, especially raw vegetables and meat. Physical handicaps can hinder food preparation and eating.

Economic factors also play a role in preventing people from eating enough. One out of every six older adults lives in poverty, which makes buying sufficient, wholesome food a difficult task.

An Unbalanced, Low-Quality Diet

Another group of adults at risk for vitamin and mineral deficiencies are those who eat enough food to feel full but eat an inadequate supply of necessary nutrients (vitamins and minerals that ensure your body's good health). Certain changes make a deficiency more likely to happen.

As a person ages, his or her daily requirement for calories decreases because of a reduction in basal metabolic rate and physical activity. In order to maintain a weight of 140 pounds, a 70-year-old must eat fewer calories than he or she did as a 40-year-old. The basal metabolic rate, which determines how many calories your body burns off while resting, can decrease as much as 15 to 20% between the ages of 30 and 75. As a result, older adults require fewer calories. Less exercise results in a loss of lean body weight with a decrease in muscle and an increase in fat.

Regular exercise is the only way to slow down or reverse this age-related process. Exercise can increase both your basal metabolic rate and the amount of muscle in your body. It can also quicken the rate at which your food is digested and used. These effects from exercise allow you to eat more food without gaining weight.

Although the number of calories needed decreases with age, nutrient needs remain about the same (unless there is a special situation, such as a physical condition or a drug, that creates a need for more). As a result, a high-quality diet becomes more essential.

One obstacle to this goal of adequate nutrition and high-quality diet is that older adults often do not shop for or prepare their own food. Eating out often makes it harder to choose a healthy diet. Being immobile or in long-term institutional care reduces control over dietary choices. Living alone is also a barrier because preparing meals for one and eating alone is not always that appealing.

Medical Problems and Drugs

Vitamin and mineral deficiencies can also be caused by medical problems, including alcohol dependence and drugs. For example, diseases of the intestine, pancreas, and liver cause decreased absorption of certain nutrients, and some chronic diseases reduce the appetite.

Certain prescription and nonprescription drugs and alcohol also cause increased requirements of certain nutrients. These are the most common drugs (see the individual drug listings for more details):

- drugs that affect the stomach or intestines, such as mineral oil and laxatives
- cholesterol-reducing drugs, such as clofibrate and cholestyramine
- antibiotics such as the cephalosporins and isoniazid
- cytotoxic drugs (drugs that cause damage to cells), such as methotrexate, colchicine, and many anticancer drugs
- anticonvulsants such as phenytoin and phenobarbital
- blood pressure drugs, such as hydrochlorothiazide, hydralazine, and furosemide
- alcohol

If you have any medical problems or use any drugs that increase the demand for certain vitamins and minerals, talk to your doctor about the best ways to increase your nutrient intake.

HOW TO PREVENT AND TREAT A VITAMIN OR MINERAL DEFICIENCY

Should people who have vitamin or mineral deficiencies take vitamin or mineral supplements? There is no simple answer to this question because of the various causes of such deficiencies. Sometimes, taking a supplement will help. But supplements are never the complete answer to anyone's nutritional problems. It is far better to address the situation that could cause the deficiency and adjust the diet than to take a supplement and do nothing more.

Steps Toward a Better Diet

Eating a well-balanced diet with plenty of variety and high-quality food is the most important way to ensure good nutrition. Here are some healthy suggestions for doing that. If you decide to make changes in your diet, make them one at a time; you will have a better chance of succeeding.

1. Decrease the amount of fat in your diet, particularly saturated fats. Most Americans eat too much fat, which contributes to heart disease, the nation's number one killer. Fat should contribute only 30% of your total daily caloric intake. You can decrease the amount of fat by:
   a. trimming fat off meat
   b. eating more fish and chicken (without the skin) instead of red meat
   c. drinking skim milk instead of whole milk and cutting down on your consumption of whole-milk dairy products
   d. eating fewer fried foods
   e. steaming or baking food instead of cooking with oils and butter

2. Decrease the amount of salt in your diet. Eating a high-salt diet contributes to high blood pressure, thereby increasing your risk of heart disease and stroke. Foods that are high in salt include processed food, condiments, and salted meats. It is possible to buy low-salt crackers, no-salt pretzels, unsalted nuts, and low-sodium canned goods and breakfast cereals.

3. Eat more fruits, vegetables, and whole grains. These are the best sources of complex carbohydrates (starches that provide fiber and essential nutrients) and are also good sources of vitamins and minerals. Carbohydrates should contribute 55% of your total daily caloric intake, with the majority of them being fruits, vegetables, and whole grains. They also provide the

best source of natural fiber, which comes from nonprocessed foods that are often more difficult to chew—raw cauliflower, broccoli, carrots, and whole-grain breads, for example. Fiber also promotes regularity (see psyllium, p. 566) and may help to significantly reduce your cholesterol level and/or blood pressure.[4]

4. Decrease the amount of simple sugars in your diet. Replace foods sweetened with refined sugar (sucrose), such as candy, ice cream, pastry, and jam, with naturally sweet foods, such as oranges and apples.

5. Decrease your alcohol intake. Drink no more than three to five alcoholic drinks a week, if not fewer.

6. Increase your fluid intake to six to eight glasses of fluids a day, especially water. Kidney function is often reduced in older adults. Drinking more fluids helps the kidneys function better and also promotes regularity. However, first ask your doctor if you need to restrict your fluid intake.

7. Eat a wide variety of foods. A wide variety of wholesome foods will provide all the nutrients you need. It's not too late to try new foods and get into new habits if your diet has been limited. Change your eating habits a little bit at a time and soon you will notice a difference. If you want to change your diet to get more of a specific nutrient, there is a list of good dietary sources of the individual vitamins and minerals at the end of this section.

WHO NEEDS VITAMIN AND MINERAL SUPPLEMENTS?

Having said that eating good food is the best and only sure way to improve your nutritional health, it should be added that for particular groups of older adults, taking vitamin and mineral supplements may be entirely reasonable and, at times, necessary:

1. People who eat fewer than 1,500 calories a day.

2. People who are institutionalized.

3. People with certain chronic diseases, including alcoholism, as well as liver, kidney, and intestinal diseases.

4. People who take drugs that interfere with absorption of or increase the excretion of nutrients.

5. People with a specific diagnosed nutritional deficiency or those who are in a high-risk group for developing a deficiency. For example, postmenopausal women should take calcium to prevent osteoporosis and strict vegetarians who do not eat eggs or milk products should take vitamin B_{12}.

People who fit into these categories may require either a supplement of a specific nutrient or a multivitamin supplement with or without minerals. Either way, supplementation should be started only after discussion with and approval by your doctor and consideration of a dietary solution to the problem.

TAKING VITAMIN AND MINERAL SUPPLEMENTS AS "INSURANCE"

What about people who do not fall into these categories? For example, what if you eat an inadequate diet and find it hard to make changes toward a healthy diet? Many people in this situation take a vitamin and mineral supplement to provide adequate "insurance" for their diets. Is this a good idea? One needs to look at both sides of the issue. Supplements cannot provide "insurance" from a poor diet because vitamin and mineral deficiencies are not the only problems resulting from eating an unbalanced diet and may not even be the most important ones.

A diet high in fat, cholesterol, and salt, for example, contributes to heart disease. A diet low in fiber causes constipation and irregularity of bowel movements and contributes to development of diverticulitis, a disease of the intestine that can result in bleeding of the intestine. A vitamin and mineral supplement will not insure against any of these problems. Only changes in your diet can help you to prevent such diseases. Relying on supplements for insurance can give you a false sense of security about your diet. We all have met people who eat a poor diet and justify it by saying, "Well, at least I'm taking vitamins." This false sense of security may remove any incentive to improve diet.

What if you want to take a supplement anyway? There is no strong medical evidence of benefit from supplements when a specific deficiency does not exist, although it is a fact that people take them for peace of mind.

On the other hand, there is no evidence that a regular multivitamin supplement, with or without minerals, taken in a dose less than or equal to the recommended dietary allowance (RDA) is detrimental to your health. This does not hold true, however, for doses that far exceed the RDA (megadoses) of vitamins and minerals. If you decide to use a supplement, there are a few things that you should know.

GUIDELINES FOR SELECTING VITAMIN AND MINERAL SUPPLEMENTS

Be rational about selecting a supplement. If you are not at risk for a specific vitamin or mineral deficiency, choose a basic multivitamin plus mineral supplement. Taking specific pills for specific vitamins is a marketing tactic designed to make supplements more expensive. The average multivitamin pill with close to 100% of the RDA of each of the vitamins is less expensive.

Read the mineral contents on the label if you are concerned about increasing your intake of minerals. Most multivitamin supplements with minerals contain close to 100% of the RDA for vitamins but not for minerals. Mineral deficiency is actually more common than vitamin deficiency, despite what advertising might say. In older postmenopausal women, for example, calcium deficiency is a major health problem. We concur with the National Institutes of Health's recommendation of 1,000 to 1,500 milligrams of calcium a day. If you cannot get this amount through your diet, take a calcium supplement (see p. 816), either alone or in combination with a vitamin supplement.

Do not buy a supplement that contains nutrients for which there are no known requirements or "new" vitamins, such as lecithin, carnitine, and inositol. Supporters of these supplements argue that we do not know all of what the human body really needs. Within the last 15 years, however, people with intestinal problems have been living successfully on injected solutions of protein, carbohydrates, fats, and established vitamins. If there were any unknown nutrients needed, this information would be known by now.

Buy the least expensive supplements. Many products are horrendously overpriced, being marked up to 1,000% over cost! Money that you overspend on supplements is money taken away from buying wholesome food. There is no benefit to be gained from a "natural" supplement versus a synthetic supplement. Brand-name vitamins are no better than generic versions. Buy the generics, which will work exactly the same as the more expensive name brands.

RECOMMENDED DIETARY ALLOWANCES (RDA)— WHAT THEY REALLY MEAN

There is no need to take vitamin or mineral doses above the recommended dietary allowances. The National Academy of Sciences is the organization that sets the recommended dietary allowance (RDA) for each vitamin and mineral, and this allowance varies for males, females, and different age groups. Because they are designed to account for differences between older and younger adults, the RDAs are the most appropriate ones for an older adult to use.

There is a prevailing myth that the RDA is no more than the amount of a vitamin or mineral that is needed to prevent deficiencies. This is not the case. When an RDA is set, the committee first decides how much of a vitamin or mineral the average person needs, and then raises this number to cover the needs of 98% of the healthy population. **This number is set at a level that is often two to three times higher than people's needs, resulting in a significant safety margin—the government's own "insurance" for your health.**

Because of this built-in safety margin, the vast majority of people do not even need to get 100% of the RDA, as it is defined by the RDA committee. Thus, there is no need to take vitamin or mineral supplements that go beyond the RDA.

You may be familiar with two other guidelines, the U.S. recommended daily allowance (USRDA) and the minimum daily requirement (MDR). Neither of these guidelines is as appropriate as the RDA, especially for older adults. The Food and Drug Administration sets a single USRDA, which is largely based on the RDA for teenage boys. This allowance is not appropriate for older adults, since it does not account for age differences. Most vitamin supplements will state on the label what percent of the USRDA they provide. The MDR was a forerunner of the USRDA and is now out of date.

THE MYTH OF MEGADOSE

There is a great deal of advertising that promotes the unproven benefits of taking "mega-doses" of vitamins and minerals—supplements well beyond the RDA. Sensational claims of health and well-being are made for mega-doses—they will "add vitality to your health," "restore the luster to your skin," and "perk up your sex life." When looked at critically, these claims just don't stand up. You will see, throughout the profiles in this chapter on specific vitamins and minerals, the results of carefully conducted studies that find practically all of the claimed benefits for megadoses are not valid.

To understand what vitamins or minerals can or cannot do, one must first understand their function in the human body. For the most part, a vitamin is a part of an enzyme (protein) that helps the enzyme perform certain chemical functions in the body. For example, many B vitamins help enzymes convert food into energy. Minerals act similarly. Calcium builds bones and also helps enzymes perform their functions. Iron is an essential element of red blood cells and helps them carry oxygen from the lungs to the tissues.

Vitamin functions were originally determined through vitamin deficiency diseases in people who were deprived of certain kinds of food for long periods of time. For instance, sailors often developed scurvy, a disease with such symptoms as bleeding into joints, poor healing of wounds, and emotional changes. It was determined that scurvy resulted from vitamin C deficiency when it was discovered that the sailors' symptoms dramatically disappeared once they ate citrus fruits.

The vitamin manufacturers take the process of deficiency diseases and vitamins one step further. For example, claims are made that vitamin C will help cure skin or emotional problems, colds, or cancer. The overwhelming majority of these problems are not caused by vitamin C deficiency, so they will not improve in the average person taking vitamin C.

The flaw in this logic can be demonstrated by substituting "food" for "vitamin" in an example of a deficiency. If you fast for a long time, you will begin to develop certain symptoms, such as muscle aches, headaches, nausea, and dizziness. These symptoms of "food" deficiency will disappear dramatically once you begin to eat again. It does not follow from this that if you have symptoms of nausea, headaches, and dizziness while eating normally, more food will cause them to go away. But this is the kind of logic most manufacturers use to make claims for the benefits of megadoses of supplements: if some is good, then more must be better, and much more must be much better.

The only way to determine a beneficial effect of a supplement is through controlled scientific experiments, in which a supplement's effects are compared with those of a placebo (dummy medication). **No extravagant claims made by manufacturers for megadoses of any vitamins have stood up to these tests.**

There are a few instances where vitamins have been determined to have specific additional benefits that have been demonstrated by rigorous scientific studies. Most of these therapeutic uses occur at doses not much greater than the RDA. They are discussed in the individual profiles that follow this section.

In addition to a lack of effectiveness, there are serious dangers associated with taking megadoses of many vitamins. People who take a mul-

---

DIETARY SOURCES OF VITAMINS AND MINERALS

VITAMINS

Folic Acid (folate)	Dried beans and nuts,* fruits, green leafy vegetables, organ meats,* whole grains, yeast
A	Beef liver,* carrots, sweet potatoes, tomatoes, green leafy vegetables, broccoli, watermelon, cantaloupe, apricots, peaches, butter,* margarine,* whole milk,* fortified skim milk
B_1 (thiamine)	Dried beans; peas; whole-grain or enriched breads and cereals; enriched or brown rice; enriched pasta, noodles, and other flour products; potatoes; pork;* beef liver;* nuts*
B_2 (riboflavin)	Milk,* enriched and whole-grain products, green leafy vegetables, meat,* fish, poultry,* eggs,* liver,* cheese*
B_3 (niacin)	Beans, peas, potatoes, enriched grain products, beef,* poultry,* pork,* liver,* nuts*
B_6 (pyridoxine)	Wheat and corn products, soybeans, lima beans, yeast, beef,* poultry,* pork,* organ meats*
B_{12} (cyanocobalamin)	Shellfish,* tongue,* fish, milk,* eggs,* cheese,* peas, beans, lentils, tofu, nuts,* beef,* poultry,* pork,* organ meats*
C	Citrus fruits (oranges, grapefruit, lemons, limes), tomatoes, strawberries, cantaloupe, cabbage, broccoli, cauliflower, potatoes, raw peppers
D	Some fatty fishes* and fish-liver oils,* vitamin D–fortified milk* and bread, eggs,* chicken livers*
E	Vegetable oils* (corn, cottonseed, soybean, safflower), wheat germ, whole-grain cereals, egg yolk*
K	Green leafy vegetables, beef,* pork*

MINERALS

Calcium	Milk,* cheese,* yogurt,* ice cream*—low-fat and nonfat dairy products can be used—canned salmon and sardines, shellfish,* broccoli, green leafy vegetables, including collards, bok choy, mustard, and turnip greens
Iron	Organ meats,* red meat,* fish, green leafy vegetables, peas, wheat germ, brewer's yeast, oysters,* dried beans and fruits

*High in fat and/or cholesterol. Keep servings of these foods to a minimum. Ideally, the calories in all of these foods together should be less than 30% of your diet.

tivitamin supplement in low doses have few risks; however, people who take high doses of certain vitamins have a risk of developing serious medical problems. Dangerous, toxic, and occasionally fatal effects have been associated with high doses of the fat-soluble vitamins A, D, E, and K. Even the water-soluble vitamin C and the B vitamins, which normally pass out of the body in your urine, can have adverse effects at high doses. Vitamin B_6 has been associated with nerve damage,[5] for example. Too much vitamin C can cause stomach cramps or diarrhea.

Some vitamins should not be taken—even in normal doses—if you use certain drugs or have certain medical problems. If you use warfarin (COUMADIN) to prevent blood clots, you should not take vitamin K; it will inhibit warfarin's ability to work. If you are B_{12} deficient and take folic acid (folate) without taking B_{12} as well, neurological symptoms can be worsened. If you are going to take any type of supplement, be sure to discuss it with your doctor before you start.

Vitamin and mineral supplements are a booming business in this country. Many people are misled by advertising into thinking that taking a supplement will help get rid of many of their health problems. But this is not the case. The most important step that you can take to maintain your nutritional well-being is to eat a healthy and well-balanced diet.

Certain older adults may need specific vitamin and mineral supplementation and should talk to their doctors about this. If you do not fall into one of these categories and still wish to take a supplement, you should follow a few rules of thumb.

First, realize that supplements are by no means the complete answer to good nutrition. Taking a supplement is not an adequate replacement for eating healthy food. If you do buy supplements there is no need to buy anything more than a regular multivitamin or a mineral supplement. Take supplements less than or

equal to the recommended dietary allowance for older adults. Try to buy the generic brands, not the expensive name brands and "natural" supplements. Finally, avoid megadoses of any supplement. They will give you no additional benefits from the supplement but will greatly increase your chances of toxic adverse effects.

NATIONAL ACADEMY OF SCIENCES RECOMMENDED DIETARY ALLOWANCES FOR ADULTS OVER 50 YEARS*

	Amount	
	Males	Females
VITAMINS		
A (Retinol)	900 mcg or 2,970 i.u.	700 mcg or 2,310 i.u.
D**	400 i.u.	600 i.u.
E	15 mg	15 mg
C	90 mg	75 mg
Thiamine (B_1)	1.2 mg	1.1 mg
Riboflavin (B_2)	1.3 mg	1.1 mg
Niacin (B_3)	16 mg	14 mg
Pyridoxine (B_6)	1.7 mg	1.5 mg
Cyanocobalamin (B_{12})	2.4 mcg	2.4 mcg
Folic Acid (folate)	400 mcg	400 mcg
MINERALS		
Calcium**	1,200 mg	1,200 mg
Phosphorus	700 mg	700 mg
Magnesium	420 mg	320 mg
Iron	8 mg	8 mg
Zinc	11 mg	8 mg
Iodine	150 mcg	150 mcg

i.u. = international units
mcg = micrograms
mg = milligrams

* From DRI (dietary reference intake) charts taken from the National Academy of Sciences Web site (www.nap.edu). All intakes are the new recommended daily allowances (RDA) except for those with double asterisks (**), which are Adequate Intakes (AI).

SUPPLEMENT PROFILES

Vitamins

Folic Acid

Folic Acid (*foe* lik *a* sid) (folate) (*foe* late)
B$_6$ (pyridoxine) (pir i *dok* sin), and B$_{12}$
(cyanocobalamin) (sye *an* oh koe *bal* a min)
FOLTX (Pamlab)

GENERIC: available
FAMILY: Vitamin Supplements

PREGNANCY AND BREAST-FEEDING WARNINGS
Vitamins taken at the level that supplies normal body needs (not megadoses) do not pose a risk to the fetus or the nursing infant.

Folic acid, also called folate or vitamin B$_9$, is essential for cell formation and growth, particularly of blood cells. It is found in several foods (see box below). A well-balanced diet with a variety of healthful foods should supply all the folic acid your body needs. The recommended dietary allowance (RDA) of folic acid for adults over 50 is 400 micrograms per day for both men and women.

It is unlikely that you would have a diet-related

FOODS HIGH IN FOLIC ACID (FOLATE)

Organ meats and nuts (both are high in cholesterol and/or fat), green vegetables, dried beans, fruits, yeast, whole grains. Cooking may destroy some folic acid.

½ cup spinach	110 micrograms folic acid
1 ounce chicken liver	108 micrograms folic acid
½ cup peanuts	60 micrograms folic acid
1 ounce shredded wheat	30 micrograms folic acid

folic acid deficiency. Rather, certain medical conditions or the long-term use of several drugs can lead to a folic acid deficiency. Alcoholism is perhaps the most common cause because alcoholics often eat an inadequate diet. Some diseases of the small intestine can also interfere with your body's absorption of folic acid, so there is less available for the body to use. Long-term treatment with drugs such as methotrexate, trimethoprim, triamterene, corticosteroids, certain painkillers, sulfasalazine, and some anticonvulsants (phenobarbital, phenytoin, and primidone) can also cause a folic acid deficiency.

If you have to increase your intake of folic acid in order to prevent or treat a deficiency, eat folate-rich foods rather than taking a vitamin supplement. (See table, p. 799.) You should only take a supplement when you have a clear need for more folic acid and when you cannot get enough from your diet. You should not take a supplement until your doctor has made sure that you do not have pernicious anemia, a disease resulting in vitamin B$_{12}$ deficiency. Folic acid supplements can hide the easily detected symptoms of pernicious anemia while allowing irreversible nervous system damage to occur undetected.

Folic acid has been shown to prevent neural tube defects, a serious type of birth defect, and as of January 1998, all grains sold in the United States contain 140 micrograms of folic acid per 100 grams (about 3 ounces). Even this amount, however, may be inadequate for prevention of neural tube defects, which occur early in pregnancy, before most women know that they are pregnant. The current recommendation is that women of childbearing age should also receive 400 micrograms of folic acid per day.[6]

"The main concern regarding ingestion of excess folic acid is the consequential masking of vitamin B$_{12}$ deficiency. A general consistency of data indicates that supplementation with 1 mg/day or less of folic acid does not mask vitamin B$_{12}$-associated anaemia in the majority of subjects, whereas supplementation with

5 mg/day or more of folic acid does. The effects of doses of between 1 and 5 mg/day are unclear. No other significant adverse effects have been associated with ingestion of folic acid. For guidance purposes only, in the general population a supplemental dose of 1 mg/day would not be expected to cause adverse effects. Assuming a maximum intake from food of approximately 0.49 mg/day, a total dose of 1.5 mg/day would not be expected to have any adverse effects."[3]

A recent randomized trial sought to find out if folic acid supplements (0.5 milligrams per day) would decrease the rate of death and cardiovascular events in people with stable coronary artery disease. After two years of folic acid supplements, there was no improvement in outcomes in those who got folic acid compared to those randomized to get standard care. The authors concluded that "low-dose folic acid supplementation should be treated with reservation" and that "the study does not seem to support the routine use of folic acid in patients with stable CAD [coronary artery disease]."[7]

If you take folic acid without a doctor's supervision, do not exceed the RDA.

The following information does not apply to the vitamin B_{12} component. See the vitamin B_{12} profile on p. 807 for information.

Before You Use This Drug

Tell your doctor if you have or have had:

- allergy to folic acid
- pernicious anemia
- pregnancy or are breast-feeding

Tell your doctor about any other drugs you take, including aspirin, herbs, vitamins, and other nonprescription products.

How to Use This Drug

- Do not share your medication with others.
- As with all drugs, it is important to take this one regularly. However, because of the

length of time required for a folic acid deficiency to occur, there is no cause for concern if a dose is missed. If you miss a dose, take it when you remember.

- Take the drug at the same time(s) each day.
- Store at room temperature with lid on tightly. Do not store in the bathroom. Do not expose to heat, moisture, or strong light. Keep out of reach of children.

Interactions with Other Drugs

The following drugs, biologics (e.g., vaccines, therapeutic antibodies), or foods are listed in *Evaluations of Drug Interactions* 2003 as causing "highly clinically significant" or "clinically significant" interactions when used together with any of the drugs in this section. In some sections with multiple drugs, the interaction may have been reported for one but not all drugs in this section, but we include the interaction because the drugs in this section are similar to one another. We have also included potentially serious interactions listed in the drug's FDA-approved professional package insert or in published medical journal articles. There may be other drugs, especially those in the families of drugs listed below, that also will react with this drug to cause severe adverse effects. Make sure to tell your doctor and pharmacist the drugs you are taking and tell them if you are taking any of these interacting drugs:

altretamine, cholestyramine, DILANTIN, HEXALEN, levodopa, LOCHOLEST, phenytoin, QUESTRAN, SINEMET.

Adverse Effects

Call your doctor immediately if you experience:

- shortness of breath
- difficulty breathing
- chest tightness
- wheezing
- reddened skin

- fever
- general weakness or discomfort
- skin rash or itching
- dependency (vitamin B_6)
- unstable walking (vitamin B_6)
- numb feet (vitamin B_6)
- hand numbness and clumsiness (vitamin B_6)

Do Not Use (Except as Occurs in Normal-Dose Multiple Vitamin Supplements)

Vitamin A (retinol) (reh-tin-ohl)
AQUASOL A (AlPharma)

FAMILY: Vitamin Supplements

PREGNANCY WARNING

Vitamins taken at the level that supplies normal body needs (not megadoses) do not pose a risk to the fetus or the nursing infant. However, fetal abnormalities have been reported in children whose mothers took excessive amounts of vitamin A during pregnancy. You should not take large doses of Vitamin A during pregnancy to avoid harm to the fetus.

BREAST-FEEDING WARNING

Vitamin A is excreted into breast milk. You should not exceed a daily amount in excess of 6,000 units to avoid harm to the nursing infant.

"Acute vitamin A toxicity in humans is rare but is more likely to occur following ingestion of high-dose supplements, rather than following high intakes of vitamin A from food. Vitamin A accumulates in the body; therefore, individuals who have regular high daily intakes of vitamin A might suffer adverse effects from chronic hypervitaminosis A. Although most manifestations of chronic vitamin A toxicity are reversible on cessation of dose, permanent damage to liver, bone, and vision and chronic muscular and skeletal pain may occur in some cases.

It is not possible to establish a safe upper level for vitamin A. There are two threads of evidence regarding potential adverse effects of vitamin A, one on teratogenicity and one on the risk of bone fracture, which suggest different levels of intake at which adverse effects may occur. Both of these ranges appear to overlap with dietary intakes of vitamin A.

A number of epidemiological studies have suggested that high doses of vitamin A may be teratogenic, that is, that they could cause malformations in the unborn child. The Expert Group on Vitamins and Minerals note and endorse the current advice that women who are pregnant or who wish to become pregnant should not take dietary supplements containing vitamin A except on medical advice.

In studies of long-term dietary intake, vitamin A has been associated with decreased bone density and increased risk of hip fracture. This finding is supported by investigations in laboratory animals in which vitamin A has been reported to affect calcium metabolism as well as to have a direct effect on bone. Other supportive epidemiological data suggest that the effect may also occur in men, since fracture risk is increased in both males and females in Scandinavian countries, where retinol intake is also higher than in southern Europe.

The risk of hip fracture is a continuous graded response associated with exposure levels that include average dietary intakes. It is not possible to identify an intake that is without some degree of risk. However, the available data indicate that total intakes greater than 1,500 micrograms (5,000 IU) per day may be inappropriate. (Note that this is only approximately twice as high as the recommended daily allowance for older adults—see p. 796.)

Data on retinol intakes from food and supplements suggest that high-level consumers of liver and liver products and/or supplements may exceed intakes at which adverse effects have been reported in the literature. It should also be noted that dietary supplements may contain 20–100% more vitamin A than is stated on the label, due to the practice of using "overages" within the food supplements industry to ensure that the product contains no less than the stated content of the vitamin throughout its shelf life. This may be particularly important given that the effect on fracture risk appears to be a graded response, with the risk of fracture increasing with increased intake."[3]

Vitamin A is necessary for growth and bone development, vision, and healthy skin. It is found in many foods (see boxes below), and a well-balanced diet with a variety of healthful foods should supply all the vitamin A that your body needs. The recommended dietary allowance (RDA) of vitamin A is 900 micrograms per day for men and 700 micrograms per day for women, corresponding to 2,970 and 2,310 international units (IU) respectively. These amounts are easily achieved through a good diet. (See boxes below.)

Vitamin A deficiency is rare, but older adults may develop this deficiency if they have certain intestinal or liver diseases, an overactive thyroid (hyperthyroidism), or diabetes. You may also develop vitamin A deficiency from an inadequate diet or if you take certain drugs such as

---

FOODS HIGH IN BETA-CAROTENE (PLANT SOURCES)

Carrots, sweet potatoes, squash, broccoli, tomatoes, green leafy vegetables, cantaloupe, apricots, peaches, margarine.

---

cholestyramine, colestipol, mineral oil, neomycin, or sucralfate. The liver stores enough vitamin A to last several months, so symptoms of a deficiency may take a few months to develop. The symptoms include night blindness and dry, cracked skin.

If you have to increase your intake of vitamin A to prevent or treat a deficiency, eat more foods that are rich in the vitamin rather than taking a vitamin supplement. You can get vitamin A from foods in two main forms. Animal sources such as liver, egg yolks, and butter provide a form of vitamin A called retinol. Plant sources such as carrots, squash, and some fruits provide a substance called beta-carotene, which your body converts into vitamin A in the body. Plant sources have several advantages over animal sources, the main one being that they are low in calories, fat, and cholesterol and high in fiber and other nutrients.

Some researchers claim that people who eat large amounts of foods containing beta-carotene have a lower risk of some types of cancer than those who eat less of these foods.[8] However, one large 12-year study found that beta-carotene supplements had no effect on the incidence of cardiovascular disease or malignancy. A second controlled clinical trial in Finnish smokers found an increased incidence of lung cancer of 18%, which was statistically significant.[6] No one should take beta-carotene supplements.

If you use vitamin A supplements despite our recommendation not to and without a doctor's supervision, do not exceed the RDA. Taking doses only slightly higher than the RDA can be risky. Unlike with some other vitamins, your

---

FOODS HIGH IN RETINOL (VITAMIN A)

Beef liver, butter, egg yolks, fish-liver oils (all four are high in cholesterol and/or fat). Freezing may destroy some vitamin A in both types of food sources.

1 large carrot	11,000 international units vitamin A
1 ounce calves' liver	9,340 international units vitamin A
½ cup cooked spinach	7,300 international units vitamin A
⅔ cup cooked broccoli	2,500 international units vitamin A
¼ cup cantaloupe	2,000 international units vitamin A
1 cup milk	300–500 international units vitamin A

body cannot eliminate excess vitamin A, so the vitamin can accumulate to dangerous, toxic levels in your body. The toxic effects of too much retinol include liver damage, weakness, increased pressure in the brain, bone and joint pain and damage, and dry, rough skin. The effects from beta-carotene are not as serious, but we nevertheless do not recommend using beta-carotene supplements either.

———

Thiamine (*thye* a min) (Vitamin B$_1$)

GENERIC: available
FAMILY: Vitamin Supplements

PREGNANCY AND BREAST-FEEDING WARNINGS
Vitamins taken at the level that supplies normal body needs (not megadoses) do not pose a risk to the fetus or the nursing infant.

Thiamine, or vitamin B$_1$, helps the body use sugars and starches (carbohydrates) effectively. It is available in several kinds of foods (see box below), and a well-balanced diet with a variety of healthful foods should supply all the thiamine that your body needs. The recommended dietary allowance (RDA) of thiamine is 1.2 milligrams per day for men over the age of 50 and 1.1 milligrams per day for women over the age of 50.

The signs of thiamine deficiency include loss of feeling on areas of the hands and feet, decreased muscle strength, personality disturbances, depression, lack of initiative, and poor memory. Thiamine deficiency is most commonly seen in alcoholics (the condition caused by a severe deficiency is called beri-beri). Alcoholics can become thiamine deficient because their diets often do not provide enough thiamine and because alcohol hinders the absorption of what thiamine they have. Chronic diarrhea can also lead to a need for more thiamine.

Thiamine is effective for treating conditions resulting from a thiamine deficiency, as in alcoholism. It has not been proven effective for treating skin problems, persistent diarrhea, fatigue, mental disorders, multiple sclerosis, ulcerative colitis, or for use as an insect repellant or appetite stimulant.[9]

If you have to increase your intake of thiamine, eat more thiamine-rich foods rather than taking a vitamin supplement. You should take a supplement only when dietary changes are inadequate to treat a deficiency.

If you take thiamine supplements without a doctor's supervision, do not take more than the RDA. Excess thiamine, beyond what is needed each day, simply passes through you and is eliminated in the urine without being used by your body.

Before You Use This Drug

Tell your doctor if you have or have had:

- allergy to thiamine
- pregnancy or are breast-feeding
- thiamine deficiency that has resulted in a brain disorder

Tell your doctor about any other drugs you take, including aspirin, herbs, vitamins, and other nonprescription products.

FOODS HIGH IN THIAMINE (VITAMIN B$_1$)

Meats (especially pork); organ meats; and nuts (all of which are high in cholesterol and/or fat); dried beans; peas; whole-grain or enriched breads and cereals; enriched or brown rice; enriched pasta, noodles, and other flour products; potatoes. Cooking destroys some thiamine.

1 loin chop	1.18 milligrams thiamine
1 ounce wheat germ	0.56 milligram thiamine
3½ ounces roast pork	0.39 milligram thiamine

How to Use This Drug

• If you miss a dose, take it as soon as you remember, but skip it if it is almost time for the next dose. **Do not take double doses.**

• Do not share your medication with others.

• Take the drug at the same time(s) each day.

• Store at room temperature with lid on tightly. Do not store in the bathroom. Do not expose to heat, moisture, or strong light. Keep out of reach of children.

Interactions with Other Drugs

Evaluations of Drug Interactions 2003 lists no drugs, biologics (e.g., vaccines, therapeutic antibodies), or foods as causing "highly clinically significant" or "clinically significant" interactions when used together with the drugs in this section. We also found no interactions in the drugs' FDA-approved professional package inserts. However, as the number of new drugs approved for marketing increases and as more experience is gained with these drugs over time, new interactions may be discovered.

Adverse Effects

Call your doctor immediately if you experience:

• coughing
• difficulty swallowing
• hives
• skin itching
• swelling of face, lips, or eyelids
• wheezing or breathing difficulty

Limited Use

Niacin (*nye* a sin) (Vitamin B$_3$)

GENERIC: available
FAMILY: Vitamin Supplements

PREGNANCY AND BREAST-FEEDING WARNINGS

Vitamins taken at the level that supplies normal body needs (not megadoses) do not pose a risk to the fetus or the nursing infant.

Niacin, also called nicotinic acid or vitamin B$_3$, and its derivative niacinamide, also called nicotinamide, are used by the body to help convert food to energy. Niacin is available in many types of foods (see box below), and a well-balanced diet with a variety of healthful foods should supply all the niacin that your body needs. The recommended dietary allowance (RDA) is 16 milligrams for men over the age of 50, and 14 milligrams for women over the age of 50.

Dietary deficiency of niacin, called pellagra, is rare. If you need to get more niacin, it is better to eat niacin-rich foods than to take a vitamin supplement. You should take niacin supplements to prevent and treat niacin deficiency only when your diet does not provide an adequate amount.

Niacin (nicotinic acid), but not niacinamide, has another use. It can be prescribed as part of a program to lower blood cholesterol or fat, which also includes a modified diet and exercise. The dose for this purpose, 300 milligrams or more, is

---

FOODS HIGH IN NIACIN (VITAMIN B$_3$)

Beef, pork, liver, eggs, nuts, poultry, milk and dairy products (all are high in cholesterol and/or fat), fish, whole-grain and enriched breads and cereals, beans, peas, potatoes. Cooking destroys some niacin.

3½ ounces calves' liver	16.5 milligrams niacin
1 cup wheat flakes	14.7 milligrams niacin
4 ounces halibut	10.4 milligrams niacin
¼ cup peanuts	10.0 milligrams niacin
3½ ounces roast turkey	7.7 milligrams niacin
1 slice whole wheat bread	6.0 milligrams niacin

much higher than the dose as a dietary supplement (10 to 20 milligrams). Taking niacin for this purpose is only an adjunct to weight reduction and exercise, not a substitute.

The adverse effects of niacin, such as blood vessel dilation, which produces intense flushing and itching of the face and upper part of the body, may limit the usefulness of this treatment. One aspirin taken 30 minutes before a dose of niacin may reduce this adverse effect.[10]

Niacin is not useful in treating schizophrenia or other mental disorders unrelated to niacin deficiency. It has not been proven effective in treating any blood vessel diseases nor in treating acne, leprosy, or motion sickness.

If you use niacin without a doctor's supervision, do not exceed the RDA. Excess niacin, beyond what is needed each day, simply passes through you and is eliminated in the urine without being used by your body. Avoid taking extended-release forms of niacin, since these may damage your liver (see p. 806).

The British Expert Group on Vitamins and Minerals has found that "Large doses of nicotinic acid [niacin] are associated with a number of adverse effects in man. These have been identified from the use of nicotinic acid in the treatment of hypercholesterolaemia. The effects reported include flushing, skin itching, nausea, vomiting and gastrointestinal disturbance. The effects are dose related and reversible on cessation of treatment. At higher intakes of nicotinic acid over long periods of time, liver dysfunction has been reported. Symptoms such as elevated liver enzymes, elevated bilirubin levels and jaundice have been observed.

"Other adverse effects reported include hyperglycaemia and adverse ophthalmological effects such as blurred vision and cystoid macular oedema. No relevant animal data have been reported and the mechanism for nicotinic acid–induced toxicity is unclear."[3]

Before You Use This Drug

Tell your doctor if you have or have had:

- allergy to niacin or niacinamide
- arterial bleeding or hemorrhage
- glaucoma
- gout
- ulcer
- liver disease
- diabetes
- low blood pressure
- pregnancy or are breast-feeding

Tell your doctor about any other drugs you take, including aspirin, herbs, vitamins, and other nonprescription products.

When You Use This Drug

- Until you know how you react to this drug, do not drive or perform other activities requiring alertness. Niacin may cause dizziness or fainting.

How to Use This Drug

- Take with food or milk; check with your doctor if stomach upset continues.
- Swallow extended-release capsules whole, or capsules may be opened and the contents mixed with applesauce, jelly, or ketchup, then swallowed without chewing.
- If you miss a dose, take it as soon as you remember, but skip the dose if it is almost time for the next dose. **Do not take double doses.**
- Do not share your medication with others.
- Take the drug at the same time(s) each day.
- Store at room temperature with lid on tightly. Do not store in the bathroom. Do not expose to heat, moisture, or strong light. Keep out of reach of children.

Interactions with Other Drugs

The following drugs, biologics (e.g., vaccines, therapeutic antibodies), or foods are listed in

Evaluations of Drug Interactions 2003 as causing "highly clinically significant" or "clinically significant" interactions when used together with any of the drugs in this section. In some sections with multiple drugs, the interaction may have been reported for one but not all drugs in this section, but we include the interaction because the drugs in this section are similar to one another. We have also included potentially serious interactions listed in the drug's FDA-approved professional package insert or in published medical journal articles. There may be other drugs, especially those in the families of drugs listed below, that also will react with this drug to cause severe adverse effects. Make sure to tell your doctor and pharmacist the drugs you are taking and tell them if you are taking any of these interacting drugs:

cholestyramine, COLESTID, colestipol, GLUCOPHAGE, lovastatin, metformin, MEVACOR, QUESTRAN.

Adverse Effects

Call your doctor immediately if you experience:

- skin rash or itching
- wheezing

Call your doctor if these symptoms continue:

- warm feeling
- skin flushing or redness, especially on face and neck
- headache

With high oral doses:

- unusually fast, slow, or irregular heartbeat
- diarrhea
- dizziness or faintness
- dryness of skin or eyes
- frequent urination
- unusual thirst

- joint pain
- side, lower back, or stomach pain
- swelling of feet or lower legs
- fever
- muscle aching or cramping
- unusual tiredness or weakness
- nausea or vomiting
- peptic ulcer
- itching

Periodic Tests

Ask your doctor which of these tests should be done periodically while you are taking this drug:

For high-dose therapy:

- blood levels of uric acid
- blood sugar levels
- liver function tests

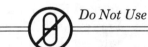

Do Not Use

ALTERNATIVE TREATMENT:
See Nonextended-release Niacin, p. 806.

Niacin (*nye* a sin) (Vitamin B$_3$)
(All Extended-Release Dosage Forms of Niacin)
NICOBID (Rhone-Poulenc Rorer)
SLO-NIACIN (Upsher-Smith)

FAMILY: Vitamin Supplements

Although niacin is useful and effective as a cholesterol-lowering drug (see p. 120), extended-release forms can cause liver damage. In the past several years, a number of studies have documented that liver toxicity, sometimes quite serious, is much more commonly associated with the extended-release form than with the crystalline or regular.[11,12]

If you are taking niacin for its lipid-lowering

effects, ask your doctor if it is the crystalline (regular) type (see p. 120). Be sure that the prescription is not changed to an extended-release preparation by a pharmacist and do not purchase slow-release pills over the counter. The doses used to lower blood lipids are much higher than the amount needed for normal metabolism, and the slow-release formulas probably promote excessive accumulation of the drug in the liver.

As can be seen in the box below, the RDA for niacin (16 milligrams for men and 14 milligrams for women) can easily be met by dietary sources.

FOODS HIGH IN NIACIN (VITAMIN B₃)

Beef, pork, liver, eggs, nuts, poultry, milk and dairy products (all are high in cholesterol and/or fat), fish, whole-grain and enriched breads and cereals, beans, peas, potatoes. Cooking destroys some niacin.

3½ ounces calves' liver	16.5 milligrams niacin
1 cup wheat flakes	14.7 milligrams niacin
4 ounces halibut	10.4 milligrams niacin
¼ cup peanuts	10.0 milligrams niacin
3½ ounces roast turkey	7.7 milligrams niacin
1 slice whole wheat bread	6.0 milligrams niacin

Limited Use

Vitamin B₁₂ (Cyanocobalamin)
(sye an oh koe *bal* a min)

GENERIC: available
FAMILY: Vitamin Supplements

PREGNANCY WARNING

Vitamins taken at the level that supplies normal body needs (not megadoses) do not pose a risk to the fetus.

BREAST-FEEDING WARNING

Vitamin B₁₂ is excreted into breast milk. No problems have been found in nursing infants of women taking the normal daily recommended amounts.

Vitamin B₁₂, also called cyanocobalamin, is essential for cell growth and normal formation of blood cells. It is found in several kinds of foods (see box below), and a well-balanced diet with a variety of healthful foods should supply all the vitamin that your body needs. The recommended dietary allowance (RDA) of vitamin B₁₂ for older adults is 2.4 micrograms per day.

Even if you do not get enough vitamin B₁₂ in your diet, a vitamin B₁₂ deficiency may take years to develop because the liver stores a vast supply of this vitamin. You may develop a deficiency from certain physical conditions or from an inadequate diet. In adults, a vitamin B₁₂ deficiency usually comes from a defect in the digestive tract's absorption of the vitamin, a condition called pernicious anemia. You may also develop a deficiency if you have had parts of your stomach or small intestine removed, which prevents the digestive tract from adequately absorbing the vitamin. In both of these cases, you need vitamin B₁₂ injections. Since plants do not contain vitamin B₁₂, strict vegetarians who do not eat eggs or milk products also need a vitamin B₁₂ supplement and can take one by mouth.

FOODS HIGH IN VITAMIN B₁₂

Tongue, beef, pork, organ meats, eggs, nuts, milk, shellfish, poultry, cheese (all may be high in cholesterol and/or fat), fish, peas, beans, lentils, tofu. Cooking is not likely to destroy vitamin B₁₂.

1 ounce beef liver	9.0–34.0 micrograms vitamin B₁₂
3½ ounces round roast	4.0 micrograms vitamin B₁₂
3½ ounces filet of sole	1.3 micrograms vitamin B₁₂
1 ounce Swiss cheese	9.0 micrograms vitamin B₁₂

Vitamin B_{12} deficiency can lead to anemia and to slow, progressive, irreversible damage to the nervous system. This damage will cause loss of feeling in the hands and feet, unsteadiness, loss of memory, confusion, and moodiness. To prevent these changes, people who require lifelong treatment with monthly B_{12} injections should be reevaluated at 6- to 12-month intervals by their doctor if they are otherwise well.[13]

Unless you have one of the conditions that require B_{12} injections, to prevent and treat a deficiency of vitamin B_{12} you should eat more food that is rich in this vitamin rather than taking a vitamin supplement. You should take a supplement only if your diet does not provide an adequate amount.

The claims made for vitamin B_{12} as a remedy for numerous conditions are unfounded. There is no evidence that supplements can provide more pep or counter depression or fatigue in people who do not have a deficiency.

Before You Use This Drug

Do not use if you have or have had:

- Leber's disease (an eye disease)

Tell your doctor if you have or have had:

- allergy to cyanocobalamin or hydroxocobalamin
- pregnancy or are breast-feeding

Tell your doctor about any other drugs you take, including aspirin, herbs, vitamins, and other nonprescription products.

How to Use This Drug

- Take at least one hour before or one hour after hot foods or liquids.
- Have follow-up blood tests every three to six months.
- If you miss a dose, take it as soon as you remember, but skip it if it is almost time for the next dose. **Do not take double doses.**

- Do not share your medication with others.
- Take the drug at the same time(s) each day.
- Store at room temperature with lid on tightly. Do not store in the bathroom. Do not expose to heat, moisture, or strong light. Keep out of reach of children.

Interactions with Other Drugs

Evaluations of Drug Interactions 2003 lists no drugs, biologics (e.g., vaccines, therapeutic antibodies), or foods as causing "highly clinically significant" or "clinically significant" interactions when used together with the drugs in this section. We also found no interactions in the drugs' FDA-approved professional package inserts. However, as the number of new drugs approved for marketing increases and as more experience is gained with these drugs over time, new interactions may be discovered.

Adverse Effects

Call your doctor if these symptoms continue:

- diarrhea
- skin itching

Periodic Tests

Ask your doctor which of these tests should be done periodically while you are taking this drug:

- blood levels of folic acid
- potassium blood tests
- vitamin B_{12} blood tests
- iron and clotting blood tests
- reticulocyte (young red blood cell) count

Limited Use

Vitamin C (ascorbic acid) (a *skor* bic *a* sid)
ARCO-CEE (Arco)
CEVI-BID (Geriatric)

GENERIC: available

FAMILY: Vitamin Supplements

PREGNANCY WARNING

Vitamins taken at the level that supplies normal body needs (not megadoses) do not pose a risk to the fetus. However, ascorbic acid crosses the placenta and, if taken in large amounts throughout pregnancy, may harm the fetus.

BREAST-FEEDING WARNING

Vitamin C is excreted into breast milk. No problems have been found in nursing infants of women taking the normal daily recommended amounts.

Ascorbic acid, also called vitamin C, helps bind cells together and promotes healing. It is found in certain fruits and vegetables (see box below), and a well-balanced diet with a variety of healthful foods should supply all the vitamin C that you need. The recommended dietary allowance (RDA) for older adults is 60 milligrams per day.

Vitamin C deficiency, known as scurvy, is rare. It is seen occasionally in people whose diet does not supply enough vitamin C—some older adults who live alone, alcoholics, and drug abusers, for example. Symptoms of scurvy include anemia, loose teeth, red and swollen gums, wounds that do not heal, and small broken blood vessels that cause tiny purplish-red spots in the skin. Scurvy is easily prevented and is treated by increasing the intake of vitamin C through diet and a supplement.

You should take a vitamin C supplement only if your diet does not supply enough to prevent and treat a vitamin C deficiency, or if your body has a special demand for more vitamin C due to surgery, smoking, or an infectious disease. Although doses that far exceed the RDA are touted as remedies for many conditions—from the common cold to cancer—research does not support such claims. There is no convincing evidence that taking supplements of vitamin C prevents any disease.[6]

One of the most common uses for large doses of vitamin C has been to prevent or lessen the severity of colds. A recent study randomized people to get a supplement containing either 30 milligrams of vitamin C (less than one-half of the recommended daily allowance) or 1 gram or 3 grams of vitamin C upon the onset of a cold and for two days subsequently. There was no difference in the duration or severity of colds in people getting 1 or 3 grams of vitamin C and those getting only 30 milligrams a day.[14]

If you use a vitamin C supplement without a doctor's supervision, do not take more than the RDA. Higher doses have few beneficial effects except in people with scurvy, and high-dose products are more expensive. Also, taking high doses of vitamin C is risky for people with a history of kidney stones and for people who use anticoagulants (drugs that prevent blood clots from forming in the blood vessels) such as warfarin (COUMADIN).[15] If you are taking high

---

FOODS HIGH IN ASCORBIC ACID (VITAMIN C)

Citrus fruits and juices (oranges, lemons, limes, grapefruit), tomatoes, strawberries, cantaloupe, cabbage, broccoli, cauliflower, potatoes, and raw peppers. Vitamin C in foods is reduced by drying, salting, and ordinary cooking. Mincing fresh vegetables and mashing potatoes also reduces the vitamin C content.

6 or 7 brussels sprouts	87 milligrams vitamin C
1 cup cauliflower	62 milligrams vitamin C
1 medium orange or	
½ cup orange juice	60 milligrams vitamin C
1 cup shredded cabbage	47 milligrams vitamin C
1 slice watermelon	42 milligrams vitamin C
½ grapefruit or ⅔ cup	
grapefruit juice	40 milligrams vitamin C
1 medium potato	30 milligrams vitamin C

doses of vitamin C and want to stop, do not stop suddenly. Reduce your dose gradually because your body needs time to adjust to the reduction.

Before You Use This Drug

Tell your doctor if you have or had:

- sensitivity to ascorbic acid or sodium ascorbate
- blood problems
- diabetes
- glucose-6-phosphate dehydrogenase deficiency
- kidney stones
- pregnancy or are breast-feeding

Tell your doctor about any other drugs you take, including aspirin, herbs, vitamins, and other nonprescription products.

When You Use This Drug

- Breakdown of tooth enamel has been reported with excessive use of chewable tablets.
- **Caution diabetics:** High doses may interfere with glucose tests.
- High doses may interfere with tests for blood in your stool.

How to Use This Drug

- If you miss a dose, take it as soon as you remember, but skip it if it is almost time for the next dose. **Do not take double doses.**
- Do not share your medication with others.
- Take the drug at the same time(s) each day.
- Take with or without food.
- Store at room temperature with lid on tightly. Do not store in the bathroom. Do not expose to heat, moisture, or strong light. Keep out of reach of children.

Interactions with Other Drugs

Evaluations of Drug Interactions 2003 lists no drugs, biologics (e.g., vaccines, therapeutic antibodies), or foods as causing "highly clinically significant" or "clinically significant" interactions when used together with the drugs in this section. We also found no interactions in the drugs' FDA-approved professional package inserts. However, as the number of new drugs approved for marketing increases and as more experience is gained with these drugs over time, new interactions may be discovered.

Adverse Effects

Call your doctor immediately if you experience:

- side or lower back pain

Call your doctor if these symptoms continue:

With oral doses greater than 1 gram a day:

- diarrhea

With oral doses greater than 600 milligrams per day:

- flushing or redness of skin
- headache
- mild increase in urination
- nausea or vomiting
- stomach cramps

Periodic Tests

Ask your doctor which of these tests should be done periodically while you are taking this drug:

- blood test for Vitamin C level

————————

Limited Use

Vitamin D
CALCIFEROL (Schwarz)

GENERIC: available
FAMILY: Vitamin Supplements

Vitamins taken at the level that supplies normal body needs (not megadoses) do not pose a risk to the fetus. However, megadoses of vitamin D have been associated with fetal malformations in animals and mental retardation and malformations in humans.

BREAST-FEEDING WARNING

Only small amounts of vitamin D are excreted into breast milk. Infants that are totally breast-fed and have little exposure to the sun may require vitamin D supplementation.

Vitamin D maintains normal blood levels of calcium and phosphate, both of which are necessary for bone growth and strength. It is available in several foods (see box below), and your body can also manufacture it (in the skin) if you are out in the sun. If you eat a well-balanced diet with a variety of healthful foods and spend some time in the sun, you should have all the vitamin D that your body needs. The recommended dietary allowance (RDA) is 400 international units per day for men and 600 per day for women.

Vitamin D deficiency in older adults prevents the body from absorbing calcium and phosphate normally. This leads to an overall decrease in bone density and weakening of the bones, called

osteomalacia. If you have to increase your intake of vitamin D, eat more foods rich in the vitamin rather than taking a vitamin pill. You should take a supplement only if your diet does not supply enough vitamin D to prevent and treat a deficiency or to treat a low blood level of calcium.

One recent randomized placebo-controlled trial involving more than 2,500 community-dwelling people aged 65–85 studied the effect of oral vitamin D_3, taken once every four months for five years, on the incidence of fractures. The group getting the vitamin D_3 had a significantly lower risk for any first fracture and for a first hip, wrist, forearm, or vertebral fracture. This approach seems promising, especially since it costs a fraction of the expensive prescription drugs discussed in Chapter 18, Drugs for Osteoporosis.[16]

The Expert Group on Vitamins and Minerals found that "Excess vitamin D may lead to hypercalcaemia [elevated calcium in the blood] and hypercalciuria [increased calcium in the urine]. Hypercalcaemia results in the deposition of calcium in soft tissues, diffuse demineralisation of bones and irreversible renal and cardiovascular toxicity. Moderate levels of vitamin D intake may enhance renal stone formation in predisposed individuals . . . Data are available from a range of human supplementation studies, but the levels of vitamin D intake at which hypercalcaemia or hypercalciuria occurs vary between studies. Likely reasons for this include differences in populations studied; for example, several of the studies are in older people, a group vulnerable to vitamin D deficiency, while other studies are in younger adults, who are not likely to be vitamin D deficient. Individuals and groups are also likely to differ in their exposure to vitamin D sources other than supplementation, such as consumption of vitamin D–fortified foods and through exposure to the sun. Excess vitamin D during gestation in rats and rabbits led to a number of adverse reproductive effects . . . long-term exposures of up to 0.025 mg/day vitamin D [1,000

FOODS HIGH IN VITAMIN D

Some fatty fishes and fish-liver oils, eggs, chicken livers, vitamin D–fortified milk (all are high in cholesterol and/or fat), and bread. Vitamin D is not affected by cooking.

½ ounce cod liver oil	1,400 international units vitamin D
3½ ounces sardines	1,380 international units vitamin D
3½ ounces salmon	300 international units vitamin D
1 egg yolk	265 international units vitamin D
1 cup vitamin D–fortified milk	100 international units vitamin D

IU] appear to be well-tolerated and may be necessary to prevent deficiency in some groups."[3] (The dose used in the study above was 100,000 IU every 120 days, or less than 1,000 IU per day.)[16]

If you use vitamin D without a doctor's supervision, do not take more than 1,000 IU per day, as recommended above. Unlike with some other vitamins, your body cannot eliminate excess vitamin D, so the vitamin can accumulate to dangerous, toxic levels. This is especially risky for people who take the heart medication digoxin (see p. 144), because vitamin D increases the adverse effects of digoxin. The signs of vitamin D toxicity are listed below. Vitamin D overdose may cause death as a result of heart, blood vessel, or kidney failure.

If your doctor has prescribed vitamin D to prevent low calcium levels, see him or her regularly to check your progress and reduce the risk of adverse effects. Tell your doctor if you are taking a calcium supplement and discuss how to best increase the amount of calcium in your diet.

Before You Use This Drug

Do not use if you have or have had:

- high level of calcium in your blood
- kidney disease
- high level of vitamin D in your blood

Tell your doctor if you have or have had:

- high sensitivity to effects of vitamin D
- heart or blood vessel disease
- high level of phosphate in your blood
- sarcoidosis
- pregnancy or are breast-feeding

Tell your doctor about any other drugs you take, including aspirin, herbs, vitamins, and other nonprescription products.

When You Use This Drug

- Avoid concurrent use of nonprescription medications or dietary supplements containing calcium, phosphorus, or vitamin D.
- Avoid use of magnesium-containing antacids.
- To avoid vitamin D toxicity, do not take more vitamin D than recommended.

How to Use This Drug

- If you miss a dose, take it as soon as you remember, but skip it if it is almost time for the next dose. **Do not take double doses.**
- Do not share your medication with others.
- Take the drug at the same time(s) each day.
- Store at room temperature with lid on tightly. Do not store in the bathroom. Do not expose to heat, moisture, or strong light. Keep out of reach of children.

Interactions with Other Drugs

The following drugs, biologics (e.g., vaccines, therapeutic antibodies), or foods are listed in *Evaluations of Drug Interactions* 2003 as causing "highly clinically significant" or "clinically significant" interactions when used together with any of the drugs in this section. In some sections with multiple drugs, the interaction may have been reported for one but not all drugs in this section, but we include the interaction because the drugs in this section are similar to one another. We have also included potentially serious interactions listed in the drug's FDA-approved professional package insert or in published medical journal articles. There may be other drugs, especially those in the families of drugs listed below, that also will react with this drug to cause severe adverse effects. Make sure to tell your doctor and pharmacist the drugs you are taking and tell them if you are taking any of these interacting drugs:

aluminum hydroxide, AMPHOJEL, DILANTIN, phenytoin.

Adverse Effects

Call your doctor immediately if you experience:

- early symptoms of vitamin D toxicity:
  - bone pain
  - constipation
  - diarrhea
  - drowsiness
  - dry mouth
  - continuing headache
  - increased thirst
  - increased frequency of urination (especially at night) or amount of urine
  - irregular heartbeat
  - appetite loss
  - metallic taste in mouth
  - muscle pain
  - nausea or vomiting
  - hives
  - unusual tiredness or weakness
- late symptoms of vitamin D toxicity:
  - bone pain
  - cloudy urine
  - redness or discharge of the eye, eyelid, or eyelid lining
  - loss of sex drive
  - calcium deposits in tissues other than bone
  - high fever
  - high blood pressure
  - eye irritation or increased sensitivity of eyes to light
  - irregular heartbeat
  - skin itching
  - drowsiness
  - appetite loss
  - muscle pain
  - nausea or vomiting
  - severe stomach pain
  - mood or mental changes

- runny nose
- weight loss

Periodic Tests

Ask your doctor which of these tests should be done periodically while you are taking this drug:

For high-dose therapy:

- blood calcium level (weekly, when therapy is started)
- liver function tests
- kidney function tests
- phosphorus blood tests
- eye exams
- parathyroid blood tests
- protein level in blood
- bone X-rays

 Do Not Use

ALTERNATIVE TREATMENT:
Eat a well-balanced diet with an adequate supply of vitamin E.

Vitamin E (alpha-tocopherol) (*al* fa to *kof* er ol)

FAMILY: Vitamin Supplements

Vitamin E is thought to work as an antioxidant, a substance that helps to protect cells from damage. It is found in many foods (see box on next page), and a well-balanced diet with a variety of healthful foods should supply all the vitamin E that your body needs. The recommended dietary allowance (RDA) of vitamin E is 15 milligrams per day for both men and women over the age of 50.

Vitamin E deficiency is extremely rare and has not been known to occur solely from an inadequate diet. It has occurred mainly in people who have certain conditions of their intes-

FOODS HIGH IN VITAMIN E

Vegetable oils (corn, cottonseed, soybean, safflower), egg yolk (all of which are high in fat and/or cholesterol), wheat germ, and whole-grain cereals. Some vitamin E may be lost in cooking.

1 ounce margarine	15 milligrams vitamin E
½ cup wheat germ	3 milligrams vitamin E
2 slices whole wheat bread	2 milligrams vitamin E

tines, pancreas, or liver that interfere with their body's ability to absorb this fat-soluble vitamin.

Vitamin E supplements have not been proven effective for treatment of beta-thalassemia, cancer, fibrocystic disease of the breast, inflammatory skin disorders, loss of hair, habitual abortion, leg cramps (intermittent claudication), menopausal syndrome, infertility, peptic ulcer, sickle cell disease, burns, porphyria, neuromuscular disorders, blood clots (thrombophlebitis), impotence, bee stings, liver spots on the hands, bursitis, diaper rash, lung toxicity from air pollution, or aging. Recent randomized, placebo-controlled studies examining a variety of alleged benefits of vitamin E are reviewed here.

A randomized placebo-controlled study of 200 IU of vitamin E supplements (the recommended daily dietary intake is about 15 IU in men, 12 in women) in well-nourished people 60 or older failed to show that vitamin E decreased the incidence of acute respiratory tract infections but showed that those people using vitamin E had a significantly increased severity of respiratory infections when they did occur compared to people getting a placebo.[17] A randomized placebo-controlled trial of vitamin E for six months failed to show any benefit for the management of symptomatic osteoarthritis of the knee.[18] Another randomized placebo-controlled trial found that vitamin E supplementation did not result in any significant improvements in heart fail-

ure or quality of life in patients with advanced heart failure.[19] In another large study of women and men 55 or older at high risk for cardiovascular events (heart attacks, strokes), the use of 400 IU of vitamin E for an average of 4.5 years had no beneficial effect on cardiovascular outcomes.[20] Another large randomized study of the use of vitamin E found that, compared to a placebo, vitamin E did not have a significant effect on the incidence of or mortality from pancreatic cancer.[21] Finally, in the ophthalmologic area, a four-year vitamin E placebo-controlled study involving people 55 to 80 years old without cataracts found that treatment with 500 IU daily did not prevent the development or slow the progression of age-related cataracts.[22]

Taking vitamin E in doses that far exceed the RDA can be harmful. Some people who have taken more than 300 milligrams have suffered muscle weakness, fatigue, headaches, nausea, high blood pressure, and increased tendency toward blood clotting.[23] A British expert group notes that "Very high doses of vitamin E have been reported to cause a few sporadic adverse effects. These include headache, fatigue, gastrointestinal distress, double vision, muscle weakness and mild creatinuria. High levels of vitamin E may also antagonise the effects of the other fat-soluble vitamins. Vitamin E also has an antiplatelet and anti-coagulant effect."[3]

Finally, a meta-analysis (statistical combining of other studies) associated high doses of vitamin E with increased total death rates.[28]

The FDA found that the available published scientific evidence demonstrates lack of a valid relationship between vitamin E supplementation, such as an increased risk of prolonged bleeding in people who routinely use nonsteroidal anti-inflammatory drugs (NSAIDs) such as ibuprofen (MOTRIN), and that this problem should be addressed in future research. At this time there is insufficient evidence to recommend the use of vitamin E for the prevention of heart attacks or for any other medical purpose.

Multivitamins (with and without Minerals)
THERAGRAN-M (Mead Johnson)
CENTRUM (Lederle)

GENERIC: available

FAMILY:　Vitamin Supplements
　　　　　Mineral Supplements

PREGNANCY AND BREAST-FEEDING WARNINGS
Vitamins taken at the level that supplies normal body needs (not megadoses) do not pose a risk to the fetus or the nursing infant.

It is estimated that 40% of adults in the United States take vitamin and mineral supplements daily.[4] Is this necessary?

Vitamin deficiencies are rare in this country. Mineral deficiencies are more common, but taking a multivitamin supplement with minerals is often not the best way to get minerals. These products either do not supply enough of the mineral you lack, or they contain other minerals that reduce your body's ability to absorb the specific mineral you need. Instead of taking such supplements, try changing your diet so that you get more of just the mineral you need, or take a specific mineral supplement. For example, if you have iron-deficiency anemia, you should be taking an iron supplement. Calcium deficiency is another example. Most multivitamin supplements with minerals do not supply enough calcium to meet the recommended dietary allowance (RDA), so taking these supplements may give you a false sense of security about your calcium intake. Changes in your diet, combined with a calcium supplement, may be the best way to increase your calcium intake. See the listings for individual minerals and vitamins for more details.

Who needs a multivitamin and mineral supplement? The following groups of older adults are at risk of vitamin deficiency and may need a supplement:

- those who eat fewer than 1,500 calories a day and may have a barely adequate vitamin intake
- those who live alone, are institutionalized, have recently been discharged from the hospital, or cannot shop for their food
- those who have certain medical problems (such as some intestinal disorders) or take certain drugs that interfere with their body's ability to absorb nutrients
- those who drink too much alcohol, which can reduce the body's supply of certain vitamins (thiamine, riboflavin, folic acid, and vitamins C and B_6)

The more of these groups you belong to, the greater your risk of having a low-calorie, unbalanced, and nutritionally deficient diet. If you have one or more of these factors, you should discuss the need for a multivitamin supplement with your doctor. Remember that a supplement will not completely make up for deficiencies in your diet, since vitamins are only a very small part of proper nutrition. Getting a good balance of protein, fat, carbohydrates, and fiber is also important, and you can only do this through a well-balanced diet.

If you don't fit into the risk categories above, should you take a supplement for "insurance"? If you are eating a well-balanced diet, there is no reason why you need one.

If you take a multivitamin supplement, don't take doses significantly higher than the recommended dietary allowance (RDA). Doses higher than the RDA will either be eliminated from your body in your urine (in the case of water-soluble vitamins such as the B vitamins and vitamin C) or will accumulate in the body tissues and cause harmful adverse effects (in the case of the fat-soluble vitamins A, D, E, and K).

When choosing a multivitamin, keep in mind that many manufacturers use the same general trademark for several products that have different formulas. Some make drastic changes in the formula of a product and keep the name the same. Read the labels and compare the contents of several products. Compare the label with the recommended dietary allowances for older adults (p. 798). There is not much logic in a formula that contains less than 50% of the RDA for some vitamins and more than 500% for others. **Choose a supplement that comes as close as possible to 100% of the RDA for each ingredient.**

Buy the least expensive supplement that meets your needs, and buy a generic version if you can. Generic products are cheaper and are just as effective as the brand-name products.

Before You Use This Drug

Tell your doctor if you have or have had:

- pregnancy or are breast-feeding

Tell your doctor about any other drugs you take, including aspirin, herbs, vitamins, and other nonprescription products.

How to Use This Drug

- If you miss a dose, take it as soon as you remember, but skip it if it is almost time for the next dose. **Do not take double doses.**
- Do not share your medication with others.
- Take the drug at the same time(s) each day.
- Store at room temperature with lid on tightly. Do not store in the bathroom. Do not expose to heat, moisture, or strong light. Keep out of reach of children.

Interactions with Other Drugs

Evaluations of Drug Interactions 2003 lists no drugs, biologics (e.g., vaccines, therapeutic antibodies), or foods as causing "highly clinically significant" or "clinically significant" interactions when used together with the drugs in this section. We also found no interactions in the drugs' FDA-approved professional package inserts. However, as the number of new drugs approved for marketing increases and as more experience is gained with these drugs over time, new interactions may be discovered.

Adverse Events

Call your doctor immediately if you experience:

- skin rash
- sores in the mouth and on the lip

Minerals

Calcium Supplements

Calcium Carbonate (*kal* see um *car* boe nate)
OS-CAL 500 (SmithKline Beecham)
CALTRATE (Lederle)

Calcium Citrate (*kal* see um *si* trate)
CITRACAL (Mission)

Calcium Gluconate (*kal* see um *glue* ko nate)

Calcium Lactate (*kal* see um *lak* tate)

GENERIC: available
FAMILY: Mineral Supplements

PREGNANCY AND BREAST-FEEDING WARNINGS

Minerals taken at the level that supplies normal body needs (not megadoses) do not pose a risk to the fetus or the nursing infant.

Calcium is a mineral that is stored in the bones and is necessary for bone growth and strength. It also benefits the nervous system, muscles, and heart. As your body ages, its ability to absorb calcium decreases, even though its need for calcium does not diminish. If you are older and also have a diet that lacks adequate calcium, both factors limit the amount of the mineral available for your body to use.

Calcium deficiency in older adults causes changes in the bones called osteomalacia and osteoporosis. Osteomalacia is an overall decrease in bone density. Osteoporosis, which occurs most frequently in thin, small-boned, or white women, is a condition in which the bones become weak, so that they are more likely to break or become deformed.

How much calcium do you need? The recommended dietary allowance (RDA) for calcium is 1,200 milligrams per day for men and women over the age of 50. We think that this is a safe and desirable intake for all adults. It will not necessarily protect you against the fractures and deformity of osteoporosis, but it may help and it is unlikely to do you any harm. We do not recommend taking more than 1,500 milligrams per day, since the greater amount has no advantages and can cause some dangerous adverse effects (see Adverse Effects).

The British Expert Group on Vitamins and Minerals concluded that "In humans, the main adverse effect associated with high levels of calcium intake is milk-alkali syndrome (MAS), resulting in hypercalcaemia [increased calcium in the blood], alkalosis and renal impairment. Symptoms can include abdominal pain, hypertension, headaches and tissue calcification. The condition has been reported in a small number of subjects taking calcium-containing medication. Previously, MAS was more common in males taking absorbable alkali and milk, but is now more common in females taking calcium-containing medication. . . . [D]oses up to 1,500 mg/day supplemental calcium would not be expected to result in any adverse effect, but higher doses could result in adverse gastrointestinal symptoms in a few people. An estimate for total calcium intakes has not been made as the effect is related to calcium in supplemental doses."[3]

The best way to get calcium is to eat foods that are rich in it (see box below). In particular, you can increase your calcium intake by drinking milk and adding liquid or powdered milk to almost any cooked food (you can use low-fat or nonfat milk if you want to keep your fat intake down). If you cannot get enough calcium from your diet, take a calcium supplement. However, if you have a history of kidney stones, do not increase your calcium intake without talking to your doctor first.

Many people, particularly women, take calcium supplements in the hope that it will decrease their risk of getting osteoporosis. While it has been shown that a diet containing adequate calcium can prevent high blood pressure, taking supplements to prevent osteoporosis is controversial. If you want to reduce your risk of osteoporosis, try quitting smoking, drinking alcohol in moderation if at all, and doing weight-bearing exercise such as walking, aerobics, jogging, dancing, tennis, or biking (although biking is less beneficial than the others).

If you decide to take a calcium supplement, some cautions are in order. You should not take calcium supplements that contain bonemeal or dolomite. The FDA reported that they might contain lead in amounts that could present a risk to older adults.[24] Furthermore, your body does not absorb all calcium supplements with equal ease. Unfortunately, it has not been determined which supplement is absorbed the best. One study showed that calcium citrate was best absorbed, but another showed that there was no significant difference in absorption among vari-

---

FOODS HIGH IN CALCIUM

Milk, liquid or powdered, including low-fat and nonfat milk, low-fat yogurt, ice cream, cheese (some are high in fat and/or cholesterol), canned salmon and sardines, shellfish, broccoli, green leafy vegetables.

1 cup plain low-fat yogurt	415 milligrams calcium
1 cup milk	300 milligrams calcium
3½ ounces canned salmon with bones	198 milligrams calcium

ous types of supplements.[24,25] Ask your pharmacist or other health professional for suggestions.

When comparing calcium supplements, you should always check how much elemental (pure) calcium they contain. Because calcium supplements contain other ingredients in addition to calcium, a 100-milligram calcium supplement tablet does not contain 100 milligrams of calcium, and a 100-milligram tablet of one supplement does not necessarily have the same amount of calcium as a 100-milligram tablet of another. Calcium carbonate is 40% calcium, calcium gluconate is 9% calcium, and calcium citrate is 24% calcium. Read the label on the container to find out the amount of elemental calcium. This is the only measurement that counts as far as your body is concerned.

Before You Use This Drug

Do not use if you have or have had:

- high level of calcium in your blood
- high level of calcium in your urine
- calcium kidney stones
- sarcoidosis

Tell your doctor if you have or have had:

- allergies to drugs
- pregnancy or are breast-feeding
- dehydrated
- electrolyte imbalance
- diarrhea
- chronic malabsorption
- kidney stones
- kidney disease
- low or no stomach acid (for calcium carbonate only)

Tell your doctor about any other drugs you take, including aspirin, herbs, vitamins, and other nonprescription products.

When You Use This Drug

- Have regular doctor visits if taking large doses or for a long period of time.

- After taking a calcium supplement, wait one to two hours before taking any other drug by mouth.
- Avoid taking this drug along with other preparations containing significant amounts of calcium, phosphate, magnesium, or vitamin D unless your doctor advises you to do so.
- Avoid taking this drug along with certain fiber-containing foods such as bran and whole-grain breads and cereals; wait one to two hours before or after taking calcium.
- *For calcium carbonate:* Take one to one and a half hours after meals.
- Avoid excessive use of alcohol, tobacco, or caffeine.
- Use only calcium products labeled "USP" (calcium carbonate)

How to Use This Drug

- If you miss a dose, take it as soon as you remember, but skip it if it is almost time for the next dose. **Do not take double doses.**
- Do not share your medication with others.
- Take the drug at the same time(s) each day.
- Take with **a full glass (eight ounces) of water** or juice (all dosage forms).
- *For chewable tablets:* chew tablets well before swallowing.
- Store at room temperature with lid on tightly. Do not store in the bathroom. Do not expose to heat, moisture, or strong light. Keep out of reach of children.

Interactions with Other Drugs

The following drugs, biologics (e.g., vaccines, therapeutic antibodies), or foods are listed in *Evaluations of Drug Interactions* 2003 as causing "highly clinically significant" or "clinically significant" interactions when used together with any of the drugs in this section. In some sections with multiple drugs, the interaction may have been reported for one but not all drugs in this section, but we include the interaction because the drugs in this section are similar to one another. We have also included potentially serious interactions listed in the drug's FDA-approved professional package insert or in published medical journal articles. There may be other drugs, especially those in the families of drugs listed below, that also will react with this drug to cause severe adverse effects. Make sure to tell your doctor and pharmacist the drugs you are taking and tell them if you are taking any of these interacting drugs:

ACHROMYCIN, AGENERASE, amprenavir, aspirin, ACTONEL, CALAN SR, CHIBROXIN, chlorothiazide, CILOXAN, CIPRO, ciprofloxacin, COVERA-HS, DIURIL, ECOTRIN, enoxacin, FLOXIN, GENUINE BAYER ASPIRIN, ISOPTIN SR, LEVAQUIN, levofloxacin, lomefloxacin, MAXAQUIN, norfloxacin, NOROXIN, OCUFLOX, ofloxacin, PANMYCIN, PENETREX, risedronate, SKELID, sparfloxacin, SUMYCIN, tetracycline, tiludronate, trovafloxacin, TROVAN, verapamil, VERELAN, ZAGAM.

Adverse Effects

Call your doctor immediately if you experience:

- drowsiness
- continuing nausea and vomiting
- weakness
- difficult or painful urination

Early symptoms of too much calcium:

- severe constipation
- dry mouth
- continuing headache
- continuing increased thirst
- irritability
- appetite loss
- mental depression
- metallic taste
- unusual tiredness or weakness

Late symptoms of too much calcium:

- confusion
- drowsiness
- high blood pressure
- increased sensitivity of eyes or skin to light
- irregular, slow, or fast heartbeat
- nausea or vomiting
- increased amount of urine or frequency of urination

Periodic Tests

Ask your doctor which of these tests should be done periodically while you are taking this drug:

- blood pressure
- blood and urine calcium levels
- electrocardiogram (ECG or EKG)
- magnesium blood test
- parathyroid blood test
- phosphate blood test
- potassium blood test
- kidney function test

Iron Supplements

Ferrous Fumarate (*fair* us *few* mar ate)
FEOSTAT (Forest)

Ferrous Gluconate (*fair* us *glue* koe nate)
FERGON (Bayer)

Ferrous Sulfate (*fair* us *sul* phate)
FEOSOL (SmithKline Beecham)
SLOW FE (Novartis)

GENERIC: available
FAMILY: Mineral Supplements

PREGNANCY AND BREAST-FEEDING WARNINGS
Minerals taken at the level that supplies normal body needs (not megadoses) do not pose a risk to the fetus or the nursing infant.

FOODS HIGH IN IRON

Organ meats, red meat, oysters (all are also high in cholesterol and/or fat), fish, green leafy vegetables, peas, brewer's yeast, wheat germ, certain dried beans and fruits. Iron from meats is absorbed an average of five times better than iron from vegetables.

3½ ounces calves' liver	14.0 milligrams iron
1 lean hamburger	3.9 milligrams iron
3½ ounces chickpeas	3.0 milligrams iron
½ cup cooked lima beans	3.0 milligrams iron

Iron is a mineral that your body needs to manufacture hemoglobin, a substance in red blood cells that carries oxygen throughout the body. A lack of iron causes anemia, a condition in which the body has too few red blood cells, too little hemoglobin, or too little blood. Iron is found in many foods (see box below), and a well-balanced diet with a variety of foods should supply all the iron that your body needs. There is no reason to take an iron supplement unless you have a low iron count or iron-deficiency anemia. The recommended dietary allowance (RDA) for adults over the age of 50 is eight milligrams per day.

Adults generally become iron-deficient from blood loss, rather than from a lack of iron in their diet. If your doctor says that you have iron-deficiency anemia, she or he must determine the site of the blood loss.

If you have iron-deficiency anemia due to blood loss, you should add iron-rich foods to your diet as well as take an iron supplement. When comparing iron supplements, you should always check how much elemental (pure) iron they contain. For example, a 324 milligram ferrous sulfate tablet contains 65 milligrams of elemental iron, while a 320 milligram ferrous gluconate tablet contains 37 milligrams of elemental iron, and a 100 milligram ferrous fumarate tablet contains 33 milligrams of elemental iron. You should start out with a supplement containing ferrous sulfate, rather than one made of ferrous gluconate or ferrous fumarate.[26]

Do not use iron supplements that also contain other minerals such as calcium and magnesium, which can interfere with your body's absorption of iron. Also, do not use enteric-coated tablets (tablets coated so they do not dissolve in your stomach) or timed-release products, because your body does not absorb them evenly. Do not take an iron supplement at the same time as eating foods high in fiber or calcium.

By two weeks after you begin to take an iron supplement, your red blood cell count should improve. If there is no improvement after three to four weeks, ask your doctor to reevaluate your situation. If you are anemic, you might need to take iron supplements for six months or longer to replenish the body's supply. If the cause of your iron deficiency is poor absorption of iron, a rare problem, you may have to take an iron supplement for longer than six months.

If you do not have a low iron count or iron-deficiency anemia, there is no reason for you to take an iron supplement. Your body saves iron and cannot get rid of extra iron except by bleeding. Taking too much iron can cause an iron overload in the body and damage to your liver, heart, or kidneys.[27]

The British Expert Group on Vitamins and Minerals has found that "For guidance purposes, a supplemental intake of approximately 17 mg/day would not be expected to produce adverse effects in the majority of people. . . . This is based on data referring to ferrous iron (Fe II), which is the form of iron used in supplements currently available in this country. A safe upper level for total iron has not been estimated, as gastrointestinal effects are associated with iron in supplements rather than in foods. The guidance value of 17 mg/day calculated above, does not apply to the small proportion of the population who have increased susceptibility to iron overload, via a mechanism of unregulated (increased) absorption from the diet, associated with the homozygous haemochromatosis genotype (estimated prevalence, approximately 0.4% in Caucasian populations)."[3]

Before You Use This Drug

Do not use if you have or have had:

- diseases of iron overload (hemochromatosis, hemosiderosis)
- thalassemia (a hereditary anemia)
- porphyria
- other anemia conditions unless accompanied by iron deficiency

Tell your doctor if you have or have had:

- asthma
- heart disease
- alcohol dependence
- allergies to drugs
- pregnancy or are breast-feeding
- disease of the intestines
- liver disease (hepatitis)
- kidney disease
- peptic ulcer
- recent blood transfusion
- rheumatoid arthritis
- sensitivity to iron

Tell your doctor about any other drugs you take, including aspirin, herbs, vitamins, and other nonprescription products.

When You Use This Drug

- Your stools will probably turn black. This is a normal side effect and no cause for concern.
- Take iron supplements one hour before or two hours after eating dairy products, eggs, coffee, tea, whole-grain breads and cereals, antacids, or calcium supplements.
- Avoid regular use of large amounts of iron supplements several times daily for more than six months unless approved by your doctor.
- Extended-release dosage forms may not release iron properly; check with your doctor if stools are not black during therapy.

- Iron supplements can stain your teeth. To prevent, reduce, or remove iron stains on your teeth:
  - Dilute liquid forms of iron preparations in water or fruit juice.
  - Use a straw (for liquid forms).
  - Place dropper doses well back on tongue (for liquid forms).
  - Brush teeth with baking soda or 3% hydrogen peroxide.

How to Use This Drug

- Take on an empty stomach, at least one hour before, or two hours after, meals. If the iron upsets your stomach, try taking it with food instead. Take with **a full glass (eight ounces) of water** or fruit juice.
- If you miss a dose, take it as soon as you remember, but skip it if it is almost time for the next dose. **Do not take double doses.**
- Do not share your medication with others.
- Take the drug at the same time(s) each day.
- Do not break, chew, or crush long-acting forms of this drug.
- *For oral suspension:* Shake well before using.
- *For chewable tablets:* Chew well before swallowing.

Interactions with Other Drugs

The following drugs, biologics (e.g., vaccines, therapeutic antibodies), or foods are listed in *Evaluations of Drug Interactions* 2003 as causing "highly clinically significant" or "clinically significant" interactions when used together with any of the drugs in this section. In some sections with multiple drugs, the interaction may have been reported for one but not all drugs in this section, but we include the interaction because the drugs in this section are similar to one another. We have also included potentially serious interactions listed in the drug's FDA-approved professional package insert or in published medical journal articles. There may be other drugs, especially those in the families of drugs listed below, that also will react with this drug to cause severe adverse effects. Make sure to tell your doctor and pharmacist the drugs you are taking and tell them if you are taking any of these interacting drugs:

ACHROMYCIN, ACTONEL, ALDOMET, AVELOX, cefdinir, CELLCEPT, CHIBROXIN, CILOXAN, CIPRO, ciprofloxacin, COMTAN, CUPRIMINE, DEPEN, enoxacin, entacapone, LARODOPA, LEVAQUIN, levodopa, levofloxacin, lomefloxacin, MAXAQUIN, methyldopa, moxifloxacin, mycophenolate, norfloxacin, NOROXIN, OMNICEF, PANMYCIN, PENETREX, penicillamine, risedronate, SINEMET, SUMYCIN, TERRAMYCIN, tetracycline, trovafloxacin, TROVAN.

Adverse Effects

Call your doctor immediately if you experience:

- abdominal or stomach pain, cramping, or soreness
- chest or throat pain, especially when swallowing
- stools containing blood

Call your doctor if these symptoms continue:

- constipation
- diarrhea
- nausea or vomiting

- darkened urine
- teeth staining
- heartburn

Signs of overdose:

- Early symptoms:
  - diarrhea, sometimes containing blood
  - fever
  - severe nausea
  - sharp stomach pain or cramping
  - severe vomiting, sometimes containing blood
- Late symptoms:
  - bluish-colored lips, fingernails, or palms of hands
  - drowsiness
  - pale, clammy skin
  - seizures
  - rapid and shallow breathing
  - unusual tiredness or weakness
  - weak and fast heartbeat

If you suspect an overdose, call this number to contact your poison control center: (800) 222-1222.

Periodic Tests

Ask your doctor which of these tests should be done periodically while you are taking this drug:

- ferritin concentration in the blood
- hemoglobin and hematocrit tests
- iron concentration in the blood
- reticulocyte (young red blood cell) counts
- total iron binding capacity (TIBC)

REFERENCES

1. US Nutrition Industry: Top 70 Supplements 1997-2002 (Chart 14). *Nutrition Business Journal* (www.nutritionbusiness.com) 2004.

2. 2005 projections are based on the assumption that change in sales from 2002 to 2005 will be the same as the change from 1999 to 2002.

3. Expert Group on Vitamins and Minerals. Safe Upper Levels for Vitamins and Minerals, 2003. Available at: http://www.foodstandards .gov.uk/multimedia/pdfs/vitmin2003.pdf.

4. Schlamowitz P, Halberg T, Warnoe O, et al. Treatment of mild to moderate hypertension with dietary fibre. *The Lancet* 1987; 2:622–3.

5. Toxic effects of vitamin overdosage. *Medical Letter on Drugs and Therapeutics* 1984; 26:73–4.

6. Vitamin supplements. *Medical Letter on Drugs and Therapeutics* 1998; 40:75–7.

7. Liem A, Reynierse-Buitenwerf GH, Zwinderman AH, et al. Secondary prevention with folic acid: Effects on clinical outcomes. *Journal of the American College of Cardiology* 2003; 41:2105–13.

8. Colditz GA, Branch LG, Lipnick RJ, et al. Increased green and yellow vegetable intake and lowered cancer deaths in an elderly population. *American Journal of Clinical Nutrition* 1985; 41:32–6.

9. *USP DI, Drug Information for the Health Care Professional*. 8th ed. Rockville, Md.: The United States Pharmacopeial Convention, Inc., 1988:2077.

10. Whelan AM, Price SO, Fowler SF, et al. The effect of aspirin on niacin-induced cutaneous reactions. *Journal of Family Practice* 1992; 34:165–8.

11. Hodis HN. Acute hepatic failure associated with the use of low-dose sustained-release niacin. *Journal of the American Medical Association* 1990; 264:181.

12. Henkin Y, Oberman A, Hurst DC, et al. Niacin revisited: Clinical observations on an important but underutilized drug. *American Journal of Medicine* 1991; 91:239–46.

13. Gilman AG, Goodman LS, Rall TW, Murad F, eds. *The Pharmacological Basis of Therapeutics*. 7th ed. New York: MacMillan, 1985:1330.

14. Audera C, Patulny RV, Sander BH, et al. Mega-dose vitamin C in treatment of the common cold: A randomised controlled trial. *Medical Journal of Australia* 2001; 175:359–62.

15. Gilman AG, Goodman LS, Rall TW, Murad F, eds. *The Pharmacological Basis of Therapeutics*. 7th ed. New York: MacMillan, 1985:1570.

16. Trivedi DP, Doll R, Khaw KT. Effect of four monthly oral vitamin D3 (cholecalciferol) supplementation on fractures and mortality in men and women living in the community: Randomised double blind controlled trial. *British Medical Journal* 2003; 326:469.

17. Graat JM, Schouten EG, Kok FJ. Effect of daily vitamin E and multivitamin-mineral supplementation on acute respiratory tract infections in elderly persons: A randomized controlled trial. *Journal of the American Medical Association* 2002; 288:715–21.

18. Brand C, Snaddon J, Bailey M, et al. Vitamin E is ineffective for symptomatic relief of knee osteoarthritis: A six month double blind, randomised, placebo controlled study. *Annals of the Rheumatic Diseases* 2001; 60:946–9.

19. Keith ME, Jeejeebhoy KN, Langer A, et al. A controlled clinical trial of vitamin E supplementation in patients with congestive heart failure. *American Journal of Clinical Nutrition* 2001; 73:219–24.

20. Yusuf S, Dagenais G, Pogue J, et al. Vitamin E supplementation and cardiovascular events in high-risk patients. The Heart Outcomes Prevention Evaluation Study Investigators. *New England Journal of Medicine* 2000; 342:154–60.

21. Rautalahti MT, Virtamo JR, Taylor PR, et al. The effects of supplementation with alpha-tocopherol and beta-carotene on the incidence and mortality of carcinoma of the pancreas in a randomized, controlled trial. *Cancer* 1999; 86:37–42.

22. McNeil JJ, Robman L, Tikellis G, et al. Vitamin E supplementation and cataract: Randomized controlled trial. *Ophthalmology* 2004; 111:75–84.

23. Roberts HJ. Perspective on vitamin E as therapy. *Journal of the American Medical Association* 1981; 246:129–31.

24. Public Citizen's Health Research Group. Osteoporosis Part II: Prevention and Treatment. *Health Letter* 1987; 3:1–7.

25. Sheikh MS, Santa Ana CA, Nicar MJ, et al. Gastrointestinal absorption of calcium from milk and calcium salts. *New England Journal of Medicine* 1987; 317:532–6.

26. AMA Department of Drugs. *AMA Drug Evaluations Annual*. Chicago: American Medical Association, 1983:797.

27. AMA Department of Drugs. *AMA Drug Evaluations Annual*. Chicago: American Medical Association, 1983:1144.

28. Miller ER, Pastor-Barriuso R, Dalal D, et al. Meta-analysis: High-dosage vitamin E supplementation may increase all-cause mortality. *Annals of Internal Medicine* 2005; 142: 37–46.

28

DIETARY AND HERBAL SUPPLEMENTS

There cannot be two kinds of medicine—conventional and alternative. There is only medicine that has been adequately tested and medicine that has not, medicine that works and medicine that may or may not work.[1]

—*New England Journal of Medicine*
editors Marcia Angell and Jerome Kassirer

Complementary and Alternative Medicine (CAM) is a catch-all term for those healing practices that fall outside of conventional medical practice. CAM includes homeopathy, acupuncture, massage, chiropractic, dietary supplements (including botanicals), meditation, and prayer.[2] Of this prodigious list, this chapter concerns only dietary supplements and is limited to the 13 with the largest sales in 2002. Dietary supplements are defined by law as products intended to supplement the diet that contain a vitamin, a mineral, an herb or other botanical, an amino acid, or "a dietary substance for use by man to supplement the diet by increasing the total dietary intake."[3] Vitamins and minerals are considered separately in Chapter 27 of this book.

Plant-based medicines are not inherently dangerous, inherently safe, nor inherently effective. *Digitalis lanata,* or foxglove, provides digoxin (LANOXIN) for treating heart conditions, and *Papaver somniferum,* the opium poppy, is the source of morphine, still one of the best pain relievers known. On the other hand, *Atropa belladonna,* or deadly nightshade, and *Strychnos nuxvomica,* the source of strychnine, are two of history's more famous poisons. A long history of use is proof of neither safety nor effectiveness.

GROWING USE OF DIETARY SUPPLEMENTS

The use of dietary supplements and other forms of CAM is widespread and growing.[4,5] One national study, based on data from 1997, estimated that two-thirds of respondents had used at least one CAM therapy in their lifetimes and that younger people were more likely to do so.[4] A very large national survey estimated that in 2002, 62% of adults used at least one CAM therapy; this number fell to 36% if prayer for health reasons was excluded.[6] The use of "nonvitamin, nonmineral, natural products" in 2002 was reported by 19% of respondents, equivalent to 38 million U.S. residents. The leading products were echinacea (40% of those who used these products in 2002), ginseng (24%), ginkgo biloba (21%), and garlic (20%). All of these products are reviewed in this chapter.

Among often-desperate cancer patients, the prevalence of dietary supplement use may be higher than in the general population, perhaps in the range of 21 to 54%.[7,8] In another study, 63% of cancer patients were believed to have used either vitamins or herbs.[8] According to the National Academy of Sciences, the sale of dietary supplements alone is now an $18 billion-a-year industry.[9]

A large amount of this use occurs below the sightlines of the medical profession. As many as one-third of cancer patients do not disclose their use of vitamins or herbs to their physicians.[7,10] We encourage all CAM users to be open about their use with their health care providers. Without this information, providers cannot interpret any benefits or adverse effects you may be experiencing.

REGULATORY STATUS OF DIETARY SUPPLEMENTS

The enormous increase in the sales of dietary supplements did not simply happen by accident. Although there are societal trends favoring products that call themselves "natural" and growing suspicion of the medical establishment by some, the growth in dietary supplement sales is in significant part the result of a single act of Congress: the 1994 Dietary Supplement Health and Education Act (DSHEA). The history of the act is instructive. In the late 1980s, an outbreak of a mysterious condition called eosinophilia-myalgia syndrome occurred among users of a supplement called L-tryptophan, an unproven insomnia remedy. The exact cause of the syndrome was never determined but is assumed to be a contaminant in batches of the supplement produced by a Japanese manufacturer. All told, over 1,500 people fell ill, with at least 37 deaths.[11]

These events strengthened the FDA's desire to regulate dietary supplements more strictly. In particular, the agency hoped to reduce misleading promotional claims being made for these products and to develop standards for Good Manufacturing Practice (GMP). The effort had the opposite effect. Dietary supplement manufacturers enlisted the aid of Senator Orrin Hatch of Utah, a state with a strong supplement industry, and solicited some 200,000 letters condemning the FDA's alleged effort to take away the citizenry's vitamins. The result was DSHEA, which left supplements less regulated than before. Supplement manufacturers have been quick to exploit the opportunity and, by judicious campaign contributions,[12] have reduced the likelihood of the statute's repeal.

DSHEA clarified that supplements were to be regulated essentially as foods, not drugs, and thus were exempt from the tougher regulation accorded to drugs. In particular, there is no requirement for companies to register either their names or their products with the government. The FDA was charged with promulgating regulations describing GMPs for dietary supplements, but a decade later these have still not been finalized. There is thus no regulation ensuring that the amount of a substance claimed to be in a supplement is actually present, or that contaminants or active drugs are not present. For each dietary supplement we discuss, we include any available published reports of contamination or instances where supplement content varied significantly from the labeled amount. In one study of products not directly evaluated in this book, 32% of Asian patent medicines examined were found to be contaminated with heavy metals (e.g., lead, arsenic, and mercury) or undeclared pharmaceuticals (e.g., chlorpheniramine [CHLOR-TRIMETON], methyltestosterone, and phenacetin, a banned painkiller).[13] In addition, the quantity of active ingredient can vary according to the particular species, what part of the plant is used, what time of year the plant is harvested, and how the ingredient is extracted from the plant. We are also particularly concerned about a subset of dietary supplements called glandulars (literally crushed organs from other animals); the possibility that supplements containing cow brain might contain the agent that causes mad cow disease has been raised.[14,15]

Supplement manufacturers wish to distinguish their products from drugs because prior to marketing, all drugs have to demonstrate their safety and effectiveness. By having their products classified as foods, supplement manufacturers evade this critical step, which can take time and money and prove unsuccessful. Thus, **no supplement has been demonstrated to be safe and effective under the standards the FDA applies to drugs.** Furthermore, while drug companies have to report any adverse events they learn about to the FDA, there is no requirement for the manufacturers of dietary supplements to do so. The Department of Health and Human Services inspector general described the system as "an inadequate safety valve" and noted that under 1% of adverse events associated with dietary supplements are reported to the FDA.[16] A classic example of this was Metabolife, a leading manufacturer of ephedra, which had 18,502 adverse reaction reports in its files, some on scraps of paper, none of which it initially reported to the FDA.[17]

If these products have never been proved safe and effective, how can they continue to be pro-moted so aggressively? The FDA makes the kind of distinction only a lawyer could love: the regulatory structure for promotions regarding dietary supplements draws on the "distinction" between health claims (not permitted) and structure/function claims (permitted). For example, a supplement manufacturer, without any supporting evidence whatsoever, can assert that its product "promotes prostate health" (a structure/function claim) but is precluded from claiming that it "treats the symptoms of an enlarged prostate" (a health claim). Of course, an older man with difficulty urinating, inability to empty the bladder, and the need to urinate at night understands that a product that "promotes prostate health" is intended to treat prostate enlargement, but Congress permits and even encourages this charade. Occasionally, a company may step over the line and make a health claim so outlandish that even the sensibilities of the Federal Trade Commission (FTC), which regulates the advertising of dietary supplements, are offended and the agency takes action, but these actions are far outweighed by misleading promotions that pass by undisturbed. For example, an FTC report on weight-loss supplements estimated that close to 40% of weight-loss advertisements in 2001, 66% of which were for dietary supplements, made at least one claim that was almost certainly false.[18]

Although the companies are not required to prove safety prior to marketing, Congress went still further by raising the bar for removing a supplement from the market due to lack of safety. The FDA can act only if it can prove a "significant or unreasonable risk of illness or injury under conditions of use suggested or recommended in the labeling."[19] This authority has been used only once, for the dangerous supplement ephedra (see p. 835), and the agency's authority to take such action has been challenged, so far unsuccessfully, in court. With the standard for removal from the market so high, the FDA has been forced to protect the public by releasing a series of warnings for certain supplements, including the following:[20]

androstenedione, an anabolic steroid
aristolochic acid, associated with kidney
    failure and urinary tract cancer
comfrey, associated with liver toxicity
kava kava, associated with liver toxicity

ASSESSING THE EFFECTIVENESS OF DIETARY SUPPLEMENTS

For centuries, the basis for establishing the effectiveness of medicines had been the health care provider's personal experience combined with an oral and written tradition whereby interventions of purported effectiveness were taught to more junior physicians and students. That was all to change. In October 1948, the *British Medical Journal* published what is arguably the first randomized, controlled trial: a study that proved that streptomycin was more effective than placebo in the treatment of tuberculosis of the lung.[21] The publication of that trial ushered in a new era in modern medicine, one in which rigorous empiricism was to supplant the personal experiences of oneself or others. Only through such methodological rigor, it was argued, could the safety and effectiveness of medicines and other interventions be determined with adequate certainty to justify exposing the public to them. Many medications (and even surgeries) that formed the core of medical practice for decades or even centuries have been debunked by these experiments.[22] Others have proved surprisingly effective.

The ideas of this movement, now carrying the soubriquet evidence-based medicine, provide the theoretical basis for this book. We apply its principles in all chapters, no less so in this one, for there is no reason to think that the movement's principles cannot and should not be applied to CAM.[2] While evidence can come in various forms, the gold standard for evidence is the randomized controlled trial.

Let us consider a hypothetical study in which we are trying to determine if a putative cholesterol-lowering drug can actually lower cholesterol. Imagine, too, that one group gets the actual drug and the other (the control group) a dummy pill that looks and tastes like the actual drug but is actually inactive (a placebo). Both groups get dietary counseling. In our study, participants are assigned by a systematic process called randomization to either the drug or placebo group, in effect by the toss of a coin; each person is as likely as any other to be assigned to drug or placebo. This ensures that the starting average cholesterols in the two groups will be about equal. Equally important, other characteristics, even those that cannot be measured, should also occur about equally in the two groups. Thus, if in the future someone discovers that, unexpectedly, eye color is a factor in determining cholesterol levels, the designer of our study will be able to say with some assurance that the number of blue-eyed people in the drug and placebo groups was about equal, even if he or she never measured eye color.

If the drug is compared to a placebo, as in our hypothetical trial, it is a special case of the randomized, controlled trial called a placebo-controlled trial. Often one is less interested in whether the putative drug is better than nothing and more interested in knowing whether it is as effective as, or even better than, established treatments. In this case, one would compare the drug to a known treatment in another kind of randomized, controlled trial called an active-controlled trial. In some cases, especially when the condition being treated is life-threatening and the existing treatments are particularly effective, randomizing volunteers to placebos would be unethical. (An ongoing concern regarding all dietary supplements, especially those that are totally ineffective, is that they might supplant more effective medications or delay effective therapy.)

But someone might criticize our trial of the cholesterol-lowering drug by arguing that if the volunteers knew they were in the placebo group they might watch their diets more carefully than those who thought they were protected by the new drug. For this reason, researchers generally purposefully do not disclose to the study volunteers which group they are in; this process is called blinding. (The volunteers are told in an informed consent form that they will not be told to which group they were assigned until after the study is completed.) In order to prevent any bias, the doctors also are not told the assignment of their patients; if they were told, perhaps they would encourage placebo patients to be more careful with their diets or to exercise more. Such a study is called a double-blind study; if it is also randomized and has a placebo control, it is called (naturally enough) a randomized, double-blind, placebo-controlled trial.

For the most part, the dietary supplements that form the core of this chapter are not being advocated for the treatment of life-threatening illnesses and in some instances the condition in question may not even have an effective treatment. Thus, we believe that each supplement considered in this chapter should have to demonstrate effectiveness (and safety) in the way the FDA requires for many drugs: by proving effectiveness in two randomized, double-blind, placebo-controlled trials.

Reading the profiles of each dietary supplement in this chapter is a bit like reliving medical history. In general, the supplements are first put forth as effective based on word of mouth or long histories of use, often by traditional groups. As demands for evidence escalate, studies are often done, though these often are not randomized, blinded, or placebo-controlled. Many of the studies collated in the oft-cited, largely unreferenced German Commission E are of this sort; these poorly conducted studies are often lauded by proponents and promoters of dietary supplements as evidence of effectiveness. By the late 1990s,

studies with the elements described above have usually been done, although even these can be poorly executed (e.g., too small, too short, too many volunteers lost to follow-up). Recently, well-conducted randomized, double-blind, placebo-controlled trials have appeared for a minority of supplements in this chapter and provide a reasonable basis for beginning to assess the safety and effectiveness of these products.

HOW THIS CHAPTER WAS COMPILED

In the other chapters of this book, we have had access to published articles describing randomized, controlled trials in medical journals, medical textbooks, the FDA-approved label, and, importantly, the detailed review of the drug (based on a review of the raw data from the sponsor's clinical trials) conducted by the FDA medical officer, at least for more recent drugs (see more detail on our methods on p. xxviii). This evidence base is far from complete for any dietary supplement. By definition, no supplement has passed an FDA safety and efficacy review (otherwise it would be a drug). This means that not only have none of these products been proved safe and effective by conventional standards, but also, in general, there has been no requirement for testing for cancer or birth defects, no studies to establish the optimal dose or dosing schedule, no chemical tests to make sure the active ingredient gets into the body consistently or is consistently present from batch to batch, and no assurance that contaminants are not present.

The dietary supplements and herbs covered in this chapter were identified using a report obtained from the *Nutrition Business Journal* that ranked the 70 top supplements by U.S. consumer sales in 2002.[23] Many of these supplements are vitamins and minerals and are considered in a separate chapter (see p. 791). The supplements reviewed in this chapter include all other supplements (other than enzymes and hormones) ranked in the top 40. Their 2002 retail sales ranged from $59 million for black cohosh to $1.4 billion for ephedra combinations.

The principal source of information for this chapter has been PubMed, the world's largest computerized database of medical journal articles. Unfortunately, this is far from foolproof. For St. John's wort (see p. 852) and glucosamine (see p. 843), in particular, there is evidence of publication bias—the selective publication of favorable results. There have been allegations of scientific misconduct leveled against some authors of published articles on dietary supplements.[24-27] Nonetheless, due to the essentially unregulated nature of these products, these published articles represent the majority of the available data.

In PubMed, we searched for articles on the effectiveness of each supplement (including common synonyms), characterized in the database as "controlled trials," and restricted ourselves to trials in humans and published in English. In contemporary medicine, the vast majority of important studies now appear in the English language literature. For the drugs reviewed for this chapter, the most recent, best-conducted studies all were published in English (there were no references in the articles we reviewed to recent pivotal trials in other languages). We then reviewed the search results, excluding small studies (generally less than 20 subjects in each study group), those evaluating products with multiple ingredients (the effect of any one ingredient cannot be determined), topical or intravenous products, and those in which the study volunteers got only one or two doses of the drug to measure acute effects. We considered only randomized studies with clinically relevant, relatively "hard" outcomes (e.g., generally not those measuring vague outcomes or only the results of blood tests) and did not consider studies of products intended to improve general well-being (as opposed to specific medical conditions) or performance in sporting activities. We collected both placebo- and active-controlled trials, but only considered the latter if the former indicated a benefit. The articles themselves had to be available either from the library of a major national medical center (electronically or in hard copy) or in hard copy at the library of the National Institutes of Health. The rare articles we could not secure through these means were considered too obscure as well as, for practical purposes, inaccessible to the general public. A second search using the supplement name and the search term "adverse events" and the same restrictions as above identified studies on interactions and adverse effects of the supplements. We also conducted separate searches using the search terms "mutagenicity" (for damage to the genes) and "carcinogenicity" (for propensity to cause cancer).

In addition to using the published medical literature, we relied on the actions and publications of several drug regulatory authorities around the world. These include the U.S. FDA, Health Canada, the Medicines Control Agency—Committee on Safety of Medicines in the United Kingdom, the Therapeutics Goods Administration in Australia, and New Zealand's Medicines and Medical Devices Safety Authority. We put particular emphasis on the views of the respected pharmacology publications *The Medical Letter,* the *Drug and Therapeutics Bulletin,* and *Prescrire International,* which do not accept any support from the pharmaceutical industry. We obtained all available meta-analyses (a statistical technique for combining multiple studies) from the Cochrane Library and searched the 2003 edition of *Evaluations of Drug Interactions* for interactions classified as "highly clinically significant" or "clinically significant." The brand names listed include all those containing the particular dietary supplement listed in the 2002 *Physicians' Desk Reference for Nonprescription Drugs and Dietary Supplements* or mentioned repeatedly in research articles.

Despite the relative paucity of information available on dietary supplements, we attempted to review these products with the same degree of skepticism that we accord all the drugs in this book. In effect, we asked: Given the available evidence, would this product have been approved as a drug by the FDA?

SUPPLEMENT PROFILES

 Do Not Use

Black Cohosh
AWARENESS FEMALE BALANCE (Amerifit)
ESTROVEN (Amerifit)
REMIFEMIN (GlaxoSmithKline)

FAMILY:	Dietary Supplements
MUTAGENICITY:	no relevant studies
CARCINOGENICITY:	see Adverse Effects below

Background

Black cohosh is a plant belonging to the buttercup family and has the botanical names *Actaea racemosa* and *Cimicifuga racemosa*. It also goes by the popular names snakeroot, rattleroot, and bugbane. The ingredients for dietary supplements are chemically extracted from the roots and rhizome.

Black cohosh is native to North America and was routinely used by Penobscot, Winnebago, and Dakota Indians for coughs, colds, rheumatism, and to increase milk production.[28] In the 19th century, black cohosh enjoyed popularity as an ingredient in a 36-proof patent medicine called Lydia Pinkham's Vegetable Compound.[29] Currently, "alternative" practitioners and some physicians prescribe black cohosh for hot flashes and other symptoms associated with menopause.

Claimed Uses

Menopausal Symptoms

The interest in black cohosh for menopausal symptoms relies in large part on the claim that the root has estrogen-like activity. However, there are conflicting studies on this issue, with recent studies usually not detecting such activity.[30]

The use of black cohosh received a boost when a committee of the American College of Obstetricians and Gynecologists reported in 2001 that it "may be helpful in the short-term ([up to] 6 months) treatment of [certain menopausal] symptoms."[31] This conclusion was, in the College's own description, "based primarily on consensus and expert opinion"; they did not cite a single randomized controlled trial to support that statement.

We identified four randomized, placebo-controlled studies of the effectiveness of black cohosh for menopausal symptoms. In the first, black cohosh had no impact upon the number or intensity of hot flashes in breast cancer patients over a two-month period.[32] Based on this study, a 1987 German study, and two randomized studies that did not have placebo groups, the National Center for Complementary and Alternative Medicine of the National Institutes of Health concluded in a 2003 report that "the currently available data are not sufficient to support a recommendation on the use of black cohosh for menopausal symptoms."[30]

We have identified three subsequent randomized, placebo-controlled studies of black cohosh for menopausal or menstrual symptoms that claimed some positive effects. In the first, black cohosh combined with two other drugs was studied to assess its effect on menstrual migraine. Consequently, the independent effect of black cohosh cannot be determined.[33] In the second, a study of hot flashes in breast cancer patients, the investigators and the patients knew who was getting black cohosh and who placebo; this can lead to bias, making study interpretation unreliable.[34] Finally, a study of the impact of black cohosh upon menopausal symptoms and bone markers was hampered by the exclusion of about one-third of the patients.[35] The latter two articles appeared in a medical journal supplement devoted almost entirely to black cohosh and sponsored by two of the herb's manufacturers. Supplements to medical journals often have promotional attributes and may not be peer-reviewed.[36]

There are inadequate data to support the claims for black cohosh's effectiveness in relieving the symptoms of menopause. Preparations tend not to be standardized, and one brand has been the subject of almost all the clinical trials. No tenable mode of action for the herb has been put forward.

Interactions with Other Drugs

Black cohosh has not been reported to interact with any drugs, but this has not been specifically studied.[30]

Adverse Effects

Adverse effects of black cohosh include stomach upset, weight gain, and headache. There are two reports in the published medical literature of liver transplants associated with the use of black cohosh.[37,38] In a randomized trial of black cohosh in rats, the supplement did not cause an increase in the rate of breast tumors, but if tumors did occur, they were more likely to have spread to the lungs in animals receiving black cohosh.[39] The National Center for Complementary and Alternative Medicine has warned about the use of black cohosh in pregnancy and by breast cancer patients.[30]

Conclusion

There is no significant evidence that black cohosh alleviates menopausal symptoms. A 12-month, randomized, placebo-controlled trial sponsored by the National Institutes of Health is currently under way but has not yet reported results.

Do Not Use

Coenzyme Q_{10} (Co Q_{10}, Q_{10}, Vitamin Q_{10}, Ubiquinone, Ubidecarenone)
ANTI-AGING DAILY PREMIUM PAK (Youngevity)
Q-GEL (Tishcon)
VITAMIST INTRA-ORAL SPRAY (Vitamist)

FAMILY:	Dietary Supplements
MUTAGENICITY:	no relevant studies
CARCINOGENICITY:	no relevant studies

Background

Coenzyme Q_{10} is unlike most other dietary supplements in this chapter in that it actually occurs naturally in humans and most mammals. Coenzymes are molecules that are needed for the functioning of enzymes; enzymes are molecules that speed up chemical reactions in the body. Coenzyme Q_{10} exists in the mitochondria of cells and is involved in chemical reactions that generate energy for cell growth and maintenance. It also functions as an antioxidant. Antioxidants neutralize so-called free radicals, which are highly reactive chemicals that can damage the DNA in genes and have been linked to cancer.[40]

Coenzyme Q_{10} is synthesized in the body and is found in all animal tissues; there is no need for healthy people eating a varied diet to supplement their food intake to obtain it. Low levels of Coenzyme Q_{10} have been detected in patients with cancer and heart failure and this has served as a rationale in and of itself for treating patients with these diseases with

Coenzyme Q_{10}. This is not logical. Cancer patients typically have low red blood cell counts and low levels of albumin in their blood; it does not follow that blood transfusions or administering albumin will cure them. As always, the best way to assess whether a chemical effectively treats a disease is to subject it to a randomized, controlled trial. The FDA has warned one Coenzyme Q_{10} manufacturer not to claim that the supplement is effective for heart disease.[41]

Claimed Uses

Cancer

Claims for the use of Coenzyme Q_{10} in cancer rest on the observation that cancer patients have low levels of the coenzyme (see above) and some clinical observations. These are either small numbers of case reports[42] or unblinded, uncontrolled studies in which selected patients taking other regimens for cancer had supposed decreases in tumor size or even cure.[43] As the National Cancer Institute notes, "No report of a *randomized clinical trial* of coenzyme Q_{10} as a treatment for cancer has been published in a peer-reviewed, scientific journal."[40]

Reduce Toxicity of Cancer Chemotherapy

The only obtainable study examining whether the administration of Coenzyme Q_{10} could reduce the heart toxicity of the chemotherapeutic agent doxorubicin (ADRIAMYCIN) is a nonrandomized study with a very high loss to follow-up,[44] which often biases the results.

Congestive Heart Failure

A number of early studies claimed that Coenzyme Q_{10} could benefit patients with congestive heart failure[45–47] or improve heart output after heart surgery.[48] However, these studies followed small numbers of patients or used mea-

sures of heart output that were vague or are no longer considered acceptable, and other early studies showed no impact of Coenzyme Q_{10}.[49]

Two more recent, better designed studies have undermined the credibility of these effectiveness claims. In one three-month study, patients with congestive heart failure randomized to Coenzyme Q_{10} had similar changes in measures of their heart function (e.g., ejection fraction, cardiac volume, quality of life) as patients randomized to placebo, although the study was small.[50] In a larger, six-month study, Coenzyme Q_{10} similarly had no effect on measures of heart function (e.g., ejection fraction, peak oxygen consumption, exercise duration).[51] The claimed effectiveness of Coenzyme Q_{10} thus remains unproven.

High Blood Pressure

Two studies claim significant blood-pressure-lowering effects for Coenzyme Q_{10}, one in a study of hypertensive patients[52] and another in those in which only the higher number is elevated (isolated systolic hypertension).[53] These studies are relatively short-term and fall well short of what the FDA would require to approve an antihypertension drug. For example, they do not explore a range of Coenzyme Q_{10} doses.

Heart Attack

A single randomized study published in 1998 claims to have shown that, among patients admitted to hospital with suspicion of a heart attack, Coenzyme Q_{10} can reduce subsequent fatal and nonfatal heart attacks.[54] However, follow-up was short, the placebo and treatment capsules were not identical, and the authors claim an unlikely 100% follow-up rate (or they are only reporting on patients they did recontact, which is not methodologically acceptable). The authors conclude that "More studies in a larger number of patients and long-term follow-up are needed to confirm our results." We were unable to locate any such study.

Diabetes

Two randomized studies claim benefits upon blood sugar control in diabetes. However, the first did not measure hemoglobin A_1C (HbA$_1$C),[52] which measures average glucose control over an approximately three-month period, and the second showed only a small improvement in HbA$_1$C but no impact upon fasting blood sugar or insulin levels.[55] Two small studies with longer follow-up showed no impact of Coenzyme Q$_{10}$ on HbA$_1$C.[56,57]

Parkinson's Disease

The only randomized, controlled trial reported a trend toward a small benefit on a scale that measured Parkinson's disease symptoms, but no impact upon the rate at which these patients with early disease began to need treatment with levodopa.[58]

Huntington's Disease

The only randomized controlled trial showed no impact of Coenzyme Q$_{10}$ on the rate of functional decline in Huntington's disease.[59]

Interactions with Other Drugs

The 2003 edition of *Evaluations of Drug Interactions* and a published medical journal article[60] list warfarin (COUMADIN) as interacting with Coenzyme Q$_{10}$.

Adverse Effects

Coenzyme Q$_{10}$ is generally well tolerated. Infrequent adverse effects have included inability to sleep, liver enzyme elevations, rashes, nausea, and abdominal pain.[40]

Conclusion

Despite the plethora of claimed uses, not a single potential indication has adequate evidence to support the clinical use of Coenzyme Q$_{10}$.

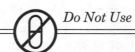 *Do Not Use*

Echinacea (Purple Coneflower, Red Sunflower, Thimbleweed, Rudbeckia)
HALLS DEFENSE MULTI-BLEND SUPPLEMENT DROPS (Pfizer)
VITAMIST INTRA-ORAL SPRAY (Vitamist)

FAMILY:	Dietary Supplements
MUTAGENICITY:	no relevant studies
CARCINOGENICITY:	no relevant studies

Background

The term echinacea, when used in the context of dietary supplements, denotes one or more of three echinacea species: *E. purpurea, E. angustifolia,* and *E. pallida.* Various echinacea preparations may contain one or more of these (the first two are most common) and the supplement may be derived from the roots, herbs, or whole plant. To complicate matters further, the chemical content of the extract varies by the season it is harvested and by the method of extraction used. Some potentially active compounds have been isolated, but a mechanism of action has never been confirmed.

The plant is a member of the daisy family and is native to North America, where Native Americans have used it since the 1600s for snakebites, wounds, tonsillitis, headache, and cold symptoms.[61,62] In the early 1900s, attention turned to use for infection, but it was eclipsed by the advent of antibiotics. In Germany, where it is marketed as a prescription drug, the supplement attracted attention as a preventive and treatment for the common cold and is widely used.

Claimed Uses

In 1998, a study that reviewed all previous randomized, controlled trials of echinacea was published.[63] The review found some positive evidence for the effectiveness of echinacea in the prevention and treatment of the common cold but acknowledged that "few recommendations can be made regarding the use of Echinacea products in practice. The heterogeneity of the available preparations and the limited quality and consistency of the evidence do not allow clear conclusions about which product might be effective in what dose and in what circumstances." Of the 16 better-quality studies in the review, all but two were conducted in Germany and only one was published in the large medical journal database MedLine.[64]

Since that time, a number of better-designed trials have been conducted. Below we summarize the data from those trials and the earlier MedLine-published trial.

Preventing the Common Cold

We identified three randomized, placebo-controlled studies of echinacea; one used an extract of *E. purpurea,* another an extract of *E. purpurea* and *E. angustifolia,* and a third did not specify. Two of the studies showed no benefit of echinacea upon the time to the first cold, the percentage that had a single cold, or the number of colds.[64,65] In a third trial, patients were randomized to echinacea or placebo and then exposed to a cold virus. The rate of clinical infections was similar between the two groups.[66]

Treating the Common Cold

Two of the prevention trials also measured the impact of echinacea upon the course of the common cold. Four treatment-only trials were also identified. Of these six studies, three evaluated a preparation with all three echinacea species and two used a formulation with only *E. purpurea* and *E. angustifolia.* The sixth study was an experimental study[65] (see above) and did not specify which forms of echinacea were studied.

The four larger, best-conducted studies, published in the best medical journals, all found no statistically significant impact of echinacea on the duration or severity of cold symptoms.[65–68] These included the experiment and the two most recently published studies, one of which is in children.[68] Two of the smaller studies did claim beneficial effects, but these studies were of poor quality. In one, which claimed the duration of a cold could be reduced by a median of three days, the study subjects in the two groups appear to have been different at the beginning of the study,[69] raising questions about whether the randomization was adequate. In the second, a very crude questionnaire evaluated the duration and severity of symptoms.[61] In addition, it is unclear that the patients in this study were properly blinded to the taste of the echinacea herbal tea that was studied.

In 2002, the authoritative *Medical Letter* reviewed the data on echinacea for both the prevention and treatment of the common cold and concluded that "there is no convincing evidence that echinacea decreases the severity or shortens the duration of an upper respiratory infection."[70]

Preventing and Treating Recurrent Genital Herpes

There is only one published randomized, placebo-controlled trial, and, despite a less than ideal follow-up of the enrolled patients, it shows no effectiveness for echinacea in reducing either the frequency or severity of genital herpes recurrences.[71] Use of the supplement for herpes prevention or treatment seems particularly unjustified, given the existence of effective therapies for that condition.

Interactions with Other Drugs

No interactions with other drugs have been reported, but this has not been studied formally. Because use of echinacea is intended to stimulate the immune system, some authors suggest avoiding the use of echinacea if the patient is taking immunosuppressive drugs.[62,72]

Adverse Effects

The most common adverse effects appear to be bad taste, stomach upset, headache, and dizziness.[72] In one randomized study, there was a statistically significant increase in rashes among echinacea-treated patients,[68] but this has not been reported in other randomized trials. Allergic reactions to echinacea, some leading to anaphylaxis, a life-threatening reaction, have been reported.[73] Some observers caution against echinacea use for longer than eight weeks or in patients with systemic progressive illnesses such as HIV infection, tuberculosis, or multiple sclerosis.[74] A study of echinacea use during pregnancy reports that the rate of major birth defects was not increased, but there were only enough patients in the study to detect a tripling or more in such defects.[75]

Conclusion

There is no convincing evidence that echinacea reduces the frequency or severity of the common cold or recurrent genital herpes.

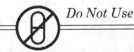

Do Not Use

Ephedra (Ma huang, Chinese ephedra, epitonin)

FAMILY: Dietary Supplements
MUTAGENICITY: stomach acid converts ephedra to a chemical[76] that damages genes[77]
CARCINOGENICITY: no relevant studies

Background

The plant species *ephedra* (also known as *ma huang,* Chinese ephedra, or epitonin) contains a number of related chemical compounds known collectively as ephedrine alkaloids. The principal active ingredient is known as ephedrine, a compound used in the 1920s as a central nervous system stimulant and as a treatment for nasal congestion and asthma. Use declined as more effective therapies for these conditions were identified.[78]

Ephedra is very closely related to the street drug amphetamine as well as phenylpropanolamine, a drug that was removed from the market due to its association with stroke.[79] All these compounds are called sympathomimetics: they increase metabolic rate, heart rate, and blood pressure. The "high" produced by these drugs makes them candidates for recreational abuse.

Claimed Uses

Other than recreational drug use, an indication not recognized by the medical profession, the primary uses of ephedra recently have been for weight loss and to enhance athletic performance. The latter is also not a medical indication (to say nothing of the ethics of drug-enhanced athletic competition); in any event, no randomized trials of ephedra itself to enhance athletic performance have been done. A meta-analysis of randomized, controlled trials concluded that "the effect of ephedra or ephedrine as it is used to promote enhanced athletic performance is unknown."[80]

For weight loss, there is not a single randomized trial that lasted longer than six months; there is, therefore, no evidence for the long-term efficacy of the ephedra alkaloids. Combining studies of ephedra and ephedrine (and including those in which caffeine, another sympathomimetic, was also administered), the weight loss due to the ephedra alkaloids was estimated at two pounds per month, a trivial amount for an obese person.[80]

Interactions with Other Drugs

The following interactions were identified from published medical journal articles and FDA documents: tramadol (ULTRAM, ULTRACET),[81] monoamine oxidase (MAO) inhibitors (e.g., phenelzine),[72] stimulants (e.g., caffeine, decongestants).[82] The 2003 edition of *Evaluations of Drug Interactions* lists metformin (GLUCOPHAGE, GLUCOVANCE, METAGLIP) and reserpine (SERPALAN) as having either "highly clinically significant" or "clinically significant" interactions with ephedrine.

Adverse Effects

The primary safety concerns with respect to ephedra have related to the cardiovascular and central nervous systems. It is no surprise that ephedra would affect the cardiovascular system. Clinical experiments have associated the supplement with heart rhythm abnormalities,[83] increased blood pressure,[84] and prolongation of an interval in the electrocardiogram (ECG or EKG) called the QT_c.[85] Prolongation of this interval is associated with increased risk for life-threatening arrhythmias; the FDA has removed drugs from the market for QT_c prolongations less severe than those described for ephedra.[85]

Ephedra has also been associated with case reports of stroke.[86] A more formal study of the risks of ephedra suggested a risk for a particular type of stroke at higher doses of ephedra, but this finding did not reach statistical significance.[87] Psychiatric effects associated with ephedra include bizarre behavior, hallucinations, paranoia, agitation, anxiety, mania, and nightmares.[88]

Additional concerns have included ephedra-induced hearing loss[89] and unrelieved, painful erections (priapism).[90] The General Accounting Office, an investigative branch of the U.S. Con-

gress, lists the following adverse effects associated with ephedra, in addition to those mentioned above: appetite loss, nausea, vomiting, urinary disturbances, sweating, insomnia, dizziness, shortness of breath, fever, tremor, muscle injury, nerve damage, severe headaches, memory loss, seizures, and dependency.[91]

As with many dietary supplements, the labels for many ephedra-containing supplements have not always accurately reflected the contents. Measured amounts of ephedra in one study ranged from 25 to 105% of the labeled amount. Many products contained other ephedra alkaloids, and there was significant lot-to-lot variation in content.[92] Public Citizen identified nine manufacturers producing 10 dietary supplements that openly advertised their products as containing synthetic ephedrine alkaloids, even though dietary supplements are not allowed to contain synthetic versions of the supplement.[93]

In addition to the clinical reports of adverse effects and the inadequate manufacturing standards, several studies systematically examined the FDA's adverse event monitoring system for cases of serious harm related to ephedra. (It is widely acknowledged that this system collects a small fraction of all events that occur, particularly for dietary supplements, because supplement manufacturers are not even required to report adverse events to the FDA.) Two non-overlapping reports covering the period from 1995 to early 1999, before the heyday of ephedra use, identified 21 deaths related to ephedra.[94,95] These reports and others led Public Citizen to call for the banning of ephedra-containing dietary supplements in September 2001. It was not until December 2003 that the FDA finally acted to do so. By then, over 155 deaths associated with the drug had been reported to the FDA, most due to heart attacks and strokes.[96] All indications are that ephedra has been by far the most injurious of all dietary supplements marketed in the United States. In FDA data from 1993 through 2001, ephedrine alkaloids accounted for 42% of all reports and 59% of all deaths for dietary supplements.[97] In another study that adjusted for the relative use of dietary supplements, ephedra was associated with a 220-fold increase in the probability of having an adverse event compared to all other dietary supplements combined.[78]

Conclusion

Years after the dangers of ephedra were recognized, the FDA has finally removed the supplement from the market.[98] Nonetheless, some stores may still have it in inventory,[99] patients may have it in their medicine chests, and the product may be available over the Internet. We recommend you not use this product and discard any pills you may have in your possession.

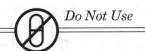 *Do Not Use*

Garlic
ANTI-AGING DAILY PREMIUM PAK
(Youngevity)
KWAI (Lichtwer)
PHYTO-VITE (Wellness)
VITAMIST INTRA-ORAL SPRAY (Vitamist)

FAMILY:	Dietary Supplements
MUTAGENICITY:	no relevant studies
CARCINOGENICITY:	no relevant studies

Background

"Garlic is as good as ten mothers," or at least so claims a documentary extolling the virtues of the plant.[100] From its role as a currency in ancient Egypt to warding off vampires in the Balkans, the plant has always been steeped in myth and mystery. Garlic, also known by its plant name *Allium sativum,* has been traced by historians to nomadic Siberian tribes 5,000

years ago who spread it to other areas.[101] But is it any good for your health?

Alliin and methiin are two chemicals in garlic of particular interest. When you crush or chop garlic, these chemicals interact with enzymes from which they are usually separated in the plant to ultimately form a class of compounds called thiosulfinates, which give garlic its characteristic flavor. (Culinary tip: the more you chop your garlic, the more the enzymes come into contact with alliin and methiin, and the more flavored your dinner.) Further exposure to oil and high temperatures produce polysulfides, which have the characteristic garlic odor. The thiosulfinates have been linked in laboratory studies to cholesterol lowering, while the polysulfides have been connected to cancer prevention.[101]

Over the millennia, garlic has been recommended as an antibacterial agent, a diuretic, and a laxative as well as for arthritis, asthma, athlete's foot, baldness, cancer, cardiovascular disease, dog and snakebites, freckles, hemorrhoids, lice, plague, thinning of the blood, toothache, tuberculosis, and wound healing. It is only in the last couple of decades that researchers have actually subjected garlic to randomized, placebo-controlled trials. This review is restricted to such trials, because they are the only reliable method for establishing the efficacy of garlic in these settings.

Claimed Uses

Cholesterol Lowering

A major review of 37 studies of the effectiveness of garlic in lowering cholesterol levels in the blood was undertaken for the Agency for Healthcare Research and Quality and published in 2000.[101] Although shorter studies (three months) typically showed small reductions in cholesterol (smaller than is often obtained with prescription cholesterol-lowering drugs), combining all eight placebo-controlled studies with at least six months of data showed no effect of garlic in total cholesterol reduction.

Since that review, four randomized, placebo-controlled trials have been conducted. Two of these showed no cholesterol-lowering effect for garlic.[102,103] In a third study, there was an apparent beneficial effect of garlic on total cholesterol in patients at high risk for preeclampsia (toxemia of pregnancy).[104] However, this study was not properly blinded (either the doctors or the patients knew who was getting garlic and who placebo) and the apparent difference was due to baseline differences between the two study groups, a difference that should not have existed if randomization had occurred properly. In the fourth study, beneficial effects upon many cholesterol-related blood measurements were reported after 12 weeks.[105] However, during the study the garlic-treated group reduced their intake of carbohydrates, fat, and alcohol more than did the placebo group, complicating study interpretation.

Studies of garlic and other strong-tasting substances are often prone to this problem, called unblinding by researchers. The problem is that both the garlic tablets and the patients consuming them have a distinctive smell and so patients can often tell (or be told by their partners) that they are in the treated group. This can lead to different dietary patterns between the two study groups, undermining the randomization. A second problem, not unique to studies of garlic, is that there are multiple formulations on the market. Because these are not standardized, it is hard to know if the results from one formulation can be applied to another. The Agency for Healthcare Research and Quality review accurately summarized other limitations in the data when it stated: "Interpreting the [cholesterol] results is best tempered by recognizing that trials often had unclear randomization processes, short durations and no [adjustment for patients who left the study]."[101]

Cancer Prevention

Claims for the effectiveness of garlic in preventing various cancers rest primarily on case-control studies: those that assess garlic intake (either in the diet or as a supplement) in people with cancer compared to those without cancer. However, such studies cannot, on their own, prove that any observed relationship between diet and cancer is causal. Patients with cancer may have diets that are different from patients without cancer in many different ways, not just with respect to garlic; they may even start taking garlic once the early symptoms of the cancer appear, producing a spurious result. Cancer patients are likely to recall their diets differently from patients without cancer. Indeed, all patients struggle to describe dietary patterns that stretch back decades.

Thus, garlic could only be recommended as a cancer preventive if it reduced the number of cases of cancer in a randomized controlled trial. In fact, for almost a decade, there has been such a study under way in China in which patients with precancerous lesions in their stomachs are randomized to various combinations of vitamins, micronutrients, and garlic or a placebo. The trial's clinical results have not yet been published.[106]

In October 2000, the Agency for Healthcare Research and Quality published a review on the subject of garlic and cancer. Here are the authors' conclusions: "Scant data, primarily from case-control studies, suggest, but do not prove, dietary garlic consumption is associated with decreased odds of laryngeal, gastric, colorectal, and endometrial cancer and adenomatous colorectal polyps. Single case-control studies suggest, but do not prove, dietary garlic consumption is not associated with breast or prostate cancer. No epidemiological study has assessed whether using particular types of garlic supplements is associated with reductions in cancer incidence. Preliminary 3-year evidence from a large cohort study suggests consumption of "any" garlic supplement does not reduce risk of breast, lung, colon, or gastric cancer."[101]

In sum, there is inadequate evidence to support garlic supplementation to reduce the risk of any kind of cancer.

High Blood Pressure

The Agency for Healthcare Research and Quality review[101] found that an effect of garlic in lowering blood pressure was usually absent, small even when present, and that no firm conclusions could be drawn due to multiple study design defects. Two subsequent randomized, controlled trials on garlic for high blood pressure showed no effect in reducing blood pressure.[102–104]

Diabetes

The Agency for Healthcare Research and Quality review[101] concluded that garlic had "no clinically significant effect" on blood sugar in patients with or without diabetes. We were unable to identify any randomized, controlled trials on garlic for hypertension published since that review.

Interactions with Other Drugs

The U.S. Food and Drug Administration has warned that garlic can increase the effectiveness of warfarin (COUMADIN), which could lead to bleeding.[107] While the warfarin label must warn of this interaction with garlic, garlic may be sold without warning of the interaction with warfarin. The 2003 edition of *Evaluations of Drug Interactions* lists saquinavir (FORTOVASE, INVIRASE) as having a "clinically significant" interaction with garlic.

Adverse Effects

Garlic may lead to bleeding abnormalities because it inhibits platelets from aggregating and hence clots from forming. There is a case of a man who developed bleeding around his spinal cord due to garlic ingestion[108] and another of bleeding after surgery.[109] Garlic can cause halitosis (bad breath) and body odor. It has been associated with intestinal gas, pain in the esophagus and abdomen, and obstruction of the small intestine, although these associations are not proven.[101]

Conclusion

There are not adequate data to support the use of garlic for cholesterol lowering, cancer prevention, hypertension, or diabetes. As an article in a leading medical journal said, "Garlic for flavour, not cardioprotection [protecting the heart]."[110]

 Do Not Use

Ginkgo Biloba (Maidenhair, EGb 761)
ANTI-AGING DAILY PREMIUM PAK
(Youngevity)
BIOLEAN FREE (Wellness)
CENTRUM PERFORMANCE COMPLETE MULTIVITAMIN MULTIMINERAL
ONE-A-DAY MEMORY AND CONCENTRATION (Bayer)
PHYTO-VITE (Wellness)
POWER CIRCULATION (Sunpower)
SATIETE (Wellness)
STEPHAN CLARITY (Wellness)
STEPHAN ELIXIR (Wellness)
SUN-CARDIO (Sunpower)
SUPPLEMENT (Wyeth)
VITAMIST INTRA-ORAL SPRAY
(Vitamist)

FAMILY:	Dietary Supplements
MUTAGENICITY:	no relevant studies
CARCINOGENICITY:	no relevant studies

Background

The ginkgo biloba or maidenhair tree is indigenous to China, Korea, and Japan but has been imported into the United States and can commonly be found in parks, residential streets, and available for sale in nurseries. To satisfy the demand for its use as a "natural therapy," it is now cultivated on an industrial scale in South Carolina, France, Korea, Japan, and China. Trees can grow up to 130 feet and live over 1,000 years; Charles Darwin referred to the tree as a "living fossil." It has distinctive bilobed leaves (hence the name) and there are separate male and female plants.

It is thought that an extract from the leaf was used in "traditional" Chinese herbal medicines. In Germany, where plant-derived remedies are particularly popular, the extract was introduced by a Dr. Schwabe in 1965 and has been approved for the treatment of dementia. The active ingredients in ginkgo biloba extract are thought to be the flavonoids, terpenoids, and terpene lactones. The most common extract is called EGb 761, but there are several others.[111,112]

Claimed Uses

A variety of theoretical pharmacological rationales have been put forth for the postulated benefits of ginkgo biloba: (1) dilation of blood vessels and consequent improved blood flow, particularly to the brain; (2) interference with platelet aggregation and prevention of clots; (3) modifying neurotransmitter systems; and (4) an antioxidant action that may curb the creation of free radicals that may injure nerve and other cells.[112] In the end, however, positing potential mechanisms for effectiveness does not suffice; for both drugs and dietary supplements, there is a need to demonstrate clinical effectiveness in properly designed studies.

Although a multitude of conditions said to be improved by ginkgo biloba have been set forth, the primary focus has been on the treatment of memory loss and dementia. (We do not review in detail studies of normal people investigating the supplement's effect on memory enhancement, but two recent randomized, placebo-controlled trials show no such effectiveness.)[113,114]

Memory Loss and Dementia

Evaluation of the very large amount of literature on this use of ginkgo biloba is hampered by several problems. Many studies are in foreign languages, do not appear in the National Library of Medicine's database, and are small or unblinded. Others involved healthy volunteers or a variety of patients carrying different or unclear diagnoses. Many studies use nonstandardized measures of mental function and these vary from study to study.

Despite these inconsistencies, there is a meta-analysis of the effect of ginkgo biloba on "cognitive impairment and dementia."[112] It is unclear that such a meta-analysis should even have been conducted, as this technique for statistically combining studies is generally reserved for similarly designed studies. The meta-analysis combined studies with different outcomes, different doses and formulations of ginkgo biloba, and different patient populations and included many short-term studies. It concluded that "there is promising evidence of improvement in cognition and function associated with Ginkgo."[112]

This conclusion does not seem supportable. As noted, the studies should probably not have been combined in the first place. Second, the studies usually conducted "completers" analyses only; this means that only patients who completed the trial (and were probably more likely to be benefiting) were included in the analyses. Most researchers agree that an "intention-to-treat" analysis, based on the patient's performance at the last study visit even if they did not complete the trial, would be an appropriate method for analyzing such trials; the FDA would doubtless not accept a "completers" analysis. Finally, even the authors of the meta-analysis concede that "the three more modern trials show inconsistent results" and call for a large trial "using modern technology" with an intention-to-treat analysis.[112]

Even these three so-called modern trials provide little support for the use of ginkgo biloba for dementia or related conditions. The first study had a 35% dropout rate and allowed patients with unsatisfactory responses in the ginkgo biloba or placebo groups to take ginkgo biloba.[115] The second study mentioned in the meta-analysis is not in the National Library of Medicine database. The most recent study made a particular effort to ensure that the placebo had a similar harsh taste to the ginkgo biloba pills and showed no statistically significant benefits.[116]

Ringing in the Ears (Tinnitus)

We were able to identify only two studies evaluating ginkgo biloba for the treatment of tinnitus. In the first, all patients were treated with intravenous ginkgo biloba before being randomized to ginkgo biloba or placebo.[117] The small effect claimed cannot be interpreted because only 37% of patients completed the study. A much larger, randomized, placebo-controlled trial did not involve any intravenous infusions and simply randomized patients to ginkgo biloba or placebo for 12 weeks.[118] The study was dependent on self-reported data from the patients. There was no evidence of ginkgo biloba effectiveness for tinnitus.

Other Claimed Uses

We identified numerous other potential uses for which only a single randomized, controlled trial had been conducted. In general, any positive finding needs to be replicated by at least one more study of adequate quality before it should gain acceptance. A single study each claimed effectiveness for ginkgo biloba against peripheral arterial disease,[119] vitiligo (patches

of light-colored skin),[120] glaucoma,[121] and schizophrenia,[122] but these studies were small, not properly randomized, and/or lacking in objective measurements of outcomes. Single studies of ginkgo biloba for cocaine dependence,[123] sexual dysfunction,[124] and winter depression[125] all showed no impact of the supplement.

Interactions with Other Drugs

The FDA has warned that ginkgo biloba can increase the effectiveness of warfarin (COUMADIN), which could lead to bleeding.[107] While the warfarin label must warn of this interaction with ginkgo biloba, ginkgo biloba may be sold without warning of the interaction with warfarin. Interactions with ginkgo biloba have also been suggested for aspirin, ticlodipine, clopidogrel, and dipyridamole.[82, 126, 127]

Adverse Effects

Like all dietary supplements, there is no assurance that the supplement actually contains the advertised ingredient. Thirteen of 14 ginkgo biloba products sampled in Hong Kong turned out to have amounts of ginkgolic acid (a known cause of allergies) higher than those recommended by the World Health Organization.[128] Another study demonstrated that the amount of ginkgo biloba released into the bloodstream by different formulations of the supplement varied widely.[129]

Although ginkgo biloba is generally well tolerated, there are multiple reports of seizures[130,131] and bleeding into the brain,[132–136] eye,[137,138] and abdomen[139] associated with use of the supplement.

Conclusion

The available data are insufficient to support the use of ginkgo biloba for improving mental function, dementia, tinnitus, or anything else. The U.S. National Institute on Aging is now sponsoring a clinical trial on the effectiveness of ginkgo biloba in the treatment of Alzheimer's disease.

——————

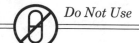 *Do Not Use*

Ginseng
BIOLEAN FREE (Wellness)
CENTRUM PERFORMANCE COMPLETE MULTIVITAMIN MULTIMINERAL SUPPLEMENT (Wyeth)
DEXATRIM RESULTS (Effcon)
5 SENG TEA (Rotta)
ONE-A-DAY ACTIVE DIETARY SUPPLEMENT (Bayer)
ONE-A-DAY ENERGY FORMULA (Bayer)
PHARMATON (Boehringer Ingelheim)
POWER REFRESH (Rotta)

FAMILY:	Dietary Supplements
MUTAGENICITY:	no relevant studies
CARCINOGENICITY:	no relevant studies

Background

Ginseng is a term applying to over 20 different species, mostly of the genus *Panax*. These include *P. ginseng* (Asian ginseng), *P. japonicus* (Japanese ginseng) and *P. quinquefolius* (American ginseng). These contain triterpene saponin glycosides called ginsenosides, which are claimed to be the source of ginseng's activity. An unrelated species, *Eleutherococci* (Siberian ginseng), does not even contain ginsenosides but often is the subject of similar health claims as the *Panax* species. The terms "red" and "white" ginseng do not refer to different plants; they refer to different methods of preparation.[140] The plants contain many different constituents and there are no generally agreed-upon standards for comparing preparations of ginseng. Thus, herbal remedies labeled "ginseng" may contain various plant extracts and vary from manufac-turer to manufacturer and within manufacturers' batches or lots. Ginseng has been used for centuries in traditional Chinese medicine "to restore and enhance well-being."[141] Other uses include enhancing mental and physical vigor, easing childbirth, and as an aphrodisiac.[142]

Claimed Uses

A plethora of vague health claims characterize the modern promotion of ginseng; indeed the genus name *Panax* appears to derive from the Latin word "panacea."[143] In this section, we generally focus only on those that correspond to claims that can be tested empirically.

We do not address claims about which only animal or test-tube evidence exists, or for which there are no accessible randomized, placebo-controlled trials (e.g., herpes infection, heart failure, hypertension, cancer). We also do not address claims of improvements in physical performance among healthy persons, although the four most recent studies of this topic reportedly show no evidence of effectiveness.[141,144]

Psychological and Motor Functions

Two randomized trials evaluated ginseng/ginkgo biloba combinations and so were not considered in this evaluation.[145,146] Another claimed cognitive and mood benefits, but only evaluated the effect of various doses of ginseng in 20 patients for no longer than six hours after a single dose.[147] The final study was not properly randomized but found no effect of various doses of a ginseng preparation upon mood after eight weeks.[142] The only accessible randomized, placebo-controlled study of this claim was small and found a statistically significant benefit for ginseng on only one of eight variables measured.[148]

Stimulation of the Immune System

Although some studies have looked at indirect measures of immune function, none has examined the clinical relevance of these findings.

Diabetes

A study claiming better blood sugar control in patients with diabetes taking ginseng is not credible because only 12 patients took each ginseng dose, follow-up was only eight weeks, and important baseline information on the patients was not provided.[149] A second small study looked only at the immediate effects of ginseng (up to two hours).[150]

Cancer

An epidemiologic study from Korea, where ginseng use is very common, showed an approximately 60% reduction in the risk of cancer overall.[151] However, the reduction occurred across multiple disparate organ systems, a finding not consistent with current understandings of how cancer is caused and prevented. Before this finding can be accepted, it would need to be replicated in another study of similar design and then confirmed in a randomized, placebo-controlled trial.

Tonic

One randomized study compared ginseng combined with multivitamins to multivitamins alone in an effort "to remedy the deterioration in quality of life in large cities." To our knowledge, this is not a recognized medical condition. The claimed benefits on quality of life may be explained by either much larger dropout rates in the control group or improper randomization.[152]

Interactions with Other Drugs

The FDA has warned that ginseng can increase the effectiveness of warfarin (COU-

MADIN), which could lead to bleeding,[107,153] including vaginal bleeding.[154] Conversely, ginseng has also been associated with clot formation on an implanted heart valve in a patient taking warfarin.[155] While the warfarin label must warn of an interaction with ginseng, ginseng may be sold without warning of the interaction with warfarin. There are also two reports of interactions between ginseng and phenelzine (NARDIL).[156,157]

Adverse Effects

Ginseng has been associated with hypertension, nervousness, insomnia, vomiting, headache, skin rashes, and nosebleeds.[62,158,159] A ginseng abuse syndrome, involving the simultaneous use of caffeine, has also been described.[160,161] Its features are hypertension, nervousness, and sleeplessness. Other reports describe estrogen-like effects for ginseng: changes in the lining of the vagina[162] and vaginal bleeding.[163]

Conclusion

In summary, ginseng is an unstandardized, highly variable preparation with extravagant claims for benefits and no scientific data to support them.

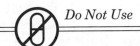

Do Not Use

Glucosamine and Chondroitin
DONA (Rotta)
MAJESTIC EARTH (American Longevity)
VITAMIST INTRA-ORAL SPRAY (Vitamist)

FAMILY:	Dietary Supplements
MUTAGENICITY:	no relevant studies
CARCINOGENICITY:	no relevant studies

Background

At the end of each of the two bones that form joints in the body is a rubbery substance called cartilage, which serves the purpose of cushioning the bone against sudden jolts. It is damage to this cartilage and the underlying bone that forms the basis of osteoarthritis, the most common arthritis of older age. The constituents of cartilage include a family of chemicals called glycosaminoglycans. The chemical glucosamine occurs naturally in the body and is a building block for the glycosaminoglycans; chondroitin is one of a particular type of glycosaminoglycan called a proteoglycan. These compounds can be derived from natural products, particularly the shells of shellfish, or they can be synthesized. In many European countries, glucosamine is regulated as a prescription drug, rather than as a dietary supplement. The FDA has warned one glucosamine manufacturer not to claim that the supplement is effective for arthritis.[41]

Claimed Uses

Glucosamine and chondroitin have been administered separately or together to treat osteoarthritis; there are even claims by some proponents that they can reverse the course of the disease, something that the standard therapy for osteoarthritis, the nonsteroidal anti-inflammatory drugs (e.g., ibuprofen, see p. 288), has never been shown to accomplish. One problem facing the advocates of glucosamine is that no human clinical data exist to confirm that glucosamine actually reaches the joint, or that it does so in adequate concentrations.[164]

Two studies have statistically combined the randomized trials on glucosamine and/or chondroitin, a technique known as meta-analysis. In the first, restricted to glucosamine, most studies showed glucosamine to be effective in osteoarthritis, but the studies were poorly designed (median design score = 2 on a 0–8 scale, where 8 is the best-designed study).[165] Among

the studies' deficiencies were short duration and lack of standardization in both diagnosis of osteoarthritis and in the measure of effectiveness. A subsequent meta-analysis found efficacy in treating osteoarthritis for glucosamine and for chondroitin.[166] However, these trials, too, were of poor methodological quality, with such major deficiencies as lack of intention-to-treat analyses (i.e., the studies included data only on those who completed the study, not on all subjects) in almost all cases and the anomalous finding that the largest and best-designed studies showed the least benefit. With the great majority of these studies either funded by the manufacturers or including authors employed by the manufacturers, the authors of the meta-analysis raised the possibility of a well-documented practice known as publication bias, in which studies showing an intervention not to be effective are simply not published.

Since these meta-analyses were published, five randomized, placebo-controlled trials of glucosamine have been conducted. (There is also a third meta-analysis reporting benefits for glucosamine and chondroitin,[167] but we prefer to review the more recent studies individually.) Three studies claim positive results. In the most widely cited, statistically significant improvements in symptom scores and on X-ray were claimed.[168] However, the improvements in symptom scores were presented in an inconsistent fashion, making interpretation difficult.[169] In fact, the scores reflecting knee function (almost all studies of glucosamine examine knee osteoarthritis only) reveal an absolute benefit for glucosamine of only 5%. The study was also unique in demonstrating, for perhaps the first time for any osteoarthritis drug, a benefit in the X-ray appearance of the knee: less narrowing of the joint, a common consequence of osteoarthritis. Again, however, the effect was very small: about 1/250th of an inch per year. In any event, the relationship between joint space narrowing and symptoms is very weak.[170] A second study, also funded by the leading glucosamine manufacturer, had similar results and limitations.[171] In the third trial, the patients did not have X-ray-confirmed diagnoses of osteoarthritis prior to the study, the number of patients was small, the glucosamine group had had osteoarthritis for longer than the placebo group, and, although reported pain scores were more improved in the glucosamine than in the placebo group, the drug had little or no impact on measures of joint function.[172] On the other hand, two somewhat smaller, well-conducted trials showed no benefit whatsoever for glucosamine compared to placebo on either pain or an array of indices of joint function.[173,174]

Three studies on chondroitin have been published since these meta-analyses, and none is sufficient to shift our view of the efficacy of these products. Two studies claim effectiveness for chondroitin, but one improperly combined the placebo groups from two separate studies[175] and the other was not designed in a manner that allowed clear comparison between chondroitin and placebo.[176] In the third, the intention-to-treat analysis does not reach statistical significance.[177]

Because of the ongoing controversy over the efficacy of these supplements,[178,179] the National Institutes of Health is conducting a six-month trial comparing glucosamine and chondroitin, alone and together, to placebo.[180] The study will examine both pain relief and the progression of osteoarthritis.

Interactions with Other Drugs

No interactions with other drugs have been reported, but this has not been studied formally.

Adverse Effects

In general, glucosamine is well tolerated. There is a case report of glucosamine raising blood sugar levels,[181] an effect also seen in animals at high doses.[182] However, a small randomized trial was not able to detect such an effect.[182] Glucosamine has been associated with an aller-

gic skin rash[183] and the combination of glucosamine and chondroitin has been associated with asthma.[184]

As for all dietary supplements, questions over the purity and consistency of commercially available formulations remain. In the National Institutes of Health trial mentioned above, such inconsistencies were so substantial that the researchers had to manufacture the supplements themselves.[179]

Conclusion

Uncertainties over the efficacy of glucosamine in the treatment of osteoarthritis remain. The evidence for chondroitin's efficacy for this condition is still weaker. We recommend that you wait until completion of the National Institutes of Health's placebo-controlled trial before considering using either supplement.

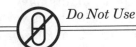 *Do Not Use*

Green Tea

FAMILY:	Dietary Supplements
MUTAGENICITY:	no relevant studies
CARCINOGENICITY:	no relevant studies

Background

If man has no tea in him, he is incapable of understanding truth and beauty.

—Japanese proverb

There is no trouble so great or grave that cannot be much diminished by a nice cup of tea.

—Bernard-Paul Heroux

If you are cold, tea will warm you. If you are too heated, it will cool you. If you are depressed, it will cheer you. If you are excited, it will calm you.

—William Gladstone

Drinking a daily cup of tea will surely starve the apothecary.

—Chinese proverb [185]

The shrub *Camellia sinensis* is the source of the three major forms of tea in the world. (For these purposes, we are excluding "teas" made from rose hips, chamomile, etc., which are considered infusions and are not made from tea leaves.) Green tea is prepared by drying and steaming the tea leaf, black tea is the same leaf but fermented, and oolong tea is partially fermented. Green tea is a popular drink in China and Japan, whereas in North America and Europe black tea is more popular. Approximately 3 billion kilograms of tea are produced and consumed annually. [186]

Green tea contains chemicals called polyphenols. These chemicals are antioxidants that block the action of free radicals, which can cause cellular and genetic damage. Antioxidants are found in many foods in addition to green tea, and certain antioxidants have been tested in large cancer prevention trials with no success. The polyphenols (flavonoids) in green tea are called catechins; these are converted into the theaflavins present in black tea during the fermentation process.

Claimed Uses

Cancer Treatment and Prevention

Green tea is unique among the supplements reviewed in this chapter in that claims for its effectiveness rest primarily on epidemiological studies. (Most other supplements reviewed in this chapter rely upon randomized clinical trials [often poorly conducted], anecdotes, or appeals to tradition or naturalness.) This alone should increase one's level of skepticism about the claims made for green tea. Although epidemiological studies are often the only way to study certain human risks (e.g., environmental or occupational exposures), no drug regulatory authority would approve a drug based on such evidence alone.

Some of the studies claiming a protective effect of green tea against a particular cancer are based on ecological studies, a particularly weak form of epidemiological study. These usually take the form of demonstrating that cancer rates are lower in areas with high consumption of green tea than in areas with lower consumption. These studies should be viewed with great caution, because such studies do not even include data on the green tea consumption of particular individuals with or without cancer. The most common kind of study has been a case-control study, in which patients with and without cancer are asked about their prior consumption of green tea. However, patients with cancer may have diets that are different from patients without cancer in many different ways, not just with respect to green tea; they may even start taking green tea once the early symptoms of the cancer appear, producing a spurious result. Cancer patients are likely to recall their diets differently than patients without cancer. Indeed, all patients struggle to describe dietary patterns that stretch back decades.

A better study (although still not one that would satisfy a drug regulatory authority) would be one in which patients are asked about their diets on a periodic basis and then are followed to see if they develop cancer. This is called a prospective study. However, the results of such studies have been mixed. For example, studies of tea consumption and stomach cancer have showed tea drinkers to be at greater risk, [187] at lower risk, [188] and at neither higher nor lower risk [189] compared to those consuming less or no tea. One study found that tea protects against pancreatic cancer, [190] but another study did not. [191] One study found that more frequent tea drinkers were at greater risk of lung cancer, [187] but another did not. [189] These studies can be difficult to interpret because of perhaps unmeasured differences between the patients who do and do not develop cancer. Conceivably the difference between black and green teas is also important.

The best way to eliminate such biases is to conduct a randomized, controlled trial, because randomization makes it very likely that the two groups will be similar in most respects. No such study has been published. The closest is an uncontrolled prospective study of 42 patients with a particular form of prostate cancer, all of whom were treated with green tea. Only one patient responded, and even this response was not sustained beyond two months. The authors concluded that "green tea, as administered in this study, does not merit further investigation in the treatment of patients with androgen independent prostate carcinoma."[192] The National Cancer Institute is conducting studies on the use of green tea for preventing skin cancer.[193]

Cholesterol Lowering

We identified two randomized, placebo-controlled trials of green tea to lower cholesterol. In the first, a small trial, neither green tea nor black tea reduced the levels of total cholesterol, the components of total cholesterol or triglycerides.[194] The second trial compared a theaflavin-enriched extract of green tea to a placebo.[195] This 12-week study showed a modest decrease in total cholesterol and LDL cholesterol ("bad cholesterol"), but no increase in HDL cholesterol ("good cholesterol") or decrease in triglycerides, compared to the placebo group. Importantly, this was not a study of green tea per se, because the extract was enriched with flavonoids characteristic of black tea. Brewed green tea has a highly variable amount of various flavonoids. Whether or not the differences claimed in this trial would be sustained, have any effect on disease outcomes, or be replicated in another study is unclear.

Interactions with Other Drugs

Interactions between green tea and anticoagulant drugs (e.g., warfarin [COUMADIN]) and other dietary supplements (including vitamin E and ginkgo biloba) have been reported. It is recommended that green tea use be discontinued at least 24 hours prior to surgery.[91]

Adverse Effects

Because green tea contains 10–80 milligrams of caffeine per cup,[196] excessive amounts may lead to insomnia, rapid heartbeat, abnormal heart rhythms, nausea, and vomiting. Green tea has also been associated with gastrointestinal distress, loss of appetite, headache, and vertigo.[91] Patients with kidney disease, overactive thyroid glands, anxiety, panic disorder, or cardiovascular disease should be cautious in their use of this supplement.[91] Green tea–induced asthma due to inhalation has also been reported in 11 patients,[197-199] five of whom simultaneously developed worsened asthma after drinking green tea.[200] According to the American Cancer Society, women who are pregnant or breast-feeding should restrict their intake of green tea.[201]

Conclusion

The health benefits of green tea remain unproven. Use it if you like the taste, but do not expect an impact on your health.

 Do Not Use

Milk Thistle
MILK THISTLE HEALTH LIVER
(DreamPharm)
RELIVE (ViriLife)
THISILYN (Legalon; Nature's Way)

FAMILY: Dietary Supplements
MUTAGENICITY: no relevant studies
CARCINOGENICITY: no relevant studies

Background

Milk thistle (*Silybum marianum*) is a plant from the aster or daisy family. Its legend dates back to biblical times; Mary is said to have sheltered Jesus in an arbor of thistle. Ancient Greek and Roman physicians and herbalists extolled its virtues, as did medieval German and 17th-century English herbalists. In the United States, the Eclectics movement, which primarily emphasized Native American herbs, advocated milk thistle for varicose veins, menstrual difficulties, and congestion of the spleen, liver, and kidneys. Over the centuries milk thistle has been recommended for a variety of other maladies, including depression, gallstones, and snakebites.[202]

Herbal products are made from the seeds of the fruit of the plant, which contain bioflavonoids, the most active of which is silybin. Milk thistle is available in a dried form as a capsule and it is also dissolved in alcohol and put into liquid form (tincture of milk thistle). Teas can also be prepared, but little of the putatively active compound dissolves in water.[202]

Claimed Uses

Modern interest in milk thistle has centered on its use for treating various liver diseases. A number of placebo-controlled trials have been conducted. However, many of these trials include patients with a variety of liver ailments and such studies are thus not included in this review. Almost all studies confined their assessments of effectiveness to measuring enzymes present in the liver called aminotransferases; these are frequently elevated in liver illnesses. However, this surrogate for liver health would be insufficient on its own for a drug to receive FDA approval. Instead, studies should focus on improvements in liver biopsies or survival (in conjunction with the amount of virus in the treatment of hepatitis C infection).

Chronic Hepatitis C Infection

Only two randomized, placebo-controlled trials have been conducted. In a 1977 German study (not reviewed directly by us but summarized in a meta-analysis[202]), before hepatitis C had been identified, silymarin, a less active bioflavonoid, was associated with a trend toward improvement in liver biopsy, but this was not evaluated statistically. In the second, which included patients with both hepatitis B and C, some blood tests improved, while others did not; biopsies and mortality were not evaluated.[203] A review of a number of complementary medicines, including milk thistle, for hepatitis C concluded that "There is no firm evidence supporting medicinal herbs for [hepatitis C virus] infection."[204] The National Center for Complementary and Alternative Medicine has concluded that "The results of scientific studies to date do not definitively find that milk thistle is beneficial in treating hepatitis C in humans."[205]

Chronic Alcoholic Liver Disease

A review conducted for the Agency for Healthcare Research and Quality identified six placebo-controlled studies of milk thistle. The studies are difficult to interpret due to ongoing alcohol consumption by the patients and due to differences in disease severity. Most of these studies showed improvement in at least one measurement (usually aminotransferases or other blood tests), but more outcomes were unaffected by the treatment and the outcome for which there was apparent effectiveness varied from study to study.[202] Two of these six studies are the only two placebo-controlled trials of milk thistle for alcoholic cirrhosis.

Summarizing the data for alcoholic liver disease as well as for other liver diseases, the Agency for Healthcare Research and Quality concluded: "Clinical efficacy for milk thistle is not clearly established. Interpretation of the evidence is hampered by poor study methods and/or poor quality of reporting in publications. Problems in study design include heterogeneity in etiology and extent of liver disease, small sample sizes, and variation in formulation, dosing, and duration of milk thistle therapy."[202]

Interactions with Other Drugs

No interactions with other drugs have been reported, but this has not been studied formally.

Adverse Effects

Milk thistle has been generally well tolerated. It has been associated with a laxative effect, nausea, and abdominal discomfort. Milk thistle can also produce allergic reactions in patients allergic to plants in the same family (daisy, ragweed, chrysanthemum, and marigold).[205]

Conclusion

While there are a number of placebo-controlled trials of milk thistle in the treatment of various liver diseases, their overall quality is very poor and is not sufficient to support the supplement's use. The National Center for Complementary and Alternative Medicine is sponsoring a clinical trial of milk thistle in the treatment of hepatitis C. At present, use of the supplement for hepatitis C seems particularly unjustified, given the existence of effective therapies for that condition.[206]

 Do Not Use

Morinda citrifolia (Noni, Nono, Nonu, Ba Ji Tian, Nhau)
PREMIUM HAWAIIAN NONI JUICE (Youngevity)
TAHITIAN NONI LIQUID (Tahitian Noni International)

FAMILY:	Dietary Supplements
MUTAGENICITY:	no relevant studies
CARCINOGENICITY:	no relevant studies

Background

Noni is the common name for *Morinda citrifolia,* the Indian mulberry or cheese fruit tree that grows wild on tropical islands such as Samoa, Tonga, Tahiti, and Hawaii. The noni plant is a small evergreen tree found in coastal areas and in forested areas as high as 1,300 feet above sea level. It has large, bright green elliptical leaves and bears a fruit that changes from green to yellow to white as it matures. The bark is used to make a reddish purple and brown dye that is used in batik. But it is the fruit that has attracted most attention. Its promotors claim that noni has been used as an herbal remedy for over 2,000 years in Polynesia.[207,208] Because it has a foul odor and taste, it is typically mixed with grape or other juices and consumed as a liquid. Hair care products, diet aids, and skin care lotions containing noni are also available.

Many of noni's claims rest on the work of Dr. Ralph Heineke, who claims that noni contains proxeronine, which is converted to xeronine in the body. It is xeronine that is claimed to cause the multiple health benefits assumed by noni supporters. There is no scientific proof for this hypothesis. More recently, the primary proponent of noni has been Dr. Neil Solomon, a former health commissioner of Maryland, who surrendered his license to practice medicine in Maryland after several of his female patients accused him of sexual misconduct.[209] He has authored a number of books with titles such as *The Noni Phenomenon* and *Noni Juice the Tropical Fruit with 101 Medicinal Uses.*[210]

Both Dr. Heineke and Dr. Solomon endorse the noni product of Tahitian Noni International,[211,212] which is the market leader. The company markets its product as "An exotic health discovery from French Polynesia," and its label features a bare-chested local male with a mohawk haircut eating the fruit.

Claimed Uses

Among the supplements reviewed for this chapter, noni bears the distinction of having the broadest claims and the weakest scientific evidence. Although a reference to a randomized, controlled trial appears in one published article,[208] we have not been able to locate a published version of this trial. The claims for noni efficacy are thus made on the basis of test tube studies,[208,213] which do not even remotely approach the standards for approval of the FDA, and Dr. Solomon's book.

The book, which describes noni as having "miraculous health benefits," lists noni's main attributes as increasing body energy, alleviating pain, inhibiting cancer and precancer, acting as an anti-inflammatory and antihistamine, regulating sleep, temperature, and mood, and its antibacterial properties.[214] Supporting evidence for these claims appears to rest in part on a review of effectiveness claims made by "over 15,000" noni patients. Dr. Solomon reports that from 51% (multiple sclerosis) to 90% (increasing energy) of patients derived benefit from noni. He adds: "The majority of Noni users who did not get optimal results failed to do so because they took a lesser dose and/or took it a lesser amount of time than recommended."[214] Collecting anecdotes from self-selected users does not remotely approach any reasonable standard of efficacy.

Interactions with Other Drugs

No interactions with other drugs have been reported, but this has not been studied formally.

Adverse Effects

Noni juice contains potassium at levels comparable to those found in orange juice and so the product should not be used in patients with kidney disease.[215]

Conclusion

Noni is a newly popular herbal product about which little is known and for which acceptable research absent. There is no scientific evidence for the wide array of health claims made for the product.

 Do Not Use

Saw Palmetto *(Serenoa repens; Serenoa serrulata; Sabal serrulata)*
ONE-A-DAY PROSTATE HEALTH (Bayer)
PERMIXON (Pierre Fabre)
POWER LASTING (Sunpower)

FAMILY:	Dietary Supplements
MUTAGENICITY:	no relevant studies
CARCINOGENICITY:	no relevant studies

Background

Saw palmetto is the popular name for an extract of the dried berry of the dwarf palm tree *Serenoa repens* that grows in the southeastern United States. The berry is rich in fatty acids and sitosterols, and the latter are thought to constitute the active ingredient. It is especially popular in Europe but has enjoyed increased attention in the United States over the past decade.

Claimed Uses

Benign Prostatic Hyperplasia

Benign prostatic hyperplasia (BPH) is a condition in which the prostate gland, which provides liquid components of seminal fluid, becomes enlarged. The condition is distinct from prostate cancer; hence the designation "benign." The urethra is the tube that carries urine out of the body; because it passes through the prostate, if that gland becomes enlarged (hyperplastic), it might block or restrict the passage of urine, resulting in incomplete emptying of the bladder. The symptoms of BPH vary, but the most common ones involve changes or problems with urination, such as a hesitant, interrupted, weak stream; urgency and leaking or dribbling; and more frequent urination, especially at night.

Saw palmetto has been promoted to relieve the symptoms of BPH. The primary evidence for this claim is a meta-analysis (a statistical combining of other studies) based on randomized, controlled trials. This meta-analysis was first published in 1998[216] but has since been updated online.[217] The most recent review concludes that saw palmetto provides "mild to moderate improvement in urinary symptoms and flow measures." (Another, less extensive meta-analysis covering many of the same trials reached a similar conclusion but is not analyzed in detail here.[218]) It claims effectiveness similar to finasteride (PROSCAR) (see p. 494), with fewer adverse effects.

Closer examination of the available data does not support this conclusion. First, of 21 studies included in the meta-analysis, only six used an accepted symptom scale and five of these six did not have a placebo control and/or tested herbal combinations that included saw palmetto, making it impossible to ascribe any effect to saw palmetto itself. Such products should not be included in meta-analyses. Second, the studies were of short duration, with three-quarters of studies lasting 13 weeks or less.

Third, most of the data in the meta-analysis come from old, poorly conducted studies published in inaccessible journals. Of the 21 studies, just one involved saw palmetto only, had a placebo control, and was published in an acces-sible journal after 1987.[219] This study showed an improvement of 2.2 points on a 36-point scale (6%) over placebo after six months. Saw palmetto had no impact upon urinary flow rates, a more objective measure of drug effectiveness.

More fundamentally, no saw palmetto study has ever shown an impact upon the development of urinary obstruction or upon the need for surgery to relieve the symptoms of BPH. In contrast, such evidence does exist for finasteride.[220] The National Institutes of Health is currently conducting a randomized, placebo-controlled trial of saw palmetto in relieving the symptoms of BPH.[221]

Interactions with Other Drugs

No interactions with other drugs have been reported, but this has not been studied formally.

Adverse Effects

Headache, gastrointestinal upset, high blood pressure, impotence, and decreased sex drive have been reported in patients taking saw palmetto.[222] Saw palmetto has been associated with a case of severe bleeding into the brain following surgery.[223] A product called PC Spes contained saw palmetto as well as seven other herbs and was used to treat prostate cancer, despite never being subjected to a controlled trial.[224] It was shown to have estrogen-like activity and to depress prostate-specific antigen (PSA) levels, which could interfere with detection and treatment-monitoring for prostate cancer.[225] It was removed from the market in 2002, as it was contaminated with the anticoagulant warfarin (COUMADIN).[226] Earlier, several lots of the preparation had been contaminated with the nonsteroidal anti-inflammatory drug indomethacin (INDOCIN) (see p. 295) and diethylstilbestrol (DES), a known carcinogen and cause of birth defects.[227]

Conclusion

There is no convincing evidence that saw palmetto is effective for treating BPH. Moreover, there are other medications with proven effectiveness for BPH.

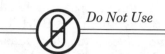

Do Not Use

St. John's Wort (Hypericum, Goatweed, The Lord God's Wonder Plant, Witch's Herb)
SATIETE (Wellness)
SUN BEAUTY (Sunpower)
VITAMIST INTRA-ORAL SPRAY (Mayor)

FAMILY:	Dietary Supplements
MUTAGENICITY:	causes gene damage in experimental studies[228]
CARCINOGENICITY:	no relevant studies

Background

St. John's wort is a common name for the flowering plant *Hypericum perforatum*. It has a five-pointed yellow flower and is common in the United States and Europe, where it is often regarded as a weed. There are claims that Hippocrates himself prescribed it. Over the centuries, use has focused on repairing nerve damage and, when applied topically, promoting wound healing. Modern use is primarily for the treatment of depression, particularly in Germany. The plant contains a number of putative active ingredients including anthracene derivatives (especially hypericin and pseudohypericin), flavonoids, and hyperforin.[229] These constituents will vary from batch to batch and plant to plant, so it is hard to standardize and make a uniform product. Dosages also vary from study to study and, in practice, from doctor to doctor.

Claimed Uses

There are probably more studies that have been done on St. John's wort than on any other supplement reviewed in this chapter. As for most other supplements, there is a tendency over time for the quality of the studies to improve and for the studies to be more likely to fail to show effectiveness.

By the late 1990s, dozens of randomized, controlled trials of St. John's wort for depression had been published. These have been summarized in a series of meta-analyses, a statistical technique for combining the results of many studies, which generally concluded that St. John's wort is more effective than placebo.[230–233] However, we find their conclusions unconvincing. The great majority of studies were of very short duration (no more than six weeks) and many had no placebo controls, used poor statistical analyses, included only patients who completed the study (this omits people more likely to have not benefited from the drug or have suffered adverse effects), utilized unclear diagnostic criteria for depression, or were plagued by publication bias (the selective publication of positive findings). Meta-analyses are only as good as the individual studies that go into them, and these studies were generally weak. These meta-analyses included some studies that compared St. John's wort to other antidepressants and generally concluded that their efficacies were similar. However, the comparator drugs were invariably the older tricyclic antidepressants (see p. 196) and the doses used were typically on the low end of (or even below) approved doses, so the trials were biased in favor of St. John's wort from the start.

Since these meta-analyses, five randomized, placebo-controlled trials have been conducted, three funded by St. John's wort manufacturers, one funded by a company that makes both antidepressants and St. John's wort, and a fifth funded by the National Institutes of Health. The three funded by the St. John's wort manufacturers reported greater effectiveness than placebo, although the improvement on the main study outcome due to the drug itself was always less than the improvement that occurred with no treatment at all.[234–236] In two of the three studies, the benefit over placebo was quite modest. The most prominent of these three studies also included the tricyclic antidepressant imipramine (TOFRANIL) (see p. 196) in a third study group, in addition to a group treated with St. John's wort and the placebo group.[235] St. John's wort was reported to be at least as effective as imipramine. However, as in previous studies comparing St. John's wort to other antidepressants, the authors used a low dose of imipramine. Moreover, the dose of St. John's wort used was considerably higher than that recommended for many St. John's wort formulations available in the United States today.[237] This underscores the problem of lack of standardization of this product (and other dietary supplements). Such standardization would occur if the supplement were actually reviewed by the FDA, as it does for drugs.

It is of some interest that of the first approximately 30 studies of St. John's wort, literally all reported a benefit for the supplement.[238] This is remarkable, because even established antidepressants cannot be shown to be superior to placebo in up to 35% of trials,[239] suggesting either remarkable efficacy, inadequate study design and conduct, or selective publication of positive results for St. John's wort. In the last several years, however, two well-designed studies have been reported, one funded by a neutral body and the other by a company manufacturing St. John's wort and antidepressants.

In the first, patients were randomized to either St. John's wort or placebo and the authors concluded that St. John's wort "was not effective for treatment of major depression" and that "there currently is no credible evidence to support the efficacy of St John's wort for people with depression."[238] A second study, published in the *Journal of the American Medical Associa-*

tion (as was the first study), also found no difference between St. John's wort and placebo.[240] This study had an added twist: the selective serotonin reuptake inhibitor (SSRI) sertraline (ZOLOFT) (see p. 190) was also little better than placebo. As noted above, not infrequently even effective antidepressants are no more effective than placebo in clinical trials. This leaves two possible interpretations for this study's results regarding St. John's wort: either St. John's wort is ineffective (because it was no more effective than placebo) or the study was inadequately designed (because it could not distinguish sertraline from placebo). Either way, the study certainly shows no evidence for the efficacy of St. John's wort. The authors conclude that the use of St. John's wort, even in patients with mild depression, "cannot be supported until trials show clear evidence of efficacy."[240]

Interactions with Other Drugs

St. John's wort is notorious for being associated with drug interactions with a wide array of drugs, more than for most prescription drugs. In part this is because, depending how it is administered, St. John's wort can both inhibit and activate cytochrome P450, a key enzyme system involved in processing drugs.[241] While the FDA has required some drugs that interact with St. John's wort to carry warnings of that danger, supplements containing St. John's wort itself are not required to do so. Moreover, the FDA has not been as rigorous as its counterpart in Britain, the Committee on Safety of Medicines, in warning about these interactions. In February 2000, the committee listed a number of drugs that interact with St. John's wort.[242] We combined that list with those listed in *Evaluations of Drug Interactions* 2003 as being "clinically significant" or "highly clinically significant," as well as with reports in the medical literature[241,243,244] to yield the following list: ADALAT, ALLEGRA, AMERGE, amitriptyline, carbamazepine, CAMPTOSAR, CELEXA, citalopram, COMTAN, COUMADIN, CRIXIVAN, cyclosporine, digoxin, DILANTIN, ELAVIL, entacapone, fexofenadine, fluoxetine, fluvoxamine, GENGRAF, IMITREX, indinavir, indoramin, irinotecan, LANOXIN, LUVOX, MAXALT, MERIDIA, midazolam, naratriptan, NEORAL, nevirapine, nifedipine, oral contraceptives, paroxetine, PAXIL, phenobarbital, PROCARDIA, PROZAC, rizatriptan, SANDIMMUNE, sertraline, sevoflurane, sibutramine, simvastatin, sumatriptan, TASMAR, TEGRETOL, THEO-DUR, theophylline, tolcapone, tyramine, ULTANE, VERSED, VIRAMUNE, warfarin, ZOCOR, zolmitriptan, ZOLOFT, ZOMIG. Even though St. John's wort has been better evaluated for its propensity to interact with other drugs than any other supplement, a recent review indicates that even this evidence base is weak.[245]

Adverse Effects

St. John's wort is generally well tolerated. The most common adverse effects include gastrointestinal symptoms, fatigue, dizziness, headache, and dry mouth.[241] However, St. John's wort has also been associated with a number of serious adverse reactions. These include the induction of mania or similar conditions,[246–249] hypertension,[251] and skin and nerve reactions,

some related to sun exposure.[252–254] St. John's wort has also been implicated in causing the array of symptoms known as serotonin syndrome, which includes mental status changes, agitation, muscle spasms, sweating, tremor, and fever.[255,256]

Conclusion

While there are many studies claiming to demonstrate a benefit for St. John's wort in the treatment of depression, the most recent, best-conducted studies do not show any evidence of effectiveness. When combined with the significant interactions and adverse effects associated with this supplement and the lack of standardization of the product, we cannot endorse its use. In Ireland, where St. John's wort used to be available over the counter, health authorities switched it to prescription-only status in 2000 because medical claims were being made for it.[257] (This effectively banned the product, because no prescription form of St. John's wort had been licensed.) This suggests the right approach for a dietary supplement: all products that have a proven beneficial effect on the body should be regulated similarly. They should be considered drugs.

REFERENCES

1. Angell M, Kassirer JP. Alternative medicine—the risks of untested and unregulated remedies. *New England Journal of Medicine* 1998; 339:839–41.

2. Miller FG, Emanuel EJ, Rosenstein DL, et al. Ethical issues concerning research in complementary and alternative medicine. *Journal of the American Medical Association* 2004; 291:599–604.

3. 21 U.S.C. 321(ff).

4. Kessler RC, Davis RB, Foster DF, et al. Long-term trends in the use of complementary and alternative medical therapies in the United States. *Annals of Internal Medicine* 2001; 135:262–8.

5. Eisenberg DM, Davis RB, Ettner SL, et al. Trends in alternative medicine use in the United States, 1990–1997: Results of a follow-up national survey. *Journal of the American Medical Association* 1998; 280:1569–75.

6. Barnes PM, Powell-Griner E, McFann K, Nahin R. Complementary and Alternative Medicine Use Among Adults: United States, 2002. Advance Data from Vital and Health Statistics 343: May 27, 2004. Available at: http://www.cdc.gov/nchs/data/ad/ad343.pdf.

7. Ashikaga T, Bosompra K, O'Brien P, et al. Use of complimentary and alternative medicine by breast cancer patients: Prevalence, patterns and communication with physicians. *Supportive Care in Cancer* 2002; 10:542–8.

8. Bernstein BJ, Grasso T. Prevalence of complementary and alternative medicine use in cancer patients. *Oncology* 2001; 15:1267–72.

9. Institute of Medicine and National Research Council, Committee on the Framework for Evaluating the Statety of Dietary Supplements. *Dietary Supplements: A Framework for Evaluating Safety*, April 1, 2004.

10. Richardson MA, Sanders T, Palmer JL, et al. Complementary/alternative medicine use in a comprehensive cancer center and the implications for oncology. *Journal of Clinical Oncology* 2000; 18:2505–14.

11. Center for Food Safety and Applied Nutrition. Information Paper on L-tryptophan and 5-hydroxy-L-tryptophan, 2001. Available at: http://vm.cfsan.fda.gov/~dms/ds-tryp1.html.

12. Wolfe SM. Letter to HHS Secretary Tommy Thompson urging him to direct the FDA to open a criminal investigation of Metabolife (HRG Publication #1635), August 15, 2002. Available at: http://www.citizen.org/publications/release.cfm?ID=7193.

13. Ko RJ. Adulterants in Asian patent medicines. *New England Journal of Medicine* 1998; 339:847.

14. Norton SA. Raw animal tissues and dietary supplements. *New England Journal of Medicine* 2000; 343:304–5.

15. Lurie P. Testimony before the Consumer Affairs, Foreign Commerce and Tourism Subcommittee concerning Bovine Spongiform Encephalopathy (BSE), otherwise known as "Mad Cow Disease" (HRG Publication #1563), April 4, 2001. Available at: http://www.citizen.org/publications/release.cfm?ID=6756.

16. Department of Health and Human Services, Office of the Inspector General. Adverse Event Reporting for Dietary Supplements: An Inadequate Safety Valve. OEI-01-00-00180, April 2001. Available at: http://oig.hhs.gov/oei/reports/oei-01-00-00180.pdf.

17. Shekelle PG, Morton S, Maglione M, et al. Ephedra and Ephedrine for Weight Loss and Athletic Performance Enhancement: Clinical Efficacy and Side Effects. Evidence Report/Technology Assessment No. 76 (Prepared by Southern California Evidence-based Practice Center, RAND, under Contract No. 290-97-0001, Task Order No. 9). AHRQ Publication No. 03-E022, Rockville, Md.: Agency for Healthcare Research and Quality: 2003. Available at: http://www.fda.gov/OHRMS/DOCKETS/98fr/95n-0304-bkg0003-ref07-01-index.htm.

18. Cleland RL, Gross WC, Koss LD, Daynard M, Muoio KM. Weight-Loss Advertising: An Analysis of Current Trends. Federal Trade Commission Staff Report, September 2002. Available at: http://www.ftc.gov/bcp/reports/weightloss.pdf.

19. 21 U.S.C. 342(f)(1)(A).

20. Center for Food Safety and Applied Nutrition. Dietary Supplements: Warnings and Safety Information, June 5, 2004. Available at: http://www.cfsan.fda.gov/~dms/ds-warn.html.

21. Medical Research Council. Streptomycin treatment of pulmonary tuberculosis. *British Medical Journal* 1948; 2:769–82.

22. Fifty years of randomised controlled trials. *British Medical Journal* 1998; 317:0.

23. US Nutrition Industry: Top 70 Supplements 1997-2002 (Chart 14). *Nutrition Business Journal* 2004. Available at: http://www.nutritionbusiness.com.

24. Chandra RK. Effect of vitamin and trace-element supplementation on cognitive function in elderly subjects. *Nutrition* 2001; 17:709–12.

25. Roberts S, Sternberg S. Do nutritional supplements improve cognitive function in the elderly? *Nutrition* 2003; 19:976–8.

26. Shenkin SD, Whiteman MC, Pattie A, et al. Supplementation and the elderly: Dramatic results? *Nutrition* 2002; 18:364–5.

27. Brody JE. A top scientist's research is under attack. *New York Times,* May 6, 2004:A31.

28. Mahady GB, Fabricant D, Chadwick LR, et al. Black cohosh: An alternative therapy for menopause? *Nutrition and Clinical Care* 2002; 5:283–9.

29. Black cohosh. UC Berkeley Wellness Letter, February 2001. Available at: http://www.berkeleywellness.com/html/ds/dsBlackCohosh.php.

30. Office of Dietary Supplements. Questions and answers about black cohosh and the symptoms of menopause, October 3, 2003. Available at: http://ods.od.nih.gov/factsheets/blackcohosh.html.

31. American College of Obstetrics and Gynecology. Use of botanicals for management of menopausal symptoms, June 2001. Available at: http://www.acog.org/from_home/publications/misc/pb028.htm.

32. Jacobson JS, Troxel AB, Evans J, et al. Randomized trial of black cohosh for the treatment of hot flashes among women with a history of breast cancer. *Journal of Clinical Oncology* 2001; 19:2739–45.

33. Burke BE, Olson RD, Cusack BJ. Randomized, controlled trial of phytoestrogen in the prophylactic treatment of menstrual migraine. *Biomedical Pharmacotherapy* 2002; 56:283–8.

34. Hernandez MG, Pluchino S. Cimicifuga racemosa for the treatment of hot flushes in women surviving breast cancer. *Maturitas* 2003; 44(suppl 1):S59–65.

35. Wuttke W, Seidlova-Wuttke D, Gorkow C. The Cimicifuga preparation BNO 1055 vs. conjugated estrogens in a double-blind placebo-controlled study: Effects on menopause symptoms and bone markers. *Maturitas* 2003; 44(suppl 1):S67–77.

36. Bero LA, Galbraith A, Rennie D. The publication of sponsored symposiums in medical journals. *New England Journal of Medicine* 1992; 327:1135–40.

37. Whiting PW, Clouston A, Kerlin P. Black cohosh and other herbal remedies associated with acute hepatitis. *Medical Journal of Australia* 2002; 177:440–3.

38. Lontos S, Jones RM, Angus PW, et al. Acute liver failure associated with the use of herbal preparations containing black cohosh. *Medical Journal of Australia* 2003; 179:390–1.

39. Davis V, Jayo MJ, Hardy ML, et al. Effects of black cohosh on mammary tumor development and progression in MMTV-neu transgenic mice. *Proceedings of the American Association for Cancer Research* 2003; 44:Abstract R910.

40. National Cancer Institute. Coenzyme Q10, July 9, 2003. Available at: http://www.cancer.gov/cancertopics/pdq/cam/coenzymeQ10.

41. Food and Drug Administration. Notice of Violation of Section 201(g)(1) of the Federal Food, Drug, and Cosmetic Act [21 USC 321(g)(1)], July 7, 2004.

42. Folkers K, Brown R, Judy WV, et al. Survival of cancer patients on therapy with coenzyme Q10. *Biochemical and Biophysical Research Communications* 1993; 192:241–5.

43. Lockwood K, Moesgaard S, Hanioka T, et al. Apparent partial remission of breast cancer in 'high risk' patients supplemented with nutritional antioxidants, essential fatty acids and coenzyme Q10. *Molecular Aspects of Medicine* 1994; 15(suppl)s231–40.

44. Cortes EP, Gupta M, Chou C, et al. Adriamycin cardiotoxicity: Early detection by systolic time interval and possible prevention by coenzyme Q10. *Cancer Treatment Reports* 1978; 62:887–91.

45. Munkholm H, Hansen HH, Rasmussen K. Coenzyme Q10 treatment in serious heart failure. *Biofactors* 1999; 9:285–9.

46. Morisco C, Trimarco B, Condorelli M. Effect of coenzyme Q10 therapy in patients with congestive heart failure: A long-term multicenter randomized study. *Clinical Investigations* 1993; 71:S134–6.

47. Langsjoen PH, Vadhanavikit S, Folkers K. Response of patients in classes III and IV of cardiomyopathy to therapy in a blind and crossover trial with coenzyme Q10. *Proceedings of the National Academy of Sciences of the United States of America* 1985; 82:4240–4.

48. Tanaka J, Tominaga R, Yoshitoshi M, et al. Coenzyme Q10: The prophylactic effect on low cardiac output following cardiac valve replacement. *Annals of Thoracic Surgery* 1982; 33:145–51.

49. Permanetter B, Rossy W, Klein G, et al. Ubiquinone (coenzyme Q10) in the long-term treatment of idiopathic dilated cardiomyopathy. *European Heart Journal* 1992; 13:1528–33.

50. Watson PS, Scalia GM, Galbraith A, et al. Lack of effect of coenzyme Q on left ventricular function in patients with congestive heart failure. *Journal of the American College of Cardiology* 1999; 33:1549–52.

51. Khatta M, Alexander BS, Krichten CM, et al. The effect of coenzyme Q10 in patients with congestive heart failure. *Annals of Internal Medicine* 2000; 132:636–40.

52. Singh RB, Niaz MA, Rastogi SS, et al. Effect of hydrosoluble coenzyme Q10 on blood pressures and insulin resistance in hypertensive patients with coronary artery disease. *Journal of Human Hypertension* 1999; 13:203–8.

53. Burke BE, Neuenschwander R, Olson RD. Randomized, double-blind, placebo-controlled trial of coenzyme Q10 in isolated systolic hypertension. *Southern Medical Journal* 2001; 94:1112–7.

54. Singh RB, Wander GS, Rastogi A, et al. Randomized, double-blind placebo-controlled trial of coenzyme Q10 in patients with acute myocardial infarction. *Cardiovascular Drugs and Therapy* 1998; 12:347–53.

55. Hodgson JM, Watts GF, Playford DA, et al. Coenzyme Q10 improves blood pressure and glycaemic control: A controlled trial in subjects with type 2 diabetes. *European Journal of Clinical Nutrition* 2002; 56:1137–42.

56. Eriksson JG, Forsen TJ, Mortensen SA, et al. The effect of coenzyme Q10 administration on metabolic control in patients with type 2 diabetes mellitus. *Biofactors* 1999; 9:315–8.

57. Henriksen JE, Andersen CB, Hother-Nielsen O, et al. Impact of ubiquinone (coenzyme Q10) treatment on glycaemic control, insulin requirement and well-being in patients with Type 1 diabetes mellitus. *Diabetic Medicine* 1999; 16:312–8.

58. Shults CW, Oakes D, Kieburtz K, et al. Effects of coenzyme Q10 in early Parkinson disease: Evidence of slowing of the functional decline. *Archives of Neurology* 2002; 59:1541–50.

59. A randomized, placebo-controlled trial of coenzyme Q10 and remacemide in Huntington's disease. *Neurology* 2001; 57:397–404.

60. Scott GN, Elmer GW. Update on natural product—drug interactions. *American Journal of Health System Pharmacy* 2002; 59:339–47.

61. Lindenmuth GF, Lindenmuth EB. The efficacy of echinacea compound herbal tea preparation on the severity and duration of upper respiratory and flu symptoms: A randomized, double-blind placebo-controlled study. *Journal of Alternative and Complementary Medicine* 2000; 6:327–34.

62. Hodges PJ, Kam PC. The peri-operative implications of herbal medicines. *Anaesthesia* 2002; 57:889–99.

63. Melchart D, Linde K, Fischer P, et al. Echinacea for preventing and treating the common cold. *Cochrane Database of Systematic Reviews* 2000:CD000530.

64. Melchart D, Walther E, Linde K, et al. Echinacea root extracts for the prevention of upper respiratory tract infections: A double-blind, placebo-controlled randomized trial. *Archives of Family Medicine* 1998; 7:541–5.

65. Grimm W, Muller HH. A randomized controlled trial of the effect of fluid extract of Echinacea purpurea on the incidence and severity of colds and respiratory infections. *American Journal of Medicine* 1999; 106:138–43.

66. Turner RB, Riker DK, Gangemi JD. Ineffectiveness of echinacea for prevention of experimental rhinovirus colds. *Antimicrobial Agents and Chemotherapy* 2000; 44:1708–9.

67. Barrett BP, Brown RL, Locken K, et al. Treatment of the common cold with unrefined echinacea. A randomized, double-blind, placebo-controlled trial. *Annals of Internal Medicine* 2002; 137:939–46.

68. Taylor JA, Weber W, Standish L, et al. Efficacy and safety of echinacea in treating upper respiratory tract infections in children: A randomized controlled trial. *Journal of the American Medical Association* 2003; 290:2824–30.

69. Schulten B, Bulitta M, Ballering-Bruhl B, et al. Efficacy of Echinacea purpurea in patients with a common cold. A placebo-controlled, randomised, double-blind clinical trial. *Arzneimittelforschung* 2001; 51:563–8.

70. Echinacea for prevention and treatment of upper respiratory infections. *Medical Letter on Drugs and Therapeutics* 2002; 44:29–30.

71. Vonau B, Chard S, Mandalia S, et al. Does the extract of the plant Echinacea purpurea influence the clinical course of recurrent genital herpes? *International Journal of STD & AIDS* 2001; 12:154–8.

72. Ang-Lee MK, Moss J, Yuan CS. Herbal medicines and perioperative care. *Journal of the American Medical Association* 2001; 286:208–16.

73. Mullins RJ, Heddle R. Adverse reactions associated with echinacea: The Australian experience. *Annals of Allergy Asthma and Immunology* 2002; 88:42–51.

74. Ernst E. The risk-benefit profile of commonly used herbal therapies: Ginkgo, St. John's Wort, Ginseng, Echinacea, Saw Palmetto, and Kava. *Annals of Internal Medicine* 2002; 136:42–53.

75. Gallo M, Sarkar M, Au W, et al. Pregnancy outcome following gestational exposure to echinacea: A prospective controlled study. *Archives of Internal Medicine* 2000; 160:3141–3.

76. Tricker AR, Wacker CD, Preussmann R. Nitrosation products from the plant Ephedra altissima and their potential endogenous formation. *Cancer Letters* 1987; 35:199–206.

77. Tricker AR, Wacker CD, Preussmann R. 2-(N-nitroso-N-methylamino)propiophenone, a direct acting bacterial mutagen found in nitrosated Ephedra altissima tea. *Toxicology Letters* 1987; 38:45–50.

78. Bent S, Tiedt TN, Odden MC, et al. The relative safety of ephedra compared with other herbal products. *Annals of Internal Medicine* 2003; 138:468–71.

79. Kernan WN, Viscoli CM, Brass LM, et al. Phenylpropanolamine and the risk of hemorrhagic stroke. *New England Journal of Medicine* 2000; 343:1826–32.

80. Shekelle PG, Hardy ML, Morton SC, et al. Efficacy and safety of ephedra and ephedrine for weight loss and athletic performance: A meta-analysis. *Journal of the American Medical Association* 2003; 289:1537–45.

81. Do Not Use! Tramadol with acetaminophen (Ultracet). *Worst Pills, Best Pills News* 2001; 7:75–7.

82. Cupp MJ. Herbal remedies: Adverse effects and drug interactions. *American Family Physician* 1999; 59:1239–45.

83. Gardner SF, Franks AM, Gurley BJ, et al. Effect of a multicomponent, ephedra-containing dietary supplement (Metabolife 356) on Holter monitoring and hemostatic parameters in healthy volunteers. *American Journal of Cardiology* 2003; 91:1510–3, A9.

84. Haller CA, Jacob P III, Benowitz NL. Pharmacology of ephedra alkaloids and caffeine after single-dose dietary supplement use. *Clinical Pharmacology and Therapeutics* 2002; 71:421–32.

85. McBride BF, Karapanos AK, Krudysz A, et al. Electrocardiographic and hemodynamic effects of a multicomponent dietary supplement containing ephedra and caffeine: A randomized controlled trial. *Journal of the American Medical Association* 2004; 291:216–21.

86. Kaberi-Otarod J, Conetta R, Kundo KK, et al. Ischemic stroke in a user of thermadrene: A case study in alternative medicine. *Clinical Pharmacology and Therapeutics* 2002; 72:343–6.

87. Morgenstern LB, Viscoli CM, Kernan WN, et al. Use of Ephedra-containing products and risk for hemorrhagic stroke. *Neurology* 2003; 60:132–5.

88. Drugs that may cause psychiatric symptoms. *Medical Letter on Drugs and Therapeutics* 2002; 44:59–62.

89. Schweinfurth J, Pribitkin E. Sudden hearing loss associated with ephedra use. *American Journal of Health System Pharmacy* 2003; 60:375–7.

90. Munarriz R, Hwang J, Goldstein I, et al. Cocaine and ephedrine-induced priapism: Case reports and investigation of potential adrenergic mechanisms. *Urology* 2003; 62:187–92.

91. Heinrich J, United States General Accounting Office. Testimony before the Subcommittee on Oversight of Government Management, Restructuring, and the District of Columbia, Committee on Governmental Affairs, US Senate: Dietary Supplements for Weight Loss: Limited Federal Oversight Has Focused More on Marketing Than on Safety (GAO-02-985T), July 31, 2002. Available at: http://www.gao.gov/new .items/d02985t.pdf.

92. Gurley BJ, Gardner SF, Hubbard MA. Content versus label claims in ephedra-containing dietary supplements. *American Journal of Health System Pharmacy* 2000; 57:963–9.

93. Ardati A, Wolfe SM. Letter to HHS Secretary Tommy Thompson calling on the government to seize 10 products containing synthetic ephedra (HRG Publication #1608), January 31, 2002. Available at: http://www.citizen.org/publications/release.cfm?ID=7146.

94. Samenuk D, Link MS, Homoud MK, et al. Adverse cardiovascular events temporally associated with ma huang, an herbal source of ephedrine. *Mayo Clinic Proceedings* 2002; 77:12–6.

95. Haller CA, Benowitz NL. Adverse cardiovascular and central nervous system events associated with dietary supplements containing ephedra alkaloids. *New England Journal of Medicine* 2000; 343:1833–8.

96. Wolfe SM. Ephedra Ban Comes Too Late; FDA Should Have Acted Much Sooner, December 30, 2003. Available at: http://www .citizen.org/pressroom/release.cfm?ID=1617.

97. Wolfe SM. Statement before the National Academy of Sciences on the Framework for Evaluating the Safety of Dietary Supplements (HRG Publication #1594), October 11, 2001. Available at: http://www .citizen.org/publications/release.cfm?ID=7091.

98. Food and Drug Administration. Final Rule Declaring Dietary Supplements Containing Ephedrine Alkaloids Adulterated Because They Present an Unreasonable Risk, February 11, 2004.

99. CBS 2 Special Report. Ephedra For Sale, July 12, 2004. Available at: http://www.cbsnewyork.com.

100. Blank L. *Garlic Is as Good as Ten Mothers.* Flower Films, 1980.

101. Mulrow C, Lawrence V, Ackerman R, et al. *Garlic: Effects on Cardiovascular Risks and Disease, Protective Effects Against Cancer, and Clinical Adverse Effects.* Evidence Report/Technology Assessment Number 20: Rockville, Md.: Agency for Healthcare Research and Quality, 2004. Available at: http://hstat.nlm.nih.gov/hq/Hquest/screen/ DirectAccess/db/3572.

102. Gardner CD, Chatterjee LM, Carlson JJ. The effect of a garlic preparation on plasma lipid levels in moderately hypercholesterolemic adults. *Atherosclerosis* 2001; 154:213–20.

103. Zhang XH, Lowe D, Giles P, et al. A randomized trial of the effects of garlic oil upon coronary heart disease risk factors in trained male runners. *Blood Coagulation and Fibrinolysis* 2001; 12:67–74.

104. Ziaei S, Hantoshzadeh S, Rezasoltani P, et al. The effect of garlic tablet on plasma lipids and platelet aggregation in nulliparous pregnants at high risk of preeclampsia. *European Journal of Obstetrics, Gynecology, and Reproductive Biology* 2001; 99:201–6.

105. Kannar D, Wattanapenpaiboon N, Savige GS, et al. Hypocholesterolemic effect of an enteric-coated garlic supplement. *Journal of the American College of Nutrition* 2001; 20:225–31.

106. You WC, Chang YS, Heinrich J, et al. An intervention trial to inhibit the progression of precancerous gastric lesions: Compliance, serum micronutrients and S-allyl cysteine levels, and toxicity. *European Journal of Cancer Prevention* 2001; 10:257–63.

107. Food and Drug Administration. Summary of safety-related drug labeling changes approved by the Center for Drug Evaluation and Research (CDER), May 2002, July 3, 2002. Available at: http://www .fda.gov/medwatch/SAFETY/2002/may02.htm#coumad.

108. Rose KD, Croissant PD, Parliament CF, et al. Spontaneous spinal epidural hematoma with associated platelet dysfunction from excessive garlic ingestion: A case report. *Neurosurgery* 1990; 26:880–2.

109. German K, Kumar U, Blackford HN. Garlic and the risk of TURP bleeding. *British Journal of Urology* 1995; 76:518.

110. Beaglehole R. Garlic for flavour, not cardioprotection. *The Lancet* 1996; 348:1186–7.

111. Gold PE, Cahill L, Wenk GL. The lowdown on Ginkgo biloba. *Scientific American* 2003; 288:86–91. Available at: http://www.sciam .com/article.cfm?articleID=0005D1A1-2400-1E64-A98A809EC5880105 &sc=I100322.

112. Birks J, Grimley EV, Van Dongen M. Ginkgo biloba for cognitive impairment and dementia. *Cochrane Database of Systematic Reviews* 2002:CD003120.

113. Solomon PR, Adams F, Silver A, et al. Ginkgo for memory enhancement: A randomized controlled trial. *Journal of the American Medical Association* 2002; 288:835–40.

114. Moulton PL, Boyko LN, Fitzpatrick JL, et al. The effect of

Ginkgo biloba on memory in healthy male volunteers. *Physiology and Behavior* 2001; 73:659–65.

115. Le Bars PL, Katz MM, Berman N, et al. A placebo-controlled, double-blind, randomized trial of an extract of Ginkgo biloba for dementia. North American EGb Study Group. *Journal of the American Medical Association* 1997; 278:1327–32.

116. Van Dongen M, van Rossum E, Kessels A, et al. Ginkgo for elderly people with dementia and age-associated memory impairment: A randomized clinical trial. *Journal of Clinical Epidemiology* 2003; 56:367–76.

117. Morgenstern C, Biermann E. The efficacy of Ginkgo special extract EGb 761 in patients with tinnitus. *International Journal of Clinical Pharmacology and Therapeutics* 2002; 40:188–97.

118. Drew S, Davies E. Effectiveness of Ginkgo biloba in treating tinnitus: Double blind, placebo controlled trial. *British Medical Journal* 2001; 322:73.

119. Bauer U. 6-month double-blind randomised clinical trial of Ginkgo biloba extract versus placebo in two parallel groups in patients suffering from peripheral arterial insufficiency. *Arzneimittelforschung* 1984; 34:716–20.

120. Parsad D, Pandhi R, Juneja A. Effectiveness of oral Ginkgo biloba in treating limited, slowly spreading vitiligo. *Clinical and Experimental Dermatology* 2003; 28:285–7.

121. Quaranta L, Bettelli S, Uva MG, et al. Effect of Ginkgo biloba extract on preexisting visual field damage in normal tension glaucoma. *Ophthalmology* 2003; 110:359–62.

122. Zhang XY, Zhou DF, Zhang PY, et al. A double-blind, placebo-controlled trial of extract of Ginkgo biloba added to haloperidol in treatment-resistant patients with schizophrenia. *Journal of Clinical Psychiatry* 2001; 62:878–83.

123. Kampman K, Majewska MD, Tourian K, et al. A pilot trial of piracetam and ginkgo biloba for the treatment of cocaine dependence. *Addictive Behaviors* 2003; 28:437–48.

124. Kang BJ, Lee SJ, Kim MD, et al. A placebo-controlled, double-blind trial of Ginkgo biloba for antidepressant-induced sexual dysfunction. *Human Psychopharmacology* 2002; 17:279–84.

125. Lingaerde O, Foreland AR, Magnusson A. Can winter depression be prevented by Ginkgo biloba extract? A placebo-controlled trial. *Acta Psychiatrica Scandinavica* 1999; 100:62–6.

126. Griffiths J, Jordan S, Pilon K. Natural health products and adverse reactions. *Canadian Adverse Drug Reaction Newsletter* 2004; 14:2–3.

127. Izzo AA, Ernst E. Interactions between herbal medicines and prescribed drugs: A systematic review. *Drugs* 2001; 61:2163–75.

128. Chiu AE, Lane AT, Kimball AB. Diffuse morbilliform eruption after consumption of ginkgo biloba supplement. *Journal of the American Academy of Dermatology* 2002; 46:145–6.

129. Kressmann S, Biber A, Wonnemann M, et al. Influence of pharmaceutical quality on the bioavailability of active components from Ginkgo biloba preparations. *Journal of Pharmacy and Pharmacology* 2002; 54:1507–14.

130. Miwa H, Iijima M, Tanaka S, et al. Generalized convulsions after consuming a large amount of gingko nuts. *Epilepsia* 2001; 42:280–1.

131. Granger AS. Ginkgo biloba precipitating epileptic seizures. *Age and Ageing* 2001; 30:523–5.

132. Benjamin J, Muir T, Briggs K, et al. A case of cerebral haemorrhage—can Ginkgo biloba be implicated? *Postgraduate Medical Journal* 2001; 77:112–3.

133. Meisel C, Johne A, Roots I. Fatal intracerebral mass bleeding associated with Ginkgo biloba and ibuprofen. *Atherosclerosis* 2003; 167:367.

134. Vale S. Subarachnoid haemorrhage associated with Ginkgo biloba. *The Lancet* 1998; 352:36.

135. Gilbert GJ. Ginkgo biloba. *Neurology* 1997; 48:1137.

136. Matthews MK Jr. Association of Ginkgo biloba with intracerebral hemorrhage. *Neurology* 1998; 50:1933–4.

137. Fong KC, Kinnear PE. Retrobulbar haemorrhage associated with chronic Gingko biloba ingestion. *Postgraduate Medical Journal* 2003; 79:531–2.

138. Rosenblatt M, Mindel J. Spontaneous hyphema associated with ingestion of Ginkgo biloba extract. *New England Journal of Medicine* 1997; 336:1108.

139. Fessenden JM, Wittenborn W, Clarke L. Gingko biloba: A case report of herbal medicine and bleeding postoperatively from a laparoscopic cholecystectomy. *American Surgeon* 2001; 67:33–5.

140. Valli G, Giardina EG. Benefits, adverse effects and drug interactions of herbal therapies with cardiovascular effects. *Journal of the American College of Cardiology* 2002; 39:1083–95.

141. Vogler BK, Pittler MH, Ernst E. The efficacy of ginseng. A systematic review of randomised clinical trials. *European Journal of Clinical Pharmacology* 1999; 55:567–75.

142. Cardinal BJ, Engels HJ. Ginseng does not enhance psychological well-being in healthy, young adults: Results of a double-blind, placebo-controlled, randomized clinical trial. *Journal of the American Dietetic Association* 2001; 101:655–60.

143. Cheng TO. Panax (ginseng) is not a panacea. *Archives of Internal Medicine* 2000; 160:3329.

144. Bahrke MS, Morgan WR. Evaluation of the ergogenic properties of ginseng: An update. *Sports Medicine* 2000; 29:113–33.

145. Wesnes KA, Ward T, McGinty A, et al. The memory enhancing effects of a Ginkgo biloba/Panax ginseng combination in healthy middle-aged volunteers. *Psychopharmacology* 2000; 152:353–61.

146. Wesnes KA, Faleni RA, Hefting NR, et al. The cognitive, subjective, and physical effects of a ginkgo biloba/panax ginseng combination in healthy volunteers with neurasthenic complaints. *Psychopharmacology Bulletin* 1997; 33:677–83.

147. Kennedy DO, Scholey AB, Wesnes KA. Modulation of cognition and mood following administration of single doses of Ginkgo biloba, ginseng, and a ginkgo/ginseng combination to healthy young adults. *Physiology and Behavior* 2002; 75:739–51.

148. D'Angelo L, Grimaldi R, Caravaggi M, et al. A double-blind, placebo-controlled clinical study on the effect of a standardized ginseng extract on psychomotor performance in healthy volunteers. *Journal of Ethnopharmacology* 1986; 16:15–22.

149. Sotaniemi EA, Haapakoski E, Rautio A. Ginseng therapy in non-insulin-dependent diabetic patients. *Diabetes Care* 1995; 18:1373–5.

150. Vuksan V, Sievenpiper JL, Koo VY, et al. American ginseng (Panax quinquefolius L) reduces postprandial glycemia in nondiabetic subjects and subjects with type 2 diabetes mellitus. *Archives of Internal Medicine* 2000; 160:1009–13.

151. Yun TK, Choi SY. Non-organ specific cancer prevention of ginseng: A prospective study in Korea. *International Journal of Epidemiology* 1998; 27:359–64.

152. Caso MA, Vargas RR, Salas VA, et al. Double-blind study of a multivitamin complex supplemented with ginseng extract. *Drugs Under Experimental and Clinical Research* 1996; 22:323–9.

153. Janetzky K, Morreale AP. Probable interaction between warfarin and ginseng. *American Journal of Health System Pharmacy* 1997; 54:692–3.

154. Palop-Larrea V, Gonzalvez-Perales JL, Catalan-Oliver C, et al. Metrorrhagia and ginseng. *Annals of Pharmacotherapy* 2000; 34:1347–8.

155. Rosado MF. Thrombosis of a prosthetic aortic valve disclosing a hazardous interaction between warfarin and a commercial ginseng product. *Cardiology* 2003; 99:111.

156. Shader RI, Greenblatt DJ. Phenelzine and the dream machine—ramblings and reflections. *Journal of Clinical Psychopharmacology* 1985; 5:65.

157. Jones BD, Runikis AM. Interaction of ginseng with phenelzine. *Journal of Clinical Psychopharmacology* 1987; 7:201–2.

158. Miller LG. Herbal medicinals: Selected clinical considerations focusing on known or potential drug-herb interactions. *Archives of Internal Medicine* 1998; 158:2200–11.

159. D'Arcy PF. Adverse reactions and interactions with herbal medicines. Part 1. Adverse reactions. *Adverse Drug Reactions and Toxicological Reviews* 1991; 10:189–208.

160. Siegel RK. Ginseng abuse syndrome. Problems with the panacea. *Journal of the American Medical Association* 1979; 241:1614–5.

161. Siegel RK. Ginseng and high blood pressure. *Journal of the American Medical Association* 1980; 243:32.

162. Punnonen R, Lukola A. Oestrogen-like effect of ginseng. *British Medical Journal* 1980; 281:1110.

163. Greenspan EM. Ginseng and vaginal bleeding. *Journal of the American Medical Association* 1983; 249:2018.

164. Is glucosamine worth taking for osteoarthritis? *Drug and Therapeutics Bulletin* 2002; 40:81–3.

165. Towheed TE, Anastassiades TP, Shea B, et al. Glucosamine therapy for treating osteoarthritis. *Cochrane Database of Systematic Reviews* 2001:CD002946.

166. McAlindon TE, LaValley MP, Gulin JP, et al. Glucosamine and chondroitin for treatment of osteoarthritis: A systematic quality assessment and meta-analysis. *Journal of the American Medical Association* 2000; 283:1469–75.

167. Richy F, Bruyere O, Ethgen O, et al. Structural and symptomatic efficacy of glucosamine and chondroitin in knee osteoarthritis: A comprehensive meta-analysis. *Archives of Internal Medicine* 2003; 163:1514–22.

168. Reginster JY, Deroisy R, Rovati LC, et al. Long-term effects of glucosamine sulphate on osteoarthritis progression: A randomised, placebo-controlled clinical trial. *The Lancet* 2001; 357:251–6.

169. Halbekath J, Lehnert R, Wille H. Glucosamine sulphate and osteoarthritis. *The Lancet* 2001; 357:1617.

170. McAlindon T. Glucosamine for osteoarthritis: Dawn of a new era? *The Lancet* 2001; 357:247–8.

171. Pavelka K, Gatterova J, Olejarova M, et al. Glucosamine sulfate use and delay of progression of knee osteoarthritis: A 3-year, randomized, placebo-controlled, double-blind study. *Archives of Internal Medicine* 2002; 162:2113–23.

172. Braham R, Dawson B, Goodman C. The effect of glucosamine supplementation on people experiencing regular knee pain. *British Journal of Sports Medicine* 2003; 37:45–9.

173. Hughes R, Carr A. A randomized, double-blind, placebo-controlled trial of glucosamine sulphate as an analgesic in osteoarthritis of the knee. *Rheumatology* 2002; 41:279–84.

174. Rindone JP, Hiller D, Collacott E, et al. Randomized, controlled trial of glucosamine for treating osteoarthritis of the knee. *Western Journal of Medicine* 2000; 172:91–4.

175. Verbruggen G, Goemaere S, Veys EM. Systems to assess the progression of finger joint osteoarthritis and the effects of disease modifying osteoarthritis drugs. *Clinical Rheumatology* 2002; 21:231–43.

176. Morreale P, Manopulo R, Galati M, et al. Comparison of the antiinflammatory efficacy of chondroitin sulfate and diclofenac sodium in patients with knee osteoarthritis. *Journal of Rheumatology* 1996; 23:1385–91.

177. Mazieres B, Combe B, Phan VA, et al. Chondroitin sulfate in osteoarthritis of the knee: A prospective, double blind, placebo controlled multicenter clinical study. *Journal of Rheumatology* 2001; 28:173–81.

178. Chard J, Dieppe P. Glucosamine for osteoarthritis: Magic, hype, or confusion? It's probably safe—but there's no good evidence that it works. *British Medical Journal* 2001; 322:1439–40.

179. Update on glucosamine for osteoarthritis. *Medical Letter on Drugs and Therapeutics* 2001; 43:111–2.

180. National Center for Complementary and Alternative Medicine and National Institutes of Health. Questions and Answers: NIH Glucosamine/Chondroitin Arthritis Intervention Trial (GAIT), 2004. Available at: http://nccam.nih.gov/news/19972000/121100/qa.htm.

181. Chan NN, Baldeweg SE, Tan TMM, et al. Glucosamine sulphate and osteoarthritis. *The Lancet* 2001; 357:1618–9.

182. Scroggie DA, Albright A, Harris MD. The effect of glucosamine-chondroitin supplementation on glycosylated hemoglobin levels in patients with type 2 diabetes mellitus: A placebo-controlled, double-blinded, randomized clinical trial. *Archives of Internal Medicine* 2003; 163:1587–90.

183. Matheu V, Gracia Bara MT, Pelta R, et al. Immediate-hypersensitivity reaction to glucosamine sulfate. *Allergy* 1999; 54:643.

184. Tallia AF, Cardone DA. Asthma exacerbation associated with glucosamine-chondroitin supplement. *Journal of the American Board of Family Practitioners* 2002; 15:481–4.

185. The Quote Garden—Quotes about Tea, June 2, 2004. Available at: http://www.quotegarden.com/tea.html.

186. Yang CS, Landau JM. Effects of tea consumption on nutrition and health. *Journal of Nutrition* 2000; 130:2409–12.

187. Kinlen LJ, Willows AN, Goldblatt P, et al. Tea consumption and cancer. *British Journal of Cancer* 1988; 58:397–401.

188. Sun CL, Yuan JM, Lee MJ, et al. Urinary tea polyphenols in relation to gastric and esophageal cancers: A prospective study of men in Shanghai, China. *Carcinogenesis* 2002; 23:1497–1503.

189. Goldbohm RA, Hertog MG, Brants HA, et al. Consumption of black tea and cancer risk: A prospective cohort study. *Journal of the National Cancer Institute* 1996; 88:93–100.

190. Whittemore AS, Paffenbarger RS Jr., Anderson K, et al. Early precursors of pancreatic cancer in college men. *Journal of Chronic Diseases* 1983; 36:251–6.

191. Hiatt RA, Klatsky AL, Armstrong MA. Pancreatic cancer, blood glucose and beverage consumption. *International Journal of Cancer* 1988; 41:794–7.

192. Jatoi A, Ellison N, Burch PA, et al. A phase II trial of green tea in the treatment of patients with androgen independent metastatic prostate carcinoma. *Cancer* 2003; 97:1442–6.

193. NCI Fact Sheet: Tea and Cancer Prevention, December 6, 2002. Available at: http://www.cancer.gov/newscenter/content_nav.aspx?view id=afc8f2c0-f3df-4f6c-9c30-28fc15c0054e.

194. Princen HM, van Duyvenvoorde W, Buytenhek R, et al. No effect of consumption of green and black tea on plasma lipid and antioxidant levels and on LDL oxidation in smokers. *Arteriosclerosis, Thrombosis, and Vascular Biology* 1998; 18:833–41.

195. Maron DJ, Lu GP, Cai NS, et al. Cholesterol-lowering effect of a theaflavin-enriched green tea extract: A randomized controlled trial. *Archives of Internal Medicine* 2003; 163:1448–53.

196. Kaegi E. Unconventional therapies for cancer: 2. Green tea. The Task Force on Alternative Therapies of the Canadian Breast Cancer Research Initiative. *Canadian Medical Association Journal* 1998; 158:1033–5.

197. Shirai T, Reshad K, Yoshitomi A, et al. Green tea–induced asthma: Relationship between immunological reactivity, specific and

non-specific bronchial responsiveness. *Clinical and Experimental Allergy* 2003; 33:1252–5.

198. Shirai T, Sato A, Chida K, et al. Epigallocatechin gallate–induced histamine release in patients with green tea–induced asthma. *Annals of Allergy Asthma and Immunology* 1997; 79:65–9.

199. Shirai T, Sato A, Hara Y. Epigallocatechin gallate. The major causative agent of green tea–induced asthma. *Chest* 1994; 106:1801–5.

200. Shirai T, Hayakawa H, Akiyama J, et al. Food allergy to green tea. *Journal of Allergy and Clinical Immunology* 2003; 112:805–6.

201. American Cancer Society. Green tea, June 2, 2004. Available at: http://www.cancer.org/docroot/ETO/content/ETO_5_3X_Green_Tea.asp?sitearea=ETO.

202. Mulrow C, Lawrence V, Jacobs B, et al. Milk Thistle: Effects on Liver Disease and Cirrhosis and Clinical Adverse Effects. Evidence Report/Technology Assessment Number 21. Rockville, Md.: Agency for Healthcare Research and Quality, 2002. Available at: http://www.ncbi.nlm.nih.gov/books/bv.fcgi?rid=hstat1.chapter.29128.

203. Buzzelli G, Moscarella S, Giusti A, et al. A pilot study on the liver protective effect of silybin-phosphatidylcholine complex (IdB1016) in chronic active hepatitis. *International Journal of Clinical Pharmacology, Therapy, and Toxicology* 1993; 31:456–60.

204. Liu J, Manheimer E, Tsutani K, et al. Medicinal herbs for hepatitis C virus infection: A Cochrane hepatobiliary systematic review of randomized trials. *American Journal of Gastroenterology* 2003; 98:538–44.

205. National Center for Complementary and Alternative Medicine. Hepatitis C and complementary and alternative medicine: 2003 update, 2003. Available at: http://nccam.nih.gov/health/hepatitisc/.

206. Kasahara A. Treatment strategies for chronic hepatitis C virus infection. *Journal of Gastroenterology* 2000; 35:411–23.

207. Tan R. Great morinda (morinda citrifolia), 2001. Available at: http://www.naturia.per.sg/buloh/plants/morinda.htm.

208. Wang MY, West BJ, Jensen CJ, et al. Morinda citrifolia (Noni): A literature review and recent advances in Noni research. *Acta Pharmacologica Sinica* 2002; 23:1127–41.

209. Valentine PW. Sexual abuse case against ex-Md. official is closed. *Washington Post*, March 5, 1996:B2.

210. Noni Books. Available at: http://www.nonihi.com/nonibooks.html.

211. Noni Juice. Available at: http://www.nonijuice.us/whatdoctorsaresaying.htm.

212. Official Site of Tahitian Noni Juice. Available at: http://www.tahitiannoni.com/us/us_index.htm.

213. Wang MY, Su C. Cancer preventive effect of Morinda citrifolia (Noni). *Annals of the New York Academy of Sciences* 2001; 952:161–8.

214. Excerpt from *The Noni Phenomenon*. Available at: http://www.greenaus.com/noni/drsolomon.html.

215. Mueller BA, Scott MK, Sowinski KM, et al. Noni juice (Morinda citrifolia): Hidden potential for hyperkalemia? *American Journal of Kidney Diseases* 2000; 35:310–2.

216. Wilt TJ, Ishani A, Stark G, et al. Saw palmetto extracts for treatment of benign prostatic hyperplasia: A systematic review. *Journal of the American Medical Association* 1998; 280:1604–9.

217. Wilt T, Ishani A, Mac DR. Serenoa repens for benign prostatic hyperplasia. *Cochrane Database of Systematic Reviews* 2002: CD001423.

218. Boyle P, Robertson C, Lowe F, et al. Meta-analysis of clinical trials of permixon in the treatment of symptomatic benign prostatic hyperplasia. *Urology* 2000; 55:533–9.

219. Gerber GS, Kuznetsov D, Johnson BC, et al. Randomized, double-blind, placebo-controlled trial of saw palmetto in men with lower urinary tract symptoms. *Urology* 2001; 58:960–4.

220. McConnell JD, Bruskewitz R, Walsh P, et al. The effect of finasteride on the risk of acute urinary retention and the need for surgical treatment among men with benign prostatic hyperplasia. Finasteride Long-Term Efficacy and Safety Study Group. *New England Journal of Medicine* 1998; 338:557–63.

221. National Institutes of Health. Saw Palmetto Extract in Benign Prostatic Hyperplasia, 2004. Available at: http://clinicaltrials.gov/ct/gui/c/w1b/show/NCT00037154?order=1&JServSessionIdzone_ct=onyx6gr3l1.

222. Saw palmetto for benign prostatic hyperplasia. *Medical Letter on Drugs and Therapeutics* 1999; 41:18.

223. Cheema P, El Mefty O, Jazieh AR. Intraoperative haemorrhage associated with the use of extract of Saw Palmetto herb: A case report and review of literature. *Journal of Internal Medicine* 2001; 250:167–9.

224. PC Spes. *Medical Letter on Drugs and Therapeutics* 2001; 43:15–6.

225. DiPaola RS, Zhang H, Lambert GH, et al. Clinical and biologic activity of an estrogenic herbal combination (PC-SPES) in prostate cancer. *New England Journal of Medicine* 1998; 339:785–91.

226. Food and Drug Administration. 2002 Safety Alerts for Drugs, Biologics, Medical Devices, and Dietary Supplements, 2002. Available at: http://www.fda.gov/medwatch/SAFETY/2002/safety02.htm#spes.

227. Sovak M, Seligson AL, Konas M, et al. Herbal composition PC-SPES for management of prostate cancer: Identification of active principles. *Journal of the National Cancer Institute* 2002; 94:1275–81.

228. Final report on the safety assessment of Hypericum perforatum extract and Hypericum perforatum oil. *International Journal of Toxicology* 2001; 20(suppl 2):31–9.

229. Pies R. Adverse neuropsychiatric reactions to herbal and over-the-counter "antidepressants." *Journal of Clinical Psychiatry* 2000; 61:815–20.

230. Linde K, Mulrow CD. St John's wort for depression. *Cochrane Database of Systematic Reviews* 2000:CD000448.

231. Linde K, Ramirez G, Mulrow CD, et al. St John's wort for depression—an overview and meta-analysis of randomised clinical trials. *British Medical Journal* 1996; 313:253–8.

232. Williams JW Jr., Mulrow CD, Chiquette E, et al. A systematic review of newer pharmacotherapies for depression in adults: Evidence report summary. *Annals of Internal Medicine* 2000; 132:743–56.

233. Gaster B, Holroyd J. St John's wort for depression: A systematic review. *Archives of Internal Medicine* 2000; 160:152–6.

234. Kalb R, Trautmann-Sponsel RD, Kieser M. Efficacy and tolerability of hypericum extract WS 5572 versus placebo in mildly to moderately depressed patients. A randomized double-blind multicenter clinical trial. *Pharmacopsychiatry* 2001; 34:96–103.

235. Philipp M, Kohnen R, Hiller KO. Hypericum extract versus imipramine or placebo in patients with moderate depression: Randomised multicentre study of treatment for eight weeks. *British Medical Journal* 1999; 319:1534–8.

236. Lecrubier Y, Clerc G, Didi R, et al. Efficacy of St. John's wort extract WS 5570 in major depression: A double-blind, placebo-controlled trial. *American Journal of Psychiatry* 2002; 159:1361–6.

237. Hypericum extract (from St. John's wort) in the treatment of moderate depression. *Worst Pills, Best Pills News* 2000; 6:11–2.

238. Shelton RC, Keller MB, Gelenberg A, et al. Effectiveness of St John's wort in major depression: A randomized controlled trial. *Journal of the American Medical Association* 2001; 285:1978–86.

239. Morris JB, Beck AT. The efficacy of antidepressant drugs. A review of research (1958–1972). *Archives of General Psychiatry* 1974; 30:667–74.

240. Effect of Hypericum perforatum (St John's wort) in major de-

pressive disorder: A randomized controlled trial. *Journal of the American Medical Association* 2002; 287:1807–14.

241. Hammerness P, Basch E, Ulbricht C, et al. St John's wort: A systematic review of adverse effects and drug interactions for the consultation psychiatrist. *Psychosomatics* 2003; 44:271–82.

242. Breckenridge A. Message from Professor A. Breckenridge, Chairman, Committee on Safety of Medicines, February 29, 2000. Available at: http://www.mca.gov.uk/ourwork/monitorsafequalmed/safetymessages/sjwcl.pdf.

243. Sugimoto K, Ohmori M, Tsuruoka S, et al. Different effects of St John's wort on the pharmacokinetics of simvastatin and pravastatin. *Clinical Pharmacology and Therapeutics* 2001; 70:518–24.

244. Wang Z, Hamman MA, Huang SM, et al. Effect of St John's wort on the pharmacokinetics of fexofenadine. *Clinical Pharmacology and Therapeutics* 2002; 71:414–20.

245. Mills E, Montori VM, Wu P, et al. Interaction of St. John's wort with conventional drugs: Systematic review of clinical trials. *British Medical Journal* 2004; 329:27–30.

246. Nierenberg AA, Burt T, Matthews J, et al. Mania associated with St. John's wort. *Biological Psychiatry* 1999; 46:1707–8.

247. Spinella M, Eaton LA. Hypomania induced by herbal and pharmaceutical psychotropic medicines following mild traumatic brain injury. *Brain Injury* 2002; 16:359–67.

248. Barbenel DM, Yusufi B, O'Shea D, et al. Mania in a patient receiving testosterone replacement postorchidectomy taking St John's wort and sertraline. *Journal of Psychopharmacology* 2000; 14:84–6.

249. Moses EL, Mallinger AG. St. John's Wort: Three cases of possible mania induction. *Journal of Clinical Psychopharmacology* 2000; 20:115–7.

250. Zullino D, Borgeat F. Hypertension induced by St. John's Wort—a case report. *Pharmacopsychiatry* 2003; 36:32.

251. Patel S, Robinson R, Burk M. Hypertensive crisis associated with St. John's Wort. *American Journal of Medicine* 2002; 112:507–8.

252. Lane-Brown MM. Photosensitivity associated with herbal preparations of St John's wort (Hypericum perforatum). *Medical Journal of Australia* 2000; 172:302.

253. Holme SA, Roberts DL. Erythroderma associated with St John's wort. *British Journal of Dermatology* 2000; 143:1127–8.

254. Bove GM. Acute neuropathy after exposure to sun in a patient treated with St John's Wort. *The Lancet* 1998; 352:1121–2.

255. Brown TM. Acute St. John's wort toxicity. *American Journal of Emergency Medicine* 2000; 18:231–2.

256. Parker V, Wong AH, Boon HS, et al. Adverse reactions to St John's Wort. *Canadian Journal of Psychiatry,* 2001; 46:77–9.

257. McIntyre M. A review of the benefits, adverse events, drug interactions, and safety of St. John's Wort (Hypericum perforatum): The implications with regard to the regulation of herbal medicines. *Journal of Alternative and Complementary Medicine* 2000; 6:115–24.

29

PROTECTING YOURSELF AND YOUR FAMILY FROM PREVENTABLE DRUG-INDUCED INJURY

Doctors and pharmacists often blame the adverse effects of prescription drugs on patients, accusing them of improperly taking their medications. The standard solution offered by some health professionals is to get patients to better "comply" with doctors' instructions by using what are called compliance programs or strategies. (Another word for compliance is, of course, obedience.) Occasionally, the blame is also put on doctors for misprescribing and overprescribing, on pharmacists for failing to detect serious drug interactions, and only rarely on the drug industry for overselling drugs to doctors and now directly to patients through direct-to-consumer advertising. Even when it is acknowledged that health professionals are partially responsible for adverse reactions, the proposed solution is based on the assumption that the system of professional education will prepare doctors to better learn about the proper use of drugs and pharmacists to do a better job of learning about and detecting dangerous drug interactions.

While important changes need to be made in the way patients, doctors, and pharmacists perform these important tasks, they are not likely to occur without other, more primary changes. First, improved communication with your doctor is necessary. Second, you must have access to comprehensive objective information about the risks and benefits of prescription drugs written in nontechnical language distributed to you by your pharmacist with each new and refill prescription.

Communication: Activating Yourself and Your Doctor

Patients and their families and friends need to feel comfortable approaching the doctor, with the help of their pharmacist, and to begin working with the doctor to reduce the number of drugs and the dosage of drugs being used, whenever possible. In most cases, this will result not only in fewer adverse reactions, including life-threatening ones, but also in fewer drugs being used, inevitably saving money as well. Equally important, this process will improve patients' ability to properly take the drugs that are actually needed. Studies show that more drugs lead to poorer patient compliance with instructions, while fewer drugs lead to better compliance.[1]

This problem is most serious for older patients, who proportionately take a higher number of drugs than their younger counterparts, but it can be a significant problem for younger patients as well. This chapter assumes that most doctors who take care of older patients, and even many doctors who treat younger age groups, have not had adequate training in the problems of drug prescribing and rely too heavily on drug company promotion to make prescribing decisions. For example, too many doctors usually employ the same decision-making process (when to treat and what drug and dose to use) for older adults as for younger people. This too often results in their prescribing too many drugs at doses that are too high. In addition, many older people see multiple doctors—an internist, a gynecologist, and a heart specialist, for example. Communication among these physicians about what drugs are being prescribed is often deficient.

The major reason for making a sharp distinction between drugs that we label **"Do Not Use"** and the other drugs in this book is to inform patients and their physicians about the 181 drugs in the book for which there are safer alternatives, also listed herein.

"Do Not Use" Drugs

If a drug already being used or being considered for use is one of the drugs that we list in this edition as **"Do Not Use"** or **"Do Not Use for Seven Years,"** ask your doctor about alternative therapy, which could be either nondrug therapy or a safer drug. If the drug you are using is listed in this book as **"Limited Use,"** it may also be a good idea to discuss the drug with your doctor to see if a better alternative might be found.

Examples of dangerous "Do Not Use" drugs from previous editions of this book that have subsequently been taken off the market, usually long after we warned against their use in the book and/or in our monthly *Worst Pills, Best Pills News*, include the antihistamines Seldane and Hismanal, the heart drugs Posicor and Baycol, the painkillers Duract and Butazolidin, the antibiotics Zagam and Raxar, the antidepressant Serzone, and the weight reduction drugs Redux and ephedra.

"Do Not Use for Seven Years" Drugs

Nineteen drugs in this book are listed as **"Do Not Use for Seven Years."** For many years, we have warned patients not to use newly approved drugs unless they are one of the decided minority of new drugs with evidence that they provide a breakthrough beyond existing treatments. A study, involving Dr. Sidney Wolfe as one of the authors, provides clear evidence why this caution of waiting seven years is well founded. A total of 548 new chemical entities (drugs marketed for the first time in the United States) were approved in 1975–1999. By 1999, 45 drugs (8.2%) acquired one or more black-box warnings and 16 (2.9%) were withdrawn from the market. **The estimated probability of acquiring a new black-box warning or being withdrawn from the market over a period of 25 years was 20%. Half of these black-box warning changes occurred within 7 years of drug introduction; half of the withdrawals occurred within 2 years.** The article concluded that serious adverse drug reactions commonly emerge after FDA approval. The safety of new agents cannot be known with certainty until a drug has been on the market for many years.[2] This study provides the basis for our "Seven-Year Rule" concerning newly marketed drugs that are not therapeutic breakthroughs.

Therefore, one way of protecting yourself without being deprived of new, breakthrough drugs, is to say no to using newly approved drugs unless they are in the small minority of such drugs with a significant therapeutic benefit.

Although most doctors are quite willing to learn to prescribe fewer and safer drugs, this is more likely to occur if you follow the Ten Rules for Safer Drug Use outlined in this chapter and have access to objective drug information written specifically for patients. Being more assertive with your doctors or pharmacists is not only appropriate but may be an important factor in better protecting your health.

Talk to your doctor before deciding to make any changes in your prescription drugs based on information in this book.

SPECIAL PROBLEMS IN NURSING HOMES

All of the problems of dangerous misprescribing of drugs for people living in the community are even worse in many nursing homes. For example, one study found that almost 40% of nursing home residents were being given antipsychotic drugs even though only a small fraction of them actually were psychotic. Another study found that one-third of people in nursing homes were getting seven or more prescription drugs. (See p. 1 for more information on the extent of prescription drug use in nursing homes.) Most of the rules below for safer drug use apply in all situations, including the nursing home situation, but there are some differences. The main one is that for patients in nursing homes, the brown-bag session and filling out the Drug Worksheet should be done by the nursing home staff, including the nurse, doctor, and pharmacist. If you are the child, other relative, or friend of a nursing home resident, you have the right, with his or her permission, to demand and receive a completed Drug Worksheet for that person and an explanation of the reasons for each drug being used. You can obtain this information, with the help of your own pharmacist and possibly your own doctor. This will very likely help to reduce the number of drugs being given and, where appropriate, reduce the doses of drugs still judged to be necessary. By taking care of these matters, you will have made a major contribution to the health and well-being of your loved one(s) in nursing homes.

Remember—the doctor is working for you, and with you.

Ten Rules for Safer Drug Use

Rule 1: Have "Brown Bag Sessions" with Your Primary Doctor; Fill Out the Drug Worksheet Enclosed with This Book.

It is impossible to overemphasize the importance of this first and most crucial step in preventing adverse drug reactions. Whenever you go to a doctor you have not previously seen or to one with whom you have never had a brown-bag session, gather all prescription and over-the-counter drugs and dietary supplements in your medicine cabinet or anywhere else and bring them to the doctor so that a list can be made and you can start to fill out the Drug Worksheet enclosed. (See p. 865 for a sample of this worksheet that you can use.)

The purpose of the Drug Worksheet is for you and your doctor (or doctors) to keep an ongoing record of all drugs you are using, the purposes for which they are being used, adverse reactions, whether the drug is working, and other information essential to the safest and most effective use of these products.

Doctors should never prescribe a drug or renew a prescription, nor should you be willing to get a new prescription, without full, up-to-date knowledge of all drugs already being taken or likely to be taken.

Before your brown-bag session with the doctor, your pharmacist may help you to fill out some of the blanks on your Drug Worksheet.

Once you have brought in all the drugs you are taking, ask your doctor to help you fill out the Drug Worksheet. You will probably be able to fill out more of the information concerning over-the-counter drugs yourself, since doctors often do not know that you are taking them or for what purpose. The doctor will be able to help you to fill out most of the information concerning prescription drugs, at least the ones that he or she has prescribed for you.

Explanation of Items on Drug Worksheet (p. 865)

a. *Name of drug, of doctor who wrote the prescription, and date drug was started or the dosage changed:* Drugs should be listed by both

Sample Page of Drug Worksheet for Patients, Family, Doctor and Pharmacist

Name Beatrice Jones

Primary Doctor's Name Dr. Jackson

Page 1

Doctor's Telephone 555-1212

Generic Name of Drug / Brand Name of Drug	a. Doctor, date started & changes	b. Reason why prescribed or changed?	c. Dose? (Each time)	Times per day	What time of day?	d. How long should you take drug? days/weeks/months	e. Problems to watch out for which this drug can cause	f. Interactions of this drug with other drugs or food; diet recommendations	g. How are you actually taking the drug?	h. New problems or complaints since drug started (Date it began)	i. Is drug working?
Example: hydrochlorothiazide / HydroDiuril (This is an example only.)	Dr. Jackson 2/10/92	high blood pressure 180/100	12.5 mg 1/2 pill	once	morning	at least till next visit in 1 month	muscle weakness; cramps from low potassium; frequent urination common	1) Eat raisins, bananas, wheat germ & drink orange juice for potassium	most days 5-6/wk	No	No
	3/8/92	pressure still high 165/100	25 mg 1 pill	once	morning	till next visit, 2 months		2) Avoid salt	stopped 4/1— felt too weak	feeling tired 3/22/92	No
	4/15/92	pressure 165/95	12.5 mg 1/2 pill	once	morning	till next visit, 2 months		3) may lower effectiveness of diabetes drugs	every day	NONE	Yes
	Dr. Lewis 10/10/92	pressure 155/87	same	same	same	till next visit, 6 months			every day	NONE	Yes

Instructions:

1. Include all over-the-counter drugs you take as well as prescription drugs.
2. When you change doses draw a single line through the old dose.
3. Bring this with you every time you go to a doctor or pharmacist.
4. Be straightforward with your doctor and yourself about how often you take medicine and why.

brand and generic names, since both are commonly used. All drugs prescribed by all doctors should be listed. Over-the-counter drugs and the amount of alcohol, tobacco, and caffeine used should also be indicated. There are many dangerous interactions between drugs and between drugs and alcohol, so this information is extremely important in avoiding adverse drug interactions.

b. *Purpose of the drug:* Identify the reason for which each drug is being taken. Often, because physicians are frustrated at not being able to do anything else for the patient, or sometimes because the doctor believes that the patient will not be satisfied unless a pill is recommended, prescriptions are written without a valid medical reason. In one study, patients reported that one out of every four times (25.4%) they received a prescription, they were not told the purpose of the drug being prescribed.[3]

c. *Dose, frequency of use, and duration of use:* It is important to know what the dose is, how often it is supposed to be taken, at what hours, and for how long.

d. *When the drug should be stopped or the need for its use reevaluated:* For any drug, new or old, you should assume that it should be used for as short a time as possible unless there is evidence that its continued use is necessary. An exception to this is the use, for a prescribed period of time (even if you are feeling better), of antibiotics. Evaluation at least every three to six months of the need for each drug being used will reduce the number of drugs being taken. For some drugs, such as tranquilizers, sleeping pills, anti-depressants, and others, much more frequent reevaluation is necessary.

e. *Important possible adverse effects of the drug:* Because many of the most serious perceptible adverse effects of drugs are often wrongly attributed to such things as "growing old" (such as falling, memory loss, depression, and many more; see Chapter 3, p. 17), it is important for patients to know about the adverse effects of the drugs they take so they can recognize them and

report them to the doctor. In one study, researchers found that 37% of documented adverse drug reactions had not been recognized by patients and reported to their doctors, and that the majority of these patients had not been informed about possible adverse drug reactions by their doctors.[3]

f. *Important possible drug and food interactions, especially with over-the-counter drugs, and diet recommendations:* Ask your doctor which foods and other drugs taken along with your drug can interact and cause adverse effects, and ask for dietary recommendations.

g. *How you are actually taking the drug:* Always be straightforward with your doctor about whether or not you are taking your medicine and how often. Do this even if you had no defined reason for stopping. This is important because not giving your doctor this information can lead to mistaken conclusions about what dosage or drugs work.

h. *New problems or complaints noticed by the patient, friends, or family since any of the drugs listed on the worksheet have been started:* As mentioned above, patients themselves often do not notice a change, especially older adults who are inclined to blame many of their problems on aging. Friends and relatives are often the first to notice adverse drug reactions, especially ones that affect thinking or mood. An additional difficulty is that patients are often reluctant to tell their doctors that something the doctor did to try to make them better actually made them worse. The safest assumption is that any worsening of a patient's condition or any new symptom that develops after a drug is started is an adverse drug reaction until proven otherwise.

i. *In the judgment of you, your family, and your doctor, is the drug working?* Have the purposes for which the drug is being prescribed (as in [b]) been achieved?

Rule 2: Make Sure Drug Therapy Is Really Needed.

Often, drugs are prescribed to treat situational problems such as loneliness, isolation, and confusion. Whenever possible, nondrug approaches to these problems should be tried. These include hobbies, socializing with others, and getting out of the house. When a person is suffering from an understandable depression after losing a loved one, for example, support from friends, relatives, or a psychotherapist is often preferable to drugs such as antidepressants. (See discussion on proper use of antidepressant drugs for depression, p. 184.)

Nondrug therapy, such as weight loss and exercise, is preferable to drug therapy for such problems as mild high blood pressure and mild adult-onset diabetes. (See discussions of these two problems on pp. 47 and 405.) Increasing fiber and liquid in the diet is preferable to using laxatives (see p. 531). For swollen legs due to "bad" veins in the legs (not due to heart disease), wearing support hose is less expensive, safer, and probably more effective than taking heart pills or water pills.

Drugs should rarely be prescribed for anxiety or difficulty sleeping, particularly in older adults. See discussions of these problems and nondrug solutions on p. 166.

A last category of "disease" for which drug therapy is rarely, if ever, appropriate is drug-induced disease or adverse drug reactions. The proper treatment for drug-induced parkinsonism is not a second drug to treat the problem caused by the first drug, but, rather, stopping the use of the first drug.

For any condition, always talk to your doctor about whether the selected drug may cause problems (adverse effects) worse than the disease being treated. A common example of this is the extraordinary overtreatment of older people with slightly high blood pressure but without any symptoms of or problems caused by high blood pressure. (See guidelines for treatment of hypertension, p. 48.) In most cases, treatment will make the person feel worse, with no evidence of any benefit. Always consider the seriousness of the condition that your doctor is considering treating, and try to make sure that the treatment is not worse than the disease.

The guiding principle is to use as few drugs as possible, in order to reduce adverse reactions and increase the odds of properly taking the drugs that are really necessary.

Rule 3: If Drug Therapy Is Indicated, in Most Cases, Especially in Older Adults, It Is Safer to Start with a Dose That Is Lower Than the Usual Adult Dose.

More generally, start with as low a dose as possible. In other words, "Start low, go slow." A lower dose will cause fewer adverse effects, which are almost always related to dose. In the elderly, some experts suggest starting with one-third to one-half the usual adult dose for most drugs and watching for side effects, increasing the dose slowly and only if necessary to get the desired effect.

Rule 4: When Adding a New Drug, See If It Is Possible to Discontinue Another Drug.

If your doctor is considering adding a new drug, this is an opportunity to reevaluate existing drugs and eliminate those that are not absolutely essential. The possibility of an adverse drug interaction between the new drug and one of the old ones may lead to discontinuing or changing the use of a drug.

Rule 5: Stopping a Drug Is as Important as Starting It.

At least every three to six months, regularly review with your doctor the need to continue each drug being taken. For many mind-affecting drugs, such as sleeping pills, tranquilizers, and antidepressants, and for antibiotics, this reevaluation should be more frequent and sooner. The prevailing principle for doctors and patients should be to discontinue any drug unless it is essential. Many adverse drug reactions have been caused by continuing to use drugs long after they are needed. Many drugs such as antidepressants, sleeping pills, tranquilizers, and others that are prescribed for an acute problem are not needed beyond a short period and cause risks without providing benefits. Slow and careful weaning off these drugs may significantly improve the user's health. In addition to considering whether to stop the drug, you and your doctor should discuss the possibility of lowering the dose. As mentioned above, an exception to this is the use of antibiotics for the prescribed period of time, even if you are feeling better before having finished the prescribed dosage.

Rule 6: Find Out If You Are Having Any Adverse Drug Reactions.

If you develop any of the following reactions after beginning to use any drug, contact your doctor. Ask if you really need a drug in the first place and, if you do, whether a safer drug can be substituted or whether a lower dose could be used to reduce or eliminate the adverse effect. Look in Chapter 3 (p. 17) for the lists of widely used drugs that can cause each of these adverse effects.

- mental adverse drug reactions: depression, hallucinations, confusion, delirium, memory loss, impaired thinking, and insomnia
- nervous system adverse drug reactions: parkinsonism, involuntary movements of the face, arms, and legs (tardive dyskinesia), dizziness on standing, falls (which can sometimes result in hip fractures), automobile accidents that result in injury because of sedation, and sexual dysfunction
- gastrointestinal adverse drug reactions: loss of appetite, nausea, vomiting, abdominal pain, bleeding, constipation, and diarrhea

- urinary tract adverse drug reactions: difficulty urinating or loss of bladder control (incontinence)

If you or a relative or friend have any of the above problems or develop other problems after starting a new drug and are taking any of the drugs listed under the respective problem in Chapter 3, notify your doctor or tell your friend or relative to notify his or hers.

Another way to identify possible adverse drug reactions you may be having is to look up the name of your drug in the Index of Drugs, p. 901. Then turn to the page in the drug profile containing details on adverse reactions caused by the drug.

The remaining rules for safer drug use (or nonuse) were compiled from a number of lists, but particularly from the World Health Organization's General Prescribing Principles for the Elderly.[4-6] These rules, however, apply to all ages. All doctors and patients involved in drug therapy should know them.

Rule 7: Assume That Any New Symptom You Develop After Starting a New Drug May Be Caused by the Drug.

If you have a new symptom, report it to your doctor.

Rule 8: Before Leaving Your Doctor's Office or Pharmacy, Make Sure the Instructions for Taking Your Medicine Are Clear to You and a Family Member or Friend.

Regardless of how old someone is, the chance of adverse reactions is high enough that at least one other person—a spouse, child, or friend—should know about these possibilities. In the presence of such adverse reactions as confusion and memory loss, this is especially critical. For older adults, the complexities of drug use may be greater, especially for people taking more than one drug and people with physical or mental disabilities. In these cases, it is even more important to inform another person about possible adverse drug reactions.

Ask your doctor to make sure that the label on the drug states, if at all possible, the purpose for which the drug is being used. This is especially important when you are using multiple drugs but is always important as a way of increasing your and your family's or friend's participation. All information concerning the proper use of the drug should also be on the label. In addition to the label, you should get a separate instruction sheet and have it explained to you.

Rule 9: Discard All Old Drugs Carefully.

Many people are tempted to keep and reuse drugs obtained in the past, even though their condition has changed. Additional drugs used may make the earlier drugs much more dangerous. In addition, you may be tempted to give drugs, such as antibiotics, to a friend or relative who you believe may benefit from them. Resist these temptations and avoid further problems caused by using outdated drugs by throwing them away when you are done with your course of therapy.

Rule 10: Ask Your Primary Doctor to Coordinate Your Care and Drug Use.

If you see a specialist and he or she wants to start you on new medicines in addition to the ones you are on, check with your primary doctor first—usually an internist or general or family practitioner. It is equally important to use one pharmacist, if possible.

Talk to your doctor before deciding to make any changes in your prescription drugs based on information in this book.

What You Can Do: Finding Information About New Drugs

If you want information on 538 commonly used drugs, you can consult this book. For monthly updates on new drugs and newly reported adverse drug reactions, you can turn to the Public Citizen's Health Research Group newsletter, *Worst Pills, Best Pills News* (see back of book for more information). The newsletter is also available online at www.worstpills .org. But what if you are prescribed one of the flood of new drugs that are now coming on the market? In 1994 and 1995, for example, 50 new drugs were marketed in the United States, while in the following two-year period, 1996 and 1997, this number almost doubled to 92 new drugs. Although fewer drugs have been approved in recent years (an average of 22 per year have been approved from 2000 to 2003), they include many big-sellers, like Crestor (see p. 117), that should never have been approved. Where else can you go for objective drug information? Until the FDA requires the distribution of objective information written in nontechnical language, placing the risks and benefits of prescription drugs in a context meaningful for patients with each new and refill prescription, you have two choices—the nearest pharmacy or the local library. You should not turn to most sites on the Internet. Drug companies and marketing firms working for drug companies maintain Internet sites that are nothing more than a new platform for drug advertising, and as with all advertising for drugs, the benefits are overemphasized while the risks are understated.

Reading Package Inserts

For every bottle of a prescription drug delivered to the pharmacy—these usually contain a very large number of pills—the FDA requires drug companies to attach detailed written information for doctors and pharmacists about the drug's uses, adverse effects, drug interactions, and dosage recommendations. This piece of paper goes by several names; the most common is simply the package insert. Only information that has first been approved by the FDA can be included in a package insert, and it is usually the best picture we have of the risks, at the time of approval, of a new drug. FDA-approved package inserts are not routinely given out by pharmacists, but it's easy for you to get one for either a new or an old drug—just ask your pharmacist. If your pharmacist tells you that she or he can't give you the package insert because it is against the law or regulation, get a new pharmacist. For many brand-name drugs, FDA-approved inserts are available online. Simply type in the brand name of the drug followed by .com.

The package insert is written in technical language, in very small print, and you may need some help with the jargon. Despite what some paternalistic doctors and pharmacists think, there is little in the package insert about a drug's risks that can't be understood by a motivated patient.

For the elderly or others with substandard vision, reading the small print may be a bigger problem than understanding the contents of the package insert. Help on this score is available in the form of the *PDR—Physicians' Desk Reference*—a dictionary-sized, annual compilation of FDA-approved package inserts that often can be found on public library reference shelves and in bookstores. Helped along by *Dorland's Illustrated Medical Dictionary* or some other medical dictionary (also available in many public libraries and on the Internet; you can search on Google, for example, for "medical dictionary"), the average reader can usually get a general idea of the drug's indications (approved uses), contraindications (no-no's), and other potential hazards. Even if you don't fully understand the complex medical language, the *PDR* will often flash a warning that tells the

prudent reader to ask the doctor some pertinent questions. One big advantage of the book over the actual package inserts is that the print is a lot easier on the eyes. Because the *PDR* is published only once a year, however, information about the very newest drugs may be absent. Also, not all older drugs are included, and the main edition of the *PDR* does not include OTC (over-the-counter, or nonprescription) drugs, although they do publish a separate book of this information.

The information in package inserts is divided into a number of sections. Those sections of greatest importance to patients include the following:

Indications and Usage

"Indication" is the term used for a drug's FDA-approved use. The FDA has approved the drug only for the specific uses, or indications, listed in the package insert. Clinical studies and a rigorous FDA review are required to establish a drug's safety and effectiveness for a particular use. Doctors are not bound by law or regulation to prescribe drugs only for FDA-approved uses, and there may or may not be adequate scientific evidence supporting the safety and effectiveness of a drug when it is prescribed for a use not approved by the FDA.

Contraindications

These include other drugs or medical conditions with which the drug should not be used because of serious safety concerns. They may include some serious drug interactions between the drug about to be prescribed and a drug already being taken by the patient.

Adverse Reactions

The adverse drug effects listed in this section of the package insert have usually come from the clinical studies that were done before the drug was approved for sale. This is a good source of information about the adverse effects of a new drug and may be as much as we know about these risks when a drug is first marketed. However, this risk information must be placed in its proper context. The number of patients receiving a drug in clinical trials is relatively small—typically only a few thousand individuals at the most. Rare but serious adverse reactions to a drug may not be detected until years later, after large numbers of people have been exposed to the drug.

This is why we recommend that you do not take a new drug until it has been released for at least seven years (see p. xxix), unless it is one of the rare "breakthrough" drugs that offer some important documented advantage over older proven drugs. Remember, most new drugs are not breakthrough drugs.

Precautions

The precautions section of the package insert contains information about other drugs and medical conditions for which the drug should be used only if its potential benefits outweigh the risks. These situations often require special monitoring for toxicity by the doctor. In addition, this section contains information about the known drug interactions when a new drug is approved. The drug interaction information in the package insert can be lifesaving.

Dosage and Administration

Not only are the specific uses for a drug approved by the FDA, but also the dosage range and sometimes even the duration of treatment. Dosages or durations of treatment not listed in this section may or may not be safe or effective. Frequently, most of the patients studied in clinical trials are younger or middle-aged men, and information may not be available on the proper dosage of a drug for women, the elderly, or children. If special dosage information is known, it will appear in this section of the package insert.

You can ask your pharmacist for a package insert; in fact, you can do this even before you have a prescription filled. Read it over, and if you think it describes a drug you should not be taking or if you have questions about it, talk with your doctor.

You have a right to all of the information in the package insert. Assert this right; it could save your life.

Beware of Patient Information Leaflets (PILs) Routinely Distributed by Pharmacists

Ask the pharmacist for the full professional labeling instead. Remember, for many brand-name drugs, FDA-approved inserts are available online by typing in the brand name of the drug followed by .com. Many pharmacists are distributing patient information leaflets (PILs). Do not confuse these with FDA-approved package inserts for the drugs you are taking. Pharmacists' PILs are produced by commercial information vendors and printed out on pharmacists' computer systems, but there is little or no evidence supporting the completeness or quality of information contained in these leaflets. In fact, guidelines for the quality of information contained in PILs distributed by pharmacists were not established until 1996.[7] However, these guidelines are only voluntary and patients have no way of knowing if a particular PIL meets them.

The most recent, nationwide study on PILs was commissioned by the FDA and done by researchers from the University of Wisconsin.[8] From a random sample of 384 community pharmacies, a total of 1,367 PILs for four drugs were evaluated: (1) atenolol (TENORMIN), a high blood pressure drug; (2) the popular cholesterol-lowering agent atorvastatin (LIPITOR); (3) glyburide (DIABETA), used in the treatment of type-2 diabetes; and (4) nitroglycerin (NITRO-STAT), used under the tongue for chest pain (angina).

Not a single one of these 1,367 PILs met all of the nationally accepted guidelines. In fact, the highest mark in the survey went to a drug that contained 80% of the information that patients should be receiving, and the average leaflet provided only 50% of the minimum amount of information needed to enable a patient to use a drug. Incomplete drug information is misleading and thus potentially dangerous.

One of the very discouraging results were in two very important areas of PIL evaluation: *Contraindications* and *Precautions*. This information is contained in the professional product labeling. Only about one-fifth of the atenolol PILs contained 80% or more of the required information about *Contraindications*. None of the PILs for glyburide or nitroglycerin reached this level of information content. The results for *Precautions* were similar. Approximately one-fourth of the atorvastatin PILs reached the 80 to 100% level of information. The PILs for the other three drugs totally failed.

Focusing on the scientific accuracy of the PILs evaluated for the cholesterol-lowering drug atorvastatin, the findings were alarming. There were more than 53 million prescriptions dispensed for this drug in 2001. Fewer than 1% of atorvastatin PILs (0.6%) cautioned about the drug's interaction with gemfibrozil (LOPID). By contrast, atorvastatin's professional product labeling warns of increased risk of a serious adverse reaction (rhabdomyolysis) that can lead to kidney failure when the drug is used in combination with drugs like gemfibrozil.

Only one-quarter of the atorvastatin leaflets warned consumers that blood tests are needed to monitor for possible liver failure. The drug's professional product labeling recommends that function tests be performed prior to starting the drug, at 12 weeks following initiation of treatment, and after any elevation of dose, and semiannually thereafter.

These PILs currently being distributed by pharmacists are misleading and potentially dangerous because of the amount of important safety information that is omitted. In addition, some PILs have been found that contain indications, or uses for drugs, that are not FDA-approved and are also FDA-disapproved (because there is no evidence of a benefit for that particular use but there are serious safety concerns). Pharmacists' PILs should not be considered as a reliable source of information for the safe and effective use of prescription drugs.

BEWARE OF DIRECT-TO-CONSUMER ADVERTISING

Whether on television, radio, or in print ads, the main purpose of advertising is not to educate but to sell drugs. The falseness of these ads, often understating the risks and overstating the benefits, has increased because of dangerously lax FDA enforcement over prescription drug advertising. Between 1998 and 2003, there was an 85% decrease in FDA actions to stop such misleading advertisements.

REFERENCES

1. Hulka BS, Kupper LL, Cassel JC, et al. Medication use and misuse: Physician-patient discrepancies. *Journal of Chronic Diseases* 1975; 28:7–21.

2. Cavuto NJ, Woosley RL, Sale M. Pharmacies and prevention of potentially fatal drug interactions. *Journal of the American Medical Association* 1996; 275:1086–7.

3. German PS, Klein LE. Adverse drug experience among the elderly. In *Pharmaceuticals for the Elderly*. Pharmaceutical Manufacturers Association, 1986.

4. Carruthers SG. Clinical pharmacology of aging. In *Fundamentals of Geriatric Medicine*. New York: Raven Press, 1983.

5. *Drugs for the Elderly*. 2nd ed. Copenhagen, Denmark: World Health Organization, 1997.

6. Vestal RE, ed. *Drug Treatment in the Elderly*. Sydney, Australia: ADIS Health Science Press, 1984:24–6.

7. Steering Committee for the Collaborative Development of a Long-Range Action Plan for the Provision of Useful Prescription Medicine Information. Action Plan for the Provision of Useful Prescription Medicine Information, presented to Donna E. Shalala, Secretary of the Department of Health and Human Services, December 1996. Available at: http://www.fda.gov/cder/Offices/ODS/Keystone.pdf.

8. Svarstad BL, Mount JK. Evaluation of Written Prescription Information Provided in Community Pharmacies: A National Study, July 17, 2002. Available at: http://www.fda.gov/ohrms/dockets/ac/02/slides/3874S1_05_Svarstad%20.ppt.

30

SAVING MONEY WHEN BUYING PRESCRIPTION DRUGS

For many people in the United States, the price of prescription drugs is unaffordable. Many drugs cost $500, $1,000, $2,000, or more per drug and many people are taking more than one of them. Although the majority of these drugs have not yet come off patent and generic equivalents are therefore not available, the lack of the kind of price controls that exist in all other developed countries (and in the Department of Defense and the Veteran's Administration in the United States) presents an insufferable financial burden for too many people.

Five Ways to Save

There are at least five ways you can save money on the high cost of prescription drugs:

1. If appropriate, for your condition, ask your doctor to help you try a nondrug treatment first.
2. Avoid **Do Not Use** drugs.
3. Avoid **Do Not Use Until Seven Years After Release** drugs, waiting at least seven years to take any new drug unless it is one of the rare "breakthrough" drugs.
4. When you can, buy generic drugs.
5. Use Caution: Internet Purchase of Drugs and Importing Drugs from Canada

1. Nondrug Treatments

For many conditions, such as mild to moderate high blood pressure, high cholesterol, type-2 diabetes, obesity, and insomnia, changes in life-style are just as effective, safer, and less expensive than prescription drugs for many people. In fact, in many instances, nondrug interventions are recommended as the first-line treatment for these conditions before drugs are tried. (See chapters on heart drugs, diabetes drugs, mind drugs, and obesity drugs.)

It may be easier for you to take pills, but pills may not be the safest or best management for your condition, and they are certainly *much* more expensive than nondrug treatments.

2. Avoid Do Not Use Drugs

Avoiding drugs listed as **"Do Not Use"** can both save you money and help you to avoid needless drug-induced injury or death. Most of the 181 **Do Not Use** drugs in this book are listed as such because they are more dangerous than a safer alternative. Safer alternatives are listed along with all **Do Not Use** drugs, and many of the alternative drugs are available in a less expensive, generic form (see suggestion 4 on buying generic drugs below). Thus, avoiding such drugs combines reducing risks and, in a large number of cases, saving money as well.

Examples of dangerous **Do Not Use** drugs from previous editions of this book that have subsequently been taken off the market, usually long after we warned against their use in the book and/or our monthly *Worst Pills, Best Pills News,* include the antihistamines Seldane and Hismanal, the heart drugs Posicor and

Baycol, the painkillers Duract and Butazolidin, the diabetes drug Rezulin, the heartburn drug Propulsid, the antibiotics Zagam and Raxar, the antidepressant Serzone, and the weight reduction drugs Redux and ephedra.

A much smaller subset of **Do Not Use** drugs are listed as **"Do Not Use"** because—taking advantage of weaknesses in the drug patent laws—they are shameless copies of other drugs already on the market and usually available in a generic form. We discuss examples of this below.

How is such a sleight of hand possible? "Smoke and mirrors" aptly describes the technique. The smoke consists of phony "breakthrough" advertising, and the mirrors are represented by a chemical gimmick involving isomers.

We all know what advertising is, but what is an isomer? It is, chemically speaking, a molecule containing identical atoms to another molecule but differently arranged: a mirror image, to be precise. So it is with many pharmaceuticals. Many exist as equal parts of a chemically identical compound that are mirror images of each other. All of the atoms in the drug molecule are the same, only their spatial orientation is different. Separating these mirror images and selling only a single mirror image as a "new" drug is a successful business scheme, *not* a strategy to improve public health. This may be likened to selling one glove and claiming that it is as good as or better than two.

This low-class "research" activity by the pharmaceutical industry is almost always done because the patent on the first drug is about to expire and the company wants the "new" drug to compete with lower-price generic versions of the original drug. The examples that follow include several pairs of drugs, one of each pair having been approved in the United States since the mid-1990s. The older drug of the pair is the original mix of mirror images, while the new drug is only one of the mirror images. In all seven cases, the single mirror image has never been shown to be therapeutically superior to the original mixture of mirror images.

Esomeprazole (NEXIUM) and Omeprazole (PRILOSEC)

The "new purple pill" esomeprazole is really only one of the two mirror images that make up the "old purple pill" omeprazole. Despite the fact that esomeprazole was only approved by the FDA in February 2001, due to clever marketing and uncritical physicians, this drug was dispensed almost 4 million times in U.S. pharmacies by the end of 2001. The FDA physician who reviewed the data on the two drugs stated that "the sponsor's conclusion that H 199/18 [esomeprazole] has been shown to provide a significant clinical advance over omeprazole in the first-line treatment of patients with acid-related disorders is **not supported by data.**" [emphasis added][1] Esomeprazole and omeprazole are both produced by the same company, AstraZeneca Pharmaceuticals, based in Wilmington, Delaware.

Escitalopram (LEXAPRO) and Citalopram (CELEXA)

Escitalopram was approved by the FDA in August 2002, bringing to six the number of selective serotonin reuptake inhibitor (SSRI) antidepressants now on the U.S. market. It is the most recent member of the mirror-image marketing rage, being one-half of the mixture that constitutes citalopram. The other SSRIs currently available are fluoxetine (PROZAC, SARAFEM), fluvoxamine (LUVOX), paroxetine (PAXIL), and sertraline (ZOLOFT).

Both escitalopram and citalopram are produced by Forest Laboratories, Inc., of St. Louis.

The editors of *The Medical Letter on Drugs and Therapeutics* concluded in their September 30, 2002, review of the drug: "Escitalopram (LEXAPRO), the active enantiomer [one of the two mirror images] of citalopram (CELEXA), is effective for treatment of depression, but it has not been shown to be more effective, more rapid-acting or less likely to cause adverse effects, including sexual dysfunction, than citalopram or any other SSRI."[2]

We have also listed escitalopram as a **DO NOT USE** drug because for practical purposes, it is the same drug as citalopram and it has no therapeutic or safety advantage over citalopram or other SSRI antidepressants.

Dexmethylphenidate (FOCALIN) and Methylphenidate (RITALIN)

Dexmethylphenidate (FOCALIN), approved by the FDA in November 2001 for attention deficit hyperactivity disorder (ADHD), is simply one-half of the chemically identical mixture of mirror images that makes up the 40-year-old drug methylphenidate (RITALIN).

Both dexmethylphenidate and methylphenidate are produced by Novartis Pharmaceuticals of New Jersey.

Dexmethylphenidate was reviewed in the August 2002 issue of *Worst Pills, Best Pills News.* Novartis's "spin" to sell its old product as a new and better drug was to claim that "the duration of activity [of dexmethylphenidate] was statistically significantly longer . . . than methylphenidate."[3] Unfortunately, this strategy works with many health professionals and patients. But the FDA medical officer who reviewed Novartis's data wasn't fooled, saying, "This statement is misleading for several reasons."

We agreed with the conclusion of the editors of *The Medical Letter on Drugs and Therapeutics* in their May 13, 2002, review of dexmethylphenidate: "There is no evidence that dexmethylphenidate (FOCALIN) offers an advantage over any other formulation of methylphenidate (RITALIN and others). Older drugs with better established dosages and longer safety records are preferred."

Clarinex and Claritin: A New Twist—Patenting Metabolites

In addition to the "smoke and mirrors" schemes described above, another patent-ending avoidance scam involves metabolites. For example, when you swallow loratadine (CLARITIN), your body metabolizes it to desloratadine, which is actually the active form of the drug. As Schering-Plough started feeling the despair of the end of the patent on their big-selling, heavily advertised drug Claritin, the business heads there arranged for the testing and ultimate FDA approval of the main metabolite, desloratidine, and came up with the sound-alike name of Clarinex.

Not surprisingly, there is no evidence that Clarinex is any better than Claritin because Clarinex is exactly the same substance as what your body turns Claritin into when you swallow it.

A former drug company executive, who also was a physician, noted while testifying before the U.S. Senate that the pharmaceutical industry is "unique in that it can make exploitation appear a noble purpose."[4] The testimony was given over 40 years ago and is as true today as it was then. Capitalizing on their decades-old charade of nobility, the pharmaceutical industry is increasingly selling expensive "new" patented drugs that are chemically identical or nearly identical to the old drugs they replace. Remarkably, physicians prescribe them and patients pay exorbitant prices, both groups somehow believing, while being exploited, that an old drug with a new name is a therapeutic breakthrough.

3. Avoid Do Not Use Until Seven Years After Release Drugs, Waiting at Least Seven Years to Take Any New Drug Unless It Is One of the Rare "Breakthrough" Drugs

In addition to abusing the drug patent laws by gaining patents on the optimal isomers or metabolites of other drugs as described above, the industry is also quite prone to modifying just a few atoms in a complicated molecule and getting a patent on a so-called me-too drug.

The alternatives (the molecules from which they made the modification) to many of these new drugs are increasingly generically available and will therefore be less expensive; in addition, the decision not to use these drugs will also have a safety benefit in many instances.

For many years, we have warned patients not to use newly approved drugs unless they are one of the decided minority of new drugs with evidence that they are a breakthrough beyond existing treatments. A study involving Dr. Sidney Wolfe as one of the authors provides clear evidence why this caution of waiting seven years is well founded. A total of 548 new chemical entities were approved in 1975–1999. By 1999, 45 drugs (8.2%) acquired one or more black-box warnings and 16 (2.9%) were withdrawn from the market. **The estimated probability of acquiring a new black-box warning or being withdrawn from the market over a period of 25 years was 20%.**

THE HEALTH RESEARCH GROUP'S SEVEN-YEAR RULE

You should wait at least seven years from the date of release to take any new drug unless it is one of those rare "breakthrough" drugs that offers you a documented therapeutic advantage over older proven drugs. New drugs are tested in a relatively small number of people before being released, and serious adverse effects or life-threatening drug interactions may not be detected until the new drug has been taken by hundreds of thousands of people. A number of new drugs have been withdrawn within their first seven years after release. Also, warnings about serious new adverse reactions have been added to the labeling of a number of drugs, or new drug interactions have been detected, usually within the first seven years after a drug's release.

Half of these black-box warning changes occurred within 7 years of drug introduction; half of the withdrawals occurred within 2 years. The article concluded that serious adverse drug reactions commonly emerge after FDA approval. The safety of new agents cannot be known with certainty until a drug has been on the market for many years.[5] This study, as mentioned above, confirms the basis for our "Seven-Year Rule" concerning newly marketed drugs that are not therapeutic breakthroughs.

4. Buy Generic Drugs When Possible

Unless you want to waste a large amount of money—often hundreds of dollars a year—by using brand-name instead of generic drugs, you should ask for the generic version, especially if you are starting on a drug for the first time. (See table below.) One of the few bits of comparative information about prescription drugs readily accessible to consumers is the retail price of brand-name versus generic drugs. You can get this information easily by asking your pharmacist. The table starting on p. 879 was prepared by simply phoning a local pharmacy.

In 1984, generic drugs accounted for less than 19% of all prescriptions filled. Today, generic drugs represent more than 54% of all prescriptions dispensed in the United States. In addition, even though generics account for more than half of prescriptions dispensed, generics account for less than 16 cents of every dollar spent on prescription drugs.[6] Today there are more than 7,800 generic versions of the approximately 10,668 FDA-approved pharmaceuticals.[7]

Brand-name drug manufacturers have gone to extraordinary lengths to mislead doctors, pharmacists, and the public into believing that their products are produced to higher standards, and thus are safer and more effective than the same drugs produced by generic companies. These strategies have included setting up sham patient groups to lobby state legislatures to protect their brand-name drugs, and the suppression of scientific research by at least one brand-name company that showed their brand-name product was no better than those of generic companies.

The quality of prescription drugs, brand-name or generic, does not depend solely on the manufacturer but also on a strong and vigilant FDA. Both brand-name and generic drug companies are regulated by the FDA using the same standards for manufacturing facilities, quality and purity, and content of prescription drugs.

The Question of Brand-Name Quality

Many brand-name drug companies such as Warner-Lambert and its subsidiary, Parke-Davis, denigrate the quality of generic drugs in an attempt to hold market share from generics and protect profits. However, the facts about this brand-name manufacturer bear examining.

From 1990 to the end of 1995, there were a total of 64 recalls of Warner-Lambert products as listed in FDA recall reports. In 1990, there were 3 recalls, 1 in 1991, 3 in 1992, 24 in 1993, 13 in 1994, and 20 in 1995. For their brand of phenytoin (DILANTIN) alone—a drug used primarily for treating seizure disorders and one where the amount of drug in the blood is critical—there have been 12 recalls during this period. Nine of these involved problems with dissolving of the drug, which can result in an insufficient amount being absorbed by the body. More than 975,000 bottles (some of which contained 1,000 capsules) and more than 30,000 injectable doses of Dilantin were affected by these recalls.[8]

In this case, Warner-Lambert officials pleaded guilty to criminal charges for withholding important information about sloppy manufacturing practices from the FDA.

FDA Repels Attacks on Generic Drugs

As discussed above, it is in the first seven years after approval—when there is never any generic equivalent available because the patent has not yet expired, that most drugs are found to cause serious problems, not infrequently leading to their removal from the market.

Examples of such disasters, which collectively have killed hundreds of Americans and injured thousands more, have involved the arthritis drugs or painkillers Oraflex, Suprol, and Zomax; the antidepressant Merital; the high blood pressure drug Selacryn; the diet drugs Pondimin, one-half of the once popular "fen/phen" combination, and its close chemical cousin Redux; Posicor, a drug for high blood pressure and chest pain; the diabetes drug Rezulin; and the painkiller Duract. Because of the serious dangers of these 10 drugs, all were taken off the market.

But what about those drugs that have been on the market for a long enough time for the patents to have expired and that are available in both brand-name and generic versions? Which version is safer or more effective? It has always been our position that there is no difference between generic and brand-name drugs as far as the odds that there will be something found wrong with the amount of active ingredient or the purity. Over the years, there have been recalls because of these kinds of problems with both generic and brand-name drugs.

A 1990 study by FDA laboratories from all over the country found that for those classes of prescription drugs that theoretically could be most likely to pose safety or effectiveness problems if they were not manufactured properly, the generic drug met the applicable standards in virtually all cases. The classes of drugs tested included contraceptives, antibiotics, and medications prescribed for asthma, epilepsy, high blood pressure, and abnormal heart rhythms. Of the 429 samples of the 24 different drugs tested, including both brand-name and generic drugs, there were no samples tested that posed a health hazard to patients when examined for potency and, where applicable, dissolution rate and content uniformity.

The reason that these 24 different drugs were chosen is that they all have a narrow therapeutic range. This means that unlike with most kinds of drugs, for which there is a relatively large range of dosages that are both effective and relatively safe, the amount of these drugs that gets into the body must be more tightly controlled. If it is not, the drug may too easily lose its effectiveness (if the dose is too low) or become toxic (if the dose is too high).

The drugs that tested included six asthma drugs, four for treating epilepsy, four high blood pressure drugs, four drugs for treating heart arrhythmias, a birth control pill, one antibiotic, a drug for treating depression, and a so-called blood-thinning drug. In six categories of drugs,

both brand-name and generic versions were tested. In the case of the birth control pill, all of the major brand names, but no generic version, were tested.

For 23 of the 24 different drugs, there was no difference between the brand-name and the generic versions in the FDA laboratory tests for purity or quality. For aminophylline, an asthma drug that we do not recommend as a first-line treatment, five batches from two manufacturers failed to meet the FDA standards. Although none of these five batches posed a health hazard, all were recalled.[9]

Listed below are the names, both brand-name and generic, by therapeutic class, of all the drugs studied except for the birth control pill (because no generic version was studied) and aminophylline (see p. 390). As indicated in the table, many of these manufacturers have changed since the 1990 study because of mergers and acquisitions within the drug industry.

ASTHMA DRUGS

Brand Name	Generic Name	Manufacturers of Brand-Name or Generic Drugs
LUFYLLIN	dyphylline	Altana Inc., Lemmon Company, Wallace Laboratories (now Medpointe)
	isoetharine mesylate	Reedco, Inc. (not identified on Internet)
MEDIHALER, ISUPREL	isoproterenol inhaler	Abbott Laboratories, Barre-National, Inc., Sterling Drug Inc. (generic manufacturing not identified on Internet)
ALUPENT, METAPREL	metaproterenol	American Therapeutics, Inc., Boehringer Ingelheim, Pharmaceutical Basics, Inc., Sandoz Pharmaceuticals (now Dey, Morton Grove, Nephron)
CHOLEDYL	oxtriphylline	Bolar Pharmaceutical Co., Inc., Warner-Lambert Company (now Parke-Davis, Warner Chilcott)
SLO-PHYLLIN, QUIBRON-T/SR	theophylline	Banner Gelatin Products, Bristol-Myers USPNG, Central Pharmaceuticals, Cord Laboratories, Graham, DM Laboratories I, Inwood Labs, KV Pharmaceutical Co., Paco PR, Inc., Riker Labs/3M Pharmaceuticals, Rorer Pharmaceutical Corp., Schering-Plough Products, Searle & Co., Inc. (now Able, Alpharma, Monarch, Morton Grove)

(continued on page 880)

(continued from page 879)

EPILEPSY DRUGS

Brand Name	Generic Name	Manufacturers of Brand-Name or Generic Drugs
TEGRETOL	carbamazepine	Geigy Pharmaceuticals, Inwood Labs, Pharmaceutical Basics Inc., Purepac, Sidmark Laboratories, Teva Pharmaceuticals, Warner Chilcott (now Apotex, Caraco, Morton Grove, Novartis)
DILANTIN	phenytoin	Bolar Pharmaceutical Co., Inc., Lannett Company, Inc., Mason Distributors, Inc., Warner-Lambert Company, Zenith Labs Inc. (now Barr, Ivax, Mylan, Parke-Davis)
MYSOLINE	primidone	Bolar Pharmaceutical Co., Inc., Danbury Pharmacal, Inc., Lannett Company, Inc., Wyeth-Ayerst Labs (now Lannett, Watson, Xcel)
DEPAKENE	valproic acid	Abbott Laboratories, Chase Chemical Co., Pharmaceutical Basics, Inc., Scherer, RP, North America (now Banner, Copley, Par)

HIGH BLOOD PRESSURE DRUGS

CATAPRESS	clonidine	American Therapeutics, Inc., Barr Labs Inc., Boehringer Ingelheim, Bolar Pharmaceutical Co., Inc., Cord Laboratories, Danbury Pharmacal, Inc., Duramed Pharmaceuticals, Interpharm Inc., Kalipharma Inc., Lederle Laboratories, Par Pharmaceutical, Warner-Lambert (now Clonmel, Halsey, Mylan)
ESIMIL, ISMELIN	guanethidine	Bolar Pharmaceutical Co., Inc., Ciba-Geigy (generic manufacturing not identified on Internet)
LONITEN	minoxidil	Danbury Pharmacal, Inc., Par Pharmaceutical, Quantum Pharmics Ltd., Upjohn Company (now Mutual, Par, Pharmacia & Upjohn, Watson)
MINIPRESS	prazosin hydrochloride	Danbury Pharmacal, Inc., Kalipharma Inc., Mylan Pharmaceuticals, Inc., Pfizer Inc., Zenith Labs Inc. (now Clonmel, Ivax, Mylan)

ANTIARRHYTHMIC DRUGS

NORPACE	disopyramide	Barr Labs Inc., Biocraft Labs Inc., Cord Laboratories, Danbury Pharmacal, Inc., Interpharm Inc., KV Pharmaceutical Co., Searle & Co., Inc., Zenith Labs Inc. (now Ivax, Teva, Watson)
PRONESTYL	procainamide	Bolar Pharmaceutical Company, Inc., Chelsea Labs, Copley Pharmaceutical Inc., Cord Laboratories, Danbury Pharmacal, Inc., Sidmak Laboratories, Squibb Corp., Warner-Lambert, Zenith Labs Inc. (now Apothecon, Abbott, Intl)
QUINAGLUTE	quinidine gluconate	Berlex Labs, Bolar Pharmaceutical Co., Inc., Cord Laboratories, Halsey Drug Co. Inc. (now Mutual)
	quinidine sulfate	American Cyanamid Co., Barr Labs Inc., Chelsea Labs, Cord Laboratories, Danbury Pharmacal., Inc., Halsey Drug Co., Inc., Kalipharma Inc., Lannett Company, Inc., Eli Lilly and Company, Mutual Pharmaceutical Co., Private Formulations Inc., Reid-Rowell, Inc., Richlyn Labs Inc., Robins, A.H. Company, Inc., Roxane Laboratories Inc., Vitarine Pharmaceuticals, Warner-Lambert (now Clonmel, Copley, Eon)

(continued on page 881)

(continued from page 880)

ANTIBIOTIC DRUGS

Brand Name	Generic Name	Manufacturers of Brand-Name or Generic Drugs
CLEOCIN	clindamycin	Upjohn Company, Vitarine Pharmaceuticals (now Corepharma, Ranbaxy, Teva)

ANTIDEPRESSANT DRUGS

ESKALITH	lithium carbonate	Bolar Pharmaceutical Co., Inc., Pfizer Inc., Reid-Rowell, Inc., Roxane Laboratories Inc., SmithKline & French (now Able, Andrx, Barr, GlaxoSmithKline)

BLOOD-THINNER DRUGS

COUMADIN	warfarin sodium	Abbott Laboratories, Bolar Pharmaceutical Co., Inc., DuPont Pharmaceuticals, Pharmaceutical Basics, Inc. (now Barr, Bristol-Myers Squibb, Sandoz, Taro)

EXAMPLES OF SAVINGS WITH GENERIC DRUGS[10]

CONDITIONS	DRUGS (BRAND NAME/ GENERIC WHERE AVAILABLE)	DOSING (1)	RETAIL COST PER DAY (ALL BRAND) (2)	RETAIL COST PER DAY (GENERIC) (3)	GENERIC SAVINGS PER DAY ($)	GENERIC SAVINGS (% OF TOTAL SPENDING)
Asthma	(VENTOLIN/albuterol) (4)	2 puffs every 4–6 hours as needed	$1.44	$0.69	$0.75	52.3%
Hypertension	(PRINIVIL/lisinopril)	20 mg per day	$1.16	$0.60	$0.57	48.5%
Congestive Heart Failure	(LASIX/furosemide)	40 mg per day	$0.38	$0.20	$0.18	47.1%

(1) All medication is taken once per day unless otherwise noted.

(2) Prices are average retail prices in brick-and-mortar pharmacies (i.e., chain, independent, and food-store pharmacies, excluding Internet, mail-order, and long-term care pharmacies) across all payer types (cash-only, Medicaid, and other third-party payers) for the first quarter of 2004.

(3) Generic prices are calculated in the same fashion using the median price among generic manufacturers. A weighted average price would have been preferable, but no prescription volume data were available at the time by which to weight the different manufacturers.

(4) Patients using albuterol are assumed to need seven puffs on an average day.
Data Source: IMS Health, National Prescription Audit *Plus*™; first Quarter 2004; extracted April 2004; analysis conducted by the FDA.

As can be seen in the above table, over the course of a year, for drugs such as the high blood pressure drug lisinopril, which must be taken daily, the savings—365 times $.57 per day—are a hefty $208 in one year; and the savings are hundreds more for others that many people may be using.

Myths and Facts About Generic Drugs[11]

Myth: Generics take longer to act in the body.

Fact: The firm seeking to sell a generic drug must show that its drug delivers the same amount of active ingredient in the same time frame as the original product.

Myth: Generics are not as potent as brand-name drugs.

Fact: FDA requires generics to have the same quality, strength, purity, and stability as brand-name drugs.

Myth: Generics are not as safe as brand-name drugs.

Fact: FDA requires that all drugs be safe and effective and that their benefits outweigh their risks. Since generics use the same active ingredients and are shown to work the same way in the body, they have the same risk-benefit profile as their brand-name counterparts.

Myth: Brand-name drugs are made in modern manufacturing facilities, and generics are often made in substandard facilities.

Fact: The FDA won't permit drugs to be made in substandard facilities. The FDA conducts about 3,500 inspections a year in all firms to ensure standards are met. Generic firms have facilities comparable to those of brand-name firms. In fact, brand-name firms account for an estimated 50% of generic drug production. They frequently make copies of their own or other brand-name drugs but sell them without the brand name.

Myth: Generic drugs are likely to cause more side effects.

Fact: There is no evidence of this. The FDA monitors reports of adverse drug reactions and has found no difference in the rates between generic and brand-name drugs.

What Is Bioequivalence?

Generics are not required to replicate the extensive clinical trials that have already been used in the development of the original, brand-name drug. These tests usually involve a few hundred to a few thousand patients. Since the safety and efficacy of the brand-name product has already been well established in clinical testing and frequently many years of patient use, it is scientifically unnecessary, and would be unethical, to require that such extensive testing be repeated in human subjects for each generic drug that a firm wishes to market. Instead, generic applicants must scientifically demonstrate that their product is bioequivalent (i.e., performs in the same manner) to the pioneer drug.

One way scientists demonstrate bioequivalence is to measure the time it takes the generic drug to reach the bloodstream and its concentration in the bloodstream in 24 to 36 healthy, normal volunteers. This gives them the rate and extent of absorption—or bioavailability—of the generic drug, which they then compare to that of the pioneer drug. The generic version must deliver the same amount of active ingredients into a patient's bloodstream in the same amount of time as the pioneer drug.

Using bioequivalence as the basis for approving generic copies of drug products was established by the Drug Price Competition and Patent Term Restoration Act of 1984, also known as the Hatch-Waxman Act. Brand-name drugs are subject to the same bioequivalency tests as generics when their manufacturers reformulate them.

The FDA has a public obligation to investigate thoroughly all allegations of drug product defects or failures. The agency has not found any of the allegations raised thus far in the brand-name versus generic drug controversy to be valid. The FDA also has an obligation to make known to health care professionals and to the public its conclusions that false or misleading reports are being generated.

The Levothyroxine (SYNTHROID) Scandal

Boots Pharmaceuticals, which became the Knoll Pharmaceutical Company of Mt. Olive, New Jersey, in March 1995, suppressed publication of scientific research for more than two years in order to perpetuate the incorrect public impression that their brand-name version of levothyroxine (SYNTHROID) was more reliable than generic levothyroxine products from three competing companies. The cost to the American public in excessive charges for Synthroid over these two years has been estimated to be $800 million.

Research that contradicted the Boots/Knoll superiority claim was finally published in the April 16, 1997, issue of the *Journal of the American Medical Association*. It found four generic and brand-name drugs—Synthroid and the three competing levothyroxines—to be bioequivalent by current FDA standards and interchangeable without loss of therapeutic efficacy in the majority of patients for treatment of hypothyroidism (low thyroid).[12]

Knoll's predecessor, Boots, contracted with a faculty member and researchers at the University of California at San Francisco (UCSF) in 1987 for a bioequivalence study comparing Synthroid with three competitors' levothyroxine products. The company paid the researchers $250,000 to do the study. In this case, a finding of bioequivalence would justify the use of less-expensive, equally effective generic products instead of Synthroid. Boots's expectation was that the study would find Synthroid to be superior to the generics.

The contract contained a clause giving Boots veto power over publication of the study's results. The problems began in late 1990, when it became known that Synthroid and the other three levothyroxines were the same.

Over the next four years, Boots waged a calculated campaign to discredit the researchers and their work. Once it was clear that the study would not support the claim of Synthroid's superiority, Boots alleged scores of deficiencies and errors in the study. The university conducted an investigation of how the research was done and found only minor and easily correctable problems. Some members of the investigating panel found Boots's interactions with

the researchers to be "harassment" and characterized the company's actions as "deceptive and self-serving." The university concluded that the study was carefully done and complied fully with the terms of the contract.[13]

The results of the study were submitted to the *Journal of the American Medical Association* in April 1994. The study was sent to five experts for peer review and was accepted for publication in November 1994, with its publication scheduled for the January 25, 1995, issue of the journal. On January 13, 1995, the researchers suddenly withdrew the study from publication, citing as the reason "impending legal action by Boots Pharmaceuticals, Inc. against UCSF and the investigators." Because of the clause in the contract giving the company veto power over publication, UCSF said it would not defend the researchers if the study was printed without the company's permission.[13]

Then, in a move striking at the very core of ethical scientific standards, the company's senior director for medical research took the study results and, without giving credit to the UCSF researchers, published a misleading version in an obscure journal of which he was also an associate editor. The new version was used to support the company's previous assertion of Synthroid's superior reliability.

Six years after it was known that there was no difference between Synthroid and generic levothyroxine products, and more than two years after the UCSF research should have been published, the *Journal of the American Medical Association* published the research just as it would have appeared in January 1995, had it not been for Boots's interference.

To sum it all up, generic drugs are just as effective and safe as brand-name drugs. Unless you want to waste quite a bit of money, ask your pharmacist to fill your prescription with a generic drug. If the brand-name drug is not yet off patent, your pharmacist will advise you of this. See the table on p. 881 for some examples of generic savings.

5. Internet Purchase (with Caution) of Drugs and Importing Drugs from Canada

As is well known, the only reason that United States residents have increasingly turned to the Internet or to Canada as a source for drugs is that drug prices are out of control at home. Drug prices in foreign countries are often half of what they are for identical drugs in the United States. Unlike every other industrialized country, the United States refuses to negotiate drug prices or, as is done in Britain, negotiate a guaranteed profit margin for pharmaceuticals. In fact, we are in many respects going in the opposite direction; the recently passed Medicare prescription drug legislation actually prevents the Medicare program from using its massive purchasing power to negotiate lower drug prices.

Among its billions of pages, the Web contains a minigrowth industry in prescription drug sales. That much of this industry has its sights trained on the United States should be no surprise: Americans use prescription drugs heavily and, thanks to the failure of the government to restrict prices or profits (as is done in most developed countries), we pay more for them.

Some consumers have responded to drug company pricing double standards by hopping a bus and heading north to Canada, but for most people in the United States, this will not be feasible. A trip to your computer terminal, however, puts you instantly in touch with dozens of drug-selling operations, all eager for your business. But can you trust them?

The General Accounting Office (GAO), an investigative branch of Congress, recently conducted a study examining the practices of Internet pharmacy sales. The results should give pause to anyone contemplating succumbing to the allure of the less expensive products on offer on the Web.[14]

The GAO identified 13 drugs of particular interest and filed orders with 90 different pharmacies around the world; in the end, 68 drugs were received. The top-selling drugs, including Celebrex, Lipitor, and (of course!) Viagra, were generally widely available, but drugs requiring patient monitoring to protect patient safety (Accutane, Clozaril) and narcotic pain relievers (OxyContin, Percocet) were tougher to find.

All six pharmacies that accepted payments for the drug and then failed to fill the order were located outside of the United States or Canada. Not one of the 21 drugs obtained from outside the United States or Canada included a product label and only six contained warning information. Most improperly shipped drugs came from these countries as well: insulin that was not refrigerated, moisture-sensitive drugs that were not sealed, drugs hidden in compact disc cases, and drugs labeled as "dye and stain remover wax."

But the United States and Canadian sites were certainly not immune from problems. Sixteen of 18 Canadian drugs did not comply with U.S. regulations in that the packaging or labeling had not been approved by the FDA or the agency had not inspected the manufacturing plant. (These drugs may well have met the requirements of Canadian regulatory authorities, and Canadian labeling is quite similar to that in the United States.) However, all 29 U.S. and all 18 Canadian drugs proved to have the proper amount of the active ingredient, while four of the other foreign drugs did not.

Where the United States proved particularly inadequate was in requiring a prescription. Internet pharmacies are usually divided into three groups: (1) those to whom you have to mail a prescription; (2) those that have you fill out a questionnaire online and that, without ever examining you, dispense the drug; and (3) those that don't even maintain the pretense of a questionnaire and simply provide the drugs. Most states consider the latter two options to constitute an improper practice of medicine but have generally failed to discipline those physicians lending their names to such schemes. Only five of the 29 United States sites required a prescription, with the remainder requiring the online questionnaire. Three of the non-Canadian foreign sites required a questionnaire, but the remaining 18 simply mailed the drugs. In contrast, every Canadian pharmacy required a prescription from the patient's own physician, the most reputable option.

The United States government, at least, seems to suspect that illegal activity is rife in this industry. Fourteen of the 68 pharmacies (nine United States, one Canadian, and four from other foreign countries) were under investigation by either the United States FDA or the Drug Enforcement Administration for allegations including selling controlled substances without a prescription, lack of a doctor-patient relationship, selling adulterated or counterfeit drugs, smuggling, and mail fraud.

Given the way the drugs were obtained, it is difficult to make general statements about the reliability of different countries' Internet sites. The most reliable predictor of Web site quality appears to be whether or not it requires a prescription from your own doctor. Ironically, given the current focus on drug importation, the GAO data suggest that, on this measure at least (and assuming you are willing to accept Canadian regulatory standards as equivalent to those in the United States), if you're going to hop on a virtual Internet bus, it would be best if it were pointed North.

Importing Drugs from Canada

Spiraling drug prices have also driven desperate consumers to look to foreign countries, particularly Canada, to obtain prescription drugs at affordable prices. The FDA and the pharmaceutical industry have complained that such importation is unsafe, due to possible counterfeiting, poor quality manufacturing, and contamination. Counterfeits are a long-standing problem in United States health care, predating the importation debate by decades. The problem is not restricted to imports; domestically manufactured drugs are also all-too-frequently counterfeited or adulterated.

Yet, while the FDA continues to raise concern over counterfeiting, in part by producing misleading reports that exaggerate the problem or focus on the importation dimension of it alone, the agency is in fact part of the problem. A law that was designed to cut down on counterfeiting has, 17 years after it was passed, still not been implemented, thanks to industry-inspired delays at the FDA.

The absurdity of the current situation can be appreciated by analogy. If a car develops a safety problem, the manufacturer has the ability to track down each car from, for example, that model-year to inform the current owner of the problem, no matter how many times the car has been resold. Incredibly, this is not possible for pharmaceuticals.

Historically, the path from a pharmaceutical manufacturer to a consumer was relatively simple: manufacturers sold to wholesalers who sold to hospitals or pharmacists who administered medications or filled prescriptions. Over the years, this path has become circuitous. Secondary wholesalers might obtain the drugs from one of the three major (primary) wholesalers and then sell it to hospitals or pharmacists. Sometimes primary wholesalers obtain drugs from the secondary wholesalers. Occasionally, secondary wholesalers procure the drugs from the manufacturers themselves. These circuitous roots to the patient provide the opportunity for counterfeiters and other fly-by-night operators to insert themselves into the process. In the process, quality assurances may be lost as drugs are not properly stored, for example.

A document could easily circulate with the batch of drugs with each resale, greatly reducing the possibility of counterfeiting or adulteration, because the perpetrator could be more easily identified. Such a document, called a pedigree, was mandated by Congress in the Prescription Drug Marketing Act (PDMA) of 1987. Even the pharmaceutical companies support it, presumably because it would protect their brands from being tarred by counterfeit knock-offs. In 1988, the FDA issued a guidance document that laid out its interpretation of the PDMA. However, the FDA did not even propose a regulation to implement the PDMA until 1994, and a final regulation was not completed until 1999. In fact, the final regulation was very similar to the 1988 guidance. It was only at that point that complaints from the drug whole-saling industry, which claimed that the paper-work would endanger their profitability, began in earnest. Ironically, it is among these very wholesalers that the counterfeiters lurk. None-theless, the FDA has "delayed" implementation of the rule five times, most recently through December 2006. Through these accumulating stalling tactics, the FDA has so far succeeded in frustrating the intent of Congress for 17 years.

This important public health issue has thus been in limbo since 1987, with the FDA never implementing its regulations but nonetheless assailing counterfeiters and importers who are aided and abetted by the FDA's failure to regu-late. Meanwhile, the secondary wholesalers practice business as usual—all at the cost of po-tentially exposing United States patients to counterfeit and adulterated drugs.

This leaves consumers in the lurch. On the one hand, they are besieged by rising drug prices; on the other they have been abandoned by the very agency that is supposed to protect them from counterfeiters. (The increasingly pro-industry FDA apparently is seeking to pro-tect manufacturers' profits by preventing the importation of less expensive drugs, an ironic stance for an administration that claims affin-ity to free-market principles.) For now, the best course is to write your congressperson and the FDA demanding that the congressionally man-dated pedigree be implemented. If you live close to the Canadian border, a trip north to take ad-vantage of the prices secured by a government that actually protects its residents from the profiteering of the pharmaceutical industry is probably reasonable.

REFERENCES

1. Gallo-Torres HE. FDA Medical Officer Review of Nexium (esomeprazole), December 3, 2004.

2. Escitalopram (lexapro) for depression. *Medical Letter on Drugs and Therapeutics* 2002; 44:83–4.

3. Glass RL. FDA Medical Officer Review of dexmethylphenidate (Focalin), July 26, 2001.

4. Mintz M. *By Prescription Only*. Boston: Beacon Press, 1967:173.

5. Lasser KE, Allen PD, Woolhandler SJ, et al. Timing of new black-box warnings and withdrawals for prescription medications. *Journal of the American Medical Association* 2002; 287:2215–20.

6. Long D. 2003 Year in Review: Trends, Issues, Forecasts, 2004. Available at: http://www.amponline.org/Media/AMP_051904.pdf.

7. Food and Drug Administration, Center for Drug Evaluation and Research. Approved Drug Products with Therapeutic Equivalence Evaluations, Cumulative Supplement 5, May 1, 2004. Available at: http://www.fda.gov/cder/orange/supplement/cspreface.htm#1.5%20REPORT%20OF%20COUNTS%20FOR%20THE%20PRESCRIPTION%20DRUG%20PRODUCT%20LIST.

8. Wolfe SM. Statement by Sidney M. Wolfe, MD, Concerning Warner-Lambert Criminal Conviction and Poor Manufacturing Practices . . . Includes Dilantin Recalls (HRG Publication #1380), November 29, 1995. Available at: http://www.citizen.org/publications/release.cfm?ID=5555.

9. Food and Drug Administration. Survey of Narrow Therapeutic Range Drug Quality, September 12, 1990.

10. Food and Drug Administration, Center for Drug Evaluation and Research. Savings from Generic Drugs Purchased at Retail Pharmacies, May 3, 2004. Available at: http://www.fda.gov/cder/consumerinfo/savingsfromgenericdrugs.htm.

11. Food and Drug Administration, Center for Drug Evaluation and Research. FDA Ensures Equivalence of Generic Drugs, June 6, 2003. Available at: http://www.fda.gov/cder/consumerinfo/generic_equivalence.htm.

12. Dong BJ, Hauck WW, Gambertoglio JG, et al. Bioequivalence of generic and brand-name levothyroxine products in the treatment of hypothyroidism. *Journal of the American Medical Association* 1997; 277:1205–13.

13. Rennie D. Thyroid storm. *Journal of the American Medical Association* 1997; 277:1238–43.

14. General Accounting Office (GAO) Report. Internet Pharmacies: Some Pose Risks for Consumers, 2004. Available at: http://www.gao.gov/new.items/d04820.pdf.

GLOSSARY

ACE inhibitor: Angiotensin-converting enzyme inhibitor. Includes drugs such as captopril, mainly used to treat high blood pressure or heart failure.

Acetylcholine: A nervous system transmitter involved in numerous body functions. Deficiencies have been implicated in Alzheimer's disease, for example.

Acetylcholinesterase: An enzyme that breaks down acetylcholine (also known as cholinesterase).

Adrenal: A small organ located above the kidney whose functions include producing hormones to regulate immune function, inflammation, and electrolytes.

Agency for Healthcare Research and Quality (AHRQ): A federal agency with responsibility for conducting research to improve the delivery of health care in the United States.

Akathisia: Restless leg syndrome. Can be drug-induced, involving an inability to remain in a sitting position, promoting restlessness and a feeling of muscular jitters.

Akinesia: Weakness and muscular fatigue. Can be drug-induced, involving nerve problems that make patient appear listless, disinterested, and depressed. Additional problems may include infrequent blinking, slower swallowing of saliva with drooling, and a lack of facial expression.

Allergy: Hypersensitivity (overreaction) to substances such as drugs, food, and pollen.

Alpha-blocker: Any of a group of drugs (including phenoxybenzamine and phentolamine) that combine with and block the activity of an alpha adrenergic receptor and that are used especially to treat hypertension, similar to a beta-blocker.

Alzheimer's disease: A progressive deterioration of the brain resulting in impaired cognition and ability to perform daily activities.

Analgesic: A drug used to relieve pain.

Androgen: Male sex hormone.

Anemia: Decrease in red blood cells or in hemoglobin of the blood.

Angina: A disease marked by brief attacks of chest pain precipitated by deficient oxygenation of the heart muscles. It is caused by narrowed coronary arteries or a spasm of thin blood vessels.

Angiotensin converting enzyme (ACE) inhibitor: Any of a class of drugs used to treat hypertension that work by blocking an enzyme that is necessary to produce angiotensin, a substance that causes blood vessels to tighten.

Angiotensin receptor blocker: A class of drugs used to treat hypertension that work by blocking the receptor for angiotensin, a substance that causes the blood vessels to tighten.

Angiotensin II modifier: A family of high-blood-pressure-lowering drugs that includes losartan (COZAAR), valsartan (DIOVAN), and irbesartan (AVAPRO).

Antacid: A drug used to neutralize excess acid in the stomach.

Antiarrhythmic: A drug used to treat abnormal heart rhythms.

Antibiotic: A drug derived from molds or bacteria that is used to treat bacterial infections.

Anticholinergic: A drug that blocks the effects of acetylcholine, a substance produced by the body that is responsible for certain nervous system activities (parasympathetic). Drugs with anticholinergic effects (including antidepressants, antihistamines, antipsychotics, drugs for intestinal problems, antiparkinsonians) inhibit the secretion of acid in the stomach, slow the passage of food through the digestive system, inhibit the production of saliva, sweat, and bronchial secretions, and increase the heart rate and blood pressure. Adverse effects of these drugs include dry mouth, constipation, difficulty urinating, confusion, worsening of glaucoma, blurred vision, and short-term memory problems.

Anticoagulant: A drug that inhibits or slows down blood clotting.

Anticonvulsant: A drug that prevents or treats seizures (convulsions or fits).

Antidepressant: A drug used to treat mental depression.

Antiflatulent: A drug used to reduce the production of gas in the gastrointestinal system.

Antifungal: A drug used to treat infections caused by a fungus (such as ringworm, thrush, or athlete's foot).

Antihistamine: A drug used to prevent or relieve the symptoms of allergy (such as hay fever).

Antihypertensive: A drug used to lower high blood pressure.

Antioxidant: A chemical said to reduce the number of free radicals (unstable, highly reactive compounds that can damage genes).

Antiparkinsonian: A drug used to control the symptoms of Parkinson's disease.

Antiprotozoal: A drug used to treat infections caused by protozoa (tiny, one-celled animals).

Antipsychotic: Any of the powerful tranquilizers (including the phenothiazines and butyrophenones) used especially to treat psychosis and believed to act by blocking dopamine nervous receptors. Also called neuroleptic.

Antispasmodic: A drug used to reduce smooth muscle spasms (for example, stomach, intestinal, or urinary tract spasms that could lead to diarrhea or incontinence).

Antitubercular: A drug used to treat tuberculosis (TB).

Aortic stenosis: Narrowing of one of the valves (aortic valve) in the heart or of the aorta itself (one of the major blood vessels in the body).

Arthritis: A chronic disease marked by painful, stiff, swollen, and sometimes red joints.

Asthma: A chronic disorder characterized by wheezing, coughing, difficulty breathing, and a suffocating feeling. Can be caused by allergies or infections.

Attention deficit/hyperactivity disorder (ADHD): A syndrome of disordered learning and disruptive behavior characterized by symptoms of inattentiveness, hyperactivity, impulsive behavior (such as speaking out of turn), or a combination of the three. Although it begins in childhood, it can persist to adulthood. The diagnosis cannot be made without considering whether problems at home or in school may be causative.

Atypical antipsychotic: Drugs are considered atypical or novel because they have adverse effects different from the conventional antipsychotic agents. The atypical drugs are far less likely to cause extrapyramidal side effects, drug-induced involuntary movements, than are the older drugs. The atypical antipsychotic drugs may also be effective in some cases that are resistant to older drugs. Significant weight gain and induction of diabetes are adverse effects of these new drugs.

Barbiturate: A drug used to produce drowsiness and/or a hypnotic state. It can become addictive if taken for a long period of time.

Benzodiazepines: A family of drugs that are prescribed for nervousness and sleeping problems and to relax muscles and control seizures. They can be addictive if taken for an extended period of time. Adverse effects include confusion, drowsiness, hallucinations, mental depression, and impaired coordination resulting in falls and hip fractures.

Beta agonist: Any of various drugs (including albuterol and terbutaline) used to treat asthma or chronic obstructive pulmonary disease that combine with and activate a beta adrenergic receptor in order to relax the muscles around the airways.

Beta-blocker: A drug used to treat high blood pressure, angina, glaucoma, and irregular heart rhythms and to prevent migraine headaches. They work to dilate (open) the blood vessels and to decrease the number of heartbeats per minute, thereby lowering blood pressure.

Biguanide: A type of diabetes medicine that helps lower blood glucose by making sure the liver does not make too much glucose. Biguanides also lower the amount of insulin in the body.

Bisphosphonate: Drugs that bind to bone, partially preventing its breakdown. Bisphosphonates are used to both prevent and treat osteoporosis and to treat Paget's disease.

Blinded study: A study in which patients and/or investigators do not know which patients are receiving which treatments.

Bone marrow depression: The body produces new red and white blood cells by making blood cells in the bone marrow, the core of the bones. Certain types of drugs reduce the ability of the marrow to produce new blood cells, leaving fewer blood cells to circulate in the body to carry oxygen or fight infection.

Bone mineral density: A characteristic of bone measured by X-rays. It provides an estimate of how much bone is present and is one of several factors that affect the tendency of bones to break.

Bronchodilator: A drug used to open the bronchial tubes (air passages) of the lungs to increase the flow of air through them. Used by patients who have asthma, chronic bronchitis, or emphysema.

Bronchospasm: Temporary narrowing of the air passages in the lungs, decreasing the flow of air. This occurs in patients who have asthma, chronic bronchitis, or emphysema.

Calcium channel blocker: A drug used to control high blood pressure (hypertension) and heart rate and to improve blood flow to the heart. It works by lowering the calcium concentrations in certain smooth muscles in the blood vessels, causing blood vessels to dilate (open) and heart rate to decrease, thereby lowering blood pressure.

Carcinogenicity: The ability of a drug to cause cancer.

Cardiovascular system: The system that allows circulation of oxygen and blood. It consists of the heart and blood vessels.

Carotid sinus: Location of a special receptor in the carotid artery, a major blood vessel in the body, which is sensitive to changes in blood pressure.

Cephalosporin: A family of antibiotics that has antibacterial activity similar to the penicillins but can work against a wider range of infections and kill some bacteria resistant to penicillins.

Cholesterol: A fatlike substance found in blood and most tissues. Too much cholesterol is associated with such health risks as hardening of the arteries and heart attacks.

Cholesterol-lowering drug: A drug that works— by various mechanisms including blocking cholesterol synthesis and increasing cholesterol breakdown—to lower blood cholesterol levels.

Cholinergic: A drug that mimics the effects of acetylcholine, a substance produced by the body that is responsible for certain nervous system activities (parasympathetic). Drugs with cholinergic effects open (dilate) blood vessels, slow the heart, increase contractions in the gastrointestinal tract, and increase the force of contractions in the bladder.

Cholinesterase inhibitor: A drug that inhibits the enzyme that breaks down acetylcholine, resulting in more cholinergic activity.

Chronic obstructive pulmonary disease: Refers to a number of chronic lung disorders that obstruct the airways. The most common form of COPD is a combination of chronic bronchitis and emphysema, which occurs when airways in the lungs have become narrow and partly clogged with mucus and some of the air sacs deep in the lungs have been damaged.

Cirrhosis: A chronic, progressive disease of the liver characterized by scarring and destruction of liver cells. May be caused by alcohol and drugs, for example.

Coating agent: A drug that coats the stomach to treat peptic ulcer disease.

Cochrane Collaboration: A consortium of international researchers that collects clinical trials and conducts meta-analyses.

Colitis: Inflammation of the colon (large bowel).

Combination drug: A single formulation (e.g., tablet) containing two active ingredients. Drugs should not be combined unless there is some advantage to administering the two active ingredients simultaneously.

Complementary and alternative medicine (CAM): Healing practices that fall outside of conventional medical practice. CAM includes homeopathy, acupuncture, massage, chiropractic, dietary supplements (including botanicals), meditation, and prayer.

Complete blood count (CBC): An examination of the blood to detect red cell and white cell counts.

Congestive heart failure: A medical condition in which the heart does not pump adequately and fluid accumulates in the lungs and in the legs. Body tissues also do not receive an adequate blood supply.

Controlled trial: A scientific study in which the effect of a drug on one group of patients is compared to the effect of another drug (or a placebo) on another group of patients. Rarely, patients act as their own controls.

Corticosteroid: A family of drugs similar to the chemical cortisone, produced by the adrenal gland, that are used as anti-inflammatory agents and to control the body's salt/water balance if needed. A glucocorticoid is a type of corticosteroid.

Cough suppressant: Drugs such as dextromethorphan and codeine that work by "turning off" the part of the brain that controls the coughing response. Also known as antitussives.

Cutaneous: Relating to the skin.

Cyst: A sac containing gas, fluid, or semisolid material.

Decongestant: Medicines used to relieve nasal congestion that typically work by relieving the swelling in membranes that line the nose by narrowing the blood vessels that supply the nose.

Dementia: Deterioration or loss of intellectual faculties, reasoning power, will, and memory due to organic brain disease; characterized by confusion, disorientation, and stupor of varying degrees.

Depression, endogenous: Serious depression not precipitated by outside factors, such as death of spouse, job loss, etc.

Delirium: A clouded state of consciousness and confusion, marked by inattentiveness, disordered thinking, illusions, hallucinations, sleep disturbances, and movement problems.

Dementia: General mental deterioration, characterized by disorientation, memory loss, and intellectual decline.

Diabetes mellitus: Also known as sugar diabetes. A disorder in which the body cannot process sugars to produce energy, due to lack of a hormone called insulin. This leads to too much sugar in the blood (hyperglycemia) and an increased risk of coronary artery disease, kidney disease, and other problems.

Dietary supplements: Defined by law as products intended to supplement the diet that contain a vitamin, a mineral, an herb or other botanical, an amino acid, or "a dietary substance for use by man to supplement the diet by increasing the total dietary intake." These products are essentially unregulated in the United States.

Dietary Supplement Health and Education Act (DSHEA): A 1994 act of Congress that largely deregulated dietary supplements.

Diuretic: Also known as a water pill. A drug that increases the amount of urine produced, by helping the kidneys get rid of water and salt. Used in the treatment of high blood pressure and congestive heart failure.

Diverticulitis: Inflammation of a small pocket (abnormal sac) protruding outward from the lining of the intestine.

Duodenum: The portion of the gastrointestinal tract immediately next to the stomach.

Eczema: Inflammation of the skin marked by itching, redness, swelling, blistering, watery discharge, and scales.

Edema: Swelling in the body, most notably feet and legs, caused by accumulation of fluid. This may be due to diseases in the veins of the legs, heart problems, kidney problems, liver problems, anemia, or electrolyte abnormalities.

Electrolyte: Important chemicals such as sodium, potassium, calcium, magnesium, chloride, and bicarbonate, found in the body tissues and fluids.

Emphysema: Condition of the lungs characterized by swelling of the alveoli (small air cells of the lungs), causing breathlessness and difficulty breathing.

Endometriosis: Condition in which material similar to the lining of the womb (uterus) is present at other sites outside of the womb (including the pelvic cavity, intestines, and lung). This condition may cause pain and bleeding.

Enzyme: A chemical that acts on other substances to speed up a chemical reaction. Enzymes in the intestines help to break down food.

Epidemiology: A branch of public health concerned with describing the patterns of disease and establishing their causes.

Epilepsy: A chronic disorder characterized by convulsive brain dysfunction due to excessive neuronal discharge and usually associated with some alteration of consciousness.

Erectile dysfunction: Sometimes called impotence, it is the repeated inability to get or keep an erection firm enough for sexual intercourse. Erectile dysfunction does not describe other problems that interfere with sexual intercourse and reproduction, such as lack of sexual desire and problems with ejaculation or orgasm.

Ergot derivative: A family of chemicals that increase the body's ability to expend energy. This family includes drugs approved by the FDA for the treatment of Alzheimer's disease.

Esophagitis: Inflammation of the esophagus, usually due to reflux of stomach contents back up the esophagus.

Esophagus: A tube in the gastrointestinal tract connecting the mouth to the stomach.

Estrogen: One of the two principal female sex hormones.

Expectorant: A drug promoted to thin mucus in the airways so that the mucus may be coughed up more easily. None of these drugs are effective.

FDA: Food and Drug Administration. U.S. agency responsible for the safety and effectiveness of medications.

Fecal impaction: A collection of stool in the rectum or colon that is difficult to pass.

Fibrate: A class of drugs that act to decrease serum triglycerides and increase HDL cholesterol.

5-Alpha reductase inhibitor: A drug that blocks the enzyme that converts testosterone to dihydrotestosterone, another androgen, and is indicated for the treatment of symptomatic benign prostatic hyperplasia. It may also have applications as a treatment for baldness.

Fixed-ratio combination drug: A combination of two or more ingredients, each ingredient is a set amount. This means that you cannot take more or less of one ingredient without also changing the amount of the other ingredient.

Fluoroquinolone: A family of antibiotics that includes ciprofloxacin (CIPRO, CILOXAN), ofloxacin (FLOXIN, OCUFLOX), lomefloxacin (MAXAQUIN), and others.

G6PD (glucose-6-phosphate dehydrogenase) deficiency: An inherited medical condition marked by a lack of or reduced amounts of an enzyme (glucose-6-phosphate dehydrogenase) that breaks down certain sugar compounds in the body.

Gastrointestinal (GI) tract: The system responsible for the extraction of nutrients from food and the elimination of wastes. Starts at the mouth and continues as the esophagus, stomach, small intestine (duodenum, jejunum, ileum), large intestine (colon), rectum, and anus.

Gastroesophageal Reflux Disease (GERD): Reflux of stomach contents into the esophagus.

Generic: A drug whose patent has expired, allowing competing companies to make lower-cost versions.

Glaucoma: Abnormally high pressure in the eye that can lead to partial or complete loss of vision. Narrow-angle (angle-closure) glaucoma is caused by inability of the fluid in the eye to drain. Open-angle glaucoma is caused by overproduction of eye fluid.

Glitazone: A class of drugs used to treat diabetes that work by lowering the resistance to insulin in fat, live, and muscle cells and by stopping abnormalities and dysfunctions in beta cells. These drugs can cause or worsen heart failure.

Glucocorticoid: A series of hormones made in the adrenal gland used to treat asthma, bronchitis, allergies, and other breathing problems; conditions that produce inflammation, such as arthritis and other joint and muscle disorders; skin conditions; and certain cancers, hormonal disorders, and infections.

Gout: A form of arthritis caused by too much uric acid buildup in the blood, which then becomes deposited around the joints.

Heart block: Failure of the electrical conduction tissue of the heart to conduct impulses normally from one part of the heart to another, causing altered rhythm of the heartbeat. There are varying degrees of severity. Slow heartbeat with fainting, seizure, or even death can result from this abnormality.

Heartburn: The symptom of burning below the breastbone, often a sign of reflux of stomach contents into the esophagus.

Heart failure: See congestive heart failure.

Herbal product: Products manufactured from plants, generally regulated as dietary supplements.

Herpes simplex: Also known as cold sores. Inflammation of the skin, caused by a virus, resulting in groups of small, painful blisters. They may occur either around the mouth or, in the case of genital herpes, around the genitals (sex organs).

Histamine: A chemical made by the body especially during an allergic reaction. It produces dilation of small blood vessels, causing redness, localized swelling, and often itching; lowers the blood pressure; and increases secretions from the stomach, the salivary glands, and other organs.

Histamine2-blocker: Drugs that prevent the production of stomach acid and are used to treat stomach and duodenal ulcers and reflux esophagitis.

Hormone: Substance produced in one part of the body (usually a gland) that then passes into the bloodstream and is carried to other organs or tissues, where it helps them to function.

Hormone replacement therapy (HRT): The use of estrogens and/or progestins in the case of ovarian failure or, much more commonly, to treat women beginning, during, and continuing after menopause.

Hypertension: High blood pressure.

Huntington's disease: An inherited disease of the nervous system characterized by progressive dementia and involuntary movements.

Hypersensitivity: An exaggerated response to a foreign stimulus.

Hypertension: High blood pressure.

Hypoglycemia: A low blood sugar level.

Hypothermia: A condition resulting from overexposure to cold temperatures. The symptoms include shivering, cold hands and feet, and memory lapse.

Immune system: The bodily system responsible for fighting inflammation, infection, and cancer.

Incontinence: The inability to prevent loss of urine or stool.

Infection: Disease resulting from presence of certain microorganisms or matter in the body. A viral infection, such as the common cold, for example, cannot be treated other than symptomatically with drugs except for herpes, flu, or AIDS. Bacterial infections are often treated with antibiotics.

Inflammation: The body's reaction to a number of insults, including infection, trauma, and immune dysfunction.

Inhaled steroid: Corticosteroids that are inhaled to reduce the swelling of the airways within the lungs. They are taken to prevent the symptoms of asthma and are generally used by asthma sufferers who are already using a reliever inhaler more than once a day.

Insomnia: Inability to sleep.

Insulin: A hormone secreted by the pancreas that is primarily responsible for maintaining blood sugar levels.

Interaction: Increased probability of toxicity or ineffectiveness when two particular drugs are administered simultaneously. Usually caused by one drug raising or lowering the level of the other.

Irritable bowel syndrome: A condition characterized by diarrhea and/or constipation. Diagnosed only in the absence of other gastrointestinal disorders.

Ischemic colitis: A condition characterized by lack of blood flow to the colon.

Ketolide: A class of antibiotics used to treat respiratory tract infections. Telithromycin is the only ketolide currently approved by the FDA. They are similar to erythromycins.

Laxative: A drug used to encourage bowel movements. Hyperosmotic laxatives increase water content in stool, bulk-forming laxatives increase the size of the stool and stimulate the bowels to contract, stimulant laxatives directly stimulate the muscles in the gastrointestinal tract, and stool softeners soften the stool itself.

Leukotriene inhibitor: A class of drugs used to treat asthma that work by blocking leukotrienes, a group of inflammatory compounds.

Leukotriene modifier: A new family of asthma drugs that includes zafirlukast (ACCOLATE) and zileuton (ZYFLO).

Loop diuretic: A class of drugs, including furosemide and bumetanide, that are used to reduce pulmonary and peripheral edema in conditions such as congestive heart failure and renal insufficiency.

Mania: An emotional disorder characterized by euphoria, increased psychomotor activity, rapid speech, flight of ideas, decreased need for sleep, distractibility, grandiosity, and poor judgment. Mania generally occurs as part of bipolar disorder.

Meta-analysis: A statistical technique for combining multiple similarly designed research studies.

Me-too drug: Drugs that offer no significant benefit over drugs already on the market.

Migraine: A complex of symptoms that occurs periodically and is characterized by headache, vertigo, nausea, vomiting, and photophobia.

Mineral: Any homogenous inorganic material usually found in the earth's crust.

Muscle relaxant: A group of drugs that have an overall sedative effect on the body, usually prescribed to relieve lower back pain that is associated with muscle spasms.

Mutagenicity: The ability of a drug to cause genetic damage and thus, potentially, cancer.

Myasthenia gravis: A chronic disease marked by abnormal weakness, and sometimes paralysis of certain muscles.

Narcotic: A drug used to relieve pain that also may produce insensibility or stupor.

Nasal steroid: A group of topical steroids that are used to reduce inflammation in the nose that typically results from nasal allergies. Nasal steroids can help provide relief from sneezing, nasal congestion, and runny nose.

National Center for Complementary and Alternative Medicine (NCCAM): One of the institutes within the NIH (see below); responsible for research into complementary and alternative medicines.

National Institutes of Health (NIH): The U.S. government's primary funder of biomedical research.

Nervous system: The brain, spinal cord, and nerves throughout the body.

Neuroleptic malignant syndrome: A rare reaction to antipsychotic medications that includes high fever, sweating, unstable blood pressure, confusion, and muscle rigidity.

Neurological: Pertaining to the nervous system.

NMDA receptor antagonist: A drug that prevents the N-methyl-D-aspartate (NMDA) receptors in the brain from binding to glutamate. A drug in this class has been approved by the FDA for the treatment of Alzheimer's disease.

Nonnarcotic painkiller: A drug such as ibuprofen that provides pain relief without generating the stupor, alteration in behavior and mood, and potential for dependence that characterizes narcotics.

Nonsteroidal anti-inflammatory drug (NSAID): A drug (such as aspirin or ibuprofen) used to treat pain, fever, and swelling. It does not contain corticosteroids.

NSAID: See Nonsteroidal anti-inflammatory drug.

Nutritional supplements: Natural substances that are consumed in order to add to the nutrients normally ingested in the diet.

Observational study: A study in which patients are followed over time but are not randomized as in a randomized, controlled trial.

Opiate: Any preparation or derivative of opium, such as morphine or heroin.

Oral: Pertaining to the mouth.

Oral contraceptive: Birth-control pill.

Oral rehydration solution (ORS): A solution of salt, sugar, and water used to replace lost body fluids, especially in diarrhea.

Osteomalacia: Softening of the bones due to lack of vitamin D.

Osteoporosis: Loss of bone tissue that occurs most often in older women (thin, small-boned, white women, in particular), resulting in bones that are brittle and easily broken.

Pancreas: An organ located near the stomach in the abdomen responsible for secreting enzymes and hormones, particularly insulin.

Parathyroid hormone: A hormone secreted by the parathyroid glands, which are located in the neck. A synthetic version of the hormone is used to treat osteoporosis.

Parkinson's disease: Disorder of the nervous system marked by tremor (shaking), muscular rigidity, slow movements, stooped posture, salivation, and an immobile facial expression.

Parkinsonism, drug-induced: A tremor often indistinguishable from Parkinson's disease caused by a drug.

Patent: A government-issued document that, in the case of drugs, allows only the company that owns the patent to produce the drug for a period of generally 20 years from the filing of the patent.

Peptic ulcer: A localized loss of tissue, involving mainly the internal lining of areas of the digestive tract exposed to acid produced by the stomach. Usually involves the lower esophagus, the stomach, or the beginning of the small intestine (duodenum).

Phosphodiesterase inhibitor: A class of drugs used in the treatment of congestive cardiac failure that work by blocking the inactivation of cyclic AMP and act like sympathetic simulation, increasing cardiac output. Viagra also functions through its activity as a phosphodiesterase inhibitor.

Placebo: A medication without any active ingredient. Used as a control in some clinical trials.

Platelets: Small cellular fragments that circulate in the blood and are responsible for blood clotting.

Pneumonia: Disease of the lungs in which the tissue becomes inflamed, hardened, and watery. Causes include bacteria, viruses, chemical inhalation, and trauma.

Polyp: Swollen or tumorous tissues that may or may not be cancerous. They may be found in various parts of the body, such as the lining of the digestive tract, bladder, nose, or throat.

Porphyria: Rare, inherited blood disease.

Postural hypotension: A condition that can result in a decrease in blood pressure when sitting or standing, resulting in lightheadedness or fainting.

Potassium-sparing diuretic: A class of drugs commonly used to help reduce the amount of water in the body. Unlike some other diuretics, these medicines do not cause the body to lose potassium.

Progestin: Synthetic variations of the naturally occurring hormone in women's bodies called progesterone.

Prostaglandin: One of a number of hormone-like substances that participate in a wide range of body functions such as the contraction and relaxation of smooth muscle, the dilation and constriction of blood vessels, control of blood pressure, and modulation of inflammation.

Prostate: A walnut-sized gland found only in males, located deep inside the abdomen just below the bladder. The prostate gland surrounds the urethra, the canal that carries urine from the bladder. The prostate gland is responsible for producing seminal fluid, the liquid that carries sperm. It enlarges with age and can cause difficulty with starting and stopping urination.

Proton pump inhibitor: Drugs that inhibit the secretion of stomach acid and are used to treat esophageal reflux and gastrointestinal ulcers.

Psoriasis: Chronic skin condition marked by itchy, scaly, dry, red skin patches.

Psychosis: Severe mental illness marked by loss of contact with reality, often involving delusions, hallucinations, and disordered thinking.

QT interval: The interval on the electrocardiogram (EKG or ECG) between the q-wave and the t-wave. If corrected for the patient's heart rate, it is called QT_c. Many drugs, acting alone or interacting with other drugs, have the potentially hazardous effect of lengthening this interval.

Randomized trial: An experiment in which patients are assigned randomly (e.g., by a coin toss) to their treatment group.

Raynaud's syndrome: Condition marked by paleness, numbness, redness, and discomfort in the toes and fingers when they are exposed to cold. It rarely occurs in males.

Reflux: Generally refers to stomach contents backing up into the esophagus.

Salicylate: A drug used to treat rheumatism and relieve pain.

Sarcoidosis: A chronic disorder in which the lymph nodes in many parts of the body are enlarged, and small fleshy swellings develop in the lungs, liver, and spleen.

Schizophrenia: Serious mental illness (the most common type of psychosis) marked by a breakdown of the thinking process, of contact with reality, and of normal emotional responses. People with schizophrenia often have hallucinations.

Scleroderma: Persistent hardening and shrinking of the body's connective tissue.

Selective estrogen receptor modulator (SERM): A drug that mimics the effect of estrogen on bone and is thus used to treat or prevent osteoporosis.

Selective serotonin reuptake inhibitor (SSRI): Drugs such as fluoxetine (PROZAC), fluvoxamine (LUVOX), paroxetine (PAXIL), and sertraline (ZOLOFT) that increase levels of serotonin in the brain to treat depression.

Serotonin: A clinical transmitter found in many areas of the body, including the brain, where it is found in relatively high concentrations.

Sick sinus syndrome: Abnormality in the wiring system of the heart marked by periods of rapid and/or extremely slow heartbeats, which may cause fainting, chest pain, or palpitations.

Sjogren's syndrome: Condition marked by swollen glands, dryness of the mouth and often the eyes, and arthritis.

Spasm: A sudden contraction of a muscle that can cause pain and restrict movement.

Spasticity: A state of increased tone of a muscle (and an increase in the deep tendon reflexes). For example, with spasticity of the legs (spastic paraplegia) there is an increase in tone of the leg muscles so they feel tight and rigid and the knee jerk reflex is exaggerated.

Statin: This term refers to the family of cholesterol-lowering drugs that include lovastatin (MEVACOR), simvastatin (ZOCOR), fluvastatin (LESCOL), and others.

Statistical significance: A finding that reaches the conventional statistical definition of importance. Statistical significance does not assure clinical significance.

Steroid: A class of chemical compounds that includes cholesterol, sex hormones, and glucocorticoids.

Stool: Bowel movement.

Sulfa drug: A class of drugs used to treat bacterial and some fungal infections, most often used to treat urinary tract infections because they concentrate in the urine before being excreted.

Sulfonamide: An antibiotic drug derived from sulfa compounds.

Sulfonylurea: A class of drugs that are used to treat type-2 diabetes by lowering the level of blood sugar and increasing the secretion of insulin by the pancreas.

Sympathomimetic: A drug that increases blood pressure and heartbeat. It is related to the chemical adrenaline, produced naturally in the body. Also relieves nasal congestion by causing constriction of blood vessels.

Systemic lupus erythematosus: Also known as lupus or SLE. A chronic disease affecting the skin, blood vessels, and various internal organs, often accompanied by arthritis.

Tardive dyskinesia: Slow, involuntary movements of the tongue, lips, arms, and other body parts often brought on by certain drugs, especially antipsychotic drugs.

Tetracycline: A family of broad-spectrum antibiotics effective against a wide variety of organisms.

Thalassemia: An inherited blood disorder that causes anemia and is most often seen in persons of Mediterranean descent.

Thiazide diuretic: A class of drugs commonly used to treat hypertension that reduce the amount of water in the body by increasing the flow of urine. They are the first-choice drugs in treating hypertension.

Thiazolidinedione: A class of drugs used to treat type-2 diabetes by lowering blood sugar, increasing sensitivity to insulin, and lowering the amount of sugar produced by the liver. These drugs can cause or worsen heart failure.

Thromboembolism: A condition in which a blood clot (thrombus), usually in the leg or heart, is dislodged and travels through the blood (embolizes) and lodges elsewhere, usually in the lung or brain.

Thyroid: A large gland in front and on either side of the trachea that secretes thyroxine, a hormone regulating the growth of the body. Malfunctioning of the gland (hyperthyroidism, hypothyroidism) can cause medical problems.

Topical medication: A medication applied to the skin.

Toxic: Poisonous; potentially deadly.

Tranquilizer: A drug that calms and relieves anxiety, prescribed for a wide variety of conditions but used primarily to treat anxiety and insomnia. Most tranquilizers are potentially addictive.

Tricyclic antidepressant: An older class of antidepressants that work by stopping or slowing the absorption of serotonin and norepinephrine in the brain.

Tuberculosis: Also known as TB. An infectious disease, usually of the lungs, marked by fever, night sweats, weight loss, and coughing up blood.

Ulcer: Localized loss of surface tissue of the skin or mucous membrane.

Uric acid: One of the products made when protein is broken down in the body. It is normally eliminated from the body by the kidneys. Too high levels of uric acid in the body cause gout.

Urinalysis: An examination of the urine to detect abnormalities, such as sugar, protein, bacteria, or crystals, and to check the pH.

Urinary retention: Inability to urinate, resulting in the accumulation of urine in the bladder.

Urinary tract: The system that produces and then eliminates bodily wastes in the urine. It extends from the two kidneys, down the ureters into the bladder, and ends finally with elimination through the urethra.

Ventricular fibrillation: A life-threatening rapid, irregular contraction of the heart.

Vertigo: Dizziness. A sensation of irregular or whirling motion, either of oneself or of external objects. Elderly people often experience "postural vertigo" when rising from a lying or sitting position.

Vitamin: A substance found in foods that does not provide energy but is needed by the body in small amounts for normal functioning.

Wolff-Parkinson-White (WPW) syndrome: An abnormality of the heart marked by periods when the heart rate is very fast and must be controlled with medication or electrical shock to the heart (defibrillation).

Xanthine: A class of compounds including caffeine, theobromine (in tea), and the stimulant in chocolate.

U.S. Department of Health and Human Services

MEDWATCH

The FDA Safety Information and Adverse Event Reporting Program

For VOLUNTARY reporting of adverse events and product problems

Page _____ of _____

Form Approved: OMB No. 0910-0291, Expires: 03/31/05
See OMB statement on reverse.

FDA USE ONLY

Triage unit sequence #

A. PATIENT INFORMATION

1. Patient Identifier	2. Age at Time of Event: or _____ Date of Birth:	3. Sex ☐ Female ☐ Male	4. Weight _____ lbs or _____ kgs
In confidence			

B. ADVERSE EVENT OR PRODUCT PROBLEM

1. ☐ **Adverse Event** and/or ☐ **Product Problem** (e.g., defects/malfunctions)

2. **Outcomes Attributed to Adverse Event** (Check all that apply)

☐ Death: _____ (mo/day/yr)
☐ Life-threatening
☐ Hospitalization - initial or prolonged
☐ Disability
☐ Congenital Anomaly
☐ Required Intervention to Prevent Permanent Impairment/Damage
☐ Other: _____

3. **Date of Event** (mo/day/year)

4. **Date of This Report** (mo/day/year)

5. **Describe Event or Problem**

6. **Relevant Tests/Laboratory Data, Including Dates**

7. **Other Relevant History, Including Preexisting Medical Conditions** (e.g., allergies, race, pregnancy, smoking and alcohol use, hepatic/renal dysfunction, etc.)

C. SUSPECT MEDICATION(S)

1. **Name** (Give labeled strength & mfr/labeler, if known)

#1

#2

2. **Dose, Frequency & Route Used**

#1

#2

3. **Therapy Dates** (If unknown, give duration) from/to (or best estimate)

#1

#2

4. **Diagnosis for Use** (Indication)

#1

#2

5. **Event Abated After Use Stopped or Dose Reduced?**

#1 ☐ Yes ☐ No ☐ Doesn't Apply

#2 ☐ Yes ☐ No ☐ Doesn't Apply

6. **Lot #** (if known)

#1

#2

7. **Exp. Date** (if known)

#1

#2

8. **Event Reappeared After Reintroduction?**

#1 ☐ Yes ☐ No ☐ Doesn't Apply

#2 ☐ Yes ☐ No ☐ Doesn't Apply

9. **NDC#** (For product problems only)

___ - ___ - ___

10. **Concomitant Medical Products and Therapy Dates** (Exclude treatment of event)

D. SUSPECT MEDICAL DEVICE

1. **Brand Name**

2. **Type of Device**

3. **Manufacturer Name, City and State**

4. **Model #** Catalog # Serial #	Lot # Expiration Date (mo/day/yr) Other #	5. **Operator of Device** ☐ Health Professional ☐ Lay User/Patient ☐ Other: _____

6. **If Implanted, Give Date** (mo/day/yr)

7. **If Explanted, Give Date** (mo/day/yr)

8. **Is this a Single-use Device that was Reprocessed and Reused on a Patient?**
☐ Yes ☐ No

9. **If Yes to Item No. 8, Enter Name and Address of Reprocessor**

10. **Device Available for Evaluation?** (Do not send to FDA)
☐ Yes ☐ No ☐ Returned to Manufacturer on: _____ (mo/day/yr)

11. **Concomitant Medical Products and Therapy Dates** (Exclude treatment of event)

E. REPORTER (See confidentiality section on back)

1. **Name and Address**

Phone #

2. **Health Professional?** ☐ Yes ☐ No

3. **Occupation**

4. **Also Reported to:**
☐ Manufacturer
☐ User Facility
☐ Distributor/Importer

5. **If you do NOT want your identity disclosed to the manufacturer, place an "X" in this box:** ☐

FDA

Mail to: **MEDWATCH**
5600 Fishers Lane
Rockville, MD 20852-9787

-or-

FAX to:
1-800-FDA-0178

FORM FDA 3500 (12/03) Submission of a report does not constitute an admission that medical personnel or the product caused or contributed to the event.

ADVICE ABOUT VOLUNTARY REPORTING

Report adverse experiences with:

- Medications *(drugs or biologics)*
- Medical devices *(including in-vitro diagnostics)*
- Special nutritional products *(dietary supplements, medical foods, infant formulas)*
- Cosmetics
- Medication errors

Report product problems - quality, performance or safety concerns such as:

- Suspected counterfeit product
- Suspected contamination
- Questionable stability
- Defective components
- Poor packaging or labeling
- Therapeutic failures

Report SERIOUS adverse events. An event is serious when the patient outcome is:

- Death
- Life-threatening *(real risk of dying)*
- Hospitalization *(initial or prolonged)*
- Disability *(significant, persistent or permanent)*
- Congenital anomaly
- Required intervention to prevent permanent impairment or damage

Report even if:

- You're not certain the product caused the event
- You don't have all the details

How to report:

- Just fill in the sections that apply to your report
- Use section C for all products except medical devices
- Attach additional blank pages if needed
- Use a separate form for each patient
- Report either to FDA or the manufacturer *(or both)*

Confidentiality: The patient's identity is held in strict confidence by FDA and protected to the fullest extent of the law. FDA will not disclose the reporter's identity in response to a request from the public, pursuant to the Freedom of Information Act. The reporter's identity, including the identity of a self-reporter, may be shared with the manufacturer unless requested otherwise.

If your report involves a serious adverse event with a device and it occurred in a facility outside a doctor's office, that facility may be legally required to report to FDA and/or the manufacturer. Please notify the person in that facility who would handle such reporting.

Important numbers:

- 1-800-FDA-0178 -- To FAX report
- 1-800-FDA-1088 -- To report by phone or for more information
- 1-800-822-7967 -- For a VAERS form for vaccines

To Report via the Internet:

http://www.fda.gov/medwatch/report.htm

-Fold Here-   -Fold Here-

The public reporting burden for this collection of information has been estimated to average 30 minutes per response, including the time for reviewing instructions, searching existing data sources, gathering and maintaining the data needed, and completing and reviewing the collection of information. Send comments regarding this burden estimate or any other aspect of this collection of information, including suggestions for reducing this burden to:

OMB statement:
"An agency may not conduct or sponsor, and a person is not required to respond to, a collection of information unless it displays a currently valid OMB control number."

Department of Health and Human Services
Food and Drug Administration
MedWatch; HFD-410
5600 Fishers Lane
Rockville, MD 20857

Please DO NOT RETURN this form to this address.

U.S. DEPARTMENT OF HEALTH AND HUMAN SERVICES
Food and Drug Administration

FORM FDA 3500 (12/03) (Back)   Please Use Address Provided Below -- Fold in Thirds, Tape and Mail

---

DEPARTMENT OF
HEALTH & HUMAN SERVICES

Public Health Service
Food and Drug Administration
Rockville, MD 20857

Official Business
Penalty for Private Use $300

BUSINESS REPLY MAIL
FIRST CLASS MAIL   PERMIT NO. 946   ROCKVILLE MD

POSTAGE WILL BE PAID BY FOOD AND DRUG ADMINISTRATION

MEDWATCH
The FDA Safety Information and Adverse Event Reporting Program
Food and Drug Administration
5600 Fishers Lane
Rockville, MD 20852-9787

INDEX OF DRUGS AND DIETARY SUPPLEMENTS

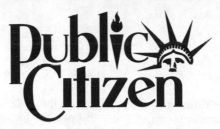

Buyers Up • Congress Watch • Critical Mass • Global Trade Watch • Health Research Group • Litigation Group
Joan Claybrook, President

Dear Friend,

It has been over 30 years since a hardy group of enterprising people came together in the nation's capital to preserve American democracy. The founders of Public Citizen showed special grit, integrity, and idealism that still serves us today.

We have always had the courage to stand up to the powerful pharmaceutical industry. But it's the support of Public Citizen members that gives us the capacity to expose the truth about dangerous drugs in *Worst Pills, Best Pills*.

In your hands, you hold just one example of the hard work we do every day on your behalf. We're using the courts, government agencies, and Congress to protect you from the voracious corporations that are exploiting consumers and waylaying the democratic process in order to increase their profits. In 2003, the drug industry spent $108.6 million on federal lobbying activities, including employing 824 lobbyists—that's more than eight lobbyists for every U.S. senator.

On your behalf, we're participating in the drug approval process by testifying on the safety and effectiveness of drugs and trying to keep dangerous drugs from being approved; petitioning and suing the Food and Drug Administration (FDA) to take dangerous drugs off the market; using the courts and the Freedom of Information Act to force the FDA to provide consumers with important drug safety and effectiveness information; and pushing the Senate Health, Education, Labor, and Pension Committee to step up its oversight of the FDA.

And that's just a few of the ways we go to battle to protect your health. We do a great deal more, as you can see on our Web site, www.citizen.org.

Public Citizen has had many successes along the way. The timeline on the following pages demonstrates how effective we are. But even with our many accomplishments in health, safety and other important areas, there is so much left to do.

I'm glad that you are protecting yourself by reading *Worst Pills, Best Pills,* but I would like to ask you to go one step further and support the necessary work of Public Citizen. Please join Public Citizen today.

Sincerely,

Joan Claybrook

Joan Claybrook

P.S. To retain our independence, Public Citizen does not accept government or corporate funds. Our support comes from individual members, foundation grants, and proceeds from Public Citizen publications.

1600 20th Street NW • Washington, DC 20009-1001 • (202) 588-1000
www.citizen.org

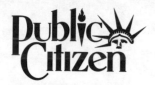

Corporations, trade associations, and other special-interest groups send lobbyists to Washington, D.C., to advance their very particular agendas. Most speak for business or industry.

Public Citizen speaks for you—
before Congress,
in the courts,
in the hallways and offices of
federal regulatory agencies.

Ralph Nader founded Public Citizen to protect the rights of citizens and give them a voice in the halls of power.

Public Citizen exposes threats to health and safety, and presses for open government and democratic decision-making. We've won important victories for consumers across an array of issues such as health care and prescription drug safety, injury prevention, access to the civil justice system, campaign finance reform, corporate subsidies and fair trade.

Join together with thousands of like-minded citizens and you can help transform many issues at the national level.

1971
■ Public Citizen petitions the FDA to ban the use of Red Dye No. 2 as food coloring, citing links to cancer and birth defects.

1972
■ Ralph Nader and Alan Morrison establish the Public Citizen Litigation Group to litigate on behalf of consumers.
■ Public Citizen asks courts to order increased disclosure of contributions to political campaigns.

1973
■ In response to Public Citizen's suit, President Nixon's firing of Watergate prosecutor Archibald Cox is ruled illegal.

1974
■ Public Citizen persuades Congress to override President Ford's veto and pass major improvements to the Freedom of Information Act.

1975
■ Public Citizen successfully lobbies Congress for energy conservation legislation, including fuel economy requirements for cars.

1976
■ The FDA bans Red Dye

No. 2 after Public Citizen's five-year campaign against the carcinogenic food dye.
■ Public Citizen petition leads to the FDA ban on use of cancer-causing chloroform in cough medicines and toothpaste.

1977
■ Public Citizen mobilizes citizens who persuade President Carter to halt construction of Clinch River breeder reactor.

1978
■ Public Citizen is instrumental in stopping the spraying of DDT in airline passenger cabins to control Japanese beetles on California-bound flights.
■ Congress passes Public Citizen's National Consumer Cooperative Bill, authorizing $300 million in seed money for consumer cooperatives.

1979
■ Public Citizen petition leads to EPA ban on the use of DBCP, a pesticide proven to cause sterility in men.
■ Public Citizen helps defeat legislation raising sugar price supports, thereby saving consumers $300 million a year.

1980
■ Public Citizen lawsuit forces government to keep records of closed-door proceedings of Chrysler bailout.
■ Public Citizen plays critical role in passage of the Superfund law, which requires cleanup of toxic waste sites without limits on liability.

1981
■ Public Citizen helps thwart President Reagan's attempts to dismantle the Clean Air Act and to diminish authority of the Consumer Product Safety Commission.

1982
■ The arthritis drug Oraflex (benoxaprofen) is withdrawn from the market after Public Citizen exposes deaths and injuries caused by the drug.
■ After an extensive Public Citizen campaign, cancer-causing urea formaldehyde is banned in home insulation.

1983
■ Public Citizen participates in landmark Supreme Court decision overturning President Reagan's revocation of auto safety standards for automatic restraints such as air bags.
■ Public Citizen wins

historic separation of powers case; Supreme Court strikes down legislative veto, affecting more than 200 statutes.

1984
■ Public Citizen wins court order forcing the EPA to recall 700,000 GM cars with faulty emission controls.
■ The FDA strengthens warning labels for anti-inflammatory drugs Butazolidin and Tandearil after Public Citizen cites serious adverse reactions.

1985
■ Public Citizen reveals the locations of more than 250 work sites nationwide where workers have been exposed to hazardous chemicals.
■ Public Citizen pressure on the FDA leads to recall of large-model Bjork-Shiley heart valve after valve fractures had been linked to 100 deaths worldwide.

1986
■ After lengthy Public Citizen campaign, the FDA requires aspirin makers to include labels warning that aspirin can cause rare Reye's syndrome in children suffering from chicken pox or flu.
■ Congress requires health

warning labels on chewing tobacco and snuff, capping Public Citizen's two-year campaign.

1987
■ Public Citizen helps persuade Congress to pass legislation restricting the time banks can hold checks.

1988
■ After seven years of litigation by Public Citizen, OSHA imposes standards for worker exposure to ethylene oxide, a cancer-causing gas used to sterilize hospital equipment.

■ Public Citizen publishes first edition of *Worst Pills, Best Pills*, a consumer guide to dangerous and ineffective drugs and their safer alternatives, selling 2 million copies over the next 10 years.

1989
■ Public Citizen obtains court order forcing the FDA to require labels warning women that high-absorbency tampons are more likely to cause toxic shock syndrome.

■ Public Citizen and Ralph Nader lead successful opposition to $45,500 congressional pay raise, forcing Congress to take a smaller raise and ban honoraria.

1990
■ Public Citizen court victory forces the Nuclear Regulatory Commission to issue mandatory training requirements for nuclear plant workers.

1991
■ Public Citizen plays key role in passage of new auto and truck safety law requiring air bags and head injury protections, and limiting the expansion of big rigs.

1992
■ Public Citizen's four-year campaign leads the FDA to restrict use of silicone gel breast implants.

■ OSHA imposes standard to protect workers from cadmium, linked to lung cancer and kidney damage, after Public Citizen wins court order.

1993
■ Public Citizen wins landmark court victory preventing destruction of electronic records of the White House under Presidents Reagan, Bush, and Clinton.

1994
■ Public Citizen helps to enlist nearly 100 cosponsors for single-payer health care reform bill modeled after the Canadian system.

■ Public Citizen helps win legislation protecting consumers from home equity scams.

1995
■ Congressional gift ban and lobbying registration reform enacted after major Public Citizen campaign.

■ Public Citizen successfully defends tobacco industry whistleblower who released key documents to Congress and the FDA, against civil damages and criminal contempt charges.

1996
■ Public Citizen wins Supreme Court decision upholding the right of people injured by federally regulated defective medical devices to sue for compensation.

■ Public Citizen forges historic settlement to secure release of Nixon's White House tapes after 15 years of litigation.

1997
■ Public Citizen exposes and helps force redesign of unethical AIDS research in Africa, which would have denied known effective treatment to HIV-positive pregnant women.

■ Public Citizen report finds that many of the more than 500 U.S. physicians disciplined for sex abuse or misconduct are still practicing.

1998
■ Public Citizen wins passage of legislation mandating safer air bags to protect women and children.

■ Public Citizen plays key role in organizing health and safety coalition that successfully opposes $368 billion tobacco industry settlement that would have immunized industry from future liability.

1999
■ Public Citizen leads global coalition to organize massive, landmark demonstrations in Seattle against the unaccountable, undemocratic World Trade Organization.

■ Public Citizen works successfully to pass major truck safety legislation, which creates the new Federal Motor Carrier Safety Administration to replace ineffective Office of Motor Carriers.

2000
■ Public Citizen petition leads to ban of diabetes drug Rezulin after 63 deaths from liver toxicity.

■ Public Citizen, spearheading a coalition of auto safety advocates, wins new federal legislation to strengthen safety in wake of hundreds of deaths and

injuries caused by rollover crashes involving Firestone tires and Ford Explorers.

2001
■ Public Citizen wins passage of legislation to beef up inspections of Mexican trucks entering United States under NAFTA.

■ Public Citizen wins appellate court ruling protecting privacy rights of Internet users who anonymously post comments critical of corporations.

■ Consumer Product Safety Commission bans lead-wick candles after lengthy campaign by Public Citizen.

2002
■ Congress passes first major campaign finance reform since Watergate era—banning "soft money" and regulating phony "issue ads"—following decadelong battle by Public Citizen and allies.

■ Public Citizen successfully sues Bush administration to win release of Reagan administration records under Presidential Records Act.

2003
■ FDA bans the dietary supplement ephedra two years after Public Citizen petitions for its removal and after 155 deaths.

■ Public Citizen research and lobbying plays critical role in defeating federal legislation that would unfairly restrict damages awarded to the seriously injured victims of medical malpractice.

2004
■ Public Citizen exposes the failure of seat belts in automobile rollover crashes and campaigns for new auto safety legislation.

To Find Public Citizen's Top-Selling Health Publications and Other Information about Our Work, Visit
www.worstpills.org

Featuring:

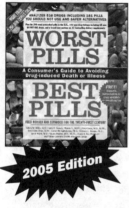

Worst Pills, Best Pills
2005 Edition

Written and edited by Public Citizen's Health Research Group

Protect yourself from dangerous drugs with this handy reference guide. With one in five new drugs requiring a new, post-approval black-box warning or being taken off the market, you can no longer be sure that your medications won't harm you. *Worst Pills, Best Pills* is the ideal guide because it tells you which drugs you should avoid and why. 180 drugs are listed as "DO NOT USE" and there are many safer alternatives to these.   **$19.95**

Order Your Friend a Copy of This Book!

**Special Introductory Offer!
$10 for 12 months**

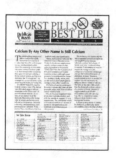

Worst Pills, Best Pills News
Annual subscription

Written and edited by Public Citizen's Health Research Group

Subscribe to *Worst Pills, Best Pills News* and get 12 issues packed full of breaking news on drugs and dietary supplements. This important information will help protect you from unsafe or ineffective medications. And our warnings often come many months, sometimes years, before dangerous drugs are withdrawn from the market.   **$10**

Public Citizen offers publications on a variety of issues. To find out about other Public Citizen products or to purchase these publications, visit our online store at
www.citizen.org.

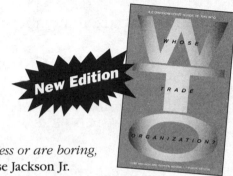
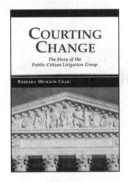

Support the Work of
Public Citizen
By Joining <u>Today</u>!

As a Public Citizen member, you'll enjoy many exclusive benefits, including:

• 6 issues of *Public Citizen News*

Public Citizen News, published bimonthly, will keep you informed about the efforts that Public Citizen makes on your behalf. *Public Citizen News* is **FREE** with a membership gift of $20 or more.

• 1 year of Public Citizen's *Health Letter*

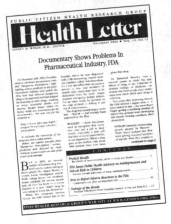

Public Citizen's *Health Letter*, edited by the renowned consumer health advocate Sidney M. Wolfe, M.D., contains vital information that will assist you in making important health decisions. The *Health Letter* and *Public Citizen News* are **FREE** with a generous annual membership gift of $35 or more.

• Member Discounts on Books, Reports, and Briefings Published by Public Citizen

<u>Plus You'll Receive:</u>

- Satisfaction in lending your voice to Public Citizen's fight for a responsible government and a healthier, safer future for all.

- Pride in being an active citizen who cares about the vitality and well-being of our democracy.

To join the fight, check the Public Citizen membership box
on the order form on the back page and
include a generous contribution of $20 or more.

Or visit us at:
www.citizen.org/join/wpbp2005

ORDER FORM

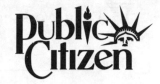

Return to:　　1600 20th Street, NW, Washington, DC 20009-1001
www.citizen.org

Publications from Public Citizen

Qty.	Item	Description	Price	Subtotal
	F6686	**Worst Pills, Best Pills** 2005 ed.	$19.95	
	G9004	**Courting Change:** *The Story of the Public Citizen Litigation Group*	$15*	
	E9011	**Whose Trade Organization?:** *A Comprehensive Guide to the WTO* (2004)	$23*	
Subtotal (1)				

* Shipping and handling included in price.

Public Citizen Membership/Newsletter Subscription

	Price	Subtotal
Basic Membership (includes *Public Citizen News*)	$20	
Combination Membership with *Health Letter*	$35	
Special Introductory subscription to *Worst Pills, Best Pills News* for 12 months	$10	
I want to help even more with an additional contribution		
Subtotal (2)		
Add (1) and (2)	TOTAL	

Ordered By:

Name_____

Address

_____

_____

City _____ State _____ Zip _____

E-mail _____

Phone number (___)_____

Please use an additional sheet of paper for gift orders.

_____

❑ Payment enclosed (check or money order payable to "Public Citizen")

❑ Charge to credit card ❑ VISA ❑ MC ❑ AMEX ❑ Discover

Credit Card #_____

Exp. Date_____

Signature_____

U.S. orders only. Please allow 6–8 weeks for delivery.

B5WPBP

℞ Drug Worksheet for Patients, Family, Doctor and Pharmacist©

Name _____ **Page** _____

Primary Doctor's Name _____ **Doctor's Telephone** _____

Generic Name of Drug — — — — — Brand Name of Drug	Doctor, date started & changes	Reason why prescribed or changed?	Dose? (Each time)	Times per day	What time of day?	How long should you take drug? days/ weeks/ months

Instructions:
1. Include all drugs you take including aspirin, herbs, vitamins and other nonprescription products as well as prescription drugs.
2. When you change doses draw a single line through the old dose.
3. Bring this with you every time you go to a doctor or pharmacist.
4. Be straightforward with your doctor and yourself about how often you take medicine and why.

See sample worksheet, *Worst Pills, Best Pills*, p. 865.

Problems to watch out for which this drug can cause	Interactions of this drug with other drugs or food; diet recommendations	How are you actually taking the drug?	New problems or complaints since drug started (Date it began)	Is drug working?

℞ Drug Worksheet for Patients, Family, Doctor and Pharmacist©, continued

Name _____ **Page** _____

Primary Doctor's Name _____ **Doctor's Telephone** _____

Generic Name of Drug — — — — Brand Name of Drug	Doctor, date started & changes	Reason why prescribed or changed?	Dose? (Each time)	Times per day	What time of day?	How long should you take drug? days/ weeks/ months
— — — — — —						
— — — — — —						
— — — — — —						
— — — — — —						
— — — — — —						

Problems to watch out for which this drug can cause	Interactions of this drug with other drugs or food; diet recommendations	How are you actually taking the drug?	New problems or complaints since drug started (Date it began)	Is drug working?